Electronic British National Formulary

The British National Formulary in now produced from a database from which a typesetting file is output every six months in order to print each new edition of the BNF. From the same database, an "electronic book" is also produced which can be viewed on any modern personal computer (PC).

This "stand-alone" version of the electronic BNF (eBNF) retains the familiar pocket book form of the BNF on the computer screen, but the Adobe™ Acrobat™ software used to view the eBNF provides powerful additional facilities. For example, a click on an entry in the contents list or index will immediately access the required page. Where a drug interaction warning is given in the text, a click on the word "interactions" in the text provides immediate access to the appropriate drug in the interactions section of the BNF. There are also various ways in which the electronic text can be searched. An electronic adverse reaction form is also included.

The annual subscription for the eBNF will be £199.00 (two electronic editions), and the price includes basic Adobe™ Acrobat ™ software.

SAMPLE DISKS OF THE eBNF ARE AVAILABLE FOR £5.00

Technical requirements: *The eBNF would occupy about 20 Mbytes of disk space. Windows is the preferred platform, but there are versions of Adobe™ Acrobat™ software which operate in DOS. The operating software will require a minimum of 4 Mbytes for Windows and at least 3 Mbytes in DOS. The preferred distribution for the eBNF will be on CD-ROM which will require the PC to have a CD-ROM player (currently costing from £100 upwards). Alternatively, the eBNF may be supplied on about 15 disks.*

To order, simply complete the form below and post the card to the freepost address overleaf.

ORDER FORM

❏ Please supply me with_____sample disk(s) from the "stand-alone" **electronic BNF** at £5.00 each (including postage and packing).

My PC operates on: ❏ Windows ❏ DOS ❏ Macintosh System 7

❏ Please enroll me for_____subscriptions to the "stand alone" **electronic BNF** at £199.00* per annum. (This includes two electronic versions of the BNF, Adobe™ Acrobat™ software, postage/ packing, and access to a "helpline").

❏ Please supply on CD-ROM

❏ Please supply on 15 floppy disks. PC operating ❏ Windows ❏ DOS

❏ Please send me an illustrated brochure of the **electronic BNF**

Name:

Full postal address:

Postcode:

My credit card number is

Expiry date

My cheque / money order for £   **is enclosed** *(made payable to The Pharmaceutical Press)*

Signature

Companies in EC member states (excluding the UK) must supply VAT identify

If the address for your credit card account is not the same as tha
* Price shown applies to U.K. only. Price may vary in other countries ❏ *F*

D0307377

2

Kate Rowan
The Pharmaceutical Press,
FREEPOST WC 1124
London SE1 1BR

BRITISH NATIONAL FORMULARY

September 1994

BRITISH NATIONAL FORMULARY

Number 28
(September 1994)

British Medical Association
and
Royal Pharmaceutical Society of Great Britain

Copies may be obtained through any bookseller or, in case of difficulty, direct from the publishers:

British Medical Association
Tavistock Square
London WC1H 9JP, England

The Pharmaceutical Press
Royal Pharmaceutical Society of Great Britain
1 Lambeth High Street
London SE1 7JN, England

ISBN: 0 85369 258 0. ISSN: 0260–535X

The text for this edition was generated from an in-house database (designed by Quartet Software Ltd). Typeset from disk by Create Publishing Services Ltd, Bath, Avon BA2 3DZ, printed and bound by The Bath Press, Bath, Avon BA2 3BL.

Joint Formulary Committee
1994–95

Contents

APPENDIXES AND INDEXES

Arrangement of Information

Guidance on prescribing
This part includes information on prescription writing, controlled drugs and dependence, prescribing for children and the elderly, and prescribing in terminal care. Advice is given on the reporting of adverse reactions.

Emergency treatment of poisoning
The main intention of this chapter is to provide information on the management of acute poisoning when first seen in the home, although aspects of hospital-based treatment are mentioned.

Classified notes on drugs and preparations
The main text consists of classified notes on drugs and preparations. These notes are divided into 15 chapters, each of which is related to a particular system of the human body or to an aspect of medical care. Each chapter is then divided into sections which begin with appropriate *notes for prescribers*. These notes are intended to provide information to doctors, pharmacists, nurses, and other health professionals to facilitate the selection of suitable treatment. The notes are followed by details of relevant drugs and preparations.

DRUGS appear under pharmacopoeial or other non-proprietary titles. When there is an *appropriate current monograph* (Medicines Act 1968, Section 65) preference is given to a name at the head of that monograph; otherwise a British Approved Name (BAN), if available, is used. If the International Non-proprietary Name (INN) differs from the British Approved Name it follows the title in brackets.

PREPARATIONS usually follow immediately after the drug which is their main ingredient. They are printed in text-sized type but those considered by the Committee to be less suitable for prescribing are described in smaller type. Small type is also used for the entries describing foods for special diets, stoma and urinary appliances, and wound management products. Preparations are included under a non-proprietary title if:
   (a) they are marketed under such a title,
   (b) they are not otherwise prescribable under the NHS, or
   (c) they may be prepared extemporaneously.
If proprietary preparations are of a distinctive colour this is stated, but flavour is not usually mentioned.
   In the case of compound preparations the indications, cautions, contra-indications, side-effects, and interactions of all constituents should be taken into account in prescribing.

PREPARATIONS NOT AVAILABLE FOR NHS PRESCRIPTION. The symbol NHS has been placed against those preparations included in the BNF that are not prescribable under the NHS. Those prescribable only for specific disorders have a foot-note specifying the condition(s) for which the preparation remains available. Prescribers are reminded that some preparations which are not *prescribable* by brand name under the NHS may nevertheless be *dispensed* using the brand name in question providing that the prescription has been written in the form of an appropriate non-proprietary name.

PRESCRIPTION-ONLY MEDICINES The symbol PoM has been placed against those preparations that are available only on medical or dental prescription. For more detailed information see *Medicines, Ethics and Practice*, No. 12, London, Pharmaceutical Press, 1994 (and subsequent editions as available). The symbol **CD** indicates that the preparation is subject to the prescription requirements of the Misuse of Drugs Act. For regulations governing prescriptions for such preparations see pages 7–9.

PRICES have been calculated from the basic cost used in pricing NHS prescriptions dispensed in February 1994 or later, see p. 1 for further details.

Appendixes and indexes
The appendixes include information on interactions, liver disease, renal impairment, pregnancy, breast-feeding, intravenous additives, borderline substances, appliances, and cautionary and advisory labels for dispensed medicines. They are designed for use in association with the main body of the text.
   The Dental Practitioners' List and the Nurse Prescribers' List are also included in this section. The indexes consist of the Index of Manufacturers and the Main Index.

Preface

This edition of the BNF is the first to be produced both as a pocket book version and as an identical electronic version. Much work has gone into the production of the electronic BNF and the Joint Formulary Committee acknowledges above all the invaluable work of Quartet Software Ltd, represented by P. L. Berkin, P. D. Johnson and B. Thomas, who designed the software. Thanks are also due to C. Gordon and I. Herbert for advice on the implications of the electronic BNF as a tool for decision support. The work involved in the transfer into a database of the many thousands of words that constitute the BNF has required immense vigilance to guarantee the continuing integrity of its text; this has entailed numerous additional checks and a very large amount of additional proof-reading. Grateful thanks are therefore due to the people who gave so much of their time to assist with this project, including E. J. Aitchison, J. Batson, M. Davis, L. Desson, C. Dewse, K. Eager, B. M. Ecclestone, S. E. Ellmers, L. M. Ferrow, M. J. Gilmour, J. V. Littler, R. McLarney, P. M. Mason, P. J. Rushworth, and S. B. Williamson; their unfailing diligence has contributed enormously to the success of the conversion.

The Joint Formulary Committee also acknowledges the help of individuals and organisations that provided information or advised on specific matters. The principal contributors for this edition were D. G. Arkell, C. G. Barnes, D. N. Bateman, L Beeley, R. H. Behrens, R. J. Buckley, I. Burgess, A.J. Camm, C. M. Castleden, D. A. Chamberlain, B. T. Colvin, C. Diamond, R. Dinwiddie, A. J. Duxbury, H. M. Elliston, A. M. Geddes, A. H. Ghodse, E. C. Gordon-Smith, M. W. Greaves, I. A. Greer, J. Guillebaud, C. H. Hawkes, M. J. S. Langman, T. H. Lee, P. N. Leigh, M. W. McNicol, G. M. Mead, D. J. Oliver, R. E. Pounder, L. E. Ramsay, P. A. Routledge, R. S. Sawers, M. C. Sheppard, S. D. Shorvon, A. Tattersfield, R. N. Thin, G. R. Thompson, M. D. Vickers, D. G. Waller, D. A. Warrell, P. Watkins, G. B. Wyatt. The Committee also wishes to express its thanks to J. E. F. Reynolds and staff, for valuable access to the *Martindale* data bank and files. The Committee also wishes to express its thanks to correspondents in the pharmaceutical industry who provided information and made numerous comments on points of detail, to colleagues who have advised members of the Committee and the editorial staff on specific matters, and T. M. Roberts for clerical assistance. Finally, the Committee would like to thank those doctors, pharmacists, nurses, and others who sent comments and suggestions.

It was with regret that the Committee learned of the death of Mr M. J. Tarr, who had advised on Appendix 6 (intravenous additives) since 1989.

The BNF is intended for rapid reference and cannot contain all the information necessary for prescribing and dispensing. It should be supplemented as necessary from specialised publications. Manufacturers' data sheets prepared in accordance with the Medicines (Data Sheet) Regulations 1972 are available for most proprietary medicines and these should also be consulted. Less detail is given in some areas such as those dealing with obstetrics, malignant disease, and anaesthesia, as it is expected that those undertaking treatment will have specialised knowledge and will consult specialist literature. Supplementary information may be available from local drug information services.

Comments and constructive criticism will be welcome, and should be sent to:
Executive Editor, British National Formulary,
c/o Royal Pharmaceutical Society of Great Britain,
1 Lambeth High Street, London SE1 7JN.

Changes

The BNF is revised twice yearly and numerous changes are made between issues. All copies of BNF No. 27 (March 1994) should therefore be withdrawn and replaced by BNF No. 28 (September 1994).

Significant changes have been made in the following sections for BNF No. 28:

Controlled drugs [new specimen prescription], p. 7

Ulcer-healing drugs [new text on *H. pylori* infection], section 1.3

Adrenoceptor stimulants [reorganisation], section 3.1.1

Hyposensitisation [new CSM advice], section 3.4.2

Anaphylaxis [new text], section 3.4.3

Pulmonary surfactants [reorganisation], section 3.5.2

Antipsychotics [advice of Royal College of Psychiatrists on doses above BNF upper limit], section 4.2

SSRIs [reorganisation], section 4.3.4

Dysmenorrhoea [new text], section 4.7.1

Migraine treatment, section 4.7.4.1

Malaria prophylaxis, section 5.4.1

Halofantrine [CSM advice], section 5.4.1

Chickenpox and corticosteroids [CSM advice], section 6.3.3

Hormone replacement therapy [reorganisation], section 6.4.1

Prostaglandins and oxytocics [new text], section 7.1.1

Hormone antagonists [reorganisation], section 8.3.4

Oral rehydration therapy, section 9.2.1.2

Azapropazone [CSM advice], section 10.1.1

NSAIDs [CSM advice], section 10.1.1

Tiaprofenic acid [CSM advice], section 10.1.1

Acne preparations [reorganisation], section 13.6.1

Immunoglobulins [reorganisation], section 14.5

Dose Changes

Preparations affected by changes in dose statements introduced into BNF No.28:
Azapropazone, p. 380

Chlorothiazide, p. 58

Cilazapril, p. 83

Co-danthramer strong suspension, p. 46

Enalapril [heart failure], p. 84

Evorel, p.288

Pabrinex, p. 370

Quinapril, p. 85

Tamoxifen [dose now in text only], p. 340

Triclofos, p. 146

Trimethoprim, p. 239

Urokinase, p. 105

Classification and Title Changes

Title Changes

Bismuth Chelate now Tripotassium Dicitratobismuthate

Cervagem now Gemeprost

Classification Changes

3.10 Systemic nasal decongestants, previously section 3.9.3

5.1.1.5 no longer exists

8.3.4 now subdivided

Electronic BNF

An electronic version of the BNF is now available on disk and CD-ROM as a stand-alone system. The BNF software displays on screen a format identical to that of the pages of the pocket book version.

This electronic version of the BNF is also available as a simple database suitable for developers to integrate into their own practice software systems.

A further phase in the development of the BNF is currently under way which involves detailed structuring of the information of the database to operate as part of an intelligent decision-support and prescribing tool. Links will be provided to patient and other records.

The electronic BNF will retain its pocket book role but in addition its data will be supplemented by links to other major publications.

New Preparations

Preparations included in appropriate sections of BNF No. 28

Alec
Amphosil
Benzamycin
Botox
Calcijex
Cardilate MR
Carnitor
Caverject
Cedax
Ciloxan
Combivent
Curosurf
Desmotabs
DF 118 Forte
Diftavax
Dostinex
Dovonex scalp solution
Eolarix
Esmeron
Fluarix
H-B-Vax II
HAES-steril
Irriclens
Kefadim
Kogenate
Lamictal dispersible tablets
Lipantil Micro

Medisense G2
Medisense
Micronor HRT
Motifene
MR vaccine
Optimax [re-introduced]
Oramorph SR
Orgafol
Otex
Pertussis vaccine, acellular [unlicensed]
Polytar AF
Pulmozyme
Replenine
Respacal syrup
Rubella Immunoglobulin
Salivace
Steri-Neb Ipratropium
Stilnoct
Tetabulin
Torem
Videx
Viscotears
Vividrin
Zirtek oral solution
Zoton
Zydol

Discontinued Preparations

Preparations discontinued during the compilation of BNF No. 28

Achromycin intramuscular injection
Addamel
Allbee with C
Bactrim dispersible tablets and adult suspension
Becotide for nebulisation
Bradilan
Callusolve
Cedocard IV
Centyl K
Disalcid
Durabolin
Enduron
Exolan
Ferrocap
Ferromyn
Imperacin

Intal Autohaler
Ismelin eye-drops
Limbitrol
Metamucil
Morsep
Nobrium
Petrolagar
Polybactrin
Pranoxen Continus
Quinoderm with Hydrocortisone
Rehibin
Rynacrom nasal insufflation
Schick test
SRM-Rhotard
Thalamonal
Variclene

Drug Information Services

Information on any aspect of drug therapy can be obtained, free of charge, from Regional and District Drug Information Services. Details regarding the *local* services provided within your Region can be obtained by telephoning the following numbers.

England

Birmingham		021-311 1974	Direct Line
	or	021-378 2211	Extn 2296/2297
Bristol		0272 282867	Direct Line
Guildford		0483 504312	Direct Line
Ipswich		0473 704430	Direct Line
	or	0473 704431	Direct Line
Leeds		0532 430715	Direct Line
Leicester		0533 555779	Direct Line
Liverpool		051-236 4620	Extn 2126/2127/2128
	or	051-231 6015	Direct Line
London			
Guy's Hospital		071-955 5000	Extn 3594/5892
	or	071-378 0023	Direct Line
Northwick Park Hospital		081-869 3973	Direct Line
Royal London Hospital		071-377 7487	Direct Line
	or	071-377 7489	Direct Line
Manchester		061-225 2063	Direct Line
	or	061-276 6270	Direct Line
Newcastle		091-232 1525	Direct Line
Oxford		0865 221808	Direct Line
	or	0865 221836	Direct Line
	or	0800 834203	
Southampton		0703 796908	Direct Line
	or	0703 796909	Direct Line

Northern Ireland

Belfast	0232 248095	Direct Line
Londonderry	0504 45171	Extn 3262

Scotland

Aberdeen	0224 681818	Extn 52316
Dundee	0382 60111	Extn 2351
Edinburgh	031-519 5482	Direct Line
	or 031-519 5454	Direct Line
Glasgow	041-552 4726	Direct Line
Inverness	0463 234151	Extn 288
	or 0463 220157	Direct Line

Wales

Cardiff	0222 742979	Direct Line

Poisons Information Services

Belfast	0232 240503
Birmingham	021-554 3801
Cardiff	0222 709901
Dublin	Dublin 379964 *or* Dublin 379966
Edinburgh	031-229 2477
Leeds	0532 430715 *or* 0532 923547
London	071-635 9191 *or* 071-955 5095
Newcastle	091-232 5131

Note. Some of these centres also advise on laboratory analytical services which may be of help in the diagnosis and management of a small number of cases

Guidance on Prescribing

Prices in the BNF

Basic **net prices** have been introduced into the BNF in order to provide better indications of relative cost. Where there is a choice of suitable preparations for a particular disease or condition the relative cost may be used in making a selection. It should be emphasised, however, that cost-effective prescribing must take into account other factors (such as dose frequency and duration of treatment) that affect the total cost. The use of more expensive drugs is justified if it will result in better treatment of the patient or a reduction of the length of an illness or the time spent in hospital.

Prices have generally been calculated from the basic cost used in pricing NHS prescriptions dispensed in February 1994, but where available later prices have been included; unless an original pack is available these prices are based on the largest pack size of the preparation in use in community pharmacies. The price for an extemporaneously prepared preparation has been omitted where the net cost of the ingredients used to make it would give a misleadingly low impression of the final price.

The unit of 20 is still sometimes used as a basis for comparison, but where suitable original packs are available these are priced instead.

Gross prices vary as follows:

1. Costs to the NHS are greater than the net prices quoted and include professional fees and overhead allowances;

2. Private prescription charges are calculated on a separate basis;

3. Over-the-counter sales are at retail price, as opposed to basic net price, and include VAT.

BNF prices are NOT, therefore, suitable for quoting to patients seeking private prescriptions or contemplating over-the-counter purchases.

A fuller explanation of costs to the NHS may be obtained from the Drug Tariff.
It should be noted that separate Drug Tariffs are operative in England and Wales, Scotland, and Northern Ireland. Prices in the different tariffs may vary.

PACT and SPA

PACT (Prescribing Analyses and Cost) and SPA (Scottish Prescribing Analysis) automatically provide general practitioners with information about their prescribing. The information is sent on a quarterly basis direct from the Prescription Pricing Authority (and may be obtained for individual months on request). It is now available as a 'standard report' which replaces the previous *level 1* and *level 2* reports. The previous *level 3 report* is replaced by a 'catalogue' which provides the data in a more helpful manner and is available on request for periods of one or more months.

General Guidance

Medicines should be prescribed only when they are essential, and in all cases the benefit of administering the medicine should be considered in relation to the risk involved. This is particularly important during pregnancy where the risk to both mother and fetus must be considered (for further details see Prescribing in Pregnancy, Appendix 4).

ABBREVIATION OF TITLES. In general, titles of drugs and preparations should be written *in full*. Unofficial abbreviations should not be used as they may be misinterpreted; obsolete titles, such as Mist. Expect. should not be used.

NON-PROPRIETARY TITLES. Where non-proprietary ('generic') titles are given, they should be used in prescribing. This will enable any suitable product to be dispensed, thereby saving delay to the patient and sometimes expense to the health service. The only exception is where bioavailability problems are so important that the patient should always receive the same brand; in such cases, the brand name or the manufacturer should be stated. Non-proprietary titles should **not** be invented for the purposes of prescribing generically since this can lead to confusion, particularly in the case of compound and modified-release preparations.

Titles used as headings for monographs may be used freely in Great Britain and Northern Ireland but in other countries may be subject to restriction.

Many of the non-proprietary titles used in this book are titles of monographs in the European Pharmacopoeia, British Pharmacopoeia or British Pharmaceutical Codex 1973. In such cases the preparations must comply with the standard (if any) in the appropriate publication, as required by the Medicines Act (section 65).

PROPRIETARY TITLES. Names followed by the symbol ® are or have been used as proprietary names in the United Kingdom. These names may in general be applied only to products supplied by the owners of the trade marks.

DOSES. The doses stated in the BNF are intended for general guidance and represent, unless otherwise stated, the usual range of doses that are generally regarded as being suitable for adults. In general the *doses, indications, cautions, contra-indications and side-effects* in the BNF reflect those in the manufacturers' data sheets which, in turn, reflect those in the corresponding Product Licences. On the few occasions that an unlicensed drug is included in the BNF, this is now indicated in brackets after the entry. Where a use (or route) is recommended outside the licensed indication of an available product this too is indicated. It has been noted (*Drug and Therapeutics Bulletin*, 1992, *30*, 97–99) that prescribing of licensed medicines outside the recommendations of the Product Licence alters (and probably increases) the doctor's professional responsibility.

ORAL SYRINGES. Since 1 July 1992, when fractional doses are prescribed, *oral liquid medicines* are **no** longer diluted to a 5-mL dose (or multiple thereof). Instead the pharmacist supplies an **oral syringe**. The oral syringe is marked in 0.5 mL divisions from 1 to 5 mL to measure doses of less than 5 mL. The 5-mL spoon will continue in use for doses of 5 mL (or multiple thereof). The oral syringe is provided with an adaptor and an instruction leaflet.

STRENGTHS AND QUANTITIES. The strength or quantity to be contained in capsules, lozenges, tablets, etc. should be stated by the prescriber.

If a pharmacist receives an incomplete prescription for a systemically administered preparation other than a prescription for a controlled drug and considers it would not be appropriate for the patient to return to the doctor, the following procedures will apply:
(a) an attempt must always be made to contact the prescriber to ascertain the intention;
(b) if the attempt is successful the pharmacist must, where practicable, subsequently arrange for details of quantity, strength where applicable, and dosage to be inserted by the prescriber on the incomplete form;
(c) where, although the prescriber has been contacted, it has not proved possible to obtain the written intention regarding an incomplete prescription, the pharmacist may endorse the form 'p.c.' (prescriber contacted) and add details of the quantity and strength where applicable of the preparation supplied, and of the dose indicated. The endorsement should be initialled and dated by the pharmacist;
(d) where the prescriber cannot be contacted and the pharmacist has sufficient information to make a professional judgment the preparation may be dispensed. If the quantity is missing the pharmacist may supply sufficient to complete up to 5 days' treatment; except that where a combination pack (i.e. a proprietary pack containing more than one medicinal product) or oral contraceptive is prescribed by name only, the smallest pack shall be dispensed. In all cases the prescription must be endorsed 'p.n.c.' (prescriber not contacted) the quantity, the dose, and the strength (where applicable) of the preparation supplied must be indicated, and the endorsement must be initialled and dated;
(e) if the pharmacist has any doubt about exercising discretion, an incomplete prescription must be referred back to the prescriber.

ADDITIVES. Oral liquid preparations in the BNF that do not contain *fructose, glucose* or *sucrose* are labelled "sugar-free".

Where the presence of *aspartame, gluten* or *tartrazine* is specified on a data sheet this is indicated in the BNF against the preparation in question; not all data sheets provide details of additives therefore if it is essential to know this the manufacturer should be contacted.

Information is provided on *preservatives* in eye-drops. Information is also provided on *selected additives* in skin preparations (for details see section 13.1). Pressurised metered aerosols containing *chlorofluorocarbons* (CFCs) have also been identified throughout the BNF (for further comment, see p. 111)

EXTEMPORANEOUS PREPARATION. The BP direction that a preparation must be *freshly prepared* indicates that it must be made not more than 24 hours before it is issued for use. The direction that a preparation should be *recently prepared* indicates that deterioration is likely if the preparation is stored for longer than about 4 weeks at 15° to 25°.

DRUGS AND DRIVING. Prescribers should advise patients if treatment is likely to affect their ability to drive motor vehicles. This applies particularly to drugs with sedative effects and patients should be warned that these effects are increased by alcohol. See also Appendix 9.

NOTICE CONCERNING PATENTS. In the BNF certain drugs have been included notwithstanding the existence of actual or potential patent rights. In so far as such substances are protected by Letters Patent, their inclusion in this Formulary neither conveys, nor implies, licence to manufacture.

HEALTH AND SAFETY. When handling chemical or biological materials particular attention should be given to the possibility of allergy, fire, explosion, radiation, or poisoning. Some substances, including corticosteroids, antibiotics, phenothiazines, and many cytotoxics, are irritant or very potent and should be handled with caution. Contact with the skin and inhalation of dust should be avoided.

SAFETY IN THE HOME. Patients must be warned to keep all medicines out of the reach of children. All solid dose oral medicines should be dispensed either in reclosable *child-resistant containers* complying with the British Standard or in unit packaging of strip or blister type unless:

(i) they are in manufacturers' original packs so designed that transfer to a reclosable child-resistant container would be a retrograde or unnecessary procedure,
(ii) the patient is elderly or handicapped and would have difficulty in opening a child-resistant container;
(iii) the patient specifically requests otherwise.

In cases (ii) and (iii) the pharmacist should make a particular point of advising that the medicines be kept well out of the reach of children. In addition, all oral liquid medicines should be dispensed in containers fitted with appropriate *child-resistant closures*.

All patients should be advised to dispose of *unwanted medicines* by returning them to a supplier for destruction.

NAME OF MEDICINE. The name of the medicine should appear on the label unless the prescriber indicates otherwise.

1. Subject to the conditions of paragraphs 4 and 6 below, the name of the prescribed medicine is stated on the label unless the prescriber deletes the letters 'NP' which appear on NHS prescription forms.
2. The strength is also stated on the label in the case of tablets, capsules, and similar preparations that are available in different strengths.
3. If it is the wish of the prescriber that a description such as 'The Sedative Tablets' should appear on the label, the prescriber should write the desired description on the prescription form.
4. The arrangement will extend to approved names, proprietary names or titles given in the BP, BPC, BNF, or DPF. The arrangement does not apply when a prescription is written so that several ingredients are given.
5. The name written on the label is that used by the prescriber on the prescription.
6. If more than one item is prescribed on one form and the prescriber does not delete the letters 'NP', each dispensed medicine is named on the label, subject to the conditions given above in paragraph 4. If the prescriber wants only selected items on such a prescription to be so labelled this should be indicated by deleting the letters 'NP' on the form and writing 'NP' alongside the medicines to be labelled.
7. When a prescription is written other than on an NHS prescription form the name of the prescribed preparation will be stated on the label of the dispensed medicine unless the prescriber indicates otherwise.
8. The Council of the Royal Pharmaceutical Society advises that the labels of dispensed medicines should indicate the total quantity of the product dispensed in the container to which the label refers. This requirement applies equally to solid, liquid, internal, and external preparations. If a product is dispensed in more than one container, the reference should be to the amount in each container.

Scope of the BNF
The BNF is intended for the guidance of medical practitioners, pharmacists, dentists, nurses, and others who have the necessary training and experience to interpret the information it provides. It is intended as a reference for the pocket, and should be supplemented by a study of more detailed publications when required.

Security and validity of prescriptions
The Councils of the British Medical Association and the Royal Pharmaceutical Society have issued a joint statement on the security and validity of prescriptions.
In particular, prescription forms should:
(i) not be left unattended at reception desks;
(ii) not left in a car where they may be visible; and
(iii) when not in use , be kept in a locked drawer within the surgery and at home.
Where there is any doubt about the authenticity of a prescription, the pharmacist should contact the prescriber. If this is done by telephone, the number should be obtained from the directory rather than relying on the prescription form information, which may be false.

Prescription Writing

> **Shared care**
>
> In its guidelines on responsibility for pre-
> scribing between hospitals and general practi-
> tioners, the Department of Health has advised
> that legal responsibility for prescribing lies
> with the doctor who signs the prescription.

Prescriptions[1] should be written legibly in ink or
otherwise so as to be indelible[2], should be dated,
should state the full name and address of the
patient, and should be signed in ink by the
prescriber[3]. The age of the patient should
preferably be stated, and is a legal requirement in
the case of prescription-only medicines for children
under 12 years of age.

In general practice the following should be noted:

(a) For solids, quantities of 1 gram or more should
be written as 1g etc.

Quantities less than 1 gram should be written in
milligrams, e.g. 500mg, not 0.5g.

Quantities less than 1mg should be written in
micrograms, e.g. 100micrograms, not 0.1mg.

When decimals are unavoidable a zero should be
written in front of the decimal point where there is
no other figure, e.g. 0.5mL, not .5mL.

Use of the decimal point is acceptable to express
a range, e.g. 0.5 to 1g.

(b) 'Micrograms' and 'nanograms' should **not** be
abbreviated. Similarly 'units' should **not** be abbreviated.

(c) The term 'millilitre' (ml or mL)[4] is used in
medicine and pharmacy, and cubic centimetre, c.c.,
or cm^3 should not be used.

(d) Dose and dose frequency should be stated; in
the case of preparations to be taken 'as required' a
minimum dose interval should be specified.

When doses other than 5 or 10mL are prescribed
for *oral liquid preparations* the dose-volume will
be provided by means of an **oral syringe**, see p. 2
(except for preparations intended to be measured
with a pipette).

Suitable quantities:

Elixirs, Linctuses, and Paediatric
  Mixtures (5-mL dose), 50, 100, or 150mL

Adult Mixtures (10-mL dose), 200 or 300mL

Ear Drops, Eye-drops, and Nasal Drops,
  10mL (or the manufacturer's pack)

Eye Lotions, Gargles, and Mouth-washes, 200 mL

(e) For suitable quantities of dermatological preparations, see section 13.1.

(f) The names of drugs and preparations should be
written clearly and **not** abbreviated, using
approved titles **only**.

(g) The symbol 'NP' on NHS forms should be
deleted if it is required that the name of the preparation should not appear on the label. For full
details see p. 3.

(h) The quantity to be supplied may be stated by
indicating the number of days of treatment required
in the box provided on NHS forms. In most cases
the exact amount will be supplied. This does not
apply to items directed to be used as required—if
the dose and frequency are not given the quantity to
be supplied needs to be stated.

When several items are ordered on one form the
box can be marked with the number of days of
treatment providing the quantity is added for any
item for which the amount cannot be calculated.

(i) Although directions should preferably be in
English without abbreviation, it is recognised
that some Latin abbreviations are used (for details
see Inside Back Cover).

(j) A prescription for a preparation that has been
withdrawn or needs to be specially imported for a
named patient should be handwritten. The name of
the preparation should be endorsed with the prescriber's signature and the letters 'WD' (withdrawn
or specially-imported drug); there may be considerable delay in obtaining a withdrawn medicine.

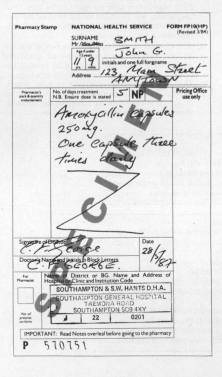

1. The above recommendations are acceptable for
prescription-only medicines (PoM). For items marked
CD see also Controlled Drugs and Drug Dependence p.
7.

2. It is permissible to issue carbon copies of NHS prescriptions as long as they are signed in ink.

3. Computer-generated facsimile signatures do not meet
the legal requirement.

4. The use of capital 'L' in mL is a printing convention
throughout the BNF; both mL and ml are recognised
abbreviations for SI units.

Computer-issued Prescriptions

For computer-issued prescriptions the following recommendations of the Joint Computing Group of the General Medical Services Committee and the Royal College of General Practitioners should also be noted:

1. The computer must print out the date[1], the patient's surname, one forename, other initials, and address, and may also print out the patient's title. The age of children under 12 years must be printed in the box available; a facility may exist to print out the age of older children and adults as well.

2. The doctor's name[2] must be printed at the bottom of the prescription form; this will be the name of the doctor responsible for the prescription (who will normally sign it). The doctor's surgery address, reference number, and Family Health Services Authority (FHSA)[3] are also necessary. In addition, the surgery telephone number should be printed.

3. When prescriptions are to be signed by trainees, assistants, locums, or deputising doctors, the name of the doctor printed at the bottom of the form must still be that of the responsible principal. To avoid difficulties for the pharmacist checking the prescription, the name of the signing doctor may be printed in the signature box, to be signed over on prescribing.

4. Names of medicines must come from a dictionary held in the computer memory, to provide a check on the spelling and ensure that the name is written in full. The computer can be programmed to recognise both the non-proprietary and the proprietary name of a particular drug and to print out the preferred choice, but must not print out both names. For medicines not in the dictionary, separate checking mechanisms are required—the user must be warned that no check was possible and the entire prescription must be entered in the lexicon.

5. The dictionary may contain information on the usual doses, formulations, and (where relevant) pack sizes to produce standard predetermined prescriptions for common preparations, and to provide a check on the validity of an individual prescription on entry.

6. The prescription must be printed in English without abbreviation; information may be entered or stored in abbreviated form. The dose must be in numbers, the frequency in words, and the quantity in numbers in brackets, thus: 40mg four times daily (112).

It must also be possible to prescribe by indicating the length of treatment required, see (h) above.

7. The BNF recommendations should be followed as in (a), (b), (c), (d), and (e) above.

8. Checks may be incorporated to ensure that all the information required for dispensing a particular drug has been filled in. Instructions such as 'as directed' should be avoided. For the instruction 'when required' the maximum daily dose should normally be specified.

9. Numbers and codes used in the system for organising and retrieving data must never appear on the form.

10. Supplementary warnings or advice should be written in full, should not interfere with the clarity of the prescription itself, and should be in line with any warnings or advice in the BNF; numerical codes should not be used.

11. A mechanism (such as printing a series of non-specific characters) may be incorporated to cancel out unused space, or wording such as 'no more items on this prescription' may be added after the last item. Otherwise the doctor should delete the space manually.

12. To avoid forgery the computer may print on the form the number of items to be dispensed (somewhere separate from the box for the pharmacist). The number of items per form need be limited only by the ability of the printer to produce clear and well-demarcated instructions with sufficient space for each item and a spacer line before each fresh item.

13. Handwritten alterations should only be made in exceptional circumstances—it is preferable to print out a new prescription. Any alterations that are made must be written in the doctor's own handwriting and countersigned.

14. Prescriptions for controlled drugs cannot be produced by a printer[4]. If there is a record of such a prescription in the computer, it must not be printed. Instead the computer may print out a blank form with the doctor's name[1] and other details printed at the bottom.

15. The strip of paper on the side of the FP10[5](Comp) may be used for various purposes but care should be taken to avoid including confidential information. It may be advisable for the patient's name to appear at the top, but this should be preceded by 'confidential'.

16. In rural dispensing practices prescription requests (or details of medicines dispensed) will normally be entered in one surgery. The prescriptions (or dispensed medicines) may then need to be delivered to another surgery or location; if possible the computer should hold up to 10 alternatives.

Generic names of **compound preparations** which appear in the BNF are those approved by the British Pharmacopoeia Commission; whenever possible they reflect the names of the active ingredients.

Prescribers should avoid creating their own compound names for the purposes of generic prescribing; such names do not have an approved definition and can be misinterpreted.

Special care should be taken to avoid errors when prescribing compound preparations; in particular the hyphen in the prefix 'co-' should be retained.

Special care should also be taken to avoid creating generic names for **modified-release** preparations where the use of these names could lead to confusion between formulations with different lengths of action.

---

1. The exemption for own handwriting regulations for phenobarbitone does not apply to the date; a computer-generated date need not be deleted but the date must also be added by the prescriber.
2. Except in Scotland where it does not appear.
3. Health Board in Scotland.
4. Except in the case of phenobarbitone (but see also foot-note 1) or where the prescriber has been exempted from handwriting requirements, for details see Controlled Drugs and Drug Dependence p. 7.
5. GP10 in Scotland.

Emergency Supply of PoM at Patient's Request[1]

The Medicines (Products Other Than Veterinary Drugs) (Prescription Only) Order 1983, as amended, allows exemptions from the Prescription Only requirements for emergency supply to be made by a person lawfully conducting a retail pharmacy business provided:

(a) that the pharmacist has interviewed the person requesting the prescription-only medicine and is satisfied:
(i) that there is immediate need for the prescription-only medicine and that it is impracticable in the circumstances to obtain a prescription without undue delay;
(ii) that treatment with the prescription-only medicine has on a previous occasion been prescribed by a doctor[2] for the person requesting it;
(iii) as to the dose which it would be appropriate for the person to take;
(b) that no greater quantity shall be supplied than will provide five days' treatment except when the prescription-only medicine is:
(i) an ointment, cream, or preparation for the relief of asthma in an aerosol dispenser when the smallest pack can be supplied;
(ii) an oral contraceptive when a full cycle may be supplied;
(iii) an antibiotic in liquid form for oral administration when the smallest quantity that will provide a full course of treatment can be supplied;
(c) that an entry shall be made in the prescription book stating:
(i) the date of supply;
(ii) the name, quantity and, where appropriate, the pharmaceutical form and strength;
(iii) the name and address of the patient;
(iv) the nature of the emergency;

---

1. For emergency supply at the request of a doctor see *Medicines, Ethics and Practice*, No. 12, London, Pharmaceutical Press, 1994 (and subsequent editions as available).
2. The doctor must be a UK-registered doctor.

(d) that the container or package must be labelled to show:
(i) the date of supply;
(ii) the name, quantity and, where appropriate, the pharmaceutical form and strength;
(iii) the name of the patient;
(iv) the name and address of the pharmacy;
(v) the words 'Emergency supply'.
(e) that the prescription-only medicine is not a substance specifically excluded from the emergency supply provision, and does not contain a Controlled Drug specified in schedules 1, 2, or 3 to the Misuse of Drugs Regulations 1985 except for phenobarbitone or phenobarbitone sodium for the treatment of epilepsy: for details see *Medicines, Ethics and Practice*, No. 12, London, Pharmaceutical Press, 1994 (and subsequent editions as available).

ROYAL PHARMACEUTICAL SOCIETY'S GUIDELINES

(1) The pharmacist should consider the medical consequences, if any, of **not** supplying.
(2) The pharmacist should identify the patient by means of documentary evidence and/or personal knowledge.
(3) The doctor who prescribed on a previous occasion should be identified and contacted, if possible.
(4) The patient should be asked whether the doctor has stopped the treatment.
(5) The patient should be asked whether any other medicine is being taken at the same time to check drug interactions.
(6) An emergency supply should not be made if the item requested was prescribed previously more than six months prior to the request. Variations may be made in the case of illnesses which occur infrequently, e.g. hay fever, asthma attack, or migraine.
(7) Consideration should be given to providing less than five days' supply if this is justified.
(8) Labelling should be clear and legible and there should be some suitable identification of emergency supply entries in the prescription book.

> **Plasma concentrations** in the BNF are expressed in mass units per litre (e.g. mg/litre). The approximate equivalent in terms of amount of substance units (e.g. micromol/litre) is given in brackets.

Approximate Conversions and Units

lb	kg	stones	kg	ml	fl. oz
1	0.45	1	6.35	50	1.8
2	0.91	2	12.70	100	3.5
3	1.36	3	19.05	150	5.3
4	1.81	4	25.40	200	7.0
5	2.27	5	31.75	500	17.6
6	2.72	6	38.10	1000	35.2
7	3.18	7	44.45		
8	3.63	8	50.80		
9	4.08	9	57.15		
10	4.54	10	63.50		
11	4.99	11	69.85		
12	5.44	12	76.20		
13	5.90	13	82.55		
14	6.35	14	88.90		
		15	92.95		

Mass

1 kilogram (kg)	= 1000 grams (g)
1 gram (g)	= 1000 milligrams (mg)
1 milligram (mg)	= 1000 micrograms
1 microgram	= 1000 nanograms
1 nanogram	= 1000 picograms

Volume

1 litre	= 1000 millilitres (mL)
1 millilitre	= 1000 microlitres
1 pint	≈ 568 mL

Other units

1 kilocalorie (kcal)	= 4186.8 joules (J)
1000 kilocalories (kcal)	= 4.1868 megajoules (MJ)
1 megajoule (MJ)	= 238.8 kilocalories (kcal)
1 millimetre of mercury (mmHg)	= 133.3 pascals (Pa)
1 kilopascal (kPa)	= 7.5 mmHg (pressure)

Controlled Drugs and Drug Dependence

PRESCRIPTIONS. Preparations which are subject to the prescription requirements of the Misuse of Drugs Regulations 1985, i.e. preparations specified in schedules 2 and 3, are distinguished throughout the BNF by the symbol **CD** (Controlled Drugs). The principal legal requirements relating to medical prescriptions are listed below.

Prescriptions ordering Controlled Drugs subject to prescription requirements must be *signed* and *dated*[1] by the prescriber and specify the prescriber's *address*. The prescription must always state *in the prescriber's own handwriting*[2] in ink or otherwise so as to be indelible:

1. The name and address of the patient;
2. In the case of a preparation, the form[3] and where appropriate the strength[4] of the preparation;
3. The total quantity of the preparation, or the number of dose units, *in both words and figures;*
4. The dose.[5]

A prescription may order a Controlled Drug to be dispensed by instalments; the amount of the instalments and the intervals to be observed must be specified.[6] Prescriptions ordering 'repeats' on the same form are **not** permitted.

It is an offence for a doctor to issue an incomplete prescription and a pharmacist is **not** allowed to dispense a Controlled Drug unless all the information required by law is given on the prescription. Failure to comply with the regulations concerning the writing of prescriptions will result in inconvenience to patients and delay in supplying the necessary medicine.

DEPENDENCE AND MISUSE. The prevalence of drug dependence and misuse in Great Britain, particularly amongst young people, continues to give cause for concern to teachers, social workers, and the police, as well as doctors.

The most serious drugs of addiction are **diamorphine** (heroin), **morphine**, and the **synthetic opioids**; illicit **cocaine** is now also a problem.

Despite marked reduction in the prescribing of **amphetamines** there is concern that abuse of illicitly produced amphetamine and related compounds is widespread.

The principal **barbiturates** are now Controlled Drugs, but phenobarbitone and phenobarbitone sodium or a preparation containing either of these are exempt from the handwriting requirement but must fulfil all other controlled drug prescription requirements (**important:** the own handwriting exemption does **not** apply to the date; a computer-generated date need not be deleted but the date must also be added by the prescriber). Moreover, for the treatment of epilepsy phenobarbitone and phenobarbitone sodium are available under the emergency supply regulations (p. 6).

Cannabis (Indian hemp) has no approved medicinal use and cannot be prescribed by doctors (except under licence from the Home Secretary). Its use is illegal but has become widespread in certain sections of society. Cannabis is a mild hallucinogen seldom accompanied by a desire to increase the dose; withdrawal symptoms are unusual. **Lysergide** (lysergic acid diethylamide,

<table>
<tr><td colspan="2">

Pharmacy Stamp

NATIONAL HEALTH SERVICE FORM FP10(HP) (Revised 10/90)

SURNAME Mr./Mrs./Miss _JONES_

Age if under 13 years — initials and one full forename _Jane M_

yrs. mths. Address _23, Wide Road, Elleaslow_

Pharmacist's pack & quantity endorsement

No. of days treatment N.B. Ensure dose is stated **NP** Pricing Office use only

Diamorphine hydrochloride
30mg ampoules
Supply by 6 (six)
ampoules
60mg daily by
Subcutaneous
infusion over
24 hours.

Signature of Doctor *T. R. George* Date 25/2/94

Doctor's Name and Initials in Block Letters **C. F. GEORGE**

For Pharmacist Name of District or Special Health Authority. Name and Address of Hospital or Clinic and Institution Code

SOUTHAMPTON & S.W. HANTS D.H.A.
SOUTHAMPTON GENERAL HOSPITAL
TREMONA ROAD
SOUTHAMPTON SO9 4XY

No. of prescrs. on form J 22 0201

IMPORTANT: Read Notes overleaf before going to the pharmacy

B 060501
</td></tr>
</table>

1. A prescription is valid for 13 weeks from the date stated thereon.
2. Unless the prescriber has been specifically exempted from this requirement or unless the prescription contains no controlled drug other than phenobarbitone or phenobarbitone sodium or a preparation containing either of these. The exemption does **not** apply to the date; a computer-generated date need not be deleted but the date must also be added by the prescriber.
3. The dosage form (e.g. tablets) must be included on a Controlled Drugs prescription irrespective of whether it is implicit in the proprietary name (e.g. Tenuate Dospan®) or of whether only one form is available.
4. When more than one strength of a preparation exists the strength required must be specified.
5. The instruction 'one as directed' constitutes a dose but 'as directed' does not.
6. A special form, FP10(HP)(ad), in Scotland HBP(A), is available to doctors in NHS drug treatment centres for prescribing cocaine, dextromoramide, diamorphine, dipipanone, methadone, morphine, or pethidine by instalments for addicts. In Scotland general practitioners can prescribe by instalments on form GP10. In England and Wales forms FP10 and FP10(HP) are not suitable for this purpose but form FP10(MDA) is available. **Important:** in all cases a special licence is necessary to prescribe cocaine, diamorphine, or dipipanone for addicts except for treatment of organic disease or injury, for details see p. 9.

LSD) is a much more potent hallucinogen; its use can lead to severe psychotic states in which life may be at risk.

PRESCRIBING DRUGS LIKELY TO CAUSE DEPENDENCE OR MISUSE. The prescriber has three main responsibilities:

1. To avoid creating dependence by introducing drugs to patients without sufficient reason. In this context, the proper use of the morphine-like drugs is well understood. The dangers of other controlled drugs are less clear because recognition of dependence is not easy and its effects, and those of withdrawal, are less obvious. Perhaps the most notable result of uninhibited prescribing is that a very large number of patients in the country take tablets which do them neither much good nor much harm, but are committed to them indefinitely because they cannot readily be stopped.

2. To see that the patient does not gradually increase the dose of a drug, given for good medical reasons, to the point where dependence becomes more likely. This tendency is seen especially with hypnotics and anxiolytics (for CSM advice see section 4.1). The prescriber should keep a close eye on the amount prescribed to prevent patients from accumulating stocks that would enable them to arrange their own dosage or even that of their families and friends. A minimal amount should be prescribed in the first instance, or when seeing a new patient for the first time.

3. To avoid being used as an unwitting source of supply for addicts. Methods include visiting more than one doctor, fabricating stories, and forging prescriptions. A doctor should therefore be wary of prescribing for strangers and may be able to get information about suspected opioid addicts from the Home Office (for details see p. 9).

Patients under temporary care should be given only small supplies of drugs unless they present an unequivocal letter from their own doctors. Doctors should also remember that their own patients may be doing a collecting round with other doctors, especially in hospitals. It is sensible to decrease dosages steadily or to issue weekly or even daily prescriptions for small amounts if it is apparent that dependence is occurring.

The stealing and misuse of prescription forms could be minimised by the following precautions:

(a) do not leave unattended if called away from the consulting room or at reception desks; do not leave in a car where they may be visible; when not in use, keep in a locked drawer within the surgery and at home;

(b) draw a diagonal line across the blank part of the form under the prescription;

(c) write the quantity in words and figures when prescribing drugs prone to abuse; this is obligatory for controlled drugs (see Prescriptions, above);

(d) alterations are best avoided but if any are made they should be clear and unambiguous; add initials against altered items;

(e) if prescriptions are left for collection they should be left in a safe place in a sealed envelope.

TRAVELLING ABROAD. Prescribed drugs listed in schedules 4 and 5 to the Misuse of Drugs Regulations 1985 are not subject to import or export licensing but doctors are advised that patients intending to carry Schedule 2 and 3 drugs abroad

may require an export licence. This is dependent upon the amount of drug to be exported and further details may be obtained from the Home Office by telephoning 071-273 3806. Applications for licences should be sent to the Home Office, Drugs Branch, Queen Anne's Gate, London SW1H 9AT.

There is no standard application form but applications must be supported by a letter from a doctor giving details of:

the patient's name and current address;
the quantities of drugs to be carried;
the strength and form in which the drugs will be dispensed;
the dates of travel to and from the United Kingdom.

Ten days should be allowed for processing the application.

Individual doctors who wish to take Controlled Drugs abroad while accompanying patients, may similarly be issued with licences. Licences are not normally issued to doctors who wish to take Controlled Drugs abroad solely in case a family emergency should arise.

These import/export licences for named individuals do not have any legal status outside the UK and are only issued to comply with the Misuse of Drugs Act and facilitate passage through UK Customs control. For clearance in the country to be visited it would be necessary to approach that country's embassy or High Commission in the UK.

The Misuse of Drugs Act, 1971

This Act was passed in 1971 to provide more flexible and more comprehensive control over the misuse of drugs of all kinds than was possible under the earlier Dangerous Drugs Act. The Act as amended prohibits certain activities in relation to 'Controlled Drugs', in particular their manufacture, supply, and possession. The penalties applicable to offences involving the different drugs are graded broadly according to the *harmfulness attributable to a drug when it is misused* and for this purpose the drugs are defined in the following three classes:

Class A includes: alfentanil, cocaine, dextromoramide, diamorphine (heroin), dipipanone, lysergide (LSD), methadone, morphine, opium, pethidine, phencyclidine, and class B substances when prepared for injection

Class B includes: oral amphetamines, barbiturates, cannabis, cannabis resin, codeine, ethylmorphine, glutethimide, pentazocine, phenmetrazine, and pholcodine

Class C includes: certain drugs related to the amphetamines such as benzphetamine and chlorphentermine, buprenorphine, diethylpropion, mazindol, meprobamate, pemoline, pipradrol, and most benzodiazepines

The Misuse of Drugs Regulations 1985 define the classes of person who are authorised to supply and possess controlled drugs while acting in their professional capacities and lay down the conditions under which these activities may be carried out. In the regulations drugs are divided into five schedules each specifying the requirements governing such activities as import, export, production, supply, possession, prescribing, and record keeping which apply to them.

Schedule 1 includes drugs such as cannabis and lysergide which are not used medicinally. Possession and supply are prohibited except in accordance with Home Office authority.

Schedule 2 includes drugs such as diamorphine (heroin), morphine, pethidine, quinalbarbitone, glutethimide, amphetamine, and cocaine and are subject to the full controlled drug requirements relating to prescriptions, safe custody, the need to keep registers, etc. (unless exempted in schedule 5).

Schedule 3 includes the barbiturates (except quinalbarbitone, now schedule 2), buprenorphine, diethylpropion, mazindol, meprobamate, pentazocine, and phentermine. They are subject to the special prescription requirements (except for phenobarbitone, see p. 7) but not to the safe custody requirements (except for buprenorphine and diethylpropion) nor to the need to keep registers (although there are requirements for the retention of invoices for 2 years).

Schedule 4 includes 34 benzodiazepines and pemoline which are subject to minimal control. In particular, controlled drug prescription requirements do not apply and they are not subject to safe custody.

Schedule 5 includes those preparations which, because of their strength, are exempt from virtually all Controlled Drug requirements other than retention of invoices for two years.

Notification of Addicts

The Misuse of Drugs (Notification of and Supply to Addicts) Regulations 1973 require that any doctor who attends a person who the doctor considers or has reasonable grounds to suspect, is addicted to any of the 14 notifiable drugs (see below) shall, within seven days of the attendance, furnish in writing particulars of that person to:

Chief Medical Officer,
Home Office, Drugs Branch,
Queen Anne's Gate,
London SW1H 9AT.

The drugs to which the Regulations apply are:

Cocaine	Methadone
Dextromoramide	Morphine
Diamorphine	Opium
Dipipanone	Oxycodone
Hydrocodone	Pethidine
Hydromorphone	Phenazocine
Levorphanol	Piritramide

Note. Dipipanone is only legally available as Diconal® Tablets. These have been much misused by opioid addicts in recent years; only medical practitioners with a special licence may now prescribe them for addicts to treat addiction. Doctors and others should be suspicious of young people who ask for them, especially as temporary residents.

Particulars[1] to be notified to the Chief Medical Officer are:

Name and address
Sex
Date of birth
National Health Service number (if known)
Date of attendance
Name of drugs of addiction
Whether patient injects any drug (whether or not notifiable)

Notification must be confirmed annually in writing if the patient is still being treated by the practitioner. Notified information is incorporated in an Index of Addicts which is maintained in the Home Office and information from this is available on a confidential basis to doctors; in fact, it is good medical practice to check all new cases of addiction or suspected addiction with the Index before prescribing or supplying controlled drugs since this is a safeguard against addicts obtaining supplies simultaneously from two or more doctors. Enquiries can be made either in writing to the Chief Medical Officer or, preferably, by telephoning 071-273 2213. To keep notified information confidential, such enquiries are normally answered by means of a return telephone call. The reply will come from lay staff who are not qualified to give guidance on the clinical handling of cases; a recorded telephone service is available for out-of-office hours.

The preceding paragraph applies only to medical practitioners in England, Scotland, and Wales. In Northern Ireland notification should be sent to:

Chief Medical Officer,
Department of Health and Social Services,
Dundonald House,
Belfast BT4 3SF.
Enquiries should also be made to that Department, telephone 0232 650111 extension 229.

Prescribing of diamorphine (heroin), dipipanone, and cocaine for addicts

The Misuse of Drugs (Notification of and Supply to Addicts) Regulations 1973 also provide that only medical practitioners who hold a special licence issued by the Home Secretary may prescribe diamorphine, dipipanone (Diconal®), or cocaine for addicts; other practitioners must refer any addict who requires these drugs to a treatment centre. Whenever possible the addict will be introduced by a member of staff from the treatment centre to a pharmacist whose agreement has been obtained and whose pharmacy is conveniently sited for the patient. Prescriptions for weekly supplies will be sent to the pharmacy by post and will be dispensed on a daily basis as indicated by the doctor. If any alterations of the arrangements are requested by the addict, the portion of the prescription affected must be represcribed and not merely altered. *General practitioners and other doctors may still prescribe diamorphine, dipipanone, and cocaine for patients (including addicts) for relief of pain due to organic disease or injury without a special licence.*

For prescription-writing guidelines, see p. 7.

---

1. Only the particulars of which the doctor has knowledge need be notified immediately; the remainder may be notified at a later date. Private doctors, police surgeons and prison medical officers may continue to notify the Home Office using form HS2A/1(Rev), available from their Family Health Services Authority (FHSA) or their Health Board in Scotland.

All other doctors, including general practitioners, hospital doctors and those practising in treatment centres, should use notification forms which can be obtained from their Regional Health Authority Drugs Misuse Database administrator.

Adverse Reactions to Drugs

Any drug may produce unwanted or unexpected adverse reactions. Detection and recording of these is of vital importance. Doctors are urged to help by reporting adverse reactions to:

CSM
Freepost
London SW8 5BR
(071-627 3291)

Yellow prepaid lettercards for reporting are available from the above address or by dialling 100 and asking for 'CSM Freepost'; also, forms are bound in this book (inside back cover).

A 24-hour Freefone service is now available to all parts of the United Kingdom, for doctors seeking advice and information on adverse reactions; it may be obtained by dialling 100 and asking for 'CSM Freefone'. Outside office hours a telephone-answering machine will take messages.

The following regional centres also collect data:

CSM Mersey
Freepost
Liverpool L3 3AB
(051-236 4620 Extn 2126)

CSM Wales
Freepost
Cardiff CF4 1ZZ
(0222 744181 Direct Line)

CSM Northern
Freepost 1085
Newcastle upon Tyne
NE1 1BR
(091-232 1525 Direct Line)

CSM West Midlands
Freepost
Birmingham B15 1BR
[No telephone number]

Suspected adverse reactions to *any* therapeutic agent should be reported, including drugs (those taken for *self medication* as well as those *prescribed*), blood products, vaccines, X-ray contrast media, dental or surgical materials, intra-uterine devices, and contact lens fluids.

ADROIT

Adverse Drug Reactions On-line Information Tracking (ADROIT) has now been introduced to facilitate the monitoring of adverse drug reactions.

NEWER DRUGS. These are indicated by the sign ▼. Doctors are asked to report *all* suspected reactions (i.e. any adverse or any unexpected event, however minor, which could conceivably be attributed to the drug). Reports should be made despite uncertainty about a causal relationship, irrespective of whether the reaction is well recognized, and even if other drugs have been given concurrently.

ESTABLISHED DRUGS. Doctors are asked to report *all* serious suspected reactions, including those that are fatal, life-threatening, disabling, incapacitating, or which result in or prolong hospitalisation; they should be reported even if the effect is well recognised.

Examples include anaphylaxis, blood disorders, endocrine disturbances, effects on fertility, haemorrhage from any site, renal impairment, jaundice, ophthalmic disorders, severe CNS effects, severe skin reactions, reactions in pregnant women, and any drug interactions. Reports of serious adverse reactions are required to enable risk/benefit ratios to be compared with other drugs of a similar class. For established drugs doctors are asked not to report well-known, relatively minor side-effects, such as dry mouth with tricyclic antidepressants, constipation with opioids, or nausea with digoxin.

Special problems

Delayed drug effects. Some reactions (e.g. cancers, chloroquine retinopathy, and retroperitoneal fibrosis) may become manifest months or years after exposure. Any suspicion of such an association should be reported.

The elderly. Doctors are asked to be particularly alert to adverse reactions in the elderly.

Congenital abnormalities. When an infant is born with a congenital abnormality or there is a malformed aborted fetus doctors are asked to consider whether this might be an adverse reaction to a drug and to report all drugs (including self-medication) taken during pregnancy.

Vaccines. Doctors are asked to report all suspected reactions to both new and established vaccines. The balance between risks and benefits needs to be kept under continuous review.

Prevention of adverse reactions

Adverse reactions may be prevented as follows:

1. Never use any drug unless there is a good indication. If the patient is pregnant do not use a drug unless the need for it is imperative.
2. It is very important to recognise allergy and idiosyncrasy as causes of adverse drug reactions. Ask if the patient had previous reactions.
3. Ask if the patient is already taking other drugs *including self-medication*; remember that interactions may occur.
4. Age and hepatic or renal disease may alter the metabolism or excretion of drugs, so that much smaller doses may need to be prescribed. Pharmacogenetic factors may also be responsible for variations in the rate of metabolism, notably of isoniazid and the tricyclic antidepressants.
5. Prescribe as few drugs as possible and give very clear instructions to the elderly or any patient likely to misunderstand complicated instructions.
6. When possible use a familiar drug. With a new drug be particularly alert for adverse reactions or unexpected events.
7. If serious adverse reactions are liable to occur warn the patient.

Defective Medicines

During the manufacture or distribution of a medicine an error or accident may occur whereby the finished product does not conform to its specification. While such a defect may impair the therapeutic effect of the product and could adversely affect the health of a patient, it should **not** be confused with an Adverse Drug Reaction where the product conforms to its specification.

The Defect Medicines Report Centre operates a 24-hour service to assist with the investigation of problems arising from licensed medicinal products thought to be defective, and to co-ordinate any necessary protective action. Reports on suspect defective medicinal products should include the brand or the non-proprietary name, the name of the manufacturer or supplier, the strength and dosage form of the product, the product licence number, the batch number or numbers of the product, the nature of the defect, and an account of any action already taken in consequence. The Centre can be contacted at:

The Defect Medicines Report Centre
Medicines Control Agency
Room 1801, Market Towers
1 Nine Elms Lane
London SW8 5NQ
071-273 0574 (weekdays 8.30 am–5.30 pm)
or 071-210 5368 or 5371 (any other time)

Prescribing for Children

All children, and particularly neonates, differ from adults in their response to drugs. Special care is needed in the neonatal period (first 30 days of life) and doses should always be calculated according to weight. At this age, the risk of toxicity is increased by inefficient renal filtration, relative enzyme deficiencies, differing target organ sensitivity, and inadequate detoxifying systems causing delayed excretion. In childhood dosage should be adjusted for weight until 50 kg or puberty is reached.

Whenever possible painful intramuscular injections should be **avoided** in children.

PRESCRIPTION WRITING. Prescriptions should be written according to the guidelines in Prescription Writing (p. 4). Inclusion of age is a legal requirement in the case of prescription-only medicines for children under 12 years of age, but it is preferable to state the age for **all** prescriptions for children.

It is particularly important to state the strengths of capsules or tablets. Although liquid preparations are particularly suitable for children, many contain sucrose which encourages dental decay. When taken over a long period, sugar-free tablets and liquid medicines should be used when possible.

When a prescription for a liquid oral preparation is written and the dose ordered is smaller than 5 mL, the preparation will no longer be diluted. Instead an **oral syringe** will be supplied, for full details, see p. 2. Parents should be advised not to add any medicines to the contents of the infant's feeding bottle, since the drug may interact with the milk or other liquid in it; moreover the ingested dosage may be reduced, if the child does not drink all the contents.

Parents must be warned to keep **all** medicines out of the reach of children, see Safety in the Home, p. 3.

Rare paediatric conditions

Information on substances such as *biotin* and *sodium benzoate* used in rare metabolic conditions can be obtained from.

Drug Information Centre, Alder Hey Children's Hospital, Liverpool L12 2AP (Tel, 051-252 5381);

Pharmacy, Hospital for Sick Children, Great Ormond St, London, WC1N 3JH (Tel. 071-405 9200)

Dosage in Children

Children's doses in the BNF are stated in the individual drug entries as far as possible, except where paediatric use is not recommended or there are special hazards.

Doses are generally based on body-weight (in kilograms) or the following age ranges:

first month (neonate)
up to 1 year (infant)
1–5 years
6–12 years

Where a single dose is quoted for a given range, it applies to the middle of the age range and some extrapolation may be necessary to obtain doses for ages at the lower and upper limits of the stated range.

DOSE CALCULATION. Children's doses may be calculated from adult doses by using age, body-weight, or body-surface area, or by a combination of these factors. The most reliable methods are those based on body-surface area.

Body-weight may be used to calculate doses expressed in mg/kg. Young children may require a higher dose per kilogram than adults because of their higher metabolic rates. Other problems need to be considered. For example, calculation by body-weight in the obese child would result in much higher doses being administered than necessary; in such cases, dose should be calculated from an ideal weight, related to height and age.

Body-surface area (BSA) estimates are more accurate for calculation of paediatric doses than body-weight since many physical phenomena are more closely related to body-surface area. The average body-surface area of a 70-kilogram human is about 1.8m^2. Thus, to calculate the dose for a child the following formula may be used:

Approximate dose for patient =
$$\frac{\text{surface area of patient } (\text{m}^2)}{1.8} \times \text{adult dose}$$

The **percentage method** below may be used to calculate paediatric doses of commonly prescribed drugs that have a wide margin between the therapeutic and the toxic dose

Age	Ideal body-weight		Height		Body-surface	Percentage of adult
	kg	lb	cm	in	m²	dose
Newborn*	3.4	7.5	50	20	0.23	12.5
1 month*	4.2	9	55	22	0.26	14.5
3 months*	5.6	12	59	23	0.32	18
6 months	7.7	17	67	26	0.40	22
1 year	10	22	76	30	0.47	25
3 years	14	31	94	37	0.62	33
5 years	18	40	108	42	0.73	40
7 years	23	51	120	47	0.88	50
12 years	37	81	148	58	1.25	75
Adult						
Male	68	150	173	68	1.80	100
Female	56	123	163	64	1.60	100

* The figures relate to full term and not preterm infants who may need reduced dosage according to their clinical condition.

More precise body-surface values may be calculated from height and weight by means of a nomogram (e.g. J. Insley, *A Paediatric Vade-Mecum*, 12th Edition, London, Edward Arnold, 1990).

DOSE FREQUENCY. Doses for antibiotics are usually stated as every 6 hours. Some flexibility should be allowed in children to avoid waking them during the night. For example, the night-time dose may be given at the parent's bedtime.

Where new or potentially toxic drugs are used, the manufacturers' recommended doses should be carefully followed.

Prescribing in Terminal Care

In recent years there has been increased interest in providing better treatment and support for patients with terminal illness. The aim is to keep them as comfortable, alert, and free of pain as possible. If patients are to end their days in serenity it may also be necessary to direct attention to emotional, financial, social, or family problems. The patient's minister or the hospital chaplain may give invaluable help.

DOMICILIARY CARE. If they wish, whenever possible, patients should end their days in their own homes. Although families may at first be afraid of caring for the patient at home, they will usually do so if extra support from district nursing services and social services is provided. Families may be reassured if an assurance is given that the patient will be admitted to a hospital or hospice if they cannot cope.

HOSPITAL OR HOSPICE CARE. The most important lesson to be drawn from the experience of hospices is that both doctors and nurses must give time to listen to the patient. This gives great support and comfort to a patient who may otherwise suffer intolerable loneliness. Often problems come to light that can easily be dealt with—adjusting a blind in the late afternoon, an irritating noise to be avoided, drinks to be placed in easier reach, someone to read the newspaper, or the TV to be replaced by radio. The staff should not exclude the family from contributing to the patient's care; if prevented they may be resentful or subsequently suffer a feeling of guilt.

DRUG TREATMENT. The number of drugs should be as few as possible, for even the taking of medicine may be an effort. Oral medication is usually satisfactory unless there is severe nausea and vomiting, dysphagia, weakness, or coma, in which case parenteral medication may be necessary.

PAIN

Analgesics are always more effective in preventing the development of pain than in the relief of established pain.

The **non-opioid** analgesics **aspirin** or **paracetamol** given regularly will often make the use of opioids unnecessary. Aspirin (or other NSAIDs if preferred) may also control the pain of *bone secondaries*; naproxen, flurbiprofen, and indomethacin (see section 10.1.1) are valuable and if necessary can be given rectally. **Corticosteroids** or **radiotherapy** are also often useful for pain due to bone metastases.

Morphine is the most useful of the **opioid analgesics**. In addition to relief of pain, it confers a state of euphoria and mental detachment.

ORAL ROUTE. Morphine is given *by mouth* as an oral solution regularly every 4 hours, the initial dose depending largely on the patient's previous treatment. A dose of 5–10 mg is enough to replace a weaker analgesic (such as paracetamol or co-proxamol), but 10–20 mg or more is required to replace a strong one (comparable to morphine itself). If the first dose of morphine is no more effective than the previous analgesic it should be increased by 50%, the aim being to choose the lowest dose which prevents pain. Although a dose of 5–20 mg is usually adequate there should be no hesitation in increasing it to 30–60mg or occasionally to 90–150mg or higher if necessary. If pain occurs between doses the next dose due is increased; in the interim an additional dose is given.

Modified-release tablets of morphine (MST Continus® tablets or Oramorph® SR tablets) are an alternative to the oral solution; they have the advantage that they need only be taken every 12 hours. The starting dose of MST Continus® tablets or Oramorph® SR tablets is usually 10–20mg every 12 hours if no other analgesic (or only paracetamol) has previously been taken, but to replace a weaker opioid analgesic (such as co-proxamol) the starting dose is usually 20–30mg every 12 hours. Increments should be made to the dose, not to the frequency of administration, which should remain at every 12 hours.

The effective dose of MST Continus® tablets or Oramorph® SR tablets can alternatively be found by giving the oral solution of morphine every 4 hours in increasing doses until the pain has been controlled, and then transferring the patient to the same total 24-hour dose of morphine given as the modified-release tablet (divided into two portions for 12-hourly administration). The first dose of the modified-release tablet is given 4 hours after the last dose of the oral solution[1].

PARENTERAL ROUTE. If the patient becomes unable to swallow, the equivalent intramuscular dose of morphine is half the oral solution dose; in the case of the modified-release tablets it is half the total 24-hour dose (which is then divided into 6 portions to be given every 4 hours). **Diamorphine** is preferred for injection because being more soluble it can be given in a smaller volume. The equivalent intramuscular (or subcutaneous) dose of diamorphine is only about a quarter to a third of the oral dose of morphine; *subcutaneous infusion via syringe driver* can be useful (for details, see p.14).

RECTAL ROUTE. Morphine is also available for *rectal administration* as suppositories; alternatively **oxycodone** suppositories can be obtained on special order.

GASTRO-INTESTINAL PAIN. The pain of *bowel colic* may be reduced by loperamide 2–4 mg 4 times daily. Hyoscine hydrobromide may also be helpful, given sublingually at a dose of 300 micrograms 3 times daily as Kwells® (Roche Consumer Health) tablets. For the dose by *subcutaneous infusion* using a syringe driver, see p.14.

Gastric distension pain due to pressure on the stomach may be helped by a preparation incorporating an antacid with an antiflatulent (see section 1.1.1) and by domperidone 10 mg 3 times daily before meals.

---

1. Studies have indicated that administration of the last dose of the *oral solution* with the first dose of the *modified-release tablets* is not necessary.

MUSCLE SPASM. The pain of muscle spasm can be helped by a muscle relaxant such as diazepam 5–10 mg daily or baclofen 5–10 mg 3 times daily.

NERVE PAIN. Pain due to *nerve compression* may be reduced by a corticosteroid such as dexamethasone 8 mg daily, which reduces oedema around the tumour, thus reducing compression.

Dysaesthetic or stabbing pain resulting from *nerve irritation* may be reduced by amitriptyline 25–75 mg at night, or by carbamazepine 200 mg 3 times daily.

Nerve blocks may be considered when pain is localised to a specific area.

MISCELLANEOUS CONDITIONS

RAISED INTRACRANIAL PRESSURE. Headache due to *raised intracranial pressure* often responds to a high dose of a corticosteroid, such as dexamethasone 16 mg daily for 4 to 5 days, subsequently reduced to 4–6 mg daily if possible.

INTRACTABLE COUGH. *Intractable cough* may be relieved by moist inhalations or may require regular administration of an oral morphine hydrochloride (or sulphate) solution in an initial dose of 5 mg every 4 hours. Methadone linctus should be avoided as it has a long duration of action and tends to accumulate.

DYSPNOEA. *Dyspnoea* may be relieved by regular oral morphine hydrochloride (or sulphate) solution in carefully titrated doses, starting at 5 mg every 4 hours. Diazepam 5–10 mg daily may be helpful; a corticosteroid, such as dexamethasone 4–8 mg daily, may also be helpful if there is *bronchospasm* or *partial obstruction*.

EXCESSIVE RESPIRATORY SECRETION. *Excessive respiratory secretion* (death rattle) may be reduced by subcutaneous injection of hyoscine hydrobromide 400–600 micrograms every 4 to 8 hours. For the dose by *subcutaneous infusion* using a syringe driver, see next page.

RESTLESSNESS AND CONFUSION. *Restlessness and confusion* may require treatment with haloperidol 1–3 mg by mouth every 8 hours. Chlorpromazine 25–50 mg by mouth every 8 hours is an alternative, but causes more sedation. Methotrimeprazine is also used occasionally for restlessness. For the dose by *subcutaneous infusion* using a syringe driver, see next page.

HICCUP. *Hiccup due to gastric distension* may be helped by a preparation incorporating an antacid with an antiflatulent (see section 1.1.1). If this fails, metoclopramide 10 mg every 6 to 8 hours by mouth or by intramuscular injection can be added; if this also fails, chlorpromazine 10–25 mg every 6 to 8 hours can be tried.

ANOREXIA. *Anorexia* may be helped by prednisolone 15–30 mg daily or dexamethasone 2–4 mg daily.

Non-licensed indications or routes
Several recommendations in this section involve non-licensed indications or routes.

CONSTIPATION. *Constipation* is a very common cause of distress and is almost invariable after administration of an opioid. It should be prevented if possible by the regular administration of laxatives; a faecal softener with a peristaltic stimulant (e.g. co-danthramer), or lactulose solution with a senna preparation should be used (see sections 1.6.2 and 1.6.3).

FUNGATING GROWTH. *Fungating growth* may be treated by cleansing with a mixture of 1 part of 4% povidone-iodine skin cleanser solution and 4 parts of liquid paraffin. Oral administration of metronidazole (see section 5.1.11) may eradicate the anaerobic bacteria responsible for the odour of fungating tumours; topical application (see section 13.10.1.2) is also used.

CAPILLARY BLEEDING. *Capillary bleeding* may be reduced by applying gauze soaked in adrenaline solution (1 in 1000).

DRY MOUTH. *Dry mouth* may be associated with candidiasis which can be treated by nystatin oral suspension or pastilles, amphotericin lozenges, or miconazole oral gel after food; alternatively, fluconazole can be given by mouth (see section 5.2). Dry mouth can also be a side-effect of morphine.

PRURITUS. *Pruritus,* even when associated with *obstructive jaundice,* often responds to simple measures such as emollients. In the case of obstructive jaundice, further measures include administration of cholestyramine or an anabolic steroid, such as stanozolol 5–10 mg daily; antihistamines can be helpful (see section 3.4.1).

CONVULSIONS. Patients with *cerebral tumours* or *uraemia* may be susceptible to convulsions. Prophylactic treatment with phenytoin or carbamazepine (see section 4.8.1) should be considered. When oral medication is no longer possible, diazepam as suppositories 10–20 mg every 4 to 8 hours, or phenobarbitone by injection 50–200 mg twice daily is continued as prophylaxis. For the use of midazolam by *subcutaneous infusion* using a syringe driver, see next page.

DYSPHAGIA. A corticosteroid such as dexamethasone 8 mg daily may help, temporarily, if there is an obstruction due to *tumour*. See also under Dry Mouth.

NAUSEA AND VOMITING. *Nausea and vomiting* are very common in patients with advanced cancer. The cause should be diagnosed before treatment with anti-emetics (see section 4.6) is started.

Nausea and vomiting may also occur in the initial stages of morphine therapy but can be prevented by giving an anti-emetic such as haloperidol or prochlorperazine. An anti-emetic is usually only necessary for the first 4 or 5 days therefore fixed-combination opioid preparations containing an anti-emetic are not recommended since they lead to unnecessary anti-emetic therapy (often with undesirable drowsiness). For the administration of anti-emetics by *subcutaneous infusion* using a syringe driver, see below.

INSOMNIA. Patients with advanced cancer may not sleep because of discomfort, cramps, night sweats, joint stiffness, or fear. There should be appropriate treatment of these problems before hypnotics are used. Benzodiazepines, such as temazepam, may be useful (see section 4.1.1).

HYPERCALCAEMIA. See section 9.5.1.2.

SYRINGE DRIVERS

Although drugs can usually be administered *by mouth* to control the symptoms of advanced cancer, the parenteral route may sometimes be necessary. If the parenteral route is necessary, repeated administration of *intramuscular injections* can be difficult in a cachectic patient. This has led to the use of a portable syringe driver to give a *continuous subcutaneous infusion,* which can provide good control of symptoms with little discomfort or inconvenience to the patient.

Indications for the **parenteral route** are:

the patient is unable to take medicines by mouth owing to *nausea and vomiting, dysphagia, severe weakness,* or *coma*;

there is *malignant bowel obstruction* in patients for whom further surgery is inappropriate (avoiding the need for an intravenous infusion or for insertion of a nasogastric tube);

occasionally when the patient *does not wish* to take regular medication by mouth.

NAUSEA AND VOMITING. **Haloperidol** is given in a *subcutaneous infusion* dose of 2.5–10 mg/24 hours.

Methotrimeprazine causes sedation in about 50% of patients; it is given in a *subcutaneous infusion* dose of 25–200mg/24 hours.

Cyclizine is particularly liable to precipitate if mixed with diamorphine or other drugs (see under Mixing and Compatibility, below); it is given in a *subcutaneous infusion dose* of 150mg/24 hours.

Metoclopramide may cause skin reactions; it is given in a *subcutaneous infusion dose* of 30–60 mg /24 hours.

BOWEL COLIC OR EXCESSIVE RESPIRATORY SECRETIONS. **Hyoscine hydrobromide** effectively reduces respiratory secretions and is sedative (but occasionally causes paradoxical agitation); it is given in a *subcutaneous infusion dose* of 0.6–2.4 mg/24 hours.

Hyoscine butylbromide is effective in bowel colic, is less sedative than hyoscine hydrobromide, but is not always adequate for the control of respiratory secretions; it is given in a *subcutaneous infusion dose* of 20–60 mg /24 hours (**important:** this dose of *hyoscine butylbromide* must not be confused with the much lower dose of *hyoscine hydrobromide,* above).

RESTLESSNESS AND CONFUSION. **Haloperidol** has little sedative effect; it is given in a *subcutaneous infusion dose* of 5–30 mg/24 hours.

Methotrimeprazine has a sedative effect; it is given in a *subcutaneous infusion dose* of 50–200mg/24 hours.

Midazolam is a sedative and an antiepileptic, and is therefore suitable for a very restless patient; it is given in a *subcutaneous infusion dose* of 20–40mg/24 hours.

CONVULSIONS. If a patient has previously been receiving an antiepileptic *or* has a primary or secondary cerebral tumour *or* is at risk of convulsion (e.g. owing to uraemia) antiepileptic medication should not be stopped. **Midazolam** is the benzodiazepine antiepileptic of choice for *continuous subcutaneous infusion,* and is given in a dose of 20–40mg/24 hours.

PAIN CONTROL. **Diamorphine** is the preferred opioid since its high solubility permits a large dose to be given in a small volume (see under Mixing and Compatibility, below). The table on the next page gives the approximate doses of *morphine by mouth* (as oral solution or standard tablets or as modified-release tablets) equivalent to *diamorphine by injection* (intramuscularly or by subcutaneous infusion).

MIXING AND COMPATIBILITY. The general principle that injections should be given into separate sites (and should not be mixed) does not apply to the use of syringe drivers in terminal care. Provided that there is evidence of compatibility, selected injections can be mixed in syringe drivers. Not all types of medication can be used in a subcutaneous infusion. In particular, **chlorpromazine, prochlorperazine** and **diazepam** are **contra-indicated** as they cause skin reactions at the injection site; to a lesser extent **cyclizine** and **methotrimeprazine** may also sometimes cause local irritation.

In theory injections dissolved in **water for injections** are more likely to be associated with pain (possibly owing to their hypotonicity). The use of **physiological saline** (sodium chloride 0.9%) however increases the likelihood of precipitation when more than one drug is used; moreover subcutaneous infusion rates are so slow (0.1–0.3 mL/hour) that pain is not usually a problem when water is used as a diluent.

Diamorphine can be given by subcutaneous infusion in a strength of up to 250mg/mL; up to a strength of 40mg/mL either *water for injections* or *physiological saline* (sodium chloride 0.9%) is a suitable diluent—above that strength only *water for injections* is used (to avoid precipitation).

The following can be mixed with *diamorphine:*

Cyclizine[1]
Dexamethasone[2]
Haloperidol[3]
Hyoscine butylbromide
Hyoscine hydrobromide
Methotrimeprazine
Metoclopramide[4]
Midazolam

---

1. Cyclizine may precipitate at concentrations above 20mg/mL *or* in the presence of physiological saline *or* as the concentration of diamorphine relative to cyclizine increases; mixtures of diamorphine and cyclizine are also liable to precipitate after 24 hours.
2. Special care is needed to avoid precipitation of dexamethasone when preparing.
3. Mixtures of haloperidol and diamorphine are liable to precipitate after 24 hours if haloperidol concentration is above 2 mg/mL.
4. Under some conditions metoclopramide may become discoloured; such solutions should be discarded.

Subcutaneous infusion solution should be monitored regularly both to check for precipitation (and discoloration) and to ensure that the infusion is running at the correct rate.

PROBLEMS ENCOUNTERED WITH SYRINGE DRIVERS. The following are problems that may be encountered with syringe drivers and the action that should be taken:

if the subcutaneous infusion runs *too quickly* check the rate setting and the calculation;

if the subcutaneous infusion runs *too slowly* check the start button, the battery, the syringe driver, the cannula, and make sure that the injection site is not inflamed;

if there is an *injection site reaction* make sure that the site does not need to be changed—firmness or swelling at the site of injection is not in itself an indication for change, but pain or obvious inflammation is.

Equivalent doses of morphine sulphate by mouth (as oral solution or standard tablets *or* as modified-release tablets) *or of* diamorphine hydrochloride by intramuscular injection *or by* subcutaneous infusion

These equivalences are approximate only and may need to be adjusted according to response

ORAL MORPHINE		PARENTERAL DIAMORPHINE	
Morphine sulphate oral solution or standard tablets	Morphine sulphate modified-release tablets	Diamorphine hydrochloride by intramuscular injection	Diamorphine hydrochloride by subcutaneous infusion
every 4 hours	**every 12 hours**	**every 4 hours**	**every 24 hours**
5 mg	20 mg	2.5 mg	15 mg
10 mg	30 mg	5 mg	20 mg
15 mg	50 mg	5 mg	30 mg
20 mg	60 mg	7.5 mg	45 mg
30 mg	90 mg	10 mg	60 mg
40 mg	120 mg	15 mg	90 mg
60 mg	180 mg	20 mg	120 mg
80 mg	240 mg	30 mg	180 mg
100 mg	300 mg	40 mg	240 mg
130 mg	400 mg	50 mg	300 mg
160 mg	500 mg	60 mg	360 mg
200 mg	600 mg	70 mg	400 mg

If breakthrough pain occurs give a subcutaneous (preferable) or intramuscular injection of diamorphine equivalent to one-sixth of the total 24-hour subcutaneous infusion dose. It is kinder to give an intermittent bolus injection *subcutaneously*—absorption is smoother so that the risk of adverse effects at peak absorption is avoided (an even better method is to use a subcutaneous butterfly needle).

To minimise the risk of infection no individual subcutaneous infusion solution should be used for longer than 24 hours.

Prescribing for the Elderly

Old people, especially the very old, require special care and consideration from prescribers.

POLYPHARMACY. Elderly patients are apt to receive multiple drugs for their multiple diseases. This greatly increases the risk of drug interactions as well as other adverse reactions. Moreover, symptoms such as headache, sleeplessness, and lightheadedness which may be associated with social stress, as in widowhood, loneliness, and family dispersal can lead to further prescribing, especially of psychotropics. The use of drugs in such cases can at best be a poor substitute for effective social measures and at worst pose a serious threat from adverse reactions.

FORM OF MEDICINE. Elderly patients may have difficulty swallowing tablets; if left in the mouth, ulceration may develop. They should always be encouraged to take their tablets or capsules with enough fluid, and in some cases it may be advisable to prescribe liquid if available.

MANIFESTATIONS OF AGEING. In very old subjects, manifestations of normal ageing may be mistaken for disease and lead to inappropriate prescribing. For example, drugs such as prochlorperazine are commonly misprescribed for giddiness due to age-related loss of postural stability. Not only is such treatment ineffective but the patient may experience serious side-effects such as drug-induced parkinsonism, postural hypotension, and mental confusion.

SELF-MEDICATION. Self-medication with over-the-counter products or with drugs prescribed for a previous illness (or even for another person) may be an added complication. Discussion with relatives and a home visit may be needed to establish exactly what is being taken.

SUSCEPTIBILITY. The ageing nervous system shows increased *susceptibility* to many commonly used drugs, such as opioid analgesics, benzodiazepines, and antiparkinsonian drugs, all of which must be used with caution.

PHARMACOKINETICS

While drug distribution and metabolism may be significantly altered, the most important effect of age is reduction in renal clearance, frequently aggravated by the effects of prostatism, nephrosclerosis, or chronic urinary tract infection. Many aged patients thus possess only *limited reserves of renal function, excrete drugs slowly,* and are *highly susceptible to nephrotoxic drugs.* Acute illness may lead to rapid reduction in renal clearance, especially if accompanied by dehydration. Hence, a patient stabilised on a drug with a narrow margin between the therapeutic and the toxic dose (e.g. digoxin) may rapidly develop adverse effects in the aftermath of a myocardial infarction or a respiratory tract infection.

The net result of pharmacokinetic changes is that tissue concentrations are commonly increased by over 50%, and aged and debilitated patients may show even larger changes.

ADVERSE REACTIONS

Adverse reactions often present in the elderly in a vague and non-specific fashion. *Mental confusion* is often the presenting symptom (caused by almost any of the commonly used drugs). Other common manifestations are *constipation* (with antimuscarinics and many tranquillisers) and postural *hypotension* and *falls* (with diuretics and many psychotropics).

HYPNOTICS. Many hypnotics with long half-lives have serious hangover effects of drowsiness, unsteady gait, and even slurred speech and confusion. Those with short half-lives should be used but they too can present problems (see section 4.1.1). Short courses of hypnotics are occasionally useful for helping a patient through an acute illness or some other crisis but every effort must be made to avoid dependence.

DIURETICS. Diuretics are overprescribed in old age and should **not** be used on a long-term basis to treat simple gravitational oedema which will usually respond to increased movement, raising the legs, and support stockings. A few days of diuretic treatment may speed the clearing of the oedema but it should rarely need continued drug therapy.

NSAIDs. Bleeding associated with *aspirin* and *other NSAIDs* is more common in the elderly, and the outcome tends to be more serious. NSAIDs are also a special hazard in patients with cardiac disease or renal impairment which may again place the elderly at particular risk.

OTHER DRUGS. Other drugs which commonly cause adverse reactions are *antiparkinsonian drugs, antihypertensives, psychotropics,* and *digoxin*; the usual maintenance dose of digoxin in very old patients is 125 micrograms daily (62.5 micrograms is often inadequate, and toxicity is common in those given 250 micrograms).

Drug-induced blood disorders are much more common in the elderly. Therefore drugs with a tendency to cause bone marrow depression (e.g. *co-trimoxazole, mianserin*) should be avoided unless there is no acceptable alternative.

The elderly generally require a lower maintenance dose of *warfarin* than younger adults; once again, the outcome of bleeding tends to be more serious.

GUIDELINES

First one must always pose the question of whether a drug is indicated at all.

LIMIT RANGE. It is a sensible policy to prescribe from a limited range of drugs and to be thoroughly familiar with their effects in the elderly.

REDUCE DOSE. Dosage should generally be substantially lower than for younger patients and it is common to start with about 50% of the adult dose. Some drugs (e.g. chlorpropamide) should be avoided altogether.

REVIEW REGULARLY. Review repeat prescriptions regularly. It may be possible to stop the drug (e.g. digoxin can often be withdrawn) or it may be necessary to reduce the dose to match diminishing renal function.

SIMPLIFY. Simplify regimens. Elderly patients cannot normally cope with more than three different drugs and, ideally, these should not be given more than twice daily. In particular, regimens which call for a confusing array of dosage intervals should be avoided.

EXPLAIN CLEARLY. Write full instructions on every prescription (*including* repeat prescriptions) so that containers can be properly labelled with full directions. Avoid imprecisions like 'as directed'. Child-resistant containers may be unsuitable.

REPEATS AND DISPOSAL. Instruct patients what to do when drugs run out, and also how to dispose of any that are no longer necessary.

If these guidelines are followed most elderly people will cope adequately with their own medicines. If not then it is essential to enrol the help of a third party, usually a relative but sometimes a home help, neighbour, or a sheltered-housing warden.

Emergency Treatment of Poisoning

TOXBASE is an on-line database which provides information about routine diagnosis, treatment and management of patients exposed to drugs, household products, and industrial and agricultural chemicals. It is available via a Viewdata system to authorised users including Accident and Emergency Departments. **Important:** for more specialised information telephone the Poisons Information Centres.

TICTAC is a computer-aided tablet and capsule identification system. It is available to authorised users including Regional Drug Information Centres (see p.xiii) and Poisons Information Centres.

POISONS INFORMATION CENTRES (consult day and night)

Belfast	0232 240503
Birmingham	021-554 3801
Cardiff	0222 709901
Dublin	Dublin 379964
	or Dublin 379966
Edinburgh	031-229 2477
Leeds	0532 430715
	or 0532 923547
London	071-635 9191
	or 071-955 5095
Newcastle	091-232 5131

Note. Some of these centres also advise on laboratory analytical services which may be of help in the diagnosis and management of a small number of cases.

These notes deal with the initial management of acute poisoning in the home; brief mention only is given of hospital-based treatment. The notes are only guidelines and it is strongly recommended that **poisons information centres** (see above) be consulted in cases where there is doubt about the degree of risk or about appropriate management.

HOSPITAL ADMISSION. All patients who show features of poisoning should generally be admitted to hospital. Patients who have taken poisons with delayed actions should also be admitted, even if they appear well; delayed-action poisons include aspirin, iron, paracetamol, tricyclic antidepressants, co-phenotrope (diphenoxylate with atropine, *Lomotil®*), and paraquat; this also applies to modified-release capsules or tablets. A note should be sent of what is known and what treatment has been given.

It is often impossible to establish with certainty the identity of the poison and the size of the dose. Fortunately this is not usually important because only a few poisons (such as opioids, paracetamol, and iron) have specific antidotes and few patients require active removal of the poison. Most patients must be treated symptomatically. Nevertheless, knowledge of the type of poisoning does help in anticipating the course of events. Patients' reports may be of little help, as they may be confused or may only be able to say that they have taken an undefined amount, possibly of mixed drugs. Parents may think a child has taken something which could be poisonous and may exaggerate or underplay the risks out of anxiety or guilt. Sometimes symptoms are due to an illness such as appendicitis. Accidents can arise from a number of domestic and industrial products (the contents of which are not generally known).

General care

> The **poisons information centres** (see page 18) will provide advice on all aspects of poisoning day and night

RESPIRATION

Respiration is often impaired in unconscious patients. An obstructed airway requires immediate attention. Pull the tongue forward, remove dentures and oral secretions, hold the jaw forward, insert an oropharyngeal airway if one is available, and turn the patient semiprone. The risk of inhaling vomit is minimised with the patient positioned semiprone and head down.

Most poisons that impair consciousness also depress respiration. Assisted ventilation by mouth-to-mouth or Ambu bag inflation may be needed. Oxygen is not a substitute for adequate ventilation, though it should be given in the highest concentration possible in poisoning with carbon monoxide and irritant gases.

Respiratory stimulants do not help and are **potentially dangerous**.

BLOOD PRESSURE

Hypotension is common in severe poisoning with central nervous system depressants. A systolic blood pressure of less than 70 mmHg may lead to irreversible brain damage or renal tubular necrosis. The patient should be carried head downwards on a stretcher and nursed in this position in the ambulance. Oxygen should be given to correct hypoxia and an intravenous infusion should be set up if at all practicable. Vasopressor drugs should **not** be used.

Fluid depletion without hypotension is common after prolonged coma and after aspirin poisoning due to vomiting, sweating, and hyperpnoea.

HEART

Cardiac conduction defects and arrhythmias may occur in acute poisoning, notably with tricyclic antidepressants. Arrhythmias often respond to correction of underlying hypoxia or acidosis. Ventricular arrhythmias that have been confirmed by emergency ECG and which are causing serious hypotension may require treatment with lignocaine 50–100 mg by slow intravenous injection. Supraventricular arrhythmias are seldom life-threatening and drug treatment is best withheld until the patient reaches hospital.

BODY TEMPERATURE

Hypothermia may develop in patients of any age who have been deeply unconscious for some hours particularly following overdose with barbiturates or phenothiazines. It may be missed unless temperature is measured rectally using a low-reading rectal thermometer. It is best treated by wrapping the patient in blankets to conserve body heat. Hot-water bottles are of little value and may cause burns.

CONVULSIONS

Single short-lived convulsions do not require treatment. Diazepam, up to 10mg by slow intravenous injection, preferably in emulsion form, should be given if convulsions are protracted or recur frequently; it should not be given intramuscularly.

Removal and elimination

REMOVAL FROM THE STOMACH

The dangers of attempting to empty the stomach have to be balanced against the toxicity of the ingested poison, as assessed by the quantity ingested, the inherent toxicity of the poison, and the time since ingestion. Gastric emptying is clearly unnecessary if the risk of toxicity is small or if the patient presents too late.

Emptying the stomach by **gastric lavage** or **emesis** is of doubtful value if attempted more than 4 hours after ingestion. However, a worthwhile recovery of salicylates can be achieved up to 24 hours after ingestion and of tricyclic antidepressants (which delay gastric emptying) up to 8 hours after ingestion. The chief danger of gastric aspiration and lavage is inhalation of stomach contents, and it should **not** be attempted in drowsy or comatose patients unless there is a good enough cough reflex or the airway can be protected by a cuffed endotracheal tube. Stomach tubes should **not** be passed after corrosive poisoning.

Petroleum products are more dangerous in the lungs than in the stomach and therefore removal from the stomach is **not** advised because of the risk of inhalation.

On balance gastric lavage is seldom practicable or desirable before the patient reaches hospital.

Emesis induced by using **ipecacuanha** (Paediatric Ipecacuanha Emetic Mixture BP) tends to be used in children. It may be given safely in the home providing that the patient is fully conscious and that the poison ingested is neither a corrosive nor a petroleum distillate, and is not liable to cause rapid onset of coma or convulsions.

Salt solutions, copper sulphate, apomorphine, and mustard are dangerous and should **not** be used.

IPECACUANHA

Indications: induction of emesis in selected patients, see notes above

Cautions: avoid in poisoning with corrosive or petroleum products owing to risk of aspiration (see notes above); also avoid if risk of aspiration, in shock, or if risk of convulsions; cardiovascular disease

Side-effects: excessive vomiting and mucosal damage; cardiac effects if absorbed

Dose: see under preparation below

Ipecacuanha Emetic Mixture, Paediatric (BP)
Paediatric Ipecacuanha Emetic
Note. Paediatric Ipecacuanha Emetic Mixture is equivalent in strength to Ipecac Syrup USP
Mixture, ipecacuanha liquid extract 0.7 mL, hydrochloric acid 0.025 mL, glycerol 1 mL, syrup to 10 mL
Dose: ADULT 30 mL; CHILD 6–18 months 10 mL, older children 15 mL; the dose is followed by a tumblerful of water and repeated after 20 minutes if necessary

PREVENTION OF ABSORPTION

Given by mouth, **activated charcoal** can bind many poisons in the stomach, thereby *reducing their absorption*. The **sooner** it is given the **more effective** it is, but it may still be effective up to 4 hours after ingestion—longer in the case of modified-release preparations or of drugs with antimusarinic (anticholinergic) properties. It is safe and is particularly useful for the prevention of absorption of poisons which are toxic in small amounts, e.g. antidepressants.

For the use of charcoal in active elimination techniques, see below.

Carbomix® (Penn)
Powder, activated charcoal. Net price 50-g bottle = £11.50
Dose: reduction of absorption, 50 g; CHILD, 25 g (50 g in severe poisoning)
Active elimination, see below

Medicoal® (Torbet)
Granules, effervescent, activated charcoal 5 g/sachet. Net price 5-sachet pack = £3.76, 30-sachet pack = £18.90
Dose: reduction of absorption, initially 1–2 sachets repeated every 15–20 minutes until dose of charcoal given is 5–10 times that of poison ingested (if amount known) *or* (if amount not known) until max. 10 sachets have been given; each sachet suspended in approx. 100 mL water (volume of suspension may need to be reduced for children)

ACTIVE ELIMINATION TECHNIQUES

Repeated doses of **activated charcoal** by mouth *enhance the elimination* of some drugs after they have been absorbed; repeated doses are given after overdosage with:

Aspirin	Phenobarbitone
Carbamazepine	and other barbiturates
Dapsone	Phenytoin
Digitoxin	Quinine
Digoxin	Theophylline

The usual adult dose of activated charcoal is 50 g initially then 25 g every 4 hours.

Other techniques intended to enhance the elimination of poisons after absorption are only practicable in hospital and are only suitable for a small number of severely poisoned patients. Moreover, they only apply to a limited number of poisons. Examples include:

Forced alkaline diuresis for salicylates and phenobarbitone (but haemodialysis now preferred)
Haemodialysis for salicylates, phenobarbitone, methyl alcohol (methanol), ethylene glycol, and lithium
Haemoperfusion for medium- and short-acting barbiturates, chloral hydrate, meprobamate, and theophylline.

Specific drugs

ALCOHOL

Acute intoxication with alcohol (ethanol) is common in adults but also occurs in children. The features include ataxia, dysarthria, nystagmus, and drowsiness, which may progress to coma, with hypotension and acidosis. Aspiration of vomit is a special hazard and hypoglycaemia may occur in children and some adults. Patients are managed supportively with particular attention to maintaining a clear airway and measures to reduce the risk of aspiration of gastric contents. The blood glucose is measured and glucose given if indicated.

ANALGESICS (NON-OPIOID)

ASPIRIN. Absorption of aspirin and other salicylates may be delayed, especially if enteric-coated tablets have been taken; blood concentrations taken within the first 6 hours may therefore be misleadingly low.

The chief features of poisoning are hyperventilation, tinnitus, deafness, vasodilatation, and sweating. Coma is uncommon but indicates very severe poisoning. The associated acid-base disturbances are complex.

Gastric emptying is carried out in all cases; a worthwhile recovery of salicylates can be achieved up to 24 hours after ingestion.

Treatment must be in hospital where plasma salicylate, pH, and electrolytes can be measured. Fluid losses are replaced and forced alkaline diuresis is considered when the plasma-salicylate concentration is greater than

500 mg/litre (3.6 mmol/litre) in adults *or*
300 mg/litre (2.2 mmol/litre) in children.

NSAIDs. Mefenamic acid is the most significant member of this group encountered in overdosage. Convulsions are the most important feature of toxicity and are treated with diazepam.

Ibuprofen may cause nausea, vomiting, and tinnitus, but more serious toxicity is very uncommon. Gastric emptying is indicated if more than 100 mg/kg has been ingested within the preceding 4 hours, followed by symptomatic measures.

PARACETAMOL. As little as 10–15 g (20–30 tablets) of paracetamol may cause severe hepatocellular necrosis and, less frequently, renal tubular necrosis. Nausea and vomiting, the only early features of poisoning, usually settle within 24 hours. Persistence beyond this time, often associated with the onset of right subcostal pain and tenderness, usually indicates development of hepatic necrosis. Liver damage is maximal 3–4 days after ingestion and may lead to encephalopathy, haemorrhage, hypoglycaemia, cerebral oedema, and death.

Therefore, despite a lack of significant early symptoms, patients who have taken an overdose of paracetamol should be transferred to hospital urgently.

Gastric emptying is carried out if the overdose was taken within 4 hours of admission.

Antidotes such as **acetylcysteine** and **methionine** protect the liver if given within 10–12 hours of ingestion; acetylcysteine may also be effective up to and possibly beyond 24 hours but expert advice is **essential**.

Patients at risk of liver damage and therefore requiring treatment can be identified from a single measurement of the plasma-paracetamol concentration, related to the time from ingestion, provided this time interval is not less than 4 hours; earlier samples may be misleading. The concentration is compared against a reference line joining plots of 200 mg/litre (1.32 mmol/litre) at 4 hours and 30 mg/litre (0.2 mmol/litre) at 15 hours, on a semi-logarithmic graph. Those whose concentrations are above that line are treated either with acetylcysteine intravenously or with methionine by mouth. Patients on enzyme-inducing drugs (e.g. carbamazepine, phenobarbitone, phenytoin, rifampicin, and alcohol) may develop toxicity at **lower** plasma-paracetamol concentrations; they should receive acetylcysteine if their plasma-paracetamol concentrations are 50% or more of the standard reference line.

In remote areas, emesis should be induced if the patient presents within 4 hours of the overdose. Methionine (2.5g) should be given by mouth once vomiting has occurred; it is seldom practicable to give acetylcysteine outside hospital. Once the patient reaches hospital the need to continue treatment with the antidote will be assessed from the plasma-paracetamol concentration (related to the time from ingestion).

See also Co-proxamol, under Analgesics (opioid).

ACETYLCYSTEINE

Indications: paracetamol overdosage (see notes above)
Cautions: asthma
Side-effects: rashes, anaphylaxis
Dose: by intravenous infusion, in glucose intravenous infusion 5%, initially 150 mg/kg in 200 mL over 15 minutes, followed by 50 mg/kg in 500 mL over 4 hours, then 100 mg/kg in 1000 mL over 16 hours

PoM **Parvolex®**(Evans)
Injection, acetylcysteine 200 mg /mL. Net price course of 12 amps of 10 mL = £31.75

METHIONINE

Indications: paracetamol overdosage, see notes above
Dose: by mouth, 2.5 g initially, followed by 3 further doses of 2.5 g every 4 hours

Methionine Tablets (Evans), DL-methionine 250 mg. Net price course of 40 tabs = £11.20

ANALGESICS (OPIOID)

Opioids (narcotic analgesics) cause varying degrees of coma, respiratory depression, and pinpoint pupils. The specific antidote **naloxone** is indicated if there is coma or bradypnoea. Since naloxone is short-acting repeated injections are necessary according to the respiratory rate and depth of coma. Alternatively, it may be given by continuous intravenous infusion, the rate of administration being adjusted according to response.

CO-PROXAMOL. Combinations of dextropropoxyphene and paracetamol (co-proxamol) are frequently taken in overdosage. The initial features are those of acute opioid overdosage with coma, respiratory depression, and pinpoint pupils. Patients may die of acute cardiovascular collapse before reaching hospital (particularly if alcohol has also been consumed) unless adequately resuscitated or given **naloxone** as antidote to the dextropropoxyphene. Paracetamol hepatotoxicity may develop later and should be anticipated and treated as indicated above.

NALOXONE HYDROCHLORIDE

Indications: overdosage with opioids; for postoperative respiratory depression, see section 15.1.7
Cautions: physical dependence on opioids; cardiac irritability; naloxone is short-acting, see notes above
Dose: by intravenous injection, 0.8–2 mg repeated at intervals of 2–3 minutes to a max. of 10 mg if respiratory function does not improve (then question diagnosis); CHILD 10 micrograms/kg; subsequent dose of 100 micrograms/kg if no response

By subcutaneous or intramuscular injection, as intravenous injection but only if intravenous route not feasible (onset of action slower)

By continuous intravenous infusion, 2 mg diluted in 500 mL intravenous infusion solution at a rate adjusted according to the response

PoM **Naloxone** (Non-proprietary)
Injection, naloxone hydrochloride 400 micrograms/ mL. Net price 1-mL amp = £4.79
Available from David Bull
PoM **Min-I-Jet® Naloxone** (IMS)
Injection, naloxone hydrochloride 400 microrams/ mL. Net price 1 mL disposable syringe – £5.23; 2-mL disposable syringe = £9.74
PoM **Narcan®** (Du Pont)
Injection, naloxone hydrochloride 400 micrograms/mL, net price 1-mL amp – £4.92, 1-mL disposable syringe – £5.44; 1 mg/mL, 2-mL amp = £22.00
Neonatal preparations—see section 15.1.7

ANTIDEPRESSANTS

Tricyclic and related antidepressants cause dry mouth, coma of varying degree, hypotension, hypothermia, hyperreflexia, extensor plantar responses, convulsions, respiratory failure, cardiac conduction defects, and arrhythmias. Dilated pupils and urinary retention also occur. Metabolic acidosis may complicate severe poisoning; delirium with confusion, agitation, and visual and auditory hallucinations, is common during recovery.

Symptomatic treatment and activated charcoal by mouth may reasonably be given in the home before transfer but hospital admission is strongly advised, and supportive measures to ensure a patent airway and adequate ventilation during transfer are mandatory. Intravenous diazepam may be required for control of convulsions (preferably in emulsion form). Although arrhythmias are worrying, some will respond to correction of hypoxia and acidosis; the use of anti-arrhythmic drugs is best avoided. Diazepam given by mouth is usually adequate to sedate delirious patients but large doses may be required.

ANTIMALARIALS

Overdosage with chloroquine and hydroxychloroquine is extremely hazardous and difficult to treat. Urgent advice from a poisons information centre is essential. Life-threatening features include arrhythmias (which can have a very rapid onset) and convulsions (which can be intractable). Quinine overdosage is also a severe hazard and also calls for urgent advice from a poisons information centre.

BETA-BLOCKERS

Therapeutic overdosages with beta-blockers may cause lightheadedness, dizziness, and possibly syncope due to impaired circulation secondary to bradycardia and hypotension; heart failure may be precipitated or exacerbated. These complications are most likely in patients with pre-existing conduction system disorders or impaired myocardial function. Bradycardia is the most common arrhythmia caused by beta-blockers, but sotalol occasionally induces ventricular tachyarrhythmias (sometimes of the torsades de pointes type). The effects of massive overdosage may vary from one beta-blocker to another; propranolol overdosage in particular may cause coma and convulsions.

Acute massive overdosage must be managed in hospital and expert advice should be obtained. Maintenance of a clear airway and adequate ventilation is mandatory. An intravenous injection of atropine is required to treat bradycardia and hypotension (3 mg for an adult, 40 micrograms/kg for a child). Cardiogenic shock unresponsive to atropine is probably best treated with an intravenous injection of glucagon 50–150 micrograms/kg [unlicensed indication and dose] in glucose 5% (with precautions to protect the airway in case of vomiting). A further dose of glucagon (or an intravenous infusion) may be required if the response is not maintained. If glucagon is not available, intravenous isoprenaline or intravenous prenalterol [not on UK market] are alternatives to glucagon.

HYPNOTICS AND ANXIOLYTICS

BARBITURATES. These cause drowsiness, coma, respiratory depression, hypotension, and hypothermia. The duration and depth of cerebral depression vary greatly with the drug, the dose, and the tolerance of the patient. The severity of poisoning is often greater with a large dose of barbiturate hypnotics than with the longer-acting phenobarbitone. The majority of patients survive with supportive measures alone. Forced alkaline diuresis may be considered in severe phenobarbitone poisoning. Charcoal haemoperfusion is the treatment of choice for the small minority of patients with very severe barbitu-

rate poisoning who fail to improve, or who deteriorate despite good supportive care.

BENZODIAZEPINES. Benzodiazepines taken alone cause drowsiness, ataxia, dysarthria, and occasionally minor and short-lived depression of consciousness. They potentiate the effects of other central nervous system depressants taken concomitantly. Flumazenil, a benzodiazepine antagonist, may be used in the *differential diagnosis* of unclear cases of multiple drug overdose but expert advice is **essential**.

IRON SALTS

Iron poisoning is commonest in childhood and is usually accidental. The symptoms are nausea, vomiting, abdominal pain, diarrhoea, haematemesis, and rectal bleeding. Hypotension, coma, and hepatocellular necrosis occur later. Mortality is reduced with intensive and specific therapy with **desferrioxamine**, which chelates iron. The stomach should be emptied at once, preferably by inducing vomiting as this is quickest. Gastric lavage in hospital should follow as soon as possible, leaving a solution of 5–10 g of desferrioxamine mesylate in 50–100 mL water in the stomach. The serum-iron concentration is measured as an emergency and parenteral desferrioxamine given to chelate absorbed iron in excess of the expected iron binding capacity.

DESFERRIOXAMINE MESYLATE

Indications: removal of iron from the body in poisoning; for use in chronic iron overload, see section 9.1.3
Cautions: avoid prochlorperazine
Side-effects: pain at site of intramuscular injection, anaphylactic reactions, and hypotension when given too rapidly by intravenous injection
Dose: by mouth after gastric lavage, see notes above
By intramuscular injection, 1–2 g in 10–20 mL of water for injections every 3–12 hours; max. 6 g in 24 hours
By continuous intravenous infusion, up to 15 mg/kg/hour; max. 80 mg/kg in 24 hours

PoM **Desferal**® (Ciba)
Injection, powder for reconstitution, desferrioxamine mesylate. Net price 500-mg vial= £3.06

LITHIUM

Most cases of lithium intoxication occur as a complication of long-term therapy and are caused by reduced excretion of the drug due to a variety of factors including dehydration, deterioration of renal function, infections, and co-administration of diuretics or NSAIDs (or other drugs that interact). Acute deliberate overdoses may also occur with delayed onset of symptoms (12 hours or more) due to slow entry of lithium into the tissues and continuing absorption from modified-release formulations.

The early clinical features are non-specific and may include apathy and restlessness which could be confused with mental changes due to the patient's depressive illness. Vomiting, diarrhoea, ataxia, weakness, dysarthria, muscle twitching, and tremor may follow. Severe poisoning is associated with convulsions, coma, renal failure, electrolyte imbalance, dehydration, and hypotension.

Therapeutic lithium concentrations are within the range of 0.4–1.0mmol/litre; concentrations in excess of 2.0mmol/litre are usually associated with serious toxicity and such cases may need treatment with forced diuresis or dialysis (if there is renal failure). In acute overdosage much higher serum concentrations may be present without features of toxicity and measures to increase urine production are usually all that are necessary. Otherwise treatment is supportive with special regard to electrolyte balance, renal function, and control of convulsions.

PHENOTHIAZINES AND RELATED DRUGS

Phenothiazines cause less depression of consciousness and respiration than other sedatives. Hypotension, hypothermia, sinus tachycardia, and arrhythmias (particularly with thioridazine) may complicate poisoning. Dystonic reactions can occur with therapeutic doses, (particularly with prochlorperazine and trifluoperazine) and convulsions may occur in severe cases. Drugs to control arrhythmias and convulsions may be needed. Dystonic reactions are rapidly abolished by injection of drugs such as benztropine or procyclidine (see section 4.9.2).

STIMULANTS

AMPHETAMINES. These cause wakefulness, excessive activity, paranoia, hallucinations, and hypertension followed by exhaustion, convulsions, hyperthermia, and coma. The early stages can be controlled by chlorpromazine and, if necessary, beta-blockers. Later, tepid sponging, anticonvulsants, and artificial respiration may be needed. Amphetamine excretion can be increased by forced acid diuresis but this is seldom necessary.

COCAINE. Cocaine can be smoked, sniffed, or injected. It stimulates the central nervous system causing agitation, dilated pupils, tachycardia, hypertension, hallucinations, hypertonia, and hyperreflexia. Convulsions, coma and metabolic acidosis may develop in the worst cases. Sedation, with intravenous diazepam, may be all that is necessary (and will also control convulsions); intravenous propranolol may be indicated for severe arrhythmias (labetalol may be preferred if there is associated hypertension).

THEOPHYLLINE

Theophylline and related drugs are often prescribed as modified-release formulations and toxicity may therefore be delayed. They cause vomiting (which may be severe and intractable), agitation, restlessness, dilated pupils, and sinus tachycardia. More serious effects are haematemesis, convulsions, and supraventricular and ventricular arrhythmias. Profound hypokalaemia may develop rapidly.

The stomach should be emptied as early as possible. Elimination of theophylline may be enhanced by repeated doses of activated charcoal by mouth (see also under Active Elimination Techniques). Hypokalaemia is corrected by intravenous infusion of potassium chloride and may be so severe as to require 60 mmol/hour (high doses under ECG monitoring). Convulsions should be controlled by intravenous administration of diazepam (emulsion preferred). Sedation with diazepam may be necessary in agitated patients.

Providing the patient is **not** an asthmatic, extreme tachycardia, hypokalaemia, and hyperglycaemia may be reversed by intravenous administration of propranolol (see section 2.4).

Other poisons

> Consult poisons information services day and night—p.18.

CYANIDES

Cyanide antidotes include dicobalt edetate, given alone, and sodium nitrite, followed by sodium thiosulphate. These antidotes are held for emergency use in hospitals as well as in centres where cyanide poisoning is a risk such as factories and laboratories.

DICOBALT EDETATE

Indications: acute poisoning with cyanides

Cautions: owing to toxicity to be used only when patient tending to lose, or has lost, consciousness; not to be used as a precautionary measure

Side-effects: transient hypotension, tachycardia, and vomiting

Dose: by intravenous injection, 300 mg (20mL) over 1 minute, followed by 50 mL of glucose intravenous infusion 50%, both repeated once or twice if necessary

PoM **Kelocyanor®** (Lipha)
Injection, dicobalt edetate 15mg/mL. Net price 20-mL (300-mg) amp = £2.66

SODIUM NITRITE

Indications: poisoning with cyanides (used in conjunction with sodium thiosulphate)

Side-effects: flushing and headache due to vasodilatation

PoM **Sodium Nitrite Injection**

Injection, sodium nitrite 3% (30 mg/mL) in water for injections

Dose: 10 mL by intravenous injection over 3 minutes, followed by 25 mL of sodium thiosulphate injection 50%, by intravenous injection over 10 minutes

'Special order' [unlicensed] product: contact Martindale, Penn or regional hospital manufacturing unit

SODIUM THIOSULPHATE

Indications: poisoning with cyanides (used in conjunction with sodium nitrite)

PoM Sodium Thiosulphate Injection

Injection, sodium thiosulphate 50% (500 mg/mL) in water for injections

Dose: see above under Sodium Nitrite Injection

'Special order' [unlicensed] product: contact Martindale, Penn or regional hospital manufacturing unit

---

HEAVY METALS

Heavy metal antidotes include dimercaprol, penicillamine, and sodium calciumedetate.

DIMERCAPROL

(BAL)

Indications: poisoning by antimony, arsenic, bismuth, gold, mercury, thallium; adjunct (with sodium calciumedetate) in lead poisoning

Cautions: hypertension

Contra-indications: not indicated for iron or cadmium poisoning; severe hepatic impairment

Side-effects: hypertension, tachycardia, malaise, nausea, vomiting, lachrymation, sweating, burning sensation (mouth and eyes), constriction of throat and chest, headache, muscle spasm, abdominal pain, tingling of extremities; pyrexia in children; local pain and abscess at injection site

Dose: by intramuscular injection, 2.5–3 mg/kg every 4 hours for 2 days, 2–4 times on the 3rd day, then 1–2 times daily for 10 days or until recovery

PoM Dimercaprol Injection (Boots), dimercaprol 50 mg/mL. Net price 2-mL amp = £15.00

PENICILLAMINE

Indications: poisoning by certain toxic metal ions, particularly by copper and lead

Cautions; Contra-indications; Side-effects: see section 10.1.3

Dose: 1–2 g daily in divided doses before food until urinary lead is stabilised at less than 500 micrograms/day; CHILD 20mg/kg daily

Preparations

See section 10.1.3

SODIUM CALCIUMEDETATE

Indications: poisoning by heavy metals, especially lead

Cautions: renal impairment

Side-effects: nausea, cramp; in overdosage renal damage

Dose: by intravenous infusion, adults and children, up to 40mg/kg twice daily in sodium chloride intravenous infusion 0.9% or glucose intravenous infusion 5% for up to 5 days, repeated if necessary after 48 hours

PoM Ledclair® (Sinclair)

Injection, sodium calciumedetate 200mg/mL. Net price 5-mL amp = £4.38

NOXIOUS GASES

CARBON MONOXIDE. Carbon monoxide poisoning is now usually due to inhalation of smoke, car exhaust, or fumes caused by blocked flues or incomplete combustion of fuel gases in confined spaces. Its toxic effects are entirely due to hypoxia.

Immediate treatment is essential. The person should be removed into the fresh air, the airway cleared, and **oxygen** 100% administered as soon as available. Artificial respiration should be given as necessary and continued until adequate spontaneous breathing starts, or stopped only after persistent and efficient treatment of cardiac arrest has failed. Admission to hospital is desirable because complications may arise after a delay of hours or days. Cerebral oedema should be anticipated in severe poisoning and is treated with an intravenous infusion of mannitol (see section 2.2.5). Referral for hyperbaric oxygen treatment should be discussed with the poisons information services if the victim is or has been unconscious or has a blood carboxyhaemoglobin concentration of more than 40%.

SULPHUR DIOXIDE, CHLORINE, PHOSGENE, AMMONIA. The immediate effect of all except phosgene is coughing and choking. Pulmonary oedema, with severe breathlessness and cyanosis may develop suddenly up to 36 hours after exposure. Death may occur. Patients are kept under observation and those who develop pulmonary oedema are given corticosteroids and oxygen. Assisted ventilation may be necessary in the most serious cases.

PESTICIDES

PARAQUAT. Concentrated liquid paraquat preparations (e.g. Gramoxone®), available to farmers and horticulturists, contain 10–20% paraquat and are extremely toxic. Granular preparations, for garden use, contain only 2.5% paraquat and have caused few deaths.

Paraquat has local and systemic effects. Splashes in the eyes irritate and ulcerate the cornea and conjunctiva. Copious washing of the eye and instillation of antibacterial eye-drops, should aid healing but it may be a long process. Skin irritation, blistering, and ulceration can occur from prolonged contact both with the concentrated and dilute forms. Inhalation of spray, mist, or dust containing paraquat may cause nose bleeding and sore throat but not systemic toxicity.

Ingestion of concentrated paraquat solutions is followed by nausea, vomiting, and diarrhoea. Painful ulceration of the tongue, lips, and fauces may appear after 36 to 48 hours together with renal failure. Some days later there may be dyspnoea with pulmonary fibrosis due to proliferative alveolitis and bronchiolitis.

Treatment should be started immediately. The single most useful measure is oral administration of either **Fuller's earth** or **bentonite** to adsorb paraquat and reduce absorption. The stomach is then emptied by careful gastric lavage and 300 mL of a suspension containing 30 g of Fuller's earth and 15 g of magnesium sulphate should be left in the stomach. Further quantities of 300 mL of a 30% Fuller's earth suspension are given after 2 and after 4 hours; magnesium sulphate or mannitol is given as required to produce diarrhoea and empty the gut. Some authorities prefer regimens employing 15% Fuller's earth suspensions. **Activated charcoal** is also effective and is given in a dose of 100g by mouth if Fuller's earth or bentonite are not available immediately. Intravenous fluids and analgesics are given as necessary. Oxygen therapy should be avoided if possible since this may exacerbate damage to the lungs. Measures to enhance elimination of absorbed paraquat are probably valueless but should be discussed with the poisons information services who will also give guidance on predicting the likely outcome from plasma concentrations. Paraquat absorption can be confirmed by a simple qualitative urine test.

ORGANOPHOSPHORUS INSECTICIDES. Organophosphorus insecticides are usually supplied as powders or dissolved in organic solvents. All are absorbed through the bronchi and intact skin as well as through the gut and inhibit cholinesterase activity thereby prolonging and intensifying the effects of acetylcholine. Toxicity between different compounds varies considerably, and onset may be delayed after skin exposure.

Anxiety, restlessness, dizziness, headache, miosis, nausea, hypersalivation, vomiting, abdominal colic, diarrhoea, bradycardia, and sweating are common. Muscle weakness and fasciculation may develop and progress to generalised flaccid paralysis including the ocular and respiratory muscles. Convulsions, coma, pulmonary oedema with copious bronchial secretions, hypoxia, and arrhythmias occur in severe cases. Hyperglycaemia and glycosuria without ketonuria may also be present.

Further absorption should be prevented by emptying the stomach, removing the patient to fresh air, or removing soiled clothing and washing contaminated skin. In severe poisoning it is vital to ensure a clear airway, frequent removal of bronchial secretions, and adequate ventilation and oxygenation. **Atropine** will reverse the muscarinic effects of acetylcholine and is given in a dose of 2 mg as atropine sulphate injection (intramuscularly or intravenously according to the severity of poisoning) every 20 to 30 minutes until the skin becomes flushed and dry, the pupils dilate, and tachycardia develops.

Pralidoxime mesylate (P2S), a cholinesterase reactivator, is indicated, as an adjunct to atropine, in moderate or severe poisoning but is only effective if given within 24 hours. It may be obtained from designated centres, the names of which are held by the poisons information centres (see p.18). A dose of 1 g by intramuscular injection or, diluted with 10–15 mL water for injections, by slow intravenous injection should produce improvement in muscle power within 30 minutes but repeated doses or, in severe cases, an intravenous infusion of up to 500 mg /hour may be required.

PRALIDOXIME MESYLATE

Indications: adjunct to atropine in the treatment of organophosphorus poisoning
Cautions: renal impairment, myasthenia gravis
Contra-indications: poisoning due to carbamates and to organophosphorus compounds without anticholinesterase activity
Side-effects: drowsiness, dizziness, disturbances of vision, nausea, tachycardia, headache, hyperventilation, and muscular weakness
Dose: by intramuscular injection, 1g initially followed by 1–2 further doses if necessary; in very severe poisoning the initial dose can be doubled; usual max. 12 g in 24 hours
By slow intravenous injection (diluted to 10–15 mL with water for injections and given over 5–10 minutes), 1 g initially followed by 1–2 further doses if necessary; in very severe poisoning the initial dose can be doubled; usual max. 12 g in 24 hours
CHILD 20–60 mg /kg as required depending on severity of poisoning and response

PoM **Pralidoxime Mesylate Injection,** pralidoxime mesylate 200 mg /mL. Available as 5-mL amps (from designated centres)

SNAKE BITES AND INSECT STINGS

SNAKE BITE. Acute envenoming from snake bite is rare in the UK and the only indigenous venomous snake is the adder (*Vipera berus*). The bite may cause local and systemic effects. Local effects include pain, swelling, bruising, and tender enlargement of regional lymph nodes. Systemic effects include early transient hypotension with syncope, angioedema, abdominal colic, diarrhoea, and vomiting, with later persistent or recurrent hypotension, ECG abnormalities, spontaneous systemic bleeding, coagulopathy, adult respiratory distress syndrome, and acute renal failure. There is a small risk of fatal envenoming especially in children and the elderly.

Indications for antivenom treatment include systemic envenoming, especially hypotension (see above), vomiting, haemostatic abnormalities, polymorphonuclear leucocytosis and local envenoming if, after bites on the hand or foot, swelling extends beyond the wrist or ankle within 4 hours of the bite. Two ampoules of **Zagreb antivenom** (Regent) are diluted with 2–3 volumes of sodium chloride intravenous infusion 0.9% and given by slow intravenous injection (not more than 2 mL of diluted antivenom per minute) or by intravenous infusion. The **same dose** should be used for **adults** and **children**. The dose can be repeated in 1–2 hours if there is no clinical improvement. Adrenaline injection must be immediately to hand for treatment of anaphylactic antivenom reactions (for full details see section 3.4.3).

Antivenom is available for certain foreign snakes and spiders. For information on identification, management, and supply, telephone:
Oxford (0865) 220968
or (0865) 741166
Liverpool 051-708 9393
Liverpool (Fazakerley Hospital Pharmacy)
(supply only) 051-525 5980
London 071-635 9191

INSECT STINGS. Stings from ants, wasps, bees, and hornets cause local pain and swelling but seldom cause severe toxicity. If the sting is in the mouth or on the tongue marked swelling may cause respiratory distress. The stings from these insects are usually treated by cleaning the area, applying a cooling lotion (such as a calamine preparation), and giving an antihistamine by mouth. Bee stings should be removed by scraping them off with a finger nail or knife before cleaning the area. Anaphylactic reactions require treatment with **adrenaline**. Inhalation of adrenaline (Medihaler-epi®, see section 3.4.3) may be sufficient for mild bronchospasm, but self-administered subcutaneous adrenaline is the best first-aid treatment for patients with severe hypersensitivity. For full details of the management of anaphylaxis, see section 3.4.3.

Classified Notes on Drugs and Preparations

SPORTS COUNCIL

DOPING CLASSES AND METHODS OF THE INTERNATIONAL OLYMPIC COMMITTEE MEDICAL COMMISSION 1993

THE FOLLOWING ARE EXAMPLES OF CLASSES AND METHODS PROHIBITED IN SPORT

Classes:

STIMULANTS e.g. amphetamine*, cocaine*, ephedrine and related compounds.

NARCOTIC ANALGESICS e.g. morphine*, pethidine* and related compounds.

ANABOLIC AGENTS e.g. nandrolone, stanozolol, testosterone and related compounds.

DIURETICS e.g. frusemide, hydrochlorothiazide, triamterene and related compounds.

PEPTIDE HORMONES & ANALOGUES e.g. growth hormone, corticotrophin, chorionic gonadotrophin, erythropoietin.

Methods:

BLOOD DOPING e.g. including erythropoietin (EPO).

PHARMACOLOGICAL, CHEMICAL AND PHYSICAL MANIPULATION

Classes of drugs subject to certain restrictions:

ALCOHOL, MARIJUANA* (not prohibited but may be restricted)

LOCAL ANAESTHETICS, CORTICOSTEROIDS (except for approved treatments)

BETA BLOCKERS e.g. acebutolol, atenolol, propranolol and related compounds.

*Controlled under the Misuse of Drugs Act 1971

JUNE 1993

TREATMENT GUIDELINES:

EXAMPLES OF PERMITTED AND **PROHIBITED** SUBSTANCES

(based upon International Olympic Committee Doping Classes 1993)

ASTHMA:	ALLOWED–salbutamol inhaler, terbutaline inhaler
	BANNED– products containing sympathomimetics (e.g. ephedrine, fenoterol, isoprenaline).
COUGH:	ALLOWED–all antibiotics, steam and menthol inhalations, cough mixtures containing antihistamines.
	BANNED– products containing sympathomimetics (e.g. ephedrine, phenylpropanolamine).
DIARRHOEA:	ALLOWED– diphenoxylate, loperamide, products containing electrolytes (e.g. Dioralyte, Rehidrat).
	BANNED– products containing opioids (e.g. morphine).
HAYFEVER:	ALLOWED–antihistamines, nasal sprays containing a corticosteroid or xylometazoline, eye drops containing sodium cromoglycate.
	BANNED– products containing ephedrine, pseudoephedrine
PAIN:	ALLOWED– aspirin, ibuprofen, paracetamol.
	BANNED– products containing opioids (e.g. dextropropoxyphene) or caffeine.
VOMITING:	ALLOWED–domperidone, metoclopramide.

CODEINE IS NOW PERMITTED FOR THERAPEUTIC USE.

WARNING: THE ABOVE ARE ONLY EXAMPLES OF SUBSTANCES CURRENTLY PERMITTED OR PROHIBITED BY THE IOC. IF IN DOUBT CHECK WITH YOUR GOVERNING BODY OR WITH THE SPORTS COUNCIL. DOPING CONTROL UNIT 071-383 2244.

REMEMBER–YOU ARE RESPONSIBLE

JUNE 1993

Supplies of this card are available from :
  Doping Control Unit, Sports Council,
  Walkden House, 3–10 Melton Street,
  London NW1 2EB

Further information on substances currently permitted or prohibited can be obtained by telephoning the Doping Control Unit on:
  071-383 5667 *or*
  071-383 5411

1: Drugs acting on the
GASTRO-INTESTINAL SYSTEM

The drugs and preparations in this chapter are described under the following sections:

1.1 Antacids

Antacids are still useful for treating gastro-intestinal disease; they can often relieve symptoms in both *ulcer* and *non-ulcer dyspepsia*, and in *reflux oesophagitis*. They are best given when symptoms occur or are expected, usually between meals and at bedtime, four or more times daily; additional doses may be required to once an hour. Conventional doses e.g. 10 mL three or four times daily of liquid magnesium–aluminium antacids promote ulcer healing, but less well than antisecretory agents (section 1.3); proof of a relationship between healing and neutralising capacity is lacking. Liquid preparations are more effective than solids.

INTERACTIONS. Antacids should not be taken at the same time as other drugs as they may impair their absorption. Antacids may also damage enteric coatings designed to prevent dissolution in the stomach. See also **Appendix 1** (antacids and adsorbents).

1.1.1 Aluminium- and magnesium-containing antacids

Aluminium- and **magnesium-containing** antacids, such as magnesium carbonate, hydroxide and trisilicate, and aluminium glycinate and hydroxide, being relatively insoluble in water, are long-acting if retained in the stomach. They are suitable for most antacid purposes. Magnesium-containing antacids tend to be laxative whereas aluminium-containing antacids may be constipating. Aluminium accumulation does not appear to be a risk if renal function is normal (see also Appendix 3).

Compound preparations have no clear advantages over simpler preparations: neutralising capacity may be the same.

Complexes, such as **hydrotalcite** and **magaldrate**, confer no special advantage.

Low Na+
The words low Na+ added after some preparations indicate a sodium content of less than 1 mmol per tablet or 10-mL dose.

ALUMINIUM HYDROXIDE

Indications: dyspepsia; for use in hyperphosphataemia, see section 9.5.2.2

Cautions: see notes above; porphyria, see section 9.8.2; **interactions:** Appendix 1 (antacids and adsorbents)

Contra-indications: hypophosphataemia

Aluminium-only preparations
Aluminium Hydroxide (Non-proprietary)
Tablets, dried aluminium hydroxide 500 mg. Net price 20 = 27p
   Dose: 1–2 tablets chewed 4 times daily and at bedtime or as required
Mixture (gel), about 4% w/w Al_2O_3 in water, with a peppermint flavour. Net price 200 mL = 41p
   Dose: antacid, 5–10 mL 4 times daily between meals and at bedtime or as required; CHILD 6–12 years, up to 5 mL 3 times daily
   Note. The brand name NHS Aludrox® (Charwell) is used for aluminium hydroxide mixture; net price 200 mL = £1.07. NHS Aludrox® tablets also contain magnesium.
Alu-Cap® (3M)
Capsules, green/red, dried aluminium hydroxide 475 mg (low Na+). Net price 120-cap pack = £4.22
   Dose: antacid, 1 capsule 4 times daily and at bedtime

Co-magaldrox
Co-magaldrox is a mixture of aluminium hydroxide and magnesium hydroxide; the proportions are expressed in the form *x*/*y* where *x* and *y* are the strengths in milligrams per unit dose of magnesium hydroxide and aluminium hydroxide respectively
Maalox® (Rhône-Poulenc Rorer)
Suspension, sugar-free, co-magaldrox 195/220 (magnesium hydroxide 195 mg, dried aluminium hydroxide 220 mg/5 mL (low Na+)). Net price 500 mL = £1.90
   Dose: 5–10 mL 20 minutes–1 hour after meals and at bedtime or when required
Maalox TC® (Rhône-Poulenc Rorer)
Tablets, co-magaldrox 300/600 (magnesium hydroxide 300 mg, dried aluminium hydroxide 600 mg (low Na+)). Net price 100 = £3.51
Suspension, sugar-free, co-magaldrox 300/600 (magnesium hydroxide 300 mg, dried aluminium hydroxide 600 mg/5 mL (low Na+)). Net price 500 mL = £3.51
   Dose: antacid, 1–2 tablets chewed or 5–10 mL suspension 4 times daily 20 minutes–1 hour after meals and at bedtime or as required; duodenal ulcer, 3 tablets or 15 mL suspension 4 times daily (treatment) *or* twice daily (prevention of recurrence)

Mucogel® (Pharmax)

Suspension, sugar-free, co-magaldrox 195/220 (magnesium hydroxide 195 mg, dried aluminium hydroxide 220 mg/5 mL (low Na⁺)). Net price 500 mL = £1.91

Dose: 10–20 mL 3 times daily, 20 minutes–1 hour after meals, and at bedtime or when required

For **preparations** containing aluminium and magnesium on sale to the public and not prescribable on the NHS, see p.31

MAGNESIUM CARBONATE

Indications: dyspepsia

Cautions: renal impairment; see also notes above; **interactions:** Appendix 1 (antacids and adsorbents)

Contra-indications: hypophosphataemia

Side-effects: diarrhoea; belching due to liberated carbon dioxide

Aromatic Magnesium Carbonate Mixture, BP

(Aromatic Magnesium Carbonate Oral Suspension)

Oral suspension, light magnesium carbonate 3%, sodium bicarbonate 5%, in a suitable vehicle containing aromatic cardamom tincture. Extemporaneous preparations should be recently prepared according to the following formula: light magnesium carbonate 300 mg, sodium bicarbonate 500 mg, aromatic cardamom tincture 0.3 mL, double-strength chloroform water 5 mL, water to 10 mL. Contains about 6 mmol Na⁺/10 mL. Net price 200 mL = 50p

Dose: 10 mL 3 times daily in water

For **preparations** also containing aluminium, see previous page.

MAGNESIUM TRISILICATE

Indications: dyspepsia

Cautions; Contra-indications: see under Magnesium Carbonate

Side-effects: diarrhoea

Magnesium Trisilicate Tablets, Compound, BP

Tablets, magnesium trisilicate 250 mg, dried aluminium hydroxide 120 mg

Dose: 1–2 tablets chewed when required

Magnesium Trisilicate Mixture, BP

(Magnesium Trisilicate Oral Suspension)

Oral suspension, 5% each of magnesium trisilicate, light magnesium carbonate, and sodium bicarbonate in a suitable vehicle with a peppermint flavour. Extemporaneous preparations should be recently prepared according to the following formula: magnesium trisilicate 500 mg, light magnesium carbonate 500 mg, sodium bicarbonate 500 mg, concentrated peppermint emulsion 0.25 mL, double-strength chloroform water 5 mL, water to 10 mL. Contains about 6 mmol Na⁺/10 mL

Dose: 10 mL 3 times daily in water

Magnesium Trisilicate Oral Powder, Compound, BP

Oral powder, magnesium trisilicate 250 mg, chalk 250 mg, heavy magnesium carbonate 250 mg,

sodium bicarbonate 250 mg/g. Contains about 3 mmol Na⁺/g. Label: 13

Dose: 1–5 g in liquid when required

For **preparations** also containing aluminium, see previous page.

ALUMINIUM-MAGNESIUM COMPLEXES

HYDROTALCITE

Aluminium magnesium carbonate hydroxide hydrate

Indications: dyspepsia

Cautions: see notes above; **interactions:** Appendix 1 (antacids and adsorbents)

Hydrotalcite (Non-proprietary)

Tablets, hydrotalcite 500 mg. Net price 56-tab pack = 81p

Dose: 2 tablets chewed between meals and at bedtime; CHILD 6–12 years 1 tablet

Suspension, hydrotalcite 500 mg/5 mL. Net price 500-mL pack = £1.96

Dose: 10 mL between meals and at bedtime; CHILD 6–12 years 5 mL

Note. The brand name **NHS** Altacite® (Roussel) is used for hydrotalcite suspension and tablets; for Altacite Plus® preparations, see pp.30 and 31.

MAGALDRATE

A synthetic combination of aluminium and magnesium hydroxides and sulphuric acid

Indications: dyspepsia

Cautions: see notes above; **interactions:** Appendix 1 (antacids and adsorbents)

Magaldrate (Non-proprietary)

Suspension, magaldrate 800 mg/5 mL. Net price 100 mL = 38p

Dose: 5–10 mL after meals and at bedtime; CHILD 6–12 years 2.5–5 mL

Note. The brand name **NHS** Dynese® (Galen) is used for magaldrate suspension; it is sugar-free and low Na⁺.

ALUMINIUM- AND MAGNESIUM-CONTAINING ANTACIDS WITH ADDITIONAL INGREDIENTS

Activated dimethicone (simethicone), given alone or added to an antacid as an antifoaming agent to relieve flatulence, is of uncertain value. Alginates added as protectants against *reflux oesophagitis* may be useful, but surface anaesthetics (e.g. oxethazaine) added to improve symptom relief are of doubtful efficacy. The amount of additional ingredient or antacid in individual preparations varies widely, as does their sodium content, so that preparations may not be freely interchangeable.

Preparations containing activated dimethicone with an antacid may be useful for the relief of *hiccup in terminal care.*

Algicon® (Rhône-Poulenc Rorer)

Tablets, aluminium hydroxide-magnesium carbonate co-dried gel 360 mg, magnesium alginate 500 mg, magnesium carbonate 320 mg, potassium bicarbonate 100 mg, sucrose 1.5 g (low Na+). Net price 60-tab pack = £2.34

Dose: 1–2 tablets 4 times daily (chewed after meals and at bedtime)

Suspension, aluminium hydroxide-magnesium carbonate co-dried gel 140 mg, magnesium alginate 250 mg, magnesium carbonate 175 mg, potassium bicarbonate 50 mg/5 mL (low Na+). Net price 500 mL (lemon- or aniseed-flavoured) = £2.54

Dose: 10–20 mL 4 times daily (after meals and at bedtime)

Altacite Plus® (Roussel)

NHS *Tablets*, see p.31

Suspension, sugar-free, co-simalcite 125/500 (activated dimethicone 125 mg, hydrotalcite 500 mg)/5 mL (low Na+). Net price 500 mL = £1.85

Dose: 10 mL between meals and at bedtime when required; CHILD 8–12 years 5 mL

Asilone® (Boots)

Suspension, sugar-free, dried aluminium hydroxide 420 mg, activated dimethicone 135 mg, light magnesium oxide 70 mg/5 mL (low Na+). Net price 500 mL = £1.95

Dose: 5–10 mL after meals and at bedtime

NHS *Tablets*, see p.31

NHS *Liquid*, see p.31

Diovol® (Pharmax)

Suspension, sugar-free, aluminium hydroxide 200 mg, dimethicone 25 mg, magnesium hydroxide 200 mg/5 mL (low Na+). Net price 300 mL = £1.13

Dose: 5–10 mL when required

Gastrocote® (Boehringer Mannheim)

Tablets, alginic acid 200 mg, dried aluminium hydroxide 80 mg, magnesium trisilicate 40 mg, sodium bicarbonate 70 mg. Contains about 1 mmol Na+/tablet. Net price 100-tab pack = £3.67

Dose: 1–2 tablets chewed 4 times daily (after meals and at bedtime)

Liquid, sugar-free, peach-coloured, dried aluminium hydroxide 80 mg, magnesium trisilicate 40 mg, sodium alginate 220 mg, sodium bicarbonate 70 mg/5 mL. Contains 1.8 mmol Na+/5 mL. Net price 500 mL = £2.79

Dose: 5–15 mL 4 times daily (after meals and at bedtime)

Gastron® (Sanofi Winthrop)

Tablets, alginic acid 600 mg, dried aluminium hydroxide 240 mg, magnesium trisilicate 60 mg, sodium bicarbonate 210 mg. Contains about 3 mmol Na+/tablet. Net price 100-tab pack =£3.80

Dose: 1–2 tablets chewed 3 times daily after meals and 2 tablets at bedtime

Gaviscon® (R&C)

NHS *Gaviscon 250® and Gaviscon 500® Tablets*, see p.31

Tablets, alginic acid 500 mg, dried aluminium hydroxide 100 mg, magnesium trisilicate 25 mg, sodium bicarbonate 170 mg. Contains 2 mmol Na+/tablet. Net price 60-tab pack = £2.25

Dose: 1–2 tablets chewed after meals and at bedtime, followed by water; CHILD 1 tablet

Liquid, sugar-free, sodium alginate 250 mg, sodium bicarbonate 133.5 mg, calcium carbonate 80 mg/5 mL. Contains about 3 mmol Na+/5 mL.

Net price 100 mL (aniseed- or peppermint flavour) = 92p

Dose: 10–20 mL after meals and at bedtime; CHILD 5–10 mL

Infant Gaviscon® (R&C)

Oral powder, sugar-free, sodium alginate 225 mg, magnesium alginate 87.5 mg, dried aluminium hydroxide 112.5 mg with colloidal silica and mannitol/dose (half dual-sachet). Contains 0.92 mmol Na+/dose. Net price 15 dual-sachets (30 doses) = £2.46

Dose: INFANT under 4.5 kg 1 dose (half dual-sachet) mixed with feeds (or water in breast-fed infants) when required; over 4.5 kg 2 doses (1 dual-sachet); CHILD 2 doses (1 dual-sachet) in water after each meal

Note. Not to be used in premature infants, or where excessive water loss likely (e.g. fever, diarrhoea, vomiting, high room temperature)

IMPORTANT. Each half of the dual-sachet is identified as 'one dose'. To avoid errors prescribe as 'dual-sachet' with directions in terms of 'dose'

Maalox Plus® (Rhône-Poulenc Rorer)

NHS*Tablets*, see p.31

Suspension, sugar-free, dried aluminium hydroxide 220 mg, activated dimethicone 25 mg, magnesium hydroxide 195 mg/5 mL (low Na+). Net price 500 mL = £1.90

Dose: 5–10 mL 4 times daily (after meals and at bedtime or when required)

PoM **Mucaine®** (Wyeth)

Suspension, sugar-free, aluminium hydroxide mixture 4.75 mL, magnesium hydroxide 100 mg, oxethazaine 10 mg/5 mL. Net price 200-mL pack = 76p

Dose: 5–10 mL (without fluid) 3–4 times daily (15 minutes before meals and at bedtime or when required)

Topal® (Innovex)

Tablets, alginic acid 200 mg, dried aluminium hydroxide 30 mg, light magnesium carbonate 40 mg with lactose 220 mg, sucrose 880 mg (low Na+). Net price 42-tab pack = £1.67

Dose: 1–3 tablets chewed 4 times daily (after meals and at bedtime); CHILD half adult dose

For **preparations** containing aluminium and magnesium on sale to the public and not prescribable on the NHS, see p.31

DIMETHICONE ALONE

Infacol® (Pharmax)

Liquid, sugar-free, activated dimethicone 40 mg/mL (low Na+). Net price 50 mL = £1.54. Counselling, use of dropper

Dose: gripes, colic or wind pains, INFANT 0.5–1 mL before feeds

1.1.2   Sodium bicarbonate

Sodium bicarbonate, being soluble in water, is rapid-acting, but absorbed bicarbonate can cause alkalosis in excessive doses. Like other carbonate-containing antacids it liberates carbon dioxide which causes belching. Sodium bicarbonate and antacid preparations with a high sodium content, such as magnesium trisilicate mixture, should be avoided in patients on salt-restricted diets (in heart failure and in hepatic and renal impairment).

Indigestion **preparations** on sale to the public (not prescribable on the NHS) include:

Actal® (alexitol=aluminium), **Actonorm Gel**® (aluminium, magnesium, dimethicone, peppermint oil), **Actonorm Powder**® (see section 1.2), **Altacite**® (hydrotalcite = aluminium, magnesium), **Altacite Plus Tablets**® (co-simalcite = aluminium, magnesium, dimethicone; suspension is prescribable), **Aludrox Liquid**® (aluminium), **Aludrox Tablets**® (aluminium, magnesium), **Aluhyde**® (see section 1.2), **Andrews Antacid**® (calcium, magnesium), **APP**® (see section 1.2), **Asilone Liquid**® (aluminium, dimethicone, magnesium; suspension is prescribable), **Asilone Tablets**® (aluminium, dimethicone)

Barum Antacid® (calcium), **Bellocarb**® (see section 1.2), **Birley**® (aluminium, magnesium), **Bismag**® (magnesium, sodium bicarbonate), **Bisma-Rex**® (bismuth, calcium, magnesium, peppermint oil), **Bisodol Extra Tablets**® (calcium, magnesium, sodium bicarbonate, dimethicone), **Bisodol Heartburn Tablets**® (alginic acid, magaldrate, sodium bicarbonate),**Bisodol Powder**® (magnesium, sodium bicarbonate), **Bisodol Tablets**® (calcium, magnesium, sodium bicarbonate), **Boots Double Action Indigestion**® (aluminium, magnesium, dimethicone), **Boots Headache and Indigestion Relief**® (sodium bicarbonate, sodium carbonate, paracetamol), **Boots Indigestion Tablets**® (calcium, magnesium, sodium bicarbonate) **Carbellon**® (magnesium, charcoal, peppermint oil) **De Witt's Antacid Powder**® (calcium, magnesium, sodium bicarbonate, light kaolin, peppermint oil), **De Witt's Antacid Tablets**® (calcium, magnesium, peppermint oil), **Dijex**® (aluminium, magnesium),

Dynese® (magaldrate = aluminium, magnesium) **Gastrils**® (aluminium, magnesium), **Gaviscon 250**® **and 500**® **Tablets** (alginic acid, aluminium, magnesium, sodium bicarbonate; Gaviscon tablets are prescribable), **Gelusil**® (aluminium, magnesium)

Maalox Plus Tablets® (aluminium, magnesium, dimethicone; suspension is prescribable), **Maclean**® (aluminium, calcium, magnesium), **Magnatol**® (alexitol, magnesium, potassium bicarbonate, xanthan gum), **Milk of Magnesia Tablets**® (magnesium; liquid is prescribable), **Moorland**® (aluminium, bismuth, calcium, magnesium, light kaolin)

Novasil Plus® (aluminium, magnesium, dimethicone), **Nulacin**® (calcium, magnesium, peppermint oil; *contain* gluten)

Opas® (calcium, magnesium, sodium bicarbonate)

Pepto-Bismol® (bismuth), **Premiums**® (aluminium, calcium, magnesium, peppermint oil)

Rap-eze® (calcium), **Remegel**® (calcium), **Rennie**® (calcium, magnesium), **Rennie Gold**® (calcium), **Roter**® (bismuth, magnesium, sodium bicarbonate, frangula)

Setlers Extra® (aluminium, magnesium), **Setlers Liquid**® (aluminium, magnesium), **Setlers Tablets**® (calcium, magnesium), **Setlers Tums**® (calcium), **Simeco**® (aluminium, magnesium, dimethicone), **Sovol**® (aluminium, magnesium, dimethicone)

Unigest® (aluminium, dimothioono) **Windcheaters**® (dimethicone)

SODIUM BICARBONATE

Indications: rapid relief of dyspepsia; urinary tract, section 7.4.3; acidosis, sections 9.2.1.3 and 9.2.2

Cautions: hepatic and renal impairment; cardiac disease, pregnancy; patients on sodium-restricted diet; elderly; avoid prolonged use; **interactions:** Appendix 1 (antacids and adsorbents)

Side-effects: belching, alkalosis on prolonged use

Dose: see under preparations, below

Sodium Bicarbonate, BP, contains about 12 mmol Na⁺/g. Label: 13

Dose: 1–5 g in water when required

Sodium Bicarbonate Tablets, Compound, BP, (Soda Mint Tablets), sodium bicarbonate 300 mg. Contains about 4 mmol Na⁺/tab

Dose: 2–6 tablets sucked when required

1.1.3 Calcium- and bismuth-containing antacids

Bismuth-containing antacids (unless chelates) are best avoided because absorbed bismuth can be neurotoxic, causing encephalopathy; they tend to be constipating. Calcium-containing antacids can induce rebound acid secretion: with modest doses the clinical significance is doubtful, but prolonged high doses also cause hypercalcaemia and alkalosis, and can precipitate the milk alkali syndrome. **Interactions:** Appendix 1 (antacids and adsorbents). For **preparations** on sale to the public (not prescribable on the NHS), see above

1.2 Antispasmodics and other drugs altering gut motility

The smooth muscle relaxant properties of antimuscarinic and other antispasmodic drugs may be useful as adjunctive treatment in *non-ulcer dyspepsia*, in the *irritable bowel syndrome*, and in *diverticular disease*. The gastric antisecretory effects of conventional antimuscarinic drugs are of little practical significance since dosage is limited by atropine like side-effects. Moreover, they have been superseded by more powerful and specific antisecretory drugs, including the histamine H_2-receptor antagonists and the selective antimuscarinic pirenzepine.

The dopamine-receptor antagonist metoclopramide has a different action, tending to stimulate transit in the gut.

ANTIMUSCARINICS

The antimuscarinics (less correctly termed 'anticholinergics') can be divided into atropine and its related alkaloids (including the belladonna alkaloids), and synthetic antimuscarinics. The synthetic antimuscarinics can, in turn, be divided into **tertiary amine** (dicyclomine hydrochloride) and **quaternary ammonium compounds** (mepenzolate bromide, pipenzolate bromide, poldine methylsulphate, and propantheline bromide). Dicyclomine hydrochloride has a much less marked antimuscarinic action than atropine and may also have some direct action on smooth muscle.

Quaternary ammonium compounds are less lipid soluble than atropine and so may be less likely to cross the blood–brain barrier; they are also less well absorbed. Although central atropine-like side-effects, such as confusion, are thereby reduced, peripheral atropine-like side-effects remain common with dry mouth, difficult visual accommodation, hesitant micturition, and constipation at doses which act as gut neuromuscular relaxants or inhibitors of acid secretion. The elderly are particularly susceptible; glaucoma and urinary retention may occur.

Antimuscarinics tend to relax the oesophageal sphincter and should be avoided in patients with symptomatic reflux; all antispasmodics should be avoided in paralytic ileus. Despite these side-effects antimuscarinics are nevertheless useful in some *dyspeptics*, in the *irritable bowel syndrome*, and in *diverticular disease*. Nonselective antimuscarinics (e.g. belladonna alkaloids) are outmoded as ulcer treatments, any clinical virtues being outweighed by atropinic side-effects.

The quaternary ammonium compound, **hyoscine butylbromide** is advocated as a gastro-intestinal antispasmodic, but it is poorly absorbed; the injection is useful in endoscopy and radiology.

ATROPINE SULPHATE and BELLADONNA ALKALOIDS

Indications: see notes above; atropine sulphate, see also section 15.1.3

Cautions: elderly; urinary retention, prostatic enlargement, tachycardia, cardiac insufficiency, paralytic ileus, ulcerative colitis, and pyloric stenosis; may aggravate gastro-oesophageal reflux; pregnancy and breast-feeding; **interactions:** Appendix 1 (antimuscarinics)

Contra-indications: closed-angle glaucoma

Side-effects: dry mouth with difficulty in swallowing and thirst, dilatation of the pupils with loss of accommodation and sensitivity to light, increased intra-ocular pressure, flushing, dry skin, bradycardia followed by tachycardia, palpitations and arrhythmias, difficulty with micturition, and constipation; rarely fever, confusional states and rashes

---

Indigestion **preparations** on sale to the **public** (not prescribable on the NHS) containing belladonna and related alkaloids include:

Actonorm Powder® (atropine, aluminium, calcium, magnesium, sodium bicarbonate, peppermint oil), **Aluhyde**® (belladonna, aluminium, magnesium), **APP**® (homatropine, aluminium, bismuth, calcium, magnesium)
Bellocarb® (belladonna, magnesium)
Opazimes® (belladonna, morphine, aluminium, kaolin)

DICYCLOMINE HYDROCHLORIDE
(Dicycloverine Hydrochloride)

Indications: adjunct in gastro-intestinal disorders characterised by smooth muscle spasm

Cautions; Contra-indications; Side-effects: see under Atropine Sulphate; contra-indicated in infants under 6 months

Dose: 10–20 mg 3 times daily; CHILD 6–24 months 5–10 mg up to 3–4 times daily, 15 minutes before feeds, 2–12 years 10 mg 3 times daily

PoM ¹ **Merbentyl**® (Merrell)
Tablets, dicyclomine hydrochloride 10 mg. Net price 20 = 57p
Syrup, dicyclomine hydrochloride 10 mg/5 mL. Net price 100 mL = 86p

1. Dicyclomine hydrochloride can be sold to the public provided that the maximum single dose is 10 mg and the maximum daily dose is 60 mg

PoM **Merbentyl 20**® (Merrell)
Tablets, dicyclomine hydrochloride 20 mg. Net price 84-tab pack = £4.77

Compound preparations
Kolanticon® (Merrell)
Gel, sugar-free, dicyclomine hydrochloride 2.5 mg, dried aluminium hydroxide 200 mg, light magnesium oxide 100 mg, activated dimethicone (simethicone USP) 20 mg/5 mL. Net price 200 mL = £1.52; 500 mL = £1.90
Dose: 10–20 mL every 4 hours when required

HYOSCINE BUTYLBROMIDE

Indications: adjunct in gastro-intestinal disorders characterised by smooth muscle spasm

Cautions; Contra-indications; Side-effects: see under Atropine Sulphate and notes above; avoid in porphyria (see section 9.8.2)

Dose: by mouth, 20 mg 4 times daily; CHILD 6–12 years, 10 mg 3 times daily

By intramuscular or intravenous injection (acute spasm), 20 mg, repeated after 30 minutes if necessary

PoM ¹ **Buscopan**® (Boehringer Ingelheim)
Tablets, coated, hyoscine butylbromide 10 mg. Net price 56-tab pack = £2.59 (not recommended, see notes above)

1. Can be sold to the public provided single dose does not exceed 20 mg, daily dose does not exceed 80 mg, and pack does not contain a total of more than 240 mg. Net price 24 × 10 mg-tab pack = £1.70
Injection, hyoscine butylbromide 20 mg/mL. Net price 1-mL amp = 20p

MEPENZOLATE BROMIDE

Indications: adjunct in gastro-intestinal disorders characterised by smooth muscle spasm

Cautions; Contra-indications; Side-effects: see under Atropine Sulphate and notes above

Dose: 25–50 mg 3–4 times daily

PoM Cantil® (Boehringer Mannheim)

Tablets, yellow, scored, mepenzolate bromide 25 mg. Net price 50-tab pack = £2.68

Additives: include tartrazine

PIPENZOLATE BROMIDE

Indications: adjunct in gastro-intestinal disorders characterised by smooth muscle spasm

Cautions; Contra-indications; Side-effects: see under Atropine Sulphate and notes above

Compound preparations

PoM Piptalin® (Boehringer Mannheim)

Suspension, orange, sugar-free, pipenzolate bromide 4 mg, activated dimethicone 40 mg/5 mL. Net price 100 mL = £1.08

Dose: 10 mL 3–4 times daily before meals; CHILD up to 10 kg 2.5 mL, 10–20 kg 2.5–5 mL, 20–40 kg 5 mL, 3–4 times daily 15 minutes before meals (or feeds)

POLDINE METHYLSULPHATE

(Poldine Metilsulfate)

Indications: adjunct in gastro-intestinal disorders characterised by smooth muscle spasm

Cautions; Contra-indications; Side-effects: see under Atropine Sulphate and notes above

Dose: 2–4 mg 4 times daily

PoM Nacton® (Pharmark)

Tablets, scored, poldine methylsulphate 2 mg. Net price 112-tab pack = £12.29

Tablets forte, orange, scored, poldine methylsulphate 4 mg. Net price 112-tab pack = £21.66

PROPANTHELINE BROMIDE

Indications: adjunct in gastro-intestinal disorders characterised by smooth muscle spasm, for use in urinary frequency, see section 7.4.2

Cautions; Contra-indications; Side-effects: see under Atropine Sulphate and notes above

Dose: 15 mg 3 times daily at least 1 hour before meals and 30 mg at night, max. 120 mg daily

PoM Pro-Banthine® (Baker Norton)

Tablets, pink, s/c, propantheline bromide 15 mg. Net price 100-tab pack = £4.56. Label: 23

OTHER ANTISPASMODICS

Alverine citrate, mebeverine hydrochloride, and peppermint oil are believed to be direct relaxants of intestinal smooth muscle and may relieve pain in the *irritable bowel syndrome* and *diverticular disease*. They have no serious adverse effects but, like all antispasmodics, should be avoided in paralytic ileus. Peppermint oil occasionally causes heartburn.

ALVERINE CITRATE

Indications: adjunct in gastro-intestinal disorders characterised by smooth muscle spasm; dysmenorrhoea

Cautions: pregnancy

Contra-indications: paralytic ileus

Dose: 60–120 mg 1–3 times daily; CHILD 8–12 years, 60 mg 3 times daily

Spasmonal® (Norgine)

Capsules, blue/grey, alverine citrate 60 mg. Net price 20 = £2.18

Compound preparations

Alvercol® (Norgine)

Granules, beige, coated, sterculia 62%, alverine citrate 0.5%. Net price 500 g = £12.19. Label: 25, 27, counselling, see below

Dose: irritable bowel syndrome, 1–2 heaped 5-mL spoonfuls swallowed without chewing with water once or twice daily after meals; CHILD 6–12 years, half adult dose

COUNSELLING. Preparations that swell in contact with liquid should always be carefully swallowed with water and should not be taken immediately before going to bed

MEBEVERINE HYDROCHLORIDE

Indications: adjunct in gastro-intestinal disorders characterised by smooth muscle spasm

Cautions: paralytic ileus; avoid in porphyria (see section 9.8.2.)

PoM Colofac® (Duphar)

Tablets, s/c, mebeverine hydrochloride 135 mg. Net price 20 = £1.67.

Dose: ADULT and CHILD over 10 years, 1 tablet 3 times daily preferably 20 minutes before meals

Note. Tablets containing mebeverine hydrochloride 135 mg also available from APS, Berk (Fomac®), Cox, Evans, Generics, Hillcross, K Pharm.

Liquid, yellow, sugar-free, mebeverine hydrochloride 50 mg (as embonate)/5 mL. Net price 300 mL = £3.50.

Dose: ADULT and CHILD over 10 years, 15 mL 3 times daily preferably 20 minutes before meals

Compound preparations

PoM Fybogel Mebeverine® (R&C)

Granules, effervescent, ispaghula husk 3.5 g, mebeverine hydrochloride 135 mg/sachet. Contains 7 mmol K$^+$/sachet (caution in renal impairment). Net price 60 sachets = £15.00. Label: 13, 22, counselling, see below

Dose: irritable bowel syndrome, ADULT and CHILD over 12 years, 1 sachet in water morning and night 30 minutes before food; an additional sachet may also be taken before the midday meal if necessary

COUNSELLING. Preparations that swell in contact with liquid should always be carefully swallowed with water and should not be taken immediately before going to bed

PEPPERMINT OIL

Indications: relief of abdominal colic and distension, particularly in irritable bowel syndrome

Cautions: rarely sensitivity to menthol

Side-effects: heartburn, rarely, allergic reactions (including rash, headache, bradycardia, muscle tremor, ataxia)

LOCAL IRRITATION. Capsules should not be broken or chewed because this would release peppermint oil causing irritation of mouth or oesophagus

Colpermin® (Pharmacia)

Capsules, m/r, e/c, light blue/dark blue, green band, peppermint oil 0.2 mL. Net price 100-cap pack = £13.90. Label: 5, 22, 25

Dose: 1–2 capsules, swallowed whole with water, 3 times daily before meals for up to 2–3 months if necessary

Mintec® (Innovex)

Capsules, e/c, green/ivory, peppermint oil 0.2 mL. Net price 100-cap pack = £12.80. Label: 5, 22, 25

Dose: 1–2 capsules swallowed whole with water, 3 times daily before meals for up to 2–3 months if necessary

MOTILITY STIMULANTS

Metoclopramide is a dopamine antagonist which stimulates gastric emptying and small intestinal transit, and enhances the strength of oesophageal sphincter contraction. It is used in some patients with *non-ulcer dyspepsia*, for speeding the transit of barium during intestinal follow-through examination, and as accessory treatment for *oesophageal reflux*. Metoclopramide may induce an acute dystonic reaction, particularly in young women and children—for further details of this and other side-effects, see section 4.6.

Cisapride is a newly introduced motility stimulant believed to promote release of acetylcholine in the gut wall; it does not have dopamine-antagonist properties. It is of use in treating *oesophageal reflux* and *gastric stasis* and in the short-term management of *non-ulcer dyspepsia.*

CISAPRIDE

Indications: see under dose

Cautions: halve dose initially in hepatic and renal impairment; elderly; **interactions:** Appendix 1 (cisapride)

Contra-indications: where gastro-intestinal stimulation dangerous; pregnancy

Side-effects: abdominal cramps and diarrhoea, occasional headaches and lightheadedness; convulsions, extrapyramidal effects reported

Dose: ADULT and CHILD over 12 years

Symptoms and mucosal lesions associated with gastro-oesophageal reflux, 10 mg 3–4 times daily (12-week course recommended); maintenance treatment, 20 mg at bedtime *or* 10 mg twice daily (20 mg twice daily if initial lesions were very severe) (reduce 20-mg dose to 10 mg if severe abdominal cramps)

Symptoms of impaired gastric motility secondary to disturbed and delayed gastric emptying associated with diabetes, systemic sclerosis and autonomic neuropathy, 10 mg 3–4 times daily initially for 6 weeks (but longer treatment may be necessary)

Symptoms of dyspepsia (peptic ulcer or other lesions excluded), 10 mg 3 times daily (usual course 4 weeks)

COUNSELLING. Advise patient to take 15–30 minutes before meals and at bedtime (for night symptoms)

PoM Prepulsid® (Janssen)

Tablets, scored, cisapride (as monohydrate) 10 mg, net price 120-tab pack = £37.60. Counselling, administration, see above (also available as Alimix®)

Suspension, cisapride (as monohydrate) 5 mg / 5 mL. Net price 500 mL = £15.60. Counselling, administration, see above

METOCLOPRAMIDE HYDROCHLORIDE

Indications: see notes above; nausea and vomiting, see section 4.6

PATIENTS UNDER 20 YEARS. Use restricted to severe intractable vomiting of known cause, vomiting of radiotherapy and cytotoxics, aid to gastro-intestinal intubation, pre-medication

Contra-indications; Side-effects; Dose: see section 4.6

Preparations

See section 4.6

1.3   Ulcer-healing drugs

1.3.1	H₂-receptor antagonists
1.3.2	Selective antimuscarinics
1.3.3	Chelates and complexes
1.3.4	Prostaglandin analogues
1.3.5	Proton pump inhibitors
1.3.6	Other ulcer-healing drugs

Peptic ulceration commonly involves the stomach, duodenum, and lower oesophagus; after gastric surgery it involves the gastro-enterostomy stoma.

General measures, including stopping smoking and taking antacids, promote healing as do the use of a wide variety of antisecretory and other treatments (see sections 1.3.1–1.3.6).

HELICOBACTER PYLORI INFECTION

In the treatment of duodenal ulcer, associated infection with *Helicobacter pylori* should be eradicated, but the ideal treatment is not yet clear. Options include a two-week course of amoxycillin and metronidazole given concurrently with tripotassium dicitratobismuthate, *or alternatively* amoxycillin and metronidazole given concurrently with ranitidine, *or alternatively* amoxycillin alone given concurrently with omeprazole; if necessary clarithromycin can be substituted for amoxycillin.

Eradication of infection commonly results in long-term ulcer remission. Antibiotic-induced colitis is a possible (but uncommon) risk and *H. pylori* reinfection can occur. In the case of regimens involving tripotassium dicitratobismuthate, ranitidine or omeprazole may also be given.

A total of 4–8 weeks of antisecretory treatment (with a H_2-receptor antagonist or omeprazole) is needed for ulcer healing.

1.3.1 H₂-receptor antagonists

All H_2-receptor antagonists heal *gastric and duodenal ulcers* by reducing gastric acid output as a result of H_2-receptor blockade; like cimetidine and ranitidine, the newer ones (famotidine and nizatidine) can also be expected to relieve *peptic oesophagitis* and, in high doses, to reduce gastric acid output in the *Zollinger–Ellison syndrome*.

Maintenance treatment with half doses prevents *ulcer relapse*, but does not modify the natural course of the disease when treatment has ceased. Maintenance treatment is best suited to those with frequent severe recurrences and to the elderly who suffer ulcer complications.

Treatment of *undiagnosed dyspepsia* may be acceptable in younger patients but is undesirable in older people because the diagnosis of gastric cancer may be delayed.

Therapy can promote healing of NSAID-associated ulcers but there is no proof that the ulcer complications are prevented.

Clear proof that treatment is beneficial in *haematemesis* and *melaena* is lacking, but prophylactic use reduces the frequency of bleeding from gastroduodenal erosions in *hepatic coma*, and possibly in other conditions requiring *intensive care*. Treatment also reduces the frequency of *acid aspiration* in obstetric patients at delivery (Mendelson's syndrome).

SIDE-EFFECTS. H_2-receptor antagonists are well tolerated and side-effects are uncommon with few significant differences between available drugs. Dizziness, somnolence or fatigue, and rash have occasionally been reported with all of them, and there are rare reports of headache, liver dysfunction, and blood disorders. Other rare reports include bradycardia or AV block, confusion, interstitial nephritis (cimetidine), and urticaria and angio-edema. Cimetidine is also associated with occasional gynaecomastia and rare reports of impotence and myalgia. Causal relationships of other reports, such as pancreatitis, are unclear.

INTERACTIONS. Cimetidine retards oxidative hepatic drug metabolism by binding to microsomal cytochrome P450. It should be avoided in patients stabilised on warfarin, phenytoin, and theophylline (or aminophylline), but other interactions (see **Appendix 1**) may be of less clinical relevance. Famotidine, nizatidine, and ranitidine do not share the drug metabolism inhibitory properties of cimetidine.

CIMETIDINE

Indications: benign gastric and duodenal ulceration, stomal ulcer, reflux oesophagitis, Zollinger-Ellison syndrome, other conditions where gastric acid reduction is beneficial (see notes above and section 1.9.4)

Cautions: see notes above; renal and hepatic impairment (reduce doses, see Appendixes 2 and 3); pregnancy and breast-feeding; preferably avoid intravenous injection (infusion is preferable) particularly in high dosage (may rarely cause arrhythmias) and in cardiovascular impairment; **interactions:** Appendix 1 (histamine H_2-antagonists) and notes above

Side-effects: altered bowel habit, dizziness, rash, tiredness; reversible confusional states, reversible liver damage, headache; rarely, blood disorders (including thrombocytopenia, agranulocytosis, and aplastic anaemia), muscle or joint pain, hypersensitivity, bradycardia and AV block; interstitial nephritis and acute pancreatitis reported; gynaecomastia is also an occasional problem with cimetidine (but usually only in high dosage), and reversible impotence has also been reported (see also notes above)

Dose: by mouth, 400 mg twice daily (with breakfast and at night) *or* 800 mg at night (benign gastric and duodenal ulceration) for at least 4 weeks (6 weeks in gastric ulceration, 8 weeks in NSAID-associated ulceration); when necessary the dose may be increased to 400 mg 4 times daily or rarely (e.g. as in stress ulceration) to a max. of 2.4 g daily in divided doses; CHILD 20–30 mg/kg daily in divided doses

Maintenance, 400 mg at night *or* 400 mg morning and night

Reflux oesophagitis, 400 mg 4 times daily for 4–8 weeks

Zollinger-Ellison syndrome, 400 mg 4 times daily or occasionally more

Gastric acid reduction (prophylaxis of acid aspiration; do not use syrup), obstetrics 400 mg at start of labour, then up to 400 mg every 4 hours if required (max. of 2.4 g daily); surgical procedures 400 mg 90–120 minutes before induction of general anaesthesia

Short-bowel syndrome, 400 mg twice daily (with breakfast and at bedtime) adjusted according to response

To reduce degradation of pancreatic enzyme supplements, 0.8–1.6 g daily in 4 divided doses according to response 1–1½ hours before meals

By intramuscular injection, 200 mg every 4–6 hours; max. 2.4 g daily

By slow intravenous injection, 200 mg given over at least 2 minutes; may be repeated every 4–6 hours; if a larger dose is needed or there is cardiovascular impairment, the dose should be diluted and given over at least 10 minutes (infusion is preferable); max. 2.4 g daily

By intravenous infusion, 400 mg in 100 mL of sodium chloride 0.9% intravenous infusion infused over ½–1 hour (may be repeated every 4–6 hours) *or* by continuous infusion at an average rate of 50–100 mg/hour over 24 hours, max.

2.4 g daily; CHILD, *by intramuscular injection or slow intravenous injection or infusion*, 20–30 mg/kg daily in divided doses

PoM[1] **Cimetidine** (Non-proprietary)

Tablets, cimetidine 200 mg, net price 120-tab pack = £9.49; 400 mg, 60-tab pack = £9.76; 800 mg, 30-tab pack = £10.06

Available from APS, Ashbourne (Peptimax®), Berk (Ultec®), BHR (Phimetin®), Bioglan, Cox, CP, Eastern (Zita®), Galen (Galenamet®), K Pharm., Lagap, Norton.

1. Cimetidine can be sold to the public for adults and children over 16 years (provided packs do not contain more than 2 weeks' supply) for the short-term symptomatic relief of heartburn, dyspepsia, and hyperacidity (max. single dose 200 mg, max. daily dose 800 mg), and for the prophylactic management of nocturnal heartburn (single night-time dose 100 mg); a proprietary brand (Tagamet 100®containing cimetidine 100 mg) is on sale to the public

PoM Dyspamet® (SK&F)

Chewtab® (chewable tablets), sugar-free, cimetidine 200 mg. Net price 120-tab pack = £16.73. Counselling, chew thoroughly

Suspension, sugar-free, cimetidine 200 mg/5 mL. Contains sorbitol 2.79 g/5 mL. Net price 600 mL = £21.89

PoM Tagamet® (SK&F)

Tablets, all green, f/c, cimetidine 200 mg, net price 120-tab pack = £17.80; 400 mg, 60-tab pack = £20.56; 800 mg, 30-tab pack = £20.56

Effervescent tablets, sugar-free, cimetidine 400 mg. Contains 17.6 mmol Na⁺/tablet. Net price 60-tab pack = £18.68. Label: 13

Syrup, orange, cimetidine 200 mg/5 mL. Net price 600 mL = £25.90

Injection, cimetidine 100 mg/mL. Net price 2-mL amp = 30p

Intravenous infusion, cimetidine 4 mg/mL in sodium chloride intravenous infusion 0.9%. Net price 100-mL infusion bag = £1.86

Cimetidine with alginate

PoM Algitec® (SK&F)

Chewtab® (chewable tablets), off-white, cimetidine 200 mg, alginic acid 500 mg. Contains 2.05 mmol Na⁺/tablet. Net price 120-tab pack = £22.50. Counselling, chew thoroughly

Suspension, cimetidine 100 mg, sodium alginate 250 mg/5 mL. Contains 1.43 mmol Na⁺/5 mL. Net price 600 mL = £15.41

Dose: gastro-oesophageal reflux disease, 1 tablet chewed or 10 mL suspension 4 times daily (after meals and at bedtime), increased if necessary to 2 tablets or 20 mL suspension 4 times daily; to be taken for 4–8 weeks

FAMOTIDINE

Indications: see under Dose

Cautions: see under Cimetidine; does not inhibit hepatic microsomal drug metabolism

Side-effects: see under Cimetidine and notes above

Dose: benign gastric and duodenal ulceration, treatment, 40 mg at night for 4–8 weeks; maintenance, 20 mg at night; CHILD not recommended

Reflux oesophagitis, 20–40 mg twice daily for 6–12 weeks

Zollinger–Ellison syndrome, 20 mg every 6 hours (higher dose in those who have previously been receiving another H₂-antagonist)

PoM[1] **Pepcid®** (Morson)

Tablets, famotidine 20 mg (beige), net price 28-tab pack = £14.00; 40 mg (brown), 28-tab pack = £26.60

1. Famotidine can be sold to the public for adults and children over 16 years (provided packs do not contain more than 2 weeks' supply) for the short-term symptomatic relief of heartburn, dyspepsia, and hyperacidity (max. single dose 10 mg, max. daily dose 20 mg); a proprietary brand (Pepcid AC® containing famotidine 10 mg) is on sale to the public

NIZATIDINE

Indications: see under Dose

Cautions: see under Cimetidine; does not inhibit hepatic microsomal drug metabolism

Side-effects: see under Cimetidine and notes above; sweating also reported; rare reports of gynaecomastia

Dose: by mouth, benign gastric and duodenal ulceration, treatment, 300 mg at night *or* 150 mg twice daily for 4–8 weeks (up to 8 weeks in NSAID-associated ulceration); maintenance, 150 mg at night for up to 1 year; CHILD not recommended

Reflux oesophagitis, 150–300 mg twice daily for up to 12 weeks

By intravenous infusion, for short-term use in peptic ulcer hospital inpatients as alternative to oral route, *by intermittent intravenous infusion* over 15 minutes, 100 mg 3 times daily, *or by continuous intravenous infusion*, 10 mg/hour; max. 480 mg daily; CHILD not recommended

PoM Axid® (Lilly)

Capsules, nizatidine 150 mg (pale yellow/dark yellow), net price 30-cap pack = £11.34; 300 mg (pale yellow/brown), 30-cap pack = £21.74

Injection, nizatidine 25 mg/mL. For dilution and use as an intravenous infusion. Net price 4-mL amp = £1.09

RANITIDINE

Indications: benign gastric and duodenal ulceration, stomal ulcer, reflux oesophagitis, Zollinger–Ellison syndrome, other conditions where reduction of gastric acidity is beneficial (see notes above and section 1.9.4)

Cautions: see under Cimetidine; does not significantly inhibit hepatic microsomal drug metabolism

Side-effects: see under Cimetidine and notes above; rare reports of breast swelling and tenderness in men

Dose: by mouth, 150 mg twice daily (morning and night) *or* 300 mg at night (benign gastric and duodenal ulceration) for 4 to 8 weeks, up to 6 weeks in chronic episodic dyspepsia, and up to 8 weeks in NSAID-associated ulceration; in duodenal ulcer 300 mg can be given twice daily for 4 weeks to achieve a higher healing rate; CHILD (peptic ulcer) 2–4 mg/kg twice daily, max. 300 mg daily

Maintenance, 150 mg at night

Prophylaxis of NSAID-induced duodenal ulcer, 150 mg twice daily

Reflux oesophagitis, 150 mg twice daily *or* 300 mg at night for up to 8 weeks, or if necessary 12 weeks (moderate to severe, 150 mg 4 times daily for up to 12 weeks)

Zollinger–Ellison syndrome, 150 mg 3 times daily increased if necessary to up to 6 g daily in divided doses

Gastric acid reduction (prophylaxis of acid aspiration) in obstetrics, *by mouth*, 150 mg at onset of labour, then every 6 hours; surgical procedures, *by intramuscular or slow intravenous injection*, 50 mg 45–60 minutes before induction of anaesthesia (intravenous injection diluted to 20 mL and given over at least 2 minutes), or *by mouth*, 150 mg 2 hours before induction of anaesthesia, and also, when possible on the preceding evening

By intramuscular injection, 50 mg every 6–8 hours

By slow intravenous injection, 50 mg diluted to 20 mL and given over at least 2 minutes; may be repeated every 6–8 hours

By intravenous infusion, 25 mg/hour for 2 hours; may be repeated every 6–8 hours

Prophylaxis of stress ulceration, initial slow intravenous injection of 50 mg (as above) then *continuous infusion*, 125–250 micrograms/kg per hour (may be followed by 150 mg twice daily *by mouth* when oral feeding commences)

PoM **Zantac®** (Glaxo)

Tablets, f/c, ranitidine (as hydrochloride) 150 mg, net price 60-tab pack = £27.89; 300 mg, 30-tab pack = £27.43

Effervescent tablets, pale yellow, ranitidine (as hydrochloride) 150 mg (contains 14.3 mmol Na⁺/tablet), net price 60-tab pack = £27.88; 300 mg (contains 20.8 mmol Na⁺/tablet), 30-tab pack = £27.42. Label: 13

Note. The effervescent tablets contain aspartame (see section 9.4.1)

Syrup, sugar-free, ranitidine (as hydrochloride) 75 mg/5 mL. Net price 300 mL = £22.32

Injection, ranitidine 25 mg (as hydrochloride)/mL. Net price 2-mL amp = 64p

1.3.2   Selective antimuscarinics

Pirenzepine is a selective antimuscarinic drug which inhibits gastric acid and pepsin secretion with fewer peripheral side-effects than the drugs in section 1.2. As it does not cross the blood-brain barrier it is unlikely to have central effects. It is as effective as H₂-receptor antagonists in healing *gastric and duodenal ulcers* and may also be useful in

maintenance treatment. It has also been used in conjunction with H₂-receptor antagonists in resistant cases.

PIRENZEPINE

Indications: benign gastric and duodenal ulceration

Cautions: renal impairment

Contra-indications: prostatic enlargement, pyloric stenosis, paralytic ileus, closed-angle glaucoma; pregnancy

Side-effects: occasionally dry mouth and visual disturbances; agranulocytosis and thrombocytopenia have been reported

Dose: 50 mg twice daily, increased if necessary to a max. of 150 mg daily in 3 divided doses, for 4–6 weeks, or in resistant cases for up to 3 months.

PoM **Gastrozepin®** (Boots)

Tablets, scored, pirenzepine hydrochloride, equivalent to anhydrous pirenzepine hydrochloride, 50 mg. Net price 60 = £27.50. Label: 22

1.3.3   Chelates and complexes

Tripotassium dicitratobismuthate is a bismuth chelate effective in healing *gastric and duodenal ulcers.* It may act by a direct toxic effect on gastric *Helicobacter (Campylobacter) pylori,* or by stimulating mucosal prostaglandin or bicarbonate secretion. The healing tends to be longer lasting than with H₂-receptor antagonists but relapse still occurs and regimens are now being developed involving co-administration of antibiotics (see p.34). The bismuth content is low but absorption has been reported; encephalopathy (described with older high-dose bismuth preparations) has not been reported. Tablets are as effective as the liquid and more palatable.

Sucralfate is another effective treatment for *gastric and duodenal ulcers* and may act by protecting the mucosa from acid-pepsin attack. It is a complex of aluminium hydroxide and sulphated sucrose but has minimal antacid properties.

TRIPOTASSIUM DICITRATOBISMUTHATE
(Bismuth Chelate)

Indications: benign gastric and duodenal ulceration

Cautions: see notes above; **interactions:** Appendix 1 (tripotassium dicitratobismuthate)

Contra-indications: renal impairment, pregnancy

Side-effects: may darken tongue and blacken faeces; nausea and vomiting reported

De-Nol® (Yamanouchi)

Liquid, red, tripotassium dicitratobismuthate 120 mg/5 mL. Net price 560 mL = £20.51. Counselling, see below

Dose: adults, 10 mL twice daily *or* 5 mL 4 times daily; taken for 28 days, followed by further 28 days if necessary; maintenance not indicated but course may be repeated after interval of 1 month; CHILD, not recommended

COUNSELLING. Each dose to be diluted with 15 mL of water; twice daily dosage to be taken 30 minutes before breakfast and main evening meal; four times daily dosage to be taken as follows: one dose 30 minutes before breakfast, midday meal and main evening meal, and one dose 2 hours after main evening meal; milk should not be drunk by itself during treatment but small quantities may be taken in tea or coffee or on cereal; antacids should not be taken half an hour before or after a dose; may darken tongue and blacken faeces

De-Noltab® (Yamanouchi)

Tablets, white, tripotassium dicitratobismuthate 120 mg. Net price 112-tab pack = £29.37. Counselling, see below

Dose: adults 2 tablets twice daily *or* 1 tablet 4 times daily; taken for 28 days followed by further 28 days if necessary; maintenance not indicated but course may be repeated after interval of 1 month; CHILD, not recommended

COUNSELLING. Each dose to be swallowed with a tumblerful of water then as above under De-Nol

SUCRALFATE

Indications: benign gastric and duodenal ulceration; chronic gastritis

Cautions: renal impairment (avoid if severe, see Appendix 3); pregnancy and breast-feeding; **interactions:** Appendix 1 (sucralfate)

Side-effects: constipation; diarrhoea, nausea, indigestion, gastric discomfort, dry mouth, rash, pruritus, back pain, dizziness, insomnia, vertigo and drowsiness

Dose: 2 g twice daily (on rising and at bedtime) *or* 1 g 4 times daily 1 hour before meals and at bedtime, taken for up to 6 weeks or in resistant cases 12 weeks; max. 8 g daily

Prophylaxis of stress ulceration (suspension), 1 g 6 times daily (max. 8 g daily)

COUNSELLING. Tablets may be dispersed in 10–15 mL of water; antacids should not be taken half an hour before or after a dose

PoM Antepsin® (Wyeth)

Tablets, scored, sucralfate 1 g. Net price 100 = £8.75. Label: 5, counselling, see dose

Suspension, sucralfate, 1 g/5 mL. Net price 560 mL = £9.80. Label: 5, counselling, antacids

1.3.4   Prostaglandin analogues

Misoprostol, a synthetic prostaglandin analogue has antisecretory and protective properties, promoting *gastric and duodenal ulcer* healing. It can prevent NSAID-associated ulcers, its use being most appropriate for the frail or very elderly from whom NSAIDs cannot be withdrawn.

MISOPROSTOL

Indications: see notes above and under Dose

Cautions: conditions where hypotension might precipitate severe complications (e.g. cerebrovascular disease, cardiovascular disease)

Contra-indications: pregnancy or planning pregnancy (increases uterine tone)

Side-effects: diarrhoea (may occasionally be severe and require withdrawal, reduced by giving single doses not exceeding 200 micrograms and by avoiding magnesium-containing antacids); also reported: abdominal pain, dyspepsia, flatulence, nausea and vomiting, abnormal vaginal bleeding (including intermenstrual bleeding, menorrhagia, and postmenopausal bleeding), rashes, dizziness

Dose: benign gastric and duodenal ulceration and NSAID-associated ulceration, 800 micrograms daily (in 2–4 divided doses) with breakfast (or main meals) and at bedtime; treatment should be continued for at least 4 weeks and may be continued for up to 8 weeks if required

Prophylaxis of NSAID-induced gastric and duodenal ulcer, 200 micrograms 2–4 times daily according to condition of patient

PoM Cytotec® (Searle)

Tablets, scored, misoprostol 200 micrograms. Net price 56-tab pack = £10.40; 112-tab pack = £20.80. Label: 21

With diclofenac or naproxen

See section 10.1.1

1.3.5   Proton pump inhibitors

The proton pump inhibitors **omeprazole** and **lansoprazole** inhibit gastric acid by blocking the hydrogen-potassium adenosine triphosphatase enzyme system (the 'proton pump') of the gastric parietal cell. They are effective treatments for *gastric and duodenal ulcers* and particularly for *erosive oesophagitis*.

OMEPRAZOLE

Indications: see under Dose

Cautions: exclude malignancy; severe liver disease (see appendix 2); avoid in pregnancy and breast-feeding; **interactions:** Appendix 1 (proton pump inhibitors)

Side-effects: diarrhoea, headache (both may be severe); also nausea, constipation, flatulence, dizziness, vertigo, somnolence, malaise, insomnia and paraesthesia; rashes, urticaria, pruritus, bullous eruption, erythema multiforme, angioedema, alopecia and photosensitivity reported; muscle and joint pain, blurred vision, peripheral oedema, gynaecomastia and rarely impotence, loss of taste, stomatitis, gastro-intestinal candidiasis, leucopenia, thrombocytopenia, fever, bronchospasm, interstitial nephritis, liver enzyme changes and liver dysfunction also reported (and encephalopathy in pre-existing liver disease); reversible mental confusion, agitation, depression and hallucinations have been noted in the severely ill

Dose: benign gastric and duodenal ulcers (including those complicating NSAID therapy), 20 mg daily for 4 weeks in duodenal ulceration or 8 weeks in gastric ulceration; in severe or recurrent cases increase to 40 mg daily; maintenance for recurrent duodenal ulcer, 20 mg daily

Duodenal ulcer associated with *H. pylori*, 40 mg daily with amoxycillin 750 mg twice daily for 2 weeks

Zollinger–Ellison syndrome, initially 60 mg once daily; usual range 20–120 mg daily (above 80 mg in 2 divided doses)

Reflux oesophagitis, 20 mg daily for 4 weeks, followed by a further 4–8 weeks if not fully healed; 40 mg daily has been given for 8 weeks in reflux oesophagitis refractory to other treatment; may be continued at 20 mg daily

PoM Losec® (Astra)

Capsules, enclosing e/c granules, omeprazole 20 mg (pink/brown), net price 28-cap pack = £36.36 (also 7-cap pack, hosp. only); 40 mg (brown), 14-cap pack = £36.36 (also 7-cap pack, hosp. only). Label: 25

Note. Should be dispensed in original container (which contains a dessicant)

LANSOPRAZOLE

Indications: see under Dose

Cautions; Side-effects: see under Omeprazole

Dose: benign gastric and duodenal ulcers, 30 mg daily in the morning for 4 weeks in duodenal ulceration or 8 weeks in gastric ulceration

Reflux oesophagitis, 30 mg daily in the morning for 4 weeks, followed by a further 4 weeks if not fully healed

▼ **PoM Zoton®** (Lederle)

Capsules, lilac/purple, enclosing e/c granules, lansoprazole 30 mg. Net price 28-cap pack = £33.36, 56-cap pack = £66.72. Label: 5, 23, 25

1.3.6   Other ulcer-healing drugs

Carbenoxolone is a synthetic derivative of glycyrrhizinic acid (a constituent of liquorice).

The only oral preparation of carbenoxolone remaining on the UK market is in the form of a combination with antacids for *oesophageal ulceration and inflammation.*

However, side-effects (commonly sodium and water retention and occasionally hypokalaemia) may cause or exacerbate hypertension, oedema, cardiac failure, and muscle weakness. For these reasons other drugs are preferred; if used regular monitoring of weight, blood pressure, and electrolytes is advisable during treatment. Carbenoxolone may act by protecting the mucosal barrier from acid–pepsin attack and increasing mucosal mucin production.

Deglycyrrhizinised liquorice is free from the above side-effects but is of doubtful efficacy.

LIQUORICE, DEGLYCYRRHIZINISED

Indications: benign gastric and duodenal ulceration

Caved-S® (Pharmacia)

Tablets, brown, deglycyrrhizinised liquorice 380 mg, aluminium hydroxide mixture 100 mg, bismuth subnitrate 100 mg, magnesium carbonate 200 mg, sodium bicarb-

onate 100 mg. Net price 180-tab pack = £10.97. Label: 24

Dose: benign gastric and duodenal ulceration, treatment, 2 tablets chewed 3 times daily (for duodenal ulceration increased if necessary to 6 times daily); maintenance, 1 tablet chewed 3 times daily (gastric ulceration), 2 tablets chewed 3 times daily (duodenal ulceration); CHILD no longer recommended

Note. Caved-S® tablets contain bismuth subnitrate; long-term use should be avoided, see also section 1.1.3

CARBENOXOLONE SODIUM

Indications: benign gastric ulceration in young and middle-aged adults (see also under preparation)

Cautions: cardiac disease, hypertension, hepatic and renal disease (see contra-indications); elderly (see under preparation); not recommended in children. See also notes above; **interactions:** Appendix 1 (carbenoxolone)

Contra-indications: hypokalaemia, cardiac failure and in those receiving cardiac glycosides (unless electrolyte levels monitored weekly and measures taken to avoid hypokalaemia); hepatic and renal impairment (see Appendixes 2 and 3); pregnancy

Side-effects: sodium and water retention (provoking hypertension and cardiac failure), hypokalaemia (leading to impaired neuromuscular function and muscle damage and to renal damage if prolonged)

Compound preparation

PoM Pyrogastrone® (Sanofi Winthrop)

Tablets, chewable, carbenoxolone sodium 20 mg, alginic acid 600 mg, dried aluminium hydroxide 240 mg, magnesium trisilicate 60 mg, sodium bicarbonate 210 mg (Na+ 3 mmol/tablet). Net price 100-tab pack = £24.85. Label: 21, 24

Liquid, carbenoxolone sodium 10 mg, dried aluminium hydroxide 150 mg (Na+ 0.85 mmol, K+ 1.5 mmol)/5 mL when reconstituted with water. Net price 500 mL = £12.39. Label: 21

Dose: for oesophageal inflammation and ulceration, 1 tablet, chewed, 3 times daily after meals, and 2 at night, for 6–12 weeks or 10 mL liquid 3 times daily after meals and 20 mL at night, for 6–12 weeks; not recommended for children or for adults over 75 years

1.4   Antidiarrhoeal drugs

1.4.1   Adsorbents and bulk-forming drugs

1.4.2   Antimotility drugs

The **first line** of treatment in acute diarrhoea, as in gastro-enteritis, is prevention or treatment of fluid and electrolyte depletion. This is particularly important in infants and in frail and elderly patients. For details of **oral rehydration preparations**, see section 9.2.1.2. Severe dehydration requires immediate admission to hospital and urgent replacement of fluid and electrolytes.

Antispasmodics (section 1.2) are occasionally of value in treating abdominal cramp associated with diarrhoea but they should **not** be used for primary treatment. Antispasmodics and antiemetics should be **avoided** in young children with gastro-enteritis as they are rarely effective and have troublesome side-effects.

Antibiotics and sulphonamides are generally unnecessary in simple gastro-enteritis, even when a bacterial cause is suspected, because the complaint will usually resolve quickly without such treatment, and infective diarrhoeas in the UK are often caused by viral infections. Systemic bacterial infection does, however, need appropriate systemic treatment. **Erythromycin** (see section 5.1.5) or **ciprofloxacin** (see section 5.1.12) can be used for treating Campylobacter enteritis. For drugs for shigellosis and salmonellosis, see section 5.1, table 1. The general use of sulphonamides in treating diarrhoea of travellers is inadvisable because of the risks of rash and agranulocytosis. Poorly absorbed drugs such as dihydrostreptomycin, neomycin, and sulphaguanidine should be **avoided** altogether in gastro-intestinal infection. They prolong rather than shorten the time taken to control diarrhoea by causing masked bacterial diarrhoea, carrier states, or pseudomembranous colitis. Clioquinol should also be **avoided** as it is neurotoxic; both it and lactobacillus preparations are valueless.

1.4.1   Adsorbents and bulk-forming drugs

Adsorbents such as kaolin are **not** recommended for *acute diarrhoeas*. Bulk-forming drugs, such as ispaghula, methylcellulose, and sterculia (see section 1.6.1) are useful in controlling faecal consistency in ileostomy and colostomy, and in controlling diarrhoea associated with diverticular disease.

KAOLIN, LIGHT
Indications: diarrhoea but see notes above
Cautions: **interactions:** Appendix 1 (antacids and adsorbents)

Kaolin Mixture, BP
(Kaolin Oral Suspension)
Oral suspension, light kaolin or light kaolin (natural) 20%, and 5% each of light magnesium carbonate and sodium bicarbonate in a suitable vehicle with a peppermint flavour.
Dose: 10–20 mL every 4 hours
Kaolin-containing preparations on sale to the public include: Kaopectate® and KLN®.

1.4.2   Antimotility drugs

In *acute diarrhoeas* antimotility drugs have a very limited role as adjuncts to fluid and electrolyte replacement (see section 9.2.1.2); they are **not** recommended for acute diarrhoeas in young children.

For comments on their role in *chronic diarrhoeas* see section 1.5.

CODEINE PHOSPHATE
Indications: see notes above
Cautions; Contra-indications; Side-effects: see section 4.7.2; not recommended for children; tolerance and dependence may occur with prolonged use; **interactions:** Appendix 1 (opioid analgesics)
Dose: see under Preparations

PoM **Codeine Phosphate Tablets,** codeine phosphate 15 mg, net price 20 = 35p; 30 mg, 20 = 37p; 60 mg, 20 = £1.11. Label: 2
Dose: 30 mg 3–4 times daily (range 15–60 mg); CHILD not recommended
Note. Travellers needing to take codeine phosphate tablets abroad may require a doctor's letter explaining why they are necessary.

PoM **Diarrest®** (Galen)
Liquid, yellow, codeine phosphate 5 mg, dicyclomine hydrochloride 2.5 mg, potassium chloride 40 mg, sodium chloride 50 mg, sodium citrate 50 mg/5 mL. For diarrhoea, vomiting, and cramp. Net price 200 mL = £3.34
Dose: 20 mL 4 times daily with water; CHILD 4–5 years 5 mL, 6–9 years 10 mL, 10–13 years 15 mL but see cautions and notes above

Kaodene® (Boots)
Mixture, codeine phosphate 10 mg, light kaolin 3 g/10 mL. Net price 250 mL = £1.06
Dose: 20 mL 3–4 times daily; CHILD over 5 years 10 mL but see cautions and notes above

CO-PHENOTROPE
A mixture of diphenoxylate hydrochloride and atropine sulphate in the mass proportions 100 parts to 1 part respectively
Indications: adjunct to rehydration in acute diarrhoea (but see notes above); chronic mild ulcerative colitis
Cautions; Contra-indications; Side-effects: see notes above and under Codeine Phosphate; young children are particularly susceptible to OVERDOSAGE and symptoms may be delayed so that observation is needed for at least 48 hours after ingestion; in addition the presence of subclinical doses of atropine may give rise to the side-effects of atropine in susceptible individuals or in overdosage

PoM **Lomotil®** (Searle)
Tablets, co-phenotrope 2.5/0.025 (diphenoxylate hydrochloride 2.5 mg, atropine sulphate 25 micrograms). Net price 20 = £1.57
Dose: initially 4 tablets, followed by 2 tablets every 6 hours until diarrhoea controlled; CHILD 4–8 years 1 tablet 3 times daily, 9–12 years 1 tablet 4 times daily, 13–16 years 2 tablets 3 times daily, but see also notes above
Liquid, red, sugar-free, co-phenotrope 2.5/0.025 (diphenoxylate hydrochloride 2.5 mg, atropine sulphate 25 micrograms)/5 mL. Net price 100 mL = £3.73
Dose: initially 20 mL, followed by 10 mL every 6 hours until diarrhoea controlled; CHILD 4–8 years 5 mL 3 times daily, 9–12 years 5 mL 4 times daily, 13–16 years 10 mL 3 times daily, but see also notes above
Note. Co-phenotrope 2.5/0.025 tablets are also available from Mepra-pharm (Diarphen®)

LOPERAMIDE HYDROCHLORIDE
Indications: adjunct to rehydration in acute diarrhoea in adults and children over 4 years (but see notes above); chronic diarrhoea in adults only
Cautions; Contra-indications: see notes above and under Codeine Phosphate (except dependence)

Side-effects: abdominal cramps and skin reactions, including urticaria reported; paralytic ileus and abdominal bloating also reported

Dose: acute diarrhoea, 4 mg initially followed by 2 mg after each loose stool for up to 5 days; usual dose 6–8 mg daily; max. 16 mg daily; CHILD 4–8 years 1 mg 4 times daily for up to *3 days only*, 9–12 years 2 mg 4 times daily for up to 5 days

Chronic diarrhoea in adults, initially, 4–8 mg daily in divided doses, subsequently adjusted according to response and given in 2 divided doses for maintenance

PoM¹ **Loperamide** (Non-proprietary)
Capsules, loperamide hydrochloride 2 mg. Net price 30 = £2.21
Available from Berk (Diocaps®), Cox, Generics, Hill-cross, K Pharm., Norton, Unichem

PoM¹ **Imodium®** (Janssen)
Capsules, green/grey, loperamide hydrochloride 2 mg. Net price 30 = £2.17
Syrup, red, sugar-free, loperamide hydrochloride 1 mg/5 mL. Net price 100 mL = £1.90

1. Loperamide can be sold to the public, for adults and children over 12 years, provided it is licensed and labelled for the treatment of acute diarrhoea; proprietary brands (Arret® capsules and adult syrup and Diocalm Ultra® capsules) are on sale to the public

MORPHINE

Indications: see notes above
Cautions; Contra-indications; Side-effects: see notes above and under Codeine Phosphate, sedation and the risk of dependence are greater

Kaolin and Morphine Mixture, BP
(Kaolin and Morphine Oral Suspension)
Oral suspension, light kaolin or light kaolin (natural) 20%, sodium bicarbonate 5%, and chloroform and morphine tincture 4% in a suitable vehicle. Contains 550 to 800 micrograms of anhydrous morphine/10 mL.
Dose: 10 mL every 4 hours in water

1.5   Treatment of chronic diarrhoeas

Once tumours are ruled out individual complaints need specific treatment including dietary manipulation as well as drug treatment and the maintenance of a liberal fluid intake.

IRRITABLE BOWEL SYNDROME

Irritable bowel syndrome can present with pain, constipation, or diarrhoea, all of which may benefit from a high-fibre diet with bran or other agents which increase stool bulk (section 1.6.1) if necessary. In some patients there may be important psychological aggravating factors which respond to reassurance. Antimotility drugs such as **loperamide** may sometimes be necessary but prolonged use may aggravate the condition (section 1.4.2). Opioids such as codeine are better avoided because of the risk of dependence. Antispasmodics (section 1.2) may relieve the pain.

MALABSORPTION SYNDROMES

Individual conditions need specific treatment and also general nutritional consideration. Thus coeliac disease (gluten enteropathy) usually needs a gluten-free diet (Appendix 7) and pancreatic insufficiency needs pancreatin supplements (section 1.9.4).

ULCERATIVE COLITIS

For *acute attacks* of ulcerative colitis topical **corticosteroid** treatment such as prednisolone enemas or suppositories for localised rectal disease will induce remission; foam preparations are especially useful where patients have difficulty retaining liquid enemas. More extensive disease requires oral corticosteroid treatment and severe extensive or fulminant disease needs hospital admission and intravenous corticosteroid administration.

Sulphasalazine, a chemical combination of sulphapyridine and 5-aminosalicylic acid ('5-ASA') is useful in mild symptomatic disease requiring oral treatment; it is also available as suppositories for rectal disease. Activity resides in the 5-aminosalicylic acid moiety; sulphapyridine acts only as a carrier to the colonic site of action (but it still causes side-effects). Newer alternatives include **mesalazine** (5-aminosalicylic acid itself) and **olsalazine** (2 molecules of 5-aminosalicylic acid bonded together, separating in the lower bowel). The sulphonamide-related side-effects of suphasalazine (rashes, blood disorders, azoospermia, and lupoid syndromes) are lacking from mesalazine and olsalazine, but they retain side-effect profiles associated with the 5-aminosalicylic acid moiety (diarrhoea, salicylate hypersensitivity, and interstitial nephritis).

Corticosteroids are unsuitable for *maintenance treatment* because of side-effects. Sulphasalazine, mesalazine, and olsalazine all have value in preventing relapse and choice is related in part to their different side-effects. In resistant cases **azathioprine** (see section 8.2.1), 2 mg/kg daily, given under close supervision may be helpful [unlicensed indication].

Laxatives are required to facilitate bowel movement when proctitis is present but a high-fibre diet and bulk-forming drugs such as **methylcellulose** are more useful in adjusting faecal consistency (section 1.6.1).

Antimotility drugs such as codeine and loperamide should not be used in severe colitis as they can precipitate paralytic ileus and megacolon. They have limited value in mild disease, but treatment of the inflammation is more logical. For similar reasons antispasmodics should **not** be used in ulcerative colitis.

CROHN'S DISEASE

Treatment of Crohn's disease (particularly of colonic disease) is similar to that for ulcerative colitis. In small bowel disease **sulphasalazine** is of doubtful value. **Oral corticosteroids** (e.g. prednisolone) suppress inflammation, and **metronidazole** may be beneficial possibly through antibacterial activity. Other antibacterials should be given if specifically indicated and for managing bacterial overgrowth in the small bowel.

In both colitis and Crohn's disease general nutritional care and appropriate supplements are essential.

Cholestyramine and **aluminium hydroxide mixture** (section 1.1.1), bind unabsorbed bile salts and provide symptomatic relief of diarrhoea following ileal disease or resection, in bacterial colonisation of the small bowel, and in post-vagotomy diarrhoea.

PSEUDOMEMBRANOUS COLITIS

Pseudomembranous colitis is caused by colonisation of the colon with *Clostridium difficile* which may follow antibiotic therapy. It is usually of acute onset, but may run a chronic course; it is a particular hazard of clindamycin but few antibiotics are free of this side-effect. Oral **vancomycin** (see section 5.1.7) or **metronidazole** (see section 5.1.11) are used as specific treatment; vancomycin may be preferred for very sick patients.

DIVERTICULAR DISEASE

Diverticular disease is treated with a high-fibre diet, **bran supplements**, and **bulk-forming drugs**. **Antispasmodics** may provide symptomatic relief when colic is a problem (section 1.2). **Antibiotics** should be used only when the diverticula in the intestinal wall become infected. **Antimotility** drugs which slow intestinal motility, e.g. codeine, diphenoxylate, and loperamide could possibly exacerbate the symptoms of diverticular disease and are **contra-indicated**.

AMINOSALICYLATES

MESALAZINE

Indications: induction and maintenance of remission in ulcerative colitis

Cautions: pregnancy and breast-feeding

Contra-indications: salicylate hypersensitivity; renal impairment (nephrotoxic)

Side-effects: nausea, diarrhoea, and abdominal pain; headache; exacerbation of symptoms of colitis; rarely reversible pancreatitis, hepatitis, and interstitial nephritis; leucopenia, neutropenia, thrombocytopenia and aplastic anaemia reported; myocarditis, lupus phenomenon, fibrosing alveolitis also reported

Dose: see under preparations, below

PoM Asacol® (SK&F)

Tablets, red, e/c, mesalazine 400 mg. Net price 120-tab pack = £37.73. Label: 5, 25

Dose: acute attack, 6 tablets daily in divided doses; maintenance 3–6 tablets daily in divided doses

Foam enema, mesalazine 1 g/metered application. Net price 14 g (14 applications) with disposable applicators and plastic bags = £39.60

Dose: acute attack affecting the rectosigmoid region, 1 metered application (mesalazine 1 g) inserted into the rectum daily for 4–6 weeks

Acute attack affecting the descending colon, 2 metered applications (mesalazine 2 g) inserted into the rectum daily for 4–6 weeks

Suppositories, mesalazine 250 mg, net price 20 = £6.50; 500 mg, 10 = £6.50

Dose: 3–6 suppositories of 250 mg (max. 3 suppositories of 500 mg) daily in divided doses, with last dose at bedtime

PoM Pentasa® (Yamanouchi)

Slow Release Tablets, m/r, both scored, mesalazine 250 mg, net price 200-tab pack = £32.28; 500 mg (grey), 100-tab pack = £32.28. Counselling, administration, see dose

Dose: acute attack, 3–4 g daily (as 6–8 tablets of 500 mg) in 2–3 divided doses; maintenance, 1.5 g daily (as 6 tablets of 250 mg or 3 tablets of 500 mg) in 2–3 divided doses; tablets may be dispersed in water, but should not be chewed

Retention enema, mesalazine 1 g in 100-mL. Net price 7 × 100-mL bottle = £19.45

Dose: 100 mL enema at bedtime

Suppositories, mesalazine 1 g. Net price 28 = £44.68

Dose: acute attack, 1 suppository daily for 2–4 weeks; maintenance, 1 suppository daily

PoM Salofalk® (Thames)

Tablets, e/c, yellow, mesalazine 250 mg. Net price 100-tab pack = £17.50. Label: 5, 25

Dose: acute attack, 6 tablets daily in 3 divided doses; maintenance 3–6 tablets daily in divided doses

OLSALAZINE SODIUM

Indications: induction and maintenance of remission in ulcerative colitis

Cautions: pregnancy and breast-feeding

Contra-indications: salicylate hypersensitivity; renal impairment

Side-effects: watery diarrhoea, abdominal cramps, headache, nausea, dyspepsia, arthralgia, and rash; rarely reversible pancreatitis

Dose: acute attack, 1 g daily in divided doses increased if necessary over 1 week to max. 3 g daily (max. single dose 1 g)

Maintenance, 500 mg twice daily

PoM Dipentum® (Pharmacia)

Capsules, brown, olsalazine sodium 250 mg. Net price 20 = £4.66. Label: 21

SULPHASALAZINE

(Sulfasalazine)

Indications: induction and maintenance of remission in ulcerative colitis; active Crohn's disease; rheumatoid arthritis, see section 10.1.3

Cautions: history of allergy; hepatic and renal disease; G6PD deficiency; slow acetylator status; risk of haematological and hepatic toxicity (differential white cell, red cell and platelet counts initially and at monthly intervals for first 3 months, liver function tests at monthly intervals for first 3 months; upper gastro-intestinal side-effects common over 4 g daily; pregnancy and breast-feeding (see Appendixes 4 and 5); porphyria (see section 9.8.2)

BLOOD DISORDERS. CSM has reminded of need to warn patient to report immediately if sore throat, fever, malaise or non-specific illness develops. Treatment should be stopped immediately if suspicion or laboratory evidence of blood disorder.

Contra-indications: salicylate and sulphonamide hypersensitivity; CHILD under 2 years of age

Side-effects: nausea, vomiting, epigastric discomfort, headache, rashes; *occasionally:* fever, minor haematological abnormalities such as Heinz-body anaemia, reversible neutropenia, folate deficiency; reversible oligospermia; *rarely:* pancreatitis, hepatitis, exacerbation of colitis, thrombocytopenia, agranulocytosis, aplastic anaemia, Stevens–Johnson syndrome, neurotoxicity, photosensitisation, lupus erythematosus-like syndrome, and fibrosing alveolitis; proteinuria, crystalluria, haematuria, and nephrotic syndrome; urine may be coloured orange; some soft contact lenses may be stained

Dose: by mouth, acute attack 1–2 g 4 times daily (but see **cautions**) until remission occurs (if necessary corticosteroids may also be given), reducing to a maintenance dose of 500 mg 4 times daily; CHILD over 2 years, acute attack 40–60 mg/kg daily, maintenance dose 20–30 mg/kg daily

By rectum, in suppositories, alone or in conjunction with oral treatment 0.5–1 g morning and night after a bowel movement. As an enema, 3 g at night, retained for at least 1 hour

PoM **Sulphasalazine** (Non-proprietary)
Tablets, sulphasalazine 500 mg. Net price 100 = £7.95. Label: 14, counselling, blood disorder symptoms (see above), contact lenses may be stained
Available from APS, Berk, Cox, K Pharm., Lagap, Norton

PoM **Salazopyrin®** (Pharmacia)
Tablets, yellow, scored, sulphasalazine 500 mg. Net price 20 = £1.41. Label: 14, counselling, blood disorder symptoms (see above), contact lenses may be stained
EN-Tabs® (= tablets e/c), yellow, f/c, sulphasalazine 500 mg. Net price 125-tab pack = £12.75. Label: 5, 14, 25, counselling, blood disorder symptoms (see above), contact lenses may be stained
Suspension, yellow, sulphasalazine 250 mg/5 mL. Net price 500 mL = £16.44. Label: 14, counselling, blood disorder symptoms (see above), contact lenses may be stained
Suppositories, brown, sulphasalazine 500 mg. Net price 10 = £2.88; 50 = £13.67. Label: 14, counselling, blood disorder symptoms (see above), contact lenses may be stained
Retention enema, sulphasalazine 3 g in 100-mL single-dose disposable packs fitted with a nozzle. Net price 7 × 100 mL = £12.43. Label: 14, counselling, blood disorder symptoms (see above), contact lenses may be stained

ANION-EXCHANGE RESINS

CHOLESTYRAMINE
(Colestyramine)

Indications: diarrhoea associated with Crohn's disease, ileal resection, vagotomy, diabetic vagal neuropathy, and radiation; pruritus in liver disease, and hypercholesterolaemia, see section 2.12

Cautions; Contra-indications; Side-effects: see section 2.12

Dose: diarrhoea, after initial introduction over 3–4 week period, 12–24 g daily mixed with water, in single or divided doses, subsequently adjusted as required; max. 36 g daily

COUNSELLING. Other drugs should be taken at least 1 hour before or 4–6 hours after cholestyramine to reduce possible interference with absorption

Preparations
Section 2.12

CORTICOSTEROIDS

HYDROCORTISONE
Indications: inflammation associated with colitis, proctitis

Cautions; Contra-indications; Side-effects: systemic absorption may occur, see section 6.3.3; prolonged use should be avoided; avoid use of enemas and rectal foams in obstruction, bowel perforation, and extensive fistulas; contra-indicated in untreated infection

Dose: rectal, see under Preparations

PoM **Hydrocortisone Suppositories,** hydrocortisone or hydrocortisone acetate 25 mg in theobroma oil or other suitable basis. Net price 12 = £1.81
Dose: proctitis, 1 suppository inserted night and morning after a bowel movement

PoM **Colifoam®** (Stafford-Miller)
Foam in aerosol pack, hydrocortisone acetate 10%. Net price 25 g (14 applications) with applicator = £7.07
Dose: initially 1 metered application (125 mg hydrocortisone acetate) inserted into the rectum once or twice daily for 2–3 weeks, then once on alternate days

PREDNISOLONE
Indications: induction and maintenance of remission in ulcerative colitis, and Crohn's disease; other indications, see section 6.3.3

Cautions; Contra-indications; Side-effects: see under Hydrocortisone and section 6.3.3

Dose: by mouth, initial dose 40 mg daily, in single or divided doses, until remission occurs, followed by reducing doses

By rectum, see under Preparations

Cautionary label wordings, see inside back cover

Prices are **net**, see p.1

Oral preparations, see section 6.3.4

Rectal preparations
PoM Predenema® (Pharmax)
Retention enema, prednisolone 20 mg (as sodium metasulphobenzoate) in 100-mL single-dose disposable pack. Net price 1 (standard tube) = 80p, 1 (long tube) = £1.35
Dose: initially 1 enema at bedtime for 2–4 weeks, extending course if good response obtained
PoM Predfoam® (Pharmax)
Foam in aerosol pack, prednisolone 20 mg (as metasulphobenzoate sodium)/metered application. Net price 25 g (14 applications) with disposable applicators = £7.06
Dose: 1 metered application (containing 20 mg prednisolone) inserted into the rectum once or twice daily for 2 weeks, continued for further 2 weeks if good response
PoM Predsol® (Evans)
Retention enema, prednisolone 20 mg (as sodium phosphate) in 100-mL single-dose disposable packs fitted with a nozzle. Net price 7 = £5.24
Dose: initially 1 enema at bedtime for 2–4 weeks, extending course if good response obtained
Suppositories, prednisolone 5 mg (as sodium phosphate). Net price 10 = £1.00
Dose: proctitis and rectal complications of Crohn's disease, 1 suppository inserted night and morning after a bowel movement

---

CROMOGLYCATE

SODIUM CROMOGLYCATE
(Sodium cromoglicate)
Indications: food allergy (in conjunction with dietary restriction)
Side-effects: occasional nausea, rashes, and joint pain
Dose: 200 mg 4 times daily before meals; CHILD 2–14 years 100 mg; capsules may be swallowed whole or the contents dissolved in hot water and diluted with cold water before taking. May be increased if necessary after 2–3 weeks to a max. of 40 mg/kg daily and then reduced according to the response

PoM Nalcrom® (Fisons)
Capsules, sodium cromoglycate 100 mg. Net price 100 = £13.38. Label: 22, counselling, see dose above

1.6   Laxatives

  1.6.1   Bulk-forming drugs
  1.6.2   Stimulant laxatives
  1.6.3   Faecal softeners
  1.6.4   Osmotic laxatives

Before prescribing laxatives it is important to be sure that the patient *is* constipated and that the constipation is *not* secondary to an underlying undiagnosed complaint.

It is also important for those who complain of constipation to understand that bowel habit can vary considerably in frequency without doing harm. Some people tend to consider themselves constipated if they do not have a bowel movement each day. A useful definition of constipation is the passage of hard stools less frequently than the patient's own normal pattern and this can be explained to the patient.

Misconceptions about bowel habits have led to excessive laxative use. Abuse may lead to hypokalaemia and an atonic non-functioning colon.

Thus, laxatives should generally be **avoided** except where straining will exacerbate a condition (such as angina) or increase the risk of rectal bleeding as in haemorrhoids. Laxatives are also of value in *drug-induced constipation*, for the expulsion of *parasites* after anthelmintic treatment, and to clear the alimentary tract before *surgery and radiological procedures*. Prolonged treatment of constipation is seldom necessary except occasionally in the elderly.

CHILDREN. The use of laxatives in children is undesirable and the introduction of fruit purée into the diet may be sufficient to regulate bowel action. In infants constipation is often remedied by adjustment of the diet.

The laxatives that follow have been divided into 4 main groups (sections 1.6.1–1.6.4). This simple classification disguises the fact that some laxatives have a complex action.

1.6.1   Bulk-forming drugs

Bulk-forming drugs relieve constipation by increasing faecal mass which stimulates peristalsis; the full effect may take some days to develop and patients should be told this.

Bulk-forming drugs are of particular value in those with small hard stools, but should not be required unless fibre cannot be increased in the diet. A balanced diet, including adequate fluid intake and fibre is of value in preventing constipation.

Bulk-forming drugs are useful in the management of patients with *colostomy, ileostomy, haemorrhoids, anal fissure, chronic diarrhoea associated with diverticular disease, irritable bowel syndrome,* and *ulcerative colitis* (section 1.5). Adequate fluid intake must be maintained to avoid intestinal obstruction. Unprocessed wheat **bran**, taken with food or fruit juice, is a most effective bulk-forming preparation. Finely ground bran, though more palatable, has poorer water-retaining properties, but can be taken as bran bread or biscuits in appropriately increased quantities. Oat bran is also used.

Methylcellulose, ispaghula, and **sterculia** are useful in patients who cannot tolerate bran. Methylcellulose also acts as a faecal softener.

BRAN

Indications: see notes above
Cautions; Contra-indications; Side-effects: see under Ispaghula Husk. Calcium and iron absorption may be impaired. Avoid in gluten enteropathies and coeliac disease
Dose: see preparations below

COUNSELLING. Preparations that swell in contact with liquid should always be carefully swallowed with water and should not be taken immediately before going to bed

NHS Proctofibe® (Roussel)

Tablets, beige, f/c, fibrous grain extract 375 mg, fibrous citrus extract 94 mg. Net price 20 = 96p. Counselling, see above

Dose: ADULTS and CHILD over 3 years 4–12 tablets daily in divided doses swallowed with plenty of water *or* crushed and dispersed in water

Trifyba® (Sanofi Winthrop)

Powder, wheat fibre 80%. Net price 56 sachets containing 3.5 g = £3.28. Counselling, see below

Note. Contains gluten

Dose: 1 sachet 2–3 times daily added to food; CHILD half to one sachet 1–2 times daily added to food

COUNSELLING. At least one glass of water or other liquid should be drunk with the meal

ISPAGHULA HUSK

Indications: see notes above

Cautions: adequate fluid intake should be maintained to avoid intestinal obstruction—it may be necessary to supervise elderly or debilitated patients or those with intestinal narrowing or decreased motility

Contra-indications: intestinal obstruction, colonic atony, faecal impaction

Side-effects: flatulence, abdominal distension, gastro-intestinal obstruction or impaction; hypersensitivity reported

Dose: see preparations below

COUNSELLING. Preparations that swell in contact with liquid should always be carefully swallowed with water and should not be taken immediately before going to bed

Fybogel® (R&C)

Granules, buff, effervescent, sugar- and gluten-free, ispaghula husk 3.5 g/sachet (low Na⁺). Net price 60 sachets (plain or orange flavoured) = £4.24. Label: 13, counselling, see above

Note. Contains aspartame (see section 9.4.1)

Dose: 1 sachet in water twice daily preferably after meals; CHILD 6–12 years ½–1 level 5-mL spoonful (children under 6 years on doctor's advice only)

Isogel® (Charwell)

Granules, pink, sugar- and gluten-free, ispaghula husk 90%. Net price 300 g = £2.94. Label: 13, counselling, see above

Dose: constipation, 2 teaspoonfuls in water once or twice daily, preferably at mealtimes; CHILD 1 teaspoonful

Diarrhoea (section 1.4.1), 1 teaspoonful 3 times daily

Regulan® (Procter & Gamble)

Powder, beige, effervescent, sugar and gluten-free ispaghula husk 3.6 g/6.4-g sachet (original flavour) or 3.4 g/5.85-g sachet (orange or lemon/lime flavour). Net price 30 sachets = £2.12. Label: 13, counselling, see above

Note. The original-flavour version contains potassium 6.4 mmol/sachet; the orange and the lemon/lime-flavour versions contain potassium <1 mmol/sachet

Dose: 1 sachet in 150 mL water 1–3 times daily; CHILD 6–12 years 2.5–5 mL

METHYLCELLULOSE

Indications: see notes above

Cautions; Contra-indications; Side-effects: see under Ispaghula Husk

Dose: see preparations below

COUNSELLING. Preparations that swell in contact with liquid should always be carefully swallowed with water and should not be taken immediately before going to bed

Celevac® (Monmouth)

Tablets, pink, methylcellulose '450' 500 mg. Net price 112-tab pack = £2.45. Counselling, see above and dose

Dose: 3–6 tablets twice daily. In constipation the dose should be taken with at least 300 mL of water. In diarrhoea, ileostomy, and colostomy control, minimise liquid intake for 30 minutes before and after the dose

STERCULIA

Indications: see notes above

Cautions; Contra-indications; Side-effects: see under Ispaghula Husk

COUNSELLING. Preparations that swell in contact with liquid should always be carefully swallowed with water and should not be taken immediately before going to bed

Normacol® (Norgine)

Granules, coated, gluten-free, sterculia 62%. Net price 100 g = £1.11; 60 × 7-g sachets = £4.65. Label: 25, 27, counselling, see above

Dose: 1–2 heaped 5-mL spoonfuls, or the contents of 1–2 sachets, washed down without chewing with plenty of liquid once or twice daily after meals; CHILD 6–12 years half adult dose

Normacol Plus® (Norgine)

Granules, brown, coated, gluten-free, sterculia 62%, frangula (standardised) 8%. Net price 500 g = £5.82; 60 × 7 g sachets = £4.98. Label: 25, 27, counselling, see above

Dose: constipation and after haemorrhoidectomy, 1–2 heaped 5-mL spoonfuls or the contents of 1–2 sachets washed down without chewing with plenty of liquid once or twice daily after meals

Prefil®

See section 4.5.1

1.6.2   Stimulant laxatives

Stimulant laxatives should seldom be needed. It is important to recognise that improved mobility and the provision of time and privacy for going to the toilet may be all that is required.

The recognised stimulant laxatives include **bisacodyl** and members of the **anthraquinone** group, e.g. senna. **Docusate** sodium probably acts both as a stimulant and as a softening agent. **Danthron** has limited indications (see below) because *rodent* studies indicate potential carcinogenic risk. Powerful stimulants such as **cascara** and **castor oil** are obsolete.

Stimulant laxatives increase intestinal motility and often cause abdominal cramp. They should not be used in intestinal obstruction, and prolonged use can precipitate the onset of an atonic non-functioning colon and hypokalaemia. They should prefera-bly be avoided in children.

Glycerol suppositories act as a rectal stimulant by virtue of the mildly irritant action of glycerol.

Soft soap is a more severe irritant; the use of soft soap enema should be **avoided**, especially in pregnancy, as it may inflame the colonic mucosa.

The **parasympathomimetics** bethanechol, distig-mine, neostigmine, and pyridostigmine (see sec-tions 7.4.1 and 10.2.1) enhance parasympathetic activity in the gut and increase intestinal motility. They are rarely used for their gastro-intestinal effects. Organic obstruction of the gut must first be excluded and they should be used with caution in bowel anastomosis.

Oxyphenisatin is indicated for diagnostic proce-dures or surgery only, since it causes hepatitis in chronic use.

BISACODYL

Indications: see under Dose; tablets act in 10–12 hours; suppositories act in 20–60 minutes

Cautions; Contra-indications; Side-effects: see notes on stimulant laxatives; tablets, griping; sup-positories, local irritation

Dose: by mouth for constipation, 5–10 mg at night; occasionally necessary to increase to 15–20 mg; CHILD 5 mg

By rectum in suppositories for constipation, 10 mg in the morning; CHILD 5 mg

Before radiological procedures and surgery, 10 mg by mouth at bedtime for 2 days before examination and, if necessary, a 10-mg supposi-tory 1 hour before examination.

Bisacodyl (Non-proprietary)

Tablets, e/c, bisacodyl 5 mg. Net price 20 = 17p. Label: 5, 25

Suppositories, bisacodyl 10 mg. Net price 12 = £1.03

Paediatric suppositories, bisacodyl 5 mg. Net price 5 = 73p

Note. The brand name NHS Dulco-Lax® (Boehringer Ingelheim) is used for bisacodyl tablets, net price 20 = 90p; suppositories, 10 = £1.28; paediatric suppositories, 5 = 73p

DANTHRON

(Dantron)

Indications: only for: constipation in geriatric practice; prophylaxis and treatment of analgesic-induced constipation in terminally ill patients of all ages; constipation in cardiac failure and coro-nary thrombosis (conditions in which bowel movement must be free of strain); acts within 6–12 hours

Cautions; Contra-indications; Side-effects: see notes on stimulant laxatives; urine may be col-oured red; avoid prolonged contact with skin (as in incontinent patients) since irritation and excori-ation may occur; avoid in pregnancy and breast-feeding; *rodent* studies indicate potential carcino-genic risk

Dose: see under preparations

Co-danthramer and co-danthrusate

PoM **Co-danthramer** (Non-proprietary)

Suspension, co-danthramer 25/200 in 5 mL (dan-thron 25 mg, poloxamer '188' 200 mg/5 mL). Label: 14 (urine red)

Dose: 5–10 mL at night; CHILD 2.5–5 mL (restricted indications, see notes above)

Note. The brand name NHS Codalax® (Napp) is used for co-danthramer 25/200 in 5 mL suspension, net price 300 mL = £10.25, 1 litre = £34.18

Strong suspension, co-danthramer 75/1000 in 5 mL (danthron 75 mg, poloxamer '188' 1 g/5 mL). Label: 14 (urine red)

Dose: 5 mL at night (restricted indications, see notes above); CHILD under 12 years not recommended

Note. The brand name NHS Codalax Forte® (Napp) is used for co-danthramer 75/1000 in 5 mL suspension, net price 300 mL = £28.69, 1 litre = £95.58

PoM **Co-danthrusate** (Non-proprietary)

Capsules, co-danthrusate 50/60 (danthron 50 mg, docusate sodium 60 mg). Label: 14 (urine red)

Dose: 1–3 capsules, usually at night; CHILD 6–12 years 1 capsule (restricted indications, see notes above)

Suspension, yellow, co-danthrusate 50/60 (danthron 50 mg, docusate sodium 60 mg/5 mL). Label: 14 (urine red)

Dose: 5–15 mL at night; CHILD 6–12 years 5 mL at night (restricted indications, see notes above)

Note. The brand name NHS Normax® (Evans) is used for co-danthrusate 50/60 capsules, net price 63-cap pack = £12.24 and co-danthrusate 50/60 in 5 mL suspension, net price = £6.40

DOCUSATE SODIUM

(Dioctyl Sodium Sulphosuccinate)

Indications: constipation (oral preparations act within 1–2 days); adjunct in abdominal radiologi-cal procedures

Cautions; Contra-indications; Side-effects: see notes on stimulant laxatives; do not give with liq-uid paraffin; rectal preparations not indicated if haemorrhoids or anal fissure

Dose: by mouth, constipation, up to 500 mg daily in divided doses; CHILD over 6 months 12.5 mg 3 times daily; 2–12 years 12.5–25 mg 3 times daily (use paediatric oral solution only)

With barium meal, 400 mg

Dioctyl® (Schwarz)

Capsules, yellow/white, docusate sodium 100 mg. Net price 100-cap pack = £4.65

Oral solution 1%, sugar-free, docusate sodium 50 mg/5 mL. Net price 300-mL pack = £2.48

Paediatric oral solution, sugar-free, docusate sod-ium 12.5 mg/5 mL. Net price 125-mL pack = 97p

Rectal preparations

Fletchers' Enemette® (Pharmax)

Enema, docusate sodium 90 mg, glycerol 3.78 g/5 mL with macrogol and sorbic acid. Net price 5-mL unit = 32p

Dose: ADULT and CHILD over 3 years, 5-mL unit when required

Norgalax Micro-enema® (Norgine)

Enema, docusate sodium 120 mg in 10-g single-dose disposable packs. Net price 10-g unit = 64p

Dose: ADULT and CHILD over 12 years, 10-g unit

GLYCEROL
(Glycerin)

Indications: constipation
Dose: see below

Glycerol Suppositories, BP
(Glycerin Suppositories)

Suppositories, gelatin 140 mg, glycerol 700 mg, purified water to 1 g. Net price 12 = 54p (infant), 62p (child), 55p (adult)

Dose: 1 suppository moistened with water before use. The usual sizes are for *infants* small (1-g mould), *children* medium (2-g mould), *adults* large (4-g mould)

OXYPHENISATIN
(Oxyphenisatine)

Indications: see under Dose
Cautions; Contra-indications; Side-effects: see notes on stimulant laxatives; avoid repeated use owing to liver toxicity

Veripaque® (Sanofi Winthrop)

Enema, powder for reconstitution, oxyphenisatin 50 mg in 3 g. Net price 1 vial = £2.03

Dose: by rectum before diagnostic procedures or surgery, oxyphenisatin 50 mg dissolved in 2 litres of water given over 5–8 minutes

Adjuvant to barium enema, oxyphenisatin 50 mg mixed thoroughly with 2 litres of barium sulphate enema

SENNA

Indications: constipation; bowel evacuation before abdominal radiological procedures, endoscopy, and surgery; acts in 8–12 hours
Cautions; Contra-indications; Side-effects: see notes on stimulant laxatives

Senna Tablets, total sennosides (calculated as sennoside B) 7.5 mg. Net price 20 = 30p

Dose: 2–4 tablets, usually at night; initial dose should be low then gradually increased; CHILD over 6 years, half adult dose (on doctor's advice only)

Note. The brand name NHS Senokot® (see below) is used for Senna tablets; for those on sale to the public lower dose recommended

Manevac® (Galen)

Granules, coated, senna fruit 12.4%, ispaghula 54.2%. Net price 250 g = £3.50. Label: 25, 27, counselling, see Ispaghula Husk

Dose: 1–2 level 5-mL spoonfuls with water or warm drink after supper and, if necessary, before breakfast *or* every 6 hours in resistant cases for 1–3 days; CHILD 5–12 years 1 level 5-mL spoonful daily

Senokot® (R&C)

NHS *Tablets, see above*

Granules, brown, total sennosides (calculated as sennoside B) 15 mg/5 mL or 5.5 mg/g (one 5-mL spoonful = 2.7 g). Net price 100 g = £2.12

Dose: 5–10 mL, usually at bedtime; CHILD over 6 years 2.5–5 mL

Note. Lower dose on packs on sale to the public

Syrup, brown, total sennosides (calculated as sennoside B) 7.5 mg/5 mL. Net price 100 mL = £1.47

Dose: 10–20 mL, usually at bedtime; CHILD 2–6 years 2.5–5 mL (doctor's advice only), over 6 years 5–10 mL

Note. Lower dose on packs on sale to the public

SODIUM PICOSULPHATE
(Sodium Picosulfate)

Indications: constipation, bowel evacuation before abdominal radiological procedures, endoscopy, and surgery
Cautions; Contra-indications; Side-effects: see notes on stimulant laxatives
Dose: see below

Sodium Picosulphate Elixir, sodium picosulphate 5 mg/5 mL. Acts within 10–14 hours. Net price 100 mL = £1.45

Dose: 5–15 mL at night; CHILD 2–5 years 2.5 mL, 5–10 years 2.5–5 mL

Note. The brand name NHS Laxoberal® (Windsor) is used for sodium picosulphate elixir 5 mg/5 mL

Bowel clearance before radiography, endoscopy or surgery

Note. Low residue diet recomended for 2 days before examination and copious intake of water or other clear fluids recommended during treatment. Consider general warnings relating to bowel cleansing solutions on p. 50
Important: Not a treatment for constipation

Picolax® (Nordic)

Oral powder, sugar free, sodium picosulphate 10 mg/sachet, with magnesium citrate (for bowel evacuation before radiological procedures, endoscopy, and surgery). Net price 2 sachets = 59p. Label: 10, patient information leaflet, 13, counselling, see below

Dose: ADULT and CHILD over 9 years, 1 sachet in water in morning (before 8 a.m.) and a second in afternoon (between 2 and 4 p.m.) of day preceding procedures; CHILD 1–2 years quarter sachet morning and afternoon, 2–4 years half sachet morning and afternoon, 4–9 years 1 sachet morning and half sachet afternoon

Acts within 3 hours of first dose

COUNSELLING. Patients should be warned that heat is generated on addition to water; for this reason the powder should be added initially to 30 mL (2 tablespoonfuls) of water; after 5 minutes (when reaction complete) the solution should be further diluted to 150 mL (about a tumblerful)

OTHER STIMULANT LAXATIVES

Unstandardised preparations of cascara, frangula, rhubarb, and senna should be **avoided** as their laxative action is unpredictable. Aloes, colocynth, and jalap should be **avoided** as they have a drastic purgative action.

Phenolphthalein can cause rashes. It may colour alkaline urine pink.

Stimulant laxative preparations on sale to the public (not prescribable on the NHS) together with their significant ingredients:

Agarol® (agar, liquid paraffin, phenolphthalein), **Alophen®** (aloin, phenolphthalein) **Beechams Pills®** (aloin), **Bonomint®** (phenolphthalein), **Boots Compound Laxative®** (fig, senna), **Brooklax®** (phenolphthalein) **Califig®** (fig, senna), **Calsalettes®** (aloin), **Carters Little Pills®** (aloin, phenolphthalein), **Correctol®** (docusate, phenolphthalein) **Delax®** (liquid paraffin, phenolphthalein) **Ex-lax®** (phenolphthalein) **Fam-lax®** (phenolphthalein, rhubarb) **Juno Junipah Salts®** (juniper berry oil, sodium bicarbonate, sodium phosphate, sodium sulphate), **Juno Junipah Tablets®** (juniper berry oil, phenolphthalein, sodium chloride, sodium phosphate, sodium sulphate) **Kest®** (magnesium sulphate, phenolphthalein) **Nylax®** (bisacodyl, phenolphthalein, senna) **Potter's Cleansing Herb®** (aloes, cascara, senna) **Reguletts®** (phenolphthalein), **Rhuaka®** (cascara, rhubarb, senna) **Senlax®** (senna), **Sure-Lax®** (phenolphthalein)

1.6.3 Faecal softeners

Liquid paraffin, the classical lubricant, has disadvantages (see below). Bulk laxatives (section 1.6.1) and non-ionic surfactant 'wetting' agents e.g. docusate sodium (section 1.6.2) also have softening properties. Such drugs are useful for oral administration in the management of haemorrhoids and anal fissure; glycerol suppositories (section 1.6.2) are useful for rectal use.

Enemas containing **arachis oil** lubricate and soften impacted faeces and promote a bowel movement.

ARACHIS OIL
Indications: see notes above
Dose: see below

Fletchers' Arachis Oil Retention Enema®
(Pharmax)
Enema, arachis oil in 130-mL single-dose disposable packs. Net price 130 mL = £1.07
Dose: to soften impacted faeces, 130 mL; the enema should be warmed before use

LIQUID PARAFFIN
Indications: constipation
Cautions: CSM recommends avoid prolonged use, and has contra-indicated in children less than 3 years of age
Side-effects: anal seepage of paraffin and consequent anal irritation after prolonged use, granulomatous reactions caused by absorption of small quantities of liquid paraffin (especially from the emulsion), lipoid pneumonia, and interference with the absorption of fat-soluble vitamins
Dose: see under preparation

Liquid Paraffin Oral Emulsion, BP
Oral emulsion, liquid paraffin 5 mL, vanillin 5 mg, chloroform 0.025 mL, benzoic acid solution 0.2 mL, methylcellulose-20 200 mg, saccharin sodium 500 micrograms, water to 10 mL
Dose: 10–30 mL at night when required
COUNSELLING. Should not be taken immediately before going to bed

With phenolphthalein, see Other Stimulant Laxatives

1.6.4 Osmotic laxatives

These act by retaining fluid in the bowel by osmosis or by changing the pattern of water distribution in the faeces.

Saline purgatives such as **magnesium hydroxide** are commonly abused but are satisfactory for occasional use; adequate fluid intake should be maintained. **Magnesium salts** are useful where rapid bowel evacuation is required. **Sodium salts** should be avoided as they may give rise to sodium and water retention in susceptible individuals. **Phosphate enemas** are useful in bowel clearance before radiology, endoscopy, and surgery.

Lactulose is a semi-synthetic disaccharide which is not absorbed from the gastro-intestinal tract. It produces an osmotic diarrhoea of low faecal pH, and discourages the proliferation of ammonia-producing organisms. It is therefore useful in the treatment of *hepatic encephalopathy.* **Lactitol** is a similar disaccharide.

LACTITOL
Indications; Contra-indications; Side-effects: see under Lactulose
Dose: constipation, initially 20 g daily in a single dose with morning or evening meal, subsequently adjusted to produce one stool daily (dose of 10 g daily may be sufficient); CHILD 1–6 years 2.5–5 g, 6–12 years 5–10 g, 12–16 years 10–20 g daily, subsequently adjusted to produce one stool daily
Hepatic encephalopathy, 500–700 mg/kg daily in 3 divided doses with meals, subsequently adjusted to produce 2 soft stools daily
COUNSELLING. Powder should be mixed with food or liquid and one to two glasses of liquid should be drunk with the meal

PoM **Lactitol** (Non-proprietary)
Powder, lactitol 10 g/sachet. Net price 20-sachet pack = £2.25; 50-sachet pack = £5.62. Counselling, see above
Available from Zyma

LACTULOSE
Indications: constipation (may take up to 48 hours to act), hepatic encephalopathy (portal systemic encephalopathy)
Contra-indications: galactosaemia, intestinal obstruction
Side-effects: flatulence, cramps, and abdominal discomfort

Dose: expressed in terms of the elixir containing lactulose 3.35 g/5 mL

Constipation, initially 15 mL twice daily, gradually reduced according to patient's needs; CHILD under 1 year 2.5 mL, 1–5 years 5 mL, 6–12 years 10 mL twice daily, gradually reduced

Hepatic encephalopathy, 30–50 mL 3 times daily, subsequently adjusted to produce 2–3 soft stools daily

Lactulose (Non-proprietary)

Solution, lactulose 3.1–3.7 g/5 mL with other ketoses. Net price 200-mL pack = £1.25

Available from APS, Ashbourne (Osmolax®), Berk (Laxose®), Cox, CP, Duphar (NHS Duphalac®), Galen (Lactugal®), K Pharm., Norton

Note. A proprietary brand of lactulose 3.3 g/5 mL (Regulose®) is on sale to the public

MAGNESIUM SALTS

Indications; Dose: see under preparations

Cautions: renal impairment (risk of magnesium accumulation); hepatic impairment (see Appendix 2); elderly and debilitated; see also notes above; **interactions:** Appendix 1 (magnesium salts)

Contra-indications: acute gastro-intestinal conditions

Side-effects: colic

Magnesium citrate
Citramag® (Bioglan)

Powder, effervescent, providing when dissolved in water magnesium citrate 17.7 g/sachet. Net price 10 sachet pack = £10.09. Label 10, patient information leaflet, 13, counselling, see below

Dose: bowel evacuation before radiological examination and surgery, 1 sachet dissolved in 200 mL water and taken at 8 a.m. on day before procedure

COUNSELLING. The patient information leaflet advises that hot water is needed to make the solution and provides guidance on reconstitution; it also mentions need for high fluid, low residue diet beforehand (according to hospital advice), and explains that only clear fluids can be taken after Citramag® until procedure completed

Magnesium hydroxide
Magnesium Hydroxide Mixture, BP
(Cream of Magnesia)

Aqueous suspension containing about 8% hydrated magnesium oxide. Do not store in cold place.

Dose: constipation, 25–50 mL when required

Magnesium hydroxide with liquid paraffin
Liquid Paraffin and Magnesium Hydroxide Emulsion, BP

Oral emulsion, 25% liquid paraffin in aqueous suspension containing 6% hydrated magnesium oxide

Dose: constipation, 5–20 mL when required

Note. Liquid paraffin and magnesium hydroxide preparations on sale to the public include: NHS Cremaffin® and NHS Milpar®

Magnesium sulphate
Magnesium Sulphate. Label: 13, 23

Dose: rapid bowel evacuation (acts in 2–4 hours) 5–10 g in a tumblerful of water preferably before breakfast

Note. Magnesium sulphate is on sale to the public as Epsom Salts; NHS Andrews Liver Salts® (citric acid, magnesium sulphate, sodium bicarbonate) is also on sale to the public

PHOSPHATES (RECTAL)

Indications: rectal use in constipation; bowel evacuation before abdominal radiological procedures, endoscopy, and surgery

Cautions: see notes above

Contra-indications: acute gastro-intestinal conditions

Dose: see below

Carbalax® (Pharmax)

Suppositories, sodium acid phosphate 1.72 g in an effervescent basis. Net price 12 = £2.24

Dose: constipation, 1 suppository, inserted 30 minutes before evacuation is required; moisten with water before use; CHILD, not recommended

Fleet® Ready-to-use Enema (De Witt)

Enema, sodium acid phosphate 21.4 g, sodium phosphate 9.4 g/118 mL. Net price single-dose pack = 59p

Dose: ADULT and CHILD over 12 years, 118 mL; CHILD 3–12 years, on doctor's advice only (under 3 years not recommended)

Fletchers' Phosphate Enema® (Pharmax)

Enema, sodium acid phosphate 12.8 g, sodium phosphate 10.24 g, purified water, freshly boiled and cooled, to 128 mL (corresponds to Phosphates Enema Formula B). Net price 128 mL with standard tube = 46p, with long rectal tube = 64p

Dose: 128 mL; CHILD, over 3 years, reduced according to body weight (under 3 years not recommended)

SODIUM CITRATE (RECTAL)

Indications: rectal use in constipation

Cautions: see notes above

Contra-indications: acute gastro-intestinal conditions

Dose: see below

Micolette Micro-enema® (Cusi)

Enema, sodium citrate 450 mg, sodium lauryl sulphoacetate 45 mg, glycerol 625 mg, together with citric acid, potassium sorbate, and sorbitol in a viscous solution, in 5 mL single-dose disposable packs with nozzle. Net price 5 mL = 33p

Dose: ADULT and CHILD over 3 years, 5–10 mL

Micralax Micro-enema® (Evans)

Enema, sodium citrate 450 mg, sodium alkylsulphoacetate 45 mg, sorbic acid 5 mg, together with glycerol and sorbitol in a viscous solution in 5-mL single-dose disposable packs with nozzle. Net price 5 mL = 45p

Dose: ADULT and CHILD over 3 years, 5 mL

Relaxit Micro-enema® (Pharmacia)

Enema, sodium citrate 450 mg, sodium lauryl sulphate 75 mg, sorbic acid 5 mg, together with glycerol and sorbitol in a viscous solution in 5-mL single-dose disposable packs with nozzle. Net price 5 mL = 31p

Dose: ADULT and CHILD over 3 years, 5 mL

BOWEL CLEANSING SOLUTIONS

Bowel cleansing solutions are used before colonic surgery, colonoscopy, or radiological examination to ensure the bowel is free of solid contents. They are **not** treatments for constipation.

BOWEL CLEANSING SOLUTIONS

Indications: see above

Cautions: pregnancy; ulcerative colitis; reflux oesophagitis; impaired gag reflex; unconscious or semiconscious or possibility of regurgitation or aspiration; oral medication taken within 1 hour may not be absorbed

Contra-indications: gastro-intestinal obstruction, gastric retention, perforated bowel; toxic colitis, toxic megacolon or ileus; weight less than 20 kg

Side-effects: nausea and bloating; less frequently abdominal cramps (usually transient—reduced by taking more slowly); vomiting, anal irritation; urticaria and allergic reactions reported

Klean-Prep® (Norgine)

Oral powder, macrogol 3350 (polyethylene glycol 3350) 59 g, anhydrous sodium sulphate 5.685 g, sodium bicarbonate 1.685 g, sodium chloride 1.465 g, potassium chloride 743 mg/sachet. Contains aspartame (see section 9.4.1). Net price 4 sachets = £8.39. Label: 10, counselling

Four sachets when reconstituted with water to 4 litres provides an iso-osmotic solution for bowel cleansing before surgery, colonoscopy or radiological procedures

Dose: by mouth, 250 mL (1 tumblerful) of reconstituted solution every 10–15 minutes, or by nasogastric tube 20–30 mL/minute, until 4 litres have been consumed or watery stools are free of solid matter; CHILD not recommended

The solution from all 4 sachets should be drunk within 4–6 hours (250 mL drunk rapidly every 10–15 minutes); flavouring such as clear fruit cordials may be added if required; to facilitate gastric emptying domperidone or metoclopramide may be given 30 minutes before starting.

Alternatively the administration may be divided into two, e.g. taking the solutions from 2 sachets on the evening before examination and the remaining 2 on the morning of the examination

After reconstitution the solution should be kept in a refrigerator and discarded if unused after 24 hours

COUNSELLING. Administration and storage (see above)

1.7   Preparations for haemorrhoids

1.7.1   Soothing preparations
1.7.2   Compound preparations with corticosteroids
1.7.3   Rectal sclerosants

Anal and perianal pruritus, soreness, and excoriation are best treated by application of bland ointments and suppositories (section 1.7.1). These conditions occur commonly in patients suffering from haemorrhoids, fistulas, and proctitis. Careful local toilet as well as adjustment of the diet to avoid hard stools, and the use of bulk-forming materials such as bran (section 1.6.1) and a high residue diet are also helpful. In proctitis these measures may supplement treatment with corticosteroids or sulphasalazine (see section 1.5).

When necessary topical preparations containing **local anaesthetics** (section 1.7.1) or **corticosteroids** (section 1.7.2) are used provided perianal thrush has been excluded. Perianal thrush is best treated with **nystatin** by mouth and by local application (see sections 5.2, 7.2.2, and 13.10.2).

1.7.1   Soothing preparations

Bland soothing preparations containing mild astringents such as bismuth subgallate, zinc oxide, and hamamelis may give symptomatic relief in haemorrhoids. Many proprietary preparations also contain lubricants, vasoconstrictors, or mild antiseptics.

Topical **heparinoids** are claimed to promote the resorption of local oedema and extravasated blood.

Local anaesthetics are used to relieve pain associated with *haemorrhoids,* and *pruritus ani* but good evidence is lacking. Lignocaine ointment (see section 15.2) is used before emptying the bowel to relieve pain associated with *anal fissure.* Alternative local anaesthetics include amethocaine, cinchocaine, and pramoxine, but they are more irritant. Local anaesthetic ointments can be absorbed through the rectal mucosa therefore excessive application should be **avoided**, particularly in infants and children. They should be used for short periods only (no longer than 2 weeks) since they may cause sensitisation of the anal skin.

Anacal® (Panpharma)

Rectal ointment, laureth '9' 5%, a heparinoid 0.2%. Net price 30 g (with rectal nozzle) = £3.04

Apply 1–4 times daily; CHILD under 5 years not recommended

Suppositories, laureth '9' 50 mg, a heparinoid 4 mg. Net price 10 = £2.08

Insert 1 suppository once or twice daily; CHILD under 5 years not recommended

Anodesyn® (Seton)

Ointment, lignocaine hydrochloride 0.5%, allantoin 0.5%. Net price 25 g = £1.28

Apply night and morning and after a bowel movement; CHILD not recommended

Suppositories, lignocaine hydrochloride 10.25 mg, allantoin 10.25 mg. Net price 12 = £1.33

Insert 1 suppository night and morning and after a bowel movement; CHILD not recommended

Anusol® (W-L)

Cream, bismuth oxide 2.14%, Peru balsam 1.8%, zinc oxide 10.75%. Net price 23 g (with rectal nozzle) = £1.51

Apply night and morning and after a bowel movement; CHILD not recommended

Ointment, bismuth oxide 0.875%, bismuth subgallate 2.25%, zinc oxide 10.75%, Peru balsam 1.875%. Net price 25 g (with rectal nozzle) = £1.51

Apply night and morning and after a bowel movement; CHILD not recommended

Suppositories, bismuth oxide 24 mg, bismuth subgallate 59 mg, Peru balsam 49 mg, zinc oxide 296 mg. Net price 12 = £1.42

Insert 1 suppository night and morning and after a bowel movement; CHILD not recommended

1.7.2   Compound preparations with corticosteroids

Corticosteroids are often combined with antibiotics, local anaesthetics, and soothing agents in preparations for haemorrhoids. They are suitable for occasional short-term use after exclusion of infections, such as herpes simplex; see section 13.4 for general comments on topical corticosteroids.

Antibiotics may do little more than encourage the growth of resistant bacteria and should be avoided. See section 1.7.1 for comment on local anaesthetics.

PoM Anugesic-HC® (P-D)

Cream, benzyl benzoate 1.2%, bismuth oxide 0.875%, hydrocortisone acetate 0.5%, Peru balsam 1.85%, pramoxine hydrochloride 1%, zinc oxide 12.35%. Net price 30 g (with rectal nozzle) = £3.09

Apply night and morning and after a bowel movement; do not use for longer than 7 days; CHILD not recommended

Suppositories, benzyl benzoate 33 mg, bismuth oxide 24 mg, bismuth subgallate 59 mg, hydrocortisone acetate 5 mg, Peru balsam 49 mg, pramoxine hydrochloride 27 mg, zinc oxide 296 mg. Net price 12 = £2.24

Insert 1 suppository night and morning and after a bowel movement; do not use for longer than 7 days; CHILD not recommended

PoM Anusol-HC® (P-D)

Ointment, benzyl benzoate 1.25%, bismuth oxide 0.875%, bismuth subgallate 2.25%, hydrocortisone acetate 0.25%, Peru balsam 1.875%, zinc oxide 10.75%. Net price 30 g (with rectal nozzle) = £2.90

Apply night and morning and after a bowel movement; do not use for longer than 7 days; CHILD not recommended

Suppositories, benzyl benzoate 33 mg, bismuth oxide 24 mg, bismuth subgallate 59 mg, hydrocortisone acetate 10 mg, Peru balsam 49 mg, zinc oxide 296 mg. Net price 12 = £2.24

Additives: include tartrazine lake

Insert 1 suppository night and morning and after a bowel movement; do not use for longer than 7 days; CHILD not recommended

PoM Betnovate® (Glaxo)

Rectal ointment, betamethasone valerate 0.05%, lignocaine hydrochloride 2.5%, phenylephrine hydrochloride 0.1%. Net price 30 g (with applicator) = £1.50

Apply 2–3 times daily until inflammation subsides then once daily, externally or by rectum; do not use for longer than 7 days; CHILD not recommended

PoM Perinal® (Dermal)

Spray application, hydrocortisone 0.2%, lignocaine hydrochloride 1%. Net price 30-mL pack = £6.31

Spray twice over the affected area up to 3 times daily; do not use for longer than 1–2 weeks; CHILD not recommended

PoM Proctofoam HC® (Stafford-Miller)

Foam in aerosol pack, hydrocortisone acetate 1%, pramoxine hydrochloride 1%. Net price 24-g pack (approx. 40 applications) with applicator = £4.71

Dose: haemorrhoids and proctitis, 1 applicatorful (4–6 mg hydrocortisone acetate, 4–6 mg pramoxine hydrochloride) by rectum 2–3 times daily and after a bowel movement; CHILD not recommended

PoM Proctosedyl® (Roussel)

Ointment, cinchocaine hydrochloride 0.5%, hydrocortisone 0.5%. Net price 30 g = £6.48 (with cannula)

Apply morning and night and after a bowel movement, externally or by rectum; CHILD not recommended

Suppositories, cinchocaine hydrochloride 5 mg, hydrocortisone 5 mg. Net price 12 = £2.93

Insert 1 suppository night and morning and after a bowel movement; CHILD not recommended

PoM Scheriproct® (Schering Health)

Ointment, cinchocaine (dibucaine) hydrochloride 0.5%, prednisolone hexanoate 0.19%. Net price 30 g = £4.41

Apply twice daily for 5–7 days (3–4 times daily on 1st day if necessary), then once daily for a few days after symptoms have cleared; CHILD not recommended

Suppositories, cinchocaine (dibucaine) hydrochloride 1 mg, prednisolone hexanoate 1.3 mg. Net price 12 = £2.08

Insert 1 suppository daily after a bowel movement, for 5–7 days (in severe cases initially 2–3 times daily); CHILD not recommended

PoM Ultraproct® (Schering Health)

Ointment, cinchocaine (dibucaine) hydrochloride 0.5%, fluocortolone hexanoate 0.095%, fluocortolone pivalate 0.092%. Net price 30 g (with rectal nozzle) = £4.57

Apply twice daily for 5–7 days (3–4 times daily on 1st day if necessary), then once daily for few days after symptoms have cleared; CHILD not recommended

Suppositories, cinchocaine (dibucaine) hydrochloride 1 mg, fluocortolone hexanoate 630 micrograms, fluocortolone pivalate 610 micrograms. Net price 12 = £2.15

Insert 1 suppository daily after a bowel movement, for 5–7 days (in severe cases initially 2–3 times daily) then 1 suppository every other day for 1 week; CHILD not recommended

PoM Uniroid-HC® (Unigreg)

Ointment, cinchocaine hydrochloride 0.5%, hydrocortisone 0.5%. Net price 30 g (with applicator) = £4.43

Apply 3 times daily, preferably after a bowel movement, externally or by rectum; do not use for longer than 7 days; CHILD not recommended

Suppositories, cinchocaine hydrochloride 5 mg, hydrocortisone 5 mg. Net price 12 = £2.00

Insert 1 suppository 3 times daily, preferably after a bowel movement; do not use for longer than 7 days; CHILD not recommended

PoM Xyloproct® (Astra)

Ointment (water-miscible), aluminium acetate 3.5%, hydrocortisone acetate 0.275%, lignocaine 5%, zinc oxide 18%. Net price 30 g (with applicator) = £3.48

Apply several times daily; CHILD not recommended

Suppositories, aluminium acetate 50 mg, hydro-cortisone acetate 5 mg, lignocaine 60 mg, zinc oxide 400 mg. Net price 10 = £1.63

Insert 1 suppository at night and after a bowel movement; CHILD not recommended

1.7.3   Rectal sclerosants

Oily phenol injection is used to inject haemorrhoids particularly when unprolapsed.

PHENOL
Indications: see notes above
Side-effects: irritation, tissue necrosis

Oily Phenol Injection, BP, phenol 5% in a suitable fixed oil. Net price 5-mL amp = £4.16

Dose: 2–3 mL into the submucosal layer at the base of the pile; several injections may be given at different sites, max. total injected 10 mL at any one time

Available from Evans

1.8   Stoma care

Prescribing for patients with stoma calls for special care. The following is a brief account of some of the main points to be borne in mind.

Enteric-coated and *modified-release* preparations are **unsuitable**, particularly in patients with ileostomies, as there may not be sufficient release of the active ingredient.

Laxatives. Enemas and washouts should **not** be prescribed for patients with ileostomies as they may cause rapid and severe dehydration.

Colostomy patients may suffer from constipation and whenever possible should be treated by increasing fluid intake or dietary fibre. **Bulk-forming drugs** (section 1.6.1) should be tried. If they are insufficient, as small a dose as possible of senna (section 1.6.2) should be used.

Antidiarrhoeals. Drugs such as **loperamide, codeine phosphate,** or **co-phenotrope** (diphenoxylate with atropine) are effective. Bulk-forming drugs (section 1.6.1) may be tried but it is often difficult to adjust the dose appropriately.

Antibiotics should **not** be given for an episode of acute diarrhoea.

Antacids. The tendency to diarrhoea from magnesium salts or constipation from aluminium salts may be increased in these patients.

Diuretics should be used with caution in patients with ileostomies as they may become excessively dehydrated and potassium depletion may easily occur. It is usually advisable to use a **potassium-sparing** diuretic (see section 2.2.3).

Digoxin. Patients with a stoma are particularly susceptible to hypokalaemia if on digoxin therapy and potassium supplements or a potassium-sparing diuretic may be advisable (for comment see section 9.2.1.1).

Potassium supplements. Liquid formulations are preferred to modified-release formulations (see above).

Analgesics. Opioid analgesics (see section 4.7.2) may cause troublesome constipation in colostomy

patients. When a non-opioid analgesic is required **paracetamol** is usually suitable but anti-inflammatory analgesics may cause gastric irritation and bleeding.

Iron preparations may cause loose stools and sore skin in these patients. If this is troublesome and if iron is definitely indicated an intramuscular iron preparation (see section 9.1.1.2) should be used. Modified-release preparations should be **avoided** for the reasons given above.

Patients are usually given advice about the use of *cleansing agents, protective creams, lotions, deodorants,* or *sealants* whilst in hospital, either by the surgeon or by the health authority stoma care nurses. Voluntary organisations offer help and support to patients with stoma.

For details of **stoma appliances and associated products**, see Appendix 8

1.9   Drugs affecting intestinal secretions

1.9.1   Drugs acting on the gall bladder
1.9.2   Drugs which increase gastric acidity
1.9.3   Aprotinin
1.9.4   Pancreatin

1.9.1   Drugs acting on the gall bladder

The use of laproscopic cholecystectomy and of endoscopic biliary techniques has limited the place of the bile acids **chenodeoxycholic acid** and **urso-deoxycholic acid** in gallstone disease. They are suitable for patients not treatable by other means who have mild symptoms, unimpaired gall bladder function, and small or medium sized radiolucent stones; they are not suitable for radio-opaque stones, which are unlikely to be dissolved. Patients should preferably be supervised in hospital because radiological monitoring is required. Long-term prophylaxis may be needed after complete dissolution of the gallstones has been confirmed (preferably with cholecystograms and ultrasound on two separate occasions) as gallstones may recur in up to 25% of patients within one year of stopping treatment.

CHENODEOXYCHOLIC ACID
Indications; Cautions: see notes above
Contra-indications: do not use when stones are radio-opaque, in pregnancy (see Appendix 4), in non-functioning gall bladders, in chronic liver disease, and inflammatory diseases of the small intestine and colon
Side-effects: diarrhoea particularly initially with high dosage (reduce dose for few days), pruritus, minor hepatic abnormalities and transient rise in serum transaminases

Dose: 10–15 mg/kg daily as a single dose at bed-time *or* in divided doses for 3–24 months, depending on size of stone; treatment is continued for 3 months after stones dissolve

PoM Chendol® (CP)

Capsules, orange/white, chenodeoxycholic acid 125 mg. Net price 224-cap pack = £47.50
Tablets, orange, f/c, scored, chenodeoxycholic acid 250 mg. Net price 112-tab pack = £48.50
PoM Chenofalk® (Thames)
Capsules, chenodeoxycholic acid 250 mg. Net price 60 = £22.50
Additives: include gluten

With ursodeoxycholic acid
PoM Combidol® (CP)
Tablets, f/c, chenodeoxycholic acid 125 mg, urso-deoxycholic acid 125 mg. Net price 60-tab pack = £40.00
Dose: 2–3 tablets (patients greater than 120% of ideal body weight, 6 tablets) daily as a single dose at bedtime or in divided doses; treatment continued for up to 3 months after stones dissolve

URSODEOXYCHOLIC ACID

Indications; Cautions; Contra-indications: see under Chenodeoxycholic Acid
Side-effects: see under Chenodeoxycholic Acid; diarrhoea occurs rarely; liver changes have not been reported
Dose: 8–12 mg/kg (obese patients up to 15 mg/kg) daily as a single dose at bedtime or in divided doses, for up to 2 years; treatment is continued for 3–4 months after stones dissolve

PoM Destolit® (Merrell)
Tablets, scored, ursodeoxycholic acid 150 mg. Net price 60 = £18.92. Label: 21

PoM Ursofalk® (Thames)
Capsules, ursodeoxycholic acid 250 mg. Net price 60 = £31.50. Label: 21
Additives: include gluten

With chenodeoxycholic acid
See under Chenodeoxycholic acid

OTHER PREPARATIONS FOR BILIARY DISORDERS

A **terpene** mixture (Rowachol®) raises biliary choles-terol solubility. It is not considered to be a useful adjunct.

PoM Rowachol® (Monmouth)
Capsules, green, e/c, borneol 5 mg, camphene 5 mg, cine-ole 2 mg, menthol 32 mg, menthone 6 mg, pinene 17 mg in olive oil. Net price 50-cap pack = £7.35. Label: 22
Dose: 1–2 capsules 3 times daily before food (but see notes above)
Interactions: Appendix 1 (*Rowachol®*)

1.9.2   Drugs which increase gastric acidity

Muripsin® is used in achlorhydria and hypochlorhydria but is of uncertain value; it replaced dilute hydrochloric acid.

Muripsin® (Norgine)
Tablets, orange, f/c, glutamic acid hydrochloride 500 mg: 1 tablet ≈ 1 mL Dilute Hydrochloric Acid BP. Net price 50 = £5.15. Label: 21
Dose: 1–2 tablets with meals

1.9.3   Aprotinin

See section 2.11.

1.9.4   Pancreatin

Supplements of pancreatin are given by mouth to compensate for reduced or absent exocrine secre-tion in cystic fibrosis, and following pancreatec-tomy, total gastrectomy, or chronic pancreatitis. They assist the digestion of starch, fat, and protein.

Pancreatin is inactivated by gastric acid therefore pancreatin preparations are best taken with food (or immediately before or after food). Gastric acid secretion may be reduced by giving cimetidine or ranitidine an hour beforehand (section 1.3). Con-current use of antacids also reduces gastric acidity. The newer enteric-coated preparations such as Creon®, Nutrizym GR®, and Pancrease® deliver a higher enzyme concentration in the duodenum (pro-viding the granules are swallowed whole without chewing). Higher-strength versions are now also available. (**important:** CSM advice on p.54)

Since pancreatin is also inactivated by heat, excessive heat should be avoided if preparations are mixed with liquids or food; the resulting mixtures should not be kept for more than one hour.

Dosage is adjusted according to size, number, and consistency of stools, so that the patient thrives; extra allowance may be needed if snacks are taken between meals.

Pancreatin may irritate the skin around mouth and anus, particularly if preparations are retained in the mouth or dosage is excessive. The most frequent side-effects are gastro-intestinal including nausea, vomiting, and abdominal discomfort; hyperuric-aemia and hyperuricosuria have been associated with very high doses. Hypersensitivity reactions occur occasionally and may affect those handling the powder.

PANCREATIN

Note. The pancreatin preparations which follow are all of porcine origin

Indications; Cautions; Side-effects: see above and (for higher-strength preparations) next page

Creon® (Duphar)

Capsules, brown/yellow, enclosing buff-coloured e/c granules of pancreatin, providing: protease 210 units, lipase 8000 units, amylase 9000 units. Net price 100 = £13.33. Counselling, see dose

Dose: ADULT and CHILD initially 1–2 capsules with meals either taken whole or contents mixed with fluid or soft food (then swallowed immediately without chewing); higher doses may be required according to response

Granules, brown, e/c, pancreatin, providing: protease 1 125 units, lipase 20 000 units, amylase 22 500 units/ sachet. Net price 40-sachet pack = £13.33. Counselling, see dose

Dose: ADULT and CHILD initially 1 sachet with meals either washed down or sprinkled on soft food (then swallowed immediately without chewing); higher doses may be required according to response

Note. One sachet of Creon granules contains the equivalent of 2½ Creon capsules

Nutrizym GR® (Merck)

Capsules, green/orange, enclosing e/c pellets of pancreatin, providing minimum of: protease 650 units, lipase 10 000 units, amylase 10 000 units. Net price 100 = £13.15. Counselling, see dose

Dose: ADULT and CHILD 1–2 capsules with meals swallowed whole or contents sprinkled on soft food (then swallowed immediately without chewing); higher doses may be required according to response

Nutrizym 10® (Merck)

Capsules, red/yellow, enclosing e/c minitablets of pancreatin providing minimum of: protease 500 units, lipase 10 000 units, amylase 9000 units. Net price 100 = £13.15. Counselling, see dose

Dose: ADULT and CHILD 1–2 capsules with meals and 1 capsule with snacks, swallowed whole or contents taken with water or sprinkled on soft food (then swallowed immediately without chewing); higher doses may be required according to response

Pancrease® (Cilag)

Capsules, enclosing e/c beads of pancreatin, providing minimum of: protease 330 units, lipase 5000 units, amylase 2900 units. Net price 100 = £17.07. Counselling, see dose

Dose: ADULT and CHILD 1–2 (occasionally 3) capsules during each meal and 1 capsule with snacks swallowed whole or contents sprinkled on liquid or soft food (then swallowed immediately without chewing); higher doses may be required according to response

Pancrex® (Paines & Byrne)

Granules, pancreatin, providing minimum of: protease 300 units, lipase 5000 units, amylase 4000 units/g. Net price 300 g = £20.39. Label: 25, counselling, see dose

Dose: ADULT and CHILD 5–10 g 4 times daily with meals washed down or mixed with liquid

Pancrex V® (Paines & Byrne)

Capsules, pancreatin, providing minimum of: protease 430 units, lipase 8000 units, amylase 9000 units. Net price 100-cap pack = £5.54, 300-cap pack = £15.80. Counselling, see dose

Dose: ADULT and CHILD over 1 year 2–6 capsules 4 times daily with meals, swallowed whole or sprinkled on food; CHILD up to 1 year 1–2 capsules mixed with feeds

Capsules '125', pancreatin, providing minimum of: protease 160 units, lipase 2950 units, amylase 3300 units. Net price 300-cap pack = £9.72. Counselling, see dose

Dose: NEONATE 1–2 capsules with feeds

Tablets, e/c, s/c, pancreatin, providing minimum of: protease 110 units, lipase 1900 units, amylase 1700 units. Net price 100-tab pack = £2.67, 300-tab pack = £4.51. Label: 5, 25, counselling, see dose

Dose: ADULT and CHILD 5–15 tablets 4 times daily before meals

Tablets forte, e/c, s/c, pancreatin, providing minimum of: protease 330 units, lipase 5600 units, amylase 5000 units. Net price 100-tab pack = £4.82, 300-tab pack = £13.74. Label: 5, 25, counselling, see dose

Dose: ADULT and CHILD 6–10 tablets 4 times daily before meals

Powder, pancreatin, providing minimum of: protease 1400 units, lipase 25 000 units, amylase 30 000 units/ g. Net price 100 g = £9.75, 300 g = £24.28. Counselling, see dose

Dose: ADULT and CHILD 0.5–2 g 4 times daily washed down or mixed with liquid; NEONATE 250–500 mg with each feed

Higher-strength preparations

Following reports of fibrotic strictures of the large bowel in children aged between 3 and 13 years with cystic fibrosis the **CSM** has recommended that all patients taking **Creon® 25 000**, **Nutrizym 22®**, **Pancrease HL®**, or **Panzytrat® 25 000** should be reviewed. Unless special reasons, it would be prudent to advise patients with cystic fibrosis to change to other pancreatin preparations for the time being. As strictures have developed many months after start of high-strength (high-lipase) products, all patients who have received them should be watched carefully. If symptoms suggestive of gastro-intestinal obstruction occur, possibility of bowel stricture should be considered.

▼ Creon® 25 000 (Duphar)

Capsules, orange/yellow, enclosing brown-coloured e/c pellets of pancreatin, providing: protease (total) 1000 units [≡ protease (free) 467 units], lipase 25 000 units, amylase 18 000 units. Net price 50-cap pack = £19.50. Counselling, see dose

Dose: ADULT and CHILD initially 1 capsule with meals either taken whole or contents mixed with fluid or soft food (then swallowed immediately without chewing)

▼ Nutrizym 22® (Merck)

Capsules, red/yellow, enclosing e/c minitablets of pancreatin, providing minimum of: protease 1100 units, lipase 22 000 units, amylase 19 800 units. Net price 100-cap pack = £30.30. Counselling, see dose

Dose: ADULT and CHILD 1–2 capsules with meals and 1 capsule with snacks, swallowed whole or contents taken with water or sprinkled on soft food (then swallowed immediately without chewing)

▼ Pancrease HL® (Cilag)

Capsules, enclosing light brown e/c minitablets of pancreatin, providing minimum of: protease 1250 units, lipase 25 000 units, amylase 22 500 units. Net price 100 = £36.18. Counselling, see dose

Dose: ADULT and CHILD 1–2 capsules during each meal and 1 capsule with snacks swallowed whole or contents sprinkled on liquid or soft food (then swallowed immediately without chewing)

▼ Panzytrat® 25 000 (Knoll)

Capsules, red/clear, enclosing e/c microtablets of pancreatin providing: protease 1250 units, lipase 25 000 units, amylase 22 500 units. Net price 100-cap pack = £31.20. Counselling, see dose

Dose: ADULT 6 capsules daily; CHILD up to 18 months 2 capsules daily, over 18 months 4 capsules daily swallowed whole or contents taken with fruit juice or sprinkled on soft, preferably slightly acidic, food (e.g. fruit salad or fruit puree), then swallowed immediately without excessive chewing

2: Drugs used in the treatment of diseases of the
CARDIOVASCULAR SYSTEM

In this chapter, drug treatment is discussed under the following headings:

2.1 Positive inotropic drugs

2.1.1   Cardiac glycosides
2.1.2   Phosphodiesterase inhibitors

Positive inotropic drugs increase the force of contraction of the myocardium; for sympathomimetics with inotropic activity see section 2.7.1.

2.1.1 Cardiac glycosides

The principal actions of the cardiac glycosides are an increase in the force of myocardial contraction and a reduction in the conductivity of the heart. They are most useful in the treatment of *supraventricular tachycardias*, especially for controlling ventricular response in atrial fibrillation. *Heart failure* may also be improved, even in patients in sinus rhythm, because of changes in the availability of intracellular calcium; this action is relatively unimportant, however, compared with effects that can be achieved with diuretics and ACE inhibitors (see section 2.5.5). Except when needed to maintain satisfactory rhythm, cardiac glycosides can often be withdrawn from patients with heart failure that is well controlled, without clinical deterioration. In the elderly who are particularly susceptible to digitalis toxicity, cardiac glycosides should be used with special care in the management of heart failure without atrial fibrillation.

Loss of appetite, nausea, and vomiting are common toxic effects; sinus bradycardia, atrioventricular block, ventricular extrasystoles, and sometimes ventricular tachycardia or atrial tachycardia with block also occur—especially in the presence of underlying conducting system defects or myocardial disease. These unwanted effects depend both on the plasma concentrations of the drugs and on the sensitivity of the conducting system or myocardium, which is often increased in heart disease. Thus, no one plasma concentration can indicate toxicity reliably but the likelihood increases progressively through the range 1.5 to 3 micrograms/litre for digoxin; higher steady-state concentrations must certainly be avoided. Measurements of plasma concentration are not necessary, however, unless problems occur during maintenance treatment. Hypokalaemia predisposes to toxicity, therefore diuretics used with digoxin should either be potassium sparing or should be given with potassium supplements.

Renal function is the most important determinant of digoxin dosage, whereas elimination of digitoxin depends on metabolism by the liver. Toxicity can often be managed by discontinuing therapy and correcting hypokalaemia if appropriate; serious manifestations require urgent specialist management. Digoxin-specific antibody fragments are available for reversal of life-threatening overdosage (see next page).

Digoxin is the glycoside most commonly used. In patients with *mild failure* a loading dose is not required, and a satisfactory plasma concentration can be achieved over a period of about a week, using a dose of 125 to 250 micrograms twice a day which may then be reduced having special regard to renal function. Because it has a long half-life maintenance doses need only be given once daily (but higher doses should be divided to avoid nausea). For management of *atrial fibrillation* the maintenance dose can usually be governed by ventricular response which should not be allowed to fall below 60 beats per minute except in special and recognised circumstances, e.g. with the concomitant administration of beta-blockers.

When *very rapid control* is needed, digoxin may be given intravenously in a digitalising dose of 0.75 to 1 mg, preferably as an infusion (suggested volume 50 mL) over two or more hours (too rapid a rate of administration is associated with nausea and risk of arrhythmias); this is followed by normal maintenance therapy. The intramuscular route is not recommended, except when other methods of administration are not available.

Digitoxin has a long half-life and maintenance doses, again, need only be given once daily.

CHILDREN. The dose is based on body-weight; they require a relatively larger dose of digoxin than adults.

DIGOXIN

Indications: heart failure, supraventricular arrhythmias (particularly atrial fibrillation)

Cautions: recent infarction; sick sinus syndrome; hypothyroidism; reduce dose in the elderly and in renal impairment; avoid hypokalaemia; **interactions:** Appendix 1 (cardiac glycosides)

Contra-indications: intermittent complete heart block, second degree AV block; supraventricular arrhythmias caused by Wolff-Parkinson-White syndrome; hypertrophic obstructive cardiomyopathy (unless concomitant atrial fibrillation and heart failure — but with caution)

Side-effects: usually associated with excessive dosage, include: anorexia, nausea, vomiting, diarrhoea, abdominal pain; visual disturbances, headache, fatigue, drowsiness, confusion, delirium, hallucinations; arrhythmias, heart block; see also notes above

Dose: by mouth, rapid digitalisation, 1–1.5 mg in divided doses over 24 hours; less urgent digitalisation, 250–500 micrograms daily (higher dose divided)

Maintenance, 62.5–500 micrograms daily (higher dose divided) according to renal function and, in atrial fibrillation, on heart-rate response; usual range, 125–250 micrograms daily (elderly 125 micrograms)

For intravenous doses, see notes above

Note. For plasma concentration monitoring blood should ideally be taken at least 6 hours after a dose

PoM Digoxin (Non-proprietary)
Tablets, digoxin 62.5 micrograms, net price 20 = 8p; 125 micrograms, 20 = 6p; 250 micrograms, 20 = 8p
Injection, digoxin 250 micrograms/mL, see Lanoxin®
Paediatric injection, digoxin 100 micrograms/mL (hosp. only, available from Boots)

PoM Lanoxin® (Wellcome)
Tablets, digoxin 125 micrograms, net price 20 = 32p; 250 micrograms (scored), 20 = 32p
Injection, digoxin 250 micrograms/mL. Net price 2-mL amp = 65p

PoM Lanoxin-PG® (Wellcome)
Tablets, blue, digoxin 62.5 micrograms. Net price 20 = 32p
Elixir, yellow, digoxin 50 micrograms/mL. Do not dilute, measure with pipette. Net price 60 mL = £5.23. Counselling, use of pipette

---

DIGITOXIN

Indications: heart failure, supraventricular arrhythmias (particularly atrial fibrillation)
Cautions; Contra-indications; Side-effects: see under Digoxin
Dose: maintenance, 50–200 micrograms daily

PoM Digitoxin (Non-proprietary)
Tablets, digitoxin 100 micrograms, net price 20 = £2.73

DIGOXIN-SPECIFIC ANTIBODY

Digoxin-specific antibody fragments are indicated for the treatment of known or strongly suspected digoxin or digitoxin overdosage, where measures beyond the withdrawal of the cardiac glycoside and correction of any electrolyte abnormality are felt to be necessary (see also notes above).

PoM Digibind® (Wellcome)
Injection, powder for preparation of infusion, digoxin-specific antibody fragments (F(ab)) 40 mg. Net price per vial = £87.44 (hosp. and poisons centres only)
Dose: see data sheet

2.1.2   Phosphodiesterase inhibitors

Enoximone and milrinone are selective phosphodiesterase inhibitors which exert most of their effect on the myocardium. Sustained haemodynamic benefit has been observed after administration, but as yet there is no conclusive evidence of any beneficial effect on survival.

ENOXIMONE

Indications: congestive heart failure where cardiac output reduced and filling pressures increased
Cautions: heart failure associated with hypertrophic cardiomyopathy, stenotic or obstructive valvular disease or other outlet obstruction; monitor blood pressure, heart rate, ECG, central venous pressure, fluid and electrolyte status, platelet count, hepatic enzymes; reduce dose in renal impairment; avoid extravasation
Side-effects: ectopic beats; less frequently ventricular tachycardia or supraventricular arrhythmias (more likely in patients with pre-existing arrhythmias); hypotension; also headache, insomnia, nausea and vomiting, diarrhoea; occasionally, chills, oliguria, fever, urinary retention; upper and lower limb pain
Dose: by slow intravenous injection (rate not exceeding 12.5 mg/minute), diluted before use, initially 0.5–1 mg/kg, then 500 micrograms/kg every 30 minutes until satisfactory response or total of 3 mg/kg given; maintenance, initial dose of up to 3 mg/kg may be repeated every 3–6 hours as required
By intravenous infusion, initially 90 micrograms / kg /minute over 10–30 minutes, followed by continuous or intermittent infusion of 5–20 micrograms /kg /minute
Total dose over 24 hours should not normally exceed 24 mg /kg

PoM Perfan® (Merrell)
Injection, enoximone 5 mg/mL. For dilution before use. Net price 20-mL amp = £15.02
Note. Plastic apparatus should be used; crystal formation if glass used

---

MILRINONE

Indications: short-term treatment of severe congestive heart failure unresponsive to conventional maintenance therapy (not immediately after myocardial infarction); acute heart failure, including low output states, following heart surgery
Cautions; Side-effects: see under Enoximone; also correct hypokalaemia, monitor renal function, chest pain reported
Dose: by slow intravenous injection (over 10 minutes), diluted before use, 50 micrograms/kg followed by *intravenous infusion* at a rate of 375–750 nanograms/kg/minute, usually for up to 12 hours following surgery or for 48–72 hours in congestive heart failure; max. daily dose 1.13 mg/kg

---

PoM **Primacor®** (Sanofi Winthrop)
Injection, milrinone (as lactate) 1 mg/mL. For dilution before use. Net price 10-mL amp = £17.39

2.2 Diuretics

2.2.1 Thiazides and related diuretics
2.2.2 Loop diuretics
2.2.3 Potassium-sparing diuretics
2.2.4 Potassium-sparing diuretics with other diuretics
2.2.5 Osmotic diuretics
2.2.6 Mercurial diuretics
2.2.7 Carbonic anhydrase inhibitors
2.2.8 Diuretics with potassium

Thiazides (section 2.2.1) are used to relieve oedema due to *heart failure* and, in lower doses, to reduce *blood pressure.*

Loop diuretics (section 2.2.2) are used in pulmonary oedema due to *left ventricular failure* and in patients with *longstanding heart failure* who no longer respond to thiazides.

Combination diuretic therapy may be effective in patients with *oedema resistant to treatment with one diuretic.* For example, a loop diuretic may be combined with a potassium-sparing diuretic (section 2.2.3).

The combination of a thiazide with spironolactone is of value in *less severe heart failure* when hypokalaemia is difficult to counter or when any degree of hypokalaemia should be avoided, as in patients with a continuing tendency to life-threatening ventricular arrhythmias.

THE ELDERLY. Diuretics are overprescribed in old age and the elderly are particularly susceptible to many of their side-effects. They should not be used on a long-term basis to treat simple gravitational oedema (which will usually respond to increased movement, raising the legs, and support stockings).

POTASSIUM LOSS. Hypokalaemia may occur with both thiazide and loop diuretics, the risk of hypokalaemia depends more on duration of action than on potency and is thus greater with thiazides than with loop diuretics.

Hypokalaemia is dangerous in severe coronary artery disease and in patients also being treated with cardiac glycosides. Often the use of potassium-sparing diuretics (section 2.2.3) avoids the need to take potassium supplements.

In hepatic failure hypokalaemia caused by diuretics can precipitate encephalopathy, particularly in alcoholic cirrhosis; diuretics may also increase the risk of hypomagnesaemia in alcoholic cirrhosis, leading to arrhythmias.

Potassium supplements are seldom necessary when thiazides are used in the routine treatment of hypertension. For further comment see section 9.2.1.1.

2.2.1 Thiazides and related diuretics

Thiazides and related compounds are moderately potent diuretics; they inhibit sodium reabsorption at the beginning of the distal convoluted tubule. They act within 1 to 2 hours of oral administration and most have a duration of action of 12 to 24 hours; they are usually administered early in the day so that the diuresis does not interfere with sleep.

In the management of *hypertension* a low dose of a thiazide, e.g. bendrofluazide 2.5 mg daily, produces a maximal or near-maximal blood pressure lowering effect, with very little biochemical disturbance. Higher doses cause more marked changes in plasma potassium, uric acid, glucose, and lipids, with no advantage in blood pressure control, and should not be used. Optimum doses for the control of *heart failure* may be larger, and long-term effects are of less importance.

Bendrofluazide is widely used for mild or moderate heart failure when the patient is not desperately ill and severe pulmonary oedema is not present. It is also used for hypertension—alone in the treatment of mild hypertension or with other drugs in more severe hypertension.

Chlorthalidone, a thiazide-related compound, has a longer duration of action than the thiazides and may be given on alternate days to control oedema. It is also useful if acute retention is liable to be precipitated by a more rapid diuresis or if patients dislike the altered pattern of micturition promoted by diuretics.

Other thiazides do not offer any significant advantage over those mentioned above, and newer ones are more expensive than the longer-established thiazides.

Metolazone is particularly effective when combined with a loop diuretic (even in renal failure); profound diuresis may occur therefore the patient should be monitored carefully.

Xipamide resembles chlorthalidone structurally, and is more potent than the other thiazides.

Indapamide is also chemically related to chlorthalidone. It is claimed to lower blood pressure with less metabolic disturbance, particularly less aggravation of diabetes mellitus.

BENDROFLUAZIDE
(Bendroflumethiazide)
Indications: oedema, hypertension
Cautions: may cause hypokalaemia, aggravates diabetes and gout; may exacerbate systemic lupus erythematosus; elderly; pregnancy (see also Appendix 4) and breast-feeding; renal and hepatic impairment (avoid if severe, see Appendixes 2 and 3); see also notes above; porphyria (see section 9.8.2); **interactions:** Appendix 1 (diuretics)
Contra-indications: refractory hypokalaemia, hyponatraemia, hypercalcaemia; severe renal and hepatic impairment; symptomatic hyperuricaemia; Addison's disease
Side-effects: postural hypotension and mild gastro-intestinal effects; impotence (reversible on withdrawal of treatment); hypokalaemia (see also notes above), hypomagnesaemia, hyponatraemia,

hypercalcaemia, hypochloraemic alkalosis, hyperuricaemia, gout, hyperglycaemia, and increases in plasma cholesterol concentration; less commonly rashes, photosensitivity; blood disorders (including neutropenia and thrombocytopenia — when given in late pregnancy neonatal thrombocytopenia has been reported); pancreatitis, intrahepatic cholestasis, and hypersensitivity reactions (including pneumonitis and severe skin reactions) also reported

Dose: oedema, initially 5–10 mg in the morning, daily *or* on alternate days; maintenance 2.5–10 mg 1–3 times weekly

Hypertension, 2.5 mg in the morning; higher doses rarely necessary (see notes above)

PoM **Bendrofluazide** (Non-proprietary)

Tablets, bendrofluazide 2.5 mg, net price 20 = 9p; 5 mg, 20 = 8p

Available from APS, Berk (Berkozide®), Boots (Aprinox®), Cox, Goldshield (Neo-NaClex®, 5 mg only), Hillcross, K Pharm.

BENZTHIAZIDE

Cautions; Contra-indications; Side-effects: see under Bendrofluazide

Preparation

Ingredient of Dytide® (section 2.2.4)

CHLOROTHIAZIDE

Indications: oedema, hypertension

Cautions; Contra-indications; Side-effects: see under Bendrofluazide

Dose: oedema, initially 0.25–1 g 1–2 times daily; maintenance 0.5–1 g daily, on alternate days, or less frequently

Hypertension, 250–500 mg daily in single or divided doses; max. 1 g daily (but see also notes above)

PoM **Saluric**® (MSD)

Tablets, scored, chlorothiazide 500 mg. Net price 20 = 46p

CHLORTHALIDONE

(Chlortalidone)

Indications: oedema, hypertension; diabetes insipidus (see section 6.5.2)

Cautions; Contra-indications; Side-effects: see under Bendrofluazide

Dose: oedema, initially 50 mg in the morning *or* 100–200 mg on alternate days, reduced for maintenance if possible

Hypertension, 25 mg, increased to 50 mg if necessary, in the morning (see also notes above)

PoM **Hygroton**® (Geigy)

Tablets, yellow, scored, chlorthalidone 50 mg, net price 28-tab pack = £1.19

CLOPAMIDE

Cautions; Contra-indications; Side-effects: see under Bendrofluazide

Preparation

Ingredient of Viskaldix® (see under Pindolol, section 2.4)

CYCLOPENTHIAZIDE

Indications: oedema, hypertension

Cautions; Contra-indications; Side-effects: see under Bendrofluazide

Dose: oedema, initially 0.5–1 mg in the morning; maintenance 500 micrograms on alternate days; max. 1.5 mg daily (rarely required)

Hypertension, 250–500 micrograms in the morning (see also notes above)

PoM **Navidrex**® (Ciba)

Tablets, scored, cyclopenthiazide 500 micrograms. Net price 100-tab pack = £1.77

Additives: include gluten

HYDROCHLOROTHIAZIDE

Indications: oedema, hypertension

Cautions; Contra-indications; Side-effects: see under Bendrofluazide

Dose: oedema, initially 25–50 mg daily, reduced for maintenance if possible; severe oedema in patients unable to tolerate loop diuretics, initially 75 mg daily

Hypertension, 25 mg daily, increased to 50 mg daily if necessary (see also notes above)

ELDERLY. In some patients (especially the elderly) an initial dose of 12.5 mg daily may be sufficient

PoM **Esidrex**® (Ciba)

Tablets, both scored, hydrochlorothiazide 25 mg, net price 28-tab pack = 80p; 50 mg, 28-tab pack = £1.47

Additives: include gluten

PoM **HydroSaluric**® (MSD)

Tablets, both scored, hydrochlorothiazide 25 mg, net price 20 = 29p; 50 mg, 20 = 54p

HYDROFLUMETHIAZIDE

Indications: oedema, hypertension

Cautions; Contra-indications; Side-effects: see under Bendrofluazide

Dose: oedema, initially 50–200 mg in the morning; maintenance 25–50 mg on alternate days

Hypertension, 25–50 mg daily (see also notes above)

PoM **Hydrenox**® (Boots)

Tablets, hydroflumethiazide 50 mg. Net price 20 = 40p

INDAPAMIDE

Indications: hypertension

Cautions: renal impairment (stop if deterioration); monitor plasma potassium and urate concentrations in elderly, hyperaldosteronism, gout, or with concomitant cardiac glycosides; hyperparathyroidism (discontinue if hypercalcaemia); pregnancy and breast-feeding; **interactions:** Appendix 1 (diuretics)

Contra-indications: recent cerebrovascular accident, severe hepatic impairment

Side-effects: hypokalaemia, headache, dizziness, fatigue, muscular cramps, nausea, anorexia, diarrhoea, constipation, dyspepsia, rashes (erythema multiforme, epidermal necrolysis reported), rarely orthostatic hypotension, metabolic alkalosis, hyperglycaemia, increased plasma urate concentrations, paraesthesia, photosensitivity, impotence, renal impairment, reversible acute myopia; diuresis with doses above 2.5 mg daily

Dose: 2.5 mg daily in the morning

PoM **Natrilix**® (Servier)

Tablets, s/c, indapamide 2.5 mg. Net price 30-tab pack = £3.89, 60-tab pack = £7.63

Note. Tablets containing indapamide 2.5 mg also available from APS, Ashbourne (Indaxa 2.5®), Cox

MEFRUSIDE

Indications: oedema, hypertension

Cautions; Contra-indications; Side-effects: see under Bendrofluazide

Dose: initially 25–50 mg in the morning, increased to 75–100 mg for oedema; maintenance 25 mg daily *or* on alternate days (see also notes above)

PoM **Baycaron**® (Bayer)

Tablets, scored, mefruside 25 mg. Net price 20 – £1.41

METOLAZONE

Indications: oedema, hypertension

Cautions; Contra-indications; Side-effects: see under Bendrofluazide; also profound diuresis on concomitant administration with frusemide (monitor patient carefully)

Dose: see preparations below

PoM **Metenix 5**® (Hoechst)

Tablets, blue, metolazone 5 mg. Net price 100-tab pack = £8.53

Dose: oedema, 5–10 mg in the morning, increased if necessary to 20 mg daily in resistant oedema, max. 80 mg daily

Hypertension, initially 5 mg in the morning; maintenance 5 mg on alternate days

Low dose formulation

Note. Xuret® brand of metolazone has a much lower dose than other brands of metolazone. It must therefore be prescribed by brand name and is not interchangeable with other brands of metolazone

PoM **Xuret**® (Galen)

Tablets, metolazone 500 micrograms. Net price 56-tab pack = £7.36

Dose: mild to moderate hypertension, 1 tablet daily in the morning; increased if necessary to 2 tablets daily

POLYTHIAZIDE

Indications: oedema, hypertension

Cautions; Contra-indications; Side-effects: see under Bendrofluazide

Dose: usually 1–4 mg daily; in hypertension 500 micrograms daily may be adequate

PoM **Nephril**® (Pfizer)

Tablets, scored, polythiazide 1 mg. Net price 28-tab pack = 79p

XIPAMIDE

Indications: oedema, hypertension

Cautions; Contra-indications: see under Bendrofluazide

Side-effects: gastro-intestinal; mild dizziness

Dose: oedema, initially 40 mg in the morning, increased to 80 mg in resistant cases; maintenance 20 mg in the morning

Hypertension, 20 mg in the morning (increase to 40 mg no longer recommended)

PoM **Diurexan**® (ASTA Medica)

Tablets, scored, xipamide 20 mg. Net price 14-tab pack = £2.19

2.2.2 Loop diuretics

Loop diuretics are used in pulmonary oedema due to *left ventricular failure* and in patients with *long-standing heart failure* who no longer respond to thiazides. These drugs inhibit resorption from the ascending loop of Henle in the renal tubule and are powerful diuretics. Hypokalaemia may develop, and care is needed to avoid hypotension. If there is an enlarged prostate, urinary retention may occur; this is less likely if small doses and less potent diuretics are used initially.

Frusemide and **bumetanide** are similar in activity; both act within 1 hour of oral administration and diuresis is complete within 6 hours so that, if necessary, they can be given twice in one day without interfering with sleep. Following intravenous administration they have a peak effect within 30 minutes. The diuresis associated with these drugs is dose related. In patients with impaired renal function very large doses may occasionally be needed; in such doses both drugs can cause deafness and bumetanide can cause myalgia.

Ethacrynic acid has a similar onset and duration of action. Gastro-intestinal side-effects are more severe and deafness may occur in renal failure, especially when given intravenously.

Piretanide has properties similar to those of frusemide and bumetanide, but is promoted for the treatment of hypertension.

Cautionary label wordings, see inside back cover

FRUSEMIDE
(Furosemide)

Indications: oedema, oliguria due to renal failure

Cautions: pregnancy (see also Appendix 4) and breast-feeding; may cause hypokalaemia and hyponatraemia; aggravates diabetes mellitus and gout; liver failure, prostatic enlargement; porphyria (see section 9.8.2); **interactions:** Appendix 1 (diuretics)

Contra-indications: precomatose states associated with liver cirrhosis; renal failure with anuria

Side-effects: hyponatraemia, hypokalaemia, and hypomagnesaemia (see also section 2.2), hypochloraemic alkalosis, increased calcium excretion, hypotension; less commonly nausea, gastro-intestinal disturbances, hyperuricaemia and gout; hyperglycaemia (less common than with thiazides); temporary increase in plasma cholesterol and triglyceride concentrations; rarely rashes, photosensitivity and bone marrow depression (withdraw treatment), pancreatitis (with large parenteral doses), tinnitus and deafness (usually with large parenteral doses and rapid administration and in renal impairment)

Dose: by mouth, oedema, initially 40 mg in the morning; maintenance 20 mg daily *or* 40 mg on alternate days, increased in resistant oedema to 80 mg daily; CHILD 1–3 mg/kg daily

Oliguria, initially 250 mg daily; if necessary larger doses, increasing in steps of 250 mg, may be given every 4–6 hours to a max. of a single dose of 2 g (rarely used)

By intramuscular injection or slow intravenous injection (rate not exceeding 4 mg/minute), initially 20–50 mg; CHILD 0.5–1.5 mg/kg to a max. daily dose of 20 mg

By intravenous infusion (by syringe pump if necessary), in oliguria, initially 250 mg over 1 hour (rate not exceeding 4 mg/minute), if satisfactory urine output not obtained in the subsequent hour further 500 mg over 2 hours, then if no satisfactory response within subsequent hour, further 1 g over 4 hours, if no response obtained dialysis probably required; effective dose (up to 1 g) can be repeated every 24 hours

PoM Frusemide (Non-proprietary)

Tablets, frusemide 20 mg, net price 20 = 25p; 40 mg, 20 = 14p; 500 mg, 20 = £5.99

Various strengths available from APS, Ashbourne (Froop®), Berk (Dryptal®), Cox, CP (including Rusyde®), Hillcross, K Pharm., Norton

Oral solutions, sugar-free, frusemide 1 mg/mL available as Lasix® paediatric liquid; frusemide 4 mg, 8 mg, and 10 mg/mL available from RP Drugs (special order)

Injection, frusemide 10 mg/mL, net price 2-mL amp = 27p

Available from Evans (also 5-mL amp)

PoM Lasix® (Hoechst)

Tablets, all scored, frusemide 20 mg, net price 28-tab pack = 82p; 40 mg, 28-tab pack = £1.19; 500 mg (yellow), 20 = £11.44

Paediatric liquid, sugar-free, frusemide 1 mg/mL when reconstituted with purified water, freshly boiled and cooled, net price 150 mL = £1.10

Injection, frusemide 10 mg/mL, net price 2-mL amp = 25p; 5-mL amp = 53p; 25-mL amp = £2.21

Note. Large volume frusemide injections also available from IMS (Min-I-Jet®)

BUMETANIDE

Indications: oedema, oliguria due to renal failure

Cautions; Contra-indications: see under Frusemide (but has been used in porphyria, see section 9.8.2)

Side-effects: see under Frusemide; also myalgia (see notes above)

Dose: by mouth, 1 mg in the morning, repeated after 6–8 hours if necessary; severe cases, increased up to 5 mg or more daily

ELDERLY, 500 micrograms daily may be sufficient

By intravenous injection, 1–2 mg, repeated after 20 minutes; when *intramuscular injection* considered necessary, 1 mg initially then adjusted according to response

By intravenous infusion, 2–5 mg over 30–60 minutes

PoM Burinex® (Leo)

Tablets, both scored, bumetanide 1 mg, net price 20 = £1.11; 5 mg, 20 = £7.81

Liquid, green, sugar-free, bumetanide 1 mg/5 mL. Net price 150 mL = £3.32

Injection, bumetanide 500 micrograms/mL. Net price 2-mL amp = 40p; 4-mL amp = 69p; 10-mL amp = £1.46

ETHACRYNIC ACID
(Etacrynic Acid)

Indications: oedema, oliguria due to renal failure

Cautions; Contra-indications; Side-effects: see under Frusemide and notes above; also contra-indicated in breast-feeding; gastro-intestinal disturbances more severe; also pain on injection

Dose: by mouth, initially 50 mg daily after breakfast; effective initial range of 50–150 mg daily (max. 400 mg) can often be reduced for maintenance and given on alternate days (daily doses above 50 mg divided)

By slow intravenous injection or infusion, 50 mg, increased to 100 mg if necessary

PoM Edecrin® (MSD)

Tablets, scored, ethacrynic acid 50 mg. Net price 20 = £1.20. Label: 21

Injection, powder for reconstitution, ethacrynic acid (as sodium salt). Net price 50-mg vial = £1.26

PIRETANIDE

Indications: hypertension

Cautions; Contra-indications; Side-effects: see under Frusemide; side-effects less marked at dosage level used for hypertension

Dose: 6–12 mg in the morning with food

PoM Arelix® (Hoechst)
Capsules, m/r, green/orange, enclosing yellow pellets, piretanide 6 mg. Net price 28-cap pack = £3.61. Label: 21

TORASEMIDE
Indications: oedema, hypertension
Cautions; Contra-indications; Side-effects: see under Frusemide; avoid in pregnancy and breast-feeding
Dose: by mouth, oedema, 5 mg once daily, preferably in the morning, increased if required to 20 mg once daily; usual max. 40 mg daily
Hypertension, 2.5 mg daily, increased if necessary to 5 mg once daily
By slow intravenous injection at a rate of 4 mg/minute, 10 mg daily, increased if necessary to 20 mg daily; usual max. 40 mg daily

▼ **PoM Torem®** (Boehringer Mannheim)
Tablets, torasemide 2.5 mg, net price 28-tab pack = £4.25; 5 mg (scored), 28-tab pack = £6.23; 10 mg (scored), 28-tab pack = £9.16
Injection, torasemide 5 mg/mL, net price 2–mL amp = 40p, 4–mL amp = 74p

2.2.3 Potassium-sparing diuretics
Amiloride and **triamterene** on their own are weak diuretics. They cause retention of potassium and are therefore used as an alternative to giving potassium supplements with thiazide or loop diuretics. (See section 2.2.4 for compound preparations with thiazides or loop diuretics.)

Spironolactone is also a potassium-sparing diuretic, and potentiates thiazide or loop diuretics by antagonising aldosterone. It is of value in the treatment of the oedema of cirrhosis of the liver and is effective in oedema of heart failure, particularly when congestion has caused hepatic engorgement.

Spironolactone is also used in primary hyperaldosteronism (Conn's syndrome).

Potassium canrenoate has similar uses to spironolactone, but can be given parenterally. It is metabolised to canrenone, which is also a metabolite of spironolactone.

Potassium supplements must **not** be given with potassium-sparing diuretics.

AMILORIDE HYDROCHLORIDE
Indications: oedema, potassium conservation with thiazide and loop diuretics
Cautions: pregnancy; diabetes mellitus; elderly; **interactions:** Appendix 1 (diuretics)
Contra-indications: hyperkalaemia, renal failure
Side-effects: include gastro-intestinal disturbances, dry mouth, rashes, confusion, orthostatic hypotension, hyperkalaemia, hyponatraemia
Dose: alone, initially 10 mg daily *or* 5 mg twice daily, adjusted according to response; max. 20 mg daily
With other diuretics, congestive heart failure and hypertension, initially 5–10 mg daily
Cirrhosis with ascites, initially 5 mg daily

PoM Amiloride (Non-proprietary)
Tablets, amiloride hydrochloride 5 mg, net price 20 = 41p
Available from APS, Ashbourne (Amilospare®), Berk (Berkamil®), Cox, CP, Hillcross, K Pharm., Norton
Oral solution, sugar-free, amiloride hydrochloride 5 mg/5 mL available from RP Drugs (special order)
PoM Midamor® (Morson)
Tablets, yellow, amiloride hydrochloride 5 mg. Net price 100-tab pack = £2.05

Compound preparations with thiazide or loop diuretics, see section 2.2.4

TRIAMTERENE
Indications: oedema, potassium conservation with thiazide and loop diuretics
Cautions; Contra-indications: see under Amiloride Hydrochloride; monitor plasma urea and potassium, particularly in the elderly and in renal impairment; also may cause blue fluorescence of urine
Side-effects: include gastro-intestinal disturbances, dry mouth, rashes; slight decrease in blood pressure, hyperkalaemia; photosensitivity and blood disorders also reported; triamterene found in kidney stones
Dose: initially 150–250 mg daily, reducing to alternate days after 1 week; taken in divided doses after breakfast and lunch; lower initial dose when given with other diuretics
COUNSELLING. Urine may look slightly blue in some lights

PoM Dytac® (Pharmark)
Capsules, maroon, triamterene 50 mg. Net price 30-cap pack = £6.98. Label: 14 (see above), 21

Compound preparations with thiazides or loop diuretics, see section 2.2.4

ALDOSTERONE ANTAGONISTS

POTASSIUM CANRENOATE
Indications: oedema associated with secondary aldosteronism, liver failure, chronic decompensated heart disease
Cautions; Contra-indications; Side-effects: see under Spironolactone; nausea and vomiting may occur, particularly after high doses; pain and irritation at injection site
Dose: by slow intravenous injection or intravenous infusion, 200–400 mg daily (exceptionally 800 mg)

PoM Spiroctan-M® (Boehringer Mannheim)
Injection, potassium canrenoate 20 mg/mL. Net price 10-mL amp = 71p

SPIRONOLACTONE

Indications: oedema and ascites in cirrhosis of the liver, malignant ascites, nephrotic syndrome, congestive heart failure; primary aldosteronism

Cautions: potential human metabolic products carcinogenic in *rodents*; elderly; hepatic impairment; renal impairment (avoid if moderate to severe); monitor electrolytes (discontinue if hyperkalaemia occurs); porphyria (see section 9.8.2); **interactions:** Appendix 1 (diuretics)

Contra-indications: hyperkalaemia, hyponatraemia, severe renal impairment; pregnancy and breast-feeding; Addison's disease

Side-effects: gastro-intestinal disturbances; impotence, gynaecomastia; menstrual irregularities; lethargy, headache, confusion; rashes; hyperkalaemia (see also Cautions); hyponatraemia; hepatotoxicity, osteomalacia, and blood disorders reported

Dose: 100–200 mg daily, increased to 400 mg if required; CHILD initially 3 mg/kg daily in divided doses

PoM **Spironolactone** (Non-proprietary)

Tablets, spironolactone 25 mg, net price 20 = 49p; 50 mg, 20 = £1.54; 100 mg, 20 = £1.60

Available from APS, Ashbourne (Spirospare®), Berk (Spirolone®), Cox, Hillcross, K Pharm., Lagap (Laractone®), Norton

Oral suspensions, sugar-free, spironolactone 5 mg, 10 mg, 25 mg, and 50 mg/5 mL ml available from RP Drugs (special order)

PoM **Aldactone®** (Searle)

Tablets, all f/c, spironolactone 25 mg (buff), net price 100-tab pack = £9.88; 50 mg (off-white), 100-tab pack = £19.76; 100 mg (buff), 28-tab pack = £11.07

PoM **Spiroctan®** (Boehringer Mannheim)

Tablets, both s/c, spironolactone 25 mg (blue, contains tartrazine), net price 100-tab pack = £7.22; 50 mg (green), 100-tab pack = £13.85

Capsules, green, spironolactone 100 mg. Net price 28-cap pack = £7.56

Compound preparations with thiazides or loop diuretics, see section 2.2.4

2.2.4 Potassium-sparing diuretics with other diuretics

Although it is preferable to prescribe thiazides (section 2.2.1) and potassium-sparing diuretics (section 2.2.3) separately, the use of fixed combinations may be justified if compliance is a problem. Potassium-sparing diuretics are not usually necessary in the routine treatment of hypertension, unless hypokalaemia develops. For **interactions**, see Appendix 1 (diuretics).

Amiloride with thiazides

PoM **Co-amilozide** (Non-proprietary)

Tablets, co-amilozide 2.5/25 (amiloride hydrochloride 2.5 mg, hydrochlorothiazide 25 mg). Net price 28-tab pack = £1.94

Available from CP, Du Pont (Moduret 25®), Lagap
Dose: hypertension, oedema, 1–4 tablets, increased if necessary to a max. of 8, daily

Tablets, co-amilozide 5/50 (amiloride hydrochloride 5 mg, hydrochlorothiazide 50 mg). Net price 20 = £1.16

Available from APS, Ashbourne (Amilmaxco 5/50®), Baker Norton (Amil-Co®), Berk (Delvas®), Cox, CP, Du Pont (Moduretic®), Hillcross, K Pharm., Lagap, Norton
Dose: hypertension, oedema, 1–2 tablets, increased if necessary to max. of 4, daily

Oral solution, co-amilozide 5/50 (amiloride hydrochloride 5 mg, hydrochlorothiazide 50 mg)/5 mL. Net price 200 mL = £4.61

Available from Du Pont (Moduretic®)
Dose: as for co-amilozide 5 /50 tablets above (5 mL = 1 tablet)

PoM **Navispare®** (Ciba)

Tablets, f/c, orange, amiloride hydrochloride 2.5 mg, cyclopenthiazide 250 micrograms. Net price 28-tab pack = £1.79

Additives: include gluten
Dose: hypertension, 1–2 tablets in the morning

Amiloride with loop diuretics

PoM **Co-amilofruse** (Non-proprietary)

Tablets, co-amilofruse 2.5/20 (amiloride hydrochloride 2.5 mg, frusemide 20 mg). Net price 28-tab pack = £3.17, 56-tab pack = £6.21

Available from Rhône-Poulenc Rorer (Frumil LS®)
Dose: oedema, 1 tablet in the morning

Tablets, co-amilofruse 5/40 (amiloride hydrochloride 5 mg, frusemide 40 mg). Net price 28-tab pack = £3.12

Available from Baker Norton (Fru-Co®), Cox, Hoechst (Lasoride®), Rhône-Poulenc Rorer (Frumil®)
Dose: oedema, 1–2 tablets in the morning

Tablets, co-amilofruse 10/80 (amiloride hydrochloride 10 mg, frusemide 80 mg). Net price 28-tab pack = £7.20, 56-tab pack = £14.11

Available from Rhône-Poulenc Rorer (Frumil Forte®)
Dose: oedema, 1 tablet in the morning

PoM **Burinex A®** (Leo)

Tablets, ivory, scored, amiloride hydrochloride 5 mg, bumetanide 1 mg. Net price 28-tab pack = £3.20

Dose: oedema, 1–2 tablets daily

Triamterene with thiazides

COUNSELLING. Urine may look slightly blue in some lights

PoM **Dyazide®** (SK&F)

Tablets, peach, scored, co-triamterzide 50/25 (triamterene 50 mg, hydrochlorothiazide 25 mg). Net price 30-tab pack = £2.41. Label: 14 (see above), 21

Dose: hypertension, 1 tablet daily after breakfast; oedema, 2 tablets daily (1 after breakfast and 1 after midday meal) increased to 3 daily if necessary (2 after breakfast and 1 after midday meal); usual maintenance, 1 daily or 2 on alternate days; max. 4 daily
Note. Tablets containing co-triamterzide 50/25 (triamterene 50 mg and hydrochlorothiazide 25 mg) are also

available from Ashbourne (TriamaxCo®), Baker Norton (Triam-Co®)

PoM Dytide® (Pharmark)

Capsules, clear/maroon, triamterene 50 mg, benz-thiazide 25 mg. Net price 30-cap pack = £6.97. Label: 14 (see above), 21

Dose: oedema, initially 3 capsules daily (2 after breakfast and 1 after midday meal) for 1 week then 1 or 2 on alternate days

PoM Kalspare® (Cusi)

Tablets, orange, f/c, scored, triamterene 50 mg, chlorthalidone 50 mg. Net price 28-tab pack = £3.19. Label: 14 (see above), 21

Dose: hypertension, oedema, 1–2 tablets in the morning

Triamterene with loop diuretics

COUNSELLING. Urine may look slightly blue in some lights

PoM Frusene® (Fisons)

Tablets, yellow, scored, triamterene 50 mg, fruse-mide 40 mg. Net price 56-tab pack = £5.78. Label: 14 (see above), 21

Dose: oedema, ½–2 tablets daily

Spironolactone with thiazides

PoM Co-flumactone (Non-proprietary)

Tablets, co-flumactone 25/25 (hydroflumethiazide 25 mg, spironolactone 25 mg). Net price 100-tab pack = £16.86

Available from Baker Norton (Spiro-Co®), Searle (Aldactide 25®)

Dose: congestive heart failure, initially 4 tablets daily; range 1–8 daily

Tablets, co-flumactone 50/50 (hydroflumethiazide 50 mg, spironolactone 50 mg). Net price 28-tab pack = £8.92

Available from Baker Norton (Spiro-Co 50®, Searle Aldactide 50®)

Dose: congestive heart failure, initially 2 tablets daily; range 1–4 daily

Spironolactone with loop diuretics

PoM Lasilactone® (Hoechst)

Capsules, blue/white, spironolactone 50 mg, fruse-mide 20 mg. Net price 28-cap pack – £4.91

Dose: resistant oedema, 1–4 capsules daily

2.2.5 Osmotic diuretics

Osmotic diuretics are rarely used in heart failure as they may acutely expand the blood volume. **Mannitol** is used in cerebral oedema—a typical dose is 1 g/kg as a 20% solution given by rapid intravenous infusion.

MANNITOL

Indications: see notes above

Cautions: extravasation causes inflammation and thrombophlebitis

Contra-indications: congestive cardiac failure, pulmonary oedema

Side-effects: chills, fever

Dose: by intravenous infusion, diuresis, 50–200 g over 24 hours, preceded by a test dose of 200 mg/kg by slow intravenous injection

Cerebral oedema, see notes above

PoM Mannitol (Non-proprietary)

Intravenous infusion, mannitol 10%, 20%, and 25%

Available from Baxter (10% and 20%) and IMS (Min-I-Jet® Mannitol 25%)

2.2.6 Mercurial diuretics

They are effective diuretics but are now almost never used because of their nephrotoxicity. Mersalyl **must** be given by intramuscular injection; intravenous use may cause severe hypotension and sudden death.

MERSALYL

Indications: oedema unresponsive to other diuretics (but see notes above)

Cautions: recent myocardial infarction, treatment with cardiac glycosides, frequent extrasystoles

Contra-indications: renal impairment; pregnancy; porphyria (see section 9.8.2)

Side-effects: gastro-intestinal disturbances, allergic reactions; see also notes above

PoM Mersalyl Injection, mersalyl sodium 100 mg, theophylline 50 mg/mL

Dose: by deep intramuscular injection, 0.5–2 mL

2.2.7 Carbonic anhydrase inhibitors

Acetazolamide and dichlorphenamide are weak diuretics, and are little used for their diuretic effect. They inhibit the formation of aqueous fluid, and are used in glaucoma (see section 11.6). Although acetazolamide is used as a prophylactic measure for mountain sickness it is not a substitute for acclimatisation.

2.2.8 Diuretics with potassium

Many patients on diuretics do not need potassium supplements (see section 9.2.1.1). For many of those who do, the amount of potassium ion in combined preparations may not be enough, and for this reason their use is to be discouraged.

Diuretics with potassium and potassium-sparing diuretics should **not** usually be given together.

COUNSELLING. Modified-release potassium tablets should be swallowed whole with plenty of fluid during meals while sitting or standing

PoM Burinex K® (Leo)

Tablets, bumetanide 500 micrograms, potassium 7.7 mmol for modified release. Net price 20 = 81p. Label: 25, 27, counselling, see above

PoM Diumide-K Continus® (ASTA Medica)

Tablets, f/c, white/orange, frusemide 40 mg, potassium 8 mmol for modified release. Net price 30-tab pack = £2.53. Label: 25, 27, counselling, see above

PoM Lasikal® (Hoechst)

Tablets, white/yellow, f/c, frusemide 20 mg, potassium 10 mmol for modified release. Net price 100-tab pack = £5.31. Label: 25, 27, counselling, see above

PoM Lasix+K® (Hoechst)

Calendar pack, 30 white scored tablets, frusemide 40 mg; 60 m/r yellow tablets, potassium chloride (potassium 10 mmol). Net price = £2.97. Label: 25, 27, counselling, see above

PoM Neo-NaClex-K® (Goldshield)

Tablets, pink/white, f/c, bendrofluazide 2.5 mg, potassium 8.4 mmol for modified release. Net price 20 = £1.18. Label: 25, 27, counselling, see above

2.3   Anti-arrhythmic drugs

2.3.1   Management of arrhythmias
2.3.2   Drugs for arrhythmias

2.3.1   Management of arrhythmias

Management of an arrhythmia, apart from the treatment of associated heart failure, requires precise diagnosis of the type of arrhythmia, and electrocardiography is essential.

ECTOPIC BEATS. If spontaneous with a normal heart, these rarely require treatment beyond reassurance. If they are particularly troublesome, beta-blockers are sometimes effective and may be safer than other suppressant drugs.

ATRIAL FIBRILLATION. The ventricular rate can usually be controlled with digoxin. A beta-blocker may be added if necessary (provided ventricular function is adequate), and in some cases other classes of drugs may be appropriate. Anticoagulants may be indicated especially in valvular or myocardial disease and in the elderly (aspirin is less effective at preventing emboli and should only be considered if the risk is low).

ATRIAL FLUTTER. The ventricular rate can often be controlled with digoxin. Reversion to sinus rhythm (if indicated) is best achieved by appropriately synchronised d.c. shock, rather than by drug therapy. If the arrhythmia is long-standing a period of treatment with anticoagulants should be considered before cardioversion to avoid the complication of emboli.

PAROXYSMAL SUPRAVENTRICULAR TACHYCARDIA. In most patients this remits spontaneously or can be returned to sinus rhythm by reflex vagal stimulation with respiratory manoeuvres, prompt squatting, or pressure over one carotid sinus (**important:** pressure over carotid sinus should be restricted to monitored patients, it can be dangerous in recent ischaemia, digitalis toxicity, or the elderly).

If vagal stimulation fails, intravenous administration of adenosine is usually the treatment of choice; digitalisation or intravenous administration of a beta-blocker may also be effective. Intravenous administration of verapamil is useful for patients without myocardial or valvular disease (**important:** never in patients recently treated with beta-blockers, see p. 93). For arrhythmias that are poorly tolerated, synchronised d.c. shock usually provides rapid relief.

In cases of paroxysmal supraventricular tachycardia with block, digitalis toxicity should be suspected. In addition to stopping administration of the cardiac glycoside and giving potassium supplements, intravenous administration of a beta-blocker may be useful. Specific digoxin antibody is available if the toxicity is considered life-threatening (section 2.1.1).

ACUTE ARRHYTHMIAS AFTER MYOCARDIAL INFARCTION. It is best to do nothing in patients with a paroxysmal tachycardia or rapid irregularity of the pulse until an ECG record is obtainable. If the condition of the patient is such that death due to the arrhythmia seems possible 100 mg of lignocaine should be given intravenously. Bradycardia, particularly if complicated by hypotension, should be treated with atropine sulphate, given intravenously in an initial dose of 300 micrograms, increasing to 1 mg if necessary.

VENTRICULAR TACHYCARDIA. Drug treatment is used both for the treatment of ventricular tachycardia and for prophylaxis of recurrent attacks that merit suppression. Ventricular tachycardia requires treatment most commonly in the acute stage of myocardial infarction, but the likelihood of this and other life-threatening arrhythmias diminishes sharply over the first 24 hours after the attack, especially in patients without heart failure or shock. Lignocaine is the preferred drug for emergency use. Other drugs are best administered under specialist supervision. Very rapid ventricular tachycardia causes profound circulatory collapse and should be treated urgently with d.c. shock.

Torsades de pointes is a special form of ventricular tachycardia which tends to occur in the presence of a long QT interval (usually drug induced, but hypokalaemia, severe bradycardia, and genetic predisposition may also be implicated). The episodes are usually self-limiting, but are frequently recurrent and may cause impairment (or loss) of consciousness. If not controlled, the arrhythmia may progress to ventricular fibrillation. Intravenous infusion of magnesium sulphate (see section 9.5.1.3) is usually effective. Anti-arrhythmics (including lignocaine) may further prolong the QT interval, thus worsening the condition.

2.3.2   Drugs for arrhythmias

Anti-arrhythmic drugs can be classified clinically into those that act on supraventricular arrhythmias (e.g. verapamil), those that act on both supraventricular and ventricular arrhythmias (e.g. quinidine), and those that act on ventricular arrhythmias (e.g. lignocaine).

They can also be classified according to their effects on the electrical behaviour of myocardial cells during activity (termed 'action potential'):

Class Ia, b, c: membrane stabilising drugs (e.g. quinidine, lignocaine, flecainide respectively)
Class II: beta-blockers
Class III: amiodarone, bretylium, and sotalol (also Class II)
Class IV: calcium-channel blockers (includes verapamil but not the nifedipine group)
This latter classification (the Vaughan Williams classification) is of less clinical significance.

CAUTIONS. The negative inotropic effects of anti-arrhythmic drugs tend to be additive therefore special care should be taken if two or more are used, especially in impaired myocardial function. Most or all drugs that are effective in countering arrhythmias can also provoke them in some circumstances;

---

moreover, hypokalaemia enhances the arrhythmogenic (pro-arrhythmic) effect of many drugs.

SUPRAVENTRICULAR ARRHYTHMIAS

Adenosine is usually the treatment of choice for terminating paroxysmal supraventricular tachycardia. As it has a very short duration of action (half-life only about 8 to 10 seconds, except in those taking dipyridamole—see below), most side-effects are short lived. Unlike verapamil, adenosine may be used after a beta-blocker. Verapamil may be preferable to adenosine in asthma.

Oral administration of a **cardiac glycoside** (such as digoxin, section 2.1.1) is the treatment of choice in slowing ventricular response in cases of atrial fibrillation and atrial flutter. Intravenous digoxin, preferably infused slowly, is occasionally required if the ventricular rate needs rapid control. Ouabain acts more quickly but may be difficult to obtain since it is not on the UK market.

Verapamil (section 2.6.2) is usually effective for supraventricular tachycardias. An initial intravenous dose (**important**: serious beta-blocker interaction hazard, see p. 93) may be followed by oral treatment; hypotension may occur with larger doses. It should not be used for tachyarrhythmias where the QRS complex is wide (i.e. broad complex) unless a supraventricular origin has been established beyond reasonable doubt. It is also contra-indicated in atrial fibrillation with pre-excitation (e.g.Wolff-Parkinson-White syndrome). It should not be used in children with arrhythmias without specialist advice; some supraventricular arrhythmias in childhood can be accelerated by verapamil with dangerous consequences.

ADENOSINE

Indications: rapid reversion to sinus rhythm of paroxysmal supraventricular tachycardias, including those associated with accessory pathways (e.g. Wolff-Parkinson-White syndrome); aid to diagnosis of broad or narrow complex supraventricular tachycardias

Cautions: atrial fibrillation or flutter with accessory pathway (increased conduction down anomalous pathway may develop); **interactions:** Appendix 1 (adenosine)—**important:** interaction with dipyridamole liable to be serious

Contra-indications: second- or third-degree AV block and sick sinus syndrome (unless pacemaker fitted); asthma

Side-effects: include transient facial flush, chest pain, dyspnoea, bronchospasm, choking sensation, nausea, light-headedness; severe bradycardia reported (requiring temporary pacing); ECG may show transient rhythm disturbances

Dose: by rapid intravenous injection into central or large peripheral vein, 3 mg over 2 seconds with cardiac monitoring; if necessary followed by 6 mg after 1–2 minutes, and then by 12 mg after a further 1–2 minutes

▼ PoM **Adenocor**® (Sanofi Winthrop)
Injection, adenosine 3 mg/mL in physiological saline. Net price 2-mL vial = £4.05 (hosp. only)

CARDIAC GLYCOSIDES
Section 2.1.1

VERAPAMIL
Section 2.6.2

SUPRAVENTRICULAR AND VENTRICULAR ARRHYTHMIAS

Amiodarone is used in the treatment of tachycardia associated with the Wolff-Parkinson-White syndrome. It may only be used for the treatment of other arrhythmias when other drugs are ineffective or contra-indicated and should be initiated only under hospital or specialist supervision. These include paroxysmal supraventricular, nodal and ventricular tachycardias, atrial fibrillation and flutter, and ventricular fibrillation. Since amiodarone has a very long half-life (extending to several weeks) it only needs to be given once daily (but high doses may cause nausea unless divided). It may be given by intravenous infusion as well as by mouth, and has the advantage of causing little or no myocardial depression. Unlike oral amiodarone, intravenous amiodarone may act relatively rapidly.

Most patients taking amiodarone develop corneal microdeposits (reversible on withdrawal of treatment); these rarely interfere with vision, but drivers may be dazzled by headlights at night. Because of the possibility of phototoxic reactions, patients should be advised to shield the skin from light and to use a wide-spectrum sunscreen such as RoC Total Sunblock® (section 13.8.1) to protect against both long ultraviolet and visible light.

Amiodarone contains iodine and can cause disorders of thyroid function; both hypothyroidism and hyperthyroidism may occur. Clinical assessment is unreliable, and laboratory tests should be performed at least every 6 months. Thyroid function tests that rely on thyroxine (T4) concentrations alone may be misleading, since T4 may be raised in the absence of hyperthyroidism; therefore tri-iodothyronine (T3), T4, and thyroid-stimulating hormone (thyrotrophin, TSH) should all be measured. A raised T4 with very low or undetectable TSH concentrations suggest the development of thyroid overactivity, and a raised T3 confirms overt thyrotoxicosis. The thyrotoxicosis may be very refractory, and amiodarone should usually be withdrawn at least temporarily to help achieve control. Hypothyroidism can be treated with replacement therapy and does not call for withdrawal of amiodarone.

Pneumonitis should always be suspected if new or progressive shortness of breath or cough develops in a patient taking amiodarone. Fresh neurolog-

---

ical symptoms should raise the possibility of peripheral neuropathy (although this is rare).

Beta-blockers act as anti-arrhythmic drugs principally by attenuating the effects of the sympathetic system on automaticity and conductivity within the heart, for details see section 2.4.

Disopyramide may be given by intravenous injection to control arrhythmias after myocardial infarction (including those not responding to lignocaine), but it impairs cardiac contractility. Oral administration of disopyramide is useful but it has an antimuscarinic effect which limits its use in patients with glaucoma or prostatic hypertrophy.

Flecainide belongs to the same general class as lignocaine. It may be of value for serious symptomatic ventricular arrhythmias. It may also be indicated for junctional re-entry tachycardias. Preliminary results with paroxysmal atrial fibrillation are promising. As with quinidine it may precipitate serious arrhythmias in a small minority of patients (including those with otherwise normal hearts).

Procainamide can be given by intravenous injection to control ventricular arrhythmias, but prolonged oral use can cause a syndrome resembling systemic lupus erythematosus.

Quinidine may be effective in suppressing supraventricular and ventricular arrhythmias. It may itself precipitate rhythm disorders, and is best used on specialist advice; it can cause hypersensitivity reactions and gastro-intestinal upsets.

AMIODARONE HYDROCHLORIDE

Indications: see notes above (should be initiated in hospital or under specialist supervision)

Cautions: liver-function and thyroid-function tests required in long-term therapy (but interferes with tests of thyroid function, see notes above); heart failure; renal impairment; elderly; severe bradycardia and conduction disturbances in excessive dosage; intravenous use may cause moderate and transient fall in blood pressure (circulatory collapse precipitated by rapid administration or overdosage); porphyria (see section 9.8.2); **interactions:** Appendix 1 (amiodarone)

Contra-indications: sinus bradycardia, sino-atrial heart block; unless pacemaker fitted avoid in severe conduction disturbances or sinus node disease; thyroid dysfunction; pregnancy and breast-feeding (see also Appendixes 4 and 5); iodine sensitivity; avoid intravenous use in severe respiratory failure, circulatory collapse, severe arterial hypotension, congestive heart failure

Side-effects: reversible corneal microdeposits (sometimes with night glare), rarely impaired vision due to optic neuritis; peripheral neuropathy and myopathy (usually reversible on withdrawal); bradycardia and conduction disturbances (see Cautions); phototoxicity and rarely persistent slate-grey skin discoloration (see also notes); hypothyroidism, hyperthyroidism, diffuse pulmonary alveolitis and fibrosis, hepatitis; rarely nausea, vomiting, metallic taste, tremor, nightmares, vertigo, headache, sleeplessness, fatigue,

benign raised intracranial pressure, epididymitis; ataxia, rashes (including exfoliative dermatitis), vasculitis, thrombocytopenia, increased prothrombin time reported; anaphylaxis on rapid injection, also bronchospasm or apnoea in respiratory failure

Dose: by mouth, 200 mg 3 times daily for 1 week reduced to 200 mg twice daily for a further week; maintenance, usually 200 mg daily or the minimum required to control the arrhythmia

By intravenous infusion via caval catheter, 5 mg/kg over 20–120 minutes with ECG monitoring; max. 1.2 g in 24 hours

Note. In extreme emergency only, may be given *by slow intravenous injection* of 150–300 mg in 10–20 mL glucose 5% over at least 3 minutes with ECG monitoring (usually in intensive care unit); do not repeat for at least 15 minutes

PoM Amiodarone Hydrochloride (Non-proprietary)

Tablets, amiodarone hydrochloride 100 mg, net price 28-tab pack = £4.91; 200 mg, 28-tab pack = £8.40. Label: 11

Available from APS, Cox, Generics, Hillcross, Norton

PoM Cordarone X® (Sanofi Winthrop)

Tablets, both scored, amiodarone hydrochloride 100 mg, net price 28-tab pack = £5.00; 200 mg, 28-tab pack = £8.19. Label: 11

Injection, amiodarone hydrochloride 50 mg/mL. Net price 3-mL amp = £1.50. For dilution and use as an infusion

DISOPYRAMIDE

Indications: ventricular arrhythmias, especially after myocardial infarction; supraventricular arrhythmias

Cautions: glaucoma; heart failure (avoid if severe); prostatic enlargement; hepatic and renal impairment; elderly; pregnancy and breast-feeding; **interactions:** Appendix 1 (disopyramide)

Contra-indications: second- and third-degree heart block and sinus node dysfunction (unless pacemaker fitted); cardiogenic shock; severe uncompensated heart failure

Side-effects: gastro-intestinal irritation; myocardial depression, hypotension, atrioventricular block; antimuscarinic effects include dry mouth, blurred vision, urinary retention; psychosis, cholestatic jaundice, hypoglycaemia also reported

Dose: by mouth, 300–800 mg daily in divided doses

By slow intravenous injection, 2 mg/kg over at least 5 minutes to a max. of 150 mg, with ECG monitoring, followed immediately *either* by 200 mg *by mouth,* then 200 mg every 8 hours for 24 hours *or* 400 micrograms/kg/hour *by intravenous infusion;* max. 300 mg in first hour and 800 mg daily

PoM **Disopyramide** (Non-proprietary)

Capsules, disopyramide (as phosphate) 100 mg, net price 20 = £1.30; 150 mg, 20 = £2.22

Available from APS, CP (100 mg), Hillcross, K Pharm. (100 mg), Lagap (100 mg), Monmouth (Isomide® 100 mg), Norton (100 mg)

PoM **Rythmodan®** (Roussel)

Capsules, disopyramide 100 mg (green/beige), net price 84-cap pack = £7.53; 150 mg, 84-cap pack = £10.99

Injection, disopyramide (as phosphate) 10 mg/mL, net price 5–mL amp = 69p

Modified release
PoM **Dirythmin SA®** (Astra)

Durules® (= tablets, m/r), f/c, disopyramide (as phosphate) 150 mg. Net price 20 = £2.53. Label: 25

Dose: 300 mg every 12 hours; max. 750 mg daily

PoM **Rythmodan Retard®** (Roussel)

Tablets, m/r, scored, f/c, disopyramide (as phosphate) 250 mg. Net price 56-tab pack = £16.24. Label: 25

Dose: 250–375 mg every 12 hours

Note. Modified-release capsules containing disopyramide (as phosphate) 250 mg also available from Monmouth (Isomide® CR)

FLECAINIDE ACETATE

Indications: (should be initiated in hospital) *tablets and injection:* AV nodal reciprocating tachycardia, arrhythmias associated with Wolff-Parkinson-White syndrome and similar conditions with accessory pathways, paroxysmal atrial fibrillation in patients with disabling symptoms (arrhythmias of recent onset will respond more readily); *tablets only:* symptomatic sustained ventricular tachycardia, premature ventricular contractions and/or non-sustained ventricular tachycardia causing disabling symptoms in patients resistant to or intolerant of other therapy; *injection only:* ventricular tachyarrhythmias resistant to other treatment

Cautions: patients with pacemakers (especially those who may be pacemaker dependent because stimulation threshold may rise appreciably); avoid in sinus node dysfunction, atrial conduction defects, second-degree or greater AV block, bundle branch block or distal block unless pacing rescue available; atrial fibrillation following heart surgery; elderly; hepatic and renal impairment (see Appendixes 2 and 3); pregnancy (toxicity in *animal* studies) and breast-feeding; **interactions:** Appendix 1 (flecainide)

Contra-indications: heart failure; history of myocardial infarction and either asymptomatic ventricular ectopics or asymptomatic non-sustained ventricular tachycardia; long-standing atrial fibrillation where no attempt has been made to convert to sinus rhythm; haemodynamically significant valvular heart disease

Side-effects: dizziness, visual disturbances (corneal deposits reported); arrhythmogenic (pro-arrhythmic) effect; rarely nausea and vomiting, photosensitivity; reversible increases in liver enzymes, jaundice; ataxia, peripheral neuropathy, pulmonary fibrosis, pneumonitis also reported

Dose: by mouth, ventricular arrhythmias, 100 mg twice daily; max. 400 mg daily (usually reserved for rapid control or in heavily built patients), reduced after 3–5 days if possible

Supraventricular arrhythmias, 50 mg twice daily, increased if required to max. 300 mg daily

ELDERLY. Rate of elimination may be reduced—care on dose adjustment

By slow intravenous injection, 2 mg/kg over 10–30 minutes, max. 150 mg, with ECG monitoring; followed if required by *infusion* at a rate of 1.5 mg/kg/hour for 1 hour, subsequently reduced to 100–250 micrograms/kg/hour for up to 24 hours; max. cumulative dose in first 24 hours, 600 mg; transfer to *oral* treatment, as above

PoM **Tambocor®** (3M)

Tablets, flecainide acetate 50 mg, net price 60-tab pack = £16.28; 100 mg (scored), 60-tab pack = £23.26

Injection, flecainide acetate 10 mg/mL. Net price 15-mL amp = £4.95

PROCAINAMIDE HYDROCHLORIDE

Indications: ventricular arrhythmias, especially after myocardial infarction; atrial tachycardia

Cautions: elderly; hepatic and renal impairment, asthma, myasthenia gravis; pregnancy; **interactions:** Appendix 1 (procainamide)

Contra-indications: heart block, heart failure, hypotension; systemic lupus erythematosus; not indicated for torsades de pointes (can exacerbate); breast-feeding

Side-effects: nausea, diarrhoea, rashes, fever, myocardial depression, heart failure, lupus erythematosus-like syndrome, agranulocytosis after prolonged treatment; psychosis and angio-edema also reported

Dose: by mouth, ventricular arrhythmias, up to 50 mg/kg daily in divided doses, preferably controlled by measurement of plasma concentration (dosage intervals can range from 3–6 hours); atrial arrhythmias, higher doses may be required

By slow intravenous injection, rate not exceeding 50 mg/minute, 100 mg with ECG monitoring, repeated at 5-minute intervals until arrhythmia controlled; max. 1 g

By intravenous infusion, 500–600 mg over 25–30 minutes with ECG monitoring, followed by maintenance at rate of 2–6 mg/minute, then if necessary oral treatment as above, starting 3–4 hours after infusion

PoM **Pronestyl®** (Squibb)

Tablets, scored, procainamide hydrochloride 250 mg. Net price 100-tab pack = £4.70

Injection, procainamide hydrochloride 100 mg/mL. Net price 10-mL vial = £1.90

Modified release
PoM Procainamide Durules® (Astra)
Tablets, m/r, yellow, procainamide hydrochloride
500 mg. Net price 20 = £1.46. Label: 25
Dose: 1–1.5 g every 8 hours

QUINIDINE
Indications: suppression of supraventricular
tachycardias and ventricular arrhythmias (see
notes above)
Cautions: 200-mg test dose to detect hypersensitivity reactions; **interactions:** Appendix 1 (quinidine)
Contra-indications: heart block
Side-effects: see under Procainamide Hydrochloride; also ventricular arrhythmias, thrombocytopenia, haemolytic anaemia; rarely
granulomatous hepatitis; also cinchonism (see
Quinine, section 5.4.1)
Dose: by mouth, quinidine sulphate 200–400 mg
3–4 times daily
Note. Quinidine sulphate 200 mg ≡ quinidine bisulphate
250 mg

PoM Quinidine Sulphate (Non-proprietary)
Tablets, quinidine sulphate 200 mg; 300 mg
Note. May be difficult to obtain

Modified release
PoM Kinidin Durules® (Astra)
Tablets, m/r, f/c, quinidine bisulphate 250 mg. Net
price 100-tab pack = £11.33. Label: 25
Dose: 500 mg every 12 hours, adjusted as
required

VENTRICULAR ARRHYTHMIAS

Bretylium is only used as an anti-arrhythmic drug
in resuscitation. It is given both intramuscularly and
intravenously but can cause severe hypotension,
particularly after intravenous administration;
nausea and vomiting can occur with either route.
The intravenous route should only be used in emergency when there is doubt about absorption because
of inadequate circulation.

Lignocaine is relatively safe when used by slow
intravenous injection and should be considered first
for emergency use. Though effective in suppressing
ventricular tachycardia and reducing the risk of
ventricular fibrillation following myocardial infarction, it has not been shown to reduce mortality
when used prophylactically in this condition. In
patients with cardiac or hepatic failure doses may
need to be reduced to avoid convulsions, depression
of the central nervous system, or depression of the
cardiovascular system.

Mexiletine may be given as a slow intravenous
injection if lignocaine is ineffective; it has a similar
action. Adverse cardiovascular and central nervous
system effects may limit the dose tolerated; nausea
and vomiting may prevent an effective dose being
given by mouth.

Moracizine is a newer drug for the prophylaxis
and treatment of serious and life-threatening ventricular arrhythmias. In common with other anti-
arrhythmic drugs it may aggravate arrhythmias and
exacerbate congestive heart failure.

Phenytoin by slow intravenous injection was formerly used in ventricular arrhythmias particularly
those caused by cardiac glycosides, but this use is
now obsolete.

Propafenone is used for the prophylaxis and
treatment of ventricular arrhythmias and is undergoing evaluation in some supraventricular arrhythmias. It has complex mechanisms of action,
including weak beta-blocking activity (therefore
great caution is needed in obstructive airways disease—contra-indicated if severe).

Tocainide is an analogue of lignocaine; because
of a high incidence of blood disorders its use is limited to treatment of life-threatening symptomatic
ventricular tachyarrhythmias associated with
severely compromised left ventricular function in
patients who do not respond to other therapy or for
whom other therapy is contra-indicated.

BRETYLIUM TOSYLATE
(Bretylium Tosilate)
Indications: ventricular arrhythmias resistant to
other treatment
Cautions: do not give noradrenaline or other sympathomimetic amines; may exacerbate ventricular
arrhythmias due to cardiac glycosides; **interactions:** Appendix 1 (bretylium)
Contra-indications: phaeochromocytoma
Side-effects: hypotension, nausea and vomiting;
tissue necrosis reported after intramuscular injection (rotate sites)
Dose: by slow intravenous injection, 5–10 mg/kg
over 8–10 minutes (preferably 15–30 minutes)
with blood pressure and ECG monitoring; may be
repeated after 1–2 hours to a total dosage of
30 mg/kg (intravenous dose being diluted to
10 mg/mL in glucose 5% or sodium chloride
intravenous infusion)
Maintenance 5–10 mg/kg *by intramuscular injection, by intravenous infusion* (over 15–30 minutes) every 6–8 hours, *or* 1–2 mg/minute *by
continuous intravenous infusion*

PoM Bretylate® (Wellcome)
Injection, bretylium tosylate 50 mg/mL. Net price
10-mL amp = £19.81
PoM Min-I-Jet® Bretylium Tosylate (IMS)
Injection, bretylium tosylate 50 mg/mL. Net price
10-mL disposable syringe = £19.50

LIGNOCAINE HYDROCHLORIDE
(Lidocaine Hydrochloride)
Indications: ventricular arrhythmias, especially
after myocardial infarction
Cautions: lower doses in congestive cardiac failure, in hepatic failure, and following cardiac surgery; **interactions:** Appendix 1 (lignocaine)

Contra-indications: sino-atrial disorders, all grades of atrioventricular block, severe myocardial depression; porphyria (see section 9.8.2)

Side-effects: dizziness, paraesthesia, or drowsiness (particularly if injection too rapid); other CNS effects include confusion, respiratory depression and convulsions; hypotension and bradycardia (may lead to cardiac arrest); hypersensitivity reported

Dose: by intravenous injection, in patients without gross circulatory impairment, 100 mg as a bolus over a few minutes, followed by *infusion* of 2–4 mg/minute

PoM Lignocaine in Glucose Injection, lignocaine hydrochloride 0.1% (1 mg/mL) and 0.2% (2 mg/mL) in glucose intravenous infusion 5%. 500-mL containers
Available from Baxter

PoM Min-I-Jet® Lignocaine (IMS)
Injection, lignocaine hydrochloride 1% (10 mg/mL), net price 10-mL disposable syringe = £3.25; 2% (20 mg/mL), 5-mL disposable syringe = £2.98

PoM Xylocard® (Astra)
Injection 100 mg, lignocaine hydrochloride (anhydrous) 20 mg/mL. Net price 5-mL syringe = £1.65

MEXILETINE HYDROCHLORIDE

Indications: ventricular arrhythmias, especially after myocardial infarction

Cautions: hepatic impairment; close monitoring on initiation of therapy (including ECG, blood pressure, etc.); **interactions:** Appendix 1 (mexiletine)

Contra-indications: bradycardia, heart block

Side-effects: nausea, vomiting, constipation; bradycardia, hypotension, confusion, convulsions, psychiatric disorders, dysarthria, nystagmus, tremor; jaundice, hepatitis, and blood disorders reported; see also notes above

Dose: by mouth, initial dose 400 mg (may be increased to 600 mg if opioid analgesics also given), followed after 2 hours by 200–250 mg 3–4 times daily
By intravenous injection, 100–250 mg at a rate of 25 mg/minute with ECG monitoring followed by *infusion* of 250 mg as a 0.1% solution over 1 hour, 125 mg/hour for 2 hours, then 500 micrograms/minute

PoM Mexitil® (Boehringer Ingelheim)
Capsules, mexiletine hydrochloride 50 mg (purple/red), net price 100-cap pack = £4.95; 200 mg (red), 100-cap pack = £11.87
Injection, mexiletine hydrochloride 25 mg/mL. Net price 10-mL amp = £1.49

Modified release
PoM Mexitil PL® (Boehringer Ingelheim)
Perlongets® (= capsules, m/r, each enclosing 5 miniature tablets), turquoise/scarlet, mexiletine hydrochloride 360 mg. Net price 56-cap pack = £11.97. Label: 25
Dose: 1 capsule twice daily

MORACIZINE HYDROCHLORIDE

Indications: ventricular arrhythmias in patients with underlying cardiac disease and history of ventricular fibrillation or sustained ventricular tachycardia, or of symptomatic non-sustained ventricular tachycardia, or of disabling symptoms due to premature ventricular contraction

Cautions: sick sinus syndrome; pre-existing conduction abnormalities; congestive heart failure; hepatic and renal impairment; pregnancy and breast-feeding; **interactions:** Appendix 1 (moracizine)

Contra-indications: second-degree or greater AV block (unless paced); cardiogenic shock

Side-effects: include gastro-intestinal disturbances; dizziness, headache, fatigue, palpitations, dyspnoea; arrhythmogenic (pro-arrhythmic effect); chest pain; congestive heart failure; reversible increases in liver enzymes, jaundice; thrombocytopenia

Dose: (initiated in hospital) usually 600–900 mg daily in 3 divided doses, adjusted by steps of 150 mg daily at intervals of 3 days; max. recommended daily dose 900 mg; rapid control, initially 400–500 mg, then 200 mg every 8 hours
Note. Patients well controlled on 3 divided doses daily may be given same total daily dosage in 2 divided doses (every 12 hours)

▼ **PoM Ethmozine®** (Monmouth)
Tablets, all f/c, moracizine hydrochloride 200 mg, net price 100-tab pack = £47.93; 250 mg, 100-tab pack = £59.06, 300 mg, 100 tab pack = £71.60

PHENYTOIN SODIUM

Indications: arrhythmias (but see notes above); for use in epilepsy, see section 4.8.1

Cautions; Contra-indications; Side-effects: see section 4.8.2

Dose: arrhythmias, *by intravenous injection* via caval catheter, 3.5–5 mg/kg at a rate not exceeding 50 mg/minute, with blood pressure and ECG monitoring; repeat once if necessary (rarely used, see notes above)

Preparations
See section 4.8.2

PROPAFENONE HYDROCHLORIDE

Indications: ventricular arrhythmias

Cautions: heart failure; hepatic and renal impairment; elderly; pacemaker patients; pregnancy; great caution in obstructive airways disease owing to beta-blocking activity (contra-indicated if severe); **interactions:** Appendix 1 (propafenone)

Contra-indications: uncontrolled congestive heart failure, cardiogenic shock (except arrhythmia induced), severe bradycardia, uncontrolled electrolyte disturbances, severe obstructive pulmonary disease, marked hypotension; myasthenia gravis; unless adequately paced avoid in sinus node dysfunction, atrial conduction defects, second degree or greater AV block, bundle branch block or distal block

Side-effects: constipation, blurred vision, dry mouth (due to antimuscarinic action); dizziness, nausea and vomiting, fatigue, bitter taste, diarrhoea, headache, and allergic skin reactions reported; postural hypotension, particularly in elderly; bradycardia, sino-atrial, atrioventricular, or intraventricular blocks; arrhythmogenic (pro-arrhythmic) effect; rarely cholestasis, blood disorders, lupus syndrome, seizures; myoclonus also reported

Dose: 70 kg and over, initially 150 mg 3 times daily after food under direct hospital supervision with ECG monitoring and blood pressure control, increased at intervals of at least 3 days to 300 mg twice daily and, if necessary, to max. 300 mg 3 times daily; under 70 kg, reduce dose
ELDERLY may respond to lower doses

PoM **Arythmol**® (Knoll)
Tablets, both f/c, propafenone hydrochloride 150 mg, net price 90-tab pack = £19.48; 300 mg (scored), 60-tab pack = £19.48. Label: 21, 25

TOCAINIDE HYDROCHLORIDE

Indications: ventricular arrhythmias (restricted use—see notes above)

Cautions: weekly blood counts essential for first 12 weeks, then monthly; correct hypokalaemia; advise patients to report pulmonary symptoms; severe hepatic or renal impairment; elderly; uncompensated heart failure, bradycardia and hypotension; pregnancy (toxicity in *animal* studies); **interactions:** Appendix 1 (tocainide)

Contra-indications: second-degree or greater AV block (unless paced)

Side-effects: CNS effects including tremor, dizziness, confusion, visual hallucinations, convulsions, paraesthesia; gastro-intestinal effects including nausea and vomiting; abnormal liver-function tests (hepatitis and jaundice reported); fever and rash (including Stevens-Johnson syndrome and exfoliative dermatitis); lupus erythematosus-like syndrome; pulmonary fibrosis, interstitial pneumonitis, fibrosing alveolitis; agranulocytosis, aplastic anaemia, and thrombocytopenia—see also notes above; arrhythmogenic (pro-arrhythmic) effect

Dose: 1.2 g daily in 3 divided doses; max. 2.4 g daily

PoM **Tonocard**® (Astra)
Tablets, yellow, f/c, tocainide hydrochloride 400 mg, net price 20 = £3.35

2.4 Beta-adrenoceptor blocking drugs

Beta-adrenoceptor blocking drugs (beta-blockers) block the beta-adrenoreceptors in the heart, peripheral vasculature, bronchi, pancreas, and liver.

Many beta-blockers are now available and in general they are all equally effective. There are, however, differences between them which may affect choice in treating particular diseases or individual patients.

Intrinsic sympathomimetic activity (ISA, partial agonist activity) represents the capacity of beta-blockers to stimulate as well as to block adrenergic receptors. **Oxprenolol, pindolol,** and **acebutolol** have intrinsic sympathomimetic activity; the newer **celiprolol** also has intrinsic sympathomimetic activity (see also below); they tend to cause less bradycardia than the other beta-blockers and may also cause less coldness of the extremities.

Some beta-blockers are *lipid soluble* and some are *water soluble*. **Atenolol, celiprolol, nadolol,** and **sotalol** are the most water-soluble; they are less likely to enter the brain, and may therefore cause less sleep disturbance and nightmares. Water-soluble beta-blockers are excreted by the kidneys; they accumulate in renal impairment and dosage reduction is therefore often necessary.

Some beta-blockers have a *relatively short duration of action* and have to be given twice or three times daily. Many of these are, however, available in modified-release formulations so that in general it is not necessary to give beta-blockers more often than once daily for hypertension. For angina twice-daily treatment may sometimes be needed even with a modified-release formulation.

All beta-blockers *slow the heart* and may induce myocardial depression and precipitate heart failure. They should not therefore be given to patients who have incipient cardiac failure or those with second- or third-degree heart block. **Sotalol** may prolong the QT interval, and has occasionally caused life-threatening ventricular arrhythmias (**important:** particular care should be taken to avoid hypokalaemia in patients taking sotalol).

Beta-blockers may *precipitate asthma* and this effect can be dangerous. Some, such as **atenolol, betaxolol, bisoprolol, metoprolol,** and (to a lesser extent) **acebutolol**, have less effect on the beta$_2$ (bronchial) receptors and are, therefore, relatively *cardioselective*, but they are **not** *cardiospecific*. They have a lesser effect on airways resistance but are **not** free of this side-effect. Patients who have a tendency towards obstructive airways disease must be treated with great caution and may require to take increased doses of their beta$_2$-stimulants (e.g. salbutamol) to overcome the effect of blockade of the bronchial adrenoceptors. **Important:** see also **CSM** advice on next page.

Beta-blockers are also associated with *fatigue, coldness of the extremities* (may be less common with those with ISA, see above), and *sleep disturbances with nightmares* (may be less common with the water-soluble ones, see above).

Beta-blockers can lead to a small deterioration of *glucose tolerance* in diabetics; they also interfere with metabolic and autonomic responses to hypoglycaemia. Their use is not contra-indicated in diabetics, but cardioselective beta-blockers (see above) may be preferable and they should be avoided altogether in those with frequent episodes of hypoglycaemia.

Labetalol combines alpha- and beta-receptor blocking activity. The alpha-blocking activity in the peripheral vessels *lowers peripheral resistance*. **Celiprolol** is a relatively cardioselective beta-blocker with additional partial beta$_2$-agonist activity, and the latter property again lowers peripheral resistance. There is no evidence that these drugs have important advantages over other beta-blockers in the treatment of hypertension.

HYPERTENSION. Beta-blockers are effective *antihypertensives* but their mode of action is not understood; they reduce cardiac output, alter baroceptor reflex sensitivity, and block peripheral adrenoceptors. Some beta-blockers depress plasma renin secretion. It is possible that a central effect may also explain their mode of action. Blood pressure can usually be controlled with relatively few side-effects. In general the dose of beta-blocker does not have to be as high as originally thought. The maximum dose of **oxprenolol** and **propranolol** necessary is probably 320 mg daily. **Atenolol** can usually be given in a dose of 50 mg daily and it is no longer considered necessary to increase to 100 mg.

Combined thiazide/beta-blocker preparations may help compliance but combined preparations should only be used when blood pressure is not adequately controlled by a thiazide or a beta-blocker alone. Beta-blockers reduce, but do not abolish, the tendency for diuretics to cause hypokalaemia.

Beta-blockers can be used to control the pulse rate in patients with *phaeochromocytoma*. However, they should never be used alone as beta-blockade without concurrent alpha blockade may lead to a hypertensive crisis. For this reason phenoxybenzamine should always be used together with the beta-blocker.

ANGINA. Beta-blockers improve exercise tolerance and relieve symptoms in patients with *angina*; this effect is caused by their reduction of cardiac work. As with hypertension there is no good evidence of the superiority of any one drug, although occasionally a patient will respond better to one beta-blocker than to another. There is some evidence that sudden withdrawal may cause an exacerbation of angina therefore gradual reduction of dose is preferable when beta-blockers are to be stopped. There is a risk of precipitating heart failure when beta-blockers and verapamil are used together in established ischaemic heart disease (**important**: see p. 93.)

MYOCARDIAL INFARCTION. Several studies have shown that some beta-blockers can cause a reduction in the recurrence rate of *myocardial infarction*. However, pre-existing heart failure, hypotension, bradyarrhythmias, and obstructive airways disease render this group of drugs unsuitable in some patients who have recovered from a myocardial infarction. **Atenolol** and **metoprolol** may reduce early mortality after intravenous and subsequent oral administration in the acute phase, while **timolol** and **propranolol** have protective value when started in the early convalescent phase. The evidence relating to other beta-blockers is less convincing; some have not been tested in trials of secondary protection. It is also not known whether the protective effect of beta-blockers continues after two years; it is possible that sudden cessation may cause a rebound worsening of myocardial ischaemia.

ARRHYTHMIAS. Beta-blockers act as *anti-arrhythmic drugs* principally by attenuating the effects of the sympathetic system on automaticity and conductivity within the heart. They may be used in conjunction with digoxin to control the ventricular response in atrial fibrillation, especially in patients with thyrotoxicosis. Beta-blockers are also useful in the management of supraventricular tachycardias, and are used to control those following myocardial infarction, see above.

Esmolol is a relatively cardioselective beta-blocker with a very short duration of action, used intravenously for the short-term treatment of supraventricular arrhythmias, sinus tachycardia, or hypertension, particularly in the peri-operative period. **Sotalol**, a non-cardioselective beta-blocker with additional class III anti-arrhythmic activity, is used for prophylaxis in paroxysmal supraventricular arrhythmias (**important**: avoid hypokalaemia, see p. 76).

THYROTOXICOSIS. Beta-blockers are used in pre-operative preparation for thyroidectomy. Administration of propranolol can reverse clinical symptoms of *thyrotoxicosis* within 4 days. Routine tests of increased thyroid function remain unaltered. The thyroid gland is rendered less vascular thus making surgery easier (see section 6.2.2).

OTHER USES. Beta-blockers have been used to alleviate some symptoms of *anxiety*; probably patients with palpitations, tremor, and tachycardia respond best (see also sections 4.1.2 and 4.9.3). Beta-blockers are also used in the *prophylaxis of migraine* (see section 4.7.4.2). Beta-blockers are used topically in *glaucoma* (see section 11.6).

PROPRANOLOL HYDROCHLORIDE

Indications: see under Dose
Cautions: late pregnancy and breast-feeding (see also Appendixes 4 and 5); avoid abrupt withdrawal in angina; reduce oral dose of propranolol in liver disease; liver function deteriorates in portal hypertension; reduce initial dose in renal impairment; diabetes; myasthenia gravis; see also notes above; **interactions:** Appendix 1 (beta-blockers), **important:** verapamil interaction, see also p. 93
Contra-indications: asthma or history of obstructive airways disease (**important:** see CSM advice

below), uncontrolled heart failure, sick sinus syndrome, second or third degree heart block, cardiogenic shock

CSM ADVICE. Beta-blockers, even those with apparent cardioselectivity, should **not** be used in patients with asthma or a history of obstructive airways disease, unless no alternative treatment is available. In such cases the risk of inducing bronchospasm should be appreciated and appropriate precautions taken.

Side-effects: bradycardia, heart failure, bronchospasm, peripheral vasoconstriction, gastro-intestinal disturbances, fatigue, sleep disturbances; rare reports of rashes and dry eyes (reversible on withdrawal); overdosage: see Emergency Treatment of Poisoning, p. 22

Dose: by mouth, hypertension, initially 80 mg twice daily, increased at weekly intervals as required; maintenance 160–320 mg daily
Portal hypertension, initially 40 mg twice daily, increased to 80 mg twice daily according to heart-rate; max. 160 mg twice daily
Phaeochromocytoma (only with an alpha-blocker), 60 mg daily for 3 days before surgery; 30 mg daily in patients unsuitable for surgery
Angina, initially 40 mg 2–3 times daily; maintenance 120–240 mg daily
Arrhythmias, hypertrophic obstructive cardiomyopathy, anxiety tachycardia, and thyrotoxicosis (adjunct), 10–40 mg 3–4 times daily
Anxiety with symptoms such as palpitations, sweating, tremor, 40 mg twice daily, increased to 3 times daily if necessary
Prophylaxis after myocardial infarction, 40 mg 4 times daily for 2–3 days, then 80 mg twice daily, beginning 5 to 21 days after infarction
Migraine prophylaxis and essential tremor, initially 40 mg 2–3 times daily; maintenance 80–160 mg daily

By intravenous injection, arrhythmias and thyrotoxic crisis, 1 mg over 1 minute; if necessary repeat at 2-minute intervals; max. 10 mg (5 mg in anaesthesia)

Note. Excessive bradycardia can be countered with intravenous injection of atropine sulphate 0.6–2.4 mg in divided doses of 600 micrograms; for overdosage see Emergency Treatment of Poisoning, p. 22

PoM Propranolol (Non-proprietary)

Tablets, propranolol hydrochloride 10 mg, net price 20 = 5p; 40 mg, 20 = 7p; 80 mg, 20 = 14p; 160 mg, 20 = 25p. Label: 8

Available from APS (Apsolol®), Ashbourne (Propanix®), Berk (Berkolol®), Cox, CP (Cardinol®), DDSA (Angilol®), Hillcross, K Pharm., Norton

Oral solution (syrup), propranolol hydrochloride 5 mg/5 mL, 10 mg/5 mL and 50 mg/5 mL available from RP Drugs (special order)

PoM Inderal® (Zeneca)

Tablets, all pink, f/c, propranolol hydrochloride 10 mg, net price 100-tab pack = 89p; 40 mg, 100-tab pack = £2.40; 80 mg, 60-tab pack = £2.35. Label: 8

Injection, propranolol hydrochloride 1 mg/mL, net price 1-mL amp = 21p

Modified release
PoM Half-Inderal LA® (Zeneca)

Capsules, m/r, lavender/pink, propranolol hydrochloride 80 mg. Net price 28-cap pack = £5.40. Label: 8, 25

Note. Modified-release capsules containing propranolol hydrochloride 80 mg also available from APS, CP, Monmouth (Half-Betadur CR®), Tillomed (Half Beta-Prograne®)

PoM Inderal-LA® (Zeneca)

Capsules, m/r, lavender/pink, propranolol hydrochloride 160 mg. Net price 28-cap pack = £6.67. Label: 8, 25

Note. Modified-release capsules containing propranolol hydrochloride 160 mg also available from APS, Ashbourne (Propanix SR®), CP (Sloprolol®), Hillcross, Lagap (Bedranol SR®), Monmouth (Betadur CR®), Tillomed (Beta-Prograne®)

With diuretic
PoM Inderetic® (Zeneca)

Capsules, propranolol hydrochloride 80 mg, bendrofluazide 2.5 mg. Net price 100-cap pack = £9.74. Label: 8

Dose: hypertension, 1 capsule twice daily

PoM Inderex® (Zeneca)

Capsules, pink/grey, propranolol hydrochloride 160 mg (m/r), bendrofluazide 5 mg. Net price 28-cap pack = £7.45. Label: 8, 25

Dose: hypertension, 1 capsule daily

ACEBUTOLOL

Indications: see under Dose

Cautions; Contra-indications; Side-effects: see under Propranolol Hydrochloride

Dose: hypertension, initially 400 mg once daily *or* 200 mg twice daily, increased after 2 weeks to 400 mg twice daily if necessary
Angina, initially 400 mg once daily *or* 200 mg twice daily; 300 mg 3 times daily in severe angina; up to 1.2 g daily has been used
Arrhythmias, 0.4–1.2 g daily in 2–3 divided doses

PoM Sectral® (Rhône-Poulenc Rorer)

Capsules, acebutolol (as hydrochloride) 100 mg (buff/white), net price 84-cap pack = £6.96; 200 mg (buff/pink), 56-cap pack = £8.93. Label: 8

Tablets, f/c, acebutolol 400 mg (as hydrochloride). Net price 28-tab pack = £8.66. Label: 8

With diuretic
PoM Secadrex® (Rhône-Poulenc Rorer)

Tablets, f/c, acebutolol 200 mg (as hydrochloride), hydrochlorothiazide 12.5 mg. Net price 28-tab pack = £8.18. Label: 8

Dose: hypertension, 1 tablet daily, increased to 2 daily as a single dose if necessary

ATENOLOL

Indications: see under Dose

Cautions; Contra-indications; Side-effects: see under Propranolol Hydrochloride; reduce dose in renal impairment (25 mg tablets available)

Dose: by mouth,

Hypertension, 50 mg daily (higher doses no longer considered necessary)

Angina, 100 mg daily in 1 or 2 doses

Arrhythmias, 50–100 mg daily

By intravenous injection, arrhythmias, 2.5 mg at a rate of 1 mg/minute, repeated at 5-minute intervals to a max. of 10 mg

Note. Excessive bradycardia can be countered with intravenous injection of atropine sulphate 0.6–2.4 mg in divided doses of 600 micrograms; for overdosage see Emergency Treatment of Poisoning, p. 22

By intravenous infusion, arrhythmias, 150 micrograms/kg over 20 minutes, repeated every 12 hours if required

Early intervention within 12 hours of infarction, 5–10 mg *by slow intravenous injection,* then *by mouth* 50 mg after 15 minutes, 50 mg after 12 hours, then 100 mg daily

PoM Atenolol (Non-proprietary)

Tablets, atenolol 25 mg, net price 28-tab pack = £3.98; 50 mg, 28-tab pack = £1.44; 100 mg, 28-tab pack = £1.99. Label: 8

Various strengths available from APS, Ashbourne (Atenix®), Berk (Antipressan®), Cox, CP (Totamol®), Hillcross, K Pharm., Lagap, Norton

PoM Tenormin® (Stuart)

'25' tablets, f/c, atenolol 25 mg. Net price 28-tab pack = £4.62. Label: 8

LS tablets, orange, f/c, scored, atenolol 50 mg. Net price 28-tab pack = £5.35. Label: 8

Tablets, orange, f/c, scored, atenolol 100 mg. Net price 28-tab pack = £6.81. Label: 8

Syrup, sugar-free, atenolol 25 mg/5mL. Net price 300 mL = £8.14. Label: 8

Injection, atenolol 500 micrograms/mL. Net price 10-mL amp = £1.00 (hosp. only)

With diuretic

PoM Co-tenidone (Non-proprietary)

Tablets, co-tenidone 50/12.5 (atenolol 50 mg, chlorthalidone 12.5 mg), net price 28-tab pack = £5.65; co-tenidone 100/25 (atenolol 100 mg, chlorthalidone 25 mg), 28-tab pack = £8.29. Label: 8

Available from APS, Ashbourne (AtenixCo®), Berk (Tenchlor®), Cox, Hillcross, K Pharm.

Dose: hypertension, 1 tablet daily (but see also under Dose above)

PoM Kalten® (Stuart)

Capsules, red/ivory, atenolol 50 mg, co-amilozide 2.5/25 (anhydrous amiloride hydrochloride 2.5 mg, hydrochlorothiazide 25 mg). Net price 28-cap pack = £8.39. Label: 8

Dose: hypertension, 1 capsule daily

PoM Tenoret 50® (Stuart)

Tablets, brown, f/c, co-tenidone 50/12.5 (atenolol 50 mg, chlorthalidone 12.5 mg). Net price 28-tab pack = £5.70. Label: 8

Dose: hypertension, 1 tablet daily

PoM Tenoretic® (Stuart)

Tablets, brown, f/c, co-tenidone 100/25 (atenolol 100 mg, chlorthalidone 25 mg). Net price 28-tab pack = £8.12. Label: 8

Dose: hypertension, 1 tablet daily (but see also under Dose above)

With calcium-channel blocker

Note. Only indicated when calcium-channel blocker or beta-blocker alone proves inadequate

PoM Beta-Adalat® (Bayer)

Capsules, reddish-brown, atenolol 50 mg, nifedipine 20 mg (m/r). Net price 28-cap pack = £10.90. Label: 8, 25

Dose: hypertension, 1 capsule daily, increased if necessary to twice daily; elderly, 1 daily

Angina, 1 capsule twice daily

PoM Tenif® (Stuart)

Capsules, reddish-brown, atenolol 50 mg, nifedipine 20 mg (m/r). Net price 28-cap pack = £10.63. Label: 8, 25

Dose: hypertension, 1 capsule daily, increased if necessary to twice daily; elderly, 1 daily

Angina, 1 capsule twice daily

BETAXOLOL HYDROCHLORIDE

Indications: hypertension

Cautions; Contra-indications; Side-effects: see under Propranolol Hydrochloride; reduce dose in renal impairment

Dose: 20 mg daily (elderly patients 10 mg), increased to 40 mg if required

PoM Kerlone® (Lorex)

Tablets, f/c, scored, betaxolol hydrochloride 20 mg. Net price 28-tab pack = £7.51. Label: 8

BISOPROLOL FUMARATE

Indications: hypertension, angina

Cautions; Contra-indications; Side-effects: see under Propranolol Hydrochloride; reduce dose in hepatic and renal impairment

Dose: usual dose 10 mg daily (5 mg may be adequate in some patients); max. recommended dose 20 mg daily

PoM Emcor® (Merck)

LS Tablets, yellow, f/c, scored, bisoprolol fumarate 5 mg. Net price 28-tab pack = £7.78. Label: 8

Tablets, orange, f/c, scored, bisoprolol fumarate 10 mg. Net price 28-tab pack = £8.74. Label: 8

PoM Monocor® (Cyanamid)

Tablets, both f/c, bisoprolol fumarate 5 mg (pink), net price 28-tab pack = £7.78; 10 mg, 28-tab pack £8.74. Label: 8

With diuretic

PoM Monozide 10® (Lederle)

Tablets, f/c, bisoprolol fumarate 10 mg, hydrochlorothiazide 6.25 mg. Net price 28-tab pack = £11.20. Label: 8

Dose: hypertension, 1 tablet daily

CELIPROLOL HYDROCHLORIDE

Indications: mild to moderate hypertension

Cautions: pregnancy, breast-feeding; avoid abrupt withdrawal; hepatic and renal impairment (avoid if severe); **interactions**: Appendix 1 (beta-blockers)

Contra-indications: as for Propranolol Hydrochloride; also severe renal impairment

Side-effects: headache, dizziness, fatigue, nausea and somnolence; also bradycardia, bronchospasm

Dose: 200 mg once daily in the morning, increased to 400 mg once daily if necessary

▼ **PoM Celectol®** (Rhône-Poulenc Rorer)

Tablets, both f/c, scored, celiprolol hydrochloride 200 mg (yellow), net price 28-tab pack = £9.56; 400 mg, 28-tab pack = £13.72. Label: 8, 22

ESMOLOL HYDROCHLORIDE

Indications: short-term treatment of supraventricular arrhythmias (including atrial fibrillation, atrial flutter, sinus tachycardia); tachycardia and hypertension in peri-operative period

Cautions; Contra-indications; Side-effects: see under Propranolol Hydrochloride

Dose: by intravenous infusion, usually within range 50–200 micrograms/kg/minute (consult data sheet for details of dose titration)

PoM Brevibloc® (Du Pont)

Injection, esmolol hydrochloride 10 mg/mL, net price 10-mL vial = £5.90; 250 mg/mL (for dilution before infusion), 10-mL amp = £65.90

LABETALOL HYDROCHLORIDE

Indications: hypertension (including hypertension in pregnancy, hypertension with angina, and hypertension following acute myocardial infarction); hypertensive crisis (but see section 2.5); controlled hypotension in surgery

Cautions: late pregnancy, breast-feeding; avoid abrupt withdrawal; stop and do not restart if liver damage occurs; interferes with laboratory tests for catecholamines; **interactions**: Appendix 1 (beta-blockers)

Contra-indications: as for Propranolol Hydrochloride; also liver disease

Side-effects: postural hypotension (avoid upright position during and for 3 hours after intravenous administration), tiredness, weakness, headache, rashes, scalp tingling, difficulty in micturition, epigastric pain, nausea, vomiting; liver damage (see Cautions); rarely lichenoid rash

Dose: by mouth, initially 100 mg (50 mg in elderly) twice daily with food, increased at intervals of 14 days to usual dose of 200 mg twice daily; up to 800 mg daily in 2 divided doses (3–4 divided doses if higher); max. 2.4 g daily

By intravenous injection, 50 mg over at least 1 minute, repeated after 5 minutes if necessary; max. 200 mg

Note. Excessive bradycardia can be countered with intravenous injection of atropine sulphate 0.6–2.4 mg in divided doses of 600 micrograms; for overdosage see Emergency Treatment of Poisoning, p. 22

By intravenous infusion, 2 mg/minute; usual range 50–200 mg, higher doses in phaeochromocytoma

Hypertension of pregnancy, 20 mg/hour, doubled every 30 minutes; usual max. 160 mg/hour

Hypertension following infarction, 15 mg/hour, gradually increased to max. 120 mg/hour

PoM Labetalol Hydrochloride (Non-proprietary)

Tablets, all f/c, labetalol hydrochloride 100 mg, net price 20 = £1.18; 200 mg, 20 = £2.17; 400 mg, 20 = £3.58. Label: 8, 21

Available from APS, Cox, Hillcross, K Pharm., Norton

PoM Trandate® (DF)

Tablets, all orange, f/c, labetalol hydrochloride 50 mg, net price 56-tab pack. £5.05; 100 mg, 56-tab pack = £5.56; 200 mg, 56-tab pack = £9.02; 400 mg, 50-tab pack = £11.21. Label: 8, 21

Injection, labetalol hydrochloride 5 mg/mL. Net price 20-mL amp = £2.83

METOPROLOL TARTRATE

Indications: see under Dose

Cautions; Contra-indications; Side-effects: see under Propranolol Hydrochloride; reduce dose in hepatic impairment

Dose: by mouth, hypertension, initially 100 mg daily, maintenance 100–200 mg daily in 1–2 doses

Angina, 50–100 mg 2–3 times daily

Arrhythmias, usually 50 mg 2–3 times daily; up to 300 mg daily in divided doses if necessary

Migraine prophylaxis, 100–200 mg daily in divided doses

Thyrotoxicosis (adjunct), 50 mg 4 times daily

By intravenous injection, arrhythmias, up to 5 mg at rate 1–2 mg/minute, repeated after 5 minutes if necessary, total dose 10–15 mg

Note. Excessive bradycardia can be countered with intravenous injection of atropine sulphate 0.6–2.4 mg in divided doses of 600 micrograms; for overdosage see Emergency Treatment of Poisoning, p. 22

In surgery, 2–4 mg *by slow intravenous injection* at induction or to control arrhythmias developing during anaesthesia; 2-mg doses may be repeated to a max. of 10 mg

Early intervention within 12 hours of infarction, 5 mg *by intravenous injection* every 2 minutes to a max. of 15 mg, followed after 15 minutes by 50 mg *by mouth* every 6 hours for 48 hours; maintenance 200 mg daily in divided doses

PoM Metoprolol Tartrate (Non-proprietary)

Tablets, metoprolol tartrate 50 mg, net price 20 = 73p; 100 mg, 20 = £1.44. Label: 8

Available from APS, Ashbourne (Mepranix®), Berk (Arbralene®), Cox, Hillcross, K Pharm., Norton

PoM Betaloc® (Astra)

Tablets, both scored, metoprolol tartrate 50 mg, net price 100-tab pack = £4.59; 100 mg, 100-tab pack = £8.53. Label: 8

Injection, metoprolol tartrate 1 mg/mL. Net price 5-mL amp = 44p

PoM Lopresor® (Geigy)

Tablets, both f/c, scored, metoprolol tartrate 50 mg (pink), net price 56-tab pack = £4.24; 100 mg (blue), 56-tab pack = £7.88. Label: 8

Modified release
PoM Betaloc-SA® (Astra)

Durules® (= tablets, m/r), metoprolol tartrate 200 mg. Net price 28-tab pack = £6.51. Label: 8, 25

Dose: hypertension, angina, 200–400 mg daily; migraine, 200 mg daily

PoM Lopresor SR® (Geigy)

Tablets, m/r, yellow, f/c, metoprolol tartrate 200 mg. Net price 28-tab pack = £7.42. Label: 8, 25

Dose: hypertension, angina, 200–400 mg daily; migraine, 200 mg daily

With diuretic
PoM Co-Betaloc® (Astra)

Tablets, scored, metoprolol tartrate 100 mg, hydrochlorothiazide 12.5 mg. Net price 28-tab pack = £6.65. Label: 8

Dose: hypertension, 1–3 tablets daily in single or divided doses

PoM Co-Betaloc SA® (Astra)

Tablets, yellow, f/c, metoprolol tartrate 200 mg (m/r), hydrochlorothiazide 25 mg. Net price 28-tab pack = £8.20. Label: 8, 25

Dose: hypertension, 1 tablet daily

PoM Lopresoretic® (Geigy)

Tablets, scored, metoprolol tartrate 100 mg, chlorthalidone 12.5 mg. Net price 56-tab pack = £7.47. Label: 8

Dose: hypertension, 1–2 tablets in the morning; max. 3–4 daily in single or divided doses

NADOLOL

Indications: see under Dose

Cautions; Contra-indications; Side-effects: see under Propranolol Hydrochloride; reduce dose in renal impairment

Dose: hypertension, 80 mg daily, increased at weekly intervals if required; max. 240 mg daily

Angina, 40 mg daily, increased at weekly intervals if required; usual max. 160 mg daily

Arrhythmias, initially 40 mg daily, increased to 160 mg if required; reduce to 40 mg if bradycardia occurs

Migraine prophylaxis, initially 40 mg daily, increased by 40 mg at weekly intervals; usual maintenance dose 80–160 mg daily

Thyrotoxicosis (adjunct), 80–160 mg daily

PoM Corgard® (Sanofi Winthrop)

Tablets, both blue, nadolol 40 mg, net price 28-tab pack = £3.76; 80 mg, 28-tab pack = £5.45. Label: 8

With diuretic
PoM Corgaretic 40® (Sanofi Winthrop)

Tablets, scored, nadolol 40 mg, bendrofluazide 5 mg. Net price 28-tab pack = £5.92. Label: 8

Dose: hypertension, 1–2 tablets daily

PoM Corgaretic 80® (Sanofi Winthrop)

Tablets, scored, nadolol 80 mg, bendrofluazide 5 mg. Net price 28-tab pack = £8.47. Label: 8

Dose: hypertension, 1–2 tablets daily

OXPRENOLOL HYDROCHLORIDE

Indications: see under Dose

Cautions; Contra-indications; Side-effects: see under Propranolol Hydrochloride

Dose: hypertension, initially 80 mg twice daily, increased as required at weekly intervals; max. 480 mg daily

Angina, 40–160 mg 3 times daily

Arrhythmias, initially 20–40 mg 3 times daily, increased as necessary

Anxiety symptoms (short-term use), initially 40 mg twice daily, increased if necessary to 160 mg daily in divided doses

PoM Oxprenolol (Non-proprietary)

Tablets, all coated, oxprenolol hydrochloride 20 mg, net price 20 = 34p; 40 mg, 20 = 46p; 80 mg, 20 = 80p; 160 mg, 20 = £1.44. Label: 8

Available from APS (Apsolox®, 80-mg tablets contain tartrazine), Cox, Hillcross, K Pharm., Norton

PoM Trasicor® (Ciba)

Tablets, all f/c, oxprenolol hydrochloride 20 mg (contain gluten), net price 20 = 42p; 40 mg (contain gluten), 20 = 84p; 80 mg (beige), 56-tab pack = £4.70; 160 mg (orange), 56-tab pack = £9.41. Label: 8

Modified release
PoM Slow-Trasicor® (Ciba)

Tablets, m/r, f/c, oxprenolol hydrochloride 160 mg. Net price 28-tab pack = £5.33. Label: 8, 25

Dose: 160–480 mg daily

Note. Modified-release tablets containing oxprenolol hydrochloride 160 mg also available from Anhhourna (Oxyprenix SR®), Norton

With diuretic
PoM Trasidrex® (Ciba)

Tablets, red, s/c, co-prenozide 160/0.25 (oxprenolol hydrochloride 160 mg (m/r), cyclopenthiazide 250 micrograms). Net price 28-tab pack = £6.73. Label: 8, 25

Dose: hypertension, 1 tablet daily, increased to 2 daily as a single dose; max. 3 daily

PINDOLOL

Indications: see under Dose

Cautions; Contra-indications; Side-effects: see under Propranolol Hydrochloride; reduce dose in renal impairment

Dose: hypertension, initially 5 mg 2–3 times daily *or* 15 mg once daily, increased as required at weekly intervals; usual maintenance 15–30 mg daily; max. 45 mg daily

Angina, 2.5–5 mg up to 3 times daily

PoM Visken® (Sandoz)

Tablets, both scored, pindolol 5 mg, net price 100-tab pack = £7.27; 15 mg, 30-tab pack = £6.54. Label: 8

With diuretic
PoM Viskaldix® (Sandoz)

Tablets, scored, pindolol 10 mg, clopamide 5 mg. Net price 28-tab pack = £5.58. Label: 8

Dose: hypertension, 1 tablet daily in the morning, increased if necessary to 2 daily; max. 3 daily

SOTALOL HYDROCHLORIDE

Indications: see under Dose

Cautions; Contra-indications; Side-effects: see under Propranolol Hydrochloride; reduce dose in renal impairment; occasionally causes atypical ventricular arrhythmias (torsades de pointes)—special need to avoid hypokalaemia if given with thiazide or loop diuretic (also stop if severe or persistent diarrhoea etc.)

Dose: by mouth, hypertension and angina, initially 80 mg twice daily *or* 160 mg once daily; maintenance 160 mg daily, increased to 400–600 mg daily if necessary
Arrhythmias, 120–240 mg daily in single or divided doses
Thyrotoxicosis (adjunct), 120–240 mg daily in single or divided doses
Prophylaxis after infarction, 320 mg daily, starting 5–14 days after infarction

By slow intravenous injection, arrhythmias, 20–60 mg over 2–3 minutes with ECG monitoring, repeated if necessary with 10-minute intervals between injections; up to 100 mg over 3 minutes or longer

Note. Excessive bradycardia can be countered with intravenous injection of atropine sulphate 0.6–2.4 mg in divided doses of 600 micrograms; for overdosage see Emergency Treatment of Poisoning, p. 22

PoM Beta-Cardone® (Evans)

Tablets, all scored, sotalol hydrochloride 40 mg (green), net price 100-tab pack = £3.96; 80 mg (pink), 100-tab pack = £5.87; 200 mg, 30-tab pack = £4.15. Label: 8

PoM Sotacor® (Bristol-Myers)

Tablets, sotalol hydrochloride 80 mg, net price 28-tab pack = £3.49; 160 mg, 28-tab pack = £6.89. Label: 8

Injection, sotalol hydrochloride 10 mg/mL. Net price 4-mL amp = £1.76

With diuretic
Note. Increased risk of hypokalaemia if combined with thiazide or loop diuretic (see Cautions above)

PoM Sotazide® (Bristol-Myers)

Tablets, blue, sotalol hydrochloride 160 mg, hydrochlorothiazide 25 mg. Net price 28-tab pack = £7.12. Label: 8

Dose: hypertension, 1 tablet daily, increased to 2 daily if necessary

PoM Tolerzide® (Bristol-Myers)

Tablets, lilac, sotalol hydrochloride 80 mg, hydrochlorothiazide 12.5 mg. Net price 28-tab pack = £4.05. Label: 8

Dose: hypertension, 1 tablet daily

TIMOLOL MALEATE

Indications: see under Dose

Cautions; Contra-indications; Side-effects: see under Propranolol Hydrochloride

Dose: hypertension, initially 5 mg twice daily or 10 mg once daily; max. 60 mg daily
Angina, initially 5 mg 2–3 times daily, maintenance 15–45 mg daily
Prophylaxis after infarction, initially 5 mg twice daily, increased after 2 days to 10 mg twice daily starting 7 to 28 days after infarction
Migraine prophylaxis, 10–20 mg daily

PoM Betim® (Leo)

Tablets, scored, timolol maleate 10 mg. Net price 20 = £1.71. Label: 8

PoM Blocadren® (MSD)

Tablets, blue, scored, timolol maleate 10 mg. Net price 20 = £1.75. Label: 8

With diuretic
PoM Moducren® (Morson)

Tablets, blue, scored, timolol maleate 10 mg, co amilozide 2.5/25 (amiloride hydrochloride 2.5 mg, hydrochlorothiazide 25 mg). Net price 28-tab pack = £8.00. Label: 8

Dose: hypertension, 1–2 tablets daily as a single dose

PoM Prestim® (Leo)

Tablets, scored, timolol maleate 10 mg, bendrofluazide 2.5 mg. Net price 20 = £2.72. Label: 8

Dose: hypertension, 1–2 tablets daily; max. 4 daily

PoM Prestim Forte® (Leo)

Tablets, scored, timolol maleate 20 mg, bendrofluazide 5 mg. Net price 20 = £5.73. Label: 8

Dose: hypertension, ½–2 tablets daily in single c divided doses

2.5   Antihypertensive therapy

Antihypertensive therapy has improved the outloo for patients with high blood pressure by decreasin the frequency of stroke, heart failure, and renal fai ure: treatment also reduces the incidence of coro nary events.

All patients should be given advice on non-phar macological measures to reduce high blood pres sure, including achieving ideal body weigh avoiding high alcohol intake and high sodiu intake, and taking regular exercise. Cigarett smoking has a powerful adverse effect on cardi vascular risk in hypertensive subjects, and th importance of stopping should be emphasised.

The recommendations of the British Hypertension Society are that specific antihypertensive treatment is indicated:

Where the initial blood pressure is *systolic ≥ 200 mmHg or diastolic ≥ 110 mmHg, treat* if these values are confirmed on 3 separate occasions over 1-2 weeks (**important:** if very severe or in presence of associated conditions such as heart failure, immediate treatment needed—see also below);

Where the initial blood pressure is *systolic 160–199 mmHg or diastolic 90–109 mmHg* (or when higher initial values fall to this range) take one of the following courses of action:

— if *vascular complications or end-organ damage* (e.g. left ventricular hypertrophy, renal impairment) *or diabetes* present, **treat** if *systolic ≥ 160 mmHg or diastolic ≥ 90 mmHg* confirmed on at least 3 separate occasions;

— if *no vascular complications, no end-organ damage and no diabetes* repeat blood pressure measurements at monthly intervals for 3–6 months and **treat** if the average value during this period is *systolic ≥ 160 mmHg or diastolic ≥ 100 mmHg*;

—if the average value is *systolic < 160 mmHg and diastolic 90–99 mmHg* treatment may be withheld but continue to monitor; however **consider treatment** if sustained in this range in older patients (over 60 years), and in those with a particularly high risk of cardiovascular complications (e.g. strong family history).

The usual aim should be to reduce the diastolic pressure to below 90 mmHg and the systolic pressure to below 160 mmHg.

Malignant (or accelerated) hypertension or very severe hypertension (diastolic blood pressure > 140 mmHg) requires urgent treatment in hospital but is not an indication for parenteral antihypertensive therapy. Normally treatment should be by mouth with a beta-blocker (atenolol or labetalol) or a calcium-channel blocker (nifedipine). Within the first 24 hours the diastolic blood pressure should be reduced to 100–110 mmHg. Over the next two or three days blood pressure should be normalised by using beta-blockers, calcium-channel blockers, diuretics, vasodilators, or angiotensin-converting enzyme inhibitors. Very rapid falls in blood pressure can cause reduced cerebral perfusion leading to cerebral infarction and blindness, a reduction in renal perfusion causing a deterioration in renal function, and myocardial ischaemia. Parenteral antihypertensive drugs are, therefore, hardly ever necessary. (On the rare occasions when a parenteral antihypertensive is necessary, sodium nitroprusside by infusion is the drug of choice.)

In moderate to severe hypertension (diastolic blood pressure > 110 mmHg) or in patients with vascular complications, drugs are best added 'stepwise' until control has been achieved; an attempt can then be made to 'step down' treatment under supervision. In uncomplicated mild hypertension (diastolic blood pressure < 110 mmHg), drugs may be substituted rather than added. Whenever the blood pressure is consistently well below the target level it is reasonable to try stepping down treatment cautiously, by gradually decreasing the dose or number of drugs, under close supervision. In some patients, usually those with mild hypertension and no end organ damage, it may even be possible to withdraw treatment completely; any subsequent rise in blood pressure may be delayed for several months, therefore blood pressure should be monitored indefinitely.

The strategy for reducing blood pressure is probably best as follows:

1. *Non-drug treatment*—obesity, high alcohol intake, high salt intake, and lack of regular exercise, may elevate blood pressure and these should be corrected.

2. *Diuretic therapy.* The optimum dose of a thiazide (section 2.2.1) used to treat hypertension is the lowest possible dose; higher doses do not have a major additional anti-hypertensive effect, but do cause more metabolic side-effects. Potassium supplements or potassium-sparing diuretics are usually not necessary in the routine treatment of hypertension, but plasma potassium concentration should be checked 3 to 4 weeks after starting treatment.

3. *Beta-adrenoceptor blocking drugs* (section 2.4) are used with a thiazide where they are not effective alone.

4(a). *Calcium-channel blockers* have antihypertensive efficacy broadly similar to that of thiazides or beta-blockers. Their safety during long-term treatment is less well established; they should therefore be considered for hypertension only when thiazides and beta-blockers are contra-indicated, not tolerated, or fail to control blood pressure. There are **important** differences between calcium-channel blockers (see section 2.6.2).

4(b). *ACE inhibitors* (section 2.5.5) may cause a precipitate drop in blood pressure in patients with renal impairment and/or receiving diuretic therapy; they should be given in low initial doses and where possible diuretic therapy should be omitted for a few days before starting.

5. *Other drugs*—vasodilators (hydralazine, minoxidil), alpha-blockers (prazosin, terazosin, doxazosin), and centrally acting drugs (methyldopa) are generally reserved for patients whose blood pressure is not controlled by, or who have contra-indications to, the drugs already mentioned.

SYSTOLIC HYPERTENSION. Isolated systolic hypertension (systolic blood pressure > 160 mmHg, diastolic < 90 mmHg) is associated with an increased risk of stroke and coronary events, particularly in those over 60 years. Systolic blood pressure averaging 160 mmHg or higher over 3 to 6 months (despite appropriate non-drug treatment) should be lowered in those over 60 years, even if diastolic hypertension is absent. Patients with severe postural hypotension should not receive blood pressure lowering drugs. The regimen proven effective is a low dose of a thiazide, with addition of a beta-blocker when necessary. Isolated systolic hypertension is uncommon in younger patients but by extrapolation it seems reasonable to recommend that a threshold pressure of 160 mmHg should also be an indication for treatment.

HYPERTENSION IN PREGNANCY. It is important to control blood pressure in pregnancy. High blood pressure may be due to pre-existing essential hypertension or to pre-eclampsia. Oral methyldopa is safe in pregnancy. Beta-blockers are effective and safe in the third trimester but may cause intra-uterine growth retardation when used from earlier in pregnancy. Hydralazine by intravenous injection can be used to control hypertensive crises.

HYPERTENSION IN THE ELDERLY. Antihypertensive therapy reduces the incidence of cardiovascular complications substantially in elderly hypertensive subjects. The benefit is evident up to at least 85 years of age, and it is probably inappropriate to apply a strict age limit when coming to a decision on drug therapy. Elderly subjects who have a good outlook for longevity from other points of view should have their blood pressure lowered if they are hypertensive. The criteria for treatment are diastolic blood pressure averaging 90 mmHg or higher *or* systolic averaging 160 mmHg or higher over 3 to 6 months observation (despite appropriate non-drug treatment). A low dose of a thiazide is the clear drug of first choice, with addition of a beta-blocker when necessary.

2.5.1   Vasodilator antihypertensive drugs

These are potent drugs, especially when used in combination with a beta-blocker and a thiazide. **Important:** for a warning on the hazards of a very rapid fall in blood pressure, see section 2.5.

Diazoxide is used by intravenous injection in hypertensive emergencies.

Hydralazine given by mouth is a useful adjunct to other treatment, but when used alone causes tachycardia and fluid retention. Side-effects can be few if the dose is kept below 100 mg daily, but systemic lupus erythematosus should be suspected if there is unexplained weight loss, arthritis, or any other unexplained ill health.

Sodium nitroprusside is given by intravenous infusion to control severe hypertensive crises.

Minoxidil should be reserved for the treatment of severe hypertension resistant to other drugs. Vasodilatation is accompanied by increased cardiac output and tachycardia and the patients develop fluid retention. For this reason a beta-blocker and a diuretic (usually frusemide, in high dosage) are mandatory. Hypertrichosis is troublesome and renders this drug unsuitable for women.

Prazosin, doxazosin, and terazosin (section 2.5.4) have alpha-blocking and vasodilator properties.

DIAZOXIDE
Indications: acute treatment of severe hypertension associated with renal disease (but see section 2.5); hypoglycaemia, see section 6.1.4
Cautions: ischaemic heart disease, pregnancy, labour, impaired renal function; **interactions:** Appendix 1 (diazoxide)
Side-effects: tachycardia, hyperglycaemia, sodium and water retention

Dose: by rapid intravenous injection (less than 30 seconds), 1–3 mg/kg to max. single dose of 150 mg (see below); may be repeated after 5–15 minutes if required
Note. Single doses of 300 mg have been associated with angina and with myocardial and cerebral infarction

PoM **Eudemine®** (Link)
Injection, diazoxide 15 mg/mL. Net price 20-mL amp = £18.90

HYDRALAZINE HYDROCHLORIDE
Indications: moderate to severe hypertension, with beta-blocker and thiazide; hypertensive crisis (but see section 2.5)
Cautions: reduce initial dose in renal impairment coronary artery disease (may provoke angina, avoid after myocardial infarction until stabilised), cerebrovascular disease; over-rapid blood pressure reduction is occasionally encountered even with low parenteral doses; pregnancy (see also Appendix 4), breast-feeding; **interactions:** Appendix 1 (hydralazine)
Contra-indications: idiopathic systemic lupus erythematosus, severe tachycardia, high output heart failure, myocardial insufficiency due to mechanical obstruction, cor pulmonale, dissecting aortic aneurysm; porphyria (see section 9.8.2)
Side-effects: tachycardia, fluid retention, nausea, and vomiting; headache; systemic lupus erythematosus-like syndrome after long-term therapy with over 100 mg daily (or less in women) (see also note above); rarely rashes, fever, changes in blood count, peripheral neuritis; blood disorders reported (including haemolytic anaemia)
Dose: by mouth, 25 mg twice daily, increased to a max. of 50 mg twice daily (see notes above)
By slow intravenous injection, 5–10 mg over 20 minutes; may be repeated after 20–30 minutes (see Cautions)
By intravenous infusion, initially 200–300 micrograms/minute; maintenance usually 50–150 micrograms/minute

PoM **Hydralazine** (Non-proprietary)
Tablets, hydralazine hydrochloride 25 mg, net price 20 = 23p; 50 mg, 20 = 48p
PoM **Apresoline®** (Ciba)
Tablets, both s/c, hydralazine hydrochloride 25 mg (yellow), net price 20 = 36p; 50 mg (violet), 20 = 70p
Additives: include gluten
Injection, powder for reconstitution, hydralazine hydrochloride. Net price 20–mg amp = 32p

MINOXIDIL
Indications: severe hypertension, in addition to a diuretic and a beta-blocker
Cautions: see notes above; angina; after myocardial infarction (until stabilised); lower doses in dialysis patients; pregnancy; **interactions:** Appendix 1 (minoxidil)
Contra-indications: phaeochromocytoma; porphyria (see section 9.8.2)
Side-effects: sodium and water retention; weight gain, peripheral oedema, tachycardia, hypertrichosis, reversible rise in creatinine and blood urea nitrogen

occasionally, gastro-intestinal disturbances, breast tenderness, rashes

Dose: initially 5 mg (elderly, 2.5 mg) daily, in 1–2 doses, increased by 5–10 mg every 3 or more days; max. usually 50 mg daily

PoM **Loniten**® (Upjohn)
Tablets, all scored, minoxidil 2.5 mg, net price 100-tab pack = £12.34; 5 mg, 100-tab pack = £21.98; 10 mg, 100-tab pack = £42.62

SODIUM NITROPRUSSIDE

Indications: hypertensive crisis (but see section 2.5); controlled hypotension in surgery; acute or chronic heart failure

Cautions: hypothyroidism, severe renal impairment, ischaemic heart disease, impaired cerebral circulation, elderly; monitor blood pressure and plasma-cyanide concentration; **interactions:** Appendix 1 (nitroprusside)

WITHDRAWAL. Normal duration of treatment should not exceed 72 hours (terminate over at least 10–30 minutes to avoid rebound)

Contra-indications: severe hepatic impairment; vitamin B$_{12}$ deficiency; Leber's optic atrophy; compensatory hypertension

Side-effects: associated with over rapid reduction in blood pressure (reduce infusion rate): headache, dizziness, nausea, retching, abdominal pain, perspiration, palpitations, apprehension, retrosternal discomfort; occasionally reduced platelet count, acute transient phlebitis

CYANIDE. Side-effects caused by excessive plasma concentration of the cyanide metabolite include tachycardia, sweating, hyperventilation, arrhythmias, marked metabolic acidosis (discontinue and give antidote, see p. 23)

Dose: hypertensive crisis, in patients not already receiving antihypertensives, *by intravenous infusion,* 0.3 micrograms/kg/minute, then adjusted; usual range 0.5–6 micrograms/kg/minute (20–400 micrograms/minute); max. 8 micrograms/kg/minute—stop if not marked response in 10 minutes (if response obtained give for few hours only to avoid cyanide risk); lower doses for patients already being treated with antihypertensives

Lower doses should also be employed for controlled hypotension in surgery (max. 1.5 micrograms/kg/minute)

Heart failure, *by intravenous infusion,* initially 10–15 micrograms/minute, increased every 5–10 minutes as necessary; usual range 10–200 micrograms/minute; max. 280 micrograms/minute (4 micrograms/kg/minute)

PoM **Sodium Nitroprusside** (Non-proprietary)
Intravenous solution, sodium nitroprusside 10 mg/mL. For dilution and use as an infusion. 5-mL vial available from David Bull, CP
PoM **Nipride**® (Roche)
Infusion, sodium nitroprusside 50-mg amp (with glucose 5% for reconstitution). Net price = £3.89

2.5.2   Centrally acting antihypertensive drugs

This group is largely falling from use, but includes **methyldopa**, which has the advantage of being safe in asthmatics, in heart failure, and in pregnancy. Side-effects are minimised if the daily dose is kept below 1 g.

Clonidine has the disadvantage that sudden withdrawal may cause a hypertensive crisis. Reserpine and rauwolfia are no longer used in Britain.

CLONIDINE HYDROCHLORIDE

Indications: hypertension (for use in migraine, see section 4.7.4.2)

Cautions: must be withdrawn gradually to avoid hypertensive crisis; Raynaud's syndrome or other occlusive peripheral vascular disease; history of depression; avoid in porphyria (see section 9.8.2); **interactions:** Appendix 1 (clonidine)

DRIVING. Drowsiness may affect performance of skilled tasks (e.g. driving); effects of alcohol may be enhanced

Side-effects: dry mouth, sedation, depression, fluid retention, bradycardia, Raynaud's phenomenon, headache, dizziness, euphoria, nocturnal unrest, rash, nausea, constipation, rarely impotence

Dose: by mouth, 50–100 micrograms 3 times daily, increased every second or third day; max. daily dose usually 1.2 mg

By slow intravenous injection, 150–300 micrograms; max. 750 micrograms in 24 hours

PoM **Catapres**® (Boehringer Ingelheim)
Tablets, both scored, clonidine hydrochloride 100 micrograms, net price 100-tab pack = £7.00; 300 micrograms, 100-tab pack = £16.30. Label: 3, 8
Injection, clonidine hydrochloride 150 micrograms/mL. Net price 1-mL amp = 29p
PoM **Dixarit**® (migraine), see section 4.7.4.2

Modified release
PoM **Catapres**® **Perlongets** (Boehringer Ingelheim)
Capsules, m/r, red/yellow, clonidine hydrochloride 250 micrograms. Net price 56-cap pack = £13.89. Label: 3, 8, 25
Dose: usually 1 capsule in the evening; 2–3 capsules daily (1 morning and 1–2 evening) if necessary

METHYLDOPA

Indications: hypertension, in conjunction with diuretic; hypertensive crisis when immediate effect not necessary

Cautions: positive direct Coombs' test in up to 20% of patients (may affect blood cross-matching); interference with laboratory tests; reduce initial dose in renal impairment; blood counts and liver-function tests advised; **interactions:** Appendix 1 (methyldopa)

DRIVING. Drowsiness may affect performance of skilled tasks (e.g. driving); effects of alcohol may be enhanced

Contra-indications: history of depression, active liver disease, phaeochromocytoma; porphyria (see section 9.8.2)

Side-effects: dry mouth, sedation, depression, drowsiness, diarrhoea, fluid retention, failure of ejaculation, liver damage, haemolytic anaemia, lupus erythematosus-like syndrome, parkinsonism, rashes, nasal stuffiness

Dose: by mouth, 250 mg 2–3 times daily, gradually increased at intervals of 2 or more days; max. daily dose 3 g; ELDERLY 125 mg twice daily initially, gradually increased; max. daily dose 2 g (see also notes above)

By intravenous infusion, methyldopate hydrochloride 250–500 mg, repeated after 6 hours if required

PoM **Methyldopa** (Non-proprietary)

Tablets, coated, methyldopa (anhydrous) 125 mg, net price 20 = 35p; 250 mg, 20 = 60p; 500 mg, 20 = £1.24. Label: 3, 8

Available from APS, Ashbourne (Metalpha®), Berk (Dopamet®), Cox, CP, Hillcross, K Pharm.

PoM **Aldomet®** (MSD)

Tablets, all yellow, f/c, methyldopa (anhydrous) 125 mg, net price 20 = 34p; 250 mg, 20 = 68p; 500 mg, 20 = £1.38. Label: 3, 8

Suspension, methyldopa 250 mg/5mL. Net price 200 mL = £3.96. Label: 3, 8

Injection, methyldopate hydrochloride 50 mg/mL. Net price 5-mL amp = £2.31

With diuretic
PoM **Hydromet®** (MSD)

Tablets, pink, f/c, methyldopa (anhydrous) 250 mg, hydrochlorothiazide 15 mg. Net price 20 = £1.52. Label: 3, 8

2.5.3   Adrenergic neurone blocking drugs

These drugs prevent the release of noradrenaline from postganglionic adrenergic neurones. Guanethidine also depletes the nerve endings of noradrenaline. These drugs do not control supine blood pressure and may cause postural hypotension. For this reason they have largely fallen from use, but may be necessary with other therapy in resistant hypertension.

GUANETHIDINE MONOSULPHATE

Indications: moderate to severe hypertension that has failed to respond adequately to other antihypertensives, in conjunction with a diuretic or a vasodilator antihypertensive

Cautions: postural hypotension may cause falls in elderly; coronary or cerebral arteriosclerosis, asthma, history of peptic ulceration; pregnancy; **interactions:** Appendix 1 (adrenergic neurone blockers)

Contra-indications: phaeochromocytoma, renal failure, heart failure

Side-effects: postural hypotension, failure of ejaculation, fluid retention, nasal congestion, headache, diarrhoea, drowsiness

Dose: by mouth, 10 mg daily, increased by 10 mg at weekly intervals; usual daily dose 25–50 mg

By intramuscular injection, 10–20 mg, repeated after 3 hours if required

PoM **Ismelin®** (Ciba)

Tablets, guanethidine monosulphate 10 mg, net price 20 = 46p; 25 mg (pink), 28-tab pack = £1.44

Additives: include gluten

Injection, guanethidine monosulphate 10 mg/mL. Net price 1-mL amp = 23p

BETHANIDINE SULPHATE

Indications; Cautions; Contra-indications; Side-effects: see under Guanethidine Monosulphate (except diarrhoea)

Dose: 10 mg (elderly 5 mg) 3 times daily after food, increased by 5 mg at intervals; max. daily dose 200 mg

PoM **Bendogen®** (Lagap)

Tablets, scored, bethanidine sulphate 10 mg, net price 100-tab pack = £15.14. Label: 21

DEBRISOQUINE

Indications; Cautions; Contra-indications; Side-effects: see under Guanethidine Monosulphate (except diarrhoea)

Dose: 10 mg 1–2 times daily, increased by 10 mg every 3 days; usual range 20–60 mg daily (120 mg or higher in severe hypertension)

PoM **Declinax®** (Roche)

Tablets, scored, debrisoquine (as sulphate) 10 mg, net price 100-tab pack = £4.26

2.5.4   Alpha-adrenoceptor blocking drugs

Prazosin has post-synaptic alpha-blocking and vasodilator properties and rarely causes tachycardia. It may, however, cause a rapid reduction in blood pressure after the first dose and should be introduced with caution. **Doxazosin** and **terazosin** have properties similar to those of prazosin.

Indoramin is also an effective alpha-blocker but has many side-effects.

PROSTATIC HYPERPLASIA. Prazosin, indoramin and terazosin are also indicated for benign prostatic hyperplasia (see section 7.4.1).

ALFUZOSIN

See section 7.4.1

DOXAZOSIN

Indications: hypertension, if necessary in conjunction with thiazide or beta-blocker

Cautions: care with initial dose (postural hypotension); **interactions:** Appendix 1 (alpha-blockers)

Side-effects: postural hypotension (rarely associated with fainting); dizziness, vertigo, headache, fatigue, asthenia, oedema

Dose: 1 mg daily, increased after 1–2 weeks to 2 mg daily, and thereafter to 4 mg daily, if necessary; max. 16 mg daily

PoM **Cardura®** (Invicta)

Tablets, doxazosin (as mesylate) 1 mg, net price 28-tab pack = £10.56; 2 mg, 28-tab pack = £14.08; 4 mg, 28-tab pack = £17.60

INDORAMIN

Indications: see preparations below

Cautions: avoid alcohol (enhances rate and extent of absorption); control incipient heart failure with diuretics and digoxin; hepatic or renal impairment; elderly patients; Parkinson's disease; epilepsy (convulsions in *animal* studies); history of depression; **interactions:** Appendix 1 (alpha-blockers)

DRIVING. Drowsiness may affect performance of skilled tasks (e.g. driving); effects of alcohol may be enhanced

Contra-indications: established heart failure; patients receiving MAOIs

Side-effects: sedation; also dizziness, depression, failure of ejaculation, dry mouth, nasal congestion, extrapyramidal effects, weight gain

Dose: see preparations below

PoM **Baratol®** (Monmouth)

Tablets, both f/c, indoramin (as hydrochloride) 25 mg (blue), net price 100-tab pack = £20.91; 50 mg (green, scored), 100-tab pack = £37.08. Label: 2

Dose: hypertension, usually in conjunction with thiazide or beta-blocker, initially 25 mg twice daily, increased by 25–50 mg daily at intervals of 2 weeks; max. daily dose 200 mg in 2–3 divided doses

Prostatic hyperplasia
PoM **Doralese®:** see section 7.4.1

PRAZOSIN HYDROCHLORIDE

Indications: see under Dose

Cautions: first dose may cause collapse due to hypotension (therefore should be taken on retiring to bed); elderly; reduce initial dose in renal impairment; **interactions:** Appendix 1 (alpha-blockers)

Contra-indications: not recommended for congestive heart failure due to mechanical obstruction (e.g. aortic stenosis)

Side-effects: postural hypotension, drowsiness, weakness, dizziness, headache, lack of energy, nausea, palpitations; urinary frequency, incontinence reported

Dose: hypertension, 500 micrograms 2–3 times daily, the initial dose on retiring to bed at night (to avoid collapse, see Cautions); increased to 1 mg 2–3 times daily after 3–7 days; further increased if necessary to max. 20 mg daily

Congestive heart failure, 500 micrograms 2–4 times daily (initial dose at bedtime, see above), increasing to 4 mg daily in divided doses; maintenance 4–20 mg daily (but rarely used)

Raynaud's syndrome, initially 500 micrograms twice daily (initial dose at bedtime, see above); maintenance 1–2 mg twice daily

Benign prostatic hyperplasia, see section 7.4.1

PoM **Hypovase®** (Invicta)

Tablets, prazosin hydrochloride 500 micrograms, net price 56-tab pack = £2.64; 1 mg (orange, scored), 56-tab pack = £3.41; 2 mg (scored), 56-tab pack = £4.63; 5 mg (scored), 56-tab pack = £9.98; starter pack of 8 × 500–microgram tabs with 32 × 1–mg tabs = £3.19. Label: 3, counselling, see dose above

*Note.*Hypovase tablets for benign prostatic hyperplasia are termed Hypovase® (Benign Prostatic Hypertrophy), see section 7.4.1; prazosin tablets also available from APS, Ashbourne (Alphavase®), Cox, Hillcross, K Pharm., Norton

---

TERAZOSIN

Indications: mild to moderate hypertension

Cautions: first dose may cause collapse due to hypotension (within 30–90 minutes, therefore should be taken on retiring to bed) (may also occur with rapid dose increase); **interactions:** Appendix 1 (alpha-blockers)

Side-effects: dizziness, lack of energy, peripheral oedema; urinary frequency reported

Dose: hypertension, 1 mg at bedtime (compliance with bedtime dose important, see Cautions); dose doubled after 7 days if necessary; usual maintenance dose 2–10 mg once daily; more than 20 mg daily rarely improves efficacy

Benign prostatic hyperplasia, see section 7.4.1

PoM **Hytrin®** (Abbott)

Tablets, terazosin (as hydrochloride) 2 mg (yellow), net price 28-tab pack = £12.55; 5 mg (tan), 28-tab pack = £18.89; 10 mg (blue), 28-tab pack = £26.59: starter pack of 7 × 1–mg tabs with 21 × 2–mg tabs = £13.00. Label: 3, counselling, see dose above

PoM Hytrin BPH® (for benign prostatic hyperplasia), see section 7.4.1

PHAEOCHROMOCYTOMA

Phenoxybenzamine is a powerful alpha-blocker with many side-effects. It is used with a beta-blocker in the short-term management of severe hypertensive episodes associated with phaeochromocytoma; it is also used in the management of severe shock unresponsive to conventional therapy.

Phentolamine is a short-acting alpha-blocker used rarely as a suppression test for phaeochromocytoma.

PHENOXYBENZAMINE HYDROCHLORIDE

Indications: phaeochromocytoma (see notes above)

Cautions: elderly; congestive heart failure; severe heart disease (see also Contra-indications); cerebrovascular disease (avoid if history of cerebro vascular accident); renal impairment; carcinogenic in *animals*; pregnancy; avoid in porphyria (see section 9.8.2); avoid infusion in hypovolaemia; avoid extravasation (irritant to tissues)

Contra-indications: history of cerebrovascular accident; during recovery period after myocardial infarction (usually 3–4 weeks)

Side-effects: postural hypotension with dizziness and marked compensatory tachycardia, lassitude, nasal congestion, miosis, inhibition of ejaculation; rarely gastro-intestinal disturbances; decreased sweating and dry mouth after intravenous infusion; idiosyncratic profound hypotension within few minutes of starting infusion

Dose: by mouth, phaeochromocytoma, 10 mg daily, increased by 10 mg daily; usual dose 1–2 mg/kg daily in 2 divided doses

---

PoM Dibenyline® (Forley)

Capsules, red/white, phenoxybenzamine hydrochloride 10 mg. Net price 30-cap pack = £20.22

Injection concentrate, phenoxybenzamine hydrochloride 50 mg/mL. To be diluted before use. Net price 3 × 2-mL amp = £43.88 (hosp. only)

Dose: by intravenous infusion (preferably through large vein), phaeochromocytoma and adjunct in severe shock, 1 mg/kg daily in 200 mL physiological saline over at least 2 hours; do not repeat within 24 hours (intensive care facilities needed)

CAUTION. Owing to risk of contact sensitisation doctors, nurses, and other health workers should avoid contamination of hands

PHENTOLAMINE MESYLATE

Indications: hypertensive episodes due to phaeochromocytoma e.g. during surgery; diagnosis of phaeochromocytoma

Cautions: monitor blood pressure (avoid in hypotension), heart rate; gastritis, peptic ulcer; elderly; **interactions:** Appendix 1 (alpha-blockers)

ASTHMA. Presence of sulphites in ampoules may (especially in patients with asthma) lead to hypersensitivity (with bronchospasm and shock)

Contra-indications: hypotension; history of myocardial infarction; coronary insufficiency, angina, or other evidence of coronary artery disease

Side-effects: postural hypotension, tachycardia, dizziness; nausea and vomiting, diarrhoea, nasal congestion; also acute or prolonged hypotension, angina, chest pain, arrhythmias

Dose: hypertensive episodes, *by intravenous injection*, 2–5 mg repeated if necessary

Diagnosis of phaeochromocytoma, consult data sheet

PoM Rogitine® (Ciba)

Injection, phentolamine mesylate 10 mg/mL. Net price 1-mL amp = 27p

2.5.5   Angiotensin-converting enzyme inhibitors

(ACE inhibitors)

Angiotensin-converting enzyme inhibitors inhibit the conversion of angiotensin I to angiotensin II. They are effective and generally well tolerated.

HYPERTENSION. ACE inhibitors should be considered for hypertension when thiazides and beta-blockers are contra-indicated, not tolerated, or fail to control blood pressure. All may cause *very rapid falls of blood pressure* in some patients. Therefore where possible diuretic therapy should be stopped for a few days before initiating therapy and the first dose should preferably be given at bedtime.

HEART FAILURE. ACE inhibitors have a valuable role in heart failure when used as an adjunct to diuretics and, where appropriate, digoxin. They have been shown to improve the prognosis substantially, and in this respect are superior to regimens such as modified-release nitrates with hydralazine. Introduction of an ACE inhibitor should be considered

when heart failure is not completely controlled by frusemide 80 mg daily (or an equivalent dose of another loop diuretic). To avoid *dangerous hyperkalaemia*, any potassium-sparing diuretic should be omitted from the diuretic regimen before introducing an ACE inhibitor, changing to the loop diuretic alone; potassium supplements should also be discontinued. *Profound first-dose hypotension* may occur when ACE inhibitors are introduced to patients with heart failure who are already taking a high dose of a loop diuretic (e.g. frusemide 80 mg daily or higher). Temporary withdrawal of the loop diuretic reduces the risk, but may cause severe rebound pulmonary oedema. The ACE inhibitor should therefore be started at very low dosage (e.g. captopril 6.25 mg), with the patient recumbent and under close medical supervision, and with facilities to treat profound hypotension. In these circumstances and in other special risk groups (see below) the patient should be admitted to hospital for initiation.

INITIATION IN HOSPITAL. ACE inhibitor therapy for heart failure should be initiated under close medical supervision (in hospital *in severe heart failure*). Initiation in hospital is also recommended for patients with *mild to moderate heart failure*:

receiving multiple or high-dose diuretic therapy (e.g. more than 80 mg of frusemide daily or its equivalent);

with hypovolaemia;

with hyponatraemia (plasma sodium below 130 mmol/litre);

with pre-existing hypotension (systolic blood pressure below 90 mmHg);

with unstable heart failure;

with renal impairment (plasma creatinine above 150 micromol/litre;

receiving high-dose vasodilator therapy;

aged 70 years or more.

RENAL IMPAIRMENT. ACE inhibitors occasionally cause impairment of renal function which may progress and become severe. At particular risk are those with pre-existing renal disease or impairment, the elderly, and those with bilateral renal artery stenosis (or stenosis of the artery supplying a single functioning kidney). Concomitant treatment with NSAIDs increases the risk of renal damage, and potassium-sparing diuretics or use of potassium-containing salt substitutes increase the risk of hyperkalaemia. Renal function and electrolytes should be checked before starting an ACE inhibitor and monitored during treatment.

ACE inhibitors should be used with **particular caution** in patients with peripheral vascular disease or generalised atherosclerosis, as such patients may have clinically silent renovascular disease.

PREGNANCY. ACE inhibitors are contra-indicated in pregnancy, and should be avoided in patients who may become pregnant.

COMBINATION PRODUCTS. A number of products incorporating an ACE inhibitor with a thiazide diuretic are now available. Use of these combination products should be reserved for patients whose blood pressure has not responded to a thiazide diuretic or an ACE inhibitor alone (see also comments above).

CAPTOPRIL

Indications: mild to moderate essential hypertension alone or with thiazide therapy and severe hypertension resistant to other treatment (but see cautions and notes above); congestive heart failure (adjunct); following myocardial infarction, see dose; diabetic nephropathy (microalbuminuria greater than 30 mg/day) in insulin-dependent diabetes

Cautions: diuretics (**important:** see notes above); first doses may cause hypotension especially in patients taking diuretics, on a low-sodium diet, on dialysis, or dehydrated; monitor renal function before and during treatment; **reduce dose** in renal impairment (urinary protein estimations needed—see also notes above) but specialised role in some forms of renal disease; collagen vascular disease (see Symptom Complex under Side-effects); in dialysis patients avoid combination of ACE inhibitor therapy with use of high-flux polyacrylonitrile membranes (anaphylactoid reactions reported); breast-feeding (see Appendix 5); **interactions:** Appendix 1 (ACE inhibitors)

Contra-indications: hypersensitivity to ACE inhibitors; known or suspected renovascular disease; aortic stenosis or outflow tract obstruction; pregnancy (see notes above and Appendix 4); porphyria (see section 9.8.2)

Side-effects: hypotension (see Cautions), dizziness, headache, fatigue, asthenia, nausea (occasionally vomiting), diarrhoea (occasionally constipation), muscle cramps, persistent dry cough, throat discomfort, voice changes, taste alteration (may be associated with weight loss), stomatitis, dyspepsia, abdominal pain, renal impairment (see Cautions and notes above); hyperkalaemia (more common in renal impairment, see notes above); angioedema, urticaria, rashes (erythema multiforme and toxic epidermal necrolysis reported), and hypersensitivity reactions (see below for symptom complex), blood disorders (including thrombocytopenia, neutropenia and agranulocytosis); other side-effects reported include upper respiratory tract symptoms, hyponatraemia, tachycardia, palpitations, arrhythmias, myocardial infarction and cerebrovascular accident (possibly associated with severe hypotension), back pain, flushing, jaundice (hepatocellular or cholestatic), pancreatitis, sleep disturbances, nervousness, mood changes, paraesthesia, impotence, onycholysis, alopecia

SYMPTOM COMPLEX. A symptom complex has been reported for ACE inhibitors which may include fever, serositis, vasculitis, myalgia, arthralgia, positive antinuclear antibody, raised erythrocyte sedimentation rate,

eosinophilia, leucocytosis; rash, photosensitivity or other skin reactions may occur.

Dose: hypertension, used alone, initially 12.5 mg twice daily; if used in addition to diuretic (see notes), in elderly, or in renal impairment, initially 6.25 mg twice daily (first dose at bedtime); usual maintenance dose 25 mg twice daily; max. 50 mg twice daily (rarely 3 times daily in severe hypertension)

Heart failure (adjunct), initially 6.25–12.5 mg under close medical supervision (see notes above); usual maintenance dose 25 mg 2–3 times daily

Prophylaxis after infarction in clinically stable patients with asymptomatic or symptomatic left ventricular dysfunction (radionuclide ventriculography or echocardiography undertaken before initiation), initially 6.25 mg, starting as early as 3 days after infarction, then increased over several weeks to 150 mg daily (if tolerated) in divided doses

Diabetic nephropathy, 75–100 mg daily in divided doses; if further blood pressure reduction required, other antihypertensives may be used in conjunction with captopril; in severe renal impairment, initially 12.5 mg twice daily (if concomitant diuretic therapy required, loop diuretic rather than thiazide should be chosen)

PoM Capoten® (Squibb)

Tablets, captopril 12.5 mg (scored), net price 100 = £18.86; 25 mg, 56-tab pack = £12.03, 100-tab pack = £21.49; 50 mg (scored), 56-tab pack = £20.50, 100-tab pack = £36.61 (also available as Acepril®)

With diuretic

Note. For mild to moderate hypertension in patients stabilised on the individual components in the same proportions

PoM Capozide® (Squibb)

LS tablets, scored, captopril 25 mg, hydrochlorothiazide 12.5 mg. Net price 28-tab pack = £11.25

Tablets, scored, captopril 50 mg, hydrochlorothiazide 25 mg. Net price 28-tab pack = £14.14 (also available as Acezide®)

CILAZAPRIL

Indications: essential hypertension (but see cautions and notes above)

Cautions; Contra-indications; Side-effects: see under Captopril and notes above

Dose: initially, 1 mg once daily; usual range 1–2.5 mg once daily; if used in addition to diuretic (see notes), in elderly, or in renal impairment, initially 500 micrograms once daily; if patient also has congestive heart failure, initially 500 micrograms once daily under close medical supervision (see notes above); max. 5 mg daily

Note. If possible discontinue diuretic for 2–3 days beforehand (see also notes above)

PoM **Vascace®** (Roche)

Tablets, all f/c, cilazapril 250 micrograms (pink), net price 28-tab pack = £3.87; 500 micrograms (white), 28-tab pack = £4.10; 1 mg (yellow), 28-tab pack = £7.06; 2.5 mg (pink), 28-tab pack = £10.67; 5 mg (brown), 28-tab pack = £14.95

ENALAPRIL MALEATE

Indications: all grades of essential hypertension (but see cautions and notes above); treatment of congestive heart failure (adjunct); prevention of symptomatic heart failure and prevention of coronary ischaemic events in patients with left ventricular dysfunction

Cautions; Contra-indications; Side-effects: see under Captopril and notes above

Dose: hypertension, used alone, initially 5 mg daily; if used in addition to diuretic (see notes), in elderly patients, or in renal impairment, initially 2.5 mg daily; usual maintenance dose 10–20 mg daily; max. 40 mg daily

Heart failure (adjunct), asymptomatic left ventricular dysfunction, initially 2.5 mg daily under close medical supervision (see notes above); usual maintenance 20 mg daily in 1–2 divided doses

PoM **Innovace®** (MSD)

Tablets, enalapril maleate 2.5 mg, net price 50 = £10.00; 5 mg (scored), 28-tab pack = £7.86, 50 = £14.03; 10 mg (red), 28-tab pack = £11.03, 50 = £19.69; 20 mg (peach), 28-tab pack = £13.10, 50 = £23.40; titration pack of 11 × 2.5–mg tabs and 14 × 5–mg tabs = £6.12

With diuretic

Note. For mild to moderate hypertension in patients stabilised on the individual components in the same proportions

PoM **Innozide®** (MSD)

Tablets, yellow, scored, enalapril maleate 20 mg, hydrochlorothiazide 12.5 mg. Net price 28-tab pack = £14.56

FOSINOPRIL

Indications: essential hypertension where standard therapy ineffective or inappropriate because of adverse effects (but see cautions and notes above)

Cautions; Contra-indications; Side-effects: see under Captopril and notes above

Dose: initially 10 mg daily; usual maintenance 10–20 mg daily; max. 40 mg daily

Note. If used in addition to diuretic, discontinue diuretic several days before and resume after about 4 weeks if blood pressure inadequately controlled (if diuretic therapy cannot be stopped careful medical supervision for several hours)

PoM **Staril®** (Squibb)

Tablets, fosinopril sodium 10 mg, net price 28-tab pack = £12.04; 20 mg, 28-tab pack = £21.00

LISINOPRIL

Indications: all grades of essential hypertension (but see cautions and notes above); congestive heart failure (adjunct)

Cautions; Contra-indications; Side-effects: see under Captopril and notes above

Dose: hypertension, initially 2.5 mg daily; usual maintenance dose 10–20 mg daily; max. 40 mg daily

Note. In hypertension discontinue diuretic for 2–3 days beforehand and resume later if required (see also notes above)

Heart failure (adjunct), initially 2.5 mg daily under close medical supervision (see notes above); usual maintenance dose 5–20 mg daily

PoM **Carace®** (Du Pont)

Tablets, lisinopril 2.5 mg (blue), net price 28-tab pack = £7.64; 5 mg (scored), 28-tab pack = £9.58; 10 mg (yellow, scored), 28-tab pack = £11.83; 20 mg (orange, scored), 28-tab pack = £13.38

PoM **Zestril®** (Zeneca)

Tablets, lisinopril (as dihydrate) 2.5 mg, net price 7-tab starter pack = £1.91, 28-tab pack = £7.64; 5 mg (pink, scored), 28-tab pack = £9.58; 10 mg (pink), 28-tab pack = £11.83; 20 mg (red), 28-tab pack = £13.38

With diuretic

Note. For mild to moderate hypertension in patients stabilised on the individual components in the same proportions

PoM **Carace Plus®** (Du Pont)

Carace 10 Plus tablets, blue, lisinopril 10 mg, hydrochlorothiazide 12.5 mg. Net price 28-tab pack = £11.83

¹*Carace 20 Plus tablets,* yellow, scored, lisinopril 20 mg, hydrochlorothiazide 12.5 mg. Net price 28-tab pack = £16.93

1. Formerly called Carace Plus®

PoM **Zestoretic®** (Zeneca)

Zestoretic 10 tablets, peach, lisinopril 10 mg, hydrochlorothiazide 12.5 mg. Net price 28-tab pack = £11.83

¹*Zestoretic 20 tablets,* lisinopril 20 mg, hydrochlorothiazide 12.5 mg. Net price 28-tab pack = £13.38

1. Formerly called Zestoretic®

PERINDOPRIL

Indications: essential hypertension (but see cautions and notes above); congestive heart failure (adjunct)

Cautions; Contra-indications; Side-effects: see under Captopril and notes above

Dose: hypertension, initially 2 mg daily; usual maintenance dose 4–8 mg once daily; max. 8 mg daily

Note. In hypertension discontinue diuretic 3 days beforehand and resume later if required (see also notes above)

Heart failure (adjunct), initial dose 2 mg in the morning under close medical supervision (see notes above); usual maintenance 4 mg daily

PoM **Coversyl®** (Servier)

Tablets, perindopril tert-butylamine 2 mg, net price 30-tab pack = £9.45; 4 mg (scored), 30-tab pack = £13.65. Label: 22

QUINAPRIL

Indications: all grades of essential hypertension where standard therapy ineffective or inappropriate because of adverse effects (but see cautions and notes above); congestive heart failure (adjunct)

Cautions; Contra-indications; Side-effects: see under Captopril and notes above

Dose: hypertension, initially 10 mg once daily; with a diuretic, in elderly, or in renal impairment initially 2.5 mg daily; usual maintenance dose 20–40 mg daily in single or 2 divided doses; up to 80 mg daily has been given

Heart failure (adjunct), initial dose 2.5 mg under close medical supervision (see notes above); usual maintenance 10–20 mg daily in 2 divided doses; up to 40 mg daily has been given

PoM **Accupro®** (P-D)

Tablets, all brown, f/c, quinapril 5 mg, net price 28-tab pack = £10.30; 10 mg, 28-tab pack = £10.07; 20 mg, 28-tab pack = £9.79; 40 mg, 28-tab pack = £9.75

With diuretic

Note. For hypertension in patients stabilised on the individual components in the same proportions

PoM **Accuretic®** (P-D)

Tablets, pink, f/c, scored, quinapril 10 mg, hydrochlorothiazide 12.5 mg. Net price 28-tab pack = £9.79

RAMIPRIL

Indications: mild to moderate essential hypertension (but see cautions and notes above); following myocardial infarction in patients with clinical evidence of heart failure

Cautions; Contra-indications; Side-effects: see under Captopril and notes above

Dose: hypertension, initially 1.25 mg daily, increased at intervals of 1–2 weeks; usual range 2.5–5 mg once daily; max. 10 mg daily

Note. Discontinue diuretic for 2–3 days beforehand and resume later if required (see also notes above); patients with renal impairment or congestive heart failure require initiation under close medical supervision in hospital; close medical supervision is also required for patients with hepatic impairment

Prophylaxis after myocardial infarction (started in hospital 3 to 10 days after infarction), initially 2.5 mg twice daily, increased after 2 days to 5 mg twice daily; maintenance 2.5–5 mg twice daily

Note. If initial 2.5–mg dose not tolerated, give 1.25 mg twice daily for 2 days before increasing to 2.5 mg twice daily, then 5 mg twice daily; withdraw if 2.5 mg twice daily not tolerated

PoM **Tritace®** (Hoechst)

Capsules, ramipril 1.25 mg (yellow/white), net price 28-cap pack = £5.30; 2.5 mg (orange/white), 28-cap pack = £7.51; 5 mg (red/white), 28-cap pack = £9.55

TRANDOLAPRIL

Indications: mild to moderate essential hypertension (but see cautions and notes above)

Cautions; Contra-indications; Side-effects: see under Captopril and notes above

Dose: initially, 500 micrograms once daily, increased at intervals of 2–4 weeks; usual range 1–2 mg once daily; max. 4 mg daily

Note. If used in addition to diuretic, discontinue diuretic 2–3 days beforehand and resume later if required; patients with renal or hepatic impairment or congestive heart failure require initiation under close medical supervision

▼ PoM **Gopten®** (Knoll)

Capsules, trandolapril 500 micrograms (red/yellow), net price 14-cap pack = £4.09; 1 mg (red/orange), 28-cap pack = £10.33; 2 mg (red/red), 28-cap pack = £12.28

▼ PoM **Odrik®** (Roussel)

Capsules, trandolapril 500 micrograms (red/yellow), net price 28-cap pack = £8.19; 1 mg (red/orange), 28-cap pack = £10.34; 2 mg (red/red), 28-cap pack = £12.29

2.5.6 Ganglion-blocking drugs

TRIMETAPHAN CAMSYLATE
(Trimetaphan Camsilate)

Indications: controlled hypotension in surgery

Cautions: hepatic or renal impairment, diabetes mellitus, elderly, cerebral or coronary vascular disease, adrenal insufficiency, Addison's disease, CNS degenerative disease

Contra-indications: severe arteriosclerosis, severe cardiac disease, pyloric stenosis, pregnancy

Side-effects: tachycardia and respiratory depression (particularly with muscle relaxants), constipation, increased intra-ocular pressure, pupillary dilatation

Dose: by intravenous infusion, 3–4 mg/minute initially, then adjusted according to response

PoM **Arfonad®** (Cambridge)

Injection, trimetaphan camsylate 50 mg/mL. Net price 5-mL amp = £5.27. For dilution and use as an infusion

2.5.7 Tyrosine hydroxylase inhibitor

Metirosine inhibits the enzyme tyrosine hydroxylase, and hence the synthesis of catecholamines. It is used in the pre-operative management of phaeochromocytoma, and long term in patients unsuitable for surgery; an alpha-adrenoceptor blocking drug (e.g. phenoxybenzamine) may also be required. Metirosine should **not** be used to treat essential hypertension.

METIROSINE

Indications: see notes above

Cautions: maintain high fluid intake and adequate blood volume; may impair ability to drive or operate machinery; **interactions:** Appendix 1 (metirosine)

Side-effects: sedation; extrapyramidal symptoms; diarrhoea (may be severe); hypersensitivity reactions

Dose: initially 250 mg 4 times daily, increased to max. of 4 g daily in divided doses; doses of 2–3 g daily should be given for 5–7 days before surgery

PoM **Demser®** (MSD)

Capsules, blue, metirosine 250 mg (hosp. only). Label: 2

2.6 Nitrates and other vasodilators, and calcium-channel blockers

2.6.1	Nitrates
2.6.2	Calcium-channel blockers
2.6.3	Peripheral vasodilators
2.6.4	Cerebral vasodilators
2.6.5	Flosequinan

Most patients with *angina pectoris* are treated with beta-blockers (section 2.4) or calcium-channel blockers (section 2.6.2). However, short-acting nitrates (section 2.6.1) retain an important role both for prophylactic use before exertion and for chest pain occurring at rest. Nitrates are sometimes used as sole therapy, especially in elderly patients with infrequent symptoms.

Vasodilators are known to act in *heart failure* either by:

arteriolar dilatation which reduces both peripheral vascular resistance and left ventricular pressure at systole and results in improved cardiac output, *or* venous dilatation which results in dilatation of capacitance vessels, increase of venous pooling, and diminution of venous return to the heart (decreasing left ventricular end-diastolic pressure).

2.6.1 Nitrates

Sublingual **glyceryl trinitrate** is one of the most effective drugs for providing rapid symptomatic relief of angina, but its effect lasts only for 20 to 30 minutes. Though a potent coronary vasodilator, its principal benefit follows from a reduction in venous return which reduces left ventricular work. Unwanted effects such as flushing, headache, and postural hypotension may limit therapy, especially when angina is severe or when patients are unusually sensitive to the effects of nitrates; the 300-microgram tablet is often appropriate when glyceryl trinitrate is first used. Duration of action may be prolonged by *modified-release* preparations. The *aerosol spray* provides an alternative method of rapid relief of symptoms for those who find difficulty in dissolving sublingual preparations. The

percutaneous preparations may be useful in the prophylaxis of angina for patients who suffer attacks at rest, especially at night.

Isosorbide dinitrate is active *sublingually* and is a more stable preparation for those who only require nitrates infrequently. It is also effective by mouth for prophylaxis; although the effect is slower in onset, it may persist for several hours. Duration of action of up to 12 hours is claimed for *modified-release* preparations. The activity of isosorbide dinitrate may depend on the production of active metabolites, the most important of which is isosorbide mononitrate. **Isosorbide mononitrate** itself is also available for angina prophylaxis, though the advantages over isosorbide dinitrate have not yet been firmly established.

Glyceryl trinitrate or isosorbide dinitrate may be tried by *intravenous injection* when the sublingual form is ineffective in patients with chest pain due to myocardial infarction or severe ischaemia. Intravenous injections are also useful in the treatment of acute left ventricular failure.

TOLERANCE. Some patients on long-acting or transdermal nitrates rapidly develop tolerance (with reduced therapeutic effects). Reduction of blood-nitrate concentrations to low levels for 4 to 8 hours each day usually maintains effectiveness in such patients. If tolerance is suspected after the use of transdermal patches they should be removed for several consecutive hours in each 24 hours; in the case of modified-release tablets of isosorbide dinitrate (and conventional formulations of isosorbide mononitrate), the second of the two daily doses can be given after about 8 hours rather than after 12 hours. Conventional formulations of isosorbide mononitrate should not usually be given more than twice daily unless small doses are used; modified-release formulations of isosorbide mononitrate should only be given once daily.

GLYCERYL TRINITRATE

Indications: prophylaxis and treatment of angina; left ventricular failure

Cautions: severe hepatic or renal impairment; hypothyroidism, malnutrition, or hypothermia; recent history of myocardial infarction; metal-containing transdermal systems should be removed before cardioversion or diathermy; tolerance (see notes above); **interactions:** Appendix 1 (glyceryl trinitrate)

Contra-indications: hypersensitivity to nitrates; hypotensive conditions and hypovolaemia; hypertrophic obstructive cardiomyopathy, aortic stenosis, cardiac tamponade, constrictive pericarditis, mitral stenosis; marked anaemia, head trauma, cerebral haemorrhage, closed-angle glaucoma

Side-effects: throbbing headache, flushing, dizziness, postural hypotension, tachycardia (but paradoxical bradycardia has occurred)

INJECTION. Specific side-effects following injection (particularly if given too rapidly) include severe hypotension, nausea and retching, diaphoresis, apprehension, restlessness, muscle twitching, retrosternal discomfort, palpitations, abdominal pain, syncope; prolonged

---

administration has been associated with methaemo-globinaemia

Dose: sublingually, 0.3–1 mg, repeated as required

By mouth, 2.6–6.4 mg as modified-release tablets, 2–3 times daily; severe angina, 10 mg 3 times daily

By intravenous infusion, 10–200 micrograms/minute

Short-acting tablets and sprays

Glyceryl Trinitrate (Non-proprietary)

Sublingual tablets, glyceryl trinitrate 300 micrograms, net price 100 = £2.84; 500 micrograms, 100 = 30p; 600 micrograms, 100 = 57p. Label: 16

Note. Glyceryl trinitrate tablets should be supplied in glass containers of not more than 100 tablets, closed with a foil-lined cap, and containing no cotton wool wadding; they should be discarded after 8 weeks in use

Coro-Nitro Spray® (Boehringer Mannheim)

Aerosol spray, glyceryl trinitrate 400 micrograms/metered dose. Net price 200-dose unit = £3.28

Dose: treatment or prophylaxis of angina, spray 1–2 doses under tongue and then close mouth
Caution: flammable

Glytrin Spray® (Sterwin)

Aerosol spray, glyceryl trinitrate 400 micrograms/metered dose. Net price 200-dose unit = £3.28. Label: 10 patient information leaflet

Dose: treatment or prophylaxis of angina, spray 1–2 doses under tongue and then close mouth
Caution: flammable

GTN 300 mcg (Martindale)

Sublingual tablets, glyceryl trinitrate 300 micrograms. Net price 100 = £2.84. Label: 16

Nitrolingual Spray® (Lipha)

Aerosol spray, glyceryl trinitrate 400 micrograms/metered dose. Net price 200-dose unit = £4.36

Dose: treatment or prophylaxis of angina, spray 1–2 doses under tongue and then close mouth
Caution: flammable

Modified-release tablets

Nitrocontin Continus® (ASTA Medica)

Tablets, m/r, both pink, glyceryl trinitrate 2.6 mg, net price 100-tab pack = £3.25; 6.4 mg, 100-tab pack = £4.28. Label: 25

Suscard® (Pharmax)

Buccal tablets, m/r, glyceryl trinitrate 1 mg, net price 20 = £1.96; 2 mg, 20 = £2.84; 3 mg, 20 = £4.10; 5 mg, 20 = £5.58. Counselling, see administration below

Dose: treatment of angina, 2 mg as required (1 mg in sensitive patients), increased to 3 mg if necessary; prophylaxis 1–3 mg 3 times daily; 5 mg in severe angina
Unstable angina (adjunct), up to 5 mg with ECG monitoring
Congestive heart failure, 5 mg 3 times daily, increased to 10 mg 3 times daily in severe cases
Acute heart failure, 5 mg repeated until symptoms abate
ADMINISTRATION. Tablets are placed between upper lip and gum, and left to dissolve; vary site to reduce risk of dental caries

Sustac® (Pharmax)

Tablets, m/r, all pink, glyceryl trinitrate 2.6 mg, net price 20 = £1.19; 6.4 mg, 20 = £1.72; 10 mg, 20 = £2.39. Label: 25

Parenteral preparations

Note. Glass or polyethylene apparatus is preferable; loss of potency will occur if PVC is used

PoM Glyceryl Trinitrate (Non-proprietary)

Injection, glyceryl trinitrate 5 mg/mL. To be diluted before use. Net price 5-mL amp = £6.30; 10-mL amp = £12.60
Available from David Bull

PoM Nitrocine® (Schwarz)

Injection, glyceryl trinitrate 1 mg/mL. To be diluted before use or given undiluted with syringe pump. Net price 10-mL amp = £8.27; 50-mL bottle = £19.38

PoM Nitronal® (Lipha)

Injection, glyceryl trinitrate 1 mg/mL. To be diluted before use or given undiluted with syringe pump. Net price 5-mL vial = £2.16; 50-mL vial = £17.64

PoM Tridil® (Du Pont)

Injection, to be diluted before use, glyceryl trinitrate 500 micrograms/mL, net price 10-mL amp = £4.39; 5 mg/mL, 10-mL amp = £21.33

Transdermal preparations

Deponit® (Schwarz)

Patches, self-adhesive, transparent, glyceryl trinitrate, '*5*' *patch* (releasing approx. 5 mg/24 hours when in contact with skin), net price 30 = £19.25; '*10*' *patch* (releasing approx. 10 mg/24 hours), 30 = £21.19

ADMINISTRATION: prophylaxis of angina, apply one '5' or one '10' patch to lateral chest wall, upper arm, or shoulder; replace every 24 hours, siting replacement patch on different area; see also notes above

Minitran® (3M)

Patches, self-adhesive, transparent, glyceryl trinitrate, '*5*' *patch* (releasing approx. 5 mg/24 hours when in contact with skin), net price 30 = £15.95; '*10*' *patch* (releasing approx. 10 mg/24 hours), 30 = £17.54; '*15*' *patch* (releasing approx. 15 mg/24 hours), 30 = £22.98

ADMINISTRATION: prophylaxis of angina, apply one '5' patch to chest or upper arm; replace every 24 hours, siting replacement patch on different area; adjust dose according to response; see also notes above
Maintenance of venous patency ('5' patch only), see literature

Nitro-Dur® (Schering-Plough)

Patches, self-adhesive, buff, glyceryl trinitrate, '*0.1 mg/h*' *patch* (releasing approx. 2.5 mg/24 hours when in contact with skin), net price 28 = £11.85; '*0.2 mg/h*' *patch* (releasing approx. 5 mg/24 hours), 28 = £13.15; '*0.4 mg/h*' *patch* (releasing approx. 10 mg/24 hours), 28 = £14.56; '*0.6 mg/h*' *patch* (releasing approx. 15 mg/24 hours), 28 = £16.02

ADMINISTRATION: prophylaxis of angina, apply one '0.2 mg/h' patch to chest or upper arm; replace every 24 hours, siting replacement patch on different area; adjust dose according to response; see also notes above

---

Cautionary label wordings, see inside back cover

Percutol® (Cusi)

Ointment, glyceryl trinitrate 2%. Net price 30 g = £5.99. Counselling, see administration below

ADMINISTRATION: prophylaxis of angina, 1–2 inches of ointment measured on to Applirule, which is applied to body (usually chest, abdomen, or thigh) without rubbing in, and secured with a dressing; repeat every 3–4 hours or as required

Note. 1 inch of ointment contains glyceryl trinitrate 16.64 mg

Transiderm-Nitro® (Geigy)

Patches, self-adhesive, pink, glyceryl trinitrate, '*5*' *patch* (releasing approx. 5 mg/24 hours when in contact with skin), net price 30 = £15.95; '*10*' *patch* (releasing approx. 10 mg/24 hours), 30 = £17.54

ADMINISTRATION: prophylaxis of angina, apply one '5' or one '10' patch to lateral chest wall; replace every 24 hours, siting replacement patch on different area; max. two '10' patches daily; see also notes above

Prophylaxis of phlebitis and extravasation ('5' patch only), see literature

---

ISOSORBIDE DINITRATE

Indications: prophylaxis and treatment of angina; left ventricular failure

Cautions; Contra-indications; Side-effects: see under Glyceryl Trinitrate

Dose: sublingually, 5–10 mg

By mouth, daily in divided doses, angina 30–120 mg, left ventricular failure 40–160 mg, up to 240 mg if required

By intravenous infusion, 2–10 mg/hour; higher doses up to 20 mg/hour may be required

Short-acting tablets and sprays

Isosorbide Dinitrate (Non-proprietary)

Tablets, isosorbide dinitrate 10 mg, net price 20 = 23p; 20 mg, 20 = 42p

Available from APS, Berk, Cox, Hillcross, K Pharm., Norton

Cedocard® (Pharmacia)

Cedocard-5 tablets (sublingual or oral), scored, isosorbide dinitrate 5 mg. Net price 60-tab pack = £1.51

Note. May be taken sublingually for a rapid onset of action or orally for a slower onset of action but a longer duration

Cedocard-10 tablets, pink, scored, isosorbide dinitrate 10 mg. Net price 100-tab pack = £1.66

Cedocard-20 tablets, blue, scored, isosorbide dinitrate 20 mg. Net price 100-tab pack = £3.17

Imtack Spray® (Astra)

Aerosol spray, isosorbide dinitrate 1.25 mg/ metered dose. Net price 200-dose unit = £4.28

Dose: treatment or prophylaxis of angina, spray 1–3 doses under tongue and then close mouth

Caution: flammable

Isordil® (Monmouth)

Tablets (sublingual), pink, isosorbide dinitrate 5 mg. Net price 100-tab pack = £1.43. Label: 26

Tablets, both scored, isosorbide dinitrate 10 mg, net price 100-tab pack = £1.45; 30 mg, 100-tab pack = £3.45

Sorbichew® (Stuart)

Tablets (chewable), green, scored, isosorbide dinitrate 5 mg. Net price 100-tab pack = £1.51. Label: 24

Sorbitrate® (Stuart)

Tablets, both scored, isosorbide dinitrate 10 mg (yellow), net price 100-tab pack = £1.51; 20 mg (blue), 100-tab pack = £2.10

Modified-release preparations

Cedocard Retard® (Pharmacia)

Retard-20 tablets, m/r, yellow, scored, isosorbide dinitrate 20 mg. Net price 60-tab pack = £5.71. Label: 25

Dose: prophylaxis of angina, 1 tablet every 12 hours

Retard-40 tablets, m/r, orange-red, scored, isosorbide dinitrate 40 mg. Net price 60-tab pack = £11.09. Label: 25

Dose: prophylaxis of angina, 1–2 tablets every 12 hours

Isoket Retard® (Schwarz)

Retard-20 tablets, m/r, yellow, scored, isosorbide dinitrate 20 mg. Net price 50-tab pack = £3.24. Label: 25

Retard-40 tablets, m/r, orange, scored, isosorbide dinitrate 40 mg. Net price 50-tab pack = £7.99. Label: 25

Dose: prophylaxis of angina, 20–40 mg every 12 hours

Isordil Tembids® (Monmouth)

Capsules, m/r, blue/clear, isosorbide dinitrate 40 mg. Net price 100-cap pack = £15.54. Label: 25

Dose: prophylaxis of angina, 1 capsule 2–3 times daily

Soni-Slo® (Lipha)

Capsules, m/r, pink/clear, enclosing off-white pellets, isosorbide dinitrate 20 mg. Net price 20 = £1.19. Label: 25

Capsules, m/r, yellow/clear, enclosing off-white pellets, isosorbide dinitrate 40 mg. Net price 20 = £1.40. Label: 25

Dose: prophylaxis of angina, 40–120 mg daily in divided doses

Sorbid SA® (Stuart)

Sorbid-20 SA capsules, m/r, red/yellow, isosorbide dinitrate 20 mg. Net price 56-cap pack = £3.50. Label: 25

Dose: prophylaxis of angina, 1–2 capsules twice daily

Sorbid-40 SA capsules, m/r, red/clear, isosorbide dinitrate 40 mg. Net price 56-cap pack = £5.00. Label: 25

Dose: prophylaxis of angina, 1–2 capsules twice daily

Parenteral preparations

PoM **Isoket®** (Schwarz)

Injection 0.05%, isosorbide dinitrate 500 micrograms/mL. To be diluted before use or given undiluted with syringe pump. Net price 50-mL bottle = £10.06

Injection 0.1%, isosorbide dinitrate 1 mg/mL. To be diluted before use. Net price 10-mL amp = £3.79; 50-mL bottle = £18.81; 100-mL bottle = £25.98

Note. Glass or polyethylene infusion apparatus is preferable; loss of potency if PVC used

---

ISOSORBIDE MONONITRATE

Indications: prophylaxis and treatment of angina; adjunct in congestive heart failure

Cautions; Contra-indications; Side-effects: see under Glyceryl Trinitrate

Dose: initially 20 mg 2–3 times daily *or* 40 mg twice daily (10 mg twice daily in those who have not previously received nitrates); up to 120 mg daily in divided doses if required

Isosorbide Mononitrate (Non-proprietary)

Tablets, isosorbide mononitrate 10 mg, net price 20 = £1.14; 20 mg, 20 = £1.29; 40 mg, 20 = £2.66. Label: 25

Various strengths available from APS, Ashbourne (Isib®), Berk, Cox, CP, Hillcross, K Pharm., Lagap, Norton

Elantan® (Schwarz)

Elantan 10 tablets, scored, isosorbide mononitrate 10 mg. Net price 50 = £3.33. Label: 25

PoM *Elantan 20 tablets,* scored, isosorbide mononitrate 20 mg. Net price 50 = £4.34. Label: 25

PoM *Elantan 40 tablets,* scored, isosorbide mononitrate 40 mg. Net price 50 = £7.07. Label: 25

Ismo® (Boehringer Mannheim)

Ismo 10 tablets, isosorbide mononitrate 10 mg. Net price 60-tab pack = £3.39. Label: 25

Ismo 20 tablets, isosorbide mononitrate 20 mg. Net price 60-tab pack = £4.97. Label: 25

Starter pack, 8 tablets, isosorbide mononitrate 10 mg; 60 tablets, scored, isosorbide mononitrate 20 mg. Net price = £5.38. Label: 25

Ismo 40 tablets, isosorbide mononitrate 40 mg. Net price 100-tab pack = £13.61. Label: 25

Isotrate® (Bioglan)

Tablets, isosorbide mononitrate 20 mg. Net price 60-tab pack = £4.60. Label: 25

Monit® (Lorex)

LS Tablets, isosorbide mononitrate 10 mg. Net price 56-tab pack = £3.37. Label: 25

Tablets, scored, isosorbide mononitrate 20 mg. Net price 56-tab pack = £4.30. Label: 25

Mono-Cedocard® (Pharmacia)

Mono-Cedocard 10 tablets, orange, scored, isosorbide mononitrate 10 mg. Net price 60-tab pack = £3.68. Label: 25

Mono-Cedocard 20 tablets, scored, isosorbide mononitrate 20 mg. Net price 100-tab pack = £6.83. Label: 25

Mono-Cedocard 40 tablets, scored, isosorbide mononitrate 40 mg. Net price 60-tab pack = £9.12. Label: 25

Modified release

Elantan LA® (Schwarz)

Elantan LA 25 capsules, m/r, light pink/dark pink, enclosing white micropellets, isosorbide mononitrate 25 mg. Net price 28-cap pack = £7.00. Label: 25

Dose: prophylaxis of angina, 1 capsule in the morning, increased if necessary to 2 capsules

Elantan LA 50 capsules, m/r, pink/dark pink, enclosing white micropellets, isosorbide mononitrate 50 mg. Net price 28-cap pack = £11.30. Label: 25

Dose: prophylaxis of angina, 1 capsule daily in the morning, increased if necessary to 2 capsules

PoM **Imdur®** (Astra)

Durules® (= tablets m/r), yellow, f/c, scored, isosorbide mononitrate 60 mg. Net price 28-tab pack = £11.43. Label: 25

Dose: prophylaxis of angina, 1 tablet in the morning (half a tablet if headache occurs), increased to 2 tablets if required

Ismo Retard® (Boehringer Mannheim)

Tablets, m/r, s/c, isosorbide mononitrate 40 mg. Net price 28-tab pack = £10.24. Label: 25

Dose: prophylaxis of angina, 1 tablet daily in the morning

¹MCR-50® (Pharmacia)

Capsules, m/r, containing white micropellets, isosorbide mononitrate 50 mg. Net price 28-cap pack = £11.02. Label: 25

Dose: prophylaxis of angina, 1 capsule in the morning, increased to 2 capsules if required

1. Full product name Mono Cedocard Retard-50®

Monit SR® (Lorex)

Tablets, m/r, s/c, isosorbide mononitrate 40 mg. Net price 28-tab pack = £10.24. Label: 25

Dose: prophylaxis of angina, 1 tablet daily in the morning

PENTAERYTHRITOL TETRANITRATE
(Pentaerythrityl Tetranitrate)

Indications: prophylaxis of angina

Cautions; Contra-indications; Side-effects: see under Glyceryl Trinitrate

Mycardol® (Sanofi Winthrop)

Tablets, scored, pentaerythritol tetranitrate 30 mg. Net price 20 = 96p. Label: 22

Dose: 2 tablets 3–4 times daily

2.6.2   Calcium-channel blockers

Calcium-channel blockers (less correctly called 'calcium-antagonists') interfere with the inward displacement of calcium ions through the slow channels of active cell membranes. They influence the myocardial cells, the cells within the specialised conducting system of the heart, and the cells of vascular smooth muscle. Thus, myocardial contractility may be reduced, the formation and propagation of electrical impulses within the heart may be depressed, and coronary or systemic vascular tone may be diminished. They should usually be **avoided** in *heart failure* because they may further depress cardiac function and cause clinically significant deterioration.

Calcium-channel blockers differ in their predelic- tion for the various possible sites of action therefore their therapeutic effects are disparate, with much greater variation than those of beta-blockers. There are important differences between verapamil and the dihydropyridine calcium-channel blockers, such as nifedipine, nicardipine and isradipine.

Verapamil is used for the treatment of *angina, hypertension*, and *arrhythmias* (section 2.3.2). It reduces cardiac output, slows the heart rate, and may impair atrioventricular conduction. It may precipitate heart failure, exacerbate conduction disorders, and cause hypotension at high doses and should **not** be used with beta-blockers (see section 2.3.2). Constipation is the most common side-effect.

Nifedipine relaxes vascular smooth muscle and dilates coronary and peripheral arteries. It has more influence on vessels and less on the myocardium than does verapamil, and unlike verapamil has no anti-arrhythmic activity. It rarely precipitates heart failure because any negative inotropic effect is off-set by a reduction in left ventricular work. **Nicardipine** has similar effects to those of nifedipine and may produce less reduction of myocardial contractility. **Amlodipine** and **felodipine** also resemble nifedipine and nicardipine in their effects and do not reduce myocardial contractility. They have a longer duration of action and can be given once daily. Nifedipine, nicardipine, and amlodipine are used for the treatment of angina or hypertension. All are valuable in forms of *angina associated with coronary vasospasm*; they are useful as adjuncts to beta-blockers for patients with severe symptoms, and as alternative treatment for those who are intolerant of beta-blockers. Side-effects associated with vasodilatation such as flushing and headache (which become less obtrusive after a few days), and ankle swelling (which does not respond to diuretics) are common.

Isradipine and **lacidipine** have similar effects to those of nifedipine and nicardipine; they are only indicated for *hypertension*.

Nimodipine is related to nifedipine but the smooth muscle relaxant effect preferentially acts on cerebral arteries. Its use is confined to prevention of *vascular spasm following subarachnoid haemorrhage.*

Diltiazem is effective in most forms of *angina*; the longer-acting formulation is also used for *hypertension*. It should be used in patients for whom beta-blockers are contra-indicated or ineffective. It has a less negative inotropic effect than verapamil and significant myocardial depression occurs rarely. Nevertheless because of the risk of bradycardia it should be used with caution in association with beta-blockers.

UNSTABLE ANGINA. Calcium-channel blockers do not reduce the risk of myocardial infarction in unstable angina. Their use should be reserved for patients resistant to treatment with beta-blockers, nitrates, and anticoagulation with aspirin and intravenous heparin.

WITHDRAWAL. There is some evidence that sudden withdrawal of calcium-channel blockers may be associated with an exacerbation of angina.

AMLODIPINE BESYLATE

Indications: hypertension, prophylaxis of angina

Cautions: pregnancy and breast-feeding; hepatic impairment; **interactions:** Appendix 1 (calcium-channel blockers)

Side-effects: headache, oedema, fatigue, nausea, flushing, dizziness; gum hyperplasia, erythema multiforme reported

Dose: hypertension or angina, initially 5 mg once daily; max. 10 mg once daily

PoM Istin® (Pfizer)

Tablets, amlodipine (as besylate) 5 mg. Net price 28-tab pack = £11.85; 10 mg, 28-tab pack = £17.70

DILTIAZEM HYDROCHLORIDE

Indications: prophylaxis and treatment of angina; hypertension

Cautions: reduce dose in hepatic and renal impairment; heart failure or significantly impaired left ventricular function, mild bradycardia (avoid if severe), first degree AV block, or prolonged PR interval; porphyria (see section 9.8.2); **interactions:** Appendix 1 (calcium-channel blockers)

Contra-indications: severe bradycardia, left ventricular failure, second- or third-degree AV block (unless pacemaker fitted), sick sinus syndrome; pregnancy (toxicity in *animal* studies)

Side-effects: bradycardia, sino-atrial block, atrioventricular block, hypotension, malaise, headache, hot flushes, gastro-intestinal disturbances, oedema(notably of ankles); rarely rashes (erythema multiforme reported); altered liver function tests; hepatitis and depression reported

Dose: angina, 60 mg 3 times daily (elderly initially twice daily); increased if necessary to 360 mg daily

Longer-acting formulations, see below

PoM Diltiazem (Non-proprietary)

Tablets, m/r, diltiazem hydrochloride 60 mg. Net price 100 = £9.25. Label: 25

Available from APS, Ashbourne (Angiozem®), Berk, Cox, CP, Hillcross, K Pharm., Lagap, Norton, Thames (Britiazim®)

PoM Adizem-60® (Napp)

Tablets, m/r, f/c, diltiazem hydrochloride 60 mg. Net price 100-tab pack = £15.38. Label: 25

PoM Tildiem® (Lorex)

Tablets, m/r, off-white, diltiazem hydrochloride 60 mg. Net price 100 = £14.25. Label: 25

Longer acting

Note. To avoid confusion between these different formulations of diltiazem, prescribers should specify the brand to be dispensed

PoM Adizem-SR® (Napp)

Capsules, m/r, diltiazem hydrochloride 90 mg (white), net price 56-cap pack = £11.06; 120 mg (brown/white), 56-cap pack = £12.29; 180 mg (brown/white), 56-cap pack = £18.43. Label: 25

Tablets, m/r, f/c, scored, diltiazem hydrochloride 120 mg. Net price 56-tab pack = £18.14. Label: 25

Dose: mild to moderate hypertension, usually 120 mg twice daily (dose form not appropriate for initial dose titration)
Angina, initially 90 mg twice daily (elderly, dose form not appropriate for initial dose titration); increased to 180 mg twice daily if required

PoM Adizem-XL® (Napp)
Capsules, m/r, diltiazem hydrochloride 120 mg (pink/blue), net price 30-cap pack = £11.49; 180 mg (dark pink/blue), 30-cap pack = £13.03; 240 mg (red/blue), 30-cap pack = £14.48; 300 mg (maroon/blue), 30-cap pack = £11.49. Label: 25
Dose: angina and mild to moderate hypertension, initially 240 mg once daily, increased if necessary to 300 mg once daily; in elderly and in hepatic or renal impairment, initially 120 mg daily

PoM Dilzem SR® (Elan)
Capsules, m/r, all beige, diltiazem hydrochloride 60 mg, net price 100-cap pack = £13.50; 90 mg, 60-cap pack = £10.94; 120 mg, 60-cap pack = £12.15. Label: 25
Dose: angina and mild to moderate hypertension, initially 90 mg twice daily (elderly 60 mg twice daily); up to 180 mg twice daily may be required

PoM Dilzem XL® (Elan)
Capsules, m/r, diltiazem hydrochloride 120 mg, net price 30-cap pack = £8.10; 180 mg, 30-cap pack = £11.10; 240 mg, 30-cap pack = £11.40. Label: 25
Dose: angina and mild to moderate hypertension, initially 180 mg once daily (elderly and in hepatic and renal impairment, 120 mg once daily); if necessary may be increased to 360 mg once daily

PoM Tildiem LA® (Lorex)
Capsules, m/r, white/yellow, containing white pellets, diltiazem hydrochloride 300 mg. Net price 28-cap pack = £10.73. Label: 25
Dose: mild to moderate hypertension, 1 capsule daily before or with food (elderly, dose form not appropriate for initial dose titration)

PoM Tildiem Retard® (Lorex)
Tablets, m/r, diltiazem hydrochloride 90 mg, net price 56-tab pack = £11.06; 120 mg, 56-tab pack = £12.29. Label: 25
COUNSELLING. Tablet membrane may pass through gastro-intestinal tract unchanged, but being porous has no effect on efficacy
Dose: mild to moderate hypertension, initially 90 mg or 120 mg twice daily (elderly once daily); up to 360 mg daily may be required (elderly up to 240 mg daily)
Angina, initially 90 mg or 120 mg twice daily (elderly, dose form not appropriate for initial dose titration); up to 480 mg daily in divided doses may be required (elderly up to 240 mg daily)

FELODIPINE
Indications: hypertension
Cautions: withdraw if ischaemic pain occurs; hepatic impairment; breast-feeding; **interactions:** Appendix 1 (calcium-channel blockers)
Contra-indications: pregnancy

Side-effects: flushing, headache, palpitations, dizziness, fatigue, gravitational oedema, rash and pruritus, gum hyperplasia
Dose: initially 5 mg daily in the morning; usual maintenance 5–10 mg once daily; doses above 20 mg daily rarely needed

▼ **PoM Plendil®** (Schwarz)
Tablets, m/r, f/c, felodipine 5 mg, net price 28-tab pack = £8.12; 10 mg, 28-tab pack = £10.92. Label: 25

ISRADIPINE
Indications: hypertension
Cautions: tight aortic stenosis; sick sinus syndrome (if pacemaker not fitted); reduce dose in hepatic or renal impairment; pregnancy (may prolong labour); **interactions:** Appendix 1 (calcium-channel blockers)
Side-effects: headache, flushing, dizziness, tachycardia and palpitations, localised peripheral oedema; hypotension uncommon; rarely weight gain, fatigue, abdominal discomfort, rashes
Dose: 2.5 mg twice daily (1.25 mg twice daily in elderly, hepatic or renal impairment); increased if necessary after 3–4 weeks to 5 mg twice daily (exceptionally up to 10 mg twice daily); maintenance 2.5 or 5 mg once daily may be sufficient

PoM Prescal® (Ciba)
Tablets, yellow, scored, isradipine 2.5 mg. Net price 56-tab pack = £11.39

LACIDIPINE
Indications: hypertension
Cautions: cardiac conduction abnormalities; poor cardiac reserve; hepatic impairment; withdraw if ischaemic pain occurs shortly after initiating treatment; breast-feeding; **interactions:** Appendix 1 (calcium-channel blockers)
Contra-indications: pregnancy
Side-effects: headache, flushing, oedema, dizziness, palpitations; also asthenia, rash (including pruritus and erythema), gastro-intestinal disturbances, polyuria, chest pain (see Cautions), gingival hyperplasia
Dose: 4 mg as a single daily dose, increased if necessary after 3–4 weeks to 6 mg daily; in hepatic impairment, initially 2 mg daily; ELDERLY, initially 2 mg daily, increased if necessary to 4 mg after 4 weeks

▼ **PoM Motens®** (Boehringer Ingelheim)
Tablets, both f/c, lacidipine 2 mg, net price 28-tab pack = £10.66; 4 mg (scored), 28-tab pack = £14.50. Label: 21

NICARDIPINE HYDROCHLORIDE

Indications: prophylaxis and treatment of angina; mild to moderate hypertension

Cautions: withdraw if ischaemic pain occurs or existing pain worsens within 30 minutes of initiating treatment or increasing dose; congestive heart failure or significantly impaired left ventricular function; elderly; hepatic or renal impairment; **interactions:** Appendix 1 (calcium-channel blockers)

Contra-indications: advanced aortic stenosis; pregnancy

Side-effects: dizziness, headache, peripheral oedema, flushing, palpitations, nausea; also gastro-intestinal disturbances, drowsiness, insomnia, tinnitus, hypotension, rashes, salivation, frequency of micturition; thrombocytopenia reported

Dose: initially 20 mg 3 times daily, increased to 30 mg 3 times daily (usual range 60–120 mg daily); patients with hypertension controlled on 20–30 mg 3 times daily can be given 30–40 mg twice daily

PoM Cardene® (Syntex)

Capsules, nicardipine hydrochloride 20 mg (blue/white), net price 100-cap pack = £15.98; 30 mg (blue/pale blue), 56-cap pack = £10.38

Modified release

PoM Cardene SR® (Syntex)

Capsules, m/r, nicardipine hydrochloride 30 mg, net price 56-cap pack = £10.33; 45 mg (blue), 56-cap pack = £14.35. Label: 25

Dose: mild to moderate hypertension, initially 30 mg twice daily; usual effective dose 45 mg twice daily (range 30–60 mg twice daily)

NIFEDIPINE

Indications: prophylaxis and treatment of angina; hypertension; Raynaud's phenomenon

Cautions: withdraw if ischaemic pain occurs or existing pain worsens shortly after initiating treatment; poor cardiac reserve; heart failure or significantly impaired left ventricular function (heart failure deterioration observed); severe hypotension; reduce dose in hepatic impairment; diabetes mellitus; may inhibit labour; breast-feeding (see Appendix 5); **interactions:** Appendix 1 (calcium-channel blockers)

Contra-indications: cardiogenic shock; advanced aortic stenosis; pregnancy (toxicity in *animal* studies); porphyria (see section 9.8.2)

Side-effects: headache, flushing, dizziness, lethargy; tachycardia, palpitations: also gravitational oedema, rash (erythema multiforme reported), nausea, increased frequency of micturition, eye pain, gum hyperplasia; depression reported; telangiectasia reported

Dose: see preparations below

PoM Adalat® (Bayer)

Capsules, both orange, nifedipine 5 mg, net price 20 = £1.42; 10 mg, 20 = £1.80. Label: 21, counselling, see dose

Dose: angina and Raynaud's phenomenon, initially 10 mg (elderly and hepatic impairment, 5 mg) 3 times daily with or after food; usual maintenance 5–20 mg 3 times daily; for immediate effect in angina bite into capsule and swallow liquid

Note. Nifedipine capsules also available from APS, Ashbourne (Angiopine®), Berk, Cox, Eastern (Calcilat®), Hillcross, K Pharm., Norton

Modified release

Note. To avoid confusion between these different formulations of nifedipine, prescribers should specify the brand to be dispensed

PoM Adalat® LA (Bayer)

LA 30 tablets, m/r, pink, nifedipine 30 mg. Net price 28-tab pack = £10.36. Label: 25

LA 60 tablets, m/r, pink, nifedipine 60 mg. Net price 28-tab pack = £15.40. Label: 25

COUNSELLING. Tablet membrane may pass through gastro-intestinal tract unchanged, but being porous has no effect on efficacy

Dose: mild to moderate hypertension, 30 mg once daily; increased if necessary (dose form not appropriate for use in hepatic impairment); max. 90 mg once daily

PoM Adalat® Retard (Bayer)

Retard 10 tablets, m/r, pink, nifedipine 10 mg. Net price 56-tab pack = £8.66. Label: 21, 25

Retard 20 tablets, m/r, pink, nifedipine 20 mg. Net price 56-tab pack = £10.81. Label: 21, 25

Dose: hypertension and angina prophylaxis, 20 mg twice daily with or after food (initial titration 10 mg twice daily); usual maintenance 10–40 mg twice daily

PoM Cardilate MR® (Norton)

Tablets, m/r, brown, nifedipine 20 mg. Net price 100-tab pack = £18.35. Label: 25

Dose: hypertension and angina prophylaxis, 20 mg twice daily (dose form not appropriate for initial dose titration in hepatic impairment); max. 80 mg daily

PoM Coracten® (Evans)

Capsules, m/r, nifedipine 10 mg (grey/pink, enclosing yellow pellets), net price 60-cap pack = £7.15; 20 mg (pink/brown, enclosing yellow pellets), 60-cap pack = £9.97. Label: 25

Dose: hypertension and angina prophylaxis, one 20-mg capsule every 12 hours, adjusted within range 10–40 mg every 12 hours

PoM Nifensar XL® (Rhône-Poulenc Rorer)

Tablets, m/r, yellow, nifedipine 20 mg. Net price 28-tab pack = £7.37. Label: 21, 25

Dose: mild to moderate hypertension, initially 40 mg once daily (initially 20 mg in elderly not previously treated with nifedipine, or in renal impairment); usual maintenance dose 20–40 mg daily; max. 100 mg daily

With atenolol
Section 2.4

NIMODIPINE

Indications: prevention and treatment of ischaemic neurological deficits following subarachnoid haemorrhage

Cautions: cerebral oedema or severely raised intracranial pressure; avoid concomitant administration of nimodipine tablets and infusion, other

---

calcium-channel blockers, or beta-blockers; impaired renal function or nephrotoxic drugs; pregnancy; **interactions:** Appendix 1 (calcium-channel blockers)

Side-effects: hypotension, variation in heart-rate, flushing, headache, gastro-intestinal disorders, nausea, and feeling of warmth; thrombocytopenia and ileus reported; transient increase in liver enzymes after intravenous administration

Dose: prevention, *by mouth*, 60 mg every 4 hours (total daily dose 360 mg), starting within 4 days of subarachnoid haemorrhage and continued for 21 days

Treatment, *by intravenous infusion* via central catheter, 1 mg/hour initially, increased after 2 hours to 2 mg/hour, providing no severe decrease in blood pressure; patients with unstable blood pressure or weighing less than 70 kg, 500 micrograms/hour initially or less if necessary; treatment should start as soon as possible and should continue for at least 5 days (max. 14 days); in the event of surgical intervention during treatment continue for at least 5 days after

PoM Nimotop® (Bayer)

Tablets, yellow, f/c, nimodipine 30 mg. Net price 100-tab pack = £38.85

Intravenous infusion, nimodipine 200 micrograms/mL; also contains ethanol 20% and macrogol '400' 17%. Net price 50-mL vial (with polyethylene infusion catheter) = £13.24; 250-mL bottle = £66.20

Note. Polyethylene or polypropylene apparatus should be used; PVC should be avoided

VERAPAMIL HYDROCHLORIDE

Indications: see under Dose

Cautions: first-degree AV block; acute phase of myocardial infarction (avoid if bradycardia, hypotension, left ventricular failure); patients taking beta-blockers (**important:** see below); reduce dose in hepatic impairment; children, specialist advice only (see section 2.3.2); pregnancy and breast-feeding; **interactions:** Appendix 1 (calcium-channel blockers)

VERAPAMIL AND BETA-BLOCKERS. Verapamil should not be injected into patients recently treated with beta-blockers because of the risk of hypotension and asystole. It has been suggested that when verapamil injection has been given first, an interval of 30 minutes before giving a beta-blocker is sufficient but this too is open to doubt. It may even be hazardous to give verapamil and a beta-blocker together by mouth (should only be contemplated if myocardial function well preserved).

Contra-indications: hypotension, bradycardia, second- and third-degree AV block, sick sinus syndrome, cardiogenic shock, sino-atrial block; history of heart failure or significantly impaired left ventricular function, even if controlled by therapy; atrial flutter or fibrillation complicating Wolff-Parkinson-White syndrome; porphyria (see section 9.8.2)

Side-effects: constipation; less commonly nausea, vomiting, flushing, headache, dizziness, fatigue, ankle oedema; rarely reversible impairment of liver function, allergic reactions (erythema, pru-

ritus); rarely gynaecomastia and gingival hyperplasia after long-term treatment; after intravenous administration, hypotension, bradycardia, heart block, and asystole

Dose: by mouth, supraventricular arrhythmias (but see also Contra-indications), 40–120 mg 3 times daily

Angina, 80–120 mg 3 times daily

Hypertension, 240–480 mg daily in 2–3 divided doses

By slow intravenous injection over 2 minutes (3 minutes in elderly), 5–10 mg (preferably with ECG monitoring); in paroxysmal tachyarrhythmias a further 5 mg after 5–10 minutes if required

PoM Verapamil (Non-proprietary)

Tablets, coated, verapamil hydrochloride 40 mg, net price 20 = 23p; 80 mg, 20 = 45p; 120 mg, 20 = 69p; 160 mg, 20 = £2.00

Various strengths available from APS, Berk (Berkatens®), Cox, CP, Cusi (Geangin®), Hillcross, K Pharm., Lagap, Norton

Oral solution, sugar-free, verapamil hydrochloride 40 mg/5 mL available from RP Drugs (special order)

PoM Cordilox® (Baker Norton)

Tablets, all yellow, f/c, verapamil hydrochloride 40 mg, net price 100-tab pack = £4.57; 80 mg, 100-tab pack = £9.15; 120 mg, 100-tab pack = £13.70; 160 mg, 56-tab pack = £12.77

Injection, verapamil hydrochloride 2.5 mg/mL, net price 2-mL amp = £1.11

PoM Securon® (Knoll)

Tablets, f/c, verapamil hydrochloride 40 mg, net price 100 = £4.57; 80 mg (scored), 100 = £9.14; 120 mg (scored), 56-tab pack = £7.67, 100 = £13.69; 160 mg (scored), 56-tab pack = £10.22

Injection, verapamil hydrochloride 2.5 mg/mL. Net price 2-mL syringe = £1.08

Modified release

PoM Half Securon SR® (Knoll)

Tablets, m/r, f/c, verapamil hydrochloride 120 mg. Net price 28-tab pack = £6.82; 100-tab pack = £24.36. Label: 25

Dose: hypertension, 1 tablet daily, increased if necessary to max. 4 tablets daily (doses above 2 tablets daily as 2 divided doses)

Angina, see Securon SR® (may be used for dose titration)

PoM Securon SR® (Knoll)

Tablets, m/r, pale green, f/c, verapamil hydrochloride 240 mg. Net price 28-tab pack = £10.64. Label: 25

Dose: hypertension, 1 tablet daily, increased to twice daily if necessary (new patients, initial dose ½ tablet); angina, 1 tablet twice daily (may sometimes be reduced to once daily)

PoM Univer® (Rhône-Poulenc Rorer)

Capsules, m/r, verapamil hydrochloride 120 mg (yellow/dark blue), net price 28-cap pack = £6.83; 180 mg (yellow), 56-cap pack = £16.50; 240 mg (yellow/dark blue), 28-cap pack = £11.13. Label: 25

Dose: hypertension, 240 mg daily, max. 480 mg daily (new patients, initial dose 120 mg); angina, 360 mg daily, max. 480 mg daily

2.6.3   Peripheral vasodilators and related drugs

Most serious peripheral disorders, such as *intermittent claudication*, are now known to be due to occlusion of vessels, either by spasm or sclerotic plaques; use of vasodilators may increase blood flow at rest, but the few controlled studies carried out have shown little improvement in walking distance. Rest pain is rarely affected.

Management of *Raynaud's syndrome* includes avoidance of exposure to cold and stopping smoking. More severe symptoms may require vasodilator treatment, which is most often successful in primary Raynaud's syndrome. Nifedipine (section 2.6.2), prazosin (section 2.5.4) and thymoxamine have all been shown to be beneficial; cinnarizine, naftidrofuryl, nicotinic acid derivatives, and oxpentifylline are not established as being effective.

Vasodilator therapy is not established as being effective for *chilblains* (see section 13.14).

CINNARIZINE

Indications: peripheral vascular disease, Raynaud's syndrome

Cautions; Side-effects: see section 4.6

Dose: initially, 75 mg 3 times daily; maintenance, 75 mg 2–3 times daily

Stugeron Forte® (Janssen)

Capsules, orange/ivory, cinnarizine 75 mg. Net price 100-cap pack = £7.85. Label: 2

Stugeron®: see section 4.6

NAFTIDROFURYL OXALATE

Indications: see under preparations

Cautions: parenteral administration in cardiac insufficiency, conduction disorders (avoid in AV block), and in hepatic and renal impairment

Side-effects: nausea, epigastric pain, rash

Dose: see below

PoM **Praxilene®** (Lipha)

Capsules, pink, naftidrofuryl oxalate 100 mg. Net price 84-cap pack = £8.60. Label: 25, 27

Dose: peripheral vascular disease, 100–200 mg 3 times daily; cerebral vascular disease, 100 mg 3 times daily

Injection forte, naftidrofuryl oxalate 20 mg/mL. Net price 10-mL amp = £1.10

Dose: peripheral vascular disease only, by intravenous or intra-arterial infusion, 200 mg over at least 90 minutes, twice daily

NICOTINIC ACID DERIVATIVES

Indications: peripheral vascular disease (for hyperlipidaemia, see section 2.12)

Side-effects: flushing, dizziness, nausea, vomiting, hypotension (more frequent with nicotinic acid than derivatives); occasional diabetogenic effect reported with nicotinic acid and nicotinyl alcohol; rarely associated with nodular changes to liver (monitor on prolonged high dosage)

Hexopal® (Sanofi Winthrop)

Tablets, scored, inositol nicotinate 500 mg. Net price 20 = £4.07

Dose: 1 g 3 times daily, increased to 4 g daily if required

Tablets forte, scored, inositol nicotinate 750 mg. Net price 112-tab pack = £34.02

Dose: 1.5 g twice daily

Suspension, sugar-free, inositol nicotinate 1 g/5 mL. Net price 300 mL = £20.85

Dose: as for tablets (above)

Ronicol® (Tillomed)

Tablets, scored, nicotinyl alcohol 25 mg (as tartrate). Net price 100-tab pack = £5.55

Dose: 25–50 mg 4 times daily

Timespan® (= tablets m/r), red, s/c, nicotinyl alcohol 150 mg (as tartrate). Net price 100-tab pack = £23.70. Label: 25

Dose: 150–300 mg twice daily

OXPENTIFYLLINE
(Pentoxifylline)

Indications: peripheral vascular disease

Cautions: hypotension, coronary artery disease; avoid in porphyria (see section 9.8.2); **interactions:** Appendix 1 (oxpentifylline)

Contra-indications: cerebral haemorrhage, extensive retinal haemorrhage, acute myocardial infarction

Side-effects: gastro-intestinal disturbances, dizziness, headache; rarely flushing, tachycardia

Dose: 400 mg 2–3 times daily

PoM **Trental®** (Hoechst)

Tablets, m/r, pink, s/c, oxpentifylline 400 mg. Net price 90-tab pack = £15.11; also 250-tab pack (hosp. only). Label: 21, 25

THYMOXAMINE
(Moxisylyte)

Indications: primary Raynaud's syndrome (short-term treatment)

Cautions: diabetes mellitus

Contra-indications: active liver disease

Side-effects: nausea, diarrhoea, flushing, headache, dizziness; hepatic reactions including cholestatic jaundice and hepatitis reported to CSM

Dose: initially 40 mg 4 times daily, increased to 80 mg 4 times daily if poor initial response; discontinue after 2 weeks if no response

PoM **Opilon®** (P-D)

Tablets, yellow, f/c, thymoxamine 40 mg (as hydrochloride). Net price 120-tab pack = £28.00. Label: 21

OTHER PREPARATION USED IN PERIPHERAL VASCULAR DISEASE

Rutosides (oxerutins, Paroven®) are not vasodilators and are not generally regarded as effective preparations as capillary sealants or for the treatment of cramps; side-effects include headache, flushing, rashes, mild gastro-intestinal disturbances.

Paroven® (Zyma)

Capsules, yellow, oxerutins 250 mg. Net price 120-cap pack = £13.67

Dose: For relief of symptoms of oedema associated with chronic venous insufficiency, 500 mg twice daily

2.6.4 Cerebral vasodilators

These drugs are claimed to improve mental function. Some improvements in performance of psychological tests have been reported but the drugs have not been shown clinically to be of much benefit in dementia.

CO-DERGOCRINE MESYLATE

A mixture in equal proportions of dihydroergocornine mesylate, dihydroergocristine mesylate, and (in the ratio 2 : 1) α- and β-dihydroergocryptine mesylates
Indications: adjunct in elderly patients with mild to moderate dementia
Cautions: severe bradycardia
Side-effects: gastro-intestinal disturbances, flushing, headache, rash, nasal congestion; postural hypotension in hypertensive patients
Dose: 1.5 mg 3 times daily *or* 4.5 mg once daily

PoM **Hydergine®** (Sandoz)
Tablets, co-dergocrine mesylate 1.5 mg (scored), net price 20 = £2.16; 4.5 mg, 28-tab pack = £10.78. Label: 22

NAFTIDROFURYL OXALATE
See section 2.6.3

2.6.5 Flosequinan

Flosequinan is a direct-acting vasodilator, producing both arterial and venous vasodilatation. Its use was restricted to patients with *congestive heart failure* who were not responsive to, or were intolerant of, diuretics, ACE inhibitors, and digoxin (where appropriate). It has now been withdrawn.

2.7 Sympathomimetics

2.7.1 Inotropic sympathomimetics
2.7.2 Vasoconstrictor sympathomimetics

The properties of sympathomimetics vary according to whether they act on alpha or on beta adrenergic receptors. Adrenaline acts on both alpha and beta receptors and increases both heart rate and contractility (beta$_1$ effects); it can cause peripheral vasodilation (a beta$_2$ effect) or vasoconstriction (an alpha effect).

In *cardiac arrest* adrenaline 1 in 10 000 (1 mg per 10 mL) is recommended in a dose of 10 mL by central intravenous injection. The procedure for cardiopulmonary resuscitation is given in the algorithm (see next page) which reflects the recommendations of the European Resuscitation Council and the Resuscitation Council (UK).
For *acute anaphylaxis* see p. 133.

ADRENALINE
(Epinephrine)
Indications; Dose: see notes above
Cautions: ischaemic heart disease, diabetes mellitus, hyperthyroidism; hypertension; **interactions:** Appendix 1 (sympathomimetics)

Side-effects: anxiety, tremor, tachycardia, headache, cold extremities; in overdosage arrhythmias, cerebral haemorrhage, pulmonary oedema

PoM **Adrenaline Injection,** adrenaline 1 in 10 000 (adrenaline 100 micrograms/mL as acid tartrate). 10-mL amp.
Available from Martindale and Penn (special order); also from IMS (Min-I-Jet® Adrenaline 3- and 10-mL disposable syringes)
Note. Adrenaline Injection BP is 1 in 1000 (adrenaline 1 mg/mL, as acid tartrate), see p. 135

2.7.1 Inotropic sympathomimetics

The cardiac stimulants **dobutamine** and **dopamine** act on beta$_1$ receptors in cardiac muscle, and increase contractility with little effect on rate; they are used in cardiogenic shock. Dosage of dopamine is critical since although low doses induce vasodilatation and increase renal perfusion, higher doses (more than 5 micrograms per kg per minute) lead to vasoconstriction and may exacerbate heart failure.

Xamoterol also acts on beta$_1$ receptors but being a partial agonist it provokes only a modest stimulatory response at rest. **Important:** restricted to **mild heart failure only**, owing to deterioration in patients with moderate to severe heart failure, see p. 97

Dopexamine acts on beta$_2$ receptors in cardiac muscle to produce its positive inotropic effect; and on peripheral dopamine receptors to increase renal perfusion; it is reported not to induce vasoconstriction.

Isoprenaline is less selective and increases both heart rate and contractility; it may prevent Stokes-Adams attacks, but insertion of a pacemaker is preferable. It is now only used as a short-term emergency treatment of heart block or severe bradycardia.

DOBUTAMINE HYDROCHLORIDE
Indications: inotropic support in infarction, cardiac surgery, cardiomyopathies, septic shock, and cardiogenic shock
Cautions: severe hypotension complicating cardiogenic shock
Side-effects: tachycardia and marked increase in systolic blood pressure indicate overdosage
Dose: by intravenous infusion, 2.5–10 micrograms/kg/minute, adjusted according to response

PoM **Dobutrex®** (Lilly)
Strong sterile solution, dobutamine (as hydrochloride) 12.5 mg/mL. For dilution and use as an intravenous infusion. Net price 20-mL vial = £8.35

ADVANCED CARDIAC LIFE SUPPORT

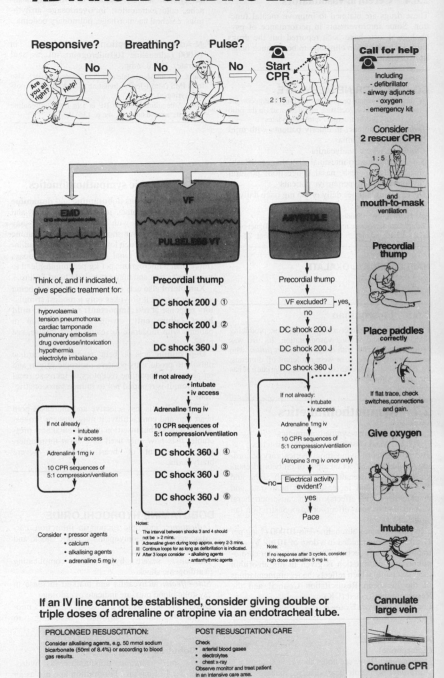

Responsive? No **Breathing?** No **Pulse?** No **Start CPR** 2:15

Call for help

Including
- defibrillator
- airway adjuncts
- oxygen
- emergency kit

Consider 2 rescuer CPR
1:5

and **mouth-to-mask** ventilation

Precordial thump

Place paddles correctly

If flat trace, check switches, connections and gain.

Give oxygen

Intubate

Cannulate large vein

Continue CPR

EMD ECG without palpable pulse

Think of, and if indicated, give specific treatment for:

hypovolaemia
tension pneumothorax
cardiac tamponade
pulmonary embolism
drug overdose/intoxication
hypothermia
electrolyte imbalance

If not already
- intubate
- iv access

Adrenaline 1mg iv

10 CPR sequences of
5:1 compression/ventilation

Consider
- pressor agents
- calcium
- alkalising agents
- adrenaline 5 mg iv

VF
PULSELESS VT

Precordial thump

DC shock 200 J ①

DC shock 200 J ②

DC shock 360 J ③

If not already
- intubate
- iv access

Adrenaline 1mg iv

10 CPR sequences of
5:1 compression/ventilation

DC shock 360 J ④

DC shock 360 J ⑤

DC shock 360 J ⑥

Notes:
I. The interval between shocks 3 and 4 should not be > 2 mins.
II. Adrenaline given during loop approx. every 2-3 mins.
III. Continue loops for as long as defibrillation is indicated.
IV. After 3 loops consider · alkalising agents · antirhythmic agents

ASYSTOLE

Precordial thump

VF excluded? — yes,

no

DC shock 200 J

DC shock 200 J

DC shock 360 J

If not already:
- intubate
- iv access

Adrenaline 1mg iv

10 CPR sequences of
5:1 compression/ventilation

(Atropine 3 mg iv *once only*)

Electrical activity evident? — no

yes

Pace

Note:
If no response after 3 cycles, consider high dose adrenaline 5 mg iv.

If an IV line cannot be established, consider giving double or triple doses of adrenaline or atropine via an endotracheal tube.

PROLONGED RESUSCITATION:
Consider alkalising agents, e.g. 50 mmol sodium bicarbonate (50ml of 8.4%) or according to blood gas results.

POST RESUSCITATION CARE
Check
- arterial blood gases
- electrolytes
- chest x-ray
Observe monitor and treat patient in an intensive care area.

European Resuscitation Council and Resuscitation Council (UK)

Reproduced with permission of the European Resuscitation Council, charts available from Laerdal Medical Ltd

DOPAMINE HYDROCHLORIDE

Indications: cardiogenic shock in infarction or cardiac surgery

Cautions: correct hypovolaemia; low dose in shock due to acute myocardial infarction—see notes above

Contra-indications: tachyarrhythmia, phaeochromocytoma

Side-effects: nausea and vomiting, peripheral vasoconstriction, hypotension, hypertension, tachycardia

Dose: by intravenous infusion, 2–5 micrograms/kg/minute initially (see notes above)

PoM **Dopamine Hydrochloride** (Non-proprietary)

Strong sterile solution, dopamine hydrochloride 40 mg/mL, net price 5-mL amp = £3.77; 160 mg/mL, 5-mL amp = £14.32. For dilution and use as an intravenous infusion

Available from David Bull

PoM **Dopamine Hydrochloride in Dextrose (Glucose) Injection** (Abbott)

Intravenous infusions (in glucose 5% intravenous infusion), dopamine hydrochloride 1.6 mg/mL, and 3.2 mg/mL. 250-mL containers (all hosp. only)

PoM **Intropin®** (Du Pont)

Strong sterile solution, dopamine hydrochloride 40 mg/mL, net price 5-mL amp or syringe = £4.68. For dilution and use as an intravenous infusion

PoM **Select-A-Jet® Dopamine** (IMS)

Strong sterile solution, dopamine hydrochloride 40 mg/mL. Net price 5-mL vial = £3.88; 10-mL vial = £7.75; 20-mL vial = £11.63. For dilution and use as an intravenous infusion

DOPEXAMINE HYDROCHLORIDE

Indications: inotropic support and vasodilator in heart failure associated with cardiac surgery

Cautions: myocardial infarction, recent angina, hypokalaemia, hyperglycaemia; correct hypovolaemia before starting, monitor blood pressure, pulse, plasma potassium, blood glucose; avoid abrupt withdrawal; **interactions:** Appendix 1 (sympathomimetics)

Contra-indications: left ventricular outlet obstruction such as hypertrophic cardiomyopathy or aortic stenosis; phaeochromocytoma, thrombocytopenia

Side-effects: increased heart rate (occasionally excessive tachycardia, particularly in atrial fibrillation), ventricular ectopic beats; also reported: nausea, vomiting, anginal pain, tremor

Dose: by intravenous infusion via caval catheter, 500 nanograms/kg/minute, may be increased to 1 microgram/kg/minute and further increased up to 6 micrograms/kg/minute in increments of 1 microgram/kg/minute at intervals of 10–15 minutes

PoM **Dopacard®** (Porton)

Strong sterile solution, dopexamine hydrochloride 10 mg/mL (1%). For dilution and use as an intravenous infusion. Net price 5-mL amp = £21.00

Note. Contact with metal in infusion apparatus should be minimised

ISOPRENALINE HYDROCHLORIDE

Indications: heart block, severe bradycardia

Cautions: ischaemic heart disease, diabetes mellitus, hyperthyroidism; **interactions:** Appendix 1 (sympathomimetics)

Side-effects: tachycardia, arrhythmias, hypotension, sweating, tremor, headache

Dose: by mouth, initially 30 mg every 6 hours, range 90–840 mg daily (but oral route rarely used)

By intravenous infusion, 0.5–10 micrograms/minute

PoM **Min-I-Jet® Isoprenaline** (IMS)

Injection, isoprenaline hydrochloride 20 micrograms/mL. Net price 10-mL disposable syringe = £3.73

PoM **Saventrine®** (Pharmax)

Tablets, isoprenaline hydrochloride 30 mg. Net price 20 = £1.67

PoM **Saventrine IV®** (Pharmax)

Strong sterile solution, isoprenaline hydrochloride 1 mg/mL. For dilution and use as an intravenous infusion. Net price 2-mL amp = 44p

XAMOTEROL

Indications: chronic mild heart failure (in patients not breathless at rest but limited by symptoms on exertion)

Cautions: withdraw if heart failure deteriorates; cardiac outflow obstruction, arrhythmias (maintain concurrent digoxin in atrial fibrillation), obstructive airways disease (withdraw if worsening, and reverse bronchospasm with inhaled bronchodilator such as salbutamol), reduce dose in renal impairment; pregnancy (toxicity in *animal* studies); **interactions:** Appendix 1 (xamoterol)

Contra-indications: moderate to severe heart failure; breast-feeding

HEART FAILURE. Patients in whom xamoterol is contra-indicated are those:

who are short of breath or fatigued at rest or limited on minimal exercise;

with resting tachycardia (>90 beats per minute) or hypotension (systolic BP <100 mmHg);

with peripheral oedema, raised jugular venous pressure, enlarged liver, or third heart sound;

with (or with history of) acute pulmonary oedema;

who require treatment with frusemide in dose in excess of 40 mg daily (or equivalent);

who require ACE inhibitor treatment

Side-effects: gastro-intestinal disturbances, headache, dizziness, bronchospasm, hypotension;

also reported: chest pain, palpitations, muscle cramp, rashes

Dose: 200 mg daily for 1 week, then 200 mg twice daily

IMPORTANT. Treatment should be started in hospital after full assessment of severity of heart failure by exercise test

PoM **Corwin**® (Stuart)
Tablets, yellow, f/c, xamoterol (as fumarate) 200 mg. Net price 56-tab pack = £25.94

2.7.2   Vasoconstrictor sympathomimetics

Vasoconstrictor sympathomimetics raise blood pressure transiently by acting on alpha-adrenergic receptors to constrict peripheral vessels. They are sometimes used as an emergency method of elevating blood pressure. They may also be used in general and spinal anaesthesia to control blood pressure.

The danger of vasoconstrictors is that although they raise blood pressure they do so at the expense of perfusion of vital organs such as the kidney. Further, in many patients with shock the peripheral resistance is already high, and to raise it further is unhelpful. Thus the use of vasoconstrictors in the treatment of shock is to be generally **deprecated**. The use of plasma substitutes, or of inotropic agents such as dopamine or dobutamine (section 2.7.1) is more appropriate. Treatment of the underlying condition is obviously important.

Spinal and epidural anaesthesia may result in sympathetic block with resultant hypotension. Management may include intravenous fluids (which are also given prophylactically in obstetrics), oxygen, elevation of the legs, and injection of a pressor drug such as ephedrine or methoxamine. As well as constricting peripheral vessels ephedrine also accelerates the heart rate (by acting on beta receptors). Use is made of this dual action of **ephedrine** to manage associated bradycardia (although intravenous injection of atropine sulphate 400 to 600 micrograms may also be required if bradycardia persists). When the hypotension occurs in association with tachycardia the pure alpha-adrenergic stimulant action of **methoxamine** is more appropriate.

EPHEDRINE HYDROCHLORIDE

Indications: see under Dose
Cautions: hyperthyroidism, diabetes mellitus, ischaemic heart disease, hypertension, elderly; may cause acute retention in prostatic hypertrophy; **interactions:** Appendix 1 (sympathomimetics)
Side-effects: tachycardia, anxiety, restlessness, insomnia; also tremor, arrhythmias, dry mouth,

cold extremities; acute retention in prostatic hypertrophy
Dose: reversal of hypotension from spinal or epidural anaesthesia, *by slow intravenous injection* of a solution containing ephedrine hydrochloride 3 mg/mL, 3–6 mg repeated every 3–4 minutes to max. 30 mg (but more than 9 mg rarely required)
Prevention of hypotension from spinal anaesthesia, *by intramuscular injection,* 15–30 mg

PoM **Ephedrine Hydrochloride** (Non-proprietary)
Injection, ephedrine hydrochloride 30 mg/mL. For dilution before intravenous administration. 1-mL amp [unlicensed]

METARAMINOL

Indications: acute hypotension
Cautions;   Contra-indications: see under Noradrenaline Acid Tartrate
Side-effects: tachycardia, arrhythmias, reduced renal blood flow
Dose: by intravenous infusion, 15–100 mg in 500 mL, adjusted according to response

PoM **Aramine**® (MSD)
Injection, metaraminol 10 mg (as tartrate)/mL. Net price 1-mL amp = 57p

METHOXAMINE HYDROCHLORIDE

Indications: hypotension in anaesthesia
Cautions: hyperthyroidism; pregnancy; **interactions:** Appendix 1 (sympathomimetics)
Contra-indications: severe coronary or cardiovascular disease
Side-effects: headache, hypertension, bradycardia
Dose: by intramuscular injection, 5–20 mg
By slow intravenous injection, 5–10 mg (rate 1 mg/minute)

PoM **Vasoxine**® (Wellcome)
Injection, methoxamine hydrochloride 20 mg/mL. Net price 1-mL amp = 52p

NORADRENALINE ACID TARTRATE
(Norepinephrine Bitartrate)
Indications: acute hypotension, cardiac arrest
Cautions: extravasation at injection site may cause necrosis; **interactions:** Appendix 1 (sympathomimetics)
Contra-indications: myocardial   infarction, pregnancy
Side-effects: headache, palpitations, bradycardia
Dose: by intravenous infusion into large vein, of a solution containing noradrenaline acid tartrate 8 micrograms/mL (equivalent to noradrenaline base 4 micrograms/mL) at an initial rate of 2 to 3 mL/minute, adjusted according to response
By rapid intravenous or intracardiac injection, 0.5 to 0.75 mL of a solution containing noradrenaline acid tartrate 200 micrograms/mL (equivalent to noradrenaline base 100 micrograms/mL)

PoM **Levophed®** (Sanofi Winthrop)
Strong sterile solution, noradrenaline acid tartrate
2 mg/mL (equivalent to noradrenaline base 1 mg/
mL). For dilution and use as an intravenous infusion. Net price 2-mL amp = £1.01; 4-mL amp =
£1.50
Special injection, noradrenaline acid tartrate
200 micrograms/mL (equivalent to noradrenaline
base 100 micrograms/mL). Net price 2-mL amp =
98p

PHENYLEPHRINE HYDROCHLORIDE
Indications: acute hypotension
Cautions;   Contra-indications: see   under
Noradrenaline Acid Tartrate; also contra-indicated in severe hypertension and hyperthyroidism
Side-effects: hypertension with headache, palpitations, vomiting; tachycardia or reflex bradycardia; tingling and coolness of skin
Dose: by subcutaneous or intramuscular injection,
5 mg
By slow intravenous injection, 100–500 micrograms
By intravenous infusion, 5–20 mg in 500 mL,
adjusted according to response

PoM **Phenylephrine Injection 1%** (Boots)
Injection, phenylephrine hydrochloride 10 mg/mL.
Net price 1-mL amp = £2.40

2.8   Anticoagulants and protamine

2.8.1	Parenteral anticoagulants
2.8.2	Oral anticoagulants
2.8.3	Protamine sulphate

The main use of anticoagulants is to prevent thrombus formation or extension of an existing thrombus
in the slower-moving venous side of the circulation,
where the thrombus consists of a fibrin web
enmeshed with platelets and red cells. They are
therefore widely used in the prevention and treatment of *deep-vein thrombosis in the legs.*

Anticoagulants are of less use in preventing
thrombus formation in arteries, for in faster-flowing
vessels thrombi are composed mainly of platelets
with little fibrin. They are used to prevent thrombi
forming on *prosthetic heart valves.*

2.8.1   Parenteral anticoagulants

HEPARIN

Heparin initiates anticoagulation rapidly but has a
short duration of action. It is now often referred to
as being **standard** or **unfractionated heparin** to
distinguish it from the **low molecular weight
heparins** (see next page), which have a longer
duration of action.

TREATMENT. For the initial treatment of *deep-vein
thrombosis and pulmonary embolism* heparin is

given as an *intravenous loading dose* , followed by
continuous intravenous infusion (using an infusion
pump) or by *intermittent subcutaneous injection*;
the use of *intermittent intravenous injection* is no
longer recommended. An oral anticoagulant (usually warfarin, see section 2.8.2) is started at the
same time as the heparin (which needs to be continued for at least 3 days, until the oral anticoagulant
has taken effect). Laboratory monitoring is essential—preferably on a daily basis, determination of
the APTT (activated partial thromboplastin time)
being the most widely used technique. Heparin is
also used in regimens for the management of *myocardial infarction* (see also section 2.10), the management of *unstable angina pectoris*, and the
management of *acute peripheral arterial occlusion.*

PROPHYLAXIS. In patients undergoing *general surgery*, low-dose heparin by subcutaneous injection is
widely advocated to *prevent postoperative deep-vein thrombosis and pulmonary embolism* in 'high
risk' patients (i.e. those with obesity, malignant disease, history of deep-vein thrombosis or pulmonary
embolism, patients over 40, or those with an established thrombophilic disorder or who are undergoing large or complicated surgical procedures);
laboratory monitoring is not required with this
standard prophylactic regimen. To combat the
increased risk in *major orthopaedic surgery* an
adjusted dose regimen may be used (with monitoring) or *low molecular weight heparin* (see next
page) may be selected.

EXTRACORPOREAL CIRCUITS. Heparin is also used
in the maintenance of extracorporeal circuits in
cardiopulmonary bypass and *haemodialysis.*

HAEMORRHAGE. If haemorrhage occurs it is usually
sufficient to withdraw heparin, but if rapid reversal
of the effects of heparin is required, protamine sulphate (section 2.8.3) is a specific antidote (but only
partially reverses the effects of low molecular
weight heparins).

HEPARIN
Indications: see under Dose
Cautions: hepatic and renal impairment (avoid if
severe); pregnancy; **interactions:** Appendix 1
(heparin)
THROMBOCYTOPENIA. Clinically important thrombocytopenia is immune-mediated, and does not usually
develop until after 6 to 10 days; it may be complicated
by thrombosis. The CSM has recommended platelet
counts for patients receiving heparin for longer than 5
days (and that heparin should be stopped immediately in
those who develop thrombocytopenia). Alternatives for
patients requiring continued anticoagulation are low
molecular weight heparins (but cross reactivity may
occur), a heparinoid (such as danaparoid), warfarin, epoprostenol, or ancrod [named-patient basis].
Contra-indications: haemophilia and other haemorrhagic disorders, thrombocytopenia, peptic
ulcer, recent cerebral haemorrhage, severe hypertension, severe liver disease (including oesophageal varices), renal failure, after major trauma
or recent surgery (especially to eye or nervous
system), hypersensitivity to heparin

Side-effects: haemorrhage (see notes above), skin necrosis, thrombocytopenia (see Cautions), hypersensitivity reactions (including urticaria, angioedema, and anaphylaxis); osteoporosis after prolonged use (and rarely alopecia)

Dose:

Treatment of deep-vein thrombosis and pulmonary embolism, *by intravenous injection,* loading dose of 5000 units (10 000 units in severe pulmonary embolism) followed by continuous *infusion* of 1000–2000 units/hour *or* by *subcutaneous injection* of 15 000 units every 12 hours (laboratory monitoring essential — preferably on a daily basis)

SMALL ADULT OR CHILD, lower loading dose *then*, 15–25 units/kg/hour *by intravenous infusion, or* 250 units/kg every 12 hours by *subcutaneous injection*

Unstable angina, acute peripheral arterial occlusion, as intravenous regimen for deep-vein thrombosis and pulmonary embolism, above

Prophylaxis of deep-vein thrombosis and pulmonary embolism, *by subcutaneous injection,* 5000 units 2 hours before surgery (see notes above), then every 8–12 hours for 7 days or until patient is ambulant (monitoring not needed); during pregnancy (with monitoring), 5000–10 000 units every 12 hours (**important:** not intended to cover prevention of prosthetic heart valve thrombosis in pregnancy which calls for separate specialist management)

MYOCARDIAL INFARCTION. For the prevention of *coronary re-occlusion after thrombolysis* heparin is used in a variety of regimens according to locally agreed protocols

For the prevention of *mural thrombosis* heparin is considered effective when given by *subcutaneous injection* of 12 500 units every 12 hours for at least 10 days

Note. Doses above reflect the guidelines of the British Society for Haematology; for doses of the low molecular weight heparins, p 100–101

PoM Heparin Injection (heparin sodium)
1000 units/mL, net price 1-mL amp = 21p; 5-mL amp = 69p; 5-mL vial = 54p
5000 units/mL, net price 1-mL amp = 33p; 5-mL amp = 98p; 5-mL vial = £1.46
25 000 units/mL, net price 1-mL amp = 86p; 5-mL vial = £6.43

PoM Calciparine® (Sanofi Winthrop)
Injection (subcutaneous only), heparin calcium 25 000 units/mL. Net price 0.2-mL syringe = 68p; 0.5-mL syringe = £1.46; 0.8-mL syringe = £1.76

PoM Minihep® (Leo)
Injection (subcutaneous only), heparin sodium 25 000 units/mL. Net price 0.2-mL amp = 41p

PoM Minihep Calcium® (Leo)
Injection (subcutaneous only), heparin calcium 25 000 units/mL. Net price 0.2-mL amp = 44p

PoM Monoparin® (CP)
Injection, heparin sodium (mucous) 1000 units/mL, net price 1-mL amp = 18p; 5-mL amp = 54p; 10-mL amp = 72p; 5000 units/mL, 1-mL amp = 36p; 5-mL amp = 98p; 25 000 units/mL, 0.2-mL amp = 44p, 1-mL amp = £1.09

PoM Monoparin Calcium® (CP)
Injection, heparin calcium 25 000 units/mL. Net price 0.2-mL amp = 47p

PoM Multiparin® (CP)
Injection, heparin sodium (mucous) 1000 units/mL, net price 5-mL vial = 46p; 5000 units/mL, 5-mL vial = 92p; 25 000 units/mL, 5-mL vial = £3.84

PoM Pump-Hep® (Leo)
Injection, heparin sodium (mucous) 1000 units/mL. Net price 5-mL amp = 39p; 10-mL amp = 64p; 20-mL amp = 95p

PoM Unihep® (Leo)
Injection, heparin sodium (mucous) 1000 units/mL, net price 1-mL amp = 13p; 5000 units/mL, 1-mL amp = 27p; 10 000 units/mL, 1-mL amp = 44p; 25 000 units/mL, 1-mL amp = £1.04

PoM Uniparin® (CP)
Injection (subcutaneous only), heparin sodium 25 000 units/mL. Net price 0.2-mL syringe = 55p; 0.4-mL syringe (Uniparin Forte®) = £1.53

PoM Uniparin Calcium® (CP)
Injection (subcutaneous only), heparin calcium 25 000 units/mL. Net price 0.2-mL syringe = 55p; 0.5-mL syringe = £1.50

LOW MOLECULAR WEIGHT HEPARINS

There is evidence that the low molecular weight heparins, **dalteparin**, **enoxaparin**, and **tinzaparin**, are as effective and as safe as unfractionated heparin in the prevention of venous thrombo-embolism; in orthopaedic practice they are probably more effective. They have a longer duration of action than unfractionated heparin; *once-daily subcutaneous* dosage means that they are convenient to use. The standard prophylactic regimen does not require monitoring.

HAEMORRHAGE. See under Heparin.

DALTEPARIN

Indications: see notes above and under preparations

Cautions; Contra-indications; Side-effects: see under Heparin

PoM Fragmin® (Pharmacia)
Injection, dalteparin sodium 2500 units/mL, net price 4-mL amp (10 000 units) = £5.36; 10 000 units/mL, 1-mL amp (10 000 units) = £5.36; 12 500 units/mL, 0.2-mL syringe (2500 units) = £1.95; 25 000 units/mL, 0.2-mL syringe (5000 units) = £2.96
Dose: prophylaxis of deep-vein thrombosis, *by subcutaneous injection, moderate risk,* 2500 units 1–2 hours before surgery then 2500 units every 24 hours for 5 days; *high risk,* 2500 units 1–2 hours before surgery, then 2500 units 12 hours later, then 5000 units every 24 hours for 5 days

---

ENOXAPARIN

Indications: see notes above and under preparations

Cautions; Contra-indications; Side-effects: see under Heparin

PoM **Clexane**® (Rhône-Poulenc Rorer)

Injection, enoxaparin 100 mg/mL. Net price 0.2-mL syringe (20 mg) = £3.55; 0.4-mL syringe (40 mg) = £4.73

Dose: prophylaxis of deep-vein thrombosis, *by subcutaneous injection, moderate risk,* 20 mg (2000 units) 1–2 hours before surgery then 20 mg (2000 units) every 24 hours for 7–10 days; *high risk,* 40 mg (4000 units) 12 hours before surgery then 40 mg (4000 units) every 24 hours for 7–10 days

TINZAPARIN

Indications: see notes above and under preparations

Cautions; Contra-indications; Side-effects: see under Heparin

▼ PoM **Innohep**® (Leo)

Injection, tinzaparin 3500 units/0.3-mL syringe, net price 1 syringe = £3.12; 5000 units/0.5-mL ampoule, 1 amp = £2.97

Dose: prophylaxis of deep-vein thrombosis, *by subcutaneous injection,* general surgery, 3500 units 2 hours before surgery, then 3500 units every 24 hours for 7–10 days; orthopaedic surgery (high risk), 50 units/kg 2 hours before surgery, then 50 units/kg every 24 hours for 7–10 days

▼ PoM **Logiparin**® (Novo Nordisk)

Injection, tinzaparin 2500 units/syringe, net price 1 syringe = £3.61; 3500 units/syringe, 1 syringe = £4.83; 4500 units/syringe, 1 syringe = £4.83

Dose: prophylaxis of deep-vein thrombosis, *by subcutaneous injection,* general surgery, 3500 units 2 hours before surgery, then 3500 units every 24 hours for 7–10 days; orthopaedic surgery, patients under 60 kg, 2500 units 2 hours before surgery then 2500 units every 24 hours for 7–10 days; 60–80 kg, 3500 units 2 hours before surgery then every 24 hours as above; over 80 kg 4500 units 2 hours before surgery then every 24 hours as above

HEPARINOIDS

Danaparoid is a heparinoid used for prophylaxis of deep-vein thrombosis in patients undergoing general or orthopaedic surgery. Providing there is no evidence of cross-sensitivity, it may also have a role in patients who develop thrombocytopenia in association with heparin.

DANAPAROID SODIUM

(Org 10172)

Indications: prophylaxis of deep vein thrombosis in general and orthopaedic surgery

Cautions: hepatic and renal imapirment (avoid if severe); pregnancy and breast-feeding

ASTHMA. Presence of sulphite in ampoules may (especially in patients with asthma) lead to hypersensitivity (with bronchospasm and shock)

Contra-indications: see under Heparin; cross-reactivity to heparin-induced thrombocytopenia

Side-effects: haemorrhage (see notes above); thrombocytopenia (may be cross-sensitivity with heparin); hypersensitivity reactions (including rash); liver enzyme changes; osteoporosis with excessive dosage; bruising or pain at injection site

Dose: *by subcutaneous injection,* 750 units 1–4 hours before surgery, then twice daily for 7–10 days

Note. If patient cannot be operated on immediately (e.g. after hip fracture), twice daily administration may be initiated, providing the last pre-operative dose is given not later than 1 hour before surgery

▼ PoM **Orgaran**® (Organon)

Injection, danaparoid sodium 1250 units/mL, net price 0.6-mL amp (750 units) = £3.49

HEPARIN FLUSHES

For maintaining catheter patency sodium chloride injection 0.9% is as effective as heparin flushes for up to 48 hours, and is therefore recommended for cannulas intended to be in place for 48 hours or less. Heparin flushes are recommended for cannulas intended to be in place for longer than 48 hours.

PoM **Canusal**® (CP)

Solution, heparin sodium 100 units/mL. Net price 2-mL amp = 29p. To maintain patency of catheters, cannulas, etc., 200 units flushed through every 4 hours or as required. Not for therapeutic use

PoM **Hep-Flush**® (Leo)

Solution, heparin sodium 100 units/mL. Net price 2-mL amp = 25p; 10-mL vial = £1.27. To maintain patency of catheters, cannulas, etc., 200 units flushed through every 4–8 hours. Not for therapeutic use

PoM **Heplok**® (Leo)

Solution, heparin sodium 10 units/mL. Net price 5-mL amp = 29p. To maintain patency of catheters, cannulas, etc., 10–50 units flushed through every 4 hours. Not for therapeutic use

PoM **Hepsal**® (CP)

Solution, heparin sodium 10 units/mL. Net price 5-mL amp = 25p. To maintain patency of catheters, cannulas, etc., 50 units flushed through every 4 hours or as required. Not for therapeutic use

ANCROD

Ancrod reduces plasma fibrinogen by cleavage of fibrin but is not in common use. It is available from Knoll (Arvin®) on 'named patient' basis only.

EPOPROSTENOL

Epoprostenol (prostacyclin) can be given to inhibit platelet aggregation during renal dialysis either alone or with heparin. Since its half-life is only about 3 minutes it must be given by continuous intravenous infusion. It is a potent vasodilator and therefore its side-effects include flushing, headache, and hypotension.

EPOPROSTENOL

Indications: see notes above
Cautions: anticoagulant monitoring required when given with heparin
Side-effects: see notes above; also bradycardia, pallor, sweating with higher doses
Dose: see manufacturer's literature

PoM **Flolan®** (Wellcome)
Infusion, powder for reconstitution, epoprostenol (as sodium salt). Net price 500-microgram vial (with diluent) = £103.86

2.8.2   Oral anticoagulants

Oral anticoagulants antagonise the effects of vitamin K, and take at least 48 to 72 hours for the anticoagulant effect to develop fully; if an immediate effect is required, heparin must be given concomitantly.

The main indication for oral anticoagulant therapy is *deep-vein thrombosis.* Patients with *pulmonary embolism* should also be treated, as should those with *atrial fibrillation who are at risk of embolisation,* and those with *prosthetic heart valves* (to prevent emboli developing on the valves); antiplatelet drugs may also be useful in these patients.

Oral anticoagulants should not be used in cerebral thrombosis or peripheral arterial occlusion, but may be of value in patients with *transient brain ischaemic attacks* whether due to carotid or vertebrobasilar arterial disease; if these patients also have severe hypertension anticoagulants are contraindicated, and antiplatelet drugs are an alternative (section 2.9).

Warfarin is the drug of choice; **nicoumalone** and **phenindione** are seldom used.

Whenever possible, the base-line prothrombin time should be determined before the initial dose is given.

The usual adult induction dose of warfarin is 10 mg[1] daily for 2 days (higher doses no longer recommended). The subsequent maintenance dose depends upon the prothrombin time (reported as INR[2]); the currently recommended therapeutic ranges are:
INR 2–2.5 for prophylaxis of deep-vein thrombosis including surgery on high-risk patients;
INR 2–3 for prophylaxis in hip surgery and fractured femur operations, for treatment of deep-vein thrombosis, pulmonary embolism, systemic embolism, prevention of venous thrombo-embolism in myocardial infarction, mitral stenosis with embolism, transient ischaemic attacks, atrial fibrillation, and tissue prosthetic heart valves;
INR 3–4.5 for recurrent deep-vein thrombosis and pulmonary embolism, arterial disease including myocardial infarction, and mechanical prosthetic heart valves.
It is essential that the INR be determined:
daily or on alternate days in early days of treatment, *then* at longer intervals (depending on response) *then* up to every 8 weeks
The daily maintenance dose[3] of warfarin is usually 3 to 9 mg (taken at the **same time** each day).

The main adverse effect of all oral anticoagulants is haemorrhage. Omission of dosage with checking of the INR is essential. The following recommendations of the British Society for Haematology are based on the result of the INR and the clinical state:
Life-threatening haemorrhage—immediately give phytomenadione (vitamin K₁) 5 mg by slow intravenous injection and a concentrate of factors II, IX, X (with factor VII concentrate if available). If no concentrate is available, fresh frozen plasma should be infused (approximately 1 litre for an adult) but this may not be as effective
Less severe haemorrhage e.g. haematuria and epistaxis—withhold warfarin for one or more days and consider giving phytomenadione (vitamin K₁) 0.5–2 mg[4] by slow intravenous injection
INR 4.5–7 without haemorrhage—withhold warfarin for 1 or 2 days then review
INR >7 without haemorrhage—withhold warfarin and consider giving phytomenadione (vitamin K₁) 500 micrograms by slow intravenous injection
Unexpected bleeding at therapeutic levels[5]—investigate possibility of underlying cause e.g. unsuspected renal or alimentary tract pathology

PREGNANCY. Oral anticoagulants are teratogenic and should not be given in the first trimester of pregnancy. Women at risk of pregnancy should be warned of this danger since stopping warfarin before the sixth week of gestation may largely avoid the risk of fetal abnormality. Oral anticoagulants cross the placenta with risk of placental or fetal haemorrhage, especially during the last few weeks of pregnancy and at delivery. Therefore, if at all possible, oral anticoagulants should be avoided in pregnancy, especially in the first and third trimesters. Difficult decisions may have to be made, particularly in women with prosthetic heart valves or with a history of recurrent venous thrombosis or pulmonary embolism.

Anticoagulant treatment booklets must be carried by patients, and are available from:

England:	Scottish Office
HMSO	Health Department
Broadway	Room 64
Chadderton	St. Andrew's House
Oldham	Edinburgh EH1 3DH
Lancs OL9 6QH	
	Northern Ireland Office
Wales:	Central Services Agency
Room 106	27 Adelaide St
Royal Pharmaceutical	Belfast BT2 8FH
Society of Great Britain	

Booklets giving advice for patients on anticoagulant treatment may be given to patients at the discretion of the doctor or pharmacist.

1. Less than 10 mg if base-line prothrombin time prolonged, if liver-function tests abnormal, or if patient in cardiac failure, on parenteral feeding, less than average body weight, or over 80 years of age.
2. The International Normalised Ratio (INR) has now replaced the British Ratio (BR).
3. Change in patient's clinical condition, particularly associated with liver disease, intercurrent illness, or drug administration, necessitates more frequent testing. See also **interactions,** Appendix 1 (warfarin). Major changes in diet (especially involving vegetables) may also affect warfarin control.
4. Usually 1 mg adequate and should be given if INR greater than desired; higher doses will prevent oral anticoagulants from acting for several days or even weeks.
5. Should always be investigated regardless of INR since even if patients over-anticoagulated bleeding generally has an additional underlying cause.

WARFARIN SODIUM

Indications: prophylaxis of embolisation in rheumatic heart disease and atrial fibrillation; prophylaxis after insertion of prosthetic heart valve; prophylaxis and treatment of venous thrombosis and pulmonary embolism; transient ischaemic attacks

Cautions: hepatic or renal disease, recent surgery; **interactions:** Appendix 1 (warfarin)

Contra-indications: pregnancy (see notes above), peptic ulcer, severe hypertension, bacterial endocarditis

Side-effects: haemorrhage

Dose: see notes above

PoM Marevan® (Goldshield)

Tablets, brown, scored, warfarin sodium 1 mg. Net price 20 = 15p. Label: 10 anticoagulant card

Tablets, blue, scored, warfarin sodium 3 mg. Net price 20 = 18p. Label: 10 anticoagulant card

Tablets, pink, scored, warfarin sodium 5 mg. Net price 20 = 28p. Label: 10 anticoagulant card

PoM Warfarin WBP (Boehringer Ingelheim)

Tablets, brown, scored, warfarin sodium 1 mg. Net price 20 = 9p. Label: 10 anticoagulant card

Tablets, blue, scored, warfarin sodium 3 mg. Net price 20 = 10p. Label: 10 anticoagulant card

Tablets, pink, scored, warfarin sodium 5 mg. Net price 20 = 16p. Label: 10 anticoagulant card

NICOUMALONE

(Acenocoumarol)

Indications; Cautions; Contra-indications; Side-effects: see under Warfarin Sodium; avoid breast-feeding

Dose: 8–12 mg on 1st day; 4–8 mg on 2nd day; maintenance dose usually 1–8 mg daily

PoM Sinthrome® (Geigy)

Tablets, nicoumalone 1 mg. Net price 20 = 38p. Label: 10 anticoagulant card

PHENINDIONE

Indications: prophylaxis of embolisation in rheumatic heart disease and atrial fibrillation; prophylaxis after insertion of prosthetic heart valve; prophylaxis and treatment of venous thrombosis and pulmonary embolism

Cautions; Contra-indications; Side-effects: see under Warfarin Sodium; also hypersensitivity reactions including rashes, fever, leucopenia, agranulocytosis, diarrhoea, renal and hepatic damage; urine coloured pink; avoid breast-feeding; **interactions:** Appendix 1 (phenindione)

Dose: 200 mg on 1st day; 100 mg on 2nd day; maintenance dose usually 50–150 mg daily

PoM Dindevan® (Goldshield)

Tablets, phenindione 10 mg, net price 20 = 91p; 25 mg (green), 20 = £1.25; 50 mg, 20 = £1.61. Label: 10 anticoagulant card, 14 (urine pink)

2.8.3   Protamine sulphate

Although protamine sulphate is used to counteract overdosage with heparin, if used in excess it has an anticoagulant effect.

PROTAMINE SULPHATE

(Protamine Sulfate)

Indications; Cautions: see above

Side-effects: flushing, hypotension, bradycardia

Dose: by slow intravenous injection, 1 mg neutralises 100 units heparin (mucous) or 80 units heparin (lung) when given within 15 minutes; if longer time, less protamine required as heparin rapidly excreted; max. 50 mg

PoM Protamine Sulphate (Non-proprietary)

Injection, protamine sulphate 10 mg/mL. Net price 5-mL amp = 98p; 10-mL amp = £1.75

Available from Boots, CP (Prosulf®), Evans

2.9   Antiplatelet drugs

By decreasing platelet aggregation, these drugs may inhibit thrombus formation on the arterial side of the circulation, where thrombi are formed by platelet aggregation and anticoagulants have little effect. Antiplatelet drugs have little effect in venous thromboembolism. **Dipyridamole** is used by mouth as an adjunct to oral anticoagulation for prophylaxis of thromboembolism associated with prosthetic heart valves.

Encouraging results have been obtained using **aspirin** 75–300 mg daily for the *secondary* prevention of thrombotic cerebrovascular or cardiovascular disease. Aspirin has also been shown to reduce mortality when given in a dose of 150 mg daily for a month after myocardial infarction. Low doses of aspirin (such as 75 or 100 mg daily) are also given following bypass surgery.

For use of epoprostenol, see section 2.8.1.

ASPIRIN (antiplatelet)

(Acetylsalicylic Acid)

Indications: prophylaxis of cerebrovascular disease or myocardial infarction (see notes above)

Cautions: asthma; uncontrolled hypertension; pregnancy (but see Appendix 4); **interactions:** Appendix 1 (aspirin)

Contra-indications: children under 12 years and in breast-feeding (Reye's syndrome, see section 4.7.1); active peptic ulceration; haemophilia and other bleeding disorders

Side-effects: bronchospasm; gastro-intestinal haemorrhage (occasionally major), also other haemorrhage (e.g. subconjunctival)

Dose: see notes above

Aspirin (Non-proprietary)

Dispersible tablets, aspirin 75 mg, net price 20 = 5p; 300 mg, see section 4.7.1. Label: 13, 21, 32

Angettes 75® (Bristol-Myers)

Tablets, aspirin 75 mg. Net price 56-tab pack = £1.88. Label: 32

Cautionary label wordings, see inside back cover

Caprin®: see section 4.7.1

Disprin CV® (R&C)

Tablets, both m/r, aspirin 100 mg, net price 28-tab pack = £1.68; 300 mg, 28-tab pack = £1.99. Label: 25, 32

Nu-Seals® Aspirin (Lilly)

Tablets, e/c, aspirin 75 mg, net price 56-tab pack = £3.09; 300 mg, see section 4.7.1. Label: 5, 25, 32

Note. Tablets may be chewed at diagnosis for rapid absorption

DIPYRIDAMOLE

Indications: see notes above

Cautions: rapidly worsening angina, aortic stenosis, recent myocardial infarction; may exacerbate migraine, hypotension; **interactions:** Appendix 1 (dipyridamole)—**important**: interaction with adenosine liable to be serious

Side-effects: nausea, diarrhoea, throbbing headache, hypotension

Dose: by mouth, 300–600 mg daily in 3–4 divided doses before food

By intravenous injection, diagnostic only, see manufacturer's literature

PoM **Dipyridamole** (Non-proprietary)

Tablets, coated, dipyridamole 25 mg, net price 20 = 40p; 100 mg, 20 = £1.06. Label: 22

Available from APS, Ashbourne (Cerebrovase®), Berk (Modaplate®), Cox, Hillcross, K Pharm., Lagap, Norton

PoM **Persantin®** (Boehringer Ingelheim)

Tablets, both s/c, dipyridamole 25 mg (orange), net price 84-tab pack = £1.78; 100 mg, 84-tab pack = £4.95. Label: 22

Injection, dipyridamole 5 mg/mL. Net price 2-mL amp = 11p

2.10   Fibrinolytic drugs

Fibrinolytic drugs act as thrombolytics by activating plasminogen to form plasmin, which degrades fibrin and so breaks up thrombi.

Streptokinase is used in the treatment of *life-threatening venous thrombosis,* and in *pulmonary embolism,* but treatment must be started rapidly.

Urokinase is currently used for *thrombolysis in the eye* and in *arteriovenous shunts.* It has the advantage of being non-immunogenic.

The value of thrombolytic drugs for the treatment of *myocardial infarction* has been established. **Streptokinase, alteplase,** and **anistreplase** have all been shown to reduce mortality when given by the intravenous route with comparable efficacy. The potential for benefit lessens as the delay from the onset of major symptoms increases, but the value of treatment within the first 12 hours is reasonably well established. Knowledge of the role of adjuvant therapy is also incomplete, but in the case of streptokinase the reduction in mortality by aspirin has been shown to be additive whilst immediate heparin is necessary to obtain full efficacy from alteplase. Thrombolytic drugs are indicated for any patient with acute myocardial infarction for whom the benefit is believed to outweigh the risk of treat-

ment. Trials have shown that the benefit is greatest in those with ECG changes that include ST segment elevation and in those with anterior infarction. Patients should not be excluded on account of age alone because mortality in this group is high and the percentage reduction in mortality is the same as in younger patients.

CAUTIONS. Risk of bleeding from venepuncture or invasive procedures, any external chest compression, pregnancy, possibility of pre-existing thrombus as in abdominal aneurysm or enlarged left atrium with atrial fibrillation (risk of dissolution of clot and subsequent embolisation), recent or concurrent anticoagulant therapy.

CONTRA-INDICATIONS. Recent haemorrhage, trauma, or surgery (including dental extraction), coagulation defects, bleeding diatheses, history of cerebrovascular disease especially recent events or with any residual disability, recent symptoms of possible peptic ulceration, heavy vaginal bleeding, severe hypertension, pulmonary disease with cavitation, acute pancreatitis, diabetic retinopathy, severe liver disease, oesophageal varices. In the case of streptokinase or anistreplase, previous allergic reactions to either drug, or therapy with either drug from 5 days to 12 months or more previously.

SIDE-EFFECTS. Side-effects of thrombolytics are mainly nausea and vomiting and bleeding. Back pain has been reported. Bleeding is usually limited to the site of injection, but intracerebral haemorrhage or bleeding from other sites may occur. Serious bleeding calls for discontinuation of the thrombolytic and may require administration of coagulation factors and antifibrinolytic drugs (aprotinin or tranexamic acid). Streptokinase and anistreplase may cause allergic reactions and anaphylaxis has been reported (for details of management see Allergic Emergencies, section 3.4.3). Guillain-Barré syndrome has been reported rarely after streptokinase treatment.

ALTEPLASE

(rt-PA, tissue-type plasminogen activator)

Indications: acute myocardial infarction (see notes above)

Cautions; Contra-indications; Side-effects: see notes above

Dose: by intravenous injection, 10 mg over 1–2 minutes, followed by *intravenous infusion* of 50 mg over 1 hour, then 40 mg over the subsequent 2 hours (total dose 100 mg over 3 hours); treatment should be initiated within 6 hours; patients weighing less than 67 kg should receive a total dose of 1.5 mg/kg according to the above schedule

PoM **Actilyse®** (Boehringer Ingelheim)

Injection, powder for reconstitution, alteplase 20 mg (11.6 mega units)/vial, net price per vial (with diluent and transfer device) = £200.00; 50 mg (29 mega units)/vial, pack of 2 vials (with diluent, transfer device, and infusion bag) = £816.00

ANISTREPLASE
(APSAC)

Indications: acute myocardial infarction (see notes above)

Cautions; Contra-indications; Side-effects: see notes above

Dose: by intravenous injection, 30 units over 4–5 minutes; treatment should be initiated as soon as possible and preferably within 6 hours

PoM **Eminase®** (Beecham)
Injection, powder for reconstitution, anistreplase. Net price 30-unit vial = £495.00 (also available in injection pack with 5-mL amp water for injections and disposable syringe and needle)

STREPTOKINASE

Indications: deep-vein thrombosis, pulmonary embolism, acute arterial thromboembolism, thrombosed arteriovenous shunts; acute myocardial infarction (see notes above)

Cautions; Contra-indications; Side-effects: see notes above

Dose: by intravenous infusion, 250 000 units over 30 minutes, then 100 000 units every hour for up to 24–72 hours according to condition (see data sheet)
Myocardial infarction, 1 500 000 units over 60 minutes followed by aspirin 150 mg daily *by mouth* for at least 4 weeks (see data sheet)

PoM **Kabikinase®** (Pharmacia)
Injection, powder for reconstitution, streptokinase; net price 250 000-unit vial = £15.00; 750 000-unit vial = £40.00; 1.5 million-unit vial = £85.00

PoM **Streptase®** (Hoechst)
Injection, powder for reconstitution, streptokinase; net price 250 000-unit vial = £15.36; 750 000-unit vial = £40.26; 1.5 million-unit vial = £80.52 (hosp. only)

UROKINASE

Indications: thrombosed arteriovenous shunts and intravenous cannulas; thrombolysis in the eye; deep-vein thrombosis, pulmonary embolism, peripheral vascular occlusion

Cautions; Contra-indications; Side-effects: see notes above

Dose: by instillation into arteriovenous shunt, 5000–25 500 International units in 2–3 mL sodium chloride injection 0.9%

By intravenous infusion 4400 International units/kg over 10 minutes, then 4400 units/kg/hour for 12 hours in pulmonary embolism or 12–24 hours in deep-vein thrombosis; for bolus injection for pulmonary embolism consult data sheet
Peripheral vascular occlusion, consult data sheet
Intra-ocular administration, 5000 International units in 2 mL sodium chloride injection 0.9%

PoM **Ukidan®** (Serono)
Injection, powder for reconstitution, urokinase; net price 5000 International unit vial = £7.88; 25 000 International unit vial = £27.71; 100 000 International unit vial = £60.00

PoM **Urokinase** (Leo)
Injection, powder for reconstitution, urokinase; net price 5000 International unit vial = £9.75; 25 000 International unit vial = £27.79

2.11 Antifibrinolytic drugs and haemostatics

Fibrin dissolution can be impaired by the administration of **tranexamic acid**, which inhibits plasminogen activation and fibrinolysis. It may be useful when haemorrhage cannot be staunched, e.g. in prostatectomy, dental extraction in haemophiliacs, or menorrhagia; it may also be used in hereditary angioedema and in streptokinase overdose.

Desmopressin (see section 6.5.2) is used in the management of mild to moderate haemophilia.

Aprotinin is a proteolytic enzyme inhibitor acting on plasmin and kallidinogenase (kallikrein). It is indicated for patients at high risk of major blood loss during and after open heart surgery with extracorporeal circulation and for patients in whom optimal blood conservation during open heart surgery is an absolute priority; it is also indicated for the treatment of life-threatening haemorrhage due to hyperplasminaemia (occasionally observed during the mobilisation and dissection of malignant tumours, in acute promyelocytic leukaemia, and following thrombolytic therapy).

Ethamsylate reduces capillary bleeding in the presence of a normal number of platelets. It does not act by fibrin stabilisation, but probably by correcting abnormal platelet adhesion.

APROTININ

Indications: see notes above

Side-effects: occasionally hypersensitivity reactions and localised thrombophlebitis

Dose: by slow intravenous injection or infusion
Open heart surgery, loading dose, 2 000 000 units (200 mL) after induction of anaesthesia and before sternotomy, *by slow intravenous injection* initially 50 000 units (5 mL) over several minutes (to detect allergy), remainder *by intravenous infusion* over 20 minutes; maintenance dose, *by intravenous infusion* 500 000 units (50 mL) every hour until end of operation (or early postoperative period in septic endocarditis); pump prime, 2 000 000 units (200 mL) in priming volume of extracorporeal circuit; in septic endocarditis 3 000 000 units (300 mL) added to pump prime
Hyperplasminaemia, *by slow intravenous injection or by infusion* initially, 500 000 units (50 mL) to 1 000 000 units (100 mL) at max. rate 10 mL/min; followed if necessary by 200 000 units (20 mL) every hour until bleeding stops

PoM Trasylol® (Bayer)
Injection, aprotinin 10 000 kallikrein inactivator units/mL. Net price 50-mL vial = £20.53
Note. Aprotinin injection containing 10 000 kallikrein inactivator units/mL also available from Paines & Byrne

ETHAMSYLATE
(Etamsylate)
Indications: see under preparations
Contra-indications: porphyria (see section 9.8.2)
Side-effects: nausea, headache, rashes
Dose: see below

PoM Dicynene® (Delandale)
Tablets, scored, ethamsylate 500 mg, net price 100-tab pack = £22.13
Dose: short-term treatment of blood loss in menorrhagia, 500 mg 4 times daily during menstruation
Injection, ethamsylate 125 mg/mL. Net price 2-mL amp = 82p
Dose: prophylaxis and treatment of periventricular haemorrhage in low birth-weight infants, by intramuscular or intravenous injection, 12.5 mg/kg every 6 hours
IMPORTANT. The ampoules currently available contain a total of 250 mg in 2 mL volume therefore **small fraction only** required for neonatal use

TRANEXAMIC ACID
Indications: see notes above
Cautions: reduce dose in renal impairment; massive haematuria (avoid if risk of ureteric obstruction); regular eye examinations and liver function tests in long-term treatment of hereditary angioedema
Note. Requirement for regular eye examinations during long-term treatment is based on unsatisfactory evidence
Contra-indications: thromboembolic disease
Side-effects: nausea, vomiting, diarrhoea (reduce dose); giddiness on rapid intravenous injection
Dose: by mouth, 1–1.5 g 2–4 times daily
By slow intravenous injection, 0.5–1 g 3 times daily

PoM Cyklokapron® (Pharmacia)
Tablets, f/c, scored, tranexamic acid 500 mg. Net price 60-tab pack = £13.61
Syrup, tranexamic acid 500 mg/5 mL. Net price 300 mL = £15.60
Injection, tranexamic acid 100 mg/mL. Net price 5-mL amp = £1.35

BLOOD PRODUCTS

FACTOR VIII FRACTION, DRIED
(Human Antihaemophilic Fraction, Dried)
A concentrate prepared from pooled plasma from suitable human donors
Indications: control of haemorrhage in haemophilia A
Cautions: intravascular haemolysis after large or frequently repeated doses in patients with blood groups A, B, or AB
Side-effects: allergic reactions including chills, fever; hyperfibrinogenaemia occurred after massive doses with earlier products but less likely

since fibrinogen content has now been substantially reduced
Available from Alpha (Alpha VIII), Armour (Monoclate-P®), Bayer (Kogenate®), BPL (8SM®, 8Y®), SNBTS (High Potency Factor VIII Concentrate)

FACTOR VIII INHIBITOR BYPASSING FRACTION
Preparations with factor VIII inhibitor bypassing activity are prepared from human plasma
Human Factor VIII Inhibitor Bypassing Fraction (*FEIBA*, Immuno) is used in patients with factor VIII inhibitors
Note. A porcine preparation of antihaemophilic factor for patients with inhibitors to human factor VIII is available from Porton (Hyate C®)

FACTOR IX FRACTION, DRIED
Factor IX fraction is prepared from pooled human plasma and may also contain clotting factors II, VII, and X.
Indications: congenital factor IX deficiency (haemophilia B)
Cautions: risk of thrombosis
Contra-indications: disseminated intravascular coagulation
Side-effects: allergic reactions, including chills, fever
Available from Alpha (Alphanine®), Armour (▼Mononine®), BPL (Dried Factor IX Fraction, Heat-Treated; ▼Replenine®), SNBTS (Human Factor IX Concentrate, Heat Treated)

FRESH FROZEN PLASMA
Fresh frozen plasma is prepared from the supernatant liquid obtained by centrifugation of one donation of whole blood
Indications: to replace coagulation factors or other plasma proteins where their concentration or functional activity is critically reduced, e.g. to reverse warfarin effect
Cautions: avoid in circulatory overload; need for compatibility
Side-effects: allergic reactions including chills, fever, bronchospasm; adult respiratory distress syndrome
Available from Regional Blood Transfusion Services and BPL

2.12   Lipid-lowering drugs

There are a number of common conditions, some familial, in which there are very high plasma concentrations of cholesterol, or triglycerides, or both. There is evidence that therapy which lowers low density lipoprotein (LDL) cholesterol and raises high density lipoprotein (HDL) cholesterol reduces the progression of coronary atherosclerosis and may even induce regression. Lipid-lowering drugs should be reserved for patients with coronary heart disease and those at high risk of developing coronary heart disease on account of multiple risk factors or severe hyperlipidaemia inadequately controlled by a modified fat diet. Any drug therapy must be combined with strict adherence to diet, maintenance of near-ideal body weight and, if appropriate, reduction of blood pressure and cessation of smoking.

Severe hyperlipidaemia often requires combinations of lipid-lowering drugs such as an anion-exchange resin with a fibrate, an HMG CoA reductase inhibitor, or nicotinic acid. Combinations of HMG CoA reductase inhibitors with nicotinic acid or a fibrate carry an increased risk of side-effects and should be used with great caution.

ANION-EXCHANGE RESINS

Cholestyramine and **colestipol** are anion-exchange resins used in the management of hypercholesterolaemia. They act by binding bile acids, preventing their reabsorption; this promotes hepatic conversion of cholesterol into bile acids; the resultant increased LDL-receptor activity of liver cells increases the breakdown of LDL-cholesterol. Thus both compounds effectively reduce LDL-cholesterol but can aggravate hypertriglyceridaemia.

COUNSELLING. Other drugs should be taken at least 1 hour before or 4–6 hours after cholestyramine or colestipol to reduce possible interference with absorption

CHOLESTYRAMINE
(Colestyramine)

Indications: hyperlipidaemias, particularly type IIa, in patients who have not responded adequately to diet and other appropriate measures; primary prevention of coronary heart disease in men aged 35–59 years with primary hypercholesterolaemia who have not responded to diet and other appropriate measures; pruritus associated with partial biliary obstruction and primary biliary cirrhosis; diarrhoeal disorders, see section 1.5

Cautions: supplements of fat-soluble vitamins and of folic acid may be required with high doses, particularly in children; pregnancy and breast-feeding; **interactions:** Appendix 1 (cholestyramine and colestipol)

Contra-indications: complete biliary obstruction

Side-effects: nausea and vomiting, constipation or diarrhoea, heartburn, flatulence, abdominal discomfort; on prolonged use, increased bleeding tendency (due to hypoprothrombinaemia associated with vitamin K deficiency)

Dose: lipid reduction (after initial introduction over 3–4 weeks) 8–24 g daily in water in single or up to 4 divided doses; up to 36 g daily if necessary

Pruritus, 4–8 g daily in water

Diarrhoeal diseases, see section 1.5

PoM **Questran®** (Bristol-Myers)
Powder, orange, cholestyramine (anhydrous) 4 g/sachet. Net price 60-sachet pack = £21.06, 180-sachet pack = £63.19. Label: 13, counselling, avoid other drugs at same time (see notes above)

PoM **Questran A®** (Bristol-Myers)
Powder, orange, cholestyramine (anhydrous) 4 g/sachet, with aspartame. Net price 60-sachet pack = £22.11, 180-sachet pack = £66.34. Label: 13, counselling, avoid other drugs at same time (see notes above)

COLESTIPOL HYDROCHLORIDE
Indications: hyperlipidaemias, particularly type IIa, in patients who have not responded adequately to diet and other appropriate measures

Cautions; Contra-indications; Side-effects: see under Cholestyramine

Dose: 5 g 1–2 times daily in liquid increased if necessary at intervals of 1–2 months to max. of 30 g daily (in single or 2 divided doses)

PoM **Colestid®** (Upjohn)
Granules, yellow, colestipol hydrochloride 5 g/sachet. Net price 30 sachets = £12.54. Label: 13, counselling, avoid other drugs at same time (see notes above)
Colestid Orange, granules, yellow/orange, colestipol hydrochloride 5 g/sachet, with aspartame. Net price 30 sachets = £12.54. Label: 13, counselling, avoid other drugs at same time (see notes above)

CLOFIBRATE GROUP

Clofibrate, bezafibrate, ciprofibrate, fenofibrate, and **gemfibrozil** can be regarded as broad-spectrum lipid-modulating agents in that although their main action is to decrease serum triglycerides they also tend to reduce LDL-cholesterol and to raise HDL-cholesterol.

All can cause a myositis-like syndrome, especially in patients with impaired renal function. In addition, clofibrate predisposes to gallstones by increasing biliary cholesterol excretion; it is therefore only indicated in patients who have had a cholecystectomy.

BEZAFIBRATE
Indications: hyperlipidaemias of types IIa, IIb, III, IV and V in patients who have not responded adequately to diet and other appropriate measures

Cautions: renal impairment (avoid if severe — see also under Myotoxicity below); **interactions:** Appendix 1 (clofibrate group)

MYOTOXICITY. Special care needed in patients with renal disease, as progressive increases in serum creatinine concentration or failure to follow dosage guidelines may result in myotoxicity (rhabdomyolysis)

Contra-indications: severe renal or hepatic impairment, hypoalbuminaemia, primary biliary cirrhosis, gall bladder disease, nephrotic syndrome, pregnancy and breast-feeding

Side-effects: gastro-intestinal (e.g. nausea, anorexia, gastric pain), pruritus, urticaria, impotence;

also headache, dizziness, vertigo, fatigue, hair loss; myotoxicity (with myasthenia or myalgia) — special risk in renal impairment (see under Cautions)

Dose: 200 mg 3 times daily with or after food; may be reduced to 200 mg twice daily in hypertriglyceridaemia

PoM Bezalip® (Boehringer Mannheim)
Tablets, f/c, bezafibrate 200 mg. Net price 100-tab pack = £10.30. Label: 21

PoM Bezalip-Mono® (Boehringer Mannheim)
Tablets, m/r, f/c, bezafibrate 400 mg. Net price 28-tab pack = £8.50. Label: 21, 25
Dose: 1 tablet daily after food (dose form not appropriate in renal impairment)

CIPROFIBRATE

Indications: hyperlipidaemias of types IIa, IIb, III, and IV in patients who have not responded adequately to diet
Cautions; Contra-indications; Side-effects: see under Bezafibrate
Dose: initially 100 mg daily; max. 200 mg daily as a single dose

▼ **PoM Modalim®** (Sanofi Winthrop)
Tablets, scored, ciprofibrate 100 mg. Net price 28-tab pack = £13.38

CLOFIBRATE

Indications: hyperlipidaemias of types IIb, III, IV and V in patients who have not responded adequately to diet and other appropriate measures (but see also notes above)
Cautions; Contra-indications: see under Bezafibrate and notes above
Side-effects: see under Bezafibrate; also cholesterol cholelithiasis
Dose: over 65 kg, 2 g daily (50–65 kg, 1.5 g daily) in 2 or 3 divided doses

PoM Atromid-S® (Zeneca)
Capsules, red, clofibrate 500 mg. Net price 100-cap pack = £4.08. Label: 21

FENOFIBRATE

Indications: hyperlipidaemias of types IIa, IIb, III, IV, and V in patients who have not responded adequately to diet and other appropriate measures
Cautions: see under Bezafibrate
Contra-indications: severe renal or hepatic impairment, existing gall bladder disease; pregnancy and breast-feeding
Side-effects: see under Bezafibrate
Dose: initially 300 mg daily in divided doses with food, adjusted according to response within range 200–400 mg daily; CHILD 5 mg/kg daily

PoM Lipantil® (Fournier)
Capsules, fenofibrate 100 mg. Net price 84-cap pack = £19.80. Label: 21
Lipantil Micro capsules, orange, fenofibrate (micronised) 200 mg. Net price 30-cap pack = £24.40. Label: 21
Dose: initially 1 capsule daily with food (dose form not appropriate for children or in renal impairment)
Note. Improved bioavailability of micronised fenofibrate may allow a lower total daily dose than with conventional formulation

GEMFIBROZIL

Indications: hyperlipidaemias of types IIa, IIb, III, IV and V in patients who have not responded adequately to diet and other appropriate measures; primary prevention of coronary heart disease in men aged 40–55 years with hyperlipidaemias that have not responded to diet and other appropriate measures
Cautions: lipid profile, blood counts, and liver-function tests before initiating long-term treatment; renal impairment; annual eye examinations; **interactions:** Appendix 1 (clofibrate group)
Contra-indications: alcoholism, hepatic impairment, gallstones; pregnancy
Side-effects: gastro-intestinal disturbances; pruritus, urticaria, rash, headache, dizziness, blurred vision, painful extremities; rarely myalgia; impotence reported
Dose: 1.2 g daily, usually in 2 divided doses; range 0.9–1.5 g daily

PoM Lopid® (P-D)
'300' capsules, white/maroon, gemfibrozil 300 mg. Net price 100-cap pack = £26.46
'600' tablets, f/c, gemfibrozil 600 mg. Net price 56-tab pack = £29.64

NICOTINIC ACID GROUP

The value of **nicotinic acid** is limited by its side-effects, especially vasodilatation. In doses of 1.5 to 3 g daily it lowers both cholesterol and triglyceride concentrations by inhibiting synthesis; it also increases HDL-cholesterol. **Acipimox** seems to have fewer side-effects but may be less effective in its lipid-modulating capabilities.

ACIPIMOX

Indications: hyperlipidaemias of types IIa, IIb, and IV in patients who have not responded adequately to diet and other appropriate measures
Cautions: renal impairment
Contra-indications: peptic ulcer; pregnancy
Side-effects: vasodilatation, flushing, itching, rashes, erythema; occasionally, heartburn, epigastric pain, nausea, diarrhoea, headache, malaise
Dose: usually 500–750 mg daily in divided doses

PoM Olbetam® (Pharmacia)
Capsules, brown/pink, acipimox 250 mg. Net price 100-cap pack = £42.90. Label: 21

NICOTINIC ACID

Indications: see notes above

Cautions: diabetes mellitus, gout, liver disease, peptic ulcer

Contra-indications: pregnancy, breast-feeding

Side-effects: flushing, dizziness, headache, palpitations, pruritus (prostaglandin-mediated symptoms can be reduced by low initial doses taken with meals, or by taking aspirin 75 mg 30 minutes before the dose); nausea, vomiting; rarely impaired liver function and rashes

Dose: initially 100–200 mg 3 times daily (see above), gradually increased over 2–4 weeks to 1–2 g 3 times daily

Nicotinic Acid Tablets, nicotinic acid 50 mg, net price 20 = 16p. Label: 21

FISH OILS

A fish-oil preparation (Maxepa®), rich in omega-3 marine triglycerides, is useful in the treatment of severe hypertriglyceridaemia; however, it can sometimes aggravate hypercholesterolaemia.

OMEGA-3 MARINE TRIGLYCERIDES

Indications: reduction of plasma triglycerides in patients with severe hypertriglyceridaemia judged to be at special risk of ischaemic heart disease and/or pancreatitis, in conjunction with dietary and other methods (see notes above)

Side-effects: occasional nausea and belching

Dose: see under preparations below

Maxepa® (Innovex)

Capsules, 1 g (approx. 1.1 mL) concentrated fish oils containing, as percentage of total fatty acid composition, eicosapentaenoic acid 18%, docosahexaenoic acid 12%. Vitamin A content less than 100 units/g, vitamin D content less than 10 units/g. Net price 200-cap pack = £28.37. Label: 21

Dose: 5 capsules twice daily with food

Emulsion, cream-coloured, concentrated fish oils containing, as percentage of total fatty acid composition, eicosapentaenoic acid 9%, docosahexaenoic acid 6%. Vitamin A content less than 100 units/g, vitamin D content less than 10 units/g. Net price 150 mL = £11.79. Label: 21

Dose: 10 mL twice daily with food

Liquid, golden-coloured, concentrated fish oils containing, as percentage of total fatty acid composition, eicosapentaenoic acid 18% w/w, docosahexaenoic acid 12% w/w. Vitamin A content less than 100 units/g, vitamin D content less than 10 units/g. Net price 150 mL = £21.43. Label: 21

Dose: 5 mL twice daily with food

OTHER DRUGS

Probucol decreases both LDL- and HDL-cholesterol; despite the latter effect it appears to promote resolution of xanthomata. Moreover, its antioxidant properties may decrease the atherogenicity of LDL.

Simvastatin and **pravastatin** belong to a new class of drugs which competitively inhibit 3-hydroxy-3-methylglutaryl coenzyme A (HMG CoA) reductase, an enzyme that catalyses a step in cholesterol synthesis, especially in the liver. They are more potent than anion-exchange resins in lowering LDL-cholesterol but less effective than the clofibrate group in reducing triglycerides and raising HDL-cholesterol. The main side-effect is reversible myositis, which is rare except in patients also receiving cyclosporin, nicotinic acid, or gemfibrozil (careful monitoring of liver function and creatine phosphokinase should be performed if these drugs are used with an HMG CoA reductase inhibitor). **Fluvastatin** has recently also been introduced.

FLUVASTATIN

Indications; Cautions; Contra-indications; Side-effects: see under Simvastatin; **interactions:** Appendix 1 (fluvastatin)

Dose: 20–40 mg once daily in the evening

▼ PoM **Lescol®** (Sandoz)

Capsules, fluvastatin (as sodium salt) 20 mg (brown/yellow), net price 28-cap pack = £14.00; 40 mg (brown/orange), 28-cap pack = £15.90

PRAVASTATIN

Indications: primary hypercholesterolaemia (hyperlipidaemia type IIa), in patients intolerant of or not responsive to other therapy, with cholesterol concentration above 7.8 mmol/litre

Cautions; Contra-indications; Side-effects: as for Simvastatin; **interactions**: Appendix 1 (pravastatin)

Dose: usual range 10–40 mg once daily at night, adjusted at intervals of not less than 4 weeks

PoM **Lipostat®** (Squibb)

Tablets, both pink, pravastatin sodium 10 mg, net price 28-tab pack = £16.18; 20 mg, 28-tab pack = £31.09

PROBUCOL

Indications: see notes above

Cautions: ECG before treatment in patients with recent myocardial damage, ventricular arrhythmias; avoid pregnancy during and for 6 months after stopping treatment

Contra-indications: pregnancy and breast-feeding

Side-effects: generally mild and transient and mainly consist of gastro-intestinal effects such as nausea, vomiting, flatulence, diarrhoea, abdominal pain; ventricular arrhythmias and angio-edema rarely reported

Dose: 500 mg twice daily with food

PoM **Lurselle®** (Merrell)

Tablets, scored, probucol 250 mg. Net price 120-tab pack = £13.40. Label: 21

SIMVASTATIN

Indications: primary hypercholesterolaemia (hyperlipidaemia type IIa) in patients with cholesterol concentration of 6.5 mmol/litre or greater and resistant to dietary control

Cautions: monitor liver function before and during treatment; history of liver disease (avoid if active); high alcohol intake; avoid pregnancy during and for 1 month after treatment; advise patients to report muscle pain; **interactions:** Appendix 1 (simvastatin)

Contra-indications: active liver disease; pregnancy (toxicity in *animal* studies) and breast-feeding; porphyria (see section 9.8.2)

Side-effects: constipation, flatulence, headache, nausea, dyspepsia, abdominal pain, diarrhoea, fatigue, insomnia, rash, rhabdomyolysis, hepatitis reported; raised creatine phosphokinase concentrations (discontinue if markedly raised or myopathy diagnosed); angioedema reported

Dose: 10 mg daily at night, adjusted at intervals of not less than 4 weeks; usual range 10–40 mg once daily at night

PoM Zocor® (MSD)

Tablets, both f/c, simvastatin 10 mg (peach), net price 28-tab pack = £18.29; 20 mg (tan), 28-tab pack = £31.09

2.13   Local sclerosants

Ethanolamine oleate and sodium tetradecyl sulphate are used in sclerotherapy of varicose veins, and phenol is used in haemorrhoids (see section 1.7.3).

ETHANOLAMINE OLEATE

(Monoethanolamine Oleate)

Indications: sclerotherapy of varicose veins

Cautions: extravasation may cause necrosis of tissues

Contra-indications: inability to walk, acute phlebitis, oral contraceptive use, obese legs

Side-effects: allergic reactions (including anaphylaxis)

PoM Ethanolamine Oleate Injection, ethanolamine oleate 5%. Net price 5-mL amp = £1.65
Available from Evans
Dose: by slow injection into empty isolated segment of vein, 2–5 mL divided between 3–4 sites; repeated at weekly intervals

SODIUM TETRADECYL SULPHATE

Indications: sclerotherapy of varicose veins

Cautions; Contra-indications; Side-effects: see under Ethanolamine Oleate

PoM STD® (STD Pharmaceutical)

Injection, sodium tetradecyl sulphate 0.5%, net price 2-mL amp =£1.10; 1%, 2-mL amp = £1.19; 3%, 2-mL amp = £1.36, 5-mL vial = £2.45
Dose: by slow injection into empty isolated segment of vein, 0.1–1 mL according to site and condition being treated (consult manufacturer's literature)

3: Drugs used in the treatment of diseases of the
RESPIRATORY SYSTEM

In this chapter, drug treatment is described under the following headings:

The initial treatment of exacerbations of chronic bronchitis and bacterial pneumonia is indicated in section 5.1 (table 1) and the treatment of tuberculosis is discussed in section 5.1.9.

3.1 Bronchodilators

3.1.1 Adrenoceptor stimulants

(Sympathomimetics)

The selective beta$_2$-adrenoceptor stimulants (selective beta$_2$-stimulants, selective beta$_2$-agonists) (section 3.1.1.1) such as salbutamol or terbutaline (preferably given by aerosol inhalation) are the safest and most effective beta-stimulants for asthma. They are recommended over the less selective beta-adrenoceptor stimulants such as isoprenaline or orciprenaline (section 3.1.1.2), which should be avoided whenever possible.

Adrenaline (see also section 2.7) (which has both alpha- and beta-adrenoceptor stimulant properties) is used in the emergency management of allergic and anaphylactic reactions (see section 3.4.3).

3.1.1.1 SELECTIVE BETA$_2$-ADRENOCEPTOR STIMULANTS

Most *mild to moderate* attacks of asthma respond rapidly to aerosol administration of a selective beta$_2$-adrenoceptor stimulant such as salbutamol or terbutaline. If beta$_2$-adrenoceptor stimulant inhalation is needed *more than once daily* prophylactic treatment should be considered, using a stepped approach as outlined on p. 112. However in *more severe attacks* a short course of an oral corticosteroid may be necessary to bring the asthma under control (section 3.2). Treatment of patients with *severe acute asthma* or airways obstruction (see

also below) is safer in hospital where oxygen and resuscitation facilities are immediately available (see also Acute Severe Asthma table, p. 113).

Patients with *chronic bronchitis* and *emphysema* are often described as having irreversible airways obstruction, but they usually respond partially to the beta$_2$-adrenoceptor stimulant drugs or to the antimuscarinic drugs ipratropium or oxitropium (section 3.1.2).

There is some evidence that patients who use beta$_2$-adrenoceptor stimulants on an 'as required' basis show a greater improvement in their asthma than those using them on a regular basis. For patients who require beta$_2$-adrenoceptor stimulants more than once daily, preventative treatment with an inhaled corticosteroid, cromoglycate, or nedocromil, should be tried.

There are some differences between the various selective beta$_2$-adrenoceptor stimulant drugs. **Salbutamol** and **terbutaline** are available in the widest range of formulations. **Rimiterol** has a shorter duration of action than salbutamol, terbutaline and fenoterol. **Fenoterol** may be less beta$_2$-selective than salbutamol.

Salmeterol is a longer-acting beta$_2$-adrenoceptor stimulant that has recently been introduced for twice daily administration; it is **not** suitable for the relief of an acute attack (a short-acting beta$_2$-stimulant such as salbutamol should be used). Salmeterol should be added to existing corticosteroid therapy and **not** replace it.

Chronic Asthma table, see p. 112
Acute Severe Asthma table, see p. 113

INHALATION. The *pressurised aerosol inhaler*[1] is an effective and convenient method of administration for *mild to moderate* airways obstruction. The duration of action of an aerosol inhaler depends on the drug and the dose administered. With recommended doses rimiterol will usually last for 1 to 2 hours, salbutamol, terbutaline and fenoterol for 3 to 5 hours, and salmeterol for around 12 hours. Aerosol inhalation is preferred because it provides relief more rapidly and causes fewer side-effects (such as tremor and nervous tension) than tablets; this is because the drug is delivered directly to the bronchi and is therefore effective in smaller doses.

Patients should be given careful instruction on the use of their pressurised aerosol inhalers and it is important to check that they continue to use them correctly as inadequate technique may be mistaken for drug failure. In particular, it should be emphasised that they must inhale slowly and hold their breath for 10 seconds after inhalation. Most patients can be successfully taught to use pressurised aerosol

---

1. The British Medical Association has recommended that, where safety and efficacy will not be compromised, doctors should prescribe alternatives to pressurised metered dose inhalers containing chlorofluorocarbons (CFCs).

Start at **step most appropriate** to initial severity; **'rescue' course** of prednisolone at **any time** and **any step**

Adult step 1

Inhaled short-acting beta$_2$ stimulant as required (up to once daily)
Note. Move to step 2 if needed more than once daily (or night-time symptoms)

Adult step 2

Inhaled short-acting beta$_2$ stimulant as required
plus
Regular standard-dose inhaled beclomethasone or budesonide
or try
Regular cromoglycate or nedocromil (but change to inhaled corticosteroid if control not achieved)
Note. Higher dose of inhaled corticosteroid may be required to gain initial control; some adults benefit from doubling for short period to cover respiratory infection

Adult step 3

Inhaled short-acting beta$_2$ stimulant as required
plus
Regular high-dose inhaled beclomethasone or budesonide (large-volume spacer)
Note. In few who have problems with high-dose inhaled corticosteroid continue with standard-dose inhaled corticosteroid *and add* regular inhaled long-acting beta$_2$ stimulant *or* regular modified-release oral theophylline *or* may try regular cromoglycate or nedocromil
In few with disproportionately prominent night-time symptoms (despite otherwise good control with standard- or high-dose corticosteroid inhalations), a modified-release oral theophylline *or* a long-acting inhaled beta$_2$ stimulant *or* a modified-release oral beta$_2$ stimulant, may be considered for administration at night

Adult step 4

Inhaled short-acting beta$_2$ stimulant as required
with
Regular high-dose inhaled beclomethasone or budesonide (large-volume spacer)
plus sequential therapeutic trial of one or more of
Inhaled long-acting beta$_2$ stimulant
Modified-release oral theophylline
Inhaled ipratropium or oxitropium
Modified-release oral beta$_2$ stimulant
High-dose inhaled bronchodilators
Cromoglycate or nedocromil
Note. High doses of inhaled bronchodilators should only be considered if the patient does not respond to standard doses; beta$_2$ stimulants and ipratropium (or oxitropium) can be given using a nebuliser (or by multiple actuations of a metered dose inhaler with a large-volume spacer); for requirements before and when prescribing nebulisers, see p. 122

Adult step 5

Inhaled short-acting beta$_2$ stimulant as required
with
Regular high-dose inhaled beclomethasone or budesonide (large-volume spacer) *and with* one or more long-acting bronchodilators (see step 4)
plus
Regular prednisolone tablets (as single daily dose)
Note. In addition to regular prednisolone tablets, continue high-dose inhaled beclomethasone or budesonide (in exceptional cases doses exceeding 2 mg may be used); these patients should normally be referred to a hospital asthma clinic

Stepping adult down

Review treatment every 3–6 months; if control achieved stepwise reduction may be possible; in patients whose treatment was started recently at step 4 or 5 (or contained corticosteroid tablets) reduction may take place after short interval; in chronic asthma a 3–6 month period of stability should be shown before slow stepwise reduction is undertaken

Child step 1

Short-acting beta$_2$ stimulant as required (not more than once daily)
Note. Whenever possible inhaled (less effective and more side-effects when given by mouth)

Child step 2

Inhaled short-acting beta$_2$ stimulant as required
plus
Regular inhaled cromoglycate (powder or large volume spacer)
Note. Try cromoglycate for 4–6 weeks before going to step 3 (supply peak flow meter where appropriate)

Child step 3

Inhaled short-acting beta$_2$ stimulant as required
plus
Regular inhaled beclomethasone or budesonide in standard paediatric dose (large-volume spacer)
Consider for stabilisation
Soluble tablets prednisolone 1–2 mg/kg daily for 1–5 days (max. 40 mg daily)
or temporary doubling of dose of inhaled corticosteroid
Note. After 1 month assess effect on peak flow and/or symptoms and adjust dose; if control not adequate consider doubling dose of inhaled corticosteroid for 1 month (alternatively give short course of soluble prednisolone tablets by mouth or consider introducing other treatments)

Child step 4

Inhaled short-acting beta$_2$ stimulant as required
plus
Regular inhaled beclomethasone or budesonide in high paediatric dose (large-volume spacer or dry powder device)
Consider
Soluble prednisolone tablets 1–2 mg/kg daily for 1–5 days (max. 40 mg daily)
Regular inhaled long-acting beta$_2$ stimulant
Note. Long-acting beta$_2$ stimulant should probably be reserved for supplementing treatment in child already receiving cromoglycate or a corticosteroid

Child step 5a

Inhaled short-acting beta$_2$ stimulant as required
with
Regular inhaled beclomethasone or budesonide in high paediatric dose (large-volume spacer or dry powder device)
As in step 4, consider soluble tablets prednisolone *with* regular inhaled long-acting beta$_2$ stimulant
plus
Regular modified-release oral theophylline
or nebulised beta$_2$ stimulant
Note. Modified-release oral theophylline may be helpful (particularly for nocturnal symptoms), but has appreciable side-effects in up to one-third of children (plasma- and salivary-concentration monitoring recommended); similar clinical improvements, with fewer side-effects, have been shown with modified-release oral salbutamol

Child step 5b

As step 5a
plus
Prednisolone 5–10 mg on alternate days
Consider
Regular inhaled ipratropium *or* subcutaneous infusion of short-acting beta$_2$ stimulant

Stepping child down

Regularly review need for treatment; in older child use peak flow record to assess speed of withdrawal; stop cromoglycate or corticosteroid after 6–12 months of few or no symptoms (if symptoms seasonal consider stopping at end of season).

Based on tables in: British Thoracic Society, the British Paediatric Association and others. Guidelines on the Management of Asthma. *Thorax* 1993; **48** (suppl); S1–S24. Reproduced with permission of BMJ Specialist Journals

MANAGEMENT OF ACUTE SEVERE ASTHMA IN GENERAL PRACTICE

Uncontrolled asthma in adults

— Speech normal
— Pulse <110 beats/minute
— Respiration <25 breaths/minute
— Peak flow >50% of predicted or best

Treat at home but response to treatment **must** be assessed before doctor leaves

Treatment:
Nebulised salbutamol 5 mg or nebulised terbutaline 10 mg

Monitor response 15–30 minutes after nebulisation

If peak flow 50–75% of predicted or best give:
Oral prednisolone 30–60 mg
and step up usual treatment

Alternatively if peak flow >75% of predicted or best.
Step up usual treatment

Follow up
Monitor symptoms and peak flow
Set up self management plan
Review in surgery within 48 hours
Modify treatment at review according to guidelines for chronic asthma (see opposite page)

Important: regard each emergency consultation as being for **acute severe asthma** until shown otherwise

Acute severe asthma in adults

— Cannot complete sentences
— Pulse ≥110 beats/minute
— Respiration ≥25 breaths/minute
— Peak flow ≤50% of predicted or best

Seriously consider hospital admission if more than one of above features present

Treatment:
Nebulised salbutamol 5 mg or nebulised terbutaline 10 mg
Oral prednisolone 30–60 mg or i/v hydrocortisone 200 mg

Monitor response 15–30 minutes after nebulisation

If any signs of acute asthma persist:
Arrange hospital admission
While awaiting ambulance repeat nebulised beta₂ stimulant and give with nebulised ipratropium 500 micrograms
or give subcutaneous terbutaline
or give slow intravenous aminophylline 250 mg
(**important:** not if taking an oral theophylline)

Alternatively if symptoms have improved, respiration and pulse settling, and peak flow >50% of predicted or best:

Follow up:
Step up usual treatment *and* continue prednisolone
Monitor symptoms and peak flow
Set up self management plan
Review in surgery within 24 hours
Modify treatment at review (see opposite page)

Life-threatening asthma in adults

— Silent chest
— Cyanosis
— Bradycardia or exhaustion
— Peak flow <33% of predicted or best

Arrange IMMEDIATE hospital admission

Treatment:
Oral prednisolone 30–60 mg or i/v hydrocortisone 200 mg (immediately)
Oxygen-driven nebuliser in ambulance
Nebulised¹ beta₂ stimulant with nebulised ipratropium or subcutaneous terbutaline
or slow intravenous aminophylline 250 mg (**important:** not if taking an oral theophylline)

STAY WITH PATIENT UNTIL AMBULANCE ARRIVES
1. If no nebuliser available give 2 puffs of beta₂ stimulant using large-volume spacer and repeat 10 – 20 times

Important: do not give bolus aminophylline to patient already taking an oral theophylline.

Important: patients with severe or life-threatening attacks may not be distressed and may not have all these abnormalities; the presence of any should alert doctor.

Features of treatment of acute asthma in children

— short-acting beta₂ stimulant from metered dose inhaler using large-volume spacer device may be as effective as use of nebuliser; dose is one puff every few seconds until improvement occurs (max. 20 puffs), using face mask in very young child
— terbutaline may be given subcutaneously in severe episodes
— oxygen is of benefit

— a child requiring high-dose inhaled bronchodilators should also receive soluble tablets prednisolone 1–2 mg/kg (max. 40 mg) once daily for up to 5 days if necessary; child needs immediate referral to hospital if failure to respond
— aminophylline should no longer be used in children at home

Signs of acute asthma in children

Acute severe asthma:
— too breathless to talk
— too breathless to feed
— respiration ≥50 breaths/minute
— pulse ≥140 beats/minute
— peak flow ≤50% of predicted or best

Important: failure to respond adequately **at any time** requires immediate referral to hospital.

Life-threatening features:
— peak flow <33% of predicted or best
— cyanosis, silent chest, or poor respiratory effort
— fatigue or exhaustion
— agitation or reduced level of consciousness

inhalers but some patients, particularly the elderly, the arthritic, and small children are unable to use them; some patients are unable to synchronise their breathing with the administration of aerosol. For such patients a variety of *spacing devices* (see section 3.1.5) is now available. Alternatively *dry powder inhalers*, activated by the patient's inspiration, are of value; some occasionally cause coughing.

The **dose** should be stated **explicitly** in terms of the number of inhalations at one time, the frequency, and the maximum number of inhalations allowed in 24 hours. High doses of beta$_2$-stimulants can be dangerous in some patients. Excessive use is usually an indication of **inadequately treated** asthma and should be treated with preventative medication such as an inhaled corticosteroid. Patients should be advised to seek medical advice when they fail to obtain their usual degree of symptomatic relief as this usually indicates a worsening of the asthma and may require alternative medication. When patients with asthma **are not adequately controlled** with inhalation of a beta$_2$-stimulant once or twice daily, **addition of a prophylactic drug** such as a corticosteroid inhalation should be considered (see Chronic Asthma table, p.112); this is more convenient for the patient than higher doses of beta$_2$-stimulants and usually provides better overall control.

Respirator (or *nebuliser*) *solutions* of salbutamol and terbutaline are increasingly used for the treatment of *acute asthma* both in hospital and in general practice. They are administered over a period of about 15 minutes from a nebuliser, usually driven by oxygen in hospital. An electrical compressor is most suitable for domiciliary use but these are costly and not currently prescribable under the NHS. Patients with a severe attack of asthma should have oxygen if possible during nebulisation since beta-adrenoceptor stimulants can cause an increase in arterial hypoxaemia. For patients with *chronic bronchitis and hypercapnia*, however, oxygen can be dangerous, and the nebuliser should be driven by air. The dose prescribed by nebuliser is substantially higher than that prescribed by metered dose inhaler. For example, a 2.5-mL Ventolin Nebule® contains 2.5 mg of salbutamol, which is equivalent to 25 puffs from the aerosol inhaler. Patients should therefore be warned that it is dangerous to exceed the stated dose and that if they fail to respond to the usual dose of their respirator solution they should call for help. See also guidelines in section 3.1.5.

ORAL. *Oral preparations* are available for patients who cannot manage the inhaled route. They are sometimes used for children, though the inhaled route is better and most children can use one or other of the inhalation devices available. They have a slower onset but a slightly more prolonged action than the aerosol inhalers. The *modified-release* preparations may be of value in patients with *nocturnal asthma* as an alternative to the modified-release theophylline preparations (section 3.1.3).

PARENTERAL. *Intravenous*, and occasionally *subcutaneous*, injections of salbutamol and terbutaline are given for severe bronchospasm.

CHILDREN. Selective beta$_2$-adrenoceptor stimulants are useful even in children under the age of 18 months. They are most effective by the *inhaled route*, but an inhalation device may be needed (with the technique carefully checked). They are also effective *by mouth*. In severe attacks *nebulisation* using a selective beta$_2$-adrenoceptor stimulant or ipratropium is advisable (see also Asthma tables, pp.112-13).

PREGNANCY AND BREAST-FEEDING. It is particularly important that asthma should be well-controlled during pregnancy; where this is achieved asthma has no important effects on pregnancy, labour, or the fetus.

Inhalation has particular advantages as a means of drug administration during pregnancy because the therapeutic action can be achieved without the need for plasma concentrations liable to have a pharmacological effect on the fetus.

Severe exacerbations of asthma can have an adverse effect on pregnancy and should be treated promptly with conventional therapy, including oral or parenteral administration of corticosteroids and nebulisation of a selective beta$_2$-adrenoceptor stimulant; prednisolone is the preferred corticosteroid for oral administration since placental transfer is slower than with some others.

Although theophylline has been given without adverse effects during pregnancy or breast-feeding there have been occasional reports of toxicity in the fetus and neonate.

SEVERE ACUTE ASTHMA

Severe asthma can be fatal and **must** be treated promptly and energetically. It is characterised by persistent dyspnoea poorly relieved by bronchodilators, exhaustion, a high pulse rate (usually over 110/minute), and a very low peak expiratory flow. The respiration is so shallow that wheezing may be absent. Such patients should be given oxygen (if available) and a large dose of a **corticosteroid** (see section 6.3.4)—for adults hydrocortisone 200 mg (preferably as sodium succinate) intravenously or prednisolone 40 mg by mouth, children half these doses. They should also be given **salbutamol** or **terbutaline** by nebuliser with oxygen if available. For a table outlining the management of acute severe asthma, see p.113.

If there is little response the following additional treatment should be considered: **ipratropium** by nebuliser (section 3.1.2), **aminophylline** by slow intravenous injection, if the patient has not already been receiving theophylline (section 3.1.3), or change of administration of the beta$_2$-selective adrenoceptor stimulant to the intravenous route.

Further treatment of these patients is safer in hospital where resuscitation facilities are immediately available. Treatment should **never** be delayed for investigations, patients should **never** be sedated and the possibility of a pneumothorax should also be remembered.

If the patient deteriorates despite appropriate pharmacological treatment, intermittent positive pressure ventilation may be needed temporarily.

SALBUTAMOL

Indications: asthma and other conditions associated with reversible airways obstruction; premature labour, see section 7.1.3

Cautions: hyperthyroidism, myocardial insufficiency, arrhythmias, hypertension, pregnancy and breast-feeding (but appropriate to use, see notes above); intravenous administration to diabetics (monitor blood glucose; ketoacidosis reported); see also notes above; **interactions:** Appendix 1 (sympathomimetics, beta$_2$)

HYPOKALAEMIA. The CSM has advised that potentially serious hypokalaemia may result from beta$_2$-adrenoceptor stimulant therapy. Particular caution is required in severe asthma, as this effect may be potentiated by concomitant treatment with theophylline and its derivatives, corticosteroids, and diuretics, and by hypoxia. Plasma-potassium concentrations should therefore be monitored in severe asthma.

Side-effects: fine tremor (usually hands), nervous tension, headache, peripheral vasodilatation, palpitations, tachycardia (seldom troublesome when given by aerosol inhalation); rarely muscle cramps; hypokalaemia after high doses (for **CSM** advice see under Cautions above); hypersensitivity reactions including paradoxical bronchospasm, urticaria, and angioedema reported; slight pain on intramuscular injection

Dose: by mouth, 4 mg (elderly and sensitive patients initially 2 mg) 3–4 times daily; max. single dose 8 mg (but unlikely to provide much extra benefit or to be tolerated); CHILD under 2 years 100 micrograms/kg 4 times daily; 2–6 years 1–2 mg 3–4 times daily, 6–12 years 2 mg

By subcutaneous or intramuscular injection, 500 micrograms, repeated every 4 hours if necessary

By slow intravenous injection, 250 micrograms, repeated if necessary

By intravenous infusion, initially 5 micrograms/minute, adjusted according to response and heart-rate usually in range 3–20 micrograms/minute, or more if necessary

By aerosol inhalation, 100–200 micrograms (1–2 puffs); for persistent symptoms up to 3–4 times daily (but see also Chronic asthma table); CHILD 100 micrograms (1 puff), increased to 200 micrograms (2 puffs) if necessary

Prophylaxis in exercise-induced bronchospasm, 200 micrograms (2 puffs); CHILD 100 micrograms (1 puff)

By inhalation of a powder (Rotacaps®, Ventodisks®), 200–400 micrograms; for persistent symptoms up to 3–4 times daily (but see also Chronic asthma table); CHILD 200 micrograms

Prophylaxis in exercise-induced bronchospasm (*powder*), 400 micrograms; CHILD 200 micrograms

Note. Bioavailability appears to be lower, so recommended doses for dry powder inhalers are twice those in a metered inhaler

By inhalation of nebulised solution, chronic bronchospasm unresponsive to conventional therapy and severe acute asthma, 2.5 mg, repeated up to 4 times daily, increased to 5 mg if necessary; in refractory patients with severe acute asthma up to 10 mg can be given but may be associated with increased side-effects; CHILD 2.5 mg, increased to 5 mg if required

Oral

PoM Salbutamol (Non-proprietary)

Tablets, salbutamol (as sulphate) 2 mg, net price 20 = 14p; 4 mg, 20 = 25p

Available from APS, Berk (Asmaven®), Cox, CP, Hillcross, K Pharm., Norton

PoM Ventolin® (A&H)

Tablets, both pink, scored, salbutamol (as sulphate), 2 mg, net price 20 = 22p; 4 mg, 20 = 43p

Syrup, sugar-free, salbutamol 2 mg (as sulphate)/5 mL. Net price 150 mL = 67p

PoM Volmax® (DF)

Tablets, m/r, salbutamol (as sulphate) 4 mg, net price 56-tab pack = £10.55; 8 mg, 56-tab pack = £12.66. Label: 25

Dose: 8 mg twice daily; CHILD 3–12 years 4 mg twice daily

Parenteral

PoM Ventolin® (A&H)

Injection, salbutamol 50 micrograms (as sulphate)/mL. Net price 5-mL amp = 57p

Injection, salbutamol 500 micrograms (as sulphate)/mL. Net price 1-mL amp = 43p

Solution for intravenous infusion, salbutamol 1 mg (as sulphate)/mL. Dilute before use. Net price 5-mL amp = £3.08

Inhalation

COUNSELLING. Advise patients not to exceed prescribed dose and to follow manufacturer's directions; if a previously effective dose of inhaled salbutamol fails to provide at least 3 hours relief, a doctor's advice should be obtained as soon as possible

PoM Salbutamol (Non-proprietary)

Aerosol inhalation, salbutamol 100 micrograms/metered inhalation, net price 200-dose unit = £1.14

Available from APS, Ashbourne (Maxivent®), Baker Norton (Salamol®), Berk (Asmaven®), Cox, CP, K Pharm., 3M (Salbulin®), Norton

Additives: include CFC propellants

PoM Aerolin® Autohaler (3M)

Aerosol inhalation, salbutamol 100 micrograms (as sulphate)/metered inhalation. Net price 200-dose breath-actuated unit = £10.51; also 100-dose unit = £5.26 (hosp. only)

Additives: include CFC propellants

PoM Steri-Neb Salamol® (Baker Norton)

Nebuliser solution unit, salbutamol 0.1% (1 mg/mL, as sulphate), net price 20 × 2.5 mL (2.5 mg) = £3.06; 0.2% (2 mg/mL), 20 × 2.5 mL (5 mg) = £6.14. May be diluted with sterile sodium chloride 0.9%

PoM Ventodisks® (A&H)

Dry powder for inhalation, disks containing 8 blisters of salbutamol (as sulphate) 200 micrograms/blister, net price pack of 14 disks with Diskhaler® = £7.11; 14-disk refill = £6.54; 400 micrograms/blister, pack of 14 disks with Diskhaler® = £12.02; 14-disk refill = £11.45

PoM **Ventolin**® (A&H)

Aerosol inhalation, salbutamol 100 micrograms/ metered inhalation. Net price 200-dose unit = £2.30
Additives: include CFC propellants

Nebules® (for use with nebuliser), salbutamol 0.1% (1 mg/mL, as sulphate), net price 2.5 mL (2.5 mg) = 19p; 0.2% (2 mg/mL), 2.5 mL (5 mg) = 38p. May be diluted with sterile sodium chloride 0.9%

Respirator solution (for use with a nebuliser or ventilator), salbutamol 0.5% (5 mg/mL, as sulphate). Net price 20 mL = £2.71 (hosp. only). May be diluted with sterile sodium chloride 0.9%

Rotacaps® (dry powder for inhalation; for use with Ventolin Rotahaler), salbutamol (as sulphate), 200 micrograms (light-blue/clear), net price 20 = £1.06; 400 micrograms (dark-blue/clear), 20 = £1.79

Note. Capsules containing 200 or 400 micrograms salbutamol (as sulphate) as dry powder for inhalation also available as Salbutamol Cyclocaps® (Du Pont); only for use with Cyclohaler®

Inhaler devices
See section 3.1.5

TERBUTALINE SULPHATE

Indications; Cautions; Side-effects: see under Salbutamol; premature labour, see section 7.1.3

Dose: by mouth, 2.5 mg 3 times daily for 1–2 weeks, then up to 5 mg 3 times daily; CHILD 75 micrograms/kg 3 times daily; 7–15 years 2.5 mg 2–3 times daily

By subcutaneous, intramuscular, or slow intravenous injection, 250–500 micrograms up to 4 times daily; CHILD 2–15 years 10 micrograms/kg to a max. of 300 micrograms

By continuous intravenous infusion as a solution containing 3–5 micrograms/mL, 1.5–5 micrograms/minute for 8–10 hours; reduce dose for children

By aerosol inhalation, adults and children 250–500 micrograms (1–2 puffs); for persistent symptoms up to 3–4 times daily (but see also Chronic asthma table)

By inhalation of powder (Turbohaler®), 500 micrograms (1 inhalation); for persistent symptoms up to 4 times daily (but see also Chronic asthma table)

By inhalation of nebulised solution, 5–10 mg 2–4 times daily; additional doses may be necessary in severe acute asthma; CHILD, up to 3 years 2 mg, 3–6 years 3 mg; 6–8 years 4 mg, over 8 years 5 mg, 2–4 times daily

Oral and parenteral
PoM **Bricanyl**® (Astra)

Tablets, scored, terbutaline sulphate 5 mg. Net price 20 = 76p
Syrup, sugar-free, terbutaline sulphate 1.5 mg/ 5 mL. Net price 300 mL = £2.42
Injection, terbutaline sulphate 500 micrograms/ mL. Net price 1-mL amp = 28p; 5-mL amp = £1.30

PoM **Bricanyl SA**® (Astra)

Tablets, m/r, terbutaline sulphate 7.5 mg. Net price 20 = £1.59. Label: 25
Dose: 7.5 mg twice daily

PoM **Monovent**® (Lagap)

Syrup, terbutaline sulphate 1.5 mg/5 mL. Net price 300 mL = £2.25

Inhalation

COUNSELLING. Advise patients not to exceed prescribed dose and to follow manufacturer's directions; if a previously effective dose of inhaled terbutaline fails to provide at least 3 hours relief, a doctor's advice should be obtained as soon as possible; little sensation associated with use of Turbohaler®

PoM **Bricanyl**® (Astra)

Aerosol inhalation, terbutaline sulphate 250 micrograms/metered inhalation. Net price 400-dose unit = £5.31; 400-dose unit with Spacer device (collapsible extended mouthpiece) = £7.21; 400-dose refill cannister for use with Nebuhaler or Spacer inhaler = £5.21
Additives: include CFC propellants

Turbohaler® (= breath-actuated dry powder inhaler), terbutaline sulphate 500 micrograms/ inhalation. Net price 100-dose unit = £8.94

Respules® (= single-dose units for nebulisation), terbutaline sulphate 2.5 mg/mL. Net price 20 × 2-mL units = £3.67

Respirator solution (for use with a nebuliser or ventilator), terbutaline sulphate 10 mg/mL. Net price 10 mL = £1.35. Before use dilute with sterile sodium chloride 0.9%

Inhaler devices
See section 3.1.5

Chronic Asthma table, see p. 112
Acute Severe Asthma table, see p. 113

BAMBUTEROL HYDROCHLORIDE

Note. Bambuterol is a pro-drug of terbutaline

Indications: asthma and other conditions associated with reversible airways obstruction

Cautions; Side-effects: see under Salbutamol reduce dose in renal impairment; avoid in cirrhosis, severe hepatic impairment; manufacturer advises avoid in pregnancy

Dose: 20 mg once daily at bedtime if patient has previously tolerated beta$_2$-adrenoceptor stimulants; other patients, initially 10 mg once daily at bedtime, increased if necessary after 1–2 weeks to 20 mg once daily; CHILD not recommended

▼ PoM **Bambec**® (Astra)

Tablets, both scored, bambuterol hydrochloride 10 mg, net price 28-tab pack = £10.00; 20 mg, 28-tab pack = £12.00

FENOTEROL HYDROBROMIDE

Indications: reversible airways obstruction

Cautions; Side-effects: see under Salbutamol

Dose: by aerosol inhalation, 100–200 micrograms (1–2 puffs Berotec '100'); for persistent symptoms up to 3–4 times daily, and see also Berotec '200' below (but see also Chronic asthma table); CHILD 6–12 years 100 micrograms (1 puff Berotec '100')

Persistent bronchospasm not adequately controlled by Berotec '100', *by aerosol inhalation,* 200–400 micrograms (1–2 puffs Berotec '200') 1–3 times daily; not more than 400 micrograms (2 puffs Berotec '200') every 6 hours; max. 1.6 mg daily (**important:** see also Chronic asthma table); CHILD under 16 years, not recommended

PoM **Berotec®** (Boehringer Ingelheim)

'100' aerosol inhalation, fenoterol hydrobromide 100 micrograms/metered inhalation. Net price 200-dose unit = £2.36

Additives: include CFC propellants

'200' aerosol inhalation, fenoterol hydrobromide 200 micrograms/metered inhalation. Net price 200-dose unit = £2.78

Additives: include CFC propellants

Note. Only for persistent bronchospasm inadequately controlled by Berotec '100'

COUNSELLING. Advise patients not to exceed prescribed dose and to follow manufacturer's directions; if a previously effective dose of inhaled fenoterol fails to provide at least 3 hours' relief, a doctor's advice should be obtained as soon as possible

PIRBUTEROL

Indications: reversible airways obstruction

Cautions; Side-effects: see under Salbutamol

Dose: by mouth, 10–15 mg 3–4 times daily

By aerosol inhalation, 200–400 micrograms (1–2 puffs); persistent symptoms, up to 3–4 times daily (but see also Chronic Asthma table)

PoM **Exirel®** (3M)

Capsules, pirbuterol (as hydrochloride) 10 mg (turquoise/olive), net price 90-cap pack = £2.83; 15 mg (turquoise/beige), 90-cap pack = £4.23

Aerosol inhalation, pirbuterol 200 micrograms (as acetate)/metered inhalation. Net price 200-dose unit = £3.78

Additives: include CFC propellants

COUNSELLING. Advise patients not to exceed prescribed dose and to follow manufacturer's directions; if a previously effective dose of inhaled pirbuterol fails to provide at least 3 hours' relief, a doctor's advice should be obtained as soon as possible

REPROTEROL HYDROCHLORIDE

Indications: reversible airways obstruction

Cautions; Side-effects: see under Salbutamol

Dose: by aerosol inhalation, 0.5–1 mg (1–2 puffs); persistent symptoms, up to 3 times daily (but see also Chronic asthma table); CHILD 6–12 years 500 micrograms (1 puff)

PoM **Bronchodil®** (ASTA Medica)

Aerosol inhalation, reproterol hydrochloride 500 micrograms/metered inhalation. Net price 400-dose unit = £6.67

Additives: include CFC propellants

COUNSELLING. Advise patients not to exceed prescribed dose and to follow manufacturer's directions; if a previously effective dose of inhaled reproterol fails to provide at least 3 hours' relief, a doctor's advice should be obtained as soon as possible

RIMITEROL HYDROBROMIDE

Indications: reversible airways obstruction

Cautions; Side-effects: see under Salbutamol

Dose: by aerosol inhalation, adults and children 200–600 micrograms (1–3 puffs); should not be repeated in less than 30 minutes; max. 8 doses daily (but see also Chronic asthma table)

PoM **Pulmadil®** (3M)

Aerosol inhalation, rimiterol hydrobromide 200 micrograms/metered inhalation. Net price 300-dose unit = £5.06

Additives: include CFC propellants

COUNSELLING. Advise patients not to exceed prescribed dose and to follow manufacturer's directions; if a previously effective dose of inhaled rimiterol fails to provide at least 1–2 hours' relief, a doctor's advice should be obtained as soon as possible

SALMETEROL

Indications: reversible airways obstruction (including nocturnal asthma and prevention of exercise-induced bronchospasm) in patients requiring long term regular bronchodilator therapy, who should normally also be receiving regular and adequate doses of inhaled anti-inflammatory drugs (e.g. corticosteroids and/or, in children, sodium cromoglycate) or oral corticosteroids

Note. CSM has emphasised that salmeterol is not for immediate relief of acute attacks and that existing corticosteroid therapy should not be reduced or withdrawn

Cautions; Side-effects: see under Salbutamol and notes above; significant incidence of paradoxical bronchospasm

Dose: by inhalation, 50 micrograms (2 puffs or 1 blister) twice daily; up to 100 micrograms (4 puffs or 2 blisters) twice daily in more severe airways obstruction; CHILD over 4 years, 50 micrograms (2 puffs of aerosol inhaler or 1 blister) twice daily

Note. See also Chronic Asthma table

PoM **Serevent®** (A&H)

Aerosol inhalation, salmeterol (as xinafoate (= hydroxynaphthoate)) 25 micrograms/metered inhalation, net price 120-inhalation unit = £28.60

Additives: include CFC propellants

Powder for inhalation, disks containing 4 blisters of salmeterol (as xinafoate (= hydroxynaphthoate)) 50 micrograms/blister, net price pack of 14 disks with Diskhaler® = £29.97; 14-disk refill = £29.40

COUNSELLING. Advise patients not to exceed prescribed dose and to follow manufacturer's directions; if a previously effective dose of inhaled salmeterol fails to provide at least 12 hours relief, a doctor's advice should be obtained as soon as possible

TULOBUTEROL HYDROCHLORIDE

Indications: reversible airways obstruction

Cautions: see under Salbutamol; also mild renal impairment (avoid if severe); pregnancy (manufacturer states not yet established)

Contra-indications: moderate to severe renal impairment; acute liver failure, chronic liver disease

Side-effects: see under Salbutamol

Dose: 2 mg twice daily; increased if necessary to 2 mg 3 times daily; CHILD 6–10 years 0.5–1 mg twice daily; over 10 years, 1–2 mg twice daily

PoM **Brelomax®** (Abbott)

Tablets, scored, tulobuterol hydrochloride 2 mg. Net price 60-tab pack = £12.54

PoM **Respacal®** (UCB Pharma)

Tablets, f/c, scored, tulobuterol hydrochloride 2 mg. Net price 60-tab pack = £12.86

Syrup, sugar-free, tulobuterol hydrochloride1 mg/ 5 mL. Net price 150 mL = £4.48

3.1.1.2 OTHER ADRENOCEPTOR STIMULANTS

These preparations (including the partially selective orciprenaline) are now regarded as less suitable and less safe for use as bronchodilators than the selective beta$_2$-adrenoceptor stimulants, as they are more likely to cause arrhythmias and other side-effects. They should be avoided whenever possible.

Adrenaline injection (1 in 1000) is used in the emergency treatment of acute allergic and anaphylactic reactions (section 3.4.3).

EPHEDRINE HYDROCHLORIDE

Indications: reversible airways obstruction, but see notes above; nocturnal enuresis in children, see section 7.4.2

Cautions: hyperthyroidism, diabetes mellitus, ischaemic heart disease, hypertension, renal impairment, elderly; may cause acute retention in prostatic hypertrophy; interaction with MAOIs a disadvantage; **interactions:** Appendix 1 (sympathomimetics)

Side-effects: tachycardia, anxiety, restlessness, insomnia common; also tremor, arrhythmias, dry mouth, cold extremities

Dose: 3 times daily, 15–60 mg; CHILD 3 times daily, up to 1 year 7.5 mg, 1–5 years 15 mg, 6–12 years 30 mg (not recommended, see above)

Nocturnal enuresis, CHILD 7–8 years 30 mg, 9–12 years 45 mg, 13–15 years 60 mg at bedtime

PoM ¹**Ephedrine Hydrochloride** (Non-proprietary)

Tablets, ephedrine hydrochloride 15 mg, net price 20 = 44p; 30 mg, 20 = 50p; 60 mg, 20 = £1.11

Elixir, ephedrine hydrochloride 15 mg/5 mL in a suitable flavoured vehicle, containing alcohol 12%. Net price 100 mL = 72p

1. For exemptions see *Medicines, Ethics and Practice*, No. 12, London, Pharmaceutical Press, 1994 (and subsequent editions as available)

For a list of **cough and decongestant preparations on sale to the public**, including those containing ephedrine, see section 3.9.2

CAM® (Rybar)

Mixture, sugar-free, ephedrine hydrochloride 4 mg/ 5 mL. Net price 200 mL = £2.06

Dose: 20 mL 3–4 times daily; CHILD 6 months–2 years 2.5 mL, 2–4 years 5 mL, 5–12 years 10 mL, 3 times daily (but not recommended, see notes above)

ISOPRENALINE SULPHATE

Indications: reversible airways obstruction, but see notes above

Cautions; Side-effects: see under Salbutamol (section 3.1.1.1) and notes above

PoM **Medihaler-iso®** (3M)

Aerosol inhalation, isoprenaline sulphate 80 micrograms/ metered inhalation. Net price 400-dose vial = £2.43

Additives: include CFC propellants

Note. Not recommended therefore no dose stated

PoM **Medihaler-iso Forte®** (3M)

Aerosol inhalation, isoprenaline sulphate 400 micrograms/metered inhalation. Net price 400-dose vial = £2.82

Additives: include CFC propellants

Note. Not recommended therefore no dose stated

ORCIPRENALINE SULPHATE

Indications: reversible airways obstruction, but see notes above

Cautions; Side-effects: see under Salbutamol (section 3.1.1.1) and notes above

Dose: by mouth, 20 mg 4 times daily; CHILD up to 1 year 5–10 mg 3 times daily, 1–3 years 5–10 mg 4 times daily, 3–12 years 40–60 mg daily in divided doses (but not recommended, see notes above)

By aerosol inhalation, 750–1500 micrograms (1–2 puffs) repeated if necessary after not less than 30 minutes to a max. of 9 mg (12 puffs) daily; CHILD up to 6 years 750 micrograms (1 puff) up to 4 times daily, 6–12 years 750–1500 micrograms (1–2 puffs) up to 4 times daily (but not recommended, see notes above)

PoM **Alupent®** (Boehringer Ingelheim)

Tablets, scored, orciprenaline sulphate 20 mg. Net price 100-tab pack = £3.80

Syrup, sugar-free, orciprenaline sulphate 10 mg/5 mL. Net price 100 mL = 75p

Aerosol inhalation, orciprenaline sulphate 750 micrograms/metered inhalation. Net price 300-dose vial with mouthpiece = £3.22; refill vial = £2.66

Additives: include CFC propellants

COUNSELLING. Advise patients not to exceed prescribed dose and to follow manufacturer's directions

PSEUDOEPHEDRINE HYDROCHLORIDE

See section 3.10

3.1.2 Antimuscarinic bronchodilators

These drugs have traditionally been regarded as more effective in relieving bronchoconstriction associated with chronic bronchitis. **Ipratropium** may provide some bronchodilation in patients with chronic bronchitis who fail to respond to the selective beta$_2$-adrenoceptor stimulants (section 3.1.1.1). Unlike the older antimuscarinic drugs, side-effects are rare and it does not increase sputum viscosity or affect mucociliary clearance of sputum. The aerosol inhalation has a maximum effect 30–60 minutes after use; its duration of action is 3 to 6 hours and bronchodilatation can usually be maintained with treatment three times a day.

Oxitropium has been introduced recently and has a similar duration of action to that of ipratropium.

IPRATROPIUM BROMIDE

Indications: reversible airways obstruction, particularly in chronic bronchitis
Cautions: glaucoma (standard doses unlikely to be harmful but see also under nebuliser, below); prostatic hypertrophy; pregnancy
Side-effects: dry mouth occasionally reported; rarely urinary retention, constipation
Dose: see below

PoM Atrovent® (Boehringer Ingelheim)
COUNSELLING. Advise patient not to exceed prescribed dose and to follow manufacturer's directions
Aerosol inhalation, ipratropium bromide 20 micrograms/metered inhalation. Net price 200-dose unit = £4.21
Additives: include CFC propellants
Autohaler® (=breath-actuated aerosol inhaler), ipratropium bromide 20 micrograms/metered inhalation. Net price 200-dose unit = £10.43
Additives: include CFC propellants
Dose: by aerosol inhalation, 20–40 micrograms (1–2 puffs), in early treatment up to 80 micrograms (4 puffs) at a time, 3–4 times daily; CHILD up to 6 years 20 micrograms (1 puff) 3 times daily, 6–12 years 20–40 micrograms (1–2 puffs) 3 times daily
Forte aerosol inhalation, ipratropium bromide 40 micrograms/metered inhalation. Net price 200-dose unit = £5.65
Additives: include CFC propellants
Dose: by aerosol inhalation 40 micrograms (1 puff), in early treatment 80 micrograms (2 puffs), 3–4 times daily; CHILD 6–12 years 40 micrograms (1 puff) 3 times daily
Nebuliser solution, isotonic, ipratropium bromide 250 micrograms/mL (0.025%); net price 20 × 1-mL unit-dose vials (preservative-free) = £6.82; 20 × 2-mL vials = £8.00. If dilution is necessary use only sterile sodium chloride solution 0.9%
Dose: reversible airways obstruction, *by inhalation of nebulised solution,* 100–500 micrograms (0.4–2 mL of a 0.025% solution) up to 4 times daily; CHILD 3–14 years 100–500 micrograms up to 3 times daily. Dilution of solution is adjusted according to equipment and length of administration
Note. Because paradoxical bronchospasm has occurred, first dose should be inhaled under medical supervision.
GLAUCOMA. Acute angle closure glaucoma has been reported in patients given nebulised ipratropium, particularly when used in association with nebulised salbutamol. Special caution is needed and care should be taken to avoid escape from mask to patient's eyes.

PoM Steri-Neb Ipratropium® (Baker Norton)
Nebuliser solution unit, isotonic, ipratropium bromide 0.025% (250 micrograms/mL), net price 20 × 1-mL (250 micrograms) unit-dose vials (preservative free) = £6.14; 20 × 2 mL (500 micrograms) = £7.20. May be diluted with sterile sodium chloride 0.9%

Chronic Asthma table, see p.112
Acute Severe Asthma table, see p.113

OXITROPIUM BROMIDE

Indications: reversible airways obstruction, particularly in chronic bronchitis
Cautions; Side-effects: see under Ipratropium Bromide; rarely blurring of vision
Dose: by aerosol inhalation, 200 micrograms (2 puffs) 2–3 times daily

PoM Oxivent® (Boehringer Ingelheim)
Aerosol inhalation, oxitropium bromide 100 micrograms/metered inhalation. Net price 200-dose unit = £12.98
Additives: include CFC propellants
Autohaler® (= breath-actuated aerosol inhaler), oxitropium bromide 100 micrograms/metered inhalation. Net price 200-dose unit = £19.65
Additives: include CFC propellants
COUNSELLING. Advise patient not to exceed prescribed dose and to follow manufacturer's directions

---

3.1.3 Theophylline

Theophylline is used for the relief of *bronchospasm*. It may have an additive effect when used in conjunction with small doses of beta$_2$-adrenoceptor stimulants; the combination may increase the risk of side-effects, including hypokalaemia (for CSM advice see p.115).

Theophylline is metabolised in the liver and there is considerable variation in its half-life in healthy non-smokers, which is even more marked in smokers, in patients with hepatic impairment or heart failure, or if other drugs are taken concurrently. The half-life is *increased* in heart failure, cirrhosis, viral infections, and by drugs such as cimetidine, ciprofloxacin, erythromycin, and oral contraceptives. The half-life is *decreased* in smokers and in heavy drinkers, and by drugs such as phenytoin, carbamazepine, rifampicin, and barbiturates. For other interactions of theophylline see Appendix 1.

These differences in half-life are important because theophylline has a narrow margin between the therapeutic and toxic dose. In most subjects *plasma concentrations* of between 10 and 20 mg/litre are required for satisfactory bronchodilatation. Side-effects can occur with concentrations below 20 mg/litre and are common at concentrations above 30–40 mg/litre.

Theophylline modified-release preparations are usually able to produce adequate plasma concentrations for up to 12 hours. When given as a single dose at night they have a useful role in controlling *nocturnal asthma* and *early morning*

---

wheezing. There is no evidence that **choline theophyllinate** (a derivative of theophylline) is better tolerated than the modified-release preparations. The use of *rapid-release* oral theophylline preparations has declined because of the high incidence of side-effects associated with rapid absorption.

Theophylline is given by injection as **aminophylline**, a mixture of theophylline with ethylenediamine, which is 20 times more soluble than theophylline alone. Aminophylline must be given by **very slow** intravenous injection (over at least 20 minutes); it is too irritant for intramuscular use. Theophylline is also available for slow intravenous injection as a mixture with lysine.

Intravenous aminophylline may have a role in the treatment of *severe attacks of asthma* that do not respond rapidly to a nebulised beta$_2$-adrenoceptor stimulant (see also Acute Severe Asthma table, p.113). Measurement of *plasma concentrations* may be helpful, and is **essential** if aminophylline is to be given to patients who have been taking oral theophylline preparations, as serious side-effects such as convulsions and arrhythmias can occasionally occur before the appearance of other symptoms of toxicity.

Aminophylline injection was formerly also used in the treatment of left ventricular failure but has been superseded for this purpose by diuretics (see sections 2.2.1 and 2.2.2) and the opioid analgesics (see section 4.7.2). However, it may have a role in patients with heart failure who are also suffering from asthma and bronchitis, where opioids are contra-indicated, though care is needed in those with increased myocardial excitability.

Aminophylline was formerly available for *rectal administration* as suppositories but these caused proctitis and the response was unpredictable; there was a particular risk of toxicity in children.

THEOPHYLLINE

Indications: reversible airways obstruction, severe acute asthma; for guidelines see also Asthma tables (pp.112–13)

Cautions: see notes above; also liver disease, epilepsy, pregnancy and breast-feeding, cardiac disease, elderly, fever; **CSM** advice on hypokalaemia risk, p.115; avoid in porphyria (see section 9.8.2); **interactions:** Appendix 1 (theophylline)—**important**, see also below

FLUVOXAMINE INTERACTION. **CSM** advises that fluvoxamine seriously increases plasma-theophylline concentration and recommends that concomitant use should usually be avoided (or where not possible halve theophylline dose and monitor plasma-theophylline levels closely)

Side-effects: tachycardia, palpitations, nausea, gastro-intestinal disturbances, headache, insomnia, arrhythmias, and convulsions especially if given rapidly by intravenous injection; overdosage: see Emergency Treatment of Poisoning, p.23

Dose: see below

Note. Plasma theophylline concentration for optimum response 10–20 mg/litre (55–110 micromol/litre); narrow margin between therapeutic and toxic dose, see also notes above

PoM Labophylline® (LAB)

Injection, theophylline 20 mg/mL, lysine 12.2 mg/mL. Net price 10-mL amp = 31p

Dose: in patients not previously treated with xanthines, *by slow intravenous injection* (over 20 minutes) initially 200 mg, *or by intravenous infusion* 4 mg/kg; maintenance if required, 500 micrograms/kg/hour for 12 hours, then 400 micrograms/kg/hour; CHILD *by slow intravenous injection* (over 20 minutes) 4 mg/kg initially

Nuelin® (3M)

Tablets, scored, theophylline 125 mg. Net price 90-tab pack = £3.44. Label: 21

Dose: 125 mg 3–4 times daily after food, increased to 250 mg if required; CHILD 7–12 years 62.5–125 mg 3–4 times daily

Liquid, brown, theophylline hydrate 60 mg (as sodium glycinate)/5 mL. Net price 200 mL = £2.05. Label: 21

Dose: 120–240 mg 3–4 times daily after food; CHILD 2–6 years 60–90 mg, 7–12 years 90–120 mg, 3–4 times daily

Modified release

Note. The Council of the Royal Pharmaceutical Society of Great Britain advises pharmacists that if a general practitioner prescribes a modified-release, oral theophylline preparation without specifying a brand name, the pharmacist should contact the prescriber and agree the brand to be dispensed. Additionally, it is essential that a patient discharged from hospital should be maintained on the brand on which that patient was stabilised as an in-patient.

Lasma® (Pharmax)

Tablets, m/r, scored, theophylline 300 mg. Net price 20 = £1.89. Label: 25

Dose: 300 mg every 12 hours (increased after 1 week to 450 mg every 12 hours in patients over 70 kg); adjust dose by 150-mg increments as required

Total daily dose may be given as single dose at night when nocturnal symptoms predominate (daytime symptoms then controlled with inhaled bronchodilators)

Nuelin SA® (3M)

SA tablets, m/r, theophylline 175 mg. Net price 60-tab pack = £3.59. Label: 25

Dose: 175–350 mg every 12 hours; CHILD over 6 years 175 mg every 12 hours

SA 250 tablets, m/r, scored, theophylline 250 mg. Net price 60-tab pack = £5.03. Label: 25

Dose: 250–500 mg every 12 hours; CHILD over 6 years 125–250 mg every 12 hours

Slo-Phyllin® (Lipha)

Capsules, all m/r, theophylline 60 mg (white/clear, enclosing white pellets), net price 56-cap pack = £1.92; 125 mg (brown/clear, enclosing white pellets), 56-cap pack = £2.42; 250 mg (blue/clear, enclosing white pellets), 56-cap pack = £3.02. Label: 25 *or* counselling, see below

Dose: 250–500 mg every 12 hours; CHILD, every 12 hours, 2–6 years 60–120 mg, 7–12 years 125–250 mg

COUNSELLING. Swallow whole with fluid *or* swallow enclosed granules with soft food (e.g. yoghurt)

Theo-Dur® (Astra)

Tablets, m/r, both scored, theophylline 200 mg, net price 20 = £1.24; 300 mg, 20 = £1.80. Label: 25

Dose: 300 mg every 12 hours; CHILD up to 35 kg 100 mg, over 35 kg 200 mg, every 12 hours

Uniphyllin Continus® (Napp)

Tablets, m/r, both scored, theophylline 300 mg, net price 56-tab pack = £6.20; 400 mg, 56-tab pack = £7.32. Label: 25

Dose: 200 mg every 12 hours increased after 1 week to 300 mg every 12 hours; over 70 kg 300 mg every 12 hours increased after 1 week to 400 mg every 12 hours

May be appropriate to give larger evening or morning dose to achieve optimum therapeutic effect when symptoms most severe; in patients whose night- or daytime symptoms persist despite other therapy, who are not currently receiving theophylline, total daily requirement may be added as single evening or morning dose

Paediatric tablets, m/r, scored, theophylline 200 mg. Net price 56-tab pack = £4.05. Label: 25

Dose: CHILD over 5 years, maintenance, 9 mg/kg twice daily

For a list of **cough and decongestant preparations on sale to the public**, including those containing theophylline, see section 3.9.2

AMINOPHYLLINE

Note. Aminophylline is a stable mixture or combination of theophylline and ethylenediamine; the ethylenediamine confers greater solubility in water

Indications: reversible airways obstruction, severe acute asthma

Cautions; Side-effects: see under Theophylline; also allergy to ethylenediamine can cause urticaria, erythema, and exfoliative dermatitis

Dose: see below

Note. Plasma theophylline concentration for optimum response 10–20 mg/litre (55–110 micromol/litre); narrow margin between therapeutic and toxic dose, see also notes above

Aminophylline (Non-proprietary)

Tablets, aminophylline 100 mg, net price 20 = 60p. Label: 21

Dose: by mouth, 100–300 mg, 3–4 times daily, after food

PoM *Injection*, aminophylline 25 mg/mL, net price 10-mL amp = 63p

Available from Evans, IMS (Min I Jet®)

Dose: by slow intravenous injection (over 20 minutes), 250–500 mg (5 mg/kg) when necessary; maintenance, if required, in patients not previously treated with theophylline, 500 micrograms/kg/hour *by slow intravenous infusion*

CHILD, *by slow intravenous injection* (over 20 minutes), 5 mg/kg; maintenance, if required, in patients not previously treated with theophylline, 6 months–9 years 1 mg/kg/hour, 10–16 years 800 micrograms/kg/hour *by slow intravenous infusion*

Modified release (see advice on p. 120)

Pecram® (Zyma)

Tablets, m/r, yellow, aminophylline hydrate 225 mg. Net price 20 = 99p. Label: 25

Dose: 1 tablet twice daily initially, increased if necessary to 2 tablets twice daily (steady-state concentrations usually reached after 3–4 days)

Phyllocontin Continus® (Napp)

Tablets, m/r, yellow, f/c, aminophylline 225 mg. Net price 60-tab pack = £3.52. Label: 25

Dose: 1 tablet twice daily initially, increased after 1 week to 2 tablets twice daily

Forte tablets, m/r, yellow, f/c, aminophylline 350 mg. Net price 60-tab pack = £5.85. Label: 25

Note. Forte tablets are for smokers and other patients with decreased theophylline half-life (see notes above)

Paediatric tablets, m/r, yellow, aminophylline 100 mg. Net price 50-tab pack = £1.89. Label: 25

Dose: CHILD over 3 years, 6 mg/kg twice daily initially, increased after 1 week to 12 mg/kg twice daily

Note. Modified-release tablets containing aminophylline 225 mg and 350 mg also available from Ashbourne (Amnivent®)

CHOLINE THEOPHYLLINATE

Indications: reversible airways obstruction

Cautions; Side-effects: see under Theophylline

Dose: by mouth, 100–400 mg 2–4 times daily preferably after food; CHILD, 3 times daily, 3–5 years 62.5–125 mg, 6–12 years 100 mg

Note. Plasma theophylline concentration for optimum response 10–20 mg/litre (55–110 micromol/litre); narrow margin between therapeutic and toxic dose, see also notes above

Choledyl® (P-D)

Tablets, both f/c, choline theophyllinate 100 mg (pink), net price 100-tab pack = £2.20; 200 mg (yellow), 100-tab pack = £3.00

Syrup, yellow, choline theophyllinate 62.5 mg/5 mL. Net price 200 mL = £2.57

3.1.4 Compound bronchodilator preparations

Most compound bronchodilator preparations have no place in the management of patients with airways obstruction.

In general, patients are best treated with single-ingredient preparations, such as a selective beta₂-adrenoceptor stimulant (section 3.1.1.1) or ipratropium bromide (section 3.1.2), so that the dose of each drug can be adjusted. This flexibility is lost with combinations, although those in which both components are effective may occasionally have a role when compliance is a problem.

For **cautions, contra-indications** and **side-effects** see under individual monographs

PoM **Combivent®** (Boehringer Ingelheim)

Aerosol inhalation, ipratropium bromide 20 micrograms, salbutamol 100 micrograms (as sulphate)/metered inhalation. Net price 200-dose unit = £6.00

Additives: include CFC propellants

Dose: 2 puffs 4 times daily; CHILD under 12 years not recommended

PoM **Duovent**® (Boehringer Ingelheim)

Aerosol inhalation, fenoterol hydrobromide 100 micrograms, ipratropium bromide 40 micrograms/metered inhalation. Net price 200-dose unit with mouthpiece = £5.76 (extension tube also available)

Additives: include CFC propellants

Autohaler® (=breath-actuated aerosol inhaler), fenoterol hydrobromide 100 micrograms, ipratropium bromide 40 micrograms/metered inhalation. Net price 200-dose unit = £11.57

Additives: include CFC propellants

Dose: 1–2 puffs 3–4 times daily; CHILD over 6 years 1 puff 3 times daily

Nebuliser solution, isotonic, fenoterol hydrobromide 1.25 mg, ipratropium bromide 500 micrograms/4-mL vial, net price 20 unit-dose vials = £10.00

Dose: acute severe asthma or acute exacerbation of chronic asthma, *by inhalation of nebulised solution*, 1 vial (4 mL); may be repeated up to max, 4 vials in 24 hours; CHILD under 14 years, not recommended

GLAUCOMA. In addition to other potential side-effects acute angle closure glaucoma has been reported with nebulised ipratropium—for details, see p. 119

With theophylline

Note. Compound theophylline preparations on sale to the public include Anestan® tablets (theophylline, ephedrine), Do-Do® tablets (theophylline, ephedrine, caffeine), Franolyn Chesty® (theophylline, ephedrine, guaiphenesin)

PoM **Franol**® (Sanofi Winthrop)

Tablets, ephedrine hydrochloride 11 mg, theophylline 120 mg. Net price 100-tab pack = £5.81. Label: 21

Dose: 1 tablet 3 times daily; an additional tablet may be taken at bedtime for nocturnal attacks

PoM **Franol Plus**® (Sanofi Winthrop)

Tablets, ephedrine sulphate 15 mg, theophylline 120 mg. Net price 20 = £1.60. Label: 21

Dose: 1 tablet 3 times daily; an additional tablet may be taken at bedtime for nocturnal attacks

3.1.5   Peak flow meters, inhaler devices and nebulisers

PEAK FLOW METERS

Measurement of peak flow is particularly helpful for patients who are 'poor perceivers' and hence slow to detect deterioration in their asthma, and for those with moderate or severe asthma. Patients can also be encouraged to adjust some of their own treatment (within specified limits) according to changes in peak flow rate.

Mini-Wright® (Clement Clarke)

Peak flow meter, standard (60 to 800 litres/minute), net price = £6.51, low range (30 to 370 litres/minute) = £6.51, replacement mouthpiece = 38p (for adult or child)

Vitalograph® (Vitalograph)

Peak flow meter, standard (50 to 750 litres/minute), net price = £6.30, low range (25 to 280 litres/minute) = £6.30, replacement mouthpiece = 40p (for adult or child)

Wright® (Ferraris)

Pocket peak flow meter, standard (90–710 litres/minute), net price = £6.26, low range (40–370 litres/minute) = £6.26, replacement mouthpiece = 38p (for adult or child)

INHALER DEVICES

A variety of spacing devices is now available for use with metered dose inhalers. By providing a space between inhaler and mouth, they reduce the velocity of the aerosol and subsequent impaction on the oropharynx; in addition they allow more time for evaporation of the propellant so that a larger proportion of the particles can be inhaled and deposited in the lungs; also co-ordination of inspiration with actuation of the aerosol is less important. They range from the Bricanyl Spacer® (for terbutaline), a collapsible extended mouthpiece, to larger spacing devices with a one-way valve (Nebuhaler®, Volumatic®).

Spacing devices are particularly useful for patients with poor inhalation technique, for children, for patients requiring higher doses, for nocturnal asthma, and for patients prone to develop candidiasis with inhaled corticosteroids.

Cyclohaler® (Du Pont)

Breath actuated device for use with Salbutamol Cyclocaps. Net price = 76p

Fisonair®, see section 3.3

NHS Haleraid® (Glaxo)

Device to place over standard inhalers as aid to operation by patients with impaired strength in hands (e.g. with arthritis). Net price = 80p

Nebuhaler® (Astra)

Spacer inhaler, large-volume device. For use with Bricanyl and Pulmicort refill canisters. Net price = £4.63; paediatric mask also available

Rotahaler® (A&H)

Breath actuated device for use with Rotacaps. Available as Becotide Rotahaler, Ventolin Rotahaler, and Ventide Rotahaler. Net price = 78p

Spinhaler®, see section 3.3

Volumatic® (A&H)

Spacer inhaler, large-volume device. For use with Becloforte, Becotide, Flixotide, Ventide, and Ventolin inhalers. Net price = £2.75; paediatric mask also available

NEBULISERS

In England and Wales nebulisers and compressors are not available on the NHS (but they are free of VAT); some nebulisers (but not compressors) are available on form GP10A in Scotland (for details consult Scottish Drug Tariff).

Nebulisers convert a solution of a drug into an aerosol for inhalation. They are used to deliver higher doses of drug to the airways than is usual with standard inhalers. The main indications for use of a nebuliser are:

to deliver a beta-adrenoceptor stimulant or ipratropium to a patient with an *acute exacerbation* of asthma or of chronic airway obstruction;

to deliver a beta-adrenoceptor stimulant or ipratropium on a *regular basis* to a patient with severe asthma or reversible airways obstruction who has been shown to benefit from regular treatment with higher doses;

to deliver *prophylactic medication* such as cromoglycate or a corticosteroid to a patient unable to use other inhalational devices (particularly a young child);

to deliver an *antibiotic* (such as colistin) to a patient with chronic purulent infection (as in cystic fibrosis or bronchiectasis);

to deliver *pentamidine* for the prophylaxis and treatment of *Pneumocystis pneumonia* to a patient with AIDS.

Only about 10% of a nebulised solution reaches the lungs, the remainder being deposited on the mouthpiece and tubing. The extent to which the nebulised solution then deposits particles in the airways or alveoli depends on particle size. Particles with a mass median diameter of 1–5 microns are deposited in the airways and are therefore appropriate for asthma whereas a particle size of 1–2 microns is needed for alveolar deposition of pentamidine to combat pneumocystis infection. A different type of nebuliser is therefore required according to the deposition required; a different type of nebuliser may also be required according to the viscosity of the solution, antibiotic solutions usually being more viscous.

It is important for the patient to be aware that the dose of a bronchodilator given by nebulisation is usually **much higher** than that received from an aerosol inhaler; see below for British Thoracic Society guidelines.

The following are the British Thoracic Society guidelines for giving regular nebulised bronchodilators:

diagnosis should be reviewed and confirmed;

other methods of administration should be explored;

patients should be complying with corticosteroid or cromoglycate (or nedocromil) prophylaxis;

increased bronchodilatation should be obtained without unacceptable side-effects;

an initial 3-week home trial should be undertaken (with peak flow monitoring);

If prescribed:

oral and written instructions should be given to patient on method and frequency of use, action to be taken in event of asthma worsening, and when to attend for follow-up;

supervision should normally entail attendance at asthma clinic or home visits by trained asthma nurse or physiotherapist;

supervision should include evaluation of peak flow, monitoring of prescriptions, and twice yearly servicing of compressor (see also recommendations for individual compressors).

Jet nebulisers

Jet nebulisers utilise the Venturi principle for nebulisation; they are more widely used than ultrasonic nebulisers. Most jet nebulisers require an optimum gas flow rate of 6–8 litres/minute and in hospital can be driven by piped air or oxygen. Domiciliary oxygen cylinders do not provide an adequate flow rate therefore for domiciliary use an electrical compressor is used.

Important: the Department of Health has reminded users of the need to use the correct grade of tubing when connecting a nebuliser to a medical gas supply or compressor.

NHS Cirrus® (Medix)

Jet nebuliser, disposable, up to 80% tracheobronchial deposition, mass median diameter 3.5 microns at 8 litres/minute; for use with viscous and non-viscous solutions, replacement recommended every 2–3 months if used 4 times a day. Compatible with **NHS AC2000 HI FLO®**, **NHS World Traveller HI FLO®**, **NHS Econoneb®**. Net price 1 = £1.50; **NHS Micro-cirrus®** is used only for nebulising pentamidine for alveolar deposition; mass median diameter 1.2 microns at 8 litres/minute; anti-pollution kit with bacterial/viral filter is also available. Net price 1 (with medication chamber) = £3.95; 1 nebuliser set = £4.85. For use with **NHS Turbo-Neb®**

NHS Medix Nebuliser® (Medix)

Jet nebuliser, consisting of mouthpiece, tubing, and nebuliser chamber. Net price 1 = £2.80; mask kits with tubing and nebuliser chamber also available, net price 1 (adult) = £1.80; 1 (child) = £1.70

NHS System 22 Durable Sidestream® (Medic-Aid)

Jet nebuliser, non-disposable, for home use, 80% deposition, mass median diameter 3 microns at 6 litres /minute; minimal dead volume 0.5–0.75 mL, yearly replacement recommended if 4 six-minute treatments used per day. Net price 10-pack = £89.50; 2-pack baffle also available. Mostly used for thin liquids such as bronchodilators and non viscous antibiotics. Compatible with **NHS CR50®**, **NHS Freeway®**, **NHS Freeway Lite®** and **NHS Porta-Neb 50®** (depending on nebulising solution)

Note. This has been developed to replace the **NHS System 22 Acorn®**

NHS Ventstream® (Medic-Aid)

Jet nebuliser, closed-system, for use with low flow compressors, compatible with **NHS CR50®**, **NHS Porta-Neb 50®**, and **NHS Freeway Lite®** (depending on antibiotic) compressors, 80% deposition, less than 5 microns at 6 litres/minute, mass median diameter 3 microns at 6 litres/minute, replacement recommended yearly if used 3 times a day. Net price 1 with filter = £27.00; 10-pack with filter = £250.00; 1 without filter = £23.00; 10-pack without filter = £215.00, patient pack with **NHS CR 50®** compressor = £119.95

Used for nebulising antibiotics

Home compressors with nebulisers

NHS AC 2000 HI FLO® (Medix, Rüsch)

Home use, containing 1 **NHS Jet Nebuliser®** set with mouthpiece, 1 adult or 1 child mask, 1 spare medication chamber, 1 spare inlet filter, filter spanner. Used with **NHS Jet Nebuliser®** provides 8 litres/minute at 20 psi and particles below 5 microns. Mains operated. Nebulises bronchodilators and antibiotics. Net price 1 = £95.00; carrying case available

NHS Econoneb® (Medix)

Home, clinic and hospital use, used with 1 **NHS Jet Nebuliser®** set with mouthpiece, 1 adult or 1 child mask. Compatible with all types of jet nebuliser sets and also the **NHS Micro Cirrus®** nebuliser (recommended for alveolar deposition). Used with **NHS Jet Nebuliser®** provides operating flow 8 litres/minute at 20 psi; nebulises bronchodilators and antibiotics. Mains operated. Net price 1 = £85.00

NHS Freeway Lite® (Medic-Aid)
Portable, containing 1 **NHS System 22 Durable Sidestream®** reusable nebuliser, 1 adult or 1 child mask, 1 mouthpiece, 1 Coiled Duratube®, 2 filters. Net price 1 = £149.00 with carrying case. **NHS Freeway Lite Luxury®** contains additional battery. Net price 1 = £198.00
Also compatible with **NHS Ventstream®** closed system nebuliser

NHS Medi-Neb® (Timesco)
Range of compressors all supplied with adult and child mask, vapourising chamber, and PVC tubing, including: **NHS Medi-Neb Elite®**, home use, provides max. flow 10 litres/minute. Mains operated. Net price 1 = £79.95. **NHS Medi-Neb Companion®**, portable, provides max. flow 7.8 litres/minute. Mains/car battery operated. Net price 1 = £94.95 (includes car battery adaptor and carrying case). **NHS Medi-Neb Companion Plus®**, portable, provides max. flow 7 litres/minute. Mains/battery operated. Net price 1 = £139.85 (includes rechargeable battery, car battery adaptor, and carrying case). **NHS Medi-Neb Tempest**, home/hospital use, provides max. flow 13.5 litres/minute. Mains operated. Net price 1 = £89.95
All used for nebulising antibiotics and bronchodilators; generate particles within range 0.5–6 microns

NHS Porta-Neb 50® (Medic-Aid)
Portable, containing 1 **NHS System 22 Durable Sidestream®** reusable nebuliser, 1 angled flow-through mouthpiece, 1 adult or 1 child mask, 1 Duratube® supply tubing, 2 spare filters (replacement recommended every 2–3 months if used on average 3 times a day). Mains operated. Compatible for occasional use with viscous antibiotics. Operating flow 6.5 litres/minute at 14 psi. Net price 1 = £99.50; carrying case available
Also compatible with **NHS Ventstream®** closed-system nebuliser and **NHS System 22 Acorn®**

NHS Pulmo-Aide® (De Vilbiss)
Home use, containing integral filter (recommend replacement every 6–8 weeks if used 4 times a day), 1 **NHS Pulmo-Neb®** disposable nebuliser set, mouthpiece, mask, mains lead, tubing, thumb-valve. Operating flow 5–8 litres/minute at 5–9 psi (recommend replacement every 3 months if used 4 times a day) delivering 0.5–5 microns in range, 9 mL capacity. For use with bronchodilators. Net price 1 = £97.00; replacement 1 **NHS Pulmo-Neb®** set = £2.50; 5-pack = £10.00

NHS Pulmo-Aide Escort® (De Vilbiss)
Portable, containing 1 **NHS Pulmo-Neb®** disposable nebuliser set, transformer, rechargeable battery, AC to DC adapter charger, DC lead with car adapter, and carrying case. Operating flow 5.5–7 litres/minute at 12–14 psi (recommend replacement every 3 months if used 4 times a day), 9 mL capacity. For use with bronchodilators. Net price 1 = £194.00; replacement 1 **NHS Pulmo-Neb®** = £2.50; 5-pack (with mouthpiece and tubing) = £10.00

NHS World Traveller HI FLO® (Medix, Rüsch)
Portable, containing 1 **NHS Jet Nebuliser®** set with mouthpiece, 1 adult or 1 child mask, 1 spare medication chamber, 1 spare inlet filter, filter spanner. Used with **NHS Jet Nebuliser®** provides 7.5 litres/minute at 20 psi. Battery/mains operated; rechargeable battery pack available. Nebulises bronchodilators and antibiotics. Net price 1 excluding battery = £115.00; 1 with battery = £155.00; carrying case available

Compressors
NHS CR50® (Medic-Aid)
Home, clinic and hospital use, supplied with **NHS System 22 Acorn nebuliser®** provides operating flow rate of 6.5 litres/minute at 14 psi; delivers low–medium viscosity drugs; outlet filter. Mains operated.

Net price 1 = £85.00. Also compatible with **NHS Ventstream®**, and **NHS System 22 Durable Sidestream®** (depending on nebulising solution)

Ultrasonic nebulisers
Ultrasonic nebulisers produce an aerosol by ultrasonic vibration of the drug solution and therefore do not require a gas flow
NHS AeroSonic® (De Vilbiss)
Portable, containing 1 controlling unit, chamber assembly, carrying case, AC to DC adapter/charger, DC lead, 1 mouthpiece with check valve and adapter; minimum nebulisation rate 0.3 mL/minute, mass median diameter 3 microns, capacity 9 mL, 30-second cut-off. Net price 1 = £250.00
NHS Easimist® (Medix)
Portable, adjustable delivery rate to suit requirement. Battery/mains operated; rechargeable battery pack available. Nebulisation rate 0.25–1.0 mL/minute, mass median diameter 4 microns, automatic cut-off with alarm. Net price 1 = £115.00; with DC lead and carrying case = £129.00

NEBULISER DILUENT

Nebulisation may be carried out using an undiluted nebuliser solution or it may require dilution beforehand. The usual diluent is sodium chloride 0.9% (physiological saline).
PoM Steri-Neb Saline® (Baker Norton)
Solution, sodium chloride 0.9% in single-dose units of 2.5 mL. Net price 20 = £3.66

3.2   Corticosteroids

Corticosteroids have been used in asthma for many years, and the use of inhaled corticosteroids has increased so that they are now recommended for prophylactic treatment when patients are using a beta$_2$-stimulant more than once daily (see Chronic Asthma table). They have many fewer side-effects than those associated with systemic administration (see section 6.3.3).

Corticosteroids are usually of no benefit in patients with chronic bronchitis and emphysema; some patients with asthma, however, may be clinically indistinguishable from those with chronic bronchitis except that they will respond to a trial course of corticosteroids.

The action of corticosteroids is not fully understood but they probably reduce bronchial mucosal inflammation, and hence reduce oedema and secretion of mucus into the airway.

INHALATION. Corticosteroid *aerosol inhalations* must be used regularly to obtain maximum benefit; alleviation of symptoms usually occurs 3 to 7 days after initiation. **Beclomethasone dipropionate** and **budesonide** appear to be equally effective; **fluticasone propionate** has been recently introduced. If a beta$_2$-adrenoceptor stimulant is to be used at the same time as an inhaled corticosteroid it should be used first to help increase the penetration of the inhaled corticosteroid.

Patients who have been taking long-term oral corticosteroids can often be transferred to inhalation but the transfer must be done slowly, with gradual

---

reduction in dose of oral corticosteroid, and at a time when the asthma is well controlled.

High-dose aerosol inhalers are available for patients who only have a partial response to standard inhalers. The maximum doses for high-dose corticosteroid inhalers are associated with some adrenal suppression (see section 6.3.3), therefore patients on high doses should be given a 'steroid card' and may need corticosteroid cover during an episode of stress (e.g. an operation). Systemic therapy may also be necessary during episodes of infection or increased bronchoconstriction where higher doses are needed and access of inhaled drug to small airways may be reduced; patients may need a reserve supply of tablets.

Although inhaled corticosteroids have considerably fewer systemic effects than oral corticosteroids, recent evidence has shown that effects on bone metabolism can be detected following inhalation of the higher doses of beclomethasone and budesonide. Although there is no firm evidence that this may lead to increased osteoporosis in the future, it is sensible to ensure that the dose of inhaled corticosteroid is no higher than necessary to keep a patient's asthma under good control. The dose can therefore be reduced cautiously when the asthma has been well controlled for a few weeks as long as the patient knows that it is necessary to reinstate it should their asthma deteriorate or the peak flow rate fall.

Corticosteroids are better inhaled from aerosol inhalers using 'spacer devices' (see section 3.1.5). These increase airway deposition and reduce oropharyngeal deposition, resulting in a marked reduction in the incidence of candidiasis and reducing systemic absorption (so that there is less adrenal suppression); these devices are bulky, but most patients only need to use them morning and night.

Dry powder inhalers which are actuated by the patient's inhalation may be tried in patients who are unable to use the aerosol inhalers.

Suspensions for nebulisation are now also available. Beclomethasone dipropionate suspension for nebulisation (Becotide®) is relatively inefficient because of its poor solubility; only a small amount is nebulised in 15 minutes. A spacing device will allow a larger amount to be administered more effectively and can be used by some children as young as 2 years. Budesonide suspension for nebulisation (Pulmicort Respules®) is also now available, and has been shown to be effective in children.

ORAL. *Acute attacks* of asthma should be treated with short courses of oral corticosteroids starting with a high dose, e.g. prednisolone 30 to 60 mg (30 to 40 mg usually adequate) daily for a few days, gradually reduced once the attack has been controlled. Patients whose asthma has deteriorated rapidly usually respond quickly to corticosteroids, which can then be tailed down over a few days; more gradual reduction is necessary in those whose asthma has deteriorated gradually. For use of corticosteroids in the emergency treatment of *severe acute asthma* see table on p.113.

In *chronic continuing asthma*, when the response to other anti-asthma drugs has been relatively small, continued administration of oral corticosteroids may be necessary; in such cases high doses of inhaled corticosteroids should be continued so that oral requirements are reduced to a minimum. Oral corticosteroids should normally be taken as a single dose in the morning to reduce the disturbance to circadian cortisol secretion. Dosage should always be titrated to the lowest dose which controls symptoms. Regular monitored peak flow measurements often help both patient and doctor to adjust the dose optimally. Prednisolone is available as tablets of 1 mg as well as 5 mg, and the smaller tablets may conveniently be used to adjust the maintenance dosage to the minimum necessary.

Alternate-day administration has not been very successful in the management of asthma in adults as they tend to deteriorate during the second 24 hours. If an attempt is made to introduce this, pulmonary function should be monitored carefully over the 48 hours.

PARENTERAL. For the use of hydrocortisone injection in the emergency treatment of *severe acute asthma*, see Acute Severe Asthma table, p.113

BECLOMETHASONE DIPROPIONATE
(Beclometasone Dipropionate)

Indications: prophylaxis of asthma especially if not fully controlled by bronchodilators or cromoglycate

Cautions: see notes above; also active or quiescent tuberculosis; may need to reinstate systemic therapy during periods of stress or when airways obstruction or mucus prevent drug access to smaller airways

Side-effects: see notes above; also hoarseness and candidiasis of mouth or throat (usually only with large doses)

CANDIDIASIS. Candidiasis can be reduced by using spacer, see notes above, and responds to antifungal lozenges, see section 12.3.2, without discontinuation of therapy—rinsing the mouth with water (or cleaning child's teeth) after inhalation of a dose may also be helpful

Dose: see preparations below

Standard-dose inhalers
PoM **AeroBec®** (3M)
AeroBec 50 Autohaler® (aerosol inhalation), beclomethasone dipropionate 50 micrograms/ metered inhalation, net price 200-inhalation breath-actuated unit = £11.00. Label: 8, counselling, dose

Additives: include CFC propellants
AeroBec 100 Autohaler® (aerosol inhalation), beclomethasone dipropionate 100 micrograms/ metered inhalation, net price 200-inhalation breath-actuated unit = £13.50. Label: 8, counselling, dose

Additives: include CFC propellants
Dose: by aerosol inhalation, 200 micrograms twice daily *or* 100 micrograms 3–4 times daily (in more severe cases initially 600–800 micrograms daily); CHILD 50– 100 micrograms 2–4 times daily

PoM Becodisks® (A&H)

Dry powder for inhalation, beclomethasone dipropionate
100 micrograms/blister, net price 14 disks of 8 blisters with Diskhaler® = £10.99, 14-disk refill = £10.42;
200 micrograms/blister, 14 disks of 8 blisters with Diskhaler® = £20.90, 14-disk refill = £20.33;
400 micrograms/blister, 7 disks of 8 blisters with Diskhaler® = £20.90, 7-disk refill = £20.33.
Label: 8, counselling, dose

Dose: by inhalation of powder, 400 micrograms twice daily *or* 200 micrograms 3–4 times daily; CHILD 100 micrograms 2–4 times daily *or* 200 micrograms twice daily

PoM Becotide Inhaler® (A&H)

Becotide-50 aerosol inhalation, beclomethasone dipropionate 50 micrograms/metered inhalation. Net price 200-dose unit = £5.43. Label: 8, counselling, dose

Becotide-100 aerosol inhalation, beclomethasone dipropionate 100 micrograms/metered inhalation. Net price 200-dose unit = £10.32. Label: 8, counselling, dose

Becotide-200 aerosol inhalation, beclomethasone dipropionate 200 micrograms/metered inhalation. Net price 200-dose unit = £19.61. Label: 8, counselling, dose

Note. Becotide-200 not indicated for children

Dose: by aerosol inhalation, 200 micrograms twice daily *or* 100 micrograms 3–4 times daily (in more severe cases initially 600–800 micrograms daily); CHILD 50–100 micrograms 2–4 times daily *or* 100–200 micrograms twice daily

Note. Aerosol inhalers containing beclomethasone dipropionate 50 micrograms/metered inhalation and 100 micrograms/metered inhalation also available from Baker Norton (Beclazone®) and 3M (Filair®)

Additives: all include CFC propellants

PoM Becotide Rotacaps® (A&H)

Rotacaps® (dry powder for inhalation; for use with Becotide Rotahaler), beclomethasone dipropionate 100 micrograms (buff/clear), net price 100-cap pack = £7.56; 200 micrograms (brown/clear), 100-cap pack = £14.35; 400 micrograms (dark brown/clear), 100-cap pack = £27.27. Label: 8, counselling, dose

Dose: by inhalation of powder, 200 micrograms 3–4 times daily or 400 micrograms twice daily; CHILD 100 micrograms 2–4 times daily *or* 200 micrograms twice daily

High-dose inhalers
Note. High-dose inhalers not indicated for children

PoM AeroBec Forte® (3M)

Aerosol inhalation, beclomethasone dipropionate 250 micrograms/metered inhalation, net price 200-inhalation breath-actuated unit (Autohaler®) = £25.10. Label: 8, counselling, dose, 10 steroid card

Additives: include CFC propellants

Dose: by aerosol inhalation, 500 micrograms twice daily *or* 250 micrograms 4 times daily; if necessary may be increased to 500 micrograms 4 times daily

PoM Becloforte® (A&H)

Aerosol inhalation, beclomethasone dipropionate 250 micrograms/metered inhalation. Net price 200-dose unit = £23.10; net price Becloforte® VM (2 Becloforte® inhalers with Volumatic®) = £46.20. Label: 8, counselling, dose, 10 steroid card

Dose: by aerosol inhalation, 500 micrograms (2 puffs) twice daily *or* 250 micrograms (1 puff) 4 times daily; if necessary may be increased to 500 micrograms 3–4 times daily

Note. Aerosol inhalers containing beclomethasone dipropionate 250 micrograms/metered inhalation also available from Baker Norton (Beclazone®) and 3M (Filair Forte®)

Additives: all include CFC propellants

Dry powder for inhalation, disks containing 8 blisters of beclomethasone dipropionate 400 micrograms/blister, net price 14 disks with Diskhaler® = £39.70; 14-disk refill = £39.13. Label: 8, counselling, dose, 10 steroid card

Dose: by inhalation of powder, 400 micrograms twice daily; if necessary may be increased to 800 micrograms twice daily

Compound preparations
(Not recommended)

PoM Ventide® (A&H)

Aerosol inhalation, beclomethasone dipropionate 50 micrograms, salbutamol 100 micrograms/metered inhalation. Net price 200-dose unit = £6.02. Label: 8, counselling, dose

Additives: include CFC propellants

Dose: maintenance, 2 puffs 3–4 times daily; CHILD 1–2 puffs 2–4 times daily

Paediatric Rotacaps® (dry powder for inhalation; for use with Ventide Rotahaler), light grey/clear, beclomethasone dipropionate 100 micrograms, salbutamol (as sulphate) 200 micrograms. Net price 100 = £12.59. Label: 8, counselling, dose

Dose: by inhalation of powder, 1 Paediatric Rotacap® 2–4 times daily

Rotacaps® (dry powder for inhalation; for use with Ventide Rotahaler), dark grey/clear, beclomethasone dipropionate 200 micrograms, salbutamol (as sulphate) 400 micrograms. Net price 100 = £22.83. Label: 8, counselling, dose

Dose: by inhalation of powder, 1 Rotacap® 3–4 times daily

Inhaler devices
See section 3.1.5

Chronic Asthma table, see p. 112
Acute Severe Asthma table, see p. 113

BUDESONIDE

Indications; Cautions; Side-effects: see under Beclomethasone Dipropionate

Dose: see preparations below

PoM Pulmicort Inhaler® (Astra)

LS aerosol inhalation, budesonide 50 micrograms/
metered inhalation. Net price 200-dose unit with
standard or Spacer inhaler = £6.66; 200-dose
refill for use with Nebuhaler or Spacer inhaler =
£4.66. Label: 8, counselling, dose

Additives: include CFC propellants

Aerosol inhalation, budesonide 200 micrograms/
metered inhalation. Net price 200-dose unit with
standard or Spacer inhaler = £19.00; 200-dose
refill for use with Nebuhaler or Spacer inhaler =
£17.00; 100-dose unit with standard and Spacer
inhaler = £7.96 (hosp. only); 100-dose refill =
£8.44 (hosp. only). Label: 8, counselling, dose, 10
steroid card

Additives: include CFC propellants

Dose: by aerosol inhalation, 200 micrograms twice
daily; may be reduced in well-controlled asthma to not
less than 200 micrograms daily; in severe asthma dose
may be increased to 1.6 mg daily; CHILD 50–
200 micrograms twice daily; in severe asthma may be
increased to 400 micrograms twice daily

PoM Pulmicort Turbohaler® (Astra)

Turbohaler® (= breath-actuated dry powder
inhaler), budesonide 100 micrograms/inhalation,
net price 200-dose unit = £18.50;
200 micrograms/inhalation, 100-dose unit =
£18.50; 400 micrograms/inhalation, 50-dose unit
=£18.50. Label: 8, counselling, dose, 10 steroid
card

Note. Little sensation associated with use

Dose: by inhalation of powder, when starting treatment,
during periods of severe asthma, and while reducing or
discontinuing oral corticosteroids, 0.2–1.6 mg daily in
divided doses; in less severe cases 200–800 micrograms
daily; CHILD 200–800 micrograms daily in divided
doses (800 micrograms daily in severe asthma)

PoM Pulmicort Respules® (Astra)

Repsules® (= single-dose units for nebulisation),
budesonide 250 micrograms/mL, net price 20 × 2-
mL unit = £32.00; 500 micrograms/mL, 20 × 2
mL unit = £44.64. May be diluted up to 50% with
sterile physiological saline. Label: 8, counselling,
dose, 10 steroid card

Dose: by inhalation of nebulised suspension, when starting treatment, during periods of severe asthma, and
while reducing or discontinuing oral corticosteroids, 1–
2 mg twice daily (may be increased further in very
severe asthma); CHILD 3 months–12 years, 0.5–1 mg
twice daily

Maintenance, usually half above doses

Inhaler devices
See section 3.1.5

FLUTICASONE PROPIONATE

Indications: prophylaxis of asthma in patients
requiring bronchodilators on a daily basis, or who
are dependent on systemic corticosteroids

Cautions; Side-effects: see under Beclomethasone
Dipropionate

Dose: see preparations below

▼ **PoM Flixotide®** (A&H)

Aerosol inhalation, fluticasone propionate
25 micrograms/metered inhalation, net price 120-
dose unit = £6.86; 50 micrograms/metered inhalation, 120-dose unit = £11.43; 125 micrograms/
metered inhalation, 120-dose unit = £22.86;
250 micrograms/metered inhalation, 120-dose
unit = £36.86. Label: 8, counselling, dose; 250-
microgram strength also label 10 steroid card

Additives: include CFC propellants

Note. Flixotide 125 micrograms and 250 micrograms
inhalers not indicated for children

Dose: by aerosol inhalation, ADULT and CHILD over 16
years, 100–250 micrograms twice daily, increased
according to severity of asthma to 1 mg twice daily;
CHILD 4–16 years, 50–100 micrograms twice daily
adjusted as necessary

Dry powder for inhalation, fluticasone propionate
50 micrograms/blister, net price 14 disks of 4 blisters with Diskhaler® = £8.23, 14-disk refill =
£7.66;
100 micrograms/blister, 14 disks of 4 blisters with
Diskhaler® = £12.80, 14-disk refill = £12.23;
250 micrograms/blister, 14 disks of 4 blisters with
Diskhaler® = £24.23, 14-disk refill = £23.66;
500 micrograms/blister, 14 disks of 4 blisters with
Diskhaler® = £40.23, 14-disk refill = £39.66.
Label: 8, counselling, dose; 250- and 500-micro-
gram strength also label 10 steroid card

Note. Flixotide 250 micrograms and 500 micrograms are
not indicated for children

Dose: by inhalation of powder, ADULT and CHILD over
16 years, 100–250 micrograms twice daily, increased
according to severity of asthma to 1 mg twice daily;
CHILD 4–16 years, 50–100 micrograms twice daily
adjusted as necessary

3.3 Cromoglycate and related therapy

Regular inhalation of sodium cromoglycate can
reduce the incidence of attacks of asthma and allow
dosage reduction of bronchodilators and oral corticosteroids. In general, prophylaxis with sodium
cromoglycate is less effective in adults than
prophylaxis with corticosteroid inhalations (see
Chronic asthma table) but the fact that in the long
term corticosteroid inhalations may be associated
with more side-effects needs to be borne in mind.
Sodium cromoglycate is of no value in the treatment of acute attacks of asthma.

Sodium cromoglycate is of value in the prevention of exercise-induced asthma, a single dose
being inhaled half-an-hour beforehand.

The mode of action of sodium cromoglycate is
not completely understood. It is of particular value
in asthma with an allergic basis, but, in practice, it
is difficult to predict who will benefit, therefore it is
reasonable to try it for a period of 4 to 6 weeks in
any patient whose asthma is poorly controlled with
bronchodilators. Children seem to respond better
than adults. Dose frequency is adjusted according
to response but is usually 3 to 4 times a day initially; this may subsequently be reduced.

If inhalation of the dry powder form of sodium
cromoglycate causes bronchospasm a selective

beta$_2$-adrenoceptor stimulant such as salbutamol or terbutaline should be inhaled a few minutes beforehand. The nebuliser solution is useful for patients who cannot manage the dry powder inhaler or the aerosol.

Nedocromil has a pharmacological action similar to that of sodium cromoglycate.

SODIUM CROMOGLYCATE

(Sodium Cromoglicate)

Indications: prophylaxis of asthma

Side-effects: coughing, transient bronchospasm, and throat irritation due to inhalation of powder (see also notes above)

Dose: see preparations below

COUNSELLING. Regular use is necessary

PoM Intal® (Fisons)

Aerosol inhalation, sodium cromoglycate 5 mg/metered inhalation. Net price 112-puff unit = £16.19; 2 × 112-puff unit with spacer device (Syncroner®) = £32.38; also available with large volume spacer inhaler (Fisonair®), complete unit = £18.88. Label: 8

Additives: include CFC propellants

Dose: by aerosol inhalation, adults and children, 10 mg (2 puffs) 4 times daily initially, increased in severe cases or during periods of risk to 6–8 times daily; additional doses may also be taken before exercise; maintenance 5 mg (1 puff) 4 times daily

Note. Sodium cromoglycate 5 mg/metered inhalation also available from Baker Norton (Cromogen®, contains CFC propellants)

Spincaps®, yellow/clear, sodium cromoglycate 20 mg. Net price 112-cap pack = £12.92. Label: 8

Dose: by inhalation of powder, adults and children, 20 mg 4 times daily, increased in severe cases to 8 times daily

Spinhaler insufflator® (for use with Intal and Intal Compound Spincaps). Net price = £1.89

Nebuliser solution, sodium cromoglycate 10 mg/mL. Net price 2-mL amp = 28p. For use with power-operated nebuliser

Dose: by inhalation of nebulised solution, adults and children, 20 mg 4 times daily, increased in severe cases to 6 times daily

Note. Sodium cromoglycate 10 mg/mL also available for nebulisation in 2-mL unit doses as Steri-Neb Cromogen® (Baker Norton)

Compound preparations

Note. The compound inhalation of sodium cromoglycate with a beta-adrenoceptor stimulant is not recommended as the inhalation is liable to be used inappropriately for relief of bronchospasm rather than for its prophylactic effect

PoM Aerocrom® (Fisons)

Aerosol inhalation, sodium cromoglycate 1 mg, salbutamol (as sulphate) 100 micrograms/metered inhalation, net price 200-inhalation unit = £15.60; 200-puff unit with spacer device (Syncroner®) = £15.60. Label: 8

Additives: include CFC propellants

Dose: by aerosol inhalation, 2 inhalations 4 times daily; CHILD, not recommended

PoM Intal Compound® (Fisons)

Spincaps®, orange/clear, isoprenaline sulphate 100 micrograms, sodium cromoglycate 20 mg. Net price 112-cap pack = £10.22. Label: 8

NEDOCROMIL SODIUM

Indications: prophylaxis of asthma

Side-effects: see under Sodium Cromoglycate; also headache, nausea, vomiting, dyspepsia, abdominal pain (mild and transient); bitter taste (masked by mint flavour)

Dose: by aerosol inhalation, 4 mg (2 puffs) 4 times daily, when control achieved may be possible to reduce to twice daily; CHILD under 12 years, not recommended

COUNSELLING. Regular use is necessary

PoM Tilade® (Fisons)

Aerosol inhalation, nedocromil sodium 2 mg/metered inhalation. Net price 2 × 56-puff mint-flavoured units = £19.48; 2 × 112-puff unit with spacer device (Syncroner®) = £38.98. Label: 8

Additives: include CFC propellants

RELATED THERAPY

Antihistamines are of no value whatsoever in the treatment of bronchial asthma. **Ketotifen** is an antihistamine with an action said to resemble that of sodium cromoglycate, but it too has proved disappointing.

KETOTIFEN

Indications: see notes above

Cautions: previous anti-asthmatic treatment should be continued for a minimum of 2 weeks after initiation of ketotifen treatment; **interactions:** Appendix 1 (antihistamines)—also, avoid with oral antidiabetics (fall in thrombocyte count reported)

DRIVING. Drowsiness may affect performance of skilled tasks (e.g. driving); effects of alcohol enhanced

Side-effects: drowsiness, dry mouth, slight dizziness; CNS stimulation, weight gain also reported

Dose: 1 mg twice daily with food increased if necessary to 2 mg twice daily; initial treatment in readily sedated patients 0.5–1 mg at night; CHILD over 2 years 1 mg twice daily

PoM Zaditen® (Sandoz)

Capsules, ketotifen 1 mg (as hydrogen fumarate). Net price 60-cap pack = £8.14. Label: 2, 8, 21

Tablets, scored, ketotifen 1 mg (as hydrogen fumarate). Net price 60-tab pack = £8.14. Label: 2, 8, 21

Elixir, sugar-free, ketotifen 1 mg (as hydrogen fumarate)/5 mL. Net price 150 mL = £4.82. Label: 2, 8, 21

3.4   Antihistamines, hyposensitisation, and allergic emergencies

3.4.1   Antihistamines
3.4.2   Hyposensitisation
3.4.3   Allergic emergencies

3.4.1   Antihistamines

All antihistamines are of potential value in the treatment of *nasal allergies*, particularly seasonal (hay fever), and may be of some value in *vasomotor rhinitis*. They reduce rhinorrhoea and sneezing but are usually less effective for nasal congestion.

Oral antihistamines are also of some value in preventing *urticaria* and are used to treat *urticarial rashes, pruritus,* and *insect bites and stings*; they are also used in *drug allergies*. Injections of chlorpheniramine or promethazine are used as an adjunct to adrenaline in the emergency treatment of *angioedema* and *anaphylaxis* (section 3.4.3). For the use of antihistamines in *nausea and vomiting*, see section 4.6.

There is no evidence that any one of the older, sedative antihistamines is superior to any other and patients vary widely in their responses. They differ somewhat in duration of action and incidence of side-effects (drowsiness and antimuscarinic effects). Most are relatively short-acting but some, (e.g. promethazine) act for up to 12 hours. They all cause sedation but **promethazine, trimeprazine,** and **dimenhydrinate** may be more sedating whereas **chlorpheniramine, cyclizine,** and **mequitazine** may be less so.

Acrivastine, astemizole, cetirizine, loratadine, and **terfenadine** are newer antihistamines; they are a very major advance over the older antihistamines. They cause less sedation and psychomotor impairment because they only penetrate the blood brain barrier to a slight extent (and for this reason do not alleviate pruritus of non-allergic origin). Astemizole has a relatively slow onset of action and is more appropriate for use on a regular basis than when symptoms occur.

DISADVANTAGES OF ANTIHISTAMINES. With most of the older antihistamines drowsiness is a disadvantage; patients should be warned that their ability to drive or operate machinery may be impaired, and that the effects of alcohol may be increased. Other side-effects include headache, psychomotor impairment, antimuscarinic effects such as urinary retention, dry mouth, blurred vision, and gastrointestinal disturbances; occasional rashes and photosensitivity reactions have been reported; paradoxical stimulation may rarely occur, especially in high dosage or in children.

Other side-effects reported include palpitations and arrhythmias (see especially *astemizole* and *terfenadine*, p.130), hypersensitivity reactions (including bronchospasm, angioedema, and anaphylaxis), convulsions, sweating, myalgia, paraesthesia, blood disorders, extrapyramidal effects, tremor, liver dysfunction, sleep disturbances, depression, and hypotension.

Antihistamines should be used with caution in epilepsy, prostatic hypertrophy, glaucoma, and hepatic disease. Most antihistamines should be avoided in **porphyria,** but chlorpheniramine and cyclizine have been used (see section 9.8.2). **Interactions:** Appendix 1 (antihistamines; **important:** special problems with *astemizole* and *terfenadine*). **Pregnancy** and **breast-feeding:** Appendixes 4 and 5 (antihistamines).

NON-SEDATIVE ANTIHISTAMINES

DRIVING. Although drowsiness is rare, nevertheless patients should be advised that it can occur and may affect performance of skilled tasks (e.g. driving); excess alcohol should be avoided.

ACRIVASTINE

Indications: symptomatic relief of allergy such as hay fever, urticaria

Cautions: see notes above; pending specific studies avoid in renal impairment

Side-effects: see notes above; incidence of sedation and antimuscarinic effects low

Dose: 8 mg 3 times daily; CHILD under 12 years, not recommended

PoM **Semprex**® (Wellcome)

Capsules, acrivastine 8 mg. Net price 84-cap pack = £5.92. Counselling, driving

---

ASTEMIZOLE

Indications: symptomatic relief of allergy such as hay fever, urticaria

Cautions: see Terfenadine (Arrhythmias) and notes above

PREGNANCY. Manufacturer advises avoid in pregnancy (toxicity at high doses in *animals*) and advises that women of childbearing potential should use contraception while taking astemizole and (owing to long half-life) for several weeks after stopping

Side-effects: see notes above; weight gain occurs infrequently; incidence of sedation and antimuscarinic effects low; **important:** ventricular arrhythmias (torsades de pointes) have followed excessive dosage, for recommendations see under Terfenadine (Arrhythmias)

Dose: 10 mg daily (must **not** be exceeded); CHILD 6–12 years, 5 mg daily (must **not** be exceeded)

PoM¹**Hismanal**® (Janssen)

Tablets, scored, astemizole 10 mg. Net price 30-tab pack = £5.70. Counselling, driving

Suspension, sugar-free, astemizole 5 mg /5 mL. Net price 200 mL = £5.80. Counselling, driving

1. Can be sold to the public for the treatment of hay fever in adults and children over 12 years; another brand on sale to the public is Pollon-eze®

CETIRIZINE

Indications: symptomatic relief of allergy such as hay fever, urticaria

Cautions: see notes above; halve dose in renal impairment; incidence of sedation and antimuscarinic effects low

Side-effects: see notes above

Dose: 10 mg daily *or* 5 mg twice daily; CHILD under 6 years, not recommended

PoM ¹Zirtek® (UCB Pharma)

Tablets, f/c, scored, cetirizine hydrochloride 10 mg. Net price 30-tab pack = £8.73. Counselling, driving

Oral solution, cetirizine hydrochloride 1 mg/mL. Net price 200 mL = £14.95. Counselling, driving

1. Can be sold to the public for adults and children over 12 years provided packs do not contain more than 10 days' supply

LORATADINE

Indications: symptomatic relief of allergy such as hay fever; urticaria

Cautions; Side-effects: see notes above; incidence of sedation and antimuscarinic effects low; pregnancy (toxicity at high doses in *animals*)

Dose: 10 mg daily; CHILD 2–12 years, under 30 kg 5 mg daily, over 30 kg 10 mg daily

PoM ¹Clarityn® (Schering-Plough)

Tablets, scored, loratadine 10 mg. Net price 30-tab pack = £7.57. Counselling, driving

Syrup, yellow, loratadine 5 mg/5 mL. Net price 100 mL = £7.57. Counselling, driving

1. Can be sold to the public for adults and children over 12 years provided packs do not contain more than 10 days' supply

TERFENADINE

Indications: symptomatic relief of allergy such as hay fever, urticaria

Cautions: see notes above

ARRHYTHMIAS. Rare hazardous arrhythmias are associated with astemizole and terfenadine particularly in association with increased blood concentrations. Recommendations are: *not to exceed* recommended dose, *to avoid* in significant hepatic impairment, and *to avoid* concomitant administration of drugs that inhibit metabolism (in particular, *ketoconazole, itraconazole and other imidazole antifungals and erythromycin and other macrolides*), *to avoid* if hypokalaemia or prolonged QT interval known or suspected and *to avoid* concomitant administration of potentially antiarrhythmogenic drugs such as *anti-arrhythmics, antipsychotics, tricyclic antidepressants* and drugs liable to produce electrolyte imbalance such as *diuretics*; *if syncope occurs* the antihistamine should be discontinued and patient evaluated for potential arrhythmias

Side-effects: see notes above; incidence of sedation and antimuscarinic effects low; hair loss reported; **important:** ventricular arrhythmias

(torsades de pointes) have followed excessive dosage, see also Arrhythmias above

Dose: 60 mg twice daily *or* 120 mg in the morning; CHILD 3–6 years 15 mg twice daily; 6–12 years 30 mg twice daily

PoM ¹Triludan® (Merrell)

Tablets, scored, terfenadine 60 mg. Net price 60-tab pack = £5.66. Counselling, driving

Forte tablets, terfenadine 120 mg. Net price 7-tab pack = £2.12; 30-tab pack = £5.66. Counselling, driving

Suspension, sugar-free, terfenadine 30 mg/5 mL. Net price 200 mL = £4.13. Counselling, driving

1. Can be sold to the public for adults and children over 6 years provided packs do not contain more than 10 days' supply; other brands on sale to the public include Aller-Eze Clear® (terfenadine 60 mg), Boots Antihistamine Tablets® (terfenadine 60 mg), Boots One-a-Day Antihistamine Tablets® (terfenadine 120 mg), Histafen® (terfenadine 60 mg), Seldane® (terfenadine 120 mg), Terfex® (terfenadine 60 mg); terfenadine 60-mg tablets also available from APS, Cox, Hillcross, and Norton

SEDATIVE ANTIHISTAMINES

DRIVING. Drowsiness may affect performance of skilled tasks (e.g. driving); effects of alcohol enhanced.

AZATADINE MALEATE

Indications: symptomatic relief of allergy such as hay fever, urticaria

Cautions; Side-effects: see notes above

Dose: 1 mg, increased if necessary to 2 mg, twice daily; CHILD under 1 year not recommended, 1–6 years 250 micrograms twice daily, 6–12 years 0.5–1 mg twice daily

Optimine® (Schering-Plough)

Tablets, scored, azatadine maleate 1 mg. Net price 56-tab pack = £4.37. Label: 2

Syrup, azatadine maleate 500 micrograms/5 mL. Net price 120 mL = £1.39. Label: 2

BROMPHENIRAMINE MALEATE

Indications: symptomatic relief of allergy such as hay fever, urticaria

Cautions; Side-effects: see notes above

Dose: 4–8 mg 3–4 times daily; CHILD up to 3 years 0.4–1 mg/kg daily in 4 divided doses, 3–6 years 2 mg 3–4 times daily, 6–12 years 2–4 mg 3–4 times daily

Dimotane® (Wyeth)

Tablets, peach, scored, brompheniramine maleate 4 mg. Net price 20 = 59p. Label: 2

Elixir, yellow-green, brompheniramine maleate 2 mg/5 mL. Net price 100 mL = 71p. Label: 2

Dimotane LA® (Wyeth)

Tablets, m/r, peach, s/c, brompheniramine maleate 12 mg. Net price 20 = 89p. Label: 2, 25

Dose: 12–24 mg twice daily; CHILD 6–12 years 12 mg at bedtime, increased if necessary to 12 mg twice daily

For a list of **cough and decongestant preparations on sale to the public**, including those containing brompheniramine, see section 3.9.2.

For compound preparations containing brompheniramine and pseudoephedrine, see also section 3.10

BUCLIZINE

Ingredient of Migraleve® (see Analgesics with Antiemetics, section 4.7.4.1)

CHLORPHENIRAMINE MALEATE

(Chlorphenamine Maleate)

Indications: symptomatic relief of allergy such as hay fever, urticaria; emergency treatment of anaphylactic reactions (section 3.4.3)

Cautions; Side-effects: see notes above. Injections may be irritant and cause transitory hypotension or CNS stimulation

Dose: by mouth, 4 mg every 4–6 hours, max. 24 mg daily; CHILD under 1 year not recommended, 1–2 years 1 mg twice daily, 2–5 years 1 mg every 4–6 hours, max. 6 mg daily, 6–12 years 2 mg every 4–6 hours, max. 12 mg daily

By subcutaneous or intramuscular injection, 10–20 mg, repeated if required; max. 40 mg in 24 hours

By slow intravenous injection over 1 minute, 10–20 mg diluted in syringe with 5–10 mL blood—or with sterile sodium chloride 0.9% or water for injection [both unlicensed diluents]

Piriton® (A&H)

Tablets, ivory, chlorpheniramine maleate 4 mg. Net price 20 = 6p. Label: 2

Syrup, chlorpheniramine maleate 2 mg/5 mL. Net price 150 mL = 85p. Label: 2

PoM *Injection*, chlorpheniramine maleate 10 mg/mL. Net price 1-mL amp = 12p

Note. In addition to Piriton®, proprietary brands of chlorpheniramine maleate tablets on sale to the public include Calimal®; chlorpheniramine maleate 4 mg tablets are also available from Cox and Hillcross

For a list of **cough and decongestant preparations on sale to the public**, including those containing chlorpheniramine, see section 3.9.2

CINNARIZINE

See section 4.6

CLEMASTINE

Indications: symptomatic relief of allergy such as hay fever, urticaria

Cautions; Side-effects: see notes above

Dose: 1 mg twice daily; CHILD under 1 year not recommended, 1–3 years 250–500 micrograms twice daily; 3–6 years 500 micrograms twice daily; 6–12 years 0.5–1 mg twice daily

Tavegil® (Sandoz)

Tablets, scored, clemastine 1 mg (as hydrogen fumarate). Net price 50-tab pack = £2.05. Label: 2

Elixir, sugar-free, clemastine 500 micrograms (as hydrogen fumarate)/5 mL. Net price 150 mL = 96p. Label: 2

Note. In addition to Tavegil®, proprietary brands of clemastine hydrogen fumarate on sale to the public include Aller-Eze®; it is also on sale to the public combined with phenylpropanolamine (Aller-eze Plus®)

CYCLIZINE

See section 4.6

CYPROHEPTADINE HYDROCHLORIDE

Indications: symptomatic relief of allergy such as hay fever, urticaria

Cautions; Side-effects: see notes above; may cause weight gain

Dose: allergy, usual dose 4 mg 3–4 times daily; usual range 4–20 mg daily, max. 32 mg daily; CHILD under 2 years not recommended, 2–6 years 2 mg 2–3 times daily, max. 12 mg daily; 7–14 years 4 mg 2–3 times daily, max. 16 mg daily

Migraine, 4 mg with a further 4 mg after 30 minutes if necessary; maintenance, 4 mg every 4–6 hours

Periactin® (MSD)

Tablets, scored, cyproheptadine hydrochloride 4 mg. Net price 20 = 57p. Label: 2

Syrup, yellow, cyproheptadine hydrochloride 2 mg/5 mL. Net price 200 mL = £1.27. Label: 2

DIMENHYDRINATE

See section 4.6

DIPHENHYDRAMINE HYDROCHLORIDE

Indications: see under Preparations

Cautions; Side-effects: see notes above

Preparations

Proprietary brands of diphenhydramine hydrochloride on sale to the public to aid relief of temporary sleep disturbance in adults include Medinex® (diphenhydramine hydrochloride 10 mg/5 mL and Nytol® (diphenhydramine hydrochloride tablets 25 mg)

For a list of **cough and decongestant preparations on sale to the public**, including those containing diphenhydramine, see section 3.9.2

DIPHENYLPYRALINE HYDROCHLORIDE

Indications: symptomatic relief of allergy such as hay fever, urticaria

Cautions; Side-effects: see notes above

Preparations

For a list of **cough and decongestant preparations on sale to the public**, including those containing diphenylpyraline, see section 3.9.2

DOXYLAMINE

Ingredient of cough and decongestant preparations (section 3.9.2.) and of compound analgesics (section 4.7.1.) on sale to the public

HYDROXYZINE HYDROCHLORIDE

Indications: pruritus, anxiety (short-term)
Cautions; Side-effects: see notes above
Dose: pruritus, initially 25 mg at night increased if necessary to 25 mg 3–4 times daily; CHILD 6 months–6 years initially 5–15 mg daily increased if necessary to 50 mg daily in divided doses; over 6 years initially 15–25 mg daily increased if necessary to 50–100 mg daily in divided doses
Anxiety (adults only), 50–100 mg 4 times daily

PoM **Atarax®** (Pfizer)
Tablets, both s/c, hydroxyzine hydrochloride 10 mg (orange), net price 84-tab pack = £1.52; 25 mg (green), 28-tab pack = £1.02. Label: 2
Syrup, hydroxyzine hydrochloride 10 mg/5 mL. Net price 150-mL pack = 85p. Label: 2
PoM **Ucerax®** (UCB Pharma)
Tablets, f/c, scored, hydroxyzine hydrochloride 25 mg, net price 25-tab pack = £1.73. Label: 2
Syrup, hydroxyzine hydrochloride 10 mg/5 mL. Net price 200-mL pack = £1.91. Label: 2

KETOTOFEN

See section 3.3

MEQUITAZINE

Indications: symptomatic relief of allergy such as hay fever, urticaria
Cautions; Side-effects: see notes above
Dose: 5 mg twice daily; CHILD under 12 years, not recommended

PoM **Primalan®** (Rhône-Poulenc Rorer)
Tablets, mequitazine 5 mg. Net price 56-tab pack = £4.88. Label: 2

OXATOMIDE

Indications: symptomatic relief of allergy such as hay fever, food allergy, urticaria
Cautions; Side-effects: see notes above; drowsiness most common; increased appetite with weight gain may occur above 120 mg daily
Dose: 30 mg twice daily after food, increased if necessary to 60 mg twice daily; ELDERLY 30 mg twice daily; CHILD 5–14 years 15–30 mg twice daily
PoM **Tinset®** (Janssen)
Tablets, scored, oxatomide 30 mg. Net price 25-tab pack = £4.90. Label: 2, 21

PHENINDAMINE TARTRATE

Indications: symptomatic relief of allergy such as hay fever, urticaria
Cautions; Side-effects: see notes above; may cause mild CNS stimulation
Dose: 25–50 mg 1–3 times daily; CHILD over 10 years 25 mg 1–3 times daily

Thephorin® (Sinclair)
Tablets, s/c, phenindamine tartrate 25 mg. Net price 50-tab pack = £2.85. Label: 2

PHENIRAMINE MALEATE

Indications: symptomatic relief of allergy such as hay fever, urticaria
Cautions; Side-effects: see notes above

Daneral SA® (Hoechst)
Tablets, m/r, pink, s/c, pheniramine maleate 75 mg. Net price 30-tab pack = £2.54. Label: 2, 25
Dose: 75–150 mg at night or 75 mg night and morning
For a list of **cough and decongestant preparations on sale to the public**, including those containing pheniramine, see section 3.9.2

PROMETHAZINE HYDROCHLORIDE

Indications: symptomatic relief of allergy such as hay fever, urticaria, emergency treatment of anaphylactic reactions (section 3.4.3)
For use in premedication see section 15.1.4.1; sedation see section 4.1.1
Cautions; Side-effects: see notes above; intramuscular injection may be painful
Dose: by mouth, 25 mg at night increased to 50 mg if necessary *or* 10–20 mg 2–3 times daily; CHILD 1–5 years 5–15 mg daily (1–2 years on doctor's advice only), 5–10 years 10–25 mg daily
By deep intramuscular injection, 25–50 mg; max. 100 mg; CHILD 5–10 years 6.25–12.5 mg
By slow intravenous injection in emergencies, 25–50 mg, max. 100 mg, as a solution containing 2.5 mg/mL in water for injections

Phenergan® (Rhône-Poulenc Rorer)
Tablets, both blue, f/c, promethazine hydrochloride 10 mg, net price 56-tab pack = £1.00; 25 mg, 56-tab pack = £1.49. Label: 2
Elixir, golden, promethazine hydrochloride 5 mg/ 5 mL. Net price 100 mL = £1.12. Label: 2
PoM *Injection*, promethazine hydrochloride 25 mg/ mL. Net price 1-mL amp = 27p; 2-mL amp = 33p
Note. In addition to Phenergan®, proprietary brands of promethazine hydrochloride on sale to the public include Sominex® (promethazine hydrochloride tablets 20 mg, for occasional insomnia in adults) and Q-Mazine® (promethazine hydrochloride 5 mg/5 mL for urticaria and other skin conditions in children)
For a list of **cough and decongestant preparations on sale to the public**, including those containing promethazine, see section 3.9.2

PROMETHAZINE THEOCLATE

See section 4.6

TRIMEPRAZINE TARTRATE

(Alimemazine Tartrate)

Indications: urticaria and pruritus; premedication, see section 15.1.4.1

Cautions; Side-effects: see notes above; see also under Chlorpromazine Hydrochloride, section 4.2.1

Dose: 10 mg 2–3 times daily, in severe cases up to max. 100 mg daily has been used; ELDERLY 10 mg 1–2 times daily; CHILD over 2 years 2.5–5 mg 3–4 times daily

PoM **Vallergan®** (Rhône-Poulenc Rorer)
Tablets, blue, f/c, trimeprazine tartrate 10 mg. Net price 28-tab pack = £1.03. Label: 2
Syrup, straw coloured, trimeprazine tartrate 7.5 mg/5 mL. Net price 100 mL = £1.17. Label: 2
Syrup forte, trimeprazine tartrate 30 mg/5 mL. Net price 100 mL = £2.42. Label: 2
Note. For use of Forte Syrup see section 15.1.4.1

TRIPROLIDINE HYDROCHLORIDE

Indications: symptomatic relief of allergy such as hay fever, urticaria

Cautions; Side-effects: see notes above

Dose: see preparation

Pro-Actidil® (Wellcome)
Tablets, m/r, white/pink/blue, triprolidine hydrochloride 10 mg. Net price 20 = £5.48. Label: 2, 25
Dose: 10 mg early evening or 5–6 hours before retiring increased to 20 mg daily if symptoms very severe; CHILD under 12 years not recommended

For a list of **cough and decongestant preparations on sale to the public,** including those containing triprolidine, see section 3.9.2

3.4.2 Hyposensitisation

Except for wasp and bee sting allergy the value of specific hyposensitisation is uncertain; administration of allergen extract desensitising vaccines is associated with a significant risk of anaphylaxis, see CSM advice below. Most atopic (allergic) patients are sensitive to a wide range of allergens hence hyposensitisation with an extract of a single allergen is usually no more than partially successful.

Diagnostic skin tests are unreliable and can only be used in conjunction with a detailed history of allergen exposure.

CSM advice. After re-examination of the efficacy and safety of desensitising vaccines, the CSM has concluded that they should only be used for the following indications:
—Seasonal allergic hay fever (which has not responded to anti-allergy drugs) caused by pollens, using licensed products only—patients with *asthma* should not be treated with desensitising vaccines as they are more likely to develop severe adverse reactions.
—Hypersensitivity to wasp and bee venoms—since reactions can be life-threatening, *asthma* is not an absolute contra-indication. There is inadequate evi-

dence of benefit from other allergens such as house dust, house dust mite, animal danders and foods and they are *not* recommended. Desensitising vaccines should be avoided in pregnant women, in children under five years old, and in those taking beta-blockers.

Recent experience indicates that bronchospasm usually develops within 1 hour and anaphylaxis within 30 minutes of injection. Therefore patients need only be monitored for 1 hour after injection. However, if symptoms or signs of hypersensitivity **develop** (e.g. rash, urticaria, bronchospasm, faintness), **even when mild,** the patient should be observed until these have **completely resolved.**

For details of the management of anaphylactic shock, see section 3.4.3.

ALLERGEN EXTRACT VACCINES

Each set usually contains vials for the administration of graded amounts to patients undergoing hyposensitisation. Maintenance sets containing vials at the highest strength are also available. Manufacturer's literature must be consulted for details of allergens, vial strengths, and administration

Indications: hypersensitivity to one or more common allergens (see notes above)

Cautions: see notes above including CSM advice; manufacturers recommend that patients should be warned not to eat a heavy meal before the injection

CSM advice. The CSM has advised that facilities for cardiopulmonary resuscitation must be immediately available and patients monitored closely for one hour after each injection, for full details see above.

Contra-indications: pregnancy, febrile conditions, acute asthma

Side-effects: allergic reactions, especially in small children

Dose: by subcutaneous injection, see manufacturer's literature

Wasp and bee venom allergy preparations
PoM **Pharmalgen®** (Allerayde)
Bee venom extract (*Apis mellifera*) or wasp venom extract (*Vespula* spp.). Net price initial treatment set = £56.90 (bee), £69.75 (wasp)

3.4.3 Allergic emergencies

Adrenaline provides physiological reversal of the immediate symptoms (such as laryngeal oedema, bronchospasm, and hypotension) associated with hypersensitivity reactions such as *anaphylaxis* and *angioedema.* See below for full details of *adrenaline administration* and for *adjunctive treatment.*

ANAPHYLAXIS

Anaphylactic shock requires prompt energetic treatment of *laryngeal oedema, bronchospasm,* and *hypotension.* Atopic individuals are particularly susceptible. *Insect bites* are a recognised risk (in particular *wasp* and *bee stings*). Certain foods, including *eggs, fish, cow's milk protein,* and *nuts* (particularly *peanuts*) may also precipitate anaphylaxis. Drugs particularly associated with anaphylaxis include *blood products, vaccines, hyposensitising (allergen) preparations, antibiotics, aspirin and other NSAIDs, iron injections, heparin,* and *neuromuscular blocking drugs.* In the case of drugs, anaphylaxis is more likely after parenteral administration; resuscitation facilities must always be available for injections associated with special risk. Anaphylactic reactions may also be associated with *additives and excipients* in foods and medicines; some oils (such as arachis oil) may be contaminated with allergenic proteins from their original source—it is wise to check the full formula of preparations which may contain *allergenic fats or oils* (including those for topical application, particularly if they are intended for use in the mouth or for application to the nasal mucosa).

First-line treatment includes securing the airway, restoration of blood pressure (laying the patient flat, raising the feet), and administration of **adrenaline** injection. This is given **intramuscularly** in a dose of 0.5–1 mg (0.5–1 mL adrenaline injection 1 in 1000), repeated every 10 minutes, according to blood pressure and pulse, until improvement occurs. **Oxygen** administration is also of primary importance. An antihistamine (e.g. **chlorpheniramine**, given by slow intravenous injection in a dose of 10–20 mg, see p. 131) is a useful adjunctive treatment, given after adrenaline injection and continued for 24 to 48 hours to prevent relapse. In patients on non-cardioselective beta-blockers severe anaphylaxis may not respond to adrenaline injection, calling for addition of **salbutamol** by intravenous injection.

Continuing deterioration requires further treatment including intravenous fluids (p. 356), intravenous aminophylline (p. 121) or a nebulised beta$_2$-adrenoceptor stimulant (such as salbutamol or terbutaline, see p. 115 and p. 116); in addition to oxygen, assisted respiration and possibly emergency tracheotomy may be necessary.

An intravenous corticosteroid e.g. **hydrocortisone** (as sodium succinate) in a dose of 100–300 mg is of secondary value in the initial management of anaphylactic shock as the onset of action is delayed for several hours, but should be given *to prevent further deterioration* in severely affected patients.

When a patient is so ill that there is *doubt as to the adequacy of the circulation*, the initial injection of adrenaline may need to be given as a *dilute solution by the intravenous route*, for details of *cautions, dose* and *strength*, see under Intravenous Adrenaline, below.

Some patients with severe allergy to insect stings or foods are encouraged to carry pre-filled adrenaline syringes for *self-administration* during periods of risk; adrenaline inhalations (Medihaler-epi®) are much less effective, but may be useful for the individual without other symptoms who is beginning to develop angioedema and laryngeal oedema (**important:** for patients with previous very serious reactions *adrenaline injection is always the first line of treatment*).

ANGIOEDEMA

Angioedema is dangerous if *laryngeal oedema* is present. In this circumstance adrenaline injection and oxygen should be given as described under Anaphylaxis (see above); antihistamines and corticosteroids should also be given (see again above). Tracheal intubation and other measures may be necessary.

The administration of C$_1$ esterase inhibitor (in fresh frozen plasma or in partially purified form) may terminate acute attacks of *hereditary angioedema*, but is not practical for long-term prophylaxis.

INTRAMUSCULAR (OR SUBCUTANEOUS) ADRENALINE

The *intramuscular route* is the *first choice route* for the administration of adrenaline in the management of anaphylactic shock. Adrenaline has a rapid onset of action after intramuscular administration and in the shocked patient its absorption from the intramuscular site may be faster and more reliable than from the subcutaneous site (the intravenous route should be reserved for extreme emergency when there is doubt as to the adequacy of the circulation, for details of *cautions, dose* and *strength* see under Intravenous Adrenaline, below).

Patients should ideally be instructed in the self-administration of adrenaline by intramuscular injection, but may find it easier to cope with a pre-assembled syringe fitted with a needle suitable for administration by the subcutaneous route (see under Self-administration of Adrenaline, below).

The *main aim* when injecting adrenaline for anaphylactic shock is *speed* and the recommendations in the following table avoid the need for complex dosage calculations in children.

Volume of adrenaline injection **1 in 1000** (1 mg/mL) for **intramuscular** injection (or alternatively **subcutaneous** injection) in anaphylactic shock	
Age	Volume of adrenaline 1 in 1000
Under 1 year	0.05 mL
1 year	0.1 mL
2 years	0.2 mL[1]
3–4 years	0.3 mL[1]
5 years	0.4 mL[1]
6–12 years	0.5 mL[1]
Adult	0.5–1 mL

These doses may be repeated every 10 minutes, according to blood pressure and pulse, until improvement occurs (may be repeated several times).
1. Suitable for robust children in these age groups; for underweight children use half these doses.

INTRAVENOUS ADRENALINE (DILUTE, EXTREME CAUTION)

Where the patient is severely ill and there is real doubt about adequacy of the circulation and absorption from the intramuscular injection site, adrenaline may be given by **slow** *intravenous injection* in a dose of 500 micrograms (5 mL of the dilute 1 in 10 000 adrenaline injection) given at a rate of 100 micrograms (1 mL of the dilute 1 in 10 000 adrenaline injection) per minute, *stopping when a response has been obtained*; children can be given a dose of 10 micrograms/kg (0.1 mL of the dilute 1 in 10 000 adrenaline injection per kg) by **slow** *intra* *venous injection* over several minutes. *Constant vigilance* is needed to ensure that the *correct strength* is used; anaphylactic shock kits need to make a *very clear distinction* between the 1 in 10 000 strength and the 1 in 1000 strength. It is *also* important that, where intramuscular injection might still succeed, time should *not be wasted* seeking intravenous access.

For reference to the use of the intravenous route for *cardiac resuscitation*, see section 2.7.

INHALATION OF ADRENALINE

Adrenaline inhalation (Medihaler-epi®) is also available, but the ability to inhale during an attack may be limited. Nevertheless, it may be useful for the individual without other symptoms who is beginning to develop angioedema and laryngeal oedema (**important:** for those with previous very severe reactions *adrenaline injection* needs to remain the *first line of treatment*).

SELF-ADMINISTRATION OF ADRENALINE

Individuals who are at considerable risk of anaphylaxis need to carry adrenaline with them at all times and need to be *instructed in advance* how to inject it. In addition, the packs need to be labelled so that in the case of rapid collapse someone else is able to administer the adrenaline.

The following rules apply.

—full instruction *in advance* on injection technique;

—ensure *adequate supply* to cover time needed for ambulance to arrive.

Some patients are able to self-administer the adrenaline by the preferred *intramuscular route* (see above), but others may best be able to cope with a pre-assembled syringe fitted with a needle suitable for administration by the alternative *subcutaneous route* (if necessary by a bystander). There is no such preparation on the UK market, but one is available in the USA (Epipen®). Epipen® can be obtained in the UK on a named-patient basis from Allerayde; it consists of a fully assembled syringe and needle containing 1 mL of a solution of adrenaline 300 micrograms/mL (the strength reflecting the dose currently used in the USA); a 150-microgram strength is also available.

ADRENALINE
(Epinephrine)

Indications: emergency treatment of acute anaphylaxis; angioedema; cardiopulmonary resuscitation, section 2.7

Cautions: hyperthyroidism, diabetes mellitus, ischaemic heart disease, hypertension, elderly patients

INTERACTIONS. Severe anaphylaxis in patients on non-cardioselective beta-blockers may not respond to adrenaline injection calling for *intravenous injection of salbutamol* (see p.115). Patients on tricyclic antidepressants are considerably more susceptible to cardiac arrhythmias calling for a *much reduced* dose of

adrenaline. Other **interactions**, see Appendix 1 (sympathomimetics).

Side-effects: anxiety, tremor, tachycardia, arrhythmias, dry mouth, cold extremities

Dose: acute anaphylaxis, *by intramuscular (or subcutaneous) injection* see notes and table above
Acute anaphylaxis when there is doubt as to the adequacy of the circulation, *by intravenous injection* (dilute, extreme caution), see notes above
IMPORTANT. Intravenous route should be used with **extreme care**, see notes above

---

Intramuscular (or subcutaneous), see notes above
PoM **Adrenaline Injection, BP,** adrenaline 1 in 1000 (adrenaline 1 mg/mL as acid tartrate). Net price 0.5-mL amp = 32p; 1-mL amp = 33p
Available from Boots, Evans, Hillcross, Martindale
PoM **Min-I-Jet® Adrenaline** (IMS)
Injection, adrenaline 1 in 1000 (1 mg/mL as hydrochloride). Net price 1 mL (with 25 gauge × 0.25" needle for subcutaneous injection) = £7.37, 1 mL (with 21 gauge × 1.5" needle for intramuscular injection) = £3.91 (both disposable syringes)
PoM **Epipen®** —named-patient basis, see notes above

Intravenous (**extreme caution**, see notes above)
PoM **Adrenaline Injection,** adrenaline 1 in 10 000 (adrenaline 100 micrograms/mL as acid tartrate). 10-mL amp.
Available from Martindale and Penn (special order); also from IMS (Min-I-Jet® Adrenaline 3- and 10-mL disposable syringes)

Inhalation, see notes above
PoM **Medihaler-epi®** (3M)
Aerosol inhalation, adrenaline acid tartrate 280 micrograms/metered inhalation. Net price 400-inhalation unit = £2.43
Additives: include CFC propellants
Dose: by aerosol inhalation, adjunct to anaphylaxis treatment only, min. of 20 puffs; CHILD 10–15 puffs under adult supervision

3.5   Respiratory stimulants and pulmonary surfactants

3.5.1   Respiratory stimulants
3.5.2   Pulmonary surfactants

3.5.1   Respiratory stimulants

Respiratory stimulants (analeptic drugs) have a limited place in the treatment of ventilatory failure in patients with chronic obstructive airways disease. They are effective only when given by intravenous injection or infusion and have a short duration of action. Their use has largely been replaced by ventilatory support. However, occasionally when the latter is contra-indicated and in patients with hypercapnic respiratory failure who are becoming drowsy or comatose, respiratory stimulants in the short term may arouse patients sufficiently to co-operate and clear their secretions.

Respiratory stimulants may be harmful in respiratory failure since they stimulate non-respiratory as

---

well as respiratory muscles. They should only be given under **expert supervision** in hospital and must be combined with active physiotherapy. There is at present no oral respiratory stimulant available for long-term use in chronic respiratory failure.

Doxapram is given by continuous intravenous infusion in an initial dosage of 2 mg per minute. Frequent arterial blood gas studies and pH measurements are necessary during treatment to ensure the correct dosage.

Nikethamide (now discontinued by most suppliers) and ethamivan were formerly used as respiratory stimulants but are no longer recommended; the effective doses were close to those causing toxic effects, especially convulsions. Respiratory stimulants such as ethamivan and nikethamide have no place whatsoever in the management of asphyxia in the newborn.

DOXAPRAM HYDROCHLORIDE

Indications: ventilatory failure (see notes above)

Cautions: epilepsy, hepatic impairment; see also notes above; **interactions:** Appendix 1 (doxapram)

Contra-indications: severe hypertension, status asthmaticus, coronary artery disease, thyrotoxicosis

Side-effects: increase in blood pressure and heart rate, dizziness, perineal warmth

Dose: by intravenous infusion, 1.5–4 mg per minute according to patient's response

By intravenous injection over at least 30 seconds, 1–1.5 mg/kg repeated if necessary at intervals of 1 hour

Postoperative respiratory depression, see section 15.1.7

PoM **Dopram**® (Wyeth)
Injection, doxapram hydrochloride 20 mg/mL. Net price 5-mL amp = £2.14
Intravenous infusion, doxapram hydrochloride 2 mg/mL in glucose 5%. Net price 500-mL bottle = £22.34

ETHAMIVAN
(Etamivan)

Indications: not recommended, see notes above

Cautions: see notes above, severe hypertension

Contra-indications: epilepsy or respiratory failure due to neurological disease or drug overdose; status asthmaticus, coronary artery disease, thyrotoxicosis

Side-effects: nausea, restlessness, convulsions, dizziness, tremor, vasoconstriction, arrhythmias

Dose: by intravenous injection, 100 mg, but not recommended see notes above

PoM **Clairvan**® (Sinclair)
Injection, ethamivan 50 mg/mL (5%). Net price 2-mL amp = £3.81

3.5.2   Pulmonary surfactants

A number of pulmonary surfactants have recently been developed for the management of respiratory distress syndrome (hyaline membrane disease) in preterm infants.

BERACTANT

Indications: treatment of respiratory distress syndrome in preterm infants undergoing mechanical ventilation for respiratory distress syndrome, whose heart rate and arterial oxygenation are continuously monitored

Cautions: continuous monitoring required to avoid hyperoxaemia (due to rapid improvement in arterial oxygen concentration)

Side-effects: pulmonary haemorrhage reported

Dose: by endotracheal tube, phospholipid 100 mg/kg equivalent to a volume of 4 mL/kg, preferably within 8 hours of birth; may be repeated within 48 hours at intervals of at least 6 hours for up to 4 doses

▼ PoM **Survanta**® (Abbott)
Suspension, beractant (bovine lung extract) providing phospholipid 25 mg/mL, with lipids and proteins, Net price 8-mL vial = £306.43

COLFOSCERIL PALMITATE

Indications: as for Beractant (also prophylaxis of respiratory distress syndrome)

Cautions; Side-effects: as for Beractant; may increase incidence of pulmonary haemorrhage; obstruction of endotracheal tube by mucous secretions

Dose: by endotracheal tube, treatment, 67.5 mg/kg; if still intubated, may be repeated after 12 hours; prophylaxis, first dose soon after birth, if still intubated may be repeated 12 and 24 hours later

PoM **Exosurf Neonatal**® (Wellcome)
Suspension, colfosceril palmitate 108 mg for reconstitution with 8 mL water for injections (when reconstituted, contains 67.5 mg/5 mL). Net price per vial (with endotracheal tube connectors) = £306.43

PORACTANT ALFA

Indications: as for Beractant

Cautions; Side-effects: as for Beractant; also transient depression of cerebro-electrical activity; data sheet reports no evidence of increased risk of pulmonary haemorrhage

Dose: by endotracheal tube, 100–200 mg/kg as soon as possible after diagnosing respiratory distress syndrome; if still intubated, further doses of 100 mg/kg may be repeated after 12 and 24 hours if required; max. total dose 300–400 mg/kg

▼ PoM **Curosurf**® (Serono)
Suspension, poractant alfa (porcine lung phospholipid fraction) 80 mg/mL. Net price 1.5-mL vial = £400.00; 3-mL vial = £800.00

Abbreviations and symbols, see inside front cover

Prices are **net**, see p. 1

PUMACTANT

Indications: as for Beractant (also prophylaxis of respiratory distress syndrome)

Cautions; Side-effects: as for Beractant; obstruction of endotracheal tube

Dose: by endotracheal tube, 100 mg as soon as possible after intubation; if still intubated may be repeated after 1 hour and again at 24 hours after intubation

▼ PoM **Alec**® (Britannia)

Suspension, pumactant 100 mg (human lung phospholipid fraction) for reconstitution with 1.2 mL sterile sodium chloride 0.9%. Net price per vial (with syringe and catheter) = £150.00

3.6 Oxygen

Oxygen should be regarded as a drug. It is prescribed for hypoxaemic patients to increase alveolar oxygen tension and decrease the work of breathing necessary to maintain a given arterial oxygen tension. The concentration depends on the condition being treated; an inappropriate concentration may have serious or even lethal effects.

High concentration oxygen therapy, with concentrations of up to 60% for short periods, is safe in conditions such as pneumonia, pulmonary thromboembolism, and fibrosing alveolitis. In such conditions low arterial oxygen (P_aO_2) is usually associated with low or normal arterial carbon dioxide (P_aCO_2), therefore there is little risk of hypoventilation and carbon dioxide retention.

In severe acute asthma, the arterial carbon dioxide (P_aCO_2) is usually subnormal but as asthma deteriorates may rise steeply (particularly in children). These patients usually require high concentrations of oxygen and if the arterial carbon dioxide (P_aCO_2) remains high despite other treatment intermittent positive pressure ventilation needs to be considered urgently. Where facilities for blood gas measurements are not immediately available, for example while transferring the patient to hospital, 35% to 50% oxygen delivered through a conventional mask is recommended. Exceptionally, asthma is diagnosed in patients with a long history of chronic bronchitis and probable respiratory failure; in these patients a lower concentration (24% to 28%) may be needed to limit oxygen-induced reduction of respiratory drive.

Low concentration oxygen therapy (controlled oxygen therapy) is reserved for patients with ventilatory failure due to chronic obstructive airways disease or other causes. The concentration should not exceed 28% and in some patients a concentration above 24% may be excessive. The aim is to provide the patient with just enough oxygen to improve hypoxaemia without worsening pre-existing carbon dioxide retention and respiratory acidosis. Treatment should be initiated in hospital as repeated blood gas measurements are required to estimate the correct concentration.

DOMICILIARY OXYGEN. Oxygen should only be prescribed for patients in the home after careful evaluation in hospital by respiratory experts; it should never be prescribed on a placebo basis.

Patients should be **advised of the fire risks** when receiving oxygen therapy.

OXYGEN CYLINDERS

Oxygen is occasionally prescribed for intermittent use for episodes of hypoxaemia of short duration, for example asthma. It is important, however, that the patient does not rely on oxygen instead of obtaining medical help or taking more specific treatment.

Alternatively, intermittent oxygen may be prescribed for patients with advanced irreversible respiratory disorders to increase mobility and capacity for exercise and to ease discomfort, for example in chronic obstructive bronchitis, emphysema, widespread fibrosis, and primary or thromboembolic pulmonary hypertension. Appropriate patients may be prescribed portable equipment through the hospital service, refillable from cylinders in the home.

Under the NHS oxygen may be supplied by pharmacy contractors as cylinders. Oxygen flow can be adjusted as the cylinders are equipped with an oxygen flow meter with 'medium' (2 litres/minute) and 'high' (4 litres/minute) settings. The FHSAs have lists of pharmacy contractors who provide domiciliary oxygen services.

Patients are supplied with either constant or variable performance masks. The Intersurgical 010 28% or Ventimask Mk IV 28% are constant performance masks and provide a nearly constant supply of oxygen (28%) over a wide range irrespective of the patient's breathing pattern. The variable performance masks include the Intersurgical 005 Mask and the Venticaire Mask; the concentration of oxygen supplied to the patient varies with the rate of flow of oxygen and also with the patient's breathing pattern.

OXYGEN CONCENTRATORS

Long-term administration of oxygen (at least 15 hours daily) may prolong survival in patients with severe chronic obstructive airways disease with cor pulmonale

Department of Health guidelines suggest that this treatment should be provided for patients who fulfil the following criteria:

$P_aO_2 < 7.3$kPa; $P_aCO_2 > 6$kPa;

$FEV_1 < 1.5$ litre and FVC < 2 litre

The measurements should be stable on two occasions at least three weeks apart after the patient has received appropriate bronchodilator therapy.

Less information is available on long-term oxygen in patients with a similar degree of hypoxaemia and airflow obstruction but no hypercapnia; the Department of Health suggests that these patients should not be denied this form of treatment but the effects of long-term therapy have not yet been assessed completely.

Increased respiratory depression from low concentrations of oxygen is seldom a problem in patients with stable respiratory failure although it may occur during exacerbations; patients and relatives should be warned to call for medical help if drowsiness or confusion occur.

Oxygen concentrators are more economical for patients requiring oxygen for long periods, and in England and Wales are now prescribable on the NHS on a regional tendering basis (see below). A concentrator was formerly only provided for a patient who required oxygen for 15 hours a day but it has been found to be cost-effective to provide one for a patient requiring it for 8 hours a day (or 21 cylinders per month).

PRESCRIBING ARRANGEMENTS FOR OXYGEN CONCENTRATORS

Prescribe concentrator and accessories (face mask, nasal cannula, and humidifier) on form FP10. Specify amount of oxygen required (hours per day) and flow rate. If required, prescribe back-up oxygen set and cylinder at same time. Inform patient that the supplier will be in contact to make arrangements and that the prescription form is to be given to the person who installs the concentrator.

Inform supplier by telephone (see table below) that a concentrator has been prescribed. The supplier will send written confirmation of the order to the prescriber, the patient, and the FHSA.

Follow the same procedure if a back-up oxygen set and cylinder are required later.

FHSA regional group	Supplier
Eastern North Western London North North Wales West Midlands	De Vilbiss Health Care Ltd *to order:* Dial 0800 020202
London South (includes Kent, Surrey, and Sussex)	Omnicare Health Group Ltd *to order:* Dial 100 *and ask for:* Freephone Omnicare Oxygen
Central and South Wales Northern South Western Yorkshire (South and West) and Humberside	Oxygen Therapy Co Ltd *to order:* Dial 0800 373580

In **Scotland** refer the patient for assessment by a respiratory consultant. If the need for a concentrator is confirmed the consultant will arrange for the provision of a concentrator through the Common Services Agency.

3.7   Mucolytics

Mucolytics are often prescribed to facilitate expectoration by reducing sputum viscosity in chronic asthma and bronchitis. Few patients, however, have been shown to derive much benefit from them although they do render sputum less viscid. Steam inhalation with postural drainage, is good expectorant therapy in bronchiectasis and some chronic bronchitics.

For reference to the newly introduced dornase alfa, see below

ACETYLCYSTEINE
Indications: reduction of sputum viscosity

Side-effects: occasional gastro-intestinal irritation, headache, urticaria, tinnitus, and sensitivity

Dose: adults and children over 6 years, 200 mg in water 3 times daily, usually for 5–10 days but if necessary may be extended to 6 months or longer; CHILD up to 2 years 200 mg daily, 2–6 years 200 mg twice daily

NHS *PoM **Acetylcysteine Granules,** acetylcysteine 200 mg/sachet. Net price 30 sachets = £5.60. Label: 13

* except for abdominal complications associated with cystic fibrosis and endorsed 'SLS' ('S2B' in Scotland)

Note. The brand name NHS Fabrol® (Zyma) is used for acetylcysteine granules

CARBOCISTEINE
Indications: reduction of sputum viscosity

Side-effects: occasional gastro-intestinal irritation, rashes

Dose: 750 mg 3 times daily initially, then 1.5 g daily in divided doses; CHILD 2–5 years 62.5–125 mg 4 times daily, 6–12 years 250 mg 3 times daily

NHS *PoM **Carbocisteine Capsules,** carbocisteine 375 mg. Net price 30-cap pack = £3.12

NHS *PoM **Carbocisteine Syrup,** carbocisteine 125 mg/5 mL, net price 300 mL = £3.42; 250 mg/5 mL, 300 mL = £4.39

* except, for patients under the age of 18 years, any condition which, through damage or disease, affects the airways and has required a tracheostomy and endorsed 'SLS' ('S2B' in Scotland)

Note. The brand name NHS Mucodyne® (Rhône-Poulenc Rorer) is used for carbocisteine preparations; capsules and 250 mg/5 mL strength of syrup contain tartrazine

METHYL CYSTEINE HYDROCHLORIDE
(Mecysteine Hydrochloride)

Indications: reduction of sputum viscosity

Dose: 100–200 mg 3–4 times daily before meals reduced to 200 mg twice daily after 6 weeks; CHILD over 5 years 100 mg 3 times daily
Prophylaxis, 100–200 mg 2–3 times every other day during winter months

NHS **Visclair®** (Sinclair)

Tablets, yellow, s/c, e/c, methyl cysteine hydrochloride 100 mg. Net price 20 = £3.66. Label: 5, 22, 25

DORNASE ALFA

Dornase alfa is a genetically engineered version of a naturally occurring human enzyme which cleaves extracellular deoxyribonucleic acid (DNA). It is administered by inhalation using a jet nebuliser.

DORNASE ALFA

Phosphorylated glycosylated recombinant human deoxyribonuclease 1 (rhDNase)

Indications: management of cystic fibrosis patients with a forced vital capacity (FVC) of greater than 40% of predicted to improve pulmonary function

Cautions: pregnancy and breast-feeding (manufacturers do not recommend)

Side-effects: pharyngitis, voice changes, laryngitis, rashes, urticaria

Dose: by inhalation of nebulised solution (by jet nebuliser), 2 500 units (2.5 mg) once daily (patients over 21 years may benefit from twice daily dosage); CHILD under 5 years not recommended

▼ PoM **Pulmozyme®** (Roche)

Nebuliser solution, dornase alfa 1000 units (1 mg)/mL. Net price 2.5-mL (2 500 units) vial = £20.39

Note. For use undiluted with jet nebulisers only; ultrasonic nebulisers are unsuitable

3.8   Aromatic inhalations

Inhalations containing volatile substances such as eucalyptus oil are traditionally used and although the vapour may contain little of the additive it encourages deliberate inspiration of warm moist air which is often comforting in bronchitis; boiling water should not be used owing to the risk of scalding. Inhalations are also used for the relief of nasal obstruction in acute rhinitis or sinusitis.

CHILDREN. The use of strong aromatic decongestants (applied as rubs or to pillows) is not advised for infants under the age of 3 months. Mothers with young infants in whom nasal obstruction with mucus is a problem can readily be taught appropriate techniques of suction aspiration.

Benzoin Tincture, Compound, BP, Friars' Balsam, balsamic acids approx. 4.5%. Label: 15

Directions for use: add one teaspoonful to a pint of hot, **not** boiling, water and inhale the vapour

NHS **Menthol and Benzoin Inhalation, BP,** racemriol or levomenthol 2 g, benzoin inhalation to 100 mL. Label: 15

Directions for use: add one teaspoonful to a pint of hot, **not** boiling, water and inhale the vapour

Menthol and Eucalyptus Inhalation, BP 1980, racementhol or levomenthol 2 g, eucalyptus oil 10 mL, light magnesium carbonate 7 g, water to 100 mL

Directions for use: add one teaspoonful to a pint of hot, **not** boiling, water and inhale the vapour

NHS **Karvol®** (Crookes)

Inhalation capsules, menthol 35.55 mg, with chlorbutol, pine oils, terpineol, and thymol. Net price 10 = £1.06

Directions for use: inhale vapour from contents of 1 capsule expressed into handkerchief or a pint of hot, **not** boiling, water; avoid in infants under 3 months

3.9   Cough preparations

3.9.1   Cough suppressants
3.9.2   Expectorant and demulcent cough preparations

3.9.1   Cough suppressants

The drawbacks of prescribing cough suppressants are rarely outweighed by the benefits of treatment and only occasionally are they useful, as, for example, if sleep is disturbed by a dry cough. Cough suppressants may cause sputum retention and this may be harmful in patients with chronic bronchitis and bronchiectasis.

Opioid cough suppressants such as codeine, dextromethorphan, and pholcodine are seldom sufficiently potent to be effective in severe cough; all tend to cause constipation.

Sedative antihistamines, such as diphenhydramine, are used as the cough suppressant component of many compound cough preparations on sale to the public; all tend to cause drowsiness which may reflect their main mode of action.

CHILDREN. The use of cough suppressants containing codeine or similar opioid analgesics is not generally recommended in children and should be avoided altogether in those under 1 year of age.

CODEINE PHOSPHATE

Indications: dry or painful cough

Cautions: asthma; hepatic and renal impairment; history of drug abuse; see also notes above and section 4.7.2; **interactions:** Appendix 1 (opioid analgesics)

Contra-indications: liver disease, ventilatory failure

Side-effects: constipation, respiratory depression in sensitive patients or if given large doses

PoM[1] **Codeine Linctus, BP,** codeine phosphate 15 mg/5 mL. Net price 100 mL = 31p (diabetic, 64p)

Dose: 5–10 mL 3–4 times daily; CHILD 5–12 years, 2.5–5 mL

Available from APS, Galen (Galcodine®, sugar-free), K Pharm.

Note. BP 1993 directs that when Diabetic Codeine Linctus is prescribed, Codeine Linctus formulated with a vehicle appropriate for administration to diabetics, whether or not labelled 'Diabetic Codeine Linctus', shall be dispensed or supplied

1. Can be sold to the public provided the maximum single dose does not exceed 5 mL

Codeine Linctus, Paediatric, BP, codeine phosphate 3 mg/5 mL. Net price 100 mL = 18p
Dose: CHILD 1–5 years 5 mL 3–4 times daily
Available from Evans, Galen (Galcodine® Paediatric, sugar-free)
Note. Sugar-free versions are available
Note. BP 1993 directs that Paediatric Codeine Linctus may be prepared extemporaneously by diluting Codeine Linctus with a suitable vehicle in accordance with the manufacturer's instructions
For a list of **cough and decongestant preparations on sale to the public,** including those containing codeine, see section 3.9.2

PHOLCODINE

Indications: dry or painful cough
Cautions; Contra-indications; Side-effects: see under Codeine Phosphate

Pholcodine Linctus, BP, pholcodine 5 mg/5 mL in a suitable flavoured vehicle, containing citric acid monohydrate 1%. Net price 100 mL = 38p
Dose: 5–10 mL 3–4 times daily; CHILD 5–12 years 2.5–5 mL
Available from APS, Boehringer Ingelheim (Pavacol-D®, sugar-free), Galen (Galenphol®, sugar-free), K Pharm., Medo (NHS Pholcomed D®, sugar-free)

Pholcodine Linctus, Strong, BP, pholcodine 10 mg/5 mL in a suitable flavoured vehicle, containing citric acid monohydrate 2%. Net price 100 mL = 34p
Dose: 5 mL 3–4 times daily
Available from APS (sugar-free), K Pharm., Medo (NHS Pholcomed Diabetic Forte®, sugar-free)

Galenphol® (Galen)
Paediatric linctus, orange, sugar-free, pholcodine 2 mg/5 mL. Net price 100 mL = 17p
Dose: CHILD 1–5 years 5 mL 3 times daily; 6–12 years 5–10 mL
For a list of **cough and decongestant preparations on sale to the public,** including those containing pholcodine, see section 3.9.2

TERMINAL CARE

Diamorphine and methadone are available in linctuses to control distressful cough in terminal lung cancer although morphine is now preferred (see Terminal Care, p. 12). In other circumstances they are contra-indicated because they induce sputum retention and ventilatory failure as well as causing opioid dependence.

DIAMORPHINE HYDROCHLORIDE

Indications: cough in terminal disease
Cautions; Contra-indications; Side-effects: see notes in section 4.7.2; more potent than morphine
Dose: see below

CD Diamorphine Linctus, BPC 1973, diamorphine hydrochloride 3 mg, oxymel 1.25 mL, glycerol 1.25 mL, compound tartrazine solution 0.06 mL, syrup to 5 mL. It should be recently prepared. Label: 2
Dose: 2.5–10 mL every 4 hours

METHADONE HYDROCHLORIDE

Indications: cough in terminal disease
Cautions; Contra-indications; Side-effects: see notes in section 4.7.2; longer-acting than morphine therefore effects may be cumulative
Dose: see below

CD Methadone Linctus, methadone hydrochloride 2 mg/5 mL in a suitable vehicle with a tolu flavour. Label: 2
Dose: 2.5–5 mL every 4–6 hours, reduced to twice daily on prolonged use

MORPHINE HYDROCHLORIDE

Indications: cough in terminal disease (see also p. 13)
Cautions; Contra-indications; Side-effects: see notes in section 4.7.2
Dose: initially 5 mg every 4 hours

Preparations
See section 4.7.2

3.9.2 Expectorant and demulcent cough preparations

Expectorants are claimed to promote expulsion of bronchial secretions but there is no evidence that any drug can specifically facilitate expectoration. The assumption that sub-emetic doses of expectorants, such as ammonium chloride, ipecacuanha, and squill promote expectoration is a myth. However, a simple expectorant mixture may serve a useful placebo function and has the advantage of being inexpensive.

Demulcent cough preparations contain soothing substances such as syrup or glycerol and certainly some patients believe that such preparations relieve a dry irritating cough. Preparations such as **simple linctus** have the advantage of being harmless and inexpensive; **paediatric simple linctus** is particularly useful in children and sugar-free versions are now available.

Compound cough preparations are on sale to the public; the rationale for some is dubious.

CHILDREN. The use of cough suppressants containing codeine or similar opioid analgesics is not generally recommended in children and should be avoided altogether in those under 1 year of age.

Ammonia and Ipecacuanha Mixture, BP, ammonium bicarbonate 200 mg, liquorice liquid extract 0.5 mL, ipecacuanha tincture 0.3 mL, concentrated camphor water 0.1 mL, concentrated anise water 0.05 mL, double-strength chloroform water 5 mL, water to 10 mL. It should be recently prepared
Dose: 10–20 mL 3–4 times daily

NHS Ammonium Chloride and Morphine Mixture, BP, ammonium chloride 300 mg, ammonium bicarbonate 200 mg, chloroform and morphine tincture 0.3 mL, liquorice liquid extract 0.5 mL, water to 10 mL. It should be recently prepared. Contains 500 micrograms of anhydrous morphine in 10 mL
Dose: 10–20 mL 3–4 times daily

NHS **Ipecacuanha and Morphine Mixture, BP 1980,** ipecacuanha tincture 0.2 mL, chloroform and morphine tincture 0.4 mL, liquorice liquid extract 1 mL, water to 10 mL. It should be recently prepared. 10 mL contains 700 micrograms of anhydrous morphine

Dose: 10 mL 3–4 times daily

Simple Linctus, BP, citric acid monohydrate 2.5% in a suitable vehicle with an anise flavour. Net price 100 mL = 17p

Dose: 5 mL 3–4 times daily

Simple Linctus, Paediatric, BP, citric acid monohydrate 0.625% in a suitable vehicle with an anise flavour. Net price 100 mL = 15p

Dose: CHILD, 5–10 mL 3–4 times daily

NHS **Squill Linctus, Opiate, BP,** Gee's Linctus, equal volumes of camphorated opium tincture, squill oxymel, and tolu syrup. It contains 800 micrograms of anhydrous morphine in 5 mL

Dose: 5 mL 3–4 times daily

NHS **Tolu Linctus, Compound, Paediatric,** citric acid monohydrate 30 mg /5 mL in a suitable vehicle with a tolu flavour

Dose: CHILD, 5–10 mL 3–4 times daily

The following is a list of systemic cough and decongestant preparations on sale to the public, together with their significant ingredients.

Important: in overdose contact **Poisons Information Services** (p. 18) for full details of the ingredients.

Actifed® (pseudoephedrine, triprolidine), **Actifed Compound Linctus**® (dextromethorphan, pseudoephedrine, triprolidine), **Actifed Expectorant**® (guaiphenesin, pseudoephedrine, triprolidine), **Actifed Junior Cough Relief**® (dextromethorphan, triprolidine), **Anestan**® (ephedrine, theophylline), **Anidox Spansules**® (diphenylpyraline, phenylpropanolamine)

Baby Meltus® (dilute acetic acid), **Balm of Gilead Cough Mixture**® (Gilead extract, squill, lobelia), **Barum Cold Relief with Decongestant**® (paracetamol, phenylephrine), **Beechams Hot Lemon**®, **Hot Lemon and Honey**®, **Beechams Powders Capsules**® **with Decongestant** (paracetamol, phenylephrine), **Benylin Chesty Cough**® (ammonium chloride, diphenhydramine, menthol), **Benylin Childrens Cough**® (diphenhydramine, menthol), **Benylin with Codeine**® (codeine, diphenhydramine, menthol), **Benylin Dry Cough**® (dextromethorphan, diphenhydramine, menthol), **Benylin Mentholated**® (dextromethorphan, diphenhydramine, pseudoephedrine, menthol), **Benylin Non-drowsy for Chesty Coughs**® (guaiphenesin, menthol), **Benylin Non-drowsy for Dry Coughs**® (dextromethorphan, menthol), **Benylin Sugar-free for Children**® (diphenhydramine, menthol), **Benylin Day and Night Cold and Flu Relief**® (*day tablets,* paracetamol, phenylephrine; *night tablets,* paracetamol, diphenhydramine), **Boots Bronchial Cough Mixture**® (ammonium carbonate, ammonium chloride, guaiphenesin), **Boots Catarrh Syrup for Children**® (diphenhydramine, pseudoephedrine), **Boots Catarrh Cough Syrup**® (codeine, creosote), **Boots Cold Capsules**® (diphenylpyraline, phenylpropanolamine), **Boots Cold and Influenza Mixture**® (squill, ammonium acetate), **Boots Cold Relief Tablets**® (paracetamol, phenylephrine), **Boots Cough Linctus for Children**® (ephedrine, ipecacuanha), **Boots Cough Relief for Children**® (diphenhydramine, pholcodine), **Boots Day Cold Comfort**® (paracetamol, pholcodine, pseudoephedrine), **Boots Day-time Cough Relief**® (pholcodine), **Boots Decongestant Tablets**® (pseudoephedrine), **Boots Night-Cold Comfort**® (diphenhydramine, paracetamol, pholcodine, pseudoephedrine), **Boots Night-time Cough Relief**® (diphenhydramine, pholcodine), **Bronal**® (dextromethorphan), **Bronalin Dry Cough**® (dextromethorphan, pseudoephedrine), **Bronalin Expectorant**® (ammonium chloride, diphenhydramine), **Bronalin Paediatric**® (diphenhydramine), **Buttercup Syrup Traditional**® (squill), **Buttercup Honey and Lemon and Blackcurrant**® (ipecacuanha, menthol)

Cabdrivers® and **Cabdrivers Sugar-free**® (dextromethorphan, menthol), **Cabdrivers Junior**® (ephedrine), **Catarrh-Ex** (paracetamol, pseudoephedrine), **Coldrex Blackcurrant Powders**®, **Hot Lemon Powders**® and **Tablets**® (paracetamol, phenylephrine), **Contac 400**® (phenylpropanolamine, chlorpheniramine), **Contac CoughCaps**® (dextromethorphan),

Copholco® (pholcodine, menthol), **Covonia**® (dextromethorphan, guaiphenesin, menthol), **Covonia for Children**® (dextromethorphan, menthol), **Cupal Baby Cough**® (dilute acetic acid)

Davenol® (carbinoxamine, ephedrine, pholcodine), **Day Nurse**®, **Day Nurse Hot**® (dextromethorphan, paracetamol, phenylpropanolamine), **Dimotane Elixir**®, **Tablets**® and **Dimotane LA**® (brompheniramine), **Dimotane Expectorant**® (brompheniramine, guaiphenesin, pseudoephedrine), **Dimotane Co**® and **Dimotane Co Paediatric**® (brompheniramine, codeine, pseudoephedrine),**Dimotane Plus**® and **Dimotane Plus Paediatric**® (brompheniramine, pseudoephedrine), **Dimotapp**®, **Dimotapp Paediatric**®, and **Dimotapp LA**® (brompheniramine, phenylephrine, phenylpropanolamine), **Do-Do Expectorant**® (guaiphenesin), **Do-Do Tablets**® (ephedrine, theophylline), **Dristan Tablets**® (aspirin, chlorpheniramine, phenylephrine),)**Ecdylin**® (ammonium chloride, diphenhydramine), **ES Bronchial**® (ammonium bicarbonate, ipecacuanha, senna, squill), **Eskornade**® (diphenylpyraline, phenylpropanolamine), **Evacode**® (codeine), **Evaphol**® (pholcodine), **Expulin**® (chlorpheniramine, menthol, pholcodine, pseudoephedrine), **Expulin Dry**® (pholcodine), **Expulin Paediatric**® (chlorpheniramine, menthol, pholcodine), **Expurhin Paediatric**® (chlorpheniramine, ephedrine, menthol)

Famel® (pholcodine), **Famel Expectorant**® (guaiphenesin), **Famel Original**® (codeine, creosote), **Fennings Little Healers**® (ipecacuanha), **Fisherman's Friend Honey Cough Syrup**® (cineole, menthol, squill), **Flurex Bedtime**® (diphenhydramine, paracetamol, pseudoephedrine), **Flurex Capsules**® and **Tablets**® (paracetamol, phenylephrine), **Franolyn Expect**® (ephedrine, guaiphenesin, theophylline), **Franolyn Chesty**® (dextromethorphan)

Galcodine® (codeine), **Galcodine Paediatric**® (codeine), **Galenphol**® (pholcodine), **Galenphol Paediatric**® (pholcodine), **Galenphol Strong**® (pholcodine), **Galloway's**® (ipecacuanha, squill), **Galpseud**® (pseudoephedrine), **Galpseud Plus**® (chlorpheniramine, pseudoephedrine), **Guanor Expectorant**® (ammonium chloride, diphenhydramine, menthol)

Haymine® (chlorpheniramine, ephedrine), **Hill's Balsam Adult Expectorant**® (ipecacuanha, pholcodine), **Hill's Balsam Cough Suppressant**® (pholcodine), **Histalix**® (ammonium chloride, diphenhydramine, menthol)

Jackson's All Fours® (guaiphenesin), **Junior Lemsip**® (paracetamol, phenylephrine), **Junior Meltus Dry Cough**® (dextromethorphan, pseudoephedrine), **Junior Meltus Expectorant**® (guaiphenesin), **Junior Mucron**® (ipecacuanha, phenylpropanolamine)

Lem-Plus Capsules® (paracetamol, phenylephrine), **Lemsip Cold Relief**® **Capsules with Decongestant, Lemsip Flu Strength**®, **Lemsip Lemon**® or ,

[Continued on next page]

Cough and decongestant preparations on sale to the public [*continued*]

Blackcurrant®, **Lemsip Junior**®, **Lemsip Menthol Extra**® (all paracetamol, phenylephrine), **Lemsip Chesty Cough**® (guaiphenesin), **Lemsip Expectorant**® (ammonium chloride, diphenhydramine), **Lemsip Flu Strength Nightime**® (chlorpheniramine, dextromethorphan, paracetamol, phenylpropanolamine), **Liqufruta Honey and Lemon**®, **Blackcurrant**® (ipecacuanha, menthol), **Liqufruta Garlic**® (guaiphenesin)
Medised® (paracetamol, promethazine), **Melo**® (ipecacuanha), **Meltus Baby**® (dilute acetic acid), **Meltus Dry Cough**® (dextromethorphan, pseudoephedrine), **Meltus Expectorant**®, **Meltus Honey and Lemon**® (guaiphenesin), **Mu-Cron Tablets**® (paracetamol, phenylpropanolamine)
Night Nurse® (dextromethorphan, paracetamol, promethazine), **Nirolex**® (ephedrine, guaiphenesin, menthol), **Nirolex for Children**® (guaiphenesin),**Numark Cold Relief Capsules**® **With Decongestant** (paracetamol, phenylephrine), **Numark Cold Relief Powders**® (paracetamol), **Nurofen Cold and Flu**® (ibuprofen, pseudoephedrine), **Nurse Sykes Balsam**® (guaiphenesin)
Owbridges® (dilute acetic acid, guaiphenesin, ammonium acetate)
Pavacol D® (pholcodine), **Phensedyl Plus**® (promethazine, pholcodine, pseudoephedrine), **Pholcomed**®, **Pholcomed D**® and **Pholcomed Diabetic Forte**® (pholcodine), **Procol**® (phenylpropanolamine), **Pulmo Bailly**® (codeine, guaiacol)
Robitussin Adult® and **Junior Cough Soother**® (dextromethorphan), **Robitussin Expectorant**® (guaiphenesin), **Robitussin Expectorant Plus**® (guaiphenesin, pseudoephedrine)

Secron® (ephedrine, vinegar of ipecacuanha), **Sinutab**® (paracetamol, phenylpropanolamine), **Sinutab Nightime**® (paracetamol, phenylpropanolamine, phenyltoloxamine), **SP Cold Relief Capsules**® (paracetamol, phenylephrine), **Sudafed**® (pseudoephedrine), **Sudafed Co**® (paracetamol, pseudoephedrine), **Sudafed Expectorant**® (guaiphenesin, pseudoephedrine), **Sudafed Linctus**® (dextromethorphan, pseudoephedrine), **Sudafed Plus**® (pseudoephedrine, triprolidine)
Tancolin® (dextromethorphan), **Terpoin**® (cineole, codeine, menthol), **Throaties Family Cough Linctus**® (ipecacuanha), **Tixylix Night-time**® (pholcodine, promethazine), **Tixylix Daytime**® (pholcodine), **Tixylix Cough and Cold**® (chlorpheniramine, pholcodine, pseudoephedrine), **Triogesic**® (paracetamol, phenylpropanolamine), **Triominic**® (pheniramine, phenylpropanolamine)
Uniflu with Gregovite C® (codeine, diphenhydramine, paracetamol, phenylephrine)
Venos for Dry Coughs® and **Venos Expectorant**® (guaiphenesin), **Venos Honey and Lemon**® (ammonium chloride, ipecacuanha), **Vicks Children's Vaposyrup Dry Cough**® (dextromethorphan), **Vicks Coldcare**® (paracetamol, dextromethorphan, phenylpropanolamine), **Vicks Expectorant Cough Syrup**® (guaiphenesin), **Vicks Medinite**® (dextromethorphan, doxylamine, ephedrine, paracetamol), **Vicks Vaposyrup Chesty Cough**® (guaiphenesin), **Vicks Vaposyrup Dry Cough**® (dextromethorphan), **Vicks Vaposyrup Chesty Coughs and Nasal Congestion**® (guaiphenesin, phenylpropanolamine), **Vicks Vaposyrup Dry Coughs and Nasal Congestion**® (dextromethorphan, phenylpropanolamine)

3.10   Systemic nasal decongestants

These preparations are of doubtful value but unlike the preparations for local application (see section 12.2.2) they do not give rise to rebound nasal congestion. They contain sympathomimetics, and should therefore be **avoided** in patients with hypertension, hyperthyroidism, coronary heart disease, or diabetes, and in patients taking monoamine-oxidase inhibitors; **interactions:** Appendix 1 (sympathomimetics). Many of the preparations also contain antihistamines which may cause drowsiness and affect ability to drive or operate machinery.

For a list of cough and decongestant preparations on sale to the public, including those containing systemic nasal decongestants, see section 3.9.2 above.

PSEUDOEPHEDRINE HYDROCHLORIDE

Indications; Dose: see notes above and under preparations

Cautions; Side-effects: see under Ephedrine Hydrochloride (section 3.1.1.2)

Galpseud® (Galen)
Tablets, pseudoephedrine hydrochloride 60 mg. Net price 20 = 87p
Dose: 1 tablet 3 times daily
Linctus, orange, sugar-free, pseudoephedrine hydrochloride 30 mg/5 mL. Net price 140 mL = 96p
Dose: 10 mL 3 times daily; CHILD 2–6 years 2.5 mL, 6–12 years 5 mL

Sudafed® (Wellcome)
Tablets, red, f/c, pseudoephedrine hydrochloride 60 mg. Net price 20 = £1.17
Dose: 1 tablet 3 times daily
Elixir, red, pseudoephedrine hydrochloride 30 mg/5 mL. Net price 100 mL = 94p
Dose: 10 mL 3 times daily; CHILD 2–5 years 2.5 mL, 6–12 years 5 mL

With antihistamine
Dimotane Plus® (Wyeth)
Liquid, brown, sugar-free, brompheniramine maleate 4 mg, pseudoephedrine hydrochloride 30 mg/5 mL. Net price 100 mL = 69p. Label: 2
Dose: 10 mL 3 times daily; CHILD 2–6 years 2.5 mL, 6–12 years 5 mL
Paediatric liquid, brown, sugar-free, brompheniramine maleate 2 mg, pseudoephedrine hydrochloride 15 mg/5 mL. Net price 100 mL = 63p. Label: 1
Dose: CHILD 2–6 years 5 mL, 6–12 years 10 mL, 3 times daily

Sudafed Plus® (Wellcome)
Tablets, pseudoephedrine hydrochloride 60 mg, triprolidine hydrochloride 2.5 mg. Net price 20-tab pack = £1.30. Label: 2
Dose: 1 tablet 3 times daily
Syrup, yellow, pseudoephedrine hydrochloride 30 mg, triprolidine hydrochloride 1.25 mg/5 mL. Net price 100 mL = £1.06. Label: 2
Dose: 10 mL 3 times daily; CHILD 2–5 years 2.5 mL 3 times daily, 6–12 years 5 mL 3 times daily

---

4: Drugs acting on the
CENTRAL NERVOUS SYSTEM

In this chapter, drug treatments are discussed under the following headings:

4.1   Hypnotics and anxiolytics

Most anxiolytics ('sedatives') will induce sleep when given in large doses at night and most hypnotics will sedate when given in divided doses during the day. Prescribing of these drugs is widespread but dependence (either physical or psychological) and tolerance to their effects occurs. This may lead to difficulty in withdrawing the drug after the patient has been taking it regularly for more than a few weeks (see Dependence and Withdrawal, below). Hypnotics and anxiolytics should not therefore be prescribed indiscriminately and should, instead, be reserved for short courses to alleviate acute conditions after causal factors have been established.

Prescribing of more than one anxiolytic or hypnotic at the same time is **not** recommended. It may constitute a hazard and there is no evidence that side-effects are minimised.

Benzodiazepines are the most commonly used anxiolytics and hypnotics; they act at benzodiazepine receptors which are associated with gamma-aminobutyric acid (GABA) receptors. Barbiturates (section 4.1.3) are no longer recommended.

Benzodiazepines have fewer side-effects than barbiturates and are much less dangerous in overdosage. They are also less likely to interact with other drugs because, unlike barbiturates, they do not induce liver microsomal enzymes.

A paradoxical increase in hostility and aggression may be reported by patients taking benzodiazepines. The effects range from talkativeness and excitement, to aggressive and antisocial acts. Adjustment of the dose (up or down) usually attenuates the impulses. Increased anxiety and perceptual disorders are other paradoxical effects. Increased hostility and aggression after barbiturates and alcohol usually indicates intoxication.

DEPENDENCE AND WITHDRAWAL. The benzodiazepine withdrawal syndrome may not develop until up to 3 weeks after stopping a long-acting benzodiazepine, but may occur within a few hours in the case of a short-acting one. It is characterised by insomnia, anxiety, loss of appetite and body weight, tremor, perspiration, tinnitus, and perceptual disturbances. These symptoms may be similar to the original complaint and encourage further prescribing; some symptoms may continue for weeks or months after stopping benzodiazepines entirely.

Withdrawal of a benzodiazepine should be gradual as abrupt withdrawal may produce confusion, toxic psychosis, convulsions, or a condition resembling delirium tremens.

DRIVING. Hypnotics and anxiolytics may impair judgement and increase reaction time, and so affect ability to drive or operate machinery; they increase the effects of alcohol. Moreover the hangover effects of a night dose may impair driving on the following day.

BENZODIAZEPINE WITHDRAWAL

Benzodiazepines can be withdrawn in steps of about $\frac{1}{8}$ (range $\frac{1}{10}-\frac{1}{4}$) of their daily dose every fortnight. For patients who are taking a benzodiazepine other than diazepam, and who are unable to reduce it, a suggested withdrawal protocol involving transfer to diazepam is as follows:

1. Transfer patient to equivalent daily dose of diazepam[1] preferably taken at night

2. Reduce diazepam dose in fortnightly steps of 2 or 2.5 mg; if withdrawal symptoms occur, maintain this dose until symptoms improve

3. Reduce dose further, if necessary in smaller fortnightly steps[2]; it is better to reduce too slowly rather than too quickly

4. Stop completely; time needed for withdrawal can vary from about 4 weeks to a year or more

Counselling may help; beta-blockers should **only** be tried if other measures fail; antidepressants should **only** be used if clinical depression present; **avoid** antipsychotics (which may aggravate withdrawal symptoms)

1.   Approximate equivalent doses, diazepam 5 mg
     ≡ chlordiazepoxide 15 mg
     ≡ loprazolam 0.5–1 mg
     ≡ lorazepam 500 micrograms
     ≡ lormetazepam 0.5–1 mg
     ≡ nitrazepam 5 mg
     ≡ oxazepam 15 mg
     ≡ temazepam 10 mg
2.   Steps may be adjusted according to initial dose and duration of treatment and can range from diazepam 500 micrograms (¼ of a 2-mg tablet) to 2.5 mg

---

Cautionary label wordings, see inside back cover   Prices are **net**, see p. 1

4.1.1 Hypnotics

Before a hypnotic is prescribed the cause of the insomnia should be established and, where possible, underlying factors should be treated. However, it should be noted that some patients have unrealistic sleep expectations, and others understate their alcohol consumption which is often the cause of the insomnia.

Transient insomnia may occur in those who normally sleep well and may be due to extraneous factors such as noise, shift work, and jet lag. If a hypnotic is indicated one that is rapidly eliminated should be chosen, and only one or two doses should be given.

Short-term insomnia is usually related to an emotional problem or serious medical illness. It may last for a few weeks, and may recur; a hypnotic can be useful but should not be given for more than three weeks (preferably only one week). Intermittent use is desirable with omission of some doses. A rapidly eliminated drug is generally appropriate.

Chronic insomnia is rarely benefited by hypnotics and is more often due to mild dependence caused by injudicious prescribing. Psychiatric disorders such as anxiety, depression, and abuse of drugs and alcohol are common issues. Sleep disturbance is very common in depressive illness and early wakening is often a useful pointer. The underlying psychiatric complaint should be treated, adapting the drug regimen to alleviate insomnia. For example, amitriptyline, prescribed for depression, will also help to promote sleep if it is taken at night. Other causes of insomnia include daytime catnapping and physical causes such as pain, pruritus, and dyspnoea.

Hypnotics should **not** be prescribed indiscriminately and routine prescribing is undesirable. Ideally, they should be reserved for short courses in the acutely distressed. Tolerance to their effects develops within 3 to 14 days of continuous use and long-term efficacy cannot be assured. A major drawback of long-term use is that withdrawal causes rebound insomnia and precipitates a withdrawal syndrome (section 4.1).

Where prolonged administration is unavoidable hypnotics should be discontinued as soon as feasible and the patient warned that sleep may be disturbed for a few days before normal rhythm is re-established; broken sleep with vivid dreams and increased REM (rapid eye movement) may persist for several weeks.

CHILDREN. The prescribing of hypnotics to children, except for occasional use such as for night terrors and somnambulism (sleep-walking), is not justified.

ELDERLY. Hypnotics should be avoided in the elderly, who are at risk of becoming ataxic and confused and so liable to fall and injure themselves.

BENZODIAZEPINES

Benzodiazepines used as hypnotics include **nitrazepam**, **flunitrazepam**, and **flurazepam** which have a prolonged action and may give rise to residual effects on the following day; repeated doses tend to be cumulative.

Loprazolam, **lormetazepam**, and **temazepam** act for a shorter time and they have little or no hangover effect. Withdrawal phenomena however are more common with the short-acting benzodiazepines.

Benzodiazepine anxiolytics such as **diazepam** given as a single dose at night may also be used as hypnotics.

For general guidelines on benzodiazepine prescribing see section 4.1.2 and for benzodiazepine withdrawal see section 4.1.

NITRAZEPAM

Indications: insomnia (short-term use)

Cautions: respiratory disease, muscle weakness, history of drug or alcohol abuse, marked personality disorder, pregnancy and breast-feeding (see Appendixes 4 and 5); reduce dose in elderly and debilitated, and in hepatic and renal impairment; avoid prolonged use (and abrupt withdrawal thereafter); porphyria (see section 9.8.2); **interactions:** Appendix 1 (benzodiazepines)

DRIVING. Drowsiness may persist the next day and affect performance of skilled tasks (e.g. driving); effects of alcohol enhanced

Contra-indications: respiratory depression; acute pulmonary insufficiency; not for phobic or obsessional states, chronic psychosis

Side-effects: drowsiness and lightheadedness the next day; confusion and ataxia (especially in the elderly); amnesia may occur; dependence; see also under Diazepam (section 4.1.2); overdosage: see Emergency Treatment of Poisoning, p.22.

Dose: 5–10 mg at bedtime; ELDERLY (or debilitated) 2.5–5 mg

PoM Nitrazepam (Non-proprietary)

Tablets, nitrazepam 5 mg, net price 20 = 12p. Label: 19

Available from APS, Berk, Cox, CP, DDSA (NHS Remnos®), K Pharm., Roche (NHS Mogadon®), Unigreg (NHS Unisomnia®)

Oral suspension, nitrazepam 2.5 mg/5 mL. Net price 150 mL = £4.15. Label: 19

Available from Norgine (NHS Somnite®)

FLUNITRAZEPAM

Indications: insomnia (short-term use)
Cautions; Contra-indications; Side-effects: see under Nitrazepam
Dose: 0.5–1 mg at bedtime; max. 2 mg; ELDERLY (or debilitated) 500 micrograms (max. 1 mg); CHILD not recommended

NHS **PoM** **Rohypnol®** (Roche)
Tablets, purple, f/c, scored, flunitrazepam 1 mg. Net price 30-tab pack = £4.00. Label: 19

FLURAZEPAM

Indications: insomnia (short-term use)
Cautions; Contra-indications; Side-effects: see under Nitrazepam
Dose: 15–30 mg at bedtime; ELDERLY 15 mg; CHILD not recommended

NHS **PoM** **Dalmane®** (Roche)
Capsules, flurazepam (as hydrochloride), 15 mg (grey/yellow), net price 30-cap pack = £2.65; 30 mg (black/grey), 30-cap pack = £3.40. Label: 19

LOPRAZOLAM

Indications: insomnia (short-term use)
Cautions; Contra-indications; Side-effects: see under Nitrazepam
Dose: 1 mg at bedtime, increased to 1.5 or 2 mg if required; ELDERLY (or debilitated) 0.5–1 mg; CHILD not recommended

PoM **Loprazolam** (Non-proprietary)
Tablets, loprazolam 1 mg (as mesylate). Net price 28-tab pack = £1.30. Label: 19
Available from Roussel (previously **NHS** Dormonoct®)

LORMETAZEPAM

Indications: insomnia (short-term use)
Cautions; Contra-indications; Side-effects: see under Nitrazepam; shorter acting
Dose: 0.5–1.5 mg at bedtime; ELDERLY (or debilitated) 500 micrograms; CHILD not recommended

PoM **Lormetazepam** (Non-proprietary)
Tablets, lormetazepam 500 micrograms, net price 20 = 53p; 1 mg, 20 = 93p. Label: 19
Available from APS, Cox, Wyeth

TEMAZEPAM

Indications: insomnia (short-term use); see also section 15.1.4.1 for peri-operative use
Cautions; Contra-indications; Side-effects: see under Nitrazepam; shorter acting
Dose: 10–30 mg (severe insomnia, up to 40–60 mg) at bedtime; ELDERLY (or debilitated) 5–15 mg; CHILD not recommended

PoM **Temazepam** (Non-proprietary)
Gel-filled capsules (soft gelatin), temazepam 10 mg, net price 20 = 36p; 15 mg, 20 = 62p; 20 mg, 20 = 63p; 30 mg, 20 = £1.24. Label: 19
Available from most generic manufacturers
Note. The name **NHS** Temazepam Gelthix® is used for some gel-filled capsules
WARNING. Gel-filled capsules may be particularly subject to abuse; gangrene has followed abuse by injection

Tablets, temazepam 10 mg, net price 20 = 48p; 20 mg, 20 = 84p. Label: 19
Oral solution, temazepam 10 mg/5 mL, net price 300 mL = £9.95. Label: 19

CHLORAL AND DERIVATIVES

Chloral hydrate and derivatives are useful hypnotics for children (but the use of hypnotics in children is not usually justified). There is no convincing evidence that they are particularly useful in the elderly. **Triclofos** causes fewer gastro-intestinal upsets than chloral hydrate.

CHLORAL HYDRATE

Indications: insomnia (short-term use)
Cautions: respiratory disease, history of drug or alcohol abuse, marked personality disorder, pregnancy, breast-feeding; reduce dose in elderly and debilitated; avoid prolonged use (and abrupt withdrawal thereafter); avoid contact with skin and mucous membranes; **interactions:** Appendix 1 (chloral)
DRIVING. Drowsiness may persist the next day and affect performance of skilled tasks (e.g. driving); effects of alcohol enhanced
Contra-indications: severe cardiac disease, gastritis, marked hepatic or renal impairment
Side-effects: gastric irritation, abdominal distention and flatulence; *occasionally:* rashes, headache, ketonuria, excitement, delirium (especially in the elderly); dependence (may be associated with gastritis and renal damage) on prolonged use
Dose: insomnia, 0.5–1 g (max. 2 g) with plenty of water at bedtime; CHILD 30–50 mg/kg up to a max. single dose of 1 g

PoM **Chloral Mixture, BP**
(Chloral Oral Solution)
Mixture, chloral hydrate 10% in a suitable vehicle. Extemporaneous preparations should be recently prepared according to the following formula: chloral hydrate 1 g, syrup 2 mL, water to 10 mL. Net price 100 mL = 22p. Label: 19, 27
Dose: 5–20 mL; CHILD 1–5 years 2.5–5 mL, 6–12 years 5–10 mL, taken well diluted with water at bedtime
Important. This preparation differs from Chloral Syrup BPC 1968 which contains 20% (1 g in 5 mL; dose: 2.5–10 mL, taken well diluted with water at bedtime)

PoM **Chloral Elixir, Paediatric, BP**
(Chloral Oral Solution, Paediatric)
Elixir, chloral hydrate 4% in a suitable vehicle with a blackcurrant flavour. Extemporaneous preparations should be recently prepared according to the following formula: chloral hydrate 200 mg, water 0.1 mL, blackcurrant syrup 1 mL, syrup to 5 mL. Net price 100 mL = 72p. Label: 1, 27
Dose: up to 1 year 5 mL, taken well diluted with water at bedtime

PoM **Noctec®** (Squibb)
Capsules, red, chloral hydrate 500 mg. Net price 50-cap pack = £1.90. Label: 19, 27
Dose: 1–2 capsules with plenty of water at bedtime (max. 4 capsules); CHILD not recommended

---

Cautionary label wordings, see inside back cover

Prices are **net**, see p.1

PoM **Welldorm®** (S&N Pharm.)
Tablets, blue-purple, f/c, chloral betaine 707 mg
(≡chloral hydrate 414 mg). Net price 30-tab pack
= £2.54. Label: 19, 27
Dose: 1–2 tablets with water or milk at bedtime, max. 5
tablets (2 g chloral hydrate) daily
Elixir, red, chloral hydrate 143 mg/5 mL. Net price
150-mL pack = £2.15. Label: 19, 27
Dose: 15–45 mL (0.4–1.3 g chloral hydrate) with water
or milk, at bedtime, max. 70 mL (2 g chloral hydrate)
daily; CHILD 1–1.75 mL/kg (30–50 mg/kg chloral
hydrate), max. 35 mL (1 g chloral hydrate) daily

TRICLOFOS SODIUM
Indications: insomnia (short-term use)
Cautions; Contra-indications; Side-effects: see
under Chloral Hydrate; less gastric irritation
Dose: see under preparation below

PoM **Triclofos Oral Solution, BP**
(Triclofos Elixir)
Oral solution, triclofos sodium 500 mg/5 mL. Net
price 100 mL = £7.65. Label: 19
Available from Evans
Dose: 10–20 mL (1–2 g triclofos sodium) at bedtime;
CHILD up to 1 year 25–30 mg/kg, 1–5 years 2.5–5 mL
(250–500 mg triclofos sodium), 6–12 years 5–10 mL
(0.5–1 g triclofos sodium)

OTHER HYPNOTICS

Chlormethiazole may be a useful hypnotic for elderly patients because of its freedom from hangover but, as with all hypnotics, routine administration is undesirable and dependence occurs occasionally.

Promethazine is popular for use in children, but the use of hypnotics in children is not usually justified (see p. 145).

Zopiclone is a cyclopyrrolone and the newly introduced **zolpidem** is an imidazopyridine. Although neither are benzodiazepines both act on the same receptors (or receptor sub-types) as benzodiazepines. As with other hypnotics they should not be used for long-term treatment.

Alcohol is a poor hypnotic as its diuretic action interferes with sleep during the latter part of the night. With chronic use, alcohol disturbs sleep patterns and causes insomnia; **interactions:** Appendix 1 (alcohol).

CHLORMETHIAZOLE
(Clomethiazole)
Indications: see under Dose; status epilepticus (section 4.8.2); alcohol withdrawal (section 4.10); sedation during regional anaesthesia (section 15.1.4.1); eclampsia, see data sheet
Cautions: cardiac and respiratory disease (confusional state may indicate hypoxia); history of drug abuse; marked personality disorder; excessive sedation particularly with higher doses; hepatic impairment (especially if severe since sedation can mask hepatic coma); renal impairment; avoid prolonged use (and abrupt with-

drawal thereafter); see also section 4.10; **interactions:** Appendix 1 (chlormethiazole)
DRIVING. Drowsiness may persist the next day and affect performance of skilled tasks (e.g. driving); effects of alcohol enhanced
Contra-indications: acute pulmonary insufficiency; alcohol-dependent patients who continue to drink
Side-effects: nasal congestion and irritation (increased nasopharyngeal and bronchial secretions), conjunctival irritation, headache; rarely, paradoxical excitement, confusion, dependence, gastro-intestinal disturbances, rash, urticaria, bullous eruption, anaphylaxis, alterations in liver enzymes; intravenous infusion, see section 4.10
Dose: by mouth, severe insomnia in the elderly (short-term use), 1–2 capsules (or 5–10 mL syrup) at bedtime; CHILD not recommended
Restlessness and agitation in the elderly, 1 capsule (or 5 mL syrup) 3 times daily
Note. For an equivalent therapeutic effect 1 capsule ≡ 5 mL syrup

PoM **Heminevrin®** (Astra)
Capsules, grey-brown, chlormethiazole base 192 mg in an oily basis. Net price 60-cap pack = £4.45. Label: 19
Syrup, sugar-free, chlormethiazole edisylate 250 mg/5 mL. Net price 300-mL pack = £3.72. Label: 19
Intravenous infusion 0.8%, section 4.10

DIPHENHYDRAMINE HYDROCHLORIDE
See section 3.4.1

PROMETHAZINE HYDROCHLORIDE
Indications: night sedation and insomnia (short-term use); other indications, see sections 3.4.1, 4.6, 15.1.4.1
Cautions; Side-effects: see section 3.4.1
Dose: by mouth, 25 mg at bedtime increased to 50 mg if necessary; CHILD under 1 year not recommended, 1–5 years 15–20 mg (1–2 years on doctors advice only), 5–10 years 20–25 mg, at bedtime

Preparations
See section 3.4.1

ZOLPIDEM TARTRATE
Indications: insomnia (short-term use)
Cautions: depression, history of drug or alcohol abuse, hepatic impairment (reduce dose, avoid if severe); renal impairment; avoid prolonged use (and abrupt withdrawal thereafter); **interactions:** Appendix 1 (zolpidem)
DRIVING. Drowsiness may persist the next day and affect performance of skilled tasks (e.g. driving); effects of alcohol enhanced
Contra-indications: obstructive sleep apnoea, acute pulmonary insufficiency, respiratory

depression, myasthenia gravis, severe hepatic impairment, pregnancy and breast-feeding

Side-effects: diarrhoea, nausea, vomiting, vertigo, dizziness, headache, daytime drowsiness, asthenia; memory disturbances, nightmares, nocturnal restlessness, depression, confusion, perceptual disturbances or diplopia, tremor, ataxia, falls reported

Dose: 10 mg at bedtime; ELDERLY (or debilitated) 5 mg; CHILD not recommended

▼ PoM **Stilnoct®** (Lorex)

Tablets, f/c, zolpidem tartrate 5 mg. Net price 28-tab pack = £3.36. Label: 19

ZOPICLONE

Indications: insomnia (short-term use)

Cautions: hepatic impairment; pregnancy and breast-feeding; elderly; history of drug abuse, psychiatric illness; avoid prolonged use (and abrupt withdrawal thereafter); **interactions:** Appendix 1 (zopiclone)

DRIVING. Drowsiness may persist the next day and affect performance of skilled tasks (e.g. driving); effects of alcohol enhanced

Side-effects: bitter or metallic taste; gastro-intestinal disturbances including nausea and vomiting; irritability, confusion, depressed mood; drowsiness, dizziness, lightheadedness, and incoordination on next day; dependence; rarely urticaria and rashes; hallucinations, amnesia, and behavioural disturbances (including aggression) reported

Dose: 7.5 mg at bedtime increased to 15 mg in severe insomnia; ELDERLY initially 3.75 mg at bedtime; CHILD not recommended

PoM **Zopiclone** (Non-proprietary)

Tablets, zopiclone 7.5 mg. Label: 19
Available from Lagap

PoM **Zimovane®** (Rhône-Poulenc Rorer)

Tablets, f/c, scored, zopiclone 7.5 mg. Net price 28-tab pack = £4.48. Label: 19

4.1.2 Anxiolytics

Benzodiazepine anxiolytics can be effective in alleviating definite anxiety states and they are widely prescribed. Although there has been a tendency to prescribe these drugs to almost anyone with stress-related symptoms, unhappiness, or minor physical disease, their use in many situations is unjustified. In particular, they should not be used to treat depression, phobic or obsessional states, or chronic psychosis. In bereavement, psychological adjustment may be inhibited by benzodiazepines. In children anxiolytic treatment should be used only to relieve acute anxiety (and related insomnia) caused by fear e.g. before surgery.

Anxiolytic treatment should be limited to the lowest possible dose for the shortest possible time (see CSM advice, section 4.1). Dependence is particularly likely in patients with a history of alcohol or drug abuse and in patients with marked personality disorders.

Anxiolytics, particularly the benzodiazepines, have been termed 'minor tranquillisers'. This term is misleading because not only do they differ markedly from the antipsychotic drugs ('major tranquillisers') but their use is by no means minor. Antipsychotics, in low doses, are also sometimes used in severe anxiety for their sedative action but long-term use should be avoided in view of a possible risk of tardive dyskinesia (section 4.2.1).

BENZODIAZEPINES

Benzodiazepines are indicated for the short-term relief of severe anxiety but long-term use should be avoided (see notes above). Diazepam, alprazolam, bromazepam, chlordiazepoxide, clobazam, and clorazepate have a sustained action. Shorter-acting compounds such as **lorazepam** and **oxazepam** may be preferred in patients with hepatic impairment but they carry a greater risk of withdrawal symptoms.

Diazepam or lorazepam are very occasionally administered intravenously for the control of panic attacks. This route is the most rapid but the procedure is not without risk (section 4.8.2) and should be used only when alternative measures have failed. The intramuscular route has no advantage over the oral route.

For guidelines on benzodiazepine withdrawal, see section 4.1.

DIAZEPAM

Indications: short-term use in anxiety or insomnia, adjunct in acute alcohol withdrawal; status epilepticus and febrile convulsions see sections 4.8.2 and 4.8.3; muscle spasm see section 10.2.2; peri-operative use see section 15.1.4.1

Cautions: respiratory disease, muscle weakness, history of drug or alcohol abuse, marked personality disorder, pregnancy and breast-feeding (see Appendixes 4 and 5); reduce dose in elderly and debilitated, and in hepatic and renal impairment; avoid prolonged use (and abrupt withdrawal thereafter); special precautions for intravenous injection (section 4.8.2); porphyria (see section 9.8.2); **interactions:** Appendix 1 (benzodiazepines)

DRIVING. Drowsiness may affect performance of skilled tasks (e.g. driving); effects of alcohol enhanced

Contra-indications: respiratory depression; acute pulmonary insufficiency; not for phobic or obsessional states, not for chronic psychosis; should not be used alone in depression or in anxiety with depression

Side-effects: drowsiness and lightheadedness the next day; confusion and ataxia (especially in the elderly); amnesia may occur; dependence; paradoxical increase in aggression (see also section 4.1); *occasionally:* headache, vertigo, hypotension, salivation changes, gastro-intestinal disturbances, rashes, visual disturbances, changes in libido, urinary retention; blood disorders and jaundice reported; on intravenous injection, pain, thrombophlebitis, and rarely apnoea or hypotension; overdosage: see Emergency Treatment of Poisoning, p. 22

Dose: by mouth, anxiety, 2 mg 3 times daily increased if necessary to 15–30 mg daily in divided doses; ELDERLY (or debilitated) half adult dose

Insomnia associated with anxiety, 5–15 mg at bedtime

CHILD night terrors and somnambulism, 1–5 mg at bedtime

By intramuscular injection or slow intravenous injection (into a large vein, at a rate of not more than 5 mg/minute), for severe acute anxiety, control of acute panic attacks, and acute alcohol withdrawal, 10 mg, repeated if necessary after not less than 4 hours

Note. Only use intramuscular route when oral and intravenous routes not possible; special precautions for intravenous injection see section 4.8.2

By intravenous infusion—section 4.8.2

By rectum as rectal solution, for acute anxiety and agitation, 10 mg (elderly 5 mg), repeated after 5 minutes if necessary

CHILD febrile convulsions, see p.201

By rectum as suppositories for anxiety when oral route not appropriate, 10–30 mg (higher dose divided); dose form not appropriate for less than 10 mg

PoM Diazepam (Non-proprietary)

Tablets, diazepam 2 mg, net price 20 = 5p; 5 mg, 20 = 6p; 10 mg, 20 = 11p. Label: 2 *or* 19

Available from APS, Berk (NHS Atensine®), Cox, DDSA (NHS Tensium®), K Pharm., Rima (NHS Rimapam®), Roche (NHS Valium®)

Oral solution, diazepam 2 mg/5 mL, net price 100 mL = £1.85. Label: 2 *or* 19

Available from Cox, Lagap (NHS Dialar®), Roche (NHS Valium®)

NHS *Strong oral solution,* diazepam 5 mg/5 mL, net price 100-mL pack = £3.30. Label: 2 *or* 19

Available from Lagap (NHS Dialar®)

Injection (solution), diazepam 5 mg/mL. Do not dilute (except for intravenous infusion). Net price 2-mL amp = 31p

Available from CP, Roche (Valium®)

Injection (emulsion), diazepam 5 mg/mL. For intravenous injection or infusion. Net price 2-mL amp = 76p

Available from Dumex (Diazemuls®)

Rectal tubes (= rectal solution), diazepam 2 mg/mL, net price 2.5-mL (5-mg) tube = £1.28; 4 mg/mL, 2.5-mL (10-mg) tube = £1.63

Available from CP (Diazepam Rectubes®), Dumex (Stesolid®), Lagap

Suppositories, diazepam 10 mg, net price 5 = £5.42. Label: 2 *or* 19

Available from Sinclair (Valclair®)

ALPRAZOLAM

Indications: anxiety (short-term use)

Cautions; Contra-indications; Side-effects: see under Diazepam

Dose: 250–500 micrograms 3 times daily (elderly or debilitated 250 micrograms 2–3 times daily), increased if necessary to a total of 3 mg daily; CHILD not recommended

NHS PoM **Xanax®** (Upjohn)

Tablets, both scored, alprazolam 250 micrograms, net price 60-tab pack = £2.75; 500 micrograms (pink), 60-tab pack = £5.27. Label: 2

BROMAZEPAM

Indications: anxiety (short-term use)

Cautions; Contra-indications; Side-effects: see under Diazepam

Dose: 3–18 mg daily in divided doses; ELDERLY (or debilitated) half adult dose; max. (in exceptional circumstances in hospitalised patients) 60 mg daily in divided doses; CHILD not recommended

NHS PoM **Lexotan®** (Roche)

Tablets, both scored, bromazepam 1.5 mg (lilac), net price 60-tab pack = £5.36; 3 mg (pink), 60-tab pack = £6.79. Label: 2

CHLORDIAZEPOXIDE

Indications: anxiety (short-term use), adjunct in acute alcohol withdrawal

Cautions; Contra-indications; Side-effects: see under Diazepam

Dose: anxiety, 10 mg 3 times daily increased if necessary to 60–100 mg daily in divided doses; ELDERLY (or debilitated) half adult dose; CHILD not recommended

Note. The doses stated above refer equally to chlordiazepoxide and to its hydrochloride

PoM Chlordiazepoxide Capsules, chlordiazepoxide hydrochloride 5 mg, net price 20 = 31p; 10 mg, 20 = 37p. Label: 2

Various strengths available from APS, Cox, CP, DDSA (NHS Tropium®), K Pharm., Lagap, Norton, Roche (NHS Librium®)

PoM Chlordiazepoxide Hydrochloride Tablets, chlordiazepoxide hydrochloride 5 mg, net price 20 = 20p; 10 mg, 20 = 22p; 25 mg, 20 = 44p. Label: 2

PoM Chlordiazepoxide Tablets, chlordiazepoxide 5 mg, net price 20 = 28p; 10 mg, 20 = 35p; 25 mg, 20 = 78p. Label: 2

Available from Roche (NHS Librium®)

CLOBAZAM

Indications: anxiety (short-term use); adjunct in epilepsy

Cautions; Contra-indications; Side-effects: see under Diazepam

Dose: anxiety, 20–30 mg daily in divided doses or as a single dose at bedtime, increased in severe anxiety (in hospital patients) to a max. of 60 mg daily in divided doses; ELDERLY (or debilitated) 10–20 mg daily

Epilepsy, 20–30 mg daily; max. 60 mg daily; CHILD over 3 years, not more than half adult dose

NHS PoM¹ **Clobazam** (Non-proprietary)

Capsules, clobazam 10 mg. Net price 30-cap pack = £3.96. Label: 2 *or* 19

1. except for epilepsy and endorsed 'SLS' ('S2B' in Scotland)

Note. The brand name NHS Frisium® (Hoechst) is used for clobazam capsules

CLORAZEPATE DIPOTASSIUM

Indications: anxiety (short-term use)

Cautions; Contra-indications; Side-effects: see under Diazepam

Dose: 7.5–22.5 mg daily in 2–3 divided doses *or* a single dose of 15 mg at bedtime; ELDERLY (or debilitated) half adult dose; CHILD not recommended

NHS PoM **Tranxene®** (Boehringer Ingelheim)

Capsules, clorazepate dipotassium 7.5 mg (maroon/grey), net price 20-cap pack = £2.66; 15 mg (pink/grey), 20-cap pack = £2.78. Label: 2 *or* 19

LORAZEPAM

Indications: short-term use in anxiety or insomnia; status epilepticus (section 4.8.2); peri-operative (section 15.1.4.1)

Cautions; Contra-indications; Side-effects: see under Diazepam; short acting

Dose: by mouth, anxiety, 1–4 mg daily in divided doses; ELDERLY (or debilitated) half adult dose
Insomnia associated with anxiety, 1–2 mg at bedtime; CHILD not recommended

By intramuscular or slow intravenous injection (into a large vein), acute panic attacks, 25–30 micrograms/kg, repeated every 6 hours if necessary; CHILD not recommended

Note. Only use intramuscular route when oral and intravenous routes not possible

PoM **Lorazepam** (Non-proprietary)

Tablets, lorazepam 1 mg, net price 20 – 21p; 2.5 mg, 20 = 28p. Label: 2 *or* 19

Available from APS, Cox, CP, K Pharm., Lagap, Norton, Wyeth (NHS Ativan®)

Injection, lorazepam 4 mg/mL. Net price 1-mL amp = 40p

For intramuscular injection it should be diluted with an equal volume of water for injections or physiological saline (but only use when oral and intravenous routes not possible)

Available from Wyeth (Ativan®)

OXAZEPAM

Indications: anxiety (short-term use)

Cautions; Contra-indications; Side-effects: see under Diazepam; short acting

Dose: anxiety, 15–30 mg (elderly or debilitated 10–20 mg) 3–4 times daily; CHILD not recommended

Insomnia associated with anxiety, 15–25 mg (max. 50 mg) at bedtime; CHILD not recommended

PoM **Oxazepam** (Non-proprietary)

Tablets, oxazepam 10 mg, net price 20 = 22p; 15 mg, 20 = 24p; 30 mg, 20 = 30p. Label: 2

Available from most generic manufacturers

OTHER DRUGS FOR ANXIETY

Buspirone is thought to act at specific serotonin ($5HT_{1A}$) receptors. Response to treatment may take up to 2 weeks. It does not alleviate the symptoms of benzodiazepine withdrawal. Therefore a patient taking a benzodiazepine still needs to have the benzodiazepine withdrawn gradually; it is advisable to do this before starting buspirone. The dependence and abuse liability of buspirone has not yet been established.

Meprobamate is **less effective** than the benzodiazepines, more hazardous in overdosage, and can also induce dependence.

Beta-blockers (e.g. propranolol, oxprenolol) (see section 2.4) do not affect psychological symptoms, such as worry, tension, and fear, but they do reduce autonomic symptoms, such as palpitations, sweating, and tremor; they do not reduce non-autonomic symptoms, such as muscle tension. Beta-blockers are therefore indicated for patients with predominantly somatic symptoms; this, in turn, may prevent the onset of worry and fear. Patients with predominantly psychological symptoms may obtain no benefit.

BUSPIRONE HYDROCHLORIDE

Indications: anxiety (short-term use)

Cautions: does not alleviate benzodiazepine withdrawal (see notes above); history of hepatic or renal impairment; **interactions:** Appendix 1 (buspirone)

DRIVING. May affect performance of skilled tasks (e.g. driving); effects of alcohol may be enhanced

Contra-indications: epilepsy, severe hepatic or renal impairment, pregnancy and breast-feeding

Side-effects: nausea, dizziness, headache, nervousness, lightheadedness, excitement; rarely tachycardia, palpitations, chest pain, drowsiness, confusion, dry mouth, fatigue, and sweating

Dose: initially 5 mg 2–3 times daily, increased as necessary every 2–3 days; usual range 15–30 mg daily in divided doses; max. 45 mg daily (30 mg in elderly); CHILD not recommended

PoM **Buspar®** (Bristol-Myers)

Tablets, buspirone hydrochloride 5 mg, net price 126-tab pack = £39.31; 10 mg, 100-tab pack = £46.80. Counselling, driving

CHLORMEZANONE

Indications: short-term use in anxiety or insomnia; muscle spasm (but see section 10.2.2)

Cautions: respiratory disease, muscle weakness, history of drug or alcohol abuse, marked personality disorder, pregnancy, breast-feeding; reduce dose in elderly and debilitated, and in hepatic and renal impairment; avoid prolonged use (and abrupt withdrawal thereafter); porphyria (see section 9.8.2); **interactions:** Appendix 1 (chlormezanone)

DRIVING. Drowsiness may persist the next day and affect performance of skilled tasks (e.g. driving); effects of alcohol enhanced

Contra-indications: acute pulmonary insufficiency; respiratory depression

Side-effects: drowsiness and lethargy, dizziness, nausea, headache, dry mouth, rashes, dependence; cholestatic jaundice reported

Dose: 200 mg 3–4 times daily *or* 400 mg at bedtime; elderly patients half adult dose; CHILD not recommended

PoM **Trancopal**® (Sanofi Winthrop)

Tablets, yellow, chlormezanone 200 mg. Net price 60-tab pack = £1.50. Label: 2 *or* 19

HYDROXYZINE HYDROCHLORIDE

See section 3.4.1

MEPROBAMATE

Indications: short-term use in anxiety, but see notes above

Cautions: respiratory disease, muscle weakness, epilepsy (may induce seizures), history of drug or alcohol abuse, marked personality disorder, pregnancy; elderly and debilitated; hepatic and renal impairment; avoid prolonged use, abrupt withdrawal may precipitate convulsions; **interactions:** Appendix 1 (meprobamate)

DRIVING. Drowsiness may affect performance of skilled tasks (e.g. driving); effects of alcohol enhanced

Contra-indications: acute pulmonary insufficiency; respiratory depression; porphyria (see section 9.8.2); breast-feeding

Side-effects: see under Diazepam, but the incidence is greater and drowsiness is the most common side-effect. Also gastro-intestinal disturbances, hypotension, paraesthesia, weakness, CNS effects which include headache, paradoxical excitement, disturbances of vision; rarely agranulocytosis and rashes

Dose: 400 mg 3–4 times daily; elderly patients half adult dose or less; CHILD not recommended

CD **Equanil**® (Wyeth)

Tablets, meprobamate 200 mg, net price 20 = 15p; 400 mg (scored), 20 = 22p. Label: 2

CD **Equagesic**®

Section 4.7.1

4.1.3   Barbiturates

The intermediate-acting **barbiturates** only have a place in the treatment of severe intractable insomnia in patients already taking barbiturates; they should be avoided in the elderly. The long-acting barbiturates, phenobarbitone and methylphenobarbitone, are still sometimes of value in epilepsy (section 4.8.1) but their use as sedatives is unjustified. The very short-acting barbiturates, methohexitone and thiopentone, are used in anaesthesia (see section 15.1.1).

BARBITURATES

Indications: severe intractable insomnia in patients already taking barbiturates; see also notes above

Cautions: avoid use where possible; dependence and tolerance readily occur; abrupt withdrawal may precipitate a serious withdrawal syndrome (rebound insomnia, anxiety, tremor, dizziness, nausea, convulsions, delirium, and death); repeated doses are cumulative and may lead to excessive sedation; caution in respiratory disease, renal disease, hepatic impairment; **interactions:** Appendix 1 (barbiturates and primidone)

DRIVING. Drowsiness may persist the next day and affect performance of skilled tasks (e.g. driving); effects of alcohol enhanced

Contra-indications: insomnia caused by pain; porphyria (see section 9.8.2), pregnancy, breast-feeding; avoid in children, young adults, elderly and debilitated patients, also patients with a history of drug or alcohol abuse-

Side-effects: include hangover with drowsiness, dizziness, ataxia, respiratory depression, hypersensitivity reactions, headache, particularly in elderly; paradoxical excitement and confusion occasionally precede sleep; overdosage: see Emergency Treatment of Poisoning, p.22

Dose: see under preparations below

CD **Amytal**® (Lilly)

Tablets, amylobarbitone 50 mg, net price 20 = 39p. Label: 19

Dose: 100–200 mg at bedtime (see also contra-indications)

CD **Sodium Amytal**® (Lilly)

Capsules, both blue, amylobarbitone sodium 60 mg, net price 20 = 63p; 200 mg, 20 = £1.25. Label: 19

Dose: 60–200 mg at bedtime (see also contra-indications)

Injection, powder for reconstitution, amylobarbitone sodium. Net price 500-mg vial = £13.75. For specialised use in procedures in **expert epilepsy centres only**

Dose: by deep intramuscular injection into large muscle, preferably gluteal, (max. 5 mL at any one site) or by slow intravenous injection (max. 50 mg/minute), 0.25–1 g; max. single dose, intramuscular 500 mg, intravenous 1 g

CD **Soneryl**® (Rhône-Poulenc Rorer)

Tablets, pink, scored, butobarbitone 100 mg. Net price 56-tab pack = 71p. Label: 19

Dose: 100–200 mg at bedtime (see also contra-indications)

Quinalbarbitone

Note. Quinalbarbitone has been transferred from schedule 3 to schedule 2 of the Misuse of Drugs Regulations 1985; receipt and supply must therefore be recorded in the CD register.

CD **Seconal Sodium**® (Lilly)

Capsules, both orange, quinalbarbitone sodium 50 mg, net price 20 = £1.17; 100 mg, 20 = £1.77. Label: 19

Dose: 100 mg at bedtime (see also contra-indications)

CD **Tuinal**® (Lilly)

Capsules, orange/blue, a mixture of amylobarbitone sodium 50 mg, quinalbarbitone sodium 50 mg. Net price 20 = 74p. Label: 19

Dose: 1–2 capsules at bedtime (see also contra-indications)

Note. Prescriptions need only specify 'Tuinal capsules'

4.2 Drugs used in psychoses and related disorders

4.2.1 Antipsychotic drugs
4.2.2 Antipsychotic depot injections
4.2.3 Antimanic drugs

Advice of Royal College of Psychiatrists on doses above BNF upper limit[1]

1. Consider alternative approaches including adjuvant therapy and newer or atypical neuroleptics such as clozapine.
2. Bear in mind risk factors, including obesity— particular caution is indicated in older patients especially those over 70.
3. Consider potential for drug interactions—see **interactions:** Appendix 1 (phenothiazines and other antipsychotics).
4. Carry out ECG to exclude untoward abnormalities such as prolonged QT interval; repeat ECG periodically and reduce dose if prolonged QT interval or other adverse abnormality develops.
5. Increase dose slowly and not more often than once weekly.
6. Carry out regular pulse, blood pressure, and temperature checks; ensure that patient maintains adequate fluid intake.
7. Consider high-dose therapy to be for limited period and review regularly; abandon if no improvement after 3 months (return to standard dosage).

Important: When prescribing an antipsychotic for administration on an emergency basis it must be borne in mind that the intramuscular dose should be lower than the corresponding oral dose (owing to absence of first-pass effect), particularly if the patient is very active (increased blood flow to muscle considerably increases the rate of absorption). The prescription should specify the dose in the context of **each route** and **not** imply that the same dose can be given by mouth or by intramuscular injection. The dose should be reviewed **daily**

1. Unless otherwise stated, doses in the BNF are licensed doses—any higher dose is therefore unlicensed (for an explanation of the significance of this, see p.2).

4.2.1 Antipsychotic drugs

Antipsychotic drugs are also known as 'neuroleptics' and (misleadingly) as 'major tranquillisers'. Antipsychotic drugs generally tranquillise without impairing consciousness and without causing paradoxical excitement but they should not be regarded merely as tranquillisers. For conditions such as schizophrenia the tranquillising effect is of secondary importance.

In the short term they are used to quieten disturbed patients whatever the underlying psychopathology, which may be brain damage, mania, toxic delirium, agitated depression, or acute behavioural disturbance.

They are used to alleviate severe anxiety but this too should be a short-term measure. Some antipsychotic drugs (e.g. chlorpromazine, thioridazine, flupenthixol) also have an antidepressant effect while others may exacerbate depression (e.g. fluphenazine, pimozide, pipothiazine).

SCHIZOPHRENIA. Antipsychotic drugs relieve florid psychotic symptoms such as thought disorder, hallucinations, and delusions, and prevent relapse. Although they are usually less effective in apathetic withdrawn patients, they sometimes appear to have an activating influence. For example, chlorpromazine may restore an acutely ill schizophrenic to normal activity and social behaviour who was previously withdrawn or even mute and akinetic. Patients with acute schizophrenia generally respond better than those with chronic symptoms.

Long-term treatment of a patient with a definite diagnosis of schizophrenia may be necessary even after the first episode of illness in order to prevent the manifest illness from becoming chronic. Withdrawal of drug treatment requires careful surveillance because the patient who appears well on medication may suffer a disastrous relapse if treatment is withdrawn inappropriately. In addition the need for continuation of treatment may not become immediately evident because relapse is often delayed for several weeks after cessation of treatment.

Antipsychotic drugs are considered to act by interfering with dopaminergic transmission in the brain by blocking dopamine receptors and may give rise to the extrapyramidal effects described below, and also to hyperprolactinaemia. Antipsychotic drugs also affect cholinergic, alpha-adrenergic, histaminergic, and serotonergic receptors.

SIDE-EFFECTS. Extrapyramidal symptoms are the most troublesome. They are caused most frequently by the piperazine phenothiazines (fluphenazine, perphenazine, prochlorperazine, and trifluoperazine), the butyrophenones (benperidol, droperidol, haloperidol, and trifluperidol), and the depot preparations. They are easy to recognise but cannot be accurately predicted because they depend partly on the dose and partly on the type of drug, and on patient susceptibility. They consist of *parkinsonian symptoms* (including tremor) which may occur gradually, *dystonia* (abnormal face and body movements) which may appear after only a few doses, *akathisia* (restlessness) which may resemble an exacerbation of the condition being treated, and *tardive dyskinesia* (which usually takes longer to develop).

Parkinsonian symptoms remit if the drug is withdrawn and may be suppressed by the administration of **antimuscarinic** drugs (section 4.9.2). Routine administration of such drugs is **not** justified as not all patients are affected and because tardive dyskinesia may be unmasked or worsened by them. Furthermore, these drugs are sometimes abused for their mood-altering effects. Tardive dyskinesia is of particular concern because it may be irreversible on withdrawing therapy and treatment may be ineffective. It occurs fairly frequently in patients (especially the elderly) on long-term therapy and with high dosage, and the treatment of such patients must be carefully and regularly reviewed. Tardive dyskinesia may also occur occasionally after short-term treatment with low dosage.

Cautionary label wordings, see inside back cover

Prices are **net**, see p.1

Hypotension and *interference with temperature regulation* are dose-related side-effects and are liable to cause dangerous falls and hypothermia in the elderly; very serious consideration should be given before prescribing these drugs for patients over 70 years of age.

Neuroleptic malignant syndrome (hyperthermia, fluctuating level of consciousness, muscular rigidity and autonomic dysfunction with pallor, tachycardia, labile blood pressure, sweating, and urinary incontinence) is a rare but potentially fatal side-effect of some drugs. Drugs for which it has been reported in the UK include haloperidol, chlorpromazine, and flupenthixol decanoate. Discontinuation of drug therapy is essential as there is no proven effective treatment but bromocriptine and dantrolene have been used. The syndrome, which usually lasts for 5–10 days after drug discontinuation, may be unduly prolonged if depot preparations have been used.

Overdosage: see Emergency Treatment of Poisoning, p.23.

CLASSIFICATION OF ANTIPSYCHOTICS. The **phenothiazine** derivatives can be divided into 3 main groups.

Group 1: chlorpromazine, methotrimeprazine, and promazine, generally characterised by pronounced sedative effects and moderate antimuscarinic and extrapyramidal side-effects.

Group 2: pericyazine, pipothiazine, and thioridazine, generally characterised by moderate sedative effects, marked antimuscarinic effects, but fewer extrapyramidal side-effects than groups 1 or 3.

Group 3: fluphenazine, perphenazine, prochlorperazine, and trifluoperazine, generally characterised by fewer sedative effects, fewer antimuscarinic effects, but more pronounced extrapyramidal side-effects than groups 1 and 2.

Drugs of other chemical groups tend to resemble the phenothiazines of *group 3*. They include the **butyrophenones** (benperidol, droperidol, haloperidol, and trifluperidol); **diphenylbutylpiperidines** (fluspirilene and pimozide); **thioxanthenes** (flupenthixol and zuclopenthixol); **substituted benzamides** (sulpiride); **oxypertine**; and **loxapine**. **Clozapine** differs in that it is sedative with fewer extrapyramidal effects.

CHOICE. As indicated above, the various drugs differ somewhat in predominant actions and side-effects. Selection is influenced by the degree of sedation required and the patient's susceptibility to extrapyramidal side-effects. However, the differences between antipsychotic drugs are less important than the great variability in patient response; moreover, tolerance to these secondary effects usually develops.

Prescribing of more than one antipsychotic at the same time is **not** recommended; it may constitute a

hazard and there is no significant evidence that side-effects are minimised.

Chlorpromazine is widely used. It has a marked sedating effect and is particularly useful for treating violent patients without causing stupor. Agitated states in the elderly can be controlled without confusion, a dose of 10 to 25 mg once or twice daily usually being adequate.

Flupenthixol and **pimozide** (see CSM advice p.156) are less sedating than chlorpromazine.

Sulpiride in high doses controls florid positive symptoms, but in lower doses it has an alerting effect on apathetic withdrawn schizophrenics.

Fluphenazine, haloperidol, and **trifluoperazine** are also of value but their use is limited by the high incidence of extrapyramidal symptoms. Haloperidol may be preferred for the rapid control of hyperactive psychotic states.

Thioridazine is popular for treating the elderly as there is a reduced incidence of extrapyramidal symptoms.

Promazine is not sufficiently active by mouth to be used as an antipsychotic drug.

Clozapine is indicated only for the treatment of schizophrenia in patients unresponsive to, or intolerant of, conventional antipsychotic drugs. It is less likely to cause tardive dyskinesia but as it can cause agranulocytosis, its use is restricted to patients registered with the Clozaril Patient Monitoring Service (see under Clozapine, below).

Loxapine causes relatively little sedation; in overdosage it has a high potential for serious neurological and cardiac toxicity.

Risperidone, a recently introduced antipsychotic drug, is a benzisoxazole derivative.

OTHER USES. Nausea and vomiting (section 4.6), choreas, motor tics (section 4.9.3), and intractable hiccup (see under Chlorpromazine Hydrochloride and under Haloperidol). **Benperidol** is used in deviant antisocial sexual behaviour but its value is not established.

Equivalent doses of oral antipsychotics
These equivalences are intended **only** as an approximate guide; individual dosage instructions should **also** be checked; patients should be carefully monitored after **any** change in medication

Antipsychotic	Daily dose
Chlorpromazine	100 mg
Clozapine	50 mg
Haloperidol	2–3 mg[1]
Loxapine	10–20 mg
Pimozide	2 mg[2]
Sulpiride	200 mg
Thioridazine	100 mg
Trifluoperazine	5 mg

1. In specialist psychiatric units where very high doses are required the equivalent dose of haloperidol might be up to 10 mg
2. See also the CSM warning concerning pimozide dose, p.156

IMPORTANT. These equivalences must **not** be extrapolated beyond the max. dose for the drug.

WITHDRAWAL. Withdrawal of antipsychotic drugs after long-term therapy should always be gradual and closely monitored to avoid the risk of acute withdrawal syndromes or rapid relapse.

DOSAGE. After an initial period of stabilisation, in most patients, the long half-life of antipsychotic drugs allows the total daily oral dose to be given as a single dose. For the advice of The Royal College of Psychiatrists on doses above the BNF upper limit, see p.151.

CHLORPROMAZINE HYDROCHLORIDE

WARNING. Owing to the risk of contact sensitisation, pharmacists, nurses, and other health workers should avoid direct contact with chlorpromazine; tablets should not be crushed and solutions should be handled with care

Indications: see under Dose; antiemetic (in terminal illness), section 4.6; peri-operative use, see section 15.1.4.1

Cautions: cardiovascular and cerebrovascular disease, respiratory disease, parkinsonism, epilepsy, acute infections, pregnancy, breast-feeding, renal and hepatic impairment (avoid if severe), history of jaundice, leucopenia (blood counts if unexplained infections); hypothyroidism, myasthenia gravis, prostatic hypertrophy, closed-angle glaucoma; caution in elderly particularly in very hot or very cold weather; avoid abrupt withdrawal; patients should remain supine for 30 minutes after intramuscular injection; **interactions:** Appendix 1 (phenothiazines and other antipsychotics)

DRIVING. Drowsiness may affect performance of skilled tasks (e.g. driving); effects of alcohol enhanced

Contra-indications: coma caused by CNS depressants; bone-marrow depression; avoid in phaeochromocytoma

Side-effects: extrapyramidal symptoms (reversed by dose reduction or antimuscarinic drugs) and, on prolonged administration, occasionally tardive dyskinesia; hypothermia (occasionally pyrexia), drowsiness, apathy, pallor, nightmares, insomnia, depression, and, more rarely, agitation, EEG changes, convulsions; antimuscarinic symptoms such as dry mouth, nasal congestion, constipation, difficulty with micturition, and blurred vision; cardiovascular symptoms such as hypotension, tachycardia, and arrhythmias; ECG changes; endocrine effects such as menstrual disturbances, galactorrhoea, gynaecomastia, impotence, and weight gain; sensitivity reactions such as agranulocytosis, leucopenia, leucocytosis, and haemolytic anaemia, photosensitisation (more common with chlorpromazine than with other antipsychotics), contact sensitisation and rashes, jaundice (including cholestatic) and alterations in liver function; neuroleptic malignant syndrome; lupus erythematosus-like syndrome reported; with prolonged high dosage, corneal and lens opacities and purplish pigmentation of the skin, cornea, conjunctiva, and retina; intramuscular injection may be painful, cause hypotension and tachycardia (see Cautions), and give rise to nodule formation; overdosage: see Poisoning, p.23

Dose: by mouth,
Schizophrenia and other psychoses, mania, short-term adjunctive management of severe anxiety, psychomotor agitation, excitement, and violent or dangerously impulsive behaviour initially 25 mg 3 times daily (*or* 75 mg at night), adjusted according to response, to usual maintenance dose of 75–300 mg daily (but up to 1 g daily may be required in psychoses); ELDERLY (or debilitated) third to half adult dose; CHILD (childhood schizophrenia and autism) 1–5 years 500 micrograms/kg every 4–6 hours (max. 40 mg daily); 6–12 years third to half adult dose (max. 75 mg daily)

Intractable hiccup, 25–50 mg 3–4 times daily

By deep intramuscular injection, (for relief of acute symptoms), 25–50 mg every 6–8 hours; CHILD, as dose by mouth

By rectum in suppositories as chlorpromazine base 100 mg every 6–8 hours [unlicensed]

Note. For equivalent therapeutic effect 100 mg chlorpromazine base given *rectally* as a suppository ≡ 20–25 mg chlorpromazine hydrochloride *by intramuscular injection* ≡ 40–50 mg of chlorpromazine base or hydrochloride *by mouth*

PoM Chlorpromazine (Non-proprietary)
Tablets, coated, chlorpromazine hydrochloride 10 mg, net price 20 = 11p; 25 mg, 20 = 17p; 50 mg, 20 = 37p; 100 mg, 20 = 76p. Label: 2
Available from APS, DDSA (Chloractil®), Hillcross, Norton

Elixir, chlorpromazine hydrochloride 25 mg/5 mL. Net price 100 mL = 58p. Label: 2

Injection, chlorpromazine hydrochloride 25 mg/mL, net price 1-mL amp = 24p; 2-mL amp = 28p

Suppositories, chlorpromazine 100 mg. Label: 2
'Special order' [unlicensed] product; contact Penn or regional hospital manufacturing unit

PoM Largactil® (Rhône-Poulenc Rorer)
Tablets, all off-white, f/c, chlorpromazine hydrochloride 10 mg. Net price 56-tab pack = 32p; 25 mg, 56-tab pack = 49p; 50 mg, 56-tab pack = £1.13; 100 mg, 56 tab pack = £2.10. Label: 2

Syrup, brown, chlorpromazine hydrochloride 25 mg/5 mL. Net price 100-mL pack = 58p. Label: 2

Suspension forte, orange, sugar-free, chlorpromazine hydrochloride 100 mg (as embonate)/5 mL. Net price 100-mL pack = £1.16. Label: 2

Injection, chlorpromazine hydrochloride 25 mg/mL. Net price 2-mL amp = 27p

BENPERIDOL

Indications: control of deviant antisocial sexual behaviour (but see notes above)

Cautions; Contra-indications; Side-effects: see under Haloperidol

Dose: 0.25–1.5 mg daily in divided doses, adjusted according to the response; ELDERLY (or debilitated) initially half adult dose; CHILD not recommended

PoM Anquil® (Janssen)
Tablets, benperidol 250 micrograms. Net price 20 = £5.23. Label: 2

CLOZAPINE

Indications: schizophrenia in patients unresponsive to, or intolerant of, conventional antipsychotic drugs

Cautions: see under Chlorpromazine Hydrochloride; initiation must be in hospital in-patients, and leucocyte and differential blood counts must be normal before treatment and must be monitored weekly for first 18 weeks then at least fortnightly; avoid drugs which depress leucopoiesis such as co-trimoxazole and carbamazepine (and taper off conventional neuroleptic before starting); withdraw treatment if leucocyte count falls below 3000/mm³ or absolute neutrophil count falls below 1500/mm³; patients should report any infections; **interactions**: Appendix 1 (clozapine)

WITHDRAWAL. On planned withdrawal reduce dose gradually over 1–2 weeks to avoid risk of rebound psychosis. If abrupt withdrawal necessary observe patient carefully

Contra-indications: history of drug-induced neutropenia/agranulocytosis; bone marrow disorders; alcoholic and toxic psychoses; history of circulatory collapse or paralytic ileus; drug intoxication; coma or severe CNS depression; pregnancy and breast-feeding

Side-effects: see under Chlorpromazine Hydrochloride but more sedating and high incidence of antimuscarinic symptoms; extrapyramidal symptoms may occur less frequently; neutropenia and potentially fatal agranulocytosis, headache and dizziness, hypersalivation, urinary incontinence, priapism, pericarditis and myocarditis, and delirium; rarely circulatory collapse (but hypertension also reported), also nausea and vomiting

Dose: (close medical supervision on initiation—risk of collapse due to hypotension) 12.5 mg once or twice on first day then 25–50 mg on second day then slowly increased (if well tolerated) in steps of 25–50 mg over 14–21 days to 300 mg daily in divided doses (larger dose at night, up to 200 mg daily may be taken as a single dose at bedtime); if necessary may be further increased in steps of 50–100 mg once (preferably) or twice weekly; usual antipsychotic dose 200–450 mg daily (max. 900 mg daily); subsequent adjustment to usual maintenance of 150–300 mg; CHILD not recommended

ELDERLY AND SPECIAL RISK GROUPS. In *elderly*, 12.5 mg once on first day—subsequent adjustments restricted to 25 mg daily; in *cardiovascular disease, hepatic* or *renal impairment* or if history of *epilepsy*, 12.5 mg on first day—subsequent adjustments slowly and in small steps (if epileptic seizures (see also Cautions), suspend for 24 hours and resume at lower dose); *restarting* after *interval of more than 2 days*, 12.5 mg once or twice on first day (but may be feasible to increase more quickly than on initiation)

PoM **Clozaril®** (Sandoz)
Tablets, both yellow, scored, clozapine 25 mg, net price 84-tab pack = £37.54; 100 mg, 84-tab pack = £150.15 (hosp. only). Label: 2, 10 patient information leaflet
Note. Patient, prescriber, and supplying pharmacist must be registered with the Sandoz Clozaril Patient Monitoring Service—takes several days to do this

DROPERIDOL

Indications: see under Dose; peri-operative use, see section 15.1.4.1

Cautions; Contra-indications; Side-effects: see under Haloperidol

Dose: by mouth, tranquillisation and emergency control in mania, 5–20 mg repeated every 4–8 hours if necessary (elderly, initially half adult dose); CHILD, 0.5–1 mg daily

By intramuscular injection, up to 10 mg repeated every 4–6 hours if necessary (elderly, initially half adult dose); CHILD, 0.5–1 mg daily

By intravenous injection, 5–15 mg repeated every 4–6 hours if necessary (elderly, initially half adult dose)

Cancer chemotherapy-induced nausea and vomiting, *by intramuscular or intravenous injection,* 1–10 mg 30 minutes before starting therapy, followed by *continuous intravenous infusion* of 1–3 mg/hour *or* 1–5 mg *by intramuscular or intravenous injection* every 1–6 hours as necessary; CHILD *by intramuscular or intravenous injection,* 20–75 micrograms/kg

PoM **Droleptan®** (Janssen)
Tablets, yellow, scored, droperidol 10 mg. Net price 50-tab pack = £12.30. Label: 2
Oral liquid, sugar-free, droperidol 1 mg/mL. Net price 100-mL pack (with graduated cap) = £4.47; 500-mL pack = £21.25. Label: 2
Injection, droperidol 5 mg/mL. Net price 2-mL amp = 90p

FLUPENTHIXOL

(Flupentixol)

Indications: schizophrenia and other psychoses, particularly with apathy and withdrawal but not mania or psychomotor hyperactivity; depression, section 4.3.4

Cautions; Contra-indications; Side-effects: see under Chlorpromazine Hydrochloride but less sedating; extrapyramidal symptoms more frequent (25% of patients); avoid in senile confusional states, excitable and overactive patients; porphyria (see section 9.8.2)

Dose: initially 3–9 mg twice daily adjusted according to the response; max. 18 mg daily; ELDERLY (or debilitated) initially quarter to half adult dose; CHILD not recommended

PoM **Depixol®** (Lundbeck)
Tablets, yellow, s/c, flupenthixol 3 mg (as dihydrochloride). Net price 20 = £2.85. Label: 2
Depot injection (flupenthixol decanoate): section 4.2.2
PoM **Fluanxol®** (depression), see section 4.3.4

FLUPHENAZINE HYDROCHLORIDE

Indications: see under Dose

Cautions; Contra-indications; Side-effects: see under Chlorpromazine Hydrochloride, but less sedating and fewer antimuscarinic or hypotensive symptoms; extrapyramidal symptoms, particularly dystonic reactions and akathisia, are more frequent; avoid in depression

Dose: schizophrenia and other psychoses, mania, initially 2.5–10 mg daily in 2–3 divided doses, adjusted according to response to 20 mg daily; doses above 20 mg daily (10 mg in elderly) only with special caution; CHILD not recommended

Short-term adjunctive management of severe anxiety, psychomotor agitation, excitement, and violent or dangerously impulsive behaviour, initially 1 mg twice daily, increased as necessary to 2 mg twice daily; CHILD not recommended

PoM **Moditen**® (Sanofi Winthrop)

Tablets, all s/c, fluphenazine hydrochloride 1 mg (pink), net price 20 = £1.06; 2.5 mg (yellow), 20 = £1.33; 5 mg, 20 = £1.77. Label: 2

Depot injections (fluphenazine decanoate): section 4.2.2

HALOPERIDOL

Indications: see under Dose; motor tics, section 4.9.3

Cautions; Contra-indications; Side-effects: see under Chlorpromazine Hydrochloride but less sedating, and fewer antimuscarinic or hypotensive symptoms; pigmentation and photosensitivity reactions rare. Extrapyramidal symptoms, particularly dystonic reactions and akathisia are more frequent especially in thyrotoxic patients. Rarely weight loss. Avoid in basal ganglia disease

Dose: by mouth,

Schizophrenia and other psychoses, mania, short-term adjunctive management of psychomotor agitation, excitement, and violent or dangerously impulsive behaviour, initially 1.5–3 mg 2–3 times daily *or* 3–5 mg 2–3 times daily in severely affected or resistant patients; in resistant schizophrenia up to 100 mg (rarely 200 mg) daily may be needed; adjusted according to response to lowest effective maintenance dose (as low as 5–10 mg daily); ELDERLY (or debilitated) initially half adult dose; CHILD initially 25–50 micrograms/kg daily to a max. of 10 mg; adolescents up to 30 mg daily (exceptionally 60 mg)

Short-term adjunctive management of severe anxiety, adults 500 micrograms twice daily; CHILD not recommended

Intractable hiccup, 1.5 mg 3 times daily adjusted according to response; CHILD not recommended

By intramuscular injection, 2–10 mg, subsequent doses being given every 4–8 hours according to response (up to every hour if necessary); severely disturbed patients may require initial dose of up to 30 mg; CHILD not recommended

Nausea and vomiting, 1–2 mg

PoM **Haloperidol** (Non-proprietary)

Tablets, haloperidol 1.5 mg, net price 20 = 89p; 5 mg, 20 = £2.52; 10 mg, 20 = £4.71; 20 mg, 20 = £8.45. Label: 2

PoM **Dozic**® (RP Drugs)

Oral liquid, haloperidol 1 mg/mL, net price 100-mL pack (with pipette) = £5.00; 2 mg/mL, 100-mL pack (with pipette) = £5.10. Label: 2

PoM **Haldol**® (Janssen)

Tablets, both scored, haloperidol 5 mg (blue), net price 20 = £1.65; 10 mg (yellow), 20 = £3.21. Label: 2

Oral liquid, sugar-free, haloperidol 2 mg/mL. Net price 100-mL pack (with pipette) = £5.08. Label: 2

Oral liquid concentrate, sugar-free, haloperidol 10 mg/mL. Net price 100-mL pack = £22.27. Label: 2

Diluent purified water, freshly boiled and cooled, life of diluted concentrate 14 days. Alternatively, purified water, freshly boiled and cooled, containing 0.05% of methyl hydroxybenzoate and 0.005% of propyl hydroxybenzoate, life of diluted concentrate 2 months.

Injection, haloperidol 5 mg/mL. Net price 1-mL amp = 33p; 2-mL amp = 62p

Depot injection (haloperidol decanoate): section 4.2.2

PoM **Serenace**® (Baker Norton)

Capsules, green, haloperidol 500 micrograms. Net price 20 = 65p. Label: 2

Tablets, all scored, haloperidol 1.5 mg, net price 20 = £1.16; 5 mg (pink), 20 = £3.27; 10 mg (pale pink), 20 = £5.87; 20 mg (dark pink), 20 = £10.58. Label: 2

Oral liquid, sugar-free, haloperidol 2 mg/mL. Net price 100-mL pack = £8.77. Label: 2

Injection, haloperidol 5 mg/mL, net price 1-mL amp = 59p; 10 mg/mL, 2-mL amp = £2.03

LOXAPINE

Indications: acute and chronic psychoses

Cautions; Contra-indications: see under Chlorpromazine Hydrochloride; porphyria (see section 9.8.2)

Side-effects: see under Chlorpromazine Hydrochloride; nausea and vomiting, weight gain or loss, dyspnoea, ptosis, hyperpyrexia, flushing and headache, paraesthesia, and polydipsia also reported; no endocrine effects yet reported

Dose: initially 20–50 mg daily in 2 divided doses, increased as necessary over 7–10 days to 60–100 mg daily (max. 250 mg) in 2–4 divided doses, then adjusted to usual maintenance dose of 20–100 mg daily; CHILD not recommended

PoM **Loxapac**® (Novex)

Capsules, loxapine (as succinate) 10 mg (yellow/green), net price 100-cap pack = £9.52; 25 mg (light green/dark green), 100-cap pack = £19.05; 50 mg (blue/dark green), 100-cap pack = £34.27. Label: 2

METHOTRIMEPRAZINE

(Levomepromazine)

Indications: see under Dose

Cautions; Contra-indications; Side-effects: see under Chlorpromazine Hydrochloride but more sedating; risk of postural hypotension particularly in patients over 50 years

Dose: by mouth, schizophrenia, initially 25–50 mg daily in divided doses increased as necessary; bedpatients initially 100–200 mg daily usually in 3 divided doses, increased if necessary to 1 g daily

Adjunctive treatment in terminal care (including management of pain and associated restlessness, distress, or vomiting), 12.5–50 mg every 4–8 hours

By intramuscular injection or by intravenous injection (by intravenous injection after dilution with an equal volume of sodium chloride 0.9% injection), adjunct in terminal care, 12.5–25 mg (severe agitation up to 50 mg) every 6–8 hours if necessary

By continuous subcutaneous infusion, adjunct in terminal care (via syringe driver), 25–200 mg daily (over 24-hour period), diluted in a suitable volume of sodium chloride 0.9% injection

PoM Nozinan® (Link)
Tablets, scored, methotrimeprazine maleate 25 mg. Net price 20 = £3.00. Label: 2
Injection, methotrimeprazine hydrochloride 25 mg/mL. Net price 1-mL amp = £1.75

OXYPERTINE

Indications: see under Dose

Cautions; Contra-indications; Side-effects: see under Chlorpromazine Hydrochloride, but extrapyramidal symptoms may occur less frequently. With low doses agitation and hyperactivity occur and with high doses sedation. Occasionally photophobia may occur

Dose: schizophrenia and other psychoses, mania, short-term adjunctive management of psychomotor agitation, excitement, and violent or dangerously impulsive behaviour, initially 80–120 mg daily in divided doses adjusted according to the response; max. 300 mg daily; CHILD not recommended

Short-term adjunctive management of severe anxiety, initially 10 mg 3–4 times daily preferably after food; max. 60 mg daily; CHILD not recommended

PoM Oxypertine (Sterwin)
Capsules, oxypertine 10 mg. Net price 20 = £2.12. Label: 2
Tablets, scored, oxypertine 40 mg. Net price 20 = £6.64. Label: 2
Note. The brand name Integrin® was formerly used for oxypertine preparations

---

PERICYAZINE

Indications: see under Dose

Cautions; Contra-indications; Side-effects: see under Chlorpromazine Hydrochloride, but more sedating; hypotension commonly occurs when treatment initiated

Dose: schizophrenia and other psychoses, initially 75 mg daily in divided doses increased at weekly intervals by steps of 25 mg according to response; usual max. 300 mg daily (elderly initially 15–30 mg daily)

Short-term adjunctive management of severe anxiety, psychomotor agitation, and violent or dangerously impulsive behaviour, initially 15–30 mg (elderly 5–10 mg) daily divided into 2 doses, taking the larger dose at bedtime, adjusted according to response

CHILD (severe mental or behavioural disorders only), initially, 500 micrograms daily for 10-kg child, increased by 1 mg for each additional 5 kg to max. total daily dose of 10 mg; dose may be gradually increased according to response but maintenance should not exceed twice initial dose

PoM Neulactil® (Rhône-Poulenc Rorer)
Tablets, all yellow, scored, pericyazine 2.5 mg, net price 84-tab pack = £1.82; 10 mg, 84-tab pack = £4.91; Label: 2
Syrup forte, brown, pericyazine 10 mg/5 mL. Net price 100-mL pack = £2.38. Label: 2

PERPHENAZINE

Indications: see under Dose; anti-emetic, section 4.6

Cautions; Contra-indications; Side-effects: see under Chlorpromazine Hydrochloride, but less sedating; extrapyramidal symptoms, especially dystonia, more frequent, particularly at high dosage; not indicated for agitation and restlessness in the elderly

Dose: schizophrenia and other psychoses, mania, short-term adjunctive management of severe anxiety, psychomotor agitation, excitement, and violent or dangerously impulsive behaviour, initially 4 mg 3 times daily adjusted according to the response; max. 24 mg daily; ELDERLY quarter to half adult dose (but see Cautions); CHILD under 14 years not recommended

PoM Fentazin® (Forley)
Tablets, both s/c, perphenazine 2 mg, net price 20 = £3.30; 4 mg, 20 = £3.90. Label: 2

PIMOZIDE

Indications: see under Dose

Cautions; Contra-indications; Side-effects: see under Chlorpromazine Hydrochloride, but less sedating; contra-indicated in breast-feeding; serious arrhythmias reported (contra-indicated if history of arrhythmias or pre-existing congenital QT prolongation); following reports of sudden unexplained death, the CSM recommends ECG before treatment in all patients, periodic ECGs at doses over 16 mg daily and review of need for pimozide if repolarisation changes or arrhythmias develop (close supervision and preferably dose reduction advised); concurrent cardioactive or antipsychotic

---

drugs, or electrolyte disturbances (notably hypo-kalaemia) may predispose to cardiotoxicity

Dose: schizophrenia, initially 10 mg daily in acute conditions, adjusted according to response in increments of 2–4 mg at intervals of not less than 1 week; max. 20 mg daily; prevention of relapse, initially 2 mg daily (range 2–20 mg daily); CHILD not recommended

Monosymptomatic hypochondriacal psychosis, paranoid psychoses, initially 4 mg daily, adjusted according to response in increments of 2–4 mg at intervals of not less than 1 week; max. 16 mg daily; CHILD not recommended

Mania, hypomania, short-term adjunctive management of excitement and psychomotor agitation, initially 10 mg daily adjusted according to response in increments of 2–4 mg at intervals of not less than 1 week; max. 20 mg daily; ELDERLY half usual starting dose; CHILD not recommended

PoM Orap® (Janssen)
Tablets, all scored, pimozide 2 mg, net price 20 = £3.17; 4 mg (green), 20 = £6.13; 10 mg, 20 = £11.76. Label: 2

PROCHLORPERAZINE

Indications: see under Dose; anti-emetic, section 4.6

Cautions; Contra-indications; Side-effects: see under Chlorpromazine Hydrochloride, but less sedating; extrapyramidal symptoms, particularly dystonic reactions, more frequent; avoid in children (but see section 4.6 for use as anti-emetic)

Dose: by mouth, schizophrenia and other psychoses, mania, prochlorperazine maleate or mesylate, 12.5 mg twice daily for 7 days adjusted at weekly intervals to usual dose of 75–100 mg daily according to response; CHILD not recommended

Short-term adjunctive management of severe anxiety, 15–20 mg daily in divided doses; max. 40 mg daily; CHILD not recommended

By deep intramuscular injection, psychoses, mania, prochlorperazine mesylate 12.5–25 mg 2–3 times daily; CHILD not recommended

By rectum in suppositories, psychoses, mania, the equivalent of prochlorperazine maleate 25 mg 2–3 times daily; CHILD not recommended

Preparations
Section 4.6

PROMAZINE HYDROCHLORIDE

Indications: see under Dose

Cautions; Contra-indications; Side-effects: see under Chlorpromazine Hydrochloride

Dose: by mouth, short-term adjunctive management of psychomotor agitation, 100–200 mg 4 times daily; CHILD not recommended

Agitation and restlessness in elderly, 25–50 mg 4 times daily

By intramuscular injection, short-term adjunctive management of psychomotor agitation, 50 mg (25 mg in elderly or debilitated), repeated if necessary after 6–8 hours; CHILD not recommended

PoM Promazine (Non-proprietary)
Tablets, coated, promazine hydrochloride 50 mg, and 100 mg. Label: 2
Available from Biorex

PoM Sparine® (Wyeth)
Suspension, yellow, promazine hydrochloride 50 mg (as embonate)/5 mL. Net price 150-mL pack = £1.29. Label: 2.
Note. Not recommended for children
Injection, promazine hydrochloride 50 mg/mL. Net price 1-mL amp = 26p

RISPERIDONE

Indications: acute and chronic psychoses

Cautions; Contra-indications; Side-effects: see under Chlorpromazine Hydrochloride, but agitation may occur more frequently; dyspepsia, nausea, abdominal pain, anxiety, concentration difficulties, headache, dizziness, fatigue, and rhinitis also reported

Dose: 1 mg twice daily increased over 3 days to 3 mg twice daily; usual range 2–4 mg twice daily; doses above 5 mg twice daily only if benefit considered to outweigh risk (max. 8 mg twice daily); ELDERLY (or in hepatic or renal impairment) 500 micrograms twice daily increased to 1–2 mg twice daily; CHILD under 15 years not recommended

▼ **PoM Risperdal®** (Janssen, Organon)
Tablets, all f/c, scored, risperidone 1 mg (white), net price, 6-tab starter pack = £4.15, 20-tab pack = £13.45; 2 mg (orange), 60-tab pack = £79.56; 3 mg (yellow), 60-tab pack = £117.00; 4 mg (green), 60-tab pack = £154.44. Label: 2

SULPIRIDE

Indications: schizophrenia

Cautions; Contra-indications; Side-effects: see under Chlorpromazine Hydrochloride, but less sedating; structurally distinct from chlorpromazine hence not associated with jaundice or skin reactions; porphyria (see section 9.8.2); avoid in breast-feeding; reduce dose (preferably avoid) in renal impairment

Dose: 200–400 mg twice daily; max. 800 mg daily in patients with predominantly negative symptoms, and 2.4 g daily in patients with mainly positive symptoms; ELDERLY, initially 100–200 mg; CHILD under 14 not recommended

PoM Dolmatil® (Delandale)
Tablets, scored, sulpiride 200 mg. Net price 20 = £4.10. Label: 2

PoM Sulpitil® (Pharmacia)
Tablets, scored, sulpiride 200 mg. Net price 28-tab pack = £5.61; 112-tab pack = £22.43. Label: 2

THIORIDAZINE

Indications: see under Dose

Cautions; Contra-indications; Side-effects: see under Chlorpromazine Hydrochloride, but less sedating and extrapyramidal symptoms and hypothermia rarely occur; more likely to induce hypotension. Pigmentary retinopathy (with reduced visual acuity, brownish colouring of vision, and impaired night vision) occurs rarely with high doses—on prolonged use examinations for eye defects are required; sexual dysfunction, particularly retrograde ejaculation, may occur; porphyria (see section 9.8.2)

Dose: schizophrenia and other psychoses, mania, 150–600 mg daily (initially in divided doses); max. 800 mg daily (hospital patients only) for up to 4 weeks

Short-term adjunctive management of psychomotor agitation, excitement, violent or dangerously impulsive behaviour, 75–200 mg daily

Short-term adjunctive management of severe anxiety, and agitation and restlessness in the elderly, 30–100 mg daily

CHILD (severe mental or behavioural problems only) under 5 years 1 mg/kg daily, 5–12 years 75–150 mg daily (in severe cases, up to 300 mg daily)

PoM Thioridazine (Non-proprietary)
Tablets, coated, thioridazine hydrochloride 25 mg, net price 20 = 31p; 50 mg, 20 = 58p; 100 mg, 20 = £1.10. Label: 2
Available from DDSA (Rideril®), Norton

PoM Melleril® (Sandoz)
Tablets, all f/c, thioridazine hydrochloride 10 mg, net price 20 = 22p; 25 mg, 20 = 31p; 50 mg, 20 = 60p; 100 mg, 20 = £1.14. Label: 2
Suspension 25 mg/5 mL, thioridazine 25 mg/5 mL. Net price 500-mL = £2.98. Label: 2
Suspension 100 mg/5 mL, thioridazine 100 mg/5 mL. Net price 500-mL = £10.89. Label: 2
Note. These suspensions should not be diluted but the two preparations may be mixed with each other to provide intermediate doses
Syrup, orange, thioridazine 25 mg (as hydrochloride)/5 mL. Net price 100-mL pack = 76p. Label: 2

TRIFLUOPERAZINE
Indications: see under Dose; anti-emetic, section 4.6

Cautions; Contra-indications; Side-effects: see under Chlorpromazine Hydrochloride but less sedating, and hypotension, hypothermia, and antimuscarinic side-effects occur less frequently; extrapyramidal symptoms, particularly dystonic reactions and akathisia, are more frequent (particularly when the daily dose exceeds 6 mg); caution in children

Dose: by mouth (reduce initial doses in elderly by at least half)
Schizophrenia and other psychoses, short-term adjunctive management of psychomotor agitation, excitement, and violent or dangerously impulsive behaviour, initially 5 mg twice daily, *or* 10 mg daily in modified-release form, increased by 5 mg after 1 week, then at intervals of 3 days, according to the response; CHILD up to 12 years, initially up to 5 mg daily in divided doses, adjusted according to response, age, and bodyweight

Short-term adjunctive management of severe anxiety, 2–4 mg daily in divided doses *or* 2–4 mg daily in modified-release form, increased if necessary to 6 mg daily; CHILD 3–5 years up to 1 mg daily, 6–12 years up to 4 mg daily
By deep intramuscular injection 1–3 mg daily in divided doses to max. 6 mg daily; CHILD 50 micrograms/kg daily

PoM Trifluoperazine (Non-proprietary)
Tablets, coated, trifluoperazine (as hydrochloride) 1 mg, net price 20 = 37p; 5 mg, 20 = 52p. Label: 2.
Available from most generic manufacturers

PoM Stelazine® (SK&F)
Tablets, both blue, s/c, trifluoperazine (as hydrochloride) 1 mg, net price 20 = 42p; 5 mg, 20 = 60p. Label: 2
Spansule® (= capsules m/r), all clear/yellow, enclosing dark blue, light blue, and white pellets, trifluoperazine (as hydrochloride) 2 mg, net price 60-cap pack = £2.71; 10 mg, 30-cap pack = £1.77; 15 mg, 30-cap pack = £2.66. Label: 2, 25
Syrup, yellow, sugar-free, trifluoperazine 1 mg (as hydrochloride)/5 mL. Net price 200-mL pack = £1.65. Label: 2
Liquid concentrate, yellow, sugar-free, trifluoperazine 10 mg (as hydrochloride)/mL for dilution before use. Net price 100-mL pack = £6.13
Diluent sorbitol solution (70%) or water containing benzoic acid 0.1%, life of diluted liquid 12 weeks
Injection, trifluoperazine 1 mg (as hydrochloride)/ mL. Net price 1-mL amp = 47p

TRIFLUPERIDOL
Indications: schizophrenia and other psychoses, particularly those with manic features
Cautions; Contra-indications; Side-effects: see under Haloperidol
Dose: initially 500 micrograms daily, adjusted by 500 micrograms every 3–4 days according to response; max. 6–8 mg daily; CHILD 5–12 years initially 250 micrograms daily, adjusted according to response; max. 2 mg daily; usual maintenance 1 mg daily

PoM Triperidol® (Lagap)
Tablets, scored, trifluperidol 500 micrograms, net price 20 = £2.59. Label: 2

ZUCLOPENTHIXOL ACETATE
Indications: short-term management of acute psychosis, mania, or exacerbations of chronic psychosis
Cautions; Contra-indications; Side-effects: see under Chlorpromazine Hydrochloride; porphyria (see section 9.8.2); treatment duration should not exceed 2 weeks
Dose: by deep intramuscular injection into the gluteal muscle or lateral thigh, 50–150 mg (elderly 50–100 mg), if necessary repeated after 2–3 days (1 additional dose may be needed 1–2 days after the first injection); max. cumulative dose 400 mg per course and max. 4 injections; if maintenance treatment necessary change to an oral

antipsychotic 2–3 days after last injection, *or* to a longer acting antipsychotic depot injection given concomitantly with last injection of zuclopenthixol acetate; CHILD not recommended

PoM Clopixol Acuphase® (Lundbeck)
Injection (oily), zuclopenthixol acetate 50 mg/mL. Net price 1-mL amp = £4.95; 2-mL amp = £9.55

ZUCLOPENTHIXOL DIHYDROCHLORIDE

Indications: schizophrenia and other psychoses, particularly when associated with agitated, aggressive, or hostile behaviour

Cautions; Contra-indications; Side-effects: see under Chlorpromazine Hydrochloride; should not be used in apathetic or withdrawn states; porphyria (see section 9.8.2)

Dose: initially 20–30 mg daily in divided doses, increasing to a max. of 150 mg daily if necessary; usual maintenance dose 20–50 mg daily; CHILD not recommended

PoM Clopixol® (Lundbeck)
Tablets, all f/c, zuclopenthixol (as dihydrochloride) 2 mg (pink), net price 20 = 61p; 10 mg (light brown), 20 = £1.65; 25 mg (brown), 20 = £3.30. Label: 2
Depot injection (zuclopenthixol decanoate): section 4.2.2

4.2.2 Antipsychotic depot injections

For maintenance therapy, long-acting depot injections of antipsychotic drugs are used because they are more convenient than oral preparations and ensure better patient compliance. However, they may give rise to a higher incidence of extrapyramidal reactions than oral preparations.

ADMINISTRATION. Depot antipsychotics are administered by deep intramuscular injection at intervals of 1 to 4 weeks. Patients should first be given a small test-dose as undesirable side-effects are prolonged. In general not more than 2–3 mL of oily injection should be administered at any one site. If the dose needs to be reduced to alleviate side-effects it is important to recognise that the plasma level may not fall for some time after reducing the dose, therefore it may be a month or longer before side-effects subside.

Equivalent doses of depot antipsychotics
These equivalences are intended **only** as an approximate guide; individual dosage instructions should **also** be checked; patients should be carefully monitored after **any** change in medication

Antipsychotic	Dose (mg)	Interval
Flupenthixol decanoate	40	2 weeks
Fluphenazine decanoate	25	2 weeks
Haloperidol (as decanoate)	100	4 weeks
Pipothiazine palmitate	50	4 weeks
Zuclopenthixol decanoate	200	2 weeks

IMPORTANT. These equivalences must **not** be extrapolated beyond the max. dose for the drug

Dosage. Individual responses to neuroleptic drugs are very variable and to achieve optimum effect, dosage and dosage interval must be titrated according to the patient's response. For the advice of The Royal College of Psychiatrists on doses above the BNF upper limit, see p.151

CHOICE. There is no clear-cut division in the use of these drugs, but **zuclopenthixol** may be suitable for the treatment of agitated or aggressive patients whereas **flupenthixol** can cause over-excitement in such patients. **Fluspirilene** has a shorter duration of action than the other depot injections. The incidence of extrapyramidal reactions is similar for all these drugs.

CAUTIONS. Treatment requires careful monitoring for optimum effect; extrapyramidal symptoms occur frequently. When transferring from oral to depot therapy, dosage by mouth should be gradually phased out.

CONTRA-INDICATIONS. Do not use in children, confusional states, coma caused by CNS depressants, parkinsonism, intolerance to antipsychotics.

SIDE-EFFECTS. Pain may occur at injection site and occasionally erythema, swelling, and nodules. For side-effects of specific antipsychotics see under the relevant monograph.

FLUPENTHIXOL DECANOATE
(Flupentixol Decanoate)

Indications: maintenance in schizophrenia and other psychoses

Cautions; Contra-indications; Side-effects: see under Chlorpromazine Hydrochloride (section 4.2.1) and notes above, but it may have a mood elevating effect; extrapyramidal symptoms usually appear 1–3 days after administration and continue for about 5 days but may be delayed; an alternative antipsychotic may be necessary if symptoms such as aggression or agitation appear; porphyria (see section 9.8.2)

Dose: by deep intramuscular injection into the gluteal muscle, test dose 20 mg, then after 5–10 days 20–40 mg repeated at intervals of 2–4 weeks, adjusted according to response; max. 400 mg weekly; usual maintenance dose 50 mg every 4 weeks to 300 mg every 2 weeks; ELDERLY initially quarter to half adult dose; CHILD not recommended

PoM Depixol® (Lundbeck)
Injection (oily), flupenthixol decanoate 20 mg/mL. Net price 1-mL amp = £1.55; 1-mL syringe = £1.96; 2-mL amp = £2.60; 2-mL syringe = £3.16; 10-mL vial = £14.74

PoM **Depixol Conc.®** (Lundbeck)

Injection (oily), flupenthixol decanoate 100 mg/mL. Net price 0.5-mL amp = £3.49; 1-mL amp = £6.40; 5-mL vial = £28.27

PoM **Depixol Low Volume®** (Lundbeck)

Injection (oily), flupenthixol decanoate 200 mg/mL. Net price 1-mL amp = £19.98

FLUPHENAZINE DECANOATE

Indications: maintenance in schizophrenia and other psychoses

Cautions; Contra-indications; Side-effects: see under Chlorpromazine Hydrochloride (section 4.2.1) and notes above. Extrapyramidal symptoms usually appear a few hours after the dose has been administered and continue for about 2 days but may be delayed. Contra-indicated in severely depressed states

Dose: by deep intramuscular injection into the gluteal muscle, test dose 12.5 mg (6.25 mg in elderly), then after 4–7 days 12.5–100 mg repeated at intervals of 14–35 days, adjusted according to response; CHILD not recommended

PoM **Modecate®** (Sanofi Winthrop)

Injection (oily), fluphenazine decanoate 25 mg/mL. Net price 0.5-mL amp = £1.42; 1-mL amp = £2.46; 1-mL syringe = £2.72; 2-mL amp = £4.84; 2-mL syringe = £4.93; 10-mL vial = £23.45

Note. Fluphenazine decanoate injection also available from Berk (Decazate®), David Bull, Hillcross

PoM **Modecate Concentrate®** (Sanofi Winthrop)

Injection (oily), fluphenazine decanoate 100 mg/mL. Net price 0.5-mL amp = £4.87; 1-mL amp = £9.53

Note. Fluphenazine decanoate injection also available from Berk (Decazate®), David Bull, Hillcross

FLUSPIRILENE

Indications: maintenance in schizophrenia

Cautions; Contra-indications; Side-effects: see under Chlorpromazine Hydrochloride (section 4.2.1) and notes above, but less sedating. Extrapyramidal symptoms usually appear 6–12 hours after the dose and continue for about 48 hours but may be delayed. Common side-effects are restlessness and sweating. With prolonged use, tissue damage (subcutaneous nodules) may occur at injection site

Dose: by deep intramuscular injection, 2 mg, increased by 2 mg at weekly intervals, according to response; usual maintenance dose 2–8 mg weekly; max. 20 mg weekly; ELDERLY initially quarter to half adult dose; CHILD not recommended

PoM **Redeptin®** (SK&F)

Injection (aqueous suspension), fluspirilene 2 mg/mL. Net price 1-mL amp = 90p; 3-mL amp = £1.59; 6-mL vial = £2.76

Note. Contains povidone, caution in renal impairment

HALOPERIDOL DECANOATE

Indications: maintenance in schizophrenia and other psychoses

Cautions; Contra-indications; Side-effects: see under Haloperidol (section 4.2.1) and notes above

Dose: by deep intramuscular injection into the gluteal muscle, haloperidol (as decanoate), initially 50 mg every 4 weeks, if necessary increasing after 2 weeks by 50-mg increments to 300 mg every 4 weeks; higher doses may be needed in some patients; ELDERLY, initially 12.5–25 mg every 4 weeks; CHILD not recommended

PoM **Haldol Decanoate®** (Janssen)

Injection (oily), haloperidol (as decanoate) 50 mg/mL, net price 1-mL amp = £4.35; 100 mg/mL, 1-mL amp = £5.77

PIPOTHIAZINE PALMITATE

(Pipotiazine Palmitate)

Indications: maintenance in schizophrenia and other psychoses

Cautions; Contra-indications; Side-effects: see under Chlorpromazine Hydrochloride (section 4.2.1) and notes above

Dose: by deep intramuscular injection into the gluteal muscle, test dose 25 mg, then a further 25–50 mg after 4–7 days, then adjusted according to response at intervals of 4 weeks; usual maintenance range 50–100 mg (max. 200 mg) every 4 weeks; ELDERLY initially 5–10 mg; CHILD not recommended

PoM **Piportil Depot®** (Rhône-Poulenc Rorer)

Injection (oily), pipothiazine palmitate 50 mg/mL. Net price 1-mL amp = £6.12; 2-mL amp = £10.01

ZUCLOPENTHIXOL DECANOATE

Indications: maintenance in schizophrenia and other psychoses, particularly with aggression and agitation

Cautions; Contra-indications; Side-effects: see under Chlorpromazine Hydrochloride (section 4.2.1) and notes above, but less sedating; porphyria (see section 9.8.2)

Dose: by deep intramuscular injection into the gluteal muscle, test dose 100 mg, followed after 7–28 days by 100–200 mg or more, followed by 200–400 mg at intervals of 2–4 weeks, adjusted according to response; max. 600 mg weekly; CHILD not recommended

PoM **Clopixol®** (Lundbeck)

Injection (oily), zuclopenthixol decanoate 200 mg/mL. Net price 1-mL amp = £3.23; 10-mL vial = £28.63

PoM **Clopixol Conc.®** (Lundbeck)

Injection (oily), zuclopenthixol decanoate 500 mg/mL. Net price 1-mL amp with needle = £7.61

4.2.3   Antimanic drugs

Drugs are used in mania both to control acute attacks and also to prevent their recurrence.

ANTIPSYCHOTIC DRUGS

In an acute attack of mania, treatment with an antipsychotic drug (section 4.2.1) is usually required because it may take a few days for lithium to exert its antimanic effect. Lithium may be given concurrently with the antipsychotic drug, and treatment with the antipsychotic gradually tailed off as lithium becomes effective. Alternatively, lithium therapy may be commenced once the patient's mood has been stabilised with the antipsychotic. Haloperidol may be preferred for rapid control of acute mania. However, high doses of haloperidol, fluphenazine, or flupenthixol may be hazardous when used with lithium; irreversible toxic encephalopathy has been reported.

LITHIUM

Lithium salts are used in the *prophylaxis and treatment of mania*, in the *prophylaxis of manic-depressive illness* (bipolar illness or bipolar depression) and in the *prophylaxis of recurrent depression* (unipolar illness or unipolar depression). Lithium is unsuitable for children.

The decision to give prophylactic lithium usually requires specialist advice, and must be based on careful consideration of the likelihood of recurrence in the individual patient, and the benefit weighed against the risks. In long-term use, therapeutic concentrations have been thought to cause histological and functional changes in the kidney. The significance of such changes is not clear but is of sufficient concern to discourage long-term use of lithium unless it is definitely indicated. Patients should therefore be maintained on lithium after 3–5 years only if, on assessment, benefit persists.

PLASMA CONCENTRATIONS. Lithium salts have a narrow therapeutic/toxic ratio and should therefore not be prescribed unless facilities for monitoring plasma concentrations are available. There seem few if any reasons for preferring one or other of the salts of lithium available. Doses are adjusted to achieve plasma concentrations of 0.4 to 1.0 mmol Li+/litre (lower end of the range for maintenance therapy and elderly patients) on samples taken 12 hours after the preceding dose. It is important to determine the optimum range for each individual patient.

Overdosage, usually with plasma concentrations over 1.5 mmol Li+/litre, may be fatal and toxic effects include tremor, ataxia, dysarthria, nystagmus, renal impairment, and convulsions. If these potentially hazardous signs occur, treatment should be stopped, plasma-lithium concentrations redetermined, and steps taken to reverse lithium toxicity. In mild cases withdrawal of lithium and administration of generous amounts of sodium and fluid will reverse the toxicity. Plasma concentrations in excess of 2.0 mmol Li+/litre require emergency treatment as indicated under Emergency Treatment of Poisoning, p. 22. When toxic concentrations are reached there may be a delay of 1 or 2 days before maximum toxicity occurs.

INTERACTIONS. Lithium toxicity is made worse by sodium depletion, therefore concurrent use of diuretics (particularly thiazides) is hazardous and should be avoided. For other **interactions** with lithium, see Appendix 1 (lithium).

WITHDRAWAL. There is no evidence of a lithium withdrawal state nor of rebound psychosis on withdrawal. Nevertheless, to allay any concerns about relapse, if possible lithium should be withdrawn slowly over a period of weeks.

Lithium cards. A lithium treatment card available from pharmacies tells patients how to take lithium preparations, what to do if a dose is missed, and what side-effects to expect. It also explains why regular blood tests are important and warns that some medicines and illnesses can change lithium plasma concentrations.

Cards from NPA Services, 38–42 St. Peter's St, St. Albans, Herts AL1 3NP.

LITHIUM CARBONATE

Indications: treatment and prophylaxis of mania, manic-depressive illness, and recurrent depression (see also notes above); aggressive or self-mutilating behaviour

Cautions: measure plasma concentrations regularly (every 3 months on stabilised regimens), monitor thyroid function; maintain adequate sodium and fluid intake; avoid in renal impairment, cardiac disease, and conditions with sodium imbalance such as Addison's disease; reduction in dose or discontinuation may be necessary in diarrhoea, vomiting and intercurrent infection (especially when associated with profuse sweating); caution in pregnancy, breast-feeding, elderly patients (reduce dose), diuretic treatment, myasthenia gravis; surgery (see section 15.1); if possible avoid abrupt withdrawal (see notes above); **interactions:** Appendix 1 (lithium)

Side-effects: gastro-intestinal disturbances, fine tremor, polyuria and polydipsia; also weight gain and oedema (may respond to dose reduction). Signs of lithium intoxication are blurred vision, increasing gastro-intestinal disturbances (anorexia, vomiting, diarrhoea), muscle weakness, increasing CNS disturbances (mild drowsiness and sluggishness increasing to giddiness with ataxia, coarse tremor, lack of co-ordination, dysarthria), and require withdrawal of treatment. With severe overdosage (plasma concentrations above 2 mmol/litre) hyperreflexia and hyperextension of limbs, convulsions, toxic psychoses, syncope, oliguria, circulatory failure, coma, and occasionally, death. Goitre, raised antidiuretic hormone concentration, hypothyroidism, hypokalaemia, ECG changes, exacerbation of psoriasis, and kidney changes may also occur. See also Emergency Treatment of Poisoning, p. 22

Cautionary label wordings, see inside back cover

Dose: see under preparations below, adjusted to achieve a plasma concentration of 0.4–1.0 mmol Li⁺/litre 12 hours after the preceding dose on the fourth or seventh day of treatment, then every week until dosage has remained constant for 4 weeks and every 3 months thereafter; doses are initially divided throughout the day, but once daily administration is preferred when plasma concentrations stabilised

PoM Camcolit® (Norgine)
Camcolit 250® tablets, f/c, scored, lithium carbonate 250 mg (6.8 mmol Li⁺). Net price 20 = 58p. Label: 10 lithium card, counselling, see below
Camcolit 400® tablets, m/r, f/c, scored, lithium carbonate 400 mg (10.8 mmol Li⁺). Net price 20 = 77p. Label: 10 lithium card, 25, counselling, see above
Dose (plasma monitoring, see above):
Treatment, initially 1.5–2 g daily (elderly, 0.5–1 g daily); prophylaxis, initially 0.5–1.2 g daily (elderly, 0.5–1 g daily); CHILD not recommended
Camcolit 250® should be given in divided doses, whereas Camcolit 400® may be given in single or divided doses

PoM Liskonum® (SK&F)
Tablets, m/r, f/c, scored, lithium carbonate 450 mg (12.2 mmol Li⁺). Net price 60-tab pack = £2.82. Label: 10 lithium card, 25, counselling, see below
Dose (plasma monitoring, see above):
Treatment, initially 450–675 mg twice daily (elderly, initially 225 mg twice daily); prophylaxis, initially 450 mg twice daily (elderly, 225 mg twice daily); CHILD not recommended

PoM Phasal® (Lagap)
Tablets, m/r, lithium carbonate 300 mg (8.1 mmol Li⁺). Net price 60-tab pack = £4.10. Label: 10 lithium card, 25, counselling, see below
Dose (plasma monitoring, see above):
Treatment, initially 600 mg twice daily (elderly, 0.5–1 g daily in divided doses); prophylaxis, initially 600 mg daily; CHILD not recommended

PoM Priadel® (Delandale)
Tablets, both m/r, scored, lithium carbonate 200 mg (5.4 mmol Li⁺), net price 20 = 41p; 400 mg (10.8 mmol Li⁺), 20 = 68p. Label: 10 lithium card, 25, counselling, see below
Dose (plasma monitoring, see above):
Treatment and prophylaxis, initially 0.4–1.2 g daily as a single dose or in 2 divided doses (elderly or patients less than 50 kg, 400 mg daily); CHILD not recommended
Liquid, see under Lithium Citrate, below

COUNSELLING. Patients should maintain an adequate fluid intake and should avoid dietary changes which might reduce or increase sodium intake; lithium treatment cards are available from pharmacies (see previous page)

Note. **Different preparations vary widely in bioavailability**; a change in the preparation used requires the same precautions as initiation of treatment.

LITHIUM CITRATE

Indications; Cautions; Side-effects: see under Lithium Carbonate and notes above
Dose: see under preparations below, adjusted to achieve plasma concentrations of 0.4–1.0 mmol Li⁺/litre as described under Lithium Carbonate

PoM Li-Liquid® (RP Drugs)
Oral solution, lithium citrate 509 mg/5 mL (5.4 mmol Li⁺/5 mL), yellow, net price 100-mL pack = £4.50; 1.018 g/5 mL (10.8 mmol Li⁺/5 mL), orange, 100-mL pack = £9.00. Label: 10 lithium card, counselling, see above
Dose (plasma monitoring, see above):
Treatment and prophylaxis, initially 1.018–3.054 g daily in 2 divided doses (elderly or patients less than 50 kg, initially 509 mg twice daily); CHILD not recommended

PoM Litarex® (CP)
Tablets, m/r, lithium citrate 564 mg (6 mmol Li⁺). Net price 20 = 72p. Label: 10 lithium card, 25, counselling, see above
Dose (plasma monitoring, see above):
Treatment and prophylaxis, initially 564 mg twice daily; CHILD not recommended

PoM Priadel® (Delandale)
Tablets, see under Lithium Carbonate, above
Liquid, sugar-free, lithium citrate 520 mg/5 mL (approx. 5.4 mmol Li⁺/5 mL), net price 150-mL pack = £6.58, 300-mL pack = £13.16. Label: 10 lithium card, counselling, see above
Dose (plasma monitoring, see above):
Treatment and prophylaxis, initially 1.04–3.12 g daily in 2 divided doses (elderly or patients less than 50 kg, 520 mg twice daily); CHILD not recommended

CARBAMAZEPINE

Carbamazepine may be used for the prophylaxis of manic-depressive illness in patients unresponsive to lithium; it seems to be particularly effective in patients with rapid cycling manic-depressive illness (4 or more affective episodes per year).

CARBAMAZEPINE

Indications: prophylaxis of manic-depressive illness unresponsive to lithium; for use in epilepsy see section 4.8.1
Cautions; Contra-indications; Side-effects: see section 4.8.1
Dose: initially 400 mg daily in divided doses increased until symptoms controlled; usual range 400–600 mg daily; max. 1.6 g daily

Preparations
Section 4.8.1

4.3   Antidepressant drugs

4.3.1   Tricyclic and related antidepressant drugs
4.3.2   Monoamine-oxidase inhibitors (MAOIs)
4.3.3   Compound antidepressant preparations
4.3.4   Other antidepressant drugs

Tricyclic and related antidepressants (antidepressives) are the drugs of choice in the treatment of depressive illness, unless it is so severe that electroconvulsive therapy is immediately indicated. They are preferred to MAOIs because they are more effective antidepressants and do not show the dangerous interactions with some foods and drugs that are characteristic of the MAOIs. **Lithium** (section 4.2.3) has a mood-regulating action and is used in the treatment and prophylaxis of mania, manic depressive illness, and recurrent depression.

Prescribing more than one antidepressant at the same time is **not** recommended. It may constitute a hazard and there is no evidence that side-effects are minimised.

Mixtures of antidepressants with tranquillisers are in section 4.3.3; they are **not** recommended.

It should be noted that although anxiety is often present in depressive illness and may be the presenting symptom, the use of antipsychotics or anxiolytics may mask the true diagnosis. They should therefore be used with caution (but are useful adjuncts in agitated depression).

CSM advice (hyponatraemia). Hyponatraemia (usually in the elderly and possibly due to inappropriate secretion of antidiuretic hormone) has been associated with all types of antidepressants and should be considered in all patients who develop drowsiness, confusion or convulsions while taking an antidepressant.

MANAGEMENT. The patient's condition must be checked frequently, especially in the early weeks of treatment, to detect any suicidal tendencies. Limited quantities of antidepressant drugs should be prescribed at any one time as they are dangerous in overdosage. Some of the newer drugs seem less dangerous in overdose than the older tricyclics.

Treatment should be continued for 2 weeks before suppression of symptoms can be expected and thereafter should be maintained at the optimum level for at least another month before any attempt is made at dose reduction. Treatment should not be withdrawn prematurely, otherwise symptoms are likely to recur. The natural history of depressive illness suggests that remission usually occurs after 3 months to a year or more and some patients appear to benefit from maintenance therapy with about half the therapeutic dosage for several months to prevent relapse. In recurrent depression, prophylactic maintenance therapy may need to be continued for several years.

In patients who do not respond to antidepressants, the diagnosis, dosage, compliance, and possible continuation of psychosocial or physical aggravating causes should all be carefully reviewed; other drug treatment may be successful.

WITHDRAWAL. Gastro-intestinal symptoms of nausea, vomiting, and anorexia, accompanied by headache, giddiness, 'chills', and insomnia, and sometimes by hypomania, panic-anxiety, and extreme motor restlessness may occur if an antidepressant (particularly an MAOI) is stopped suddenly after regular administration for 8 weeks or more. Reduction in dosage should preferably be carried out gradually over a period of about 4 weeks.

4.3.1   Tricyclic and related antidepressant drugs

The term 'tricyclic' is misleading as there are now 1-, 2-, and 4-ring structured drugs with broadly similar properties.

These drugs are most effective for treating moderate to severe *endogenous depression* associated with psychomotor and physiological changes such as loss of appetite and sleep disturbances; improvement in sleep is usually the first benefit of therapy. Since there may be an interval of 2 weeks before the antidepressant action takes place electroconvulsive treatment may be required in severe depression when delay is hazardous or intolerable.

Tricyclic antidepressants are also effective in the management of *panic disorder*.

For reference to the role of some tricyclic antidepressants in some forms of neuralgia, see section 4.7.3, and in *nocturnal enuresis* in children, see section 7.4.2.

DOSAGE. About 10 to 20% of patients fail to respond to tricyclic and related antidepressant drugs and inadequate plasma concentrations may account for some of these failures. It is important to achieve plasma concentrations which are sufficiently high for effective treatment but not high enough to cause toxic effects. Low doses should be used for initial treatment in the **elderly** (see under Side-effects, below).

In most patients the long half-life of tricyclic antidepressant drugs allows **once-daily** administration, usually at night; the use of modified-release preparations is therefore unnecessary.

CHOICE. Tricyclic and related antidepressant drugs can be roughly divided into those with additional sedative properties, e.g. **amitriptyline**, and those with less e.g. **imipramine**. Agitated and anxious patients tend to respond best to the sedative compounds whereas withdrawn and apathetic patients will often obtain most benefit from less sedating compounds.

Antidepressants with **sedative** properties include amitriptyline, clomipramine, dothiepin, doxepin, maprotiline, mianserin, trazodone, and trimipramine.

Less sedative antidepressants include amoxapine, desipramine, imipramine, iprindole, lofepramine, nortriptyline, and viloxazine. Protriptyline has a **stimulant** action.

Amitriptyline may be given in divided doses or the entire daily dose may be given at night to promote sleep and avoid daytime drowsiness. **Imipramine** can also be given once daily but as it has a much less sedative action there is less need.

Imipramine and amitriptyline are well established and nevertheless safe and effective, but nevertheless have more marked antimuscarinic or cardiac side-effects than compounds such as **doxepin, lofepramine, mianserin, trazodone**, and **viloxazine**; this may be important in individual patients.

Amoxapine is related to the antipsychotic loxapine and its side-effects include tardive dyskinesia; overdosage has been associated with seizures.

SIDE-EFFECTS. *Arrhythmias* and *heart block* occasionally follow the use of tricyclic antidepressants, particularly amitriptyline, and may be a factor in the sudden death of patients with cardiac disease. They are also sometimes associated with *convulsions* (and should be prescribed with special caution in epilepsy as they lower the convulsive threshold) and *hepatic* and *haematological* reactions may occur. In particular, mianserin has been associated with haematological and hepatic reactions and maprotiline has been associated with convulsions. Patients being treated with these drugs therefore require careful supervision. In the case of **mianserin** a full **blood count** is recommended every 4 weeks during the first 3 months of treatment; subsequent clinical monitoring should continue and treatment should be stopped and a full blood count obtained if *fever, sore throat, stomatitis,* or other signs of infection develop.

Other side-effects of tricyclic and related antidepressants include *drowsiness, dry mouth, blurred vision, constipation,* and *urinary retention* (all attributed to antimuscarinic activity), and sweating. The patient should be encouraged to persist with treatment as some tolerance to these side-effects seems to develop. They are reduced if low doses are given initially and then gradually increased. This gradual introduction of treatment is particularly important in the elderly, who, because of the hypotensive effects of these drugs, are prone to attacks of *dizziness* or even *syncope.* Another side-effect to which the elderly are particularly susceptible is *hyponatraemia* (see CSM advice on p.163).

Neuroleptic malignant syndrome (section 4.2.1) may, very rarely, arise in the course of antidepressant treatment.

Overdosage: see Emergency Treatment of Poisoning, p.21.

WITHDRAWAL. If possible tricyclic and related antidepressants should be withdrawn slowly (see also section 4.3).

INTERACTIONS. A tricyclic or related antidepressant should not be started until 2 weeks after stopping an MAOI. Conversely, an MAOI should not be started until at least a week after a tricyclic or related antidepressant has been stopped. For guidance relating to the reversible monoamine oxidase inhibitor, moclobemide, see p.169. For other tricyclic antidepressant **interactions**, see Appendix 1 (antidepressants, tricyclic).

TRICYCLIC ANTIDEPRESSANTS

AMITRIPTYLINE HYDROCHLORIDE

Indications: depressive illness, particularly where sedation is required; nocturnal enuresis in children (see section 7.4.2)

Cautions: cardiac disease (particularly with arrhythmias, see Contra-indications below), epilepsy,

pregnancy and breast-feeding see Appendixes 4 and 5, elderly, hepatic impairment (avoid if severe), thyroid disease, psychoses (may aggravate mania), closed-angle glaucoma, urinary retention, concurrent electroconvulsive therapy; avoid abrupt withdrawal; also caution in anaesthesia (increased risk of arrhythmias and hypotension, see surgery section 15.1); porphyria (see section 9.8.2); see section 7.4.2 for additional nocturnal enuresis warnings; **interactions:** Appendix 1 (antidepressants, tricyclic)

DRIVING. Drowsiness may affect performance of skilled tasks (e.g. driving); effects of alcohol enhanced

Contra-indications: recent myocardial infarction, arrhythmias (particularly heart block), mania, severe liver disease

Side-effects: dry mouth, sedation, blurred vision, constipation, nausea, difficulty with micturition (due to antimuscarinic action). Other common side-effects are cardiovascular (arrhythmias, postural hypotension, tachycardia, syncope, particularly with high doses), sweating, tremor, rashes, behavioural disturbances (particularly children), hypomania, confusion (particularly elderly), interference with sexual function, blood sugar changes; increased appetite and weight gain (occasionally weight loss). Less common include, black tongue, paralytic ileus, convulsions, agranulocytosis, leucopenia, eosinophilia, purpura, thrombocytopenia, hyponatraemia (may be due to inappropriate antidiuretic hormone secretion) see CSM advice, p.163, and jaundice; overdosage: see Emergency Treatment of Poisoning, p.21

Dose: by mouth, depression, initially 50–75 mg (elderly and adolescents 25–50 mg) daily in divided doses *or* as a single dose at bedtime increased gradually as necessary to max. 150–200 mg; usual maintenance 50–100 mg daily; CHILD under 16 years not recommended for depression

Nocturnal enuresis, CHILD 7–10 years 10–20 mg, 11–16 years 25–50 mg at night; max. period of treatment (including gradual withdrawal) 3 months—full physical examination before further course

By intramuscular or intravenous injection, 10–20 mg 4 times daily; CHILD not recommended

PoM **Amitriptyline** (Non-proprietary)

Tablets, coated, amitriptyline hydrochloride 10 mg, net price 20 = 14p; 25 mg, 20 = 9p; 50 mg, 20 = 34p. Label: 2

Available from APS, Berk (Domical®), Cox, DDSA (Elavil®), K Pharm.

PoM **Lentizol**® (P-D)

Capsules, m/r, both enclosing white pellets, amitriptyline hydrochloride 25 mg (pink), net price 100-cap pack = £4.61; 50 mg (pink/red), 100-cap pack = £8.56. Label: 2, 25

PoM **Tryptizol**® (Morson)

Tablets, all f/c, amitriptyline hydrochloride 10 mg (blue), net price 20 = 11p; 25 mg (yellow), 20 = 8p; 50 mg (brown), 20 = 35p. Label: 2

Capsules, m/r, orange, amitriptyline hydrochloride 75 mg. Net price 20 = £1.07. Label: 2, 25

Mixture, pink, sugar-free, amitriptyline 10 mg (as embonate)/5 mL. Net price 200-mL pack = £1.87. Label: 2
Injection, amitriptyline hydrochloride 10 mg/mL. Net price 10-mL vial = 54p

AMOXAPINE

Indications: depressive illness
Cautions; Contra-indications; Side-effects: see under Amitriptyline Hydrochloride; tardive dyskinesia reported; menstrual irregularities, breast enlargement, and galactorrhoea reported in women
Dose: initially 100–150 mg daily in divided doses *or* as a single dose at bedtime increased as necessary to max. 300 mg daily; usual maintenance 150–250 mg daily; ELDERLY initially 25 mg twice daily increased as necessary after 5–7 days to max. 50 mg 3 times daily; CHILD under 16 years not recommended

PoM **Asendis**® (Novex)
Tablets, amoxapine 25 mg, net price 20 = £2.18; 50 mg (orange, scored), 20 = £3.63; 100 mg (blue, scored), 20 = £6.05; 150 mg (scored), 20 = £9.02. Label: 2

CLOMIPRAMINE HYDROCHLORIDE

Indications: depressive illness, phobic and obsessional states; adjunctive treatment of cataplexy associated with narcolepsy
Cautions; Contra-indications; Side-effects: see under Amitriptyline Hydrochloride. Postural hypotension may occur on intravenous infusion
Dose: by mouth, initially 10 mg daily, increased gradually as necessary to 30–150 mg (elderly 75 mg) in divided doses *or* as a single dose at bedtime; max. 250 mg daily; usual maintenance 30–50 mg daily (severe cases 50–100 mg daily); CHILD not recommended
Phobic and obsessional states, initially 25 mg daily (elderly 10 mg daily) increased over 2 weeks to 100–150 mg daily; CHILD not recommended
By intramuscular injection, initially 25–50 mg daily, increased by 25 mg daily to 100–150 mg daily; CHILD not recommended
By intravenous infusion, initially to assess tolerance, 25–50 mg, then usually about 100 mg daily for 7–10 days; CHILD not recommended

PoM **Clomipramine** (Non-proprietary)
Capsules, clomipramine hydrochloride 10 mg, net price 20 = 61p; 25 mg, 20 = £1.22; 50 mg, 20 = £2.24. Label: 2
Available from APS, Cox, Generics, Hillcross, K Pharm., Norton
PoM **Anafranil**® (Geigy)
Capsules, clomipramine hydrochloride 10 mg (yellow/caramel), net price 84-cap pack = £2.76; 25 mg (orange/caramel), 84-cap pack = £5.43; 50 mg (grey/caramel), 56-cap pack = £6.89. Label: 2

Syrup, clomipramine hydrochloride 25 mg/5 mL. Net price 150-mL pack = £6.18. Label: 2
Injection, clomipramine hydrochloride 12.5 mg/mL. Net price 2-mL amp = 40p
PoM **Anafranil SR**® (Geigy)
Tablets, m/r, pink, f/c, clomipramine hydrochloride 75 mg. Net price 28-tab pack = £6.86. Label: 2, 25

DESIPRAMINE HYDROCHLORIDE

Indications: depressive illness
Cautions; Contra-indications; Side-effects: see under Amitriptyline Hydrochloride, but less sedating
Dose: 75 mg daily in divided doses *or* as a single dose at bedtime, increased as necessary to a usual max. of 200 mg (in resistant depression max. 300 mg daily with plasma concentration monitoring); ELDERLY initially 25 mg daily then about half usual adult dose; ADOLESCENT about half usual adult dose; CHILD not recommended

PoM **Pertofran**® (Ciba)
Tablets, pink, s/c, desipramine hydrochloride 25 mg. Net price 84-tab pack = £2.99. Label: 2

DOTHIEPIN HYDROCHLORIDE
(Dosulepin Hydrochloride)
Indications: depressive illness, particularly where sedation is required
Cautions; Contra-indications; Side-effects: see under Amitriptyline Hydrochloride
Dose: initially 75 mg (elderly 50–75 mg) daily in divided doses *or* as a single dose at bedtime, increased gradually as necessary to 150 mg daily (elderly 75 mg may be sufficient); up to 225 mg daily in some circumstances (e.g. hospital use); CHILD not recommended

PoM **Dothiepin** (Non-proprietary)
Capsules, dothiepin hydrochloride 25 mg, net price 20 = 86p. Label: 2
Available from APS, Ashbourne (Dothapax®), Berk (Prepadine®), Cox, Evans, Generics, Hillcross, K Pharm., Norton
Tablets, dothiepin hydrochloride 75 mg, net price 28-tab pack = £3.50. Label: 2
Available from APS, Ashbourne (Dothapax®), Berk (Prepadine®), Cox, Generics, Hillcross, K Pharm., Norton
PoM **Prothiaden**® (Boots)
Capsules, red/brown, dothiepin hydrochloride 25 mg. Net price 20 = £1.00. Label: 2
Tablets, red, s/c, dothiepin hydrochloride 75 mg. Net price 28-tab pack = £4.00. Label: 2

DOXEPIN

Indications: depressive illness, particularly where sedation is required
Cautions; Contra-indications; Side-effects: see under Amitriptyline Hydrochloride; avoid in breast-feeding (see Appendix 5)

Dose: initially 75 mg daily in 3 divided doses, increased gradually to max. 300 mg daily in divided doses; range 30–300 mg daily; up to 100 mg may be given as a single dose at bedtime; ELDERLY initially 10–50 mg daily, range of 30–50 mg daily may be adequate; CHILD not recommended

PoM **Sinequan®** (Pfizer)
Capsules, doxepin (as hydrochloride) 10 mg (orange), net price 56-cap pack = £1.21; 25 mg (orange/blue), 28-cap pack = 87p; 50 mg (blue), 28-cap pack = £1.43; 75 mg (yellow/blue), 28-cap pack = £2.26. Label: 2

IMIPRAMINE HYDROCHLORIDE

Indications: depressive illness; nocturnal enuresis in children (see section 7.4.2)
Cautions; Contra-indications; Side-effects: see under Amitriptyline Hydrochloride, but less sedating
Dose: depression, initially up to 75 mg daily in divided doses increased gradually to 150–200 mg (up to 300 mg in hospital patients); up to 150 mg may be given as a single dose at bedtime; usual maintenance 50–100 mg daily; ELDERLY initially 10 mg daily, increased gradually to 30–50 mg daily; CHILD not recommended for depression
Nocturnal enuresis, CHILD 7 years 25 mg, 8–11 years 25–50 mg, over 11 years 50–75 mg at bedtime; max. period of treatment (including gradual withdrawal) 3 months—full physical examination before further course

PoM **Imipramine** (Non-proprietary)
Tablets, coated, imipramine hydrochloride 10 mg, net price 20 = 14p; 25 mg, 20 = 13p. Label: 2
PoM **Tofranil®** (Geigy)
Tablets, both red-brown, s/c, imipramine hydrochloride 10 mg, net price 84-tab pack = £1.39; 25 mg, 84-tab pack = £2.65. Label: 2
Syrup, imipramine hydrochloride 25 mg/5 mL. Net price 150-mL pack = £2.70. Label: 2

LOFEPRAMINE

Indications: depressive illness
Cautions; Contra-indications; Side-effects: see under Amitriptyline Hydrochloride, but less sedating; hepatic disorders reported; contra-indicated in hepatic and severe renal impairment
Dose: 140–210 mg daily in divided doses; ELDERLY may respond to lower doses; CHILD not recommended

PoM **Gamanil®** (Merck)
Tablets, f/c, brown-violet, lofepramine 70 mg (as hydrochloride). Net price 56-tab pack = £10.27. Label: 2

NORTRIPTYLINE

Indications: depressive illness; nocturnal enuresis in children (see section 7.4.2)
Cautions; Contra-indications; Side-effects: see under Amitriptyline Hydrochloride but less sedating

Dose: depression, low dose intially increased as necessary to 100 mg daily in divided doses *or* as a single dose; plasma concentration monitoring above 100 mg daily (max. 150 mg daily, in hospitalised patients); ADOLESCENT and ELDERLY 30–50 mg daily in divided doses; CHILD not recommended for depression
Nocturnal enuresis, CHILD 7 years 10 mg, 8–11 years 10–20 mg, over 11 years 25–35 mg, at night; max period of treatment (including gradual withdrawal) 3 months—full physical examination and ECG before further course

PoM **Allegron®** (Dista)
Tablets, nortriptyline (as hydrochloride) 10 mg, net price 20 = £1.01; 25 mg (orange, scored), 20 = £2.05. Label: 2
PoM **Aventyl®** (Lilly)
Capsules, both yellow/white, nortriptyline (as hydrochloride) 10 mg, net price 20 = £1.01; 25 mg, 20 = £2.05. Label: 2

PROTRIPTYLINE HYDROCHLORIDE

Indications: depressive illness, particularly with apathy and withdrawal
Cautions; Contra-indications; Side-effects: see under Amitriptyline Hydrochloride but less sedating; anxiety, agitation, tachycardia, and hypotension more common; rashes associated with photosensitisation (avoid direct sunlight); daily dose above 20 mg in elderly (increased risk of cardiovascular side-effects)
Dose: initially 10 mg 3–4 times daily (elderly 5 mg 3 times daily initially) if insomnia, last dose not after 4 p.m.; usual range 15–60 mg daily; CHILD under 16 years not recommended

PoM **Concordin®** (MSD)
Tablets, both f/c, protriptyline hydrochloride 5 mg (pink), net price 20 = 44p; 10 mg, 20 = 65p. Label: 2, 11

TRIMIPRAMINE

Indications: depressive illness, particularly where sedation is required
Cautions; Contra-indications; Side-effects: see under Amitriptyline Hydrochloride
Dose: 50–75 mg daily as a single dose 2 hours before bedtime *or* as 25 mg midday and 50 mg evening, increased as necessary to max. of 300 mg daily; usual maintenance dose 75–150 mg daily; ELDERLY 10–25 mg 3 times daily initially, half adult maintenance dose may be sufficient; CHILD not recommended

PoM **Surmontil®** (Rhône-Poulenc Rorer)
Capsules, green/white, trimipramine 50 mg (as maleate). Net price 28-cap pack = £4.51. Label: 2
Tablets, trimipramine (as maleate) 10 mg, net price 50-tab pack = £2.42; 25 mg, 50-tab pack = £4.02. Label: 2

RELATED ANTIDEPRESSANTS

IPRINDOLE

Indications: depressive illness

Cautions; Contra-indications; Side-effects: see under Amitriptyline Hydrochloride, but less sedating. Caution in liver disease; jaundice, although rare, may develop, usually in the first 21 days

Dose: initially 15–30 mg 3 times daily, increased gradually to max. 60 mg 3 times daily; usual maintenance 30 mg 3 times daily; CHILD not recommended

PoM **Prondol**® (Wyeth)

Tablets, yellow, iprindole (as hydrochloride) 15 mg, net price 20 = 42p. Label: 2

MAPROTILINE HYDROCHLORIDE

Indications: depressive illness, particularly where sedation is required

Cautions; Contra-indications; Side-effects: see under Amitriptyline Hydrochloride, antimuscarinic effects may occur less frequently but rashes common and increased risk of convulsions at higher dosage; contra-indicated if history of epilepsy

Dose: initially 25–75 mg (elderly 30 mg) daily in 3 divided doses *or* as a single dose at bedtime, increased gradually as necessary to max. 150 mg daily; CHILD not recommended

PoM **Ludiomil**® (Ciba)

Tablets, all f/c, maprotiline hydrochloride 10 mg (pale yellow), net price 28-tab pack = 84p; 25 mg (greyish-red), 28-tab pack = £1.64; 50 mg (light orange), 28-tab pack = £3.19; 75 mg (brownish-orange), 28-tab pack = £4.66. Label: 2
Additives: include gluten

MIANSERIN HYDROCHLORIDE

Indications: depressive illness, particularly where sedation is required

Cautions; Contra-indications; Side-effects: see under Amitriptyline Hydrochloride; leucopenia, agranulocytosis and aplastic anaemia (particularly in the elderly); jaundice; arthritis, arthralgia; influenza-like syndrome may occur; **blood counts needed, p.164**

Fewer and milder antimuscarinic and cardiovascular effects; **interactions:** Appendix 1 (mianserin)

Dose: initially 30–40 mg (elderly 30 mg) daily in divided doses *or* as a single dose at bedtime, increased gradually as necessary; usual dose range 30–90 mg; CHILD not recommended

PoM **Mianserin** (Non-proprietary)

Tablets, mianserin hydrochloride 10 mg, net price 20 = £1.05; 20 mg, 20 = £2.10; 30 mg, 20 = £2.90. Label: 2, 25

PoM **Bolvidon**® (Organon)

Tablets, all f/c, mianserin hydrochloride 10 mg, net price 20 = £1.16; 20 mg, 20 = £2.33; 30 mg (scored), 20 = £3.49. Label: 2, 25

PoM **Norval**® (Bencard)

Tablets, orange, f/c, mianserin hydrochloride 20 mg, net price 28-tab pack = £3.66. Label: 2, 25

TRAZODONE HYDROCHLORIDE

Indications: depressive illness, particularly where sedation is required

Cautions; Contra-indications; Side-effects: see under Amitriptyline Hydrochloride but fewer antimuscarinic and cardiovascular effects; rarely priapism; **interactions:** Appendix 1 (trazodone)

Dose: initially 150 mg (elderly 100 mg) daily in divided doses after food *or* as a single dose at bedtime; may be increased to 300 mg daily; hospital patients up to max. 600 mg daily in divided doses; CHILD not recommended

PoM **Molipaxin**® (Roussel)

Capsules, trazodone hydrochloride 50 mg (violet/green), net price 84-cap pack = £17.31; 100 mg (violet/fawn), 56-cap pack = £20.38. Label: 2, 21
Tablets, pink, f/c, trazodone hydrochloride 150 mg. Net price 28-tab pack = £11.62. Label: 2, 21
Liquid, sugar-free, trazodone hydrochloride 50 mg/5 mL. Net price 150-mL pack = £7.74. Label: 2, 21
CR tablets, m/r, blue, f/c, trazodone hydrochloride 150 mg. Net price 28-tab pack = £11.62. Label: 2, 21, 25
Dose: initially 1 tablet daily (elderly, dose form not appropriate for initial dose titration), increased if necessary to 2 tablets daily (up to 4 tablets daily in hospital patients); CHILD not recommended

VILOXAZINE HYDROCHLORIDE

Indications: depressive illness

Cautions; Contra-indications; Side-effects: see under Amitriptyline Hydrochloride, but less sedating and antimuscarinic and cardiovascular side-effects are fewer and milder; nausea and headache may occur; **interactions:** Appendix 1 (viloxazine)

Dose: 300 mg daily (preferably as 200 mg in the morning and 100 mg at midday), increased gradually as necessary; max. 400 mg daily; last dose not later than 6 p.m.; ELDERLY 100 mg daily initially, half adult maintenance dose may be sufficient; CHILD under 14 years not recommended

PoM **Vivalan**® (Zeneca)

Tablets, f/c, viloxazine 50 mg (as hydrochloride). Net price 20 = £1.23. Label: 2

4.3.2 Monoamine-oxidase inhibitors
(MAOIs)

Monoamine-oxidase inhibitors are used much less frequently than tricyclic and related antidepressants because of the dangers of dietary and drug interactions and the fact that it is easier to prescribe MAOIs when tricyclic antidepressants have been unsuccessful than vice versa. **Tranylcypromine** is the most **hazardous** of the MAOIs because of its stimulant action. The drugs of choice are **phenelzine** or **isocarboxazid** which are less stimulant and therefore safer.

Phobic patients and depressed patients with atypical, hypochondriacal, or hysterical features are said to respond best to MAOIs. However, MAOIs should be tried in any patients who are refractory to treatment with other antidepressants as there is occasionally a dramatic response. Response to treatment may be delayed for 3 weeks or more and may take an additional 1 or 2 weeks to become maximal.

WITHDRAWAL. If possible MAOIs should be withdrawn slowly (see also section 4.3).

INTERACTIONS. MAOIs inhibit monoamine oxidase, thereby causing an accumulation of amine neurotransmitters. The metabolism of some amine drugs such as indirect-acting sympathomimetics is also inhibited and their pressor action may be potentiated; the pressor effect of tyramine (in some foods, such as mature cheese, yeast extracts and fermented soya bean products) may also be dangerously potentiated.

Sympathomimetics are present in many proprietary cough mixtures and decongestant nasal drops. See Appendix 1 (MAOIs) and Treatment Card.

These interactions may cause a dangerous rise in blood pressure. An early warning symptom may be a throbbing headache. The danger of interaction persists for up to 2 weeks after treatment with MAOIs is discontinued.

Other antidepressants should **not** be started for 2 weeks after treatment with MAOIs has been stopped. Some psychiatrists use selected tricyclics in conjunction with MAOIs but this is hazardous, indeed potentially lethal, except in experienced hands and there is no evidence that the combination is more effective than when either constituent is used alone. The combination of tranylcypromine with clomipramine is particularly **dangerous**.

Conversely, an MAOI should not be started until at least 1 week after a tricyclic or related antidepressant or a serotonin-uptake inhibitor antidepressant has been stopped (2 weeks in the case of paroxetine, 5 weeks in the case of fluoxetine).

In addition, an MAOI should not be started for at least a week after a previous MAOI has been stopped (then started at a reduced dose).

For other interactions with MAOIs including those with opioid analgesics (notably pethidine), see Appendix 1 (MAOIs). For guidance on interactions relating to the reversible monoamine oxidase inhibitor, moclobemide, see p. 169.

TREATMENT CARDS. Cards which list the necessary precautions to be taken by a patient receiving an MAOI are distributed by the Royal Pharmaceutical Society and given to patients at pharmacies and clinics. In Northern Ireland they can be obtained *via* Central Services Agency, 27 Adelaide St, Belfast BT2 8FH. In the case of the reversible MAOI, moclobemide, a patient information leaflet is available in the pack.

TREATMENT CARD
Carry this card with you at all times. Show it to any doctor who may treat you other than the doctor who prescribed this medicine, and to your dentist if you require dental treatment.

INSTRUCTIONS TO PATIENTS
Please read carefully
While taking this medicine and for 14 days after your treatment finishes you must observe the following simple instructions:-

1 Do not eat CHEESE, PICKLED HERRING OR BROAD BEAN PODS.

2 Do not eat or drink BOVRIL, OXO, MARMITE or ANY SIMILAR MEAT OR YEAST EXTRACT.

3 Eat only FRESH foods and avoid food that you suspect could be stale or 'going off'.   This is especially important with meat, fish, poultry or offal. Avoid game.

4 Do not take any other MEDICINES (including tablets, capsules, nose drops, inhalations or suppositories) whether purchased by you or previously prescribed by your doctor, without first consulting your doctor or your pharmacist.

   NB *Treatment for coughs and colds, pain relievers, tonics and laxatives are medicines.*

5 Avoid alcoholic drinks and de-alcoholised (low alcohol) drinks.

Keep a careful note of any food or drink that disagrees with you, avoid it and tell your doctor.

Report any unusual or severe symptoms to your doctor and follow any other advice given by him.

M.A.O.I. Prepared by The Pharmaceutical Society and the British Medical Association on behalf of the Health Departments of the United Kingdom.

Printed in the UK for HMSO 8217411/150M/9.89/4529
Revised Sep. 1989

PHENELZINE
Indications: depressive illness

Cautions: diabetes mellitus, cardiovascular disease, epilepsy, blood disorders, concurrent electroconvulsive therapy; avoid abrupt withdrawal; severe hypertensive reactions to certain drugs and foods (see Treatment Card); avoid in elderly and agitated patients; porphyria (see section 9.8.2); pregnancy and breast-feeding; surgery (see section 15.1); **interactions:** Appendix 1 (MAOIs)

DRIVING. Drowsiness may affect performance of skilled tasks (e.g. driving)

Contra-indications: hepatic impairment (see Appendix 2), cerebrovascular disease, phaeochromocytoma

Side-effects: adverse effects commonly associated with phenelzine and other MAOIs include postural hypotension and dizziness; other common side-effects include drowsiness, headache, weakness and fatigue, dryness of mouth, constipation and other gastro-intestinal disturbances, and oedema; agitation and tremors, nervousness, arrhythmias, blurred vision, difficulty in micturition, sweating, convulsions, rashes, leucopenia, sexual disturbances, and weight gain with inappropriate appetite may also occur; psychotic episodes with hypomanic behaviour, confusion, and hallucinations, may be induced in susceptible per-

---

sons; jaundice has been reported and, on rare occasions, fatal progressive hepatocellular necrosis; peripheral neuropathy may be due to pyridoxine deficiency; for CSM advice on possible hyponatraemia, see p.163

Dose: 15 mg 3 times daily, increased if necessary to 4 times daily after 2 weeks (hospital patients, max. 30 mg 3 times daily), then reduced gradually to lowest possible maintenance dose (15 mg on alternate days may be adequate); CHILD not recommended

PoM Nardil® (P-D)

Tablets, orange, f/c, phenelzine 15 mg (as sulphate). Net price 20 = £1.33. Label: 3, 10 MAOI card

ISOCARBOXAZID

Indications: depressive illness

Cautions; Contra-indications; Side-effects: see under Phenelzine

Dose: initially up to 30 mg daily in single or divided doses increased after 4 weeks if necessary to max. 60 mg daily for up to 6 weeks under close supervision only; then reduced to usual maintenance dose 10–20 mg daily (but up to 40 mg daily may be required); CHILD not recommended

PoM Marplan® (Cambridge)

Tablets, pink, scored, isocarboxazid 10 mg. Net price 50 = £2.52. Label: 3, 10 MAOI card

TRANYLCYPROMINE

Indications: depressive illness

Cautions; Contra-indications: see under Phenelzine; also contra-indicated in hyperthyroidism

Side-effects: see under Phenelzine; insomnia if given in evening; hypertensive crises with throbbing headache requiring discontinuation of treatment occur more frequently than with other MAOIs; liver damage occurs less frequently than with phenelzine

Dose: initially 10 mg twice daily not later than 3 p.m., increasing the second daily dose to 20 mg after 1 week if necessary; doses above 30 mg daily under close supervision only; usual maintenance dose 10 mg daily; CHILD not recommended

PoM Parnate® (SK&F)

Tablets, red, s/c, tranylcypromine 10 mg (as sulphate). Net price 20 = 91p. Label: 3, 10 MAOI card

REVERSIBLE MAOIs

Moclobemide is a newly introduced antidepressant indicated for major depression only; it is reported to act by reversible inhibition of monoamine oxidase type A (it is therefore termed a RIMA).

INTERACTIONS. Moclobemide is claimed to cause less potentiation of the pressor effect of tyramine than the traditional (irreversible) MAOIs, but

patients should avoid consuming large amounts of tyramine-rich food (such as mature cheese, yeast extracts and fermented soya bean products).

The risk of drug interactions is also claimed to be less but patients still need to avoid sympathomimetics such as ephedrine, pseudoephedrine, and phenylpropanolamine. In addition, moclobemide should not be given with another antidepressant. Owing to its short duration of action no treatment-free period is required after it has been stopped but it should not be started until at least a week after a tricyclic or related antidepressant or a serotonin-uptake inhibitor antidepressant has been stopped (2 weeks in the case of paroxetine, 5 weeks in the case of fluoxetine), or for at least a week after an MAOI has been stopped. For other interactions, see Appendix 1 (moclobemide).

MOCLOBEMIDE

Indications: major depression

Cautions: avoid in agitated or excited patients (or give with sedative for up to 2–3 weeks), thyrotoxicosis, severe hepatic impairment, may provoke manic episodes in bipolar disorders, pregnancy and breast-feeding (patient information leaflet advises avoid); **interactions:** see notes above and Appendix 1 (moclobemide)

Contra-indications: acute confusional states, phaeochromocytoma

Side-effects: sleep disturbances, dizziness, nausea, headache, restlessness, agitation; confusional states reported; rarely raised liver enzymes; for CSM advice on possible hyponatraemia, see p.163

Dose: initially 300 mg daily usually in divided doses after food, adjusted according to response; usual range 150–600 mg daily; CHILD not recommended

▼ PoM Manerix® (Roche)

Tablets, yellow, f/c, scored, moclobemide 150 mg. Net price 30 tab pack = £10.50. Label: 10 patient information leaflet, 21

4.3.3 Compound antidepressant preparations

The use of preparations listed below is **not** recommended because the dosage of the individual components should be adjusted separately. Whereas antidepressants are given continuously over several months, anxiolytics are prescribed on a short-term basis.

PoM Motipress® (Sanofi Winthrop)

Tablets, yellow, s/c, fluphenazine hydrochloride 1.5 mg, nortriptyline 30 mg (as hydrochloride). Net price 28-tab pack = £2.83. Label: 2

PoM Motival® (Sanofi Winthrop)

Tablets, pink, s/c, fluphenazine hydrochloride 500 micrograms, nortriptyline 10 mg (as hydrochloride). Net price 20 = 69p. Label: 2

PoM Parstelin® (SK&F)

Tablets, green, s/c, tranylcypromine 10 mg (as sulphate), trifluoperazine 1 mg (as hydrochloride). Net price 20 = 93p. Label: 3, 10 MAOI card

Caution: contains MAOI

PoM **Triptafen**® (Forley)

Tablets, pink, s/c, amitriptyline hydrochloride 25 mg, perphenazine 2 mg. Net price 20 = £3.45. Label: 2

PoM **Triptafen-M**® (Forley)

Tablets, pink, s/c, amitriptyline hydrochloride 10 mg, perphenazine 2 mg. Net price 20 = £3.04. Label: 2

4.3.4   Other antidepressant drugs

FLUPENTHIXOL

The thioxanthene **flupenthixol** (Fluanxol®) has antidepressant properties, and low doses (1 to 3 mg daily) are given by mouth for this purpose. Its advantages over the tricyclic and related antidepressants are that, with the low doses employed, side-effects are fewer, and that overdosage is less toxic.

FLUPENTHIXOL

(Flupentixol)

Indications: depressive illness (short-term use). For use in psychoses, see section 4.2.1

Cautions: cardiovascular disease (including cardiac disorders and cerebral arteriosclerosis), senile confusional states, parkinsonism, renal and hepatic disease; avoid in excitable and overactive patients; porphyria (see section 9.8.2); **interactions**: Appendix 1 (phenothiazines and other antipsychotics)

DRIVING. Drowsiness may affect performance of skilled tasks (e.g. driving); effects of alcohol enhanced

Side-effects: restlessness, insomnia; hypomania reported; rarely dizziness, tremor, visual disturbances, headache, hyperprolactinaemia, extrapyramidal symptoms

Dose: initially 1 mg (elderly 500 micrograms) in the morning, increased after 1 week to 2 mg (elderly 1 mg) if necessary. Max. 3 mg (elderly 2 mg) daily, doses above 2 mg (elderly 1 mg) being divided in 2 portions, second dose not after 4 p. m. Discontinue if no response after 1 week at maximum dosage; CHILD not recommended

COUNSELLING. Although drowsiness may occur, can also have an alerting effect so should not be taken in the evening

PoM **Depixol**® (psychoses), see section 4.2.1

PoM **Fluanxol**® (Lundbeck)

Tablets, both red, s/c, flupenthixol (as dihydrochloride) 500 micrograms, net price 20 = 98p; 1 mg, 60-tab pack = £4.98. Label: 2, counselling, administration

TRYPTOPHAN

Tryptophan appears to benefit some patients with resistant depression when given as adjunctive therapy but tryptophan products were withdrawn following evidence of an association with the eosinophilia-myalgia syndrome; Optimax® (Merck) has now been re-introduced for patients for whom no alternative treatment is suitable.

TRYPTOPHAN

(L-Tryptophan)

Indications: restricted to use by hospital specialists *only* for patients with severe and disabling depressive illness of more than 2 years continuous duration, *only* after an adequate trial of standard antidepressant drug treatment, and *only* as an adjunct to other antidepressant medication

Cautions: eosinophilia-myalgia syndrome has been reported with tryptophan-containing products therefore close and regular surveillance required; monitor eosinophil count, haematological changes and muscle symptomatology; pregnancy and breast-feeding; **interactions:** Appendix 1 (tryptophan)

Contra-indications: history of eosinophilia-myalgia syndrome following use of tryptophan

Side-effects: drowsiness, nausea, headache, lightheadedness; eosinophilia-myalgia syndrome, see Cautions

Dose: 1 g 3 times daily; max. 6 g daily; ELDERLY lower dose may be appropriate especially where renal or hepatic impairment; CHILD not recommended

▼ PoM **Optimax**® (Merck)

Tablets, scored, tryptophan 500 mg. Net price 84-tab pack = £16.30 (hosp. only). Label: 3

Note. Patient and prescriber must be registered with the Optimax® Information and Clinical Support (OPTICS) Unit

SSRIs

Fluvoxamine, fluoxetine, paroxetine, and **sertraline** selectively inhibit the re-uptake of serotonin (5-hydroxytryptamine, 5-HT); they are termed selective serotonin re-uptake inhibitors (SSRIs) and appear to be effective antidepressants. They are less sedative than the tricyclics, with few antimuscarinic effects and with low cardiotoxicity. They do not cause weight gain. Gastro-intestinal side-effects (diarrhoea, nausea and vomiting) are dose-related; headache, restlessness and anxiety may also occur. As with the tricyclic antidepressants caution is necessary in epilepsy.

WITHDRAWAL. If possible SSRIs should be withdrawn slowly (see also section 4.3). See also next page for a CSM warning relating to paroxetine withdrawal.

INTERACTIONS. A serotonin-uptake inhibitor antidepressant should not be started until 2 weeks after stopping an MAOI. Conversely, an MAOI should not be started until at least a week after a serotonin-uptake inhibitor has been stopped (2 weeks in the case of paroxetine, 5 weeks in the case of fluoxetine). For guidance relating to the reversible monoamine oxidase inhibitor, moclobemide, see p. 169. For other serotonin-uptake inhibitor antidepressant interactions, see Appendix 1 (antidepressants, serotonin-uptake inhibitor).

FLUOXETINE

Indications: see under Dose

Cautions: cardiac disease, epilepsy (avoid if poorly controlled, discontinue if convulsions develop), concurrent electroconvulsive therapy (prolonged seizures reported), history of mania, hepatic and renal impairment (see Appendixes 2 and 3), pregnancy and breast-feeding (see Appendixes 4 and 5), diabetes mellitus, avoid abrupt withdrawal; **interactions:** Appendix 1 (antidepressants, serotonin uptake inhibitor)

DRIVING. May impair performance of skilled tasks (e.g. driving)

Side-effects: gastro-intestinal (fairly common—include nausea, vomiting, dyspepsia, abdominal pain, diarrhoea, constipation, anorexia with weight loss and possible changes in blood sugar); hypersensitivity reactions (**important:** see also below); also dry mouth, nervousness, anxiety, headache, insomnia, palpitations, tremor, confusion, dizziness, hypotension, hypomania or mania, drowsiness, asthenia, convulsions, fever, sexual dysfunction, sweating; movement disorders and dyskinesias, liver function changes (discontinue), neuroleptic malignant syndrome-like event; hyponatraemia (may be due to inappropriate antidiuretic hormone secretion), see CSM warning on p.163; also reported (no causal relationship established): aplastic anaemia, cerebrovascular accident, ecchymoses, eosinophilic pneumonia, gastro-intestinal haemorrhage, hyperprolactinaemia, haemolytic anaemia, pancreatitis, pancytopenia, suicidal ideation, thrombocytopenia, thrombocytopenic purpura, vaginal bleeding on withdrawal, violent behaviour; hair loss also reported

HYPERSENSITIVITY. Angioedema, urticaria, pruritus, and other allergic reactions including anaphylaxis have been reported (discontinue if rash occurs, may be warning of impending serious systemic reaction, possibly associated with vasculitis); pharyngitis and rarely pulmonary inflammation or fibrosis (with dyspnoea only warning sign) also reported; possible hypersensitivity signs associated with other SSRIs include arthralgia, myalgia

Dose: depressive illness, 20 mg daily; CHILD not recommended

Bulimia nervosa, 60 mg daily; CHILD not recommended

Obsessive-compulsive disorder, initially 20 mg daily, dose increase may be considered if response after several weeks, but may be increased potential for side-effects; max. 60 mg daily; CHILD not recommended

LONG DURATION OF ACTION. Account should be taken of the long half-life of fluoxetine when adjusting dosage (or in overdosage)

PoM **Prozac**® (Dista)

Capsules, green/off-white, fluoxetine (as hydrochloride) 20 mg, net price 30-cap pack = £20.77, 98-cap pack = £67.85. Counselling, driving

Liquid, fluoxetine (as hydrochloride), 20 mg/5 mL. Net price 70-mL pack = £19.39. Counselling, driving

FLUVOXAMINE MALEATE

Indications: depressive illness

Cautions; Side-effects: see under Fluoxetine; bradycardia also reported

Dose: 100–200 mg daily (up to 100 mg as single dose in evening); max. 300 mg daily in divided doses; CHILD not recommended

PoM **Faverin**® (Duphar)

Tablets, both yellow, fluvoxamine maleate 50 mg, net price 60-tab pack = £25.00; 100 mg, 30-tab pack = £25.00. Counselling, driving

PAROXETINE

Indications: depressive illness

Cautions; Side-effects: see under Fluoxetine

CSM advice. Extrapyramidal reactions (including orofacial dystonias) and withdrawal syndrome are reported to the CSM more commonly than with other SSRIs

Dose: usually 20 mg each morning, if necessary increased gradually in increments of 10 mg to max. 50 mg daily (elderly, 40 mg daily); CHILD not recommended

▼ PoM **Seroxat**® (SmithKline Beecham)

Tablets, both f/c, scored, paroxetine 20 mg (as hydrochloride), net price 30-tab pack = £27.46; 30 mg (blue), 30-tab pack = £41.19. Label: 21, counselling, driving

SERTRALINE

Indications: depressive illness

Cautions; Side-effects: see under Fluoxetine

Dose: initially 50 mg daily, increased if necessary by increments of 50 mg over several weeks to max. 200 mg daily, then reduced to usual maintenance of 50–100 mg daily; doses of 150 mg or greater should not be used for more than 8 weeks; CHILD not recommended

PoM **Lustral**® (Invicta)

Tablets, sertraline (as hydrochloride) 50 mg, net price 28-tab pack = £26.51; 100 mg, 28-tab pack = £39.77. Label: 21, counselling, driving

4.4   Central nervous system stimulants

Central nervous system stimulants have very few indications and in particular, should **not** be used to treat depression, obesity, senility, debility, or for relief of fatigue.

Caffeine is a weak stimulant present in tea and coffee. It is included in many analgesic preparations (section 4.7.1) but does not contribute to their analgesic or anti-inflammatory effect. Over-indulgence may lead to a state of anxiety.

The **amphetamines** have a limited field of usefulness and their use should be **discouraged** as they may cause dependence and psychotic states.

Patients with narcolepsy may derive benefit from treatment with amphetamines.

Amphetamines have been advocated (under specialist supervision) for the management of hyperactive children; beneficial effects have been described. However, they must be used very selectively as they retard growth and the effect of long-term therapy has not been evaluated.

Amphetamines have **no place** in the management of **depression** or **obesity**.

Pemoline is a weak central nervous system stimulant that has been advocated for the management of hyperactive children. The same general reservations apply as for amphetamines and treatment should be carried out only under specialist supervision.

DEXAMPHETAMINE SULPHATE

Indications: narcolepsy, adjunct in the management of hyperkinesia in children (under specialist supervision)

Cautions: mild hypertension (contra-indicated if moderate or severe); monitor growth in children; avoid abrupt withdrawal; porphyria (see section 9.8.2); **interactions:** Appendix 1 (sympathomimetics)

Contra-indications: cardiovascular disease or moderate to severe hypertension (caution if mild), hyperexcitable states, hyperthyroidism, history of drug abuse, glaucoma, extrapyramidal disorders, pregnancy and breast-feeding

DRIVING. May affect performance of skilled tasks (e.g. driving); effects of alcohol unpredictable

Side-effects: insomnia, restlessness, irritability, nervousness, night terrors, euphoria, tremor, dizziness, headache; dependence, tolerance, sometimes psychosis; anorexia, gastro-intestinal symptoms, growth retardation in children; dry mouth, sweating, tachycardia, palpitations, increased blood pressure; rarely cardiomyopathy reported with chronic use; overdosage: see Emergency Treatment of Poisoning, p.23

Dose: narcolepsy, 10 mg (elderly, 5 mg) daily in divided doses increased by 10 mg (elderly, 5 mg) daily at intervals of 1 week to a max. of 60 mg daily

Hyperkinesia, CHILD over 6 years 5–10 mg in the morning, increased if necessary by 5 mg at intervals of 1 week to usual max. 20 mg daily (older children have received max. 40 mg daily)

CD Dexedrine® (Evans)
Tablets, scored, dexamphetamine sulphate 5 mg. Net price 20 = 68p. Counselling, driving

PEMOLINE

Indications: adjunct in the management of hyperkinesia in children (under specialist supervision)

Cautions; Contra-indications; Side-effects: see under Dexamphetamine Sulphate; chorea, tics, mania, depression, neutropenia, and liver enzyme abnormalities also reported

Dose: CHILD over 6 years, initially 20 mg every morning increased by increments of 20 mg at intervals of 1 week to 60 mg every morning, followed, if no improvement, by gradual increase to max. 120 mg every morning

PoM **Volital®** (LAB)
Tablets, scored, pemoline 20 mg. Net price 25-tab pack = £1.10

STIMULANT WITH VITAMINS

Prolintane is contained in a preparation with vitamins; it is **not** recommended and is specifically **contra-indicated** in epilepsy and hyperthyroidism.

NHS PoM **Villescon®** (Boehringer Ingelheim)
Liquid, red, prolintane hydrochloride 2.5 mg/5 mL with vitamins B group and C. Net price 150-mL pack = 85p
Dose: 10 mL twice daily before 4 p.m. for 1–2 weeks but see notes above.

COCAINE

Cocaine is a drug of addiction which causes central nervous stimulation. Its clinical use is mainly as a topical local anaesthetic (see sections 11.7 and 15.2). It has been included in analgesic elixirs for the relief of pain in terminal care but this use is obsolete. For management of cocaine poisoning, see p.23.

4.5   Appetite suppressants

4.5.1   Bulk-forming drugs
4.5.2   Centrally acting appetite suppressants

The development of obesity appears to be multifactorial. Aggravating factors may be depression or other psychosocial problems or drug treatment.

The main treatment of the obese patient is an appropriate diet, carefully explained to the patient, with support and encouragement from the doctor. Attendance at groups (for example 'weight-watchers') helps some individuals. Drugs can play only a limited role and should never be used as the sole element of treatment; their effects tend to be disappointing.

The use of diuretics is **not** appropriate for weight reduction.

4.5.1   Bulk-forming drugs

The most commonly used bulk-forming drug is **methylcellulose**. It is claimed to reduce intake by producing feelings of satiety but there is little evidence to support this claim.

METHYLCELLULOSE

Indications: obesity; other indications, see section 1.6.1

Cautions: maintain adequate fluid intake

Contra-indications: gastro-intestinal obstruction

Side-effects: flatulence, abdominal distension, intestinal obstruction

Dose: see under preparations below

COUNSELLING. Preparations that swell in contact with liquid should always be carefully swallowed with water and should not be taken immediately before going to bed

Celevac® (Monmouth)

Tablets, pink, methylcellulose '450' 500 mg. Net price 112-tab pack = £2.45. Counselling, see above and dose

Dose: 3 tablets, chewed or crushed, with a tumblerful of liquid half an hour before food or when hungry

STERCULIA

Indications; Cautions; Contra-indications; Side-effects: see under Methylcellulose
Dose: see under preparation below

Prefil® (Norgine)

Granules, brown, coated, sugar- and gluten-free, sterculia 80%, 7 g/sachet. Net price 30-sachet pack = £4.42. Label: 22, 27, counselling, administration

Dose: one sachet followed by a tumblerful of liquid ½–1 hour before food, lower initial dose in patients accustomed to a low-residue diet; CHILD reduced dose

4.5.2   Centrally acting appetite suppressants

Centrally acting appetite suppressants are of no real value in the treatment of obesity since they do not improve the long-term outlook. They are sympathomimetics and most have a pronounced stimulant effect on the central nervous system.

Use of the amphetamine-like drugs **diethylpropion** and **phentermine** is **not** justified as any possible benefits are outweighed by the risks involved; abuse, particularly of diethylpropion, is an increasing problem.

Although **fenfluramine** is also related to amphetamine, in standard doses it has a sedative rather than a stimulant effect. Nevertheless, abuse has occurred and abrupt withdrawal may induce depression. It should preferably be avoided but may be considered for short-term adjunctive treatment in selected patients with severe obesity, given close support and supervision. It should **not** be given to patients with a past history of epilepsy, drug abuse or psychiatric illness and is **not recommended** for periods of treatment beyond 3 months. It should **not** be used for cosmetic reasons in mild to moderate obesity.

Dexfenfluramine is the dextro isomer of fenfluramine.

Thyroid hormones have no place in the treatment of obesity except in hypothyroid patients.

CHILDREN. These drugs should be avoided in children because of the possibility of growth suppression.

DEXFENFLURAMINE HYDROCHLORIDE

Indications: see notes above
Cautions; Contra-indications; Side-effects: see under Fenfluramine Hydrochloride; avoid in hepatic and renal impairment

Dose: 15 mg morning and evening, at mealtimes; max. period of treatment should not exceed 3 months; ELDERLY and CHILD not recommended

▼ **PoM Adifax®** (Servier)

Capsules, dexfenfluramine hydrochloride 15 mg, net price 60-cap pack = £8.08. Label: 2

DIETHYLPROPION HYDROCHLORIDE

Indications: not recommended, see notes above
Cautions: severe hepatic or renal impairment; cardiovascular disease (avoid if severe), avoid in peptic ulceration, prostatic hypertrophy, depression, anxiety, tension states, porphyria (see section 9.8.2); **interactions:** Appendix 1 (sympathomimetics)
DRIVING. May impair performance of skilled tasks (e.g. driving); effects of alcohol unpredictable
Contra-indications: glaucoma, hyperthyroidism, epilepsy, unstable personality, psychiatric illness, severe hypertension; history of drug abuse; pregnancy (congenital malformations reported) and breast-feeding
Side-effects: dry mouth, headache, rashes, dependence; less common, insomnia, increased nervousness, depression, psychosis, hallucinations, tachycardia, hypertension, constipation; rarely, gynaecomastia

CD Apisate® (Wyeth)

Tablets, m/r, yellow, diethylpropion hydrochloride 75 mg, thiamine hydrochloride 5 mg, pyridoxine hydrochloride 2 mg, riboflavine 4 mg, nicotinamide 30 mg. Net price 20 = 52p. Label: 25, counselling, driving
Dose: 1 tablet mid-morning; to reduce risk of dependence max. continuous period of treatment should not exceed 4–8 weeks (followed by similar period without treatment); ELDERLY and CHILD not recommended

CD Tenuate Dospan® (Merrell)

Tablets, m/r, scored, diethylpropion hydrochloride 75 mg. Net price 30-tab pack = 94p. Label: 25, counselling, driving
Dose: 1 tablet mid-morning; to reduce risk of dependence max. continuous period of treatment should not exceed 8 weeks (followed by similar period without treatment); ELDERLY and CHILD not recommended
Note. Brand name prescriptions for Tenuate Dospan must also specify the word 'tablets' (i.e. 'Tenuate Dospan Tablets').

FENFLURAMINE HYDROCHLORIDE

Indications: see notes above
Cautions: dependence reported, depression on sudden withdrawal (gradual reduction over at least a week preferable); advise patient to report immediately dyspnoea or deterioration in exercise tolerance; elderly; porphyria (see section 9.8.2); **interactions:** Appendix 1 (sympathomimetics)
DRIVING. Drowsiness may affect performance of skilled tasks (e.g. driving); effects of alcohol enhanced
Contra-indications: history of psychiatric illness (including anorexia nervosa and depression), drug or alcohol abuse; personality disorders; epilepsy; glaucoma; pregnancy and breast-feeding
Side-effects: diarrhoea and other gastro-intestinal disturbances; drowsiness, dizziness, and lethargy; also dry mouth, headache, nervousness, irritability, sleep disturbances, depression, visual disorders, hypotension, urinary frequency, impotence and loss of libido; rarely rashes, blood disorders,

pulmonary hypertension, schizophrenia-like reactions; neurotoxicity reported in *animal* studies
Dose: see below

PoM Ponderax® (Servier)
Pacaps® (= capsules m/r), clear/blue, enclosing white pellets, fenfluramine hydrochloride 60 mg. Net price 60-cap pack = £7.08. Label: 2, 25
Dose: 1 capsule daily; max. period of treatment should not exceed 3 months (see also notes above); CHILD not recommended

PHENTERMINE
Indications: not recommended, see notes above
Cautions; Contra-indications; Side-effects: see under Diethylpropion Hydrochloride
Dose: 15–30 mg before breakfast; to reduce the risk of dependence max. continuous period of treatment should not exceed 4–8 weeks (followed by similar period without treatment); ELDERLY and CHILD not recommended

CD Duromine® (3M)
Capsules, both m/r, phentermine (as resin complex) 15 mg (green/grey), net price 30-cap pack = £1.14; 30 mg (maroon/grey), 30-cap pack = £1.50. Label: 25, counselling, driving
CD Ionamin® (Lipha)
Capsules, both m/r, phentermine (as resin complex) 15 mg (grey/yellow), net price 20 = 97p; 30 mg (yellow), 20 = £1.22. Label: 25, counselling, driving

4.6 Drugs used in nausea and vertigo

Anti-emetics should be prescribed only when the cause of vomiting is known, particularly in children, otherwise the symptomatic relief that they produce may delay diagnosis. Anti-emetics are unnecessary and sometimes harmful when the cause can be treated, e.g. as in diabetic ketoacidosis, or in excessive digoxin or antiepileptic dosage.

If antinauseant drug treatment is indicated the choice of drug depends on the aetiology of vomiting.

VESTIBULAR DISORDERS

The most effective drug for the prevention of *motion sickness* is **hyoscine**. Adverse effects (drowsiness, blurred vision, dry mouth, urinary retention) are more frequent than with the antihistamines but are not generally prominent at the doses employed. **Antihistamines** are slightly less effective, but are generally better tolerated. There is no evidence that any one antihistamine is superior to another but their duration of action and incidence of adverse effects (drowsiness and antimuscarinic effects) differ. If a sedative effect is desired **promethazine** and **dimenhydrinate** are useful, but generally a slightly less sedating antihistamine such as **cyclizine** or **cinnarizine** is preferred. **Metoclopramide** and the **phenothiazines** (except the antihistamine phenothiazine promethazine), which act selectively on the chemoreceptor trigger zone, are ineffective in motion sickness.

Vertigo and nausea associated with *Ménière's disease* and *middle-ear surgery* may be difficult to treat. **Hyoscine, antihistamines,** and **phenothiazines** (such as prochlorperazine) are effective in the prophylaxis and treatment of such conditions. **Cinnarizine** and **betahistine** have been promoted as specific treatments for Ménière's disease. In the acute attack **cyclizine** or **prochlorperazine** may be given rectally or by intramuscular injection.

Treatment of vertigo in its chronic forms is seldom fully effective but antihistamines (such as dimenhydrinate) or phenothiazines (such as prochlorperazine) may help.

For advice to avoid the inappropriate prescribing of drugs (notably phenothiazines) for dizziness in the elderly, see Prescribing for the Elderly, p. 16.

VOMITING OF PREGNANCY

Nausea in the first trimester of pregnancy does **not** require drug therapy. On rare occasions if vomiting is severe, an antihistamine or a phenothiazine (e.g. promethazine) may be required. If symptoms have not settled in 24 to 48 hours then a specialist opinion should be sought.

SYMPTOMATIC RELIEF OF NAUSEA FROM UNDERLYING DISEASE

The **phenothiazines** are dopamine antagonists and act centrally by blocking the chemoreceptor trigger zone. They are of considerable value for the prophylaxis and treatment of nausea and vomiting associated with diffuse neoplastic disease, radiation sickness, and the emesis caused by drugs such as opioid analgesics, general anaesthetics, and cytotoxic drugs. **Prochlorperazine, perphenazine,** and **trifluoperazine** are less sedating than **chlorpromazine** but severe dystonic reactions sometimes occur, especially in children.

Metoclopramide is an effective anti-emetic with a spectrum of activity closely resembling that of the phenothiazines but it has a peripheral action on the gut in addition to its central effect and therefore may be superior to the phenothiazines in the emesis associated with gastroduodenal, hepatic, and biliary disease. As with the phenothiazines, metoclopramide may induce acute dystonic reactions with facial and skeletal muscle spasms and oculogyric crises. These are more common in the young (especially girls and young women) and the very old, usually occur shortly after starting treatment, and subside within 24 hours of stopping the drug. Injection of an antiparkinsonian agent such as procyclidine (see section 4.9.2) will abort attacks. The high-dose preparation of metoclopramide is of value in the prevention of nausea and vomiting associated with cytotoxic drug therapy.

Domperidone is used for the relief of nausea and vomiting, especially when associated with cytotoxic drug therapy. It has the advantage over metoclopramide and the phenothiazines of being less likely to cause central effects such as sedation and dystonic reactions because it does not readily cross the blood-brain barrier. It may be given for the treatment of levodopa- and bromocriptine-induced vomiting in parkinsonism (section 4.9.1). Domperidone acts at the chemoreceptor trigger zone and so is unlikely to be effective in motion sickness and other vestibular disorders.

Antihistamines are active in most of these conditions, but are not usually drugs of choice.

Nabilone is a synthetic cannabinoid with antiemetic properties, reported to be superior to prochlorperazine. It is beneficial in the relief of nausea and vomiting associated with cytotoxic drug therapy. Side-effects occur in most patients given standard doses.

Granisetron, ondansetron and **tropisetron** are specific $(5HT_3)$ serotonin antagonists. They have a valuable role in the management of nausea and vomiting in patients receiving cytotoxics who are unable to tolerate, or whose nausea and vomiting is not controlled by, less expensive drugs.

CYTOTOXIC CHEMOTHERAPY. For *anti-emetic regimens* used in the management of nausea and vomiting induced by cytotoxic chemotherapy, see section 8.1.

ANTIHISTAMINES

CINNARIZINE

Indications: vestibular disorders, such as vertigo, tinnitus, nausea, and vomiting in Ménière's disease; motion sickness; vascular disease, see section 2.6.3

Cautions; Side-effects: see under Cyclizine; also allergic skin reactions and fatigue; caution in hypotension (high doses); rarely, extrapyramidal symptoms in elderly on prolonged therapy; avoid in porphyria (see section 9.8.2)

Dose: vestibular disorders, 30 mg 3 times daily; CHILD 5–12 years half adult dose
Motion sickness, 30 mg 2 hours before travel then 15 mg every 8 hours during journey if necessary; CHILD 5–12 years half adult dose

Cinnarizine (Non-proprietary)
Tablets, cinnarizine 15 mg. Net price 20 = £1.07. Label: 2
Available from APS, Ashbourne (Cinazière®), Cox, Hillcross, Norton
Stugeron® (Janssen)
Tablets, scored, cinnarizine 15 mg. Net price 20 = £1.07. Label: 2
Stugeron Forte® : see section 2.6.3

CYCLIZINE

Indications: nausea, vomiting, vertigo, motion sickness, labyrinthine disorders
Cautions; Side-effects: drowsiness, occasional dry mouth and blurred vision; see also section 3.4.1 (Disadvantages of Antihistamines); cyclizine may aggravate severe heart failure and counteract the haemodynamic benefits of opioids; **interactions:** Appendix 1 (antihistamines)
DRIVING. Drowsiness may affect performance of skilled tasks (e.g. driving); effects of alcohol enhanced

Dose: by mouth, cyclizine hydrochloride 50 mg up to 3 times daily; CHILD 6–12 years 25 mg
By intramuscular or intravenous injection, cyclizine lactate 50 mg 3 times daily

Valoid® (Wellcome)
Tablets, scored, cyclizine hydrochloride 50 mg. Net price 20 = 99p. Label: 2
PoM *Injection,* cyclizine lactate 50 mg/mL. Net price 1-mL amp = 57p

DIMENHYDRINATE

Indications: nausea, vomiting, vertigo, motion sickness, labyrinthine disorders
Cautions; Side-effects: see under Cyclizine; porphyria (see section 9.8.2)
Dose: 50–100 mg 2–3 times daily; CHILD 1–6 years 12.5–25 mg, 7–12 years 25–50 mg
Motion sickness, first dose 30 minutes before journey

Dramamine® (Searle)
Tablets, scored, dimenhydrinate 50 mg, net price 100-tab pack = £5.13. Label: 2
Note. A 10-tab pack is on sale to the public for motion sickness

MECLOZINE HYDROCHLORIDE

Indications: see under preparations
Cautions; Side-effects: see under Cyclizine

Preparations

A proprietary brand of meclozine hydrochloride tablets 12.5 mg (Sea-legs®) is on sale to the public for motion sickness

PROMETHAZINE HYDROCHLORIDE

Indications: nausea, vomiting, vertigo, labyrinthine disorders, motion sickness; other indications, see sections 3.4.1, 4.1.1, 15.1.4.1
Cautions; Side-effects: see under Cyclizine but more sedating; intramuscular injection may be painful; avoid in porphyria (see section 9.8.2)
Dose: by mouth, 25–50 mg daily in single or divided doses; max. 75 mg
Motion sickness prevention, 25 mg at bedtime on night before travelling, repeat following morning if necessary; CHILD, 1–5 years, 5 mg at night and following morning (1–2 years on doctor's advice only); 5–10 years, 10 mg at night and following morning
By deep intramuscular injection, 25–50 mg when necessary; CHILD 5–10 years 6.25–12.5 mg
By slow intravenous injection, see section 3.4.1

Preparations
See section 3.4.1

PROMETHAZINE THEOCLATE

(Promethazine Teoclate)

Indications: nausea, vertigo, labyrinthine disorders, motion sickness (acts longer than the hydrochloride)

Cautions; Side-effects: see under Promethazine Hydrochloride

Dose: 25–75 mg, max. 100 mg, daily; CHILD 5–10 years, 12.5–37.5 mg daily

Motion sickness prevention, 25 mg at bedtime on night before travelling *or* 25 mg 1–2 hours before travelling; CHILD 5–10 years, half adult dose

For severe vomiting in pregnancy, 25 mg at bedtime, increased if necessary to a max. of 100 mg daily (but see also Vomiting of Pregnancy in notes above)

Avomine® (Rhône-Poulenc Rorer)

Tablets, scored, promethazine theoclate 25 mg. Net price 10-tab pack = 90p; 28-tab pack = 93p. Label: 2

PHENOTHIAZINES AND RELATED

CHLORPROMAZINE HYDROCHLORIDE

Indications: nausea and vomiting of terminal illness (where other drugs have failed or are not available); other indications, see sections 4.2.1, 15.1.4.1

Cautions; Contra-indications; Side-effects: see section 4.2.1

Dose: by mouth, 10–25 mg every 4–6 hours; CHILD 500 micrograms/kg every 4–6 hours (1–5 years max. 40 mg daily, 6–12 years max. 75 mg daily)

By deep intramuscular injection 25 mg initially then 25–50 mg every 3–4 hours until vomiting stops; CHILD 500 micrograms/kg every 6–8 hours (1–5 years max. 40 mg daily, 6–12 years max. 75 mg daily)

By rectum in suppositories, chlorpromazine 100 mg every 6–8 hours [unlicensed]

Preparations
Section 4.2.1

DROPERIDOL
Section 4.2.1

HALOPERIDOL
Section 4.2.1

METHOTRIMEPRAZINE
Section 4.2.1

PERPHENAZINE

Indications: severe nausea, vomiting (see notes above); other indications, section 4.2.1

Cautions; Contra-indications; Side-effects: see section 4.2.1; extrapyramidal symptoms may occur, particularly in young adults, elderly, and debilitated

Dose: 4 mg 3 times daily, adjusted according to response; max. 24 mg daily (chemotherapy-induced); ELDERLY quarter to half adult dose; CHILD under 14 years not recommended

Preparations
Section 4.2.1

PROCHLORPERAZINE

Indications: severe nausea, vomiting, vertigo, labyrinthine disorders (see notes above); other indications, section 4.2.1

Cautions; Contra-indications: see under Chlorpromazine Hydrochloride (section 4.2.1). Oral route only for children (avoid if less than 10 kg); elderly (see notes above)

Side-effects: see under Chlorpromazine Hydrochloride; extrapyramidal symptoms may occur, particularly in children, elderly, and debilitated

Dose: by mouth, nausea and vomiting, prochlorperazine maleate or mesylate, acute attack, 20 mg initially then 10 mg after 2 hours; prevention 5–10 mg 2–3 times daily; CHILD (over 10 kg only) 250 micrograms/kg 2–3 times daily

Labyrinthine disorders, 5 mg 3 times daily, gradually increased if necessary to 30 mg daily in divided doses, then reduced after several weeks to 5–10 mg daily; CHILD not recommended

By deep intramuscular injection, nausea and vomiting, 12.5 mg when required followed if necessary after 6 hours by an oral dose, as above; CHILD not recommended

By rectum in suppositories, nausea and vomiting, 25 mg followed if necessary after 6 hours by oral dose, as above; *or* due to migraine, 5 mg 3 times daily; CHILD not recommended

PoM **Prochlorperazine** (Non-proprietary)

Tablets, prochlorperazine maleate 5 mg, net price 20 = 67p. Label: 2

Available from Ashbourne (Prozière®), Cox, Hillcross, K Pharm., Norton

PoM **Stemetil®** (Rhône-Poulenc Rorer)

Tablets, prochlorperazine maleate 5 mg (off-white), net price 84-tab pack = £2.87; 25 mg (scored), 56-tab pack = £5.06. Label: 2

Syrup, straw-coloured, prochlorperazine mesylate 5 mg/5 mL. Net price 100-mL pack =£1.62. Label: 2

Eff sachets, granules, effervescent, sugar-free, prochlorperazine mesylate 5 mg/sachet. Net price 21-sachet pack = £3.01. Label: 2, 13

Injection, prochlorperazine mesylate 12.5 mg/mL. Net price 1-mL amp = 32p; 2-mL amp = 40p

Suppositories, prochlorperazine maleate (as prochlorperazine), 5 mg, net price 10 = £4.06; 25 mg, 10 = £5.33. Label: 2

Buccal preparation

PoM **Buccastem**® (R&C)

Tablets (buccal), pale yellow, prochlorperazine maleate 3 mg. Net price 4 × 15-tab pack = £6.90. Label: 2, counselling, administration, see under Dose below

Dose: 1–2 tablets twice daily; tablets are placed high between upper lip and gum and left to dissolve; CHILD not recommended

TRIFLUOPERAZINE

Indications: severe nausea and vomiting (see notes above); other indications, section 4.2.1

Cautions; Contra-indications; Side-effects: see section 4.2.1; extrapyramidal symptoms may occur, particularly in children, elderly, and debilitated

Dose: by mouth, 2–4 mg daily in divided doses or as a single dose of a modified-release preparation; max. 6 mg daily; CHILD 3–5 years up to 1 mg daily, 6–12 years up to 4 mg daily

By deep intramuscular injection, 1–3 mg daily in divided doses, max. 6 mg daily

Preparations

See section 4.2.1

DOMPERIDONE AND METOCLOPRAMIDE

DOMPERIDONE

Indications: see under Dose

Cautions: renal impairment; pregnancy and breast-feeding; not recommended for routine prophylaxis of post-operative vomiting or for chronic administration; **interactions:** Appendix 1 (domperidone)

Side-effects: raised prolactin concentrations (possible galactorrhoea and gynaecomastia), reduced libido reported; rashes and other allergic reactions; acute dystonic reactions reported

Dose: by mouth, acute nausea and vomiting (including nausea and vomiting induced by levodopa and bromocriptine), 10–20 mg every 4–8 hours, max. period of treatment 12 weeks; CHILD, nausea and vomiting following cytotoxic therapy or radiotherapy only, 200–400 micrograms/kg every 4–8 hours

Functional dyspepsia, 10–20 mg 3 times daily before food and 10–20 mg at night; max. period of treatment 12 weeks; CHILD not recommended

By rectum in suppositories, nausea and vomiting, 30–60 mg every 4–8 hours; CHILD over 2 years (following cytotoxic therapy or radiotherapy only), body-weight 10–15 kg max. 15 mg twice daily, body-weight 15.5–25 kg max. 30 mg twice daily, body-weight 25.5–35 kg max. 30 mg 3 times daily, body-weight 35.5–45 kg max. 30 mg 4 times daily; since dose needs to be divided throughout day, suppositories may be cut in half for younger children

PoM **Motilium**® (Sanofi Winthrop)

Tablets, f/c, domperidone 10 mg (as maleate). Net price 30-tab pack = £2.46; 100-tab pack = £8.21

Suspension, sugar-free, domperidone 5 mg/5 mL. Net price 200-mL pack = £1.80

Suppositories, domperidone 30 mg. Net price 10 = £2.65

METOCLOPRAMIDE HYDROCHLORIDE

Indications: adults, nausea and vomiting, particularly in gastro-intestinal disorders and treatment with cytotoxics or radiotherapy; gastro-intestinal—section 1.2; migraine—section 4.7.4.1

PATIENTS UNDER 20 YEARS. Use restricted to severe intractable vomiting of known cause, vomiting of radiotherapy and cytotoxics, aid to gastro-intestinal intubation, pre-medication

Cautions: hepatic and renal impairment; elderly, young adults, and children (measure dose accurately, preferably with a pipette); may mask underlying disorders such as cerebral irritation; avoid for 3–4 days following gastro-intestinal surgery, may cause acute hypertensive response in phaeochromocytoma; pregnancy and breast-feeding; porphyria (see section 9.8.2); **interactions:** Appendix 1 (metoclopramide)

Side-effects: extrapyramidal effects (especially in children/young adults), hyperprolactinaemia, occasionally tardive dyskinesia on prolonged administration; also reported, drowsiness, restlessness, diarrhoea, depression

Dose: by mouth, or by intramuscular injection or by intravenous injection over 1–2 minutes, 10 mg (5 mg in young adults 15–19 years under 60 kg) 3 times daily; CHILD up to 1 year (up to 10 kg) 1 mg twice daily, 1–3 years (10–14 kg) 1 mg 2–3 times daily, 3–5 years (15–19 kg) 2 mg 2–3 times daily, 5–9 years (20–29 kg) 2.5 mg 3 times daily, 9–14 years (30 kg and over) 5 mg 3 times daily

Note. Daily dose of metoclopramide should not normally exceed 500 micrograms/kg, particularly for children and young adults (restricted use, see above)

For radiological examinations, as a single dose 5–10 minutes before examination. 10–20 mg (10 mg in young adults 15–19 years); CHILD under 3 years 1 mg, 3–5 years 2 mg, 5–9 years 2.5 mg, 9–14 years 5 mg

PoM **Metoclopramide** (Non-proprietary)

Tablets, metoclopramide hydrochloride 10 mg, net price 20 = 52p

Available from APS, Ashbourne (Gastroflux®), Berk (Primperan®), Cox, CP, K Pharm., Lagap (Parmid®), Norton

Oral solution, metoclopramide hydrochloride 5 mg/5 mL, net price 100-mL pack = £1.74

Available from Berk (Primperan®, sugar-free), Lagap (Parmid® sugar-free), RP Drugs

Injection, metoclopramide hydrochloride 5 mg/mL, net price 2-mL amp = 17p

Available from Berk (Primperan®)

PoM **Maxolon**® (Beecham)

Tablets, scored, metoclopramide hydrochloride 10 mg. Net price 21-tab pack = £2.20, 84-tab pack = £8.53

Syrup, sugar-free, metoclopramide hydrochloride 5 mg/5 mL. Net price 200-mL pack = £3.48

Cautionary label wordings, see inside back cover

Prices are **net**, see p.1

Paediatric liquid, sugar-free, metoclopramide hydrochloride 1 mg/mL. Net price 15-mL pack with pipette = £1.37. Counselling, use of pipette
Injection, metoclopramide hydrochloride 5 mg/mL. Net price 2-mL amp = 24p

High-dose (with cytotoxic chemotherapy only)
PoM **Maxolon High Dose®** (Beecham)
Injection, metoclopramide hydrochloride 5 mg/mL. Net price 20-mL amp = £2.43.
For dilution and use as an intravenous infusion in nausea and vomiting associated with cytotoxic chemotherapy only
Dose: by continuous intravenous infusion (preferred method), initially (before starting chemotherapy), 2–4 mg/kg over 15–30 minutes, then 3–5 mg/kg over 8–12 hours; max. in 24 hours, 10 mg/kg
By intermittent intravenous infusion, initially (before starting chemotherapy), up to 2 mg/kg over at least 15 minutes then up to 2 mg/kg over at least 15 minutes every 2 hours; max. in 24 hours, 10 mg/kg

Modified-release preparations
Note. All unsuitable for patients under 20 years
PoM **Gastrobid Continus®** (Napp)
Tablets, m/r, metoclopramide hydrochloride 15 mg. Net price 56-tab pack = £10.16. Label: 25
Dose: patients over 20 years, 1 tablet twice daily
PoM **Gastromax®** (Pharmacia)
Capsules, m/r, orange/yellow, enclosing white to light beige pellets, metoclopramide hydrochloride 30 mg. Net price 28-cap pack = £11.55. Label: 22, 25
Dose: patients over 20 years, 1 capsule daily
PoM **Maxolon SR®** (Beecham)
Capsules, m/r, clear, enclosing white granules, metoclopramide hydrochloride 15 mg. Net price 56-cap pack = £9.78. Label: 25
Dose: patients over 20 years, 1 capsule twice daily

Compound preparations (for migraine), section 4.7.4.1

5HT₃ ANTAGONISTS

GRANISETRON
Indications: nausea and vomiting induced by cytotoxic chemotherapy or radiotherapy
Cautions: pregnancy and breast-feeding
Side-effects: constipation, headache, rash; transient increases in liver enzymes
Dose: by mouth, 1 mg within 1 hour before start of treatment, then 1 mg twice daily during treatment; when intravenous infusion also used, max. combined total 9 mg in 24 hours; CHILD not recommended
By intravenous injection (diluted and given over not less than 30 seconds) *or by intravenous infusion* (over 5 minutes), prevention, 3 mg (up to 2 additional 3-mg doses may be given within 24 hours); treatment, as for prevention (the two additional doses must not be given less than 10 minutes apart); max. 9 mg in 24 hours; CHILD not recommended

▼ PoM **Kytril®** (SmithKline Beecham)
Tablets, f/c, granisetron (as hydrochloride) 1 mg. Net price 10-tab pack = £91.43

Sterile solution, granisetron (as hydrochloride) 1 mg/mL, for dilution and use as injection or infusion—for details see Appendix 6, net price 3-mL amp = £36.00

ONDANSETRON
Indications: see under Dose
Cautions: pregnancy and breast-feeding; moderate or severe hepatic impairment (max. 8 mg daily)
Side-effects: constipation; headache, sensation of warmth or flushing in head and over stomach; occasional alterations in liver enzymes; hypersensitivity reactions reported; occasional transient visual disturbances following intravenous administration; chest pain and arrhythmias also reported (causal relationship not established)
Dose: moderately emetogenic chemotherapy or radiotherapy, *by mouth*, 8 mg 1–2 hours before treatment *or, by slow intravenous injection*, 8 mg immediately before treatment, *then* 8 mg *by mouth* every 12 hours for up to 5 days
Severely emetogenic chemotherapy, *by slow intravenous injection*, 8 mg immediately before treatment, followed by 8 mg at intervals of 2–4 hours for 2 further doses (*or followed by* 1 mg/hour *by continuous intravenous infusion* for up to 24 hours) *then* 8 mg *by mouth* every 12 hours for up to 5 days
alternatively, by intravenous infusion over 15 minutes, 32 mg immediately before treatment *then* 8 mg *by mouth* every 12 hours for up to 5 days
Note. Efficacy may be enhanced by addition of a single dose of dexamethasone sodium phosphate 20 mg by intravenous injection
CHILD, *by slow intravenous injection or by intravenous infusion* over 15 minutes, 5 mg/m² immediately before chemotherapy then, 4 mg *by mouth* every 12 hours for up to 5 days
Prevention and treatment of postoperative nausea and vomiting, *by mouth*, 8 mg 1 hour before anaesthesia, followed by 8 mg at intervals of 8 hours for 2 further doses
alternatively by intramuscular or by slow intravenous injection, a single dose of 4 mg at induction

▼ PoM **Zofran®** (Glaxo)
Tablets, both yellow, f/c, ondansetron (as hydrochloride) 4 mg, net price 30-tab pack = £121.50; 8 mg, 10-tab pack = £81.00
Injection, ondansetron (as hydrochloride) 2 mg/mL, net price 2-mL amp = £6.75; 4-mL amp = £13.50

TROPISETRON
Indications: nausea and vomiting induced by cytotoxic chemotherapy
Cautions: uncontrolled hypertension (has been aggravated by doses higher than recommended); pregnancy and breast-feeding
DRIVING. Dizziness or drowsiness may affect performance of skilled tasks (e.g. driving)

Side-effects: constipation, diarrhoea, abdominal pain; headache, dizziness, fatigue

Dose: by slow intravenous injection or by intravenous infusion, 5 mg shortly before chemotherapy, then 5 mg *by mouth* every morning for 5 days, CHILD not recommended

▼ PoM **Navoban®** (Sandoz)

Capsules, white/yellow, tropisetron (as hydrochloride) 5 mg, net price 5-cap pack = £63.37; 50-cap pack = £633.65. Label: 23

Injection, tropisetron (as hydrochloride), 1 mg/mL, net price 5-mL amp = £14.31

CANNABINOID

NABILONE

Indications: nausea and vomiting caused by cytotoxic chemotherapy, unresponsive to conventional anti-emetics

Cautions: severe hepatic impairment; history of psychiatric disorder; elderly; hypertension; heart disease; **interactions:** Appendix 1 (nabilone)

DRIVING. Drowsiness may affect performance of skilled tasks (e.g. driving); effects of alcohol enhanced

Side-effects: drowsiness, vertigo, euphoria, dry mouth, ataxia, visual disturbance, concentration difficulties, sleep disturbance, dysphoria, hypotension, headache and nausea; also confusion, disorientation, hallucinations, psychosis, depression, decreased coordination, tremors, tachycardia, decreased appetite, and abdominal pain

Dose: patients over 18 years, initially 1 mg twice daily, increased if necessary to 2 mg twice daily, throughout each cycle of cytotoxic therapy and, if necessary, for 48 hours after the last dose of each cycle; max. 6 mg daily given in 3 divided doses. The first dose should be taken the night before initiation of cytotoxic treatment and the second dose 1–3 hours before the first dose of cytotoxic drug; ADOLESCENT and CHILD under 18 years not recommended

PoM **Cesamet®** (Lilly)

Capsules, blue/white, nabilone 1 mg. Net price 20-cap pack = £48.04 (hosp. only). Label: 2

HYOSCINE

HYOSCINE HYDROBROMIDE

(Scopolamine Hydrobromide)

Indications: motion sickness; premedication, see section 15.1.3

Cautions: elderly; urinary retention, cardiovascular disease, gastro-intestinal obstruction, hepatic or renal impairment; porphyria (see section 9.8.2); pregnancy and breast-feeding; **interactions:** Appendix 1 (antimuscarinics)

DRIVING. Drowsiness may affect performance of skilled tasks (e.g. driving) and may persist for up to 24 hours or longer after removal: effects of alcohol enhanced

Contra-indications: closed-angle glaucoma

Side-effects: drowsiness, dry mouth, dizziness, blurred vision, difficulty with micturition

Dose: motion sickness, *by mouth,* 300 micrograms 30 minutes before start of journey followed by 300 micrograms every 6 hours if required; max. 3 doses in 24 hours; CHILD 4–10 years 75–150 micrograms, over 10 years 150–300 micrograms

Note. Proprietary brands of hyoscine tablets (Joy-rides®, Kwells®) are on sale to the public for motion sickness

Injection, see section 15.1.3

PoM **Scopoderm TTS®** (Ciba)

Patch, self-adhesive, pink, releasing hyoscine approx. 500 micrograms/72 hours when in contact with skin. Net price 2 = £2.84. Label: 19, counselling, see below

Administration: motion sickness prevention, apply 1 patch to hairless area of skin behind ear 5–6 hours before journey; replace if necessary after 72 hours, siting replacement patch behind other ear; CHILD under 10 years not recommended

COUNSELLING. Explain accompanying instructions to patient and in particular emphasise advice to wash hands after handling and to wash application site after removing, and to use one at a time

---

OTHER DRUGS FOR MÉNIÈRE'S DISEASE

Betahistine has been promoted as a specific treatment for Ménière's disease.

BETAHISTINE HYDROCHLORIDE

Indications: vertigo, tinnitus and hearing loss associated with Ménière's disease

Cautions: asthma, history of peptic ulcer; **interactions:** Appendix 1 (betahistine)

Contra-indications: phaeochromocytoma

Side-effects: gastro-intestinal disturbances; headache, rashes and pruritus reported

Dose: initially 16 mg 3 times daily, preferably with food; maintenance 24–48 mg daily; CHILD not recommended

PoM **Serc®** (Duphar)

Tablets, scored, betahistine hydrochloride 8 mg (Serc®-8), net price 120-tab pack = £10.04; 16 mg (Serc®-16), 84-tab pack = £18.03. Label: 21

4.7 Analgesics

4.7.1 Non-opioid analgesics
4.7.2 Opioid analgesics
4.7.3 Trigeminal neuralgia
4.7.4 Antimigraine drugs

For advice on pain relief in terminal care see Prescribing in Terminal Care, p. 12.

4.7.1 Non-opioid analgesics

The non-opioid drugs, aspirin and paracetamol, are particularly suitable for pain in musculoskeletal conditions, whereas the opioid analgesics are more suitable for severe visceral pain.

Aspirin is the analgesic of choice for headache, transient musculoskeletal pain, and dysmenorrhoea.

It also has anti-inflammatory properties which may be useful, and is an antipyretic. Aspirin tablets or dispersible aspirin tablets are adequate for most purposes as they act rapidly.

Gastric irritation may be a problem; it is minimised by taking the dose after food. Enteric coated preparations are available, but have a slow onset of action and are therefore unsuitable for single-dose analgesic use (though their prolonged action may be useful for night pain).

Aspirin interacts significantly with a number of other drugs and its interaction with warfarin is a **special hazard**, see **interactions:** Appendix 1 (aspirin).

Paracetamol is similar in efficacy to aspirin, but has no demonstrable anti-inflammatory activity; it is less irritant to the stomach. Overdosage with paracetamol is particularly dangerous as it may cause hepatic damage which is sometimes not apparent for 4 to 6 days. **Benorylate** is an aspirin–paracetamol ester.

Nefopam may have a place in the relief of persistent pain unresponsive to other non-opioid analgesics. It causes little or no respiratory depression, but sympathomimetic and antimuscarinic side-effects may be troublesome.

Anti-inflammatory analgesics (see section 10.1.1) are particularly useful for the treatment of patients with chronic disease accompanied by pain and inflammation. Some of them are also used in the short-term treatment of mild to moderate pain including transient musculoskeletal pain. They are also suitable for the relief of pain in *dysmenorrhoea* and to treat pain caused by *secondary bone tumours*, many of which produce lysis of bone and release prostaglandins (see Prescribing in Terminal Care, p. 12).

COMPOUND ANALGESIC PREPARATIONS

Compound analgesic preparations containing paracetamol or aspirin with a *low dose* of an opioid analgesic (e.g. 8 mg of codeine phosphate per compound tablet) are commonly used, but the advantages have not been substantiated. The low dose of the opioid may be enough to cause opioid side-effects (in particular, constipation) and can complicate the treatment of overdosage (see p. 21) yet may not provide significant additional relief of pain.

Compound analgesic preparations containing a *full dose* of the opioid component (e.g. 30 mg of codeine phosphate per compound tablet) carry the full range of opioid side-effects (including nausea, vomiting, severe constipation, drowsiness, respiratory depression, and risk of dependence on long-term administration). For details of the **side-effects, cautions** and **contra-indications** of opioid analgesics, see p. 21 (**important**: the elderly are particularly susceptible to opioid side-effects and should receive lower doses).

In general, when assessing pain, it is necessary to weigh up carefully whether there is a need for a non-opioid and an opioid analgesic to be taken simultaneously.

Caffeine is a weak stimulant that is often included, in small doses, in analgesic preparations. It does not contribute to the analgesic or anti-inflammatory effect of the preparation and may possibly aggravate the gastric irritation caused by aspirin. Moreover, in excessive dosage or on withdrawal caffeine may itself induce headache.

DYSMENORRHOEA

Use of an oral contraceptive prevents the pain of dysmenorrhoea which is generally associated with ovulatory cycles. If treatment is necessary paracetamol or an NSAID will generally provide adequate relief of pain. The vomiting and severe pain associated with dysmenorrhoea in women with endometriosis may call for an antiemetic (in addition to an analgesic). Antispasmodics (such as alverine citrate) have been advocated for dysmenorroea but the antispasmodic action does not generally provide significant relief. Hyoscine butylbromide has also been advocated for its antispasmodic action despite the fact that its absorption following oral administration is extremely poor.

ASPIRIN

(Acetylsalicylic Acid)

Indications: mild to moderate pain, pyrexia (see notes above); see also section 10.1.1; antiplatelet, see section 2.9

Cautions: asthma, allergic disease, impaired renal or hepatic function (avoid if severe), dehydration, pregnancy; G6PD-deficiency (see section 9.1.5); **interactions:** Appendix 1 (aspirin)

Contra-indications: children under 12 years and in breast-feeding (Reye's syndrome, see below); gastro-intestinal ulceration, haemophilia; not for treatment of gout

HYPERSENSITIVITY. Aspirin and other NSAIDs are **contra-indicated** in patients with a history of hypersensitivity to aspirin or any other NSAID—*which includes those* in whom attacks of *asthma, angioedema, urticaria or rhinitis* have been precipitated by aspirin or any other NSAID

REYE'S SYNDROME. Owing to an association with Reye's syndrome the CSM has recommended that aspirin-containing preparations should no longer be given to children under the age of 12 years, unless specifically indicated, e.g. for juvenile arthritis (Still's disease). It is **important** to advise families that aspirin is not a suitable medicine for children with minor illness.

Side-effects: generally mild and infrequent but high incidence of gastro-intestinal irritation with slight asymptomatic blood loss, increased bleeding time, bronchospasm and skin reactions in hypersensitive patients. Prolonged administration, see section 10.1.1. Overdosage: see Emergency Treatment of Poisoning, p. 20

Dose: 300–900 mg every 4–6 hours when necessary; max. 4 g daily; CHILD not recommended (see notes above)

Aspirin (Non-proprietary)

Tablets, aspirin 300 mg. Net price 20 = 9p. Label: 21, 32

Available from most generic manufacturers

Dispersible tablets, aspirin 300 mg, net price 20 = 9p; 75 mg, see section 2.9. Label: 13, 21, 32

Available from most generic manufacturers

Note. BP 1993 directs that when soluble aspirin tablets are prescribed, dispersible aspirin tablets shall be dispensed.

Suppositories, aspirin 300 mg, net price 10 = £7.90. Label: 32

Dose: 2–3 suppositories inserted every 4 hours when necessary (max. 12 suppositories in 24 hours); CHILD not recommended (see above)

Available from Aurum (who also supply a 150-mg strength)

Caprin® (Sinclair)

Tablets, e/c, f/c, pink, aspirin 300 mg. Net price 100-tab pack = £4.97. Label: 5, 25, 32

Disprin CV®: see section 2.9

Nu-Seals® Aspirin (Lilly)

Tablets, e/c, aspirin 300 mg, net price 100-tab pack = £5.80; 75 mg, see section 2.9. Label: 5, 25, 32

Note. Aspirin enteric-coated also available from Ashbourne (postMI®)

With codeine phosphate 8 mg

Co-codaprin (Non-proprietary)

Tablets, co-codaprin 8/400 (codeine phosphate 8 mg, aspirin 400 mg). Net price 20 = 34p. Label: 21, 32

Dose: 1–2 tablets every 4–6 hours when necessary; max. 8 tablets daily

Dispersible tablets, co-codaprin 8/400 (codeine phosphate 8 mg, aspirin 400 mg). Net price 20 = 35p. Label: 13, 21, 32

Dose: 1–2 tablets in water every 4–6 hours; max. 8 tablets daily

Available from Cox

When co-codaprin tablets or dispersible tablets are prescribed and no strength is stated tablets, or dispersible tablets, respectively, containing codeine phosphate 8 mg and aspirin 400 mg should be dispensed

Other compound preparations

PoM Aspav® (Roussel)

Dispersible tablets, aspirin 500 mg, mixed opium alkaloids (anhydrous morphine (as morphine hydrochloride) 5 mg, papaverine hydrochloride 600 micrograms, codeine hydrochloride 520 micrograms). Net price 20 = £2.04. Label: 2, 13, 21, 32

Dose: 1–2 tablets in water every 4–6 hours if necessary; max. 8 tablets daily

NHS PoM Doloxene Compound® (Lilly)

Capsules, grey/red, dextropropoxyphene napsylate 100 mg, aspirin 375 mg, caffeine 30 mg. Net price 20 = £1.84. Label: 2, 21, 32

Dose: 1 capsule 3–4 times daily; max. 4 capsules daily

NHS CD Equagesic® (Wyeth)

Tablets, pink/white/yellow, ethoheptazine citrate 75 mg, meprobamate 150 mg, aspirin 250 mg. Net price 20 = 66p. Label: 2, 21, 32

Dose: muscle pain, 1–2 tablets 3–4 times daily

NHS PoM Robaxisal Forte® (Shire)

Tablets, pink/white, scored, methocarbamol 400 mg, aspirin 325 mg. Net price 20 = £1.90. Label: 2, 21, 32

Dose: muscle pain, 2 tablets 4 times daily

For a list of preparations containing aspirin and paracetamol **on sale to the public,** see p. 183.

PARACETAMOL

Indications: mild to moderate pain, pyrexia

Cautions: hepatic and renal impairment, alcohol dependence; **interactions:** Appendix 1 (paracetamol)

Side-effects: side-effects rare, but rashes, blood disorders, and acute pancreatitis reported; **important:** liver damage (and less frequently renal damage) following overdosage, see Emergency Treatment of Poisoning, p. 20

Dose: by mouth, 0.5–1 g every 4–6 hours to a max. of 4 g daily; CHILD 2 months 60 mg for post-immunisation pyrexia; otherwise under 3 months (on doctor's advice only), 10 mg/kg (5 mg/kg if jaundiced); 3 months–1 year 60–120 mg, 1–5 years 120–250 mg, 6–12 years 250–500 mg; these doses may be repeated every 4–6 hours when necessary (max. of 4 doses in 24 hours)

For full Joint Committee on Vaccination and Immunisation recommendation on post-immunisation pyrexia, see section 14.1

Rectal route, see below

Paracetamol (Non-proprietary)

Tablets, paracetamol 500 mg. Net price 20 = 8p. Label: 29, 30

Available from APS, Cox, Evans, K Pharm., Sterling Health (NHS Panadol®)

Soluble Tablets (= Dispersible tablets), paracetamol 500 mg. Net price 60-tab pack = £1.98. Label: 13, 29, 30

Available from Sanofi Winthrop (NHS Panadol Soluble®)

Paediatric Soluble Tablets (= Paediatric dispersible tablets), paracetamol 120 mg. Net price 24-tab pack = 69p. Label: 13, 30

Available from R&C (NHS Disprol® Junior)

Paediatric Oral Solution (= Paediatric Elixir), paracetamol 120 mg/5 mL. Net price 100 mL = 37p. Label: 30

Note. Sugar-free versions are available and can be ordered by specifying 'sugar-free' on the prescription.

Available from Berk, Evans, K Pharm., RP Drugs (NHS Paldesic®), Wallace Mfg (NHS Salzone®)

Oral Suspension 120 mg/5 mL (= Paediatric Mixture), paracetamol 120 mg/5 mL. Net price 100 mL = 43p. Label: 30

Note. BP directs that when Paediatric Paracetamol Oral Suspension or Paediatric Paracetamol Mixture is prescribed Paracetamol Oral Suspension 120 mg/5 mL should be dispensed; sugar-free versions can be ordered by specifying 'sugar-free' on the prescription

Available from Cupal (Cupanol® Paediatric, sugar-free), R&C (Disprol® Paediatric, sugar-free), Sterling Health (Panadol®, sugar-free), Wellcome (Calpol® Paediatric, Calpol® Paediatric sugar-free)

Oral Suspension 250 mg/5 mL (= Mixture), paracetamol 250 mg/5 mL. Net price 100 mL = £1.57. Label: 30

Available from Cupal (NHS Cupanol® Over 6, sugar-free), Wellcome (NHS Calpol® 6 Plus)

Cautionary label wordings, see inside back cover

Suppositories, paracetamol 125 mg. Net price 10 = £10.50. Label: 30

Dose: by rectum, CHILD 1–5 years 125–250 mg (1–2 suppositories) up to 4 times daily

Available from Novex (Alvedon®)

Co-codamol 8/500

When co-codamol tablets, dispersible (or effervescent) tablets, or capsules are prescribed and no strength is stated tablets, dispersible (or effervescent) tablets, or capsules, respectively, containing codeine phosphate 8 mg and paracetamol 500 mg should be dispensed.

Co-codamol (Non-proprietary)

Tablets, co-codamol 8/500 (codeine phosphate 8 mg, paracetamol 500 mg) Net price 20 = 22p. Label: 29, 30

Dose: 1–2 tablets every 4–6 hours; max. 8 tablets daily; CHILD 6–12 years ½–1 tablet

Available from APS, Cox, Galen, (NHS Parake®), K Pharm., Norton, Sterling Health (NHS Panadeine®)

Effervescent or *dispersible tablets*, co-codamol 8/500 (codeine phosphate 8 mg, paracetamol 500 mg). Net price 20 = 59p. Label: 13, 29, 30

Dose: 1–2 tablets in water every 4–6 hours, max. 8 tablets daily; CHILD 6–12 years ½–1 tablet, max 4 daily

Available from Fisons (NHS Paracodol®), Sterwin

Note. The Drug Tariff allows tablets of co-codamol labelled 'dispersible' to be dispensed against an order for 'effervescent' and *vice versa*

Capsules, co-codamol 8/500 (codeine phosphate 8 mg, paracetamol 500 mg). Net price 30 = £1.78. Label: 29, 30

Dose: 1–2 capsules every 4 hours; max. 8 capsules daily

Available from Fisons (NHS Paracodol®)

Co-codamol 30/500

When co-codamol tablets, dispersible (or effervescent) tablets, or capsules are prescribed and no strength is stated tablets, dispersible (or effervescent) tablets, or capsules, respectively, containing codeine phosphate 8 mg and paracetamol 500 mg should be dispensed (see preparations above).

See warnings and notes on p.180 (**important**: special care in elderly—reduce dose)

PoM **Kapake®** (Galen)

Tablets, scored, co-codamol 30/500 (codeine phosphate 30 mg, paracetamol 500 mg). Net price 100-tab pack = £6.88. Label: 2, 29, 30

Dose: 1–2 tablets every 4 hours; max. 8 tablets daily; CHILD not recommended

PoM **Solpadol®** (Sanofi Winthrop)

Caplets (= tablets), co-codamol 30/500 (codeine phosphate 30 mg, paracetamol 500 mg). Net price 100-tab pack = £7.90. Label: 2, 29, 30

Dose: 2 tablets every 4 hours; max. 8 daily; CHILD not recommended

Effervescent tablets, co-codamol 30/500 (codeine phosphate 30 mg, paracetamol 500 mg). Contains 18.6 mmol Na⁺/tablet; avoid in renal impairment. Net price 100-tab pack = £9.50. Label: 2, 13, 29, 30

Dose: 2 tablets in water every 4 hours; max. 8 daily; CHILD not recommended

PoM **Tylex®** (Cilag)

Capsules, co-codamol 30/500 (codeine phosphate 30 mg, paracetamol 500 mg). Net price 100-cap pack = £8.60. Label: 2, 29, 30

Dose: 1–2 capsules every 4 hours; max. 8 capsules daily; CHILD not recommended

With dihydrocodeine tartrate 10 mg

See notes on p.180

PoM **Co-dydramol** (Non-proprietary)

Tablets, scored, co-dydramol 10/500 (dihydrocodeine tartrate 10 mg, paracetamol 500 mg). Net price 20 = 27p. Label: 21, 29, 30

Dose: 1–2 tablets every 4–6 hours; max. 8 tablets daily; CHILD not recommended

Available from APS, Cox, Galen (NHS Galake®), K Pharm., Norton, Sterwin

When co-dydramol tablets are prescribed and no strength is stated tablets containing dihydrocodeine tartrate 10 mg and paracetamol 500 mg should be dispensed.

Note. Tablets containing paracetamol 500 mg and dihydrocodeine 7.46 mg (NHS Paramol®) are on sale to the public. The name Paramol® was formerly applied to a brand of co-dydramol tablets

With dihydrocodeine tartrate 20 or 30 mg

See warnings and notes on p.180 (**important**: special care in elderly—reduce dose)

PoM **Remedeine®** (Napp)

Tablets, paracetamol 500 mg, dihydrocodeine tartrate 20 mg. Net price 112-tab pack = £12.21. Label: 2, 21, 29, 30

Dose: 1–2 tablets every 4–6 hours; max. 8 tablets daily; CHILD not recommended

Forte tablets, paracetamol 500 mg, dihydrocodeine tartrate 30 mg. Net price 56-tab pack = £7.54. Label: 2, 21, 29, 30

Dose: 1–2 tablets every 4–6 hours; max. 8 tablets daily; CHILD not recommended

Other compound preparations

See warnings and notes on p.180 (**important**: special care in elderly—reduce dose)

PoM **Co-proxamol** (Non-proprietary)

Tablets, co-proxamol 32.5/325 (dextropropoxyphene hydrochloride 32.5 mg, paracetamol 325 mg). Net price 20 = 25p. Label: 2, 10 patient information leaflet (if available), 29, 30

Dose: 2 tablets 3–4 times daily; max. 8 tablets daily; CHILD not recommended

Available from APS, Berk, Cox (NHS Cosalgesic®), Dista (NHS Distalgesic®), K Pharm., Sterwin

When co-proxamol tablets are prescribed and no strength is stated tablets containing dextropropoxyphene hydrochloride 32.5 mg and paracetamol 325 mg should be dispensed.

NHS **CD Fortagesic®** (Sanofi Winthrop)

Tablets, pentazocine 15 mg (as hydrochloride), paracetamol 500 mg. Net price 20 = £1.40. Label: 2, 21, 29, 30

Dose: 2 tablets up to 4 times daily; CHILD 7–12 years 1 tablet every 4 hours, max. 4 tablets daily

NHS PoM **Lobak®** (Sanofi Winthrop)

Tablets, scored, chlormezanone 100 mg, paracetamol 450 mg. Net price 50 = £7.67. Label: 2, 29, 30

Dose: muscle pain, 1–2 tablets 3 times daily; max. 8 tablets daily; CHILD not recommended

For a list of **preparations** containing aspirin and paracetamol **on sale to the public**, see p.183.

The following is a list of preparations on sale to the public that contain **aspirin** or **paracetamol**, **alone** or with **other ingredients**. Other significant ingredients (such as codeine) are listed, but minor ingredients (such as caffeine) are not. For details of preparations containing ibuprofen on sale to the public, see section 10.1.1.
Important: in overdose contact **Poisons Information Services** (p. 18) for full details of the ingredients

Actron® (aspirin, paracetamol), **Alka Seltzer**® (aspirin), **Anadin**® (aspirin, quinine), **Anadin All Night**® (aspirin), **Anadin Extra**®, **Anadin Extra Soluble**® (both aspirin, paracetamol), **Anadin Maximum Strength**® (aspirin), **Anadin Paracetamol**® (paracetamol), **Andrews Answer**® (paracetamol), **Angettes 75**® (aspirin), **Askit**® (aspirin, aloxiprin = polymeric product of aspirin), **Aspro**® (aspirin), **Aspro Clear**® (aspirin), **Aspro Paraclear Junior**®, **Aspro Paraclear**® (both paracetamol) **Barum Cold Relief with Decongestant**® (paracetamol, phenylephrine), **Barum Extra Power Pain Reliever**® (aspirin, paracetamol), **Bayer Aspirin**® (aspirin), **Beechams Hot Lemon**®, **Hot Lemon and Honey**®, **Hot Blackcurrant**® (all paracetamol, phenylephrine), **Beechams Powders**® (aspirin), **Beechams Powders Capsules**® **With Decongestant** (paracetamol, phenylephrine), **Beecham Aspirin**®, **Beechams Powders Tablets**® (both aspirin), **Benylin Day and Night Cold and Flu Relief**® (*day tablets*, paracetamol, phenylpropanolamine, *night tablets*, paracetamol, diphenhydramine), **Boots Cold Relief Tablets**® (paracetamol, phenylephrine), **Boots Cold Relief for Children**®, **Boots Cold Relief Hot Blackcurrant**®, **Hot Lemon**® (paracetamol), **Boots Day Cold Comfort**® (paracetamol, pholcodine, pseudoephedrine), **Boots Headache and Indigestion Relief**® (paracetamol), **Boots Night-Cold Comfort**® (diphenhydramine, paracetamol, pholcodine, pseudoephedrine), **Boots Pain Relief Syrup for Children**® and **Boots Pain Relief Tablets**® (both paracetamol), **Boots Pain Relief Plus**® (codeine, paracetamol) **Cafadol**® (paracetamol), **Calpol Extra For Adults**® (paracetamol, codeine), **Calpol Infant**®, **Calpol 6 Plus**®, **Calpol Paediatric**® (all paracetamol), **Caprin**® (aspirin), **Catarrh-Ex**® (paracetamol, pseudoephedrine), **Coda-med**® (paracetamol, codeine), **Codanin**® (paracetamol, codeine), **Codis 500**® (aspirin, codeine), **Cojene**® (aspirin, codeine), **Cold Relief Capsules (Thornton & Ross)** (paracetamol, phenylephrine), **Coldrex Blackcurrant Powders**®, **Hot Lemon Powders**®, and **Tablets**® (all paracetamol, phenylephrine), **Mrs. Cullen's**® (aspirin), **Cupanol Over 6**®, **Cupanol Under 6**® (both paracetamol) **Day Nurse**® (paracetamol, dextromethorphan, phenylpropanolamine), **De Witt's Analgesic Pills**® (paracetamol), **Disprin**®, **Disprin CV**® **Disprin Direct**® (all aspirin), **Disprin Extra**® (aspirin, paracetamol), **Disprol**®, **Disprol Infant**®, **Disprol Junior**®, **Disprol Paediatric**® (all paracetamol), **Doan's**® **Backache pills** (paracetamol, sodium salicylate), **Dristan Tablets**® (aspirin, chlorpheniramine, phenylephrine) **Elkamol**® (paracetamol), **EP**® (paracetamol, codeine) **Fanalgic**® (paracetamol), **Femigraine**® (aspirin, cyclizine), **Feminax**® (paracetamol, codeine, hyoscine), **Fennings Children's Cooling Powders**® (paracetamol), **Flu-caps**® (paracetamol, codeine), **Flurex Bedtime**® (paracetamol, diphenhydramine, pseudoephedrine), **Flurex Capsules**®

and **Tablets**® (paracetamol, phenylephrine), **Fynnon**® **Calcium Aspirin** (aspirin) **Hedex**®, **Hedex Soluble**®, **Hedex Extra**® (all paracetamol) **Infadrops**® (paracetamol) **Lem-plus Capsules**® (paracetamol, phenylephrine), **Lem-plus Powders**® (paracetamol), **Lemsip Cold Relief**® **Capsules with Decongestant**, **Lemsip Flu Strength**®, **Lemsip Lemon**® or **Blackcurrant**®, **Lemsip Junior**®, **Lemsip Menthol Extra**® (all paracetamol, phenylephrine), **Lemsip Flu Strength Nightime**® (paracetamol, chlorpheniramine, dextromethorphan, phenylpropanolamine) **Maximum Strength Aspro Clear**® (aspirin), **Medised**® (paracetamol, promethazine), **Medised Plain**®, **Medised 6+**® (both paracetamol), **Midrid**® (paracetamol, isometheptene mucate), **Migraleve**® (*pink tablets*, paracetamol, codeine, buclizine, *yellow tablets*, paracetamol, codeine), **Miradol**® (paracetamol), **Mu-Cron Tablets**® (paracetamol, phenylpropanolamine) **Night Nurse**® (paracetamol, dextromethorphan, promethazine), **Numark Cold Relief Capsules**® **With Decongestant** (paracetamol, phenylephrine), **Numark Cold Relief Powders**® (paracetamol), **Nurse Sykes' Powders**® (aspirin, paracetamol, codeine), **Nu-Seals**® **Aspirin** (aspirin) **Paldesic**® (paracetamol), **Pameton**® (paracetamol, methionine), **Panadeine**® (paracetamol, codeine), **Panadol**®, **Panadol Baby and Infant**®, **Panadol Extra**®, **Panadol Junior**® (all paracetamol), **Panadol Ultra**® (paracetamol, codeine), **Panaleve Junior**®, **Panaleve 6+**® (both paracetamol), **Panerel**® (paracetamol, codeine), **Paracets**® (paracetamol), **Paraclear Extra Strength**®, **Paraclear Junior**®, **Paraclear**® (all paracetamol), **Paracodol**® (paracetamol, codeine), **Paramin**® (paracetamol), **Paramol**® (paracetamol, dihydrocodeine), **Phensic**® (aspirin), **Placidex**® (paracetamol), **Platet**® (aspirin), **Powerin**® (aspirin, paracetamol), **Propain**® (paracetamol, codeine, diphenhydramine) **Resolve**® (paracetamol), **Rimadol**® (paracetamol) **Salzone**® (paracetamol), **Sinutab**® (paracetamol, phenylpropanolamine), **Sinutab Nightime**® (paracetamol, phenylpropanolamine, phenyltoloxamine), **Solpadeine**® (paracetamol, codeine), **SP Cold Relief Capsules**® (paracetamol, phenylephrine), **Sudafed-Co**® (paracetamol, pseudoephedrine), **Syndol**® (paracetamol, codeine, doxylamine) **Toptabs**® (aspirin), **Tramil**® (paracetamol), **Triogesic**® (paracetamol, phenylpropanolamine) **Uniflu with Gregovite** C® (paracetamol, codeine, diphenhydramine, phenylephrine) **Veganin**® (aspirin, paracetamol, codeine), **Vicks**® **Coldcare** (paracetamol, dextromethorphan, phenylpropanolamine), **Vicks Medinite**® (paracetamol, dextro-methorphan, doxylamine, ephedrine)

IBUPROFEN

Indications: fever and pain in children; see also section 10.1.1

Cautions; Contra-indications; Side-effects: see section 10.1.1

Dose: see section 10.1.1; CHILD, fever and pain, see below

Fever and pain in children

PoM Junifen Sugar Free® (Boots)

Suspension, sugar-free, ibuprofen 100 mg/5 mL, net price 150-mL pack = £2.37. Label: 21

Dose: fever and pain in children, under 1 year not recommended, 1–12 years 20 mg/kg daily in divided doses *or* 1–2 years 2.5 mL 3–4 times daily, 3–7 years 5 mL, 8–12 years 10 mL

Note. Junifen Sugar-Free® suspension also on sale to the public for fever and pain relief in children over 1 year of age

Other preparations: see section 10.1.1

KETOROLAC

See section 15.1.4.2

NSAIDs other than aspirin (p.180) and ibuprofen (above) licensed for pain now appear in section 10.1.1. They include:

BENORYLATE	**FLURBIPROFEN**
DICLOFENAC	**KETOPROFEN**
SODIUM	**MEFENAMIC ACID**
DIFLUNISAL	**NAPROXEN**
FENOPROFEN	

NEFOPAM HYDROCHLORIDE

Indications: moderate pain
Cautions: hepatic or renal disease, elderly, urinary retention; **interactions:** Appendix 1 (nefopam)
Contra-indications: convulsive disorders; not indicated for myocardial infarction
Side-effects: nausea, nervousness, urinary retention, dry mouth, lightheadedness; less frequently vomiting, blurred vision, drowsiness, sweating, insomnia, tachycardia, headache; confusion and hallucinations also reported; may colour urine (pink)
Dose: by mouth, initially 60 mg (elderly, 30 mg) 3 times daily, adjusted according to response; usual range 30–90 mg 3 times daily; CHILD not recommended
By intramuscular injection, 20 mg every 6 hours; CHILD not recommended
Note. Nefopam hydrochloride 20 mg by injection ≡ 60 mg by mouth

PoM **Acupan®** (3M)
Tablets, f/c, nefopam hydrochloride 30 mg. Net price 90-tab pack = £11.44. Label: 2, 14
Injection, nefopam hydrochloride 20 mg/mL. Net price 1-mL amp = 73p

4.7.2   Opioid analgesics

Opioid analgesics are used to relieve moderate to severe pain particularly of visceral origin. Repeated administration may cause dependence and tolerance, but this is no deterrent in the control of pain in terminal illness, for guidelines see Prescribing in Terminal Care, p.12.

SIDE-EFFECTS. Opioid analgesics share many side-effects though qualitative and quantitative differences exist. The most common include nausea, vomiting, constipation, and drowsiness. Larger doses produce respiratory depression and hypotension. Overdosage, see Emergency Treatment of Poisoning, p.21.

INTERACTIONS. See Appendix 1 (opioid analgesics) (**important**: special hazard with *pethidine and possibly other opioids* and MAOIs).

DRIVING. Drowsiness may affect performance of skilled tasks (e.g. driving); effects of alcohol enhanced.

CHOICE. **Morphine** remains the most valuable opioid analgesic for severe pain although it fre-quently causes nausea and vomiting. It is the standard against which other opioid analgesics are compared. In addition to relief of pain, morphine also confers a state of euphoria and mental detachment.

Morphine is the opioid of choice for the oral treatment of *severe pain in terminal care.* It is given regularly every 4 hours (or every 12 hours as modified-release tablets). For guidelines on dosage adjustment in terminal care, see p.12.

Buprenorphine has both opioid agonist and antagonist properties and may precipitate withdrawal symptoms, including pain, in patients dependent on other opioids. It has abuse potential and may itself cause dependence. It has a much longer duration of action than morphine and sublingually is an effective analgesic for 6 to 8 hours. Vomiting may be a problem. Unlike most opioid analgesics its effects are only partially reversed by naloxone.

Codeine is effective for the relief of mild to moderate pain but is too constipating for long-term use.

Dextromoramide is less sedating than morphine and has a short duration of action.

Dipipanone used alone is less sedating than morphine but the only preparation available contains an anti-emetic and is therefore not suitable for regular regimens in terminal care (see p.12).

Dextropropoxyphene given alone is a very mild analgesic somewhat less potent than codeine. Combinations of dextropropoxyphene with paracetamol (co-proxamol) or aspirin have little more analgesic effect than paracetamol or aspirin alone. An important disadvantage of co-proxamol is that overdosage (which may be combined with alcohol) is complicated by respiratory depression and acute heart failure due to the dextropropoxyphene and by hepatotoxicity due to the paracetamol. Rapid treatment is essential (see Emergency Treatment of Poisoning, p.21).

Diamorphine (heroin) is a powerful opioid analgesic. It may cause less nausea and hypotension than morphine. In *terminal care* the greater solubility of diamorphine allows effective doses to be injected in smaller volumes and this is important in the emaciated patient.

Dihydrocodeine has an analgesic efficacy similar to that of codeine. The dose of dihydrocodeine by mouth is usually 30 mg every 4 hours; doubling the dose to 60 mg may provide some additional pain relief but this may be at the cost of more nausea and vomiting. A 40-mg tablet is now also available.

Meptazinol is claimed to have a low incidence of respiratory depression. It has a reported length of action of 2 to 7 hours with onset within 15 minutes, but there is an incidence of nausea and vomiting.

Methadone is less sedating than morphine and acts for longer periods. In prolonged use, methadone should not be administered more often than twice daily to avoid the risk of accumulation and opioid overdosage.

Nalbuphine has a similar efficacy to that of morphine for pain relief, but may have fewer side-effects and less abuse potential. Nausea and vomiting occur less than with other opioids but respiratory depression is similar to that with morphine.

Oxycodone is used as the pectinate in suppositories (special order, Boots) for the control of *pain in terminal care*.

Pentazocine has both agonist and antagonist properties and precipitates withdrawal symptoms, including pain in patients dependent on other opioids. By injection it is more potent than dihydrocodeine or codeine, but hallucinations and thought disturbances may occur. It is not recommended and, in particular, should be avoided after myocardial infarction as it may increase pulmonary and aortic blood pressure as well as cardiac work.

Pethidine produces prompt but short-lasting analgesia; it is less constipating than morphine, but even in high doses is a less potent analgesic. It is not suitable for severe continuing pain. It is used for analgesia in labour, and in the neonate it is associated with less respiratory depression than other opioid analgesics (probably because its action is weaker).

Phenazocine is effective in severe pain and has less tendency to increase biliary pressure than other opioid analgesics. It can be administered sublingually if nausea and vomiting are a problem.

Tramadol has been recently introduced and is claimed to produce analgesia by two mechanisms: a weak central effect and an enhancement of serotoninergic and adrenergic pathways. It is reported to have fewer of the typical opioid side-effects (notably, less respiratory depression, less constipation and less addiction potential).

ADDICTS. Although caution is necessary addicts (and ex addicts) may be treated with analgesics in the same way as other people when there is a real clinical need. Doctors are reminded that they do not require a special licence to prescribe opioid analgesics for addicts for relief of pain due to organic disease or injury.

MORPHINE SALTS

Indications: see notes above; acute pulmonary oedema; peri-operative analgesia see section 15.1.4.3

Cautions: hypotension, hypothyroidism, asthma (avoid during attack), and decreased respiratory reserve; pregnancy and breast-feeding; may precipitate coma in hepatic impairment (reduce dose but many such patients tolerate morphine well); reduce dose in renal impairment, elderly and debilitated (reduce dose); dependence (severe withdrawal symptoms if withdrawn abruptly); use of cough suppressants containing opioid analgesics not generally recommended in children and should be avoided altogether in those under at least 1 year; **interactions:** Appendix 1 (opioid analgesics)

TERMINAL CARE. In the control of pain in terminal illness these cautions should not necessarily be a deterrent to the use of opioid analgesics

Contra-indications: avoid in raised intracranial pressure or head injury (in addition to interfering with respiration, affect pupillary responses vital for neurological assessment)

Side-effects: nausea and vomiting (particularly in initial stages), constipation, and drowsiness; larger doses produce respiratory depression and hypotension; other side-effects include difficulty with micturition, ureteric or biliary spasm, dry mouth, sweating, headache, facial flushing, vertigo, bradycardia, palpitations, postural hypotension, hypothermia, hallucinations, mood changes, dependence, miosis, urticaria and pruritus; overdosage: see Emergency Treatment of Poisoning, p.21

Dose: acute pain, *by subcutaneous or intramuscular injection*, 10 mg every 4 hours if necessary (15 mg for heavier well-muscled patients); CHILD up to 1 month 150 micrograms/kg, 1–12 months 200 micrograms/kg, 1–5 years 2.5–5 mg, 6–12 years 5–10 mg

By slow intravenous injection, quarter to half corresponding intramuscular dose

Patient controlled analgesia (PCA), consult hospital protocols

Myocardial infarction, *by slow intravenous injection* (2 mg/minute), 10 mg followed by a further 5–10 mg if necessary; elderly or frail patients, reduce dose by half

Acute pulmonary oedema, *by slow intravenous injection* (2 mg/minute) 5–10 mg

Chronic pain, *by mouth or by subcutaneous or intramuscular injection*, 5–20 mg regularly every 4 hours; dose may be increased according to needs; oral dose should be approximately double corresponding intramuscular dose and triple to quadruple corresponding intramuscular *diamorphine* dose (see also Prescribing in Terminal Care, p.12); *by rectum*, as suppositories, 15–30 mg regularly every 4 hours

Note. The doses stated above refer equally to morphine hydrochloride, sulphate, and tartrate; for dose of **modified-release** tablets, see next column.

Oral solutions

Note. For advice on transfer from oral solutions of morphine to modified-release preparations of morphine, see Prescribing in Terminal Care, p.12

PoM or CD Morphine Oral Solutions

Oral solutions of morphine can be prescribed by writing the formula:

Morphine hydrochloride 5 mg

Chloroform water to 5 mL

Note. The proportion of morphine hydrochloride may be altered when specified by the prescriber; if above 13 mg per 5 mL the solution becomes **CD**. For sample prescription see Controlled Drugs and Drug Dependence, p.7. It is usual to adjust the strength so that the dose volume is 5 or 10 mL.

Oramorph® (Boehringer Ingelheim)

PoM *Oramorph® oral solution*, morphine sulphate 10 mg/5 mL. Net price 100-mL pack = £2.31; 250-mL pack = £5.36; 500-mL pack = £9.70. Label: 2

PoM *Oramorph® Unit Dose Vials 10 mg* (oral vials), sugar-free, morphine sulphate 10 mg/5-mL vial, net price 25 vials = £3.31. Label: 2

CD *Oramorph® Unit Dose Vials 30 mg* (oral vials), sugar-free, morphine sulphate 30 mg/5-mL vial, net price 25 vials = £9.30. Label: 2

CD *Oramorph®* *concentrated oral solution*, sugar-free, morphine sulphate 100 mg/5 mL. Net price 30-mL pack = £6.47; 120-mL pack = £24.15 (both with calibrated dropper). Label: 2

CD *Oramorph®* *Unit Dose Vials 100 mg* (oral vials), sugar-free, morphine sulphate 100 mg/5-mL vial, net price 25 vials = £31.00. Label: 2

Tablets

CD Sevredol® (Napp)

Tablets, both f/c, scored, morphine sulphate 10 mg (blue), net price 56-tab pack = £6.31; 20 mg (pink), 56-tab pack = £12.62. Label: 2

Dose: severe pain uncontrolled by weaker opioid, 10–20 mg every 4 hours; CHILD 3–5 years, 5 mg; 6–12 years, 5–10 mg

Modified release

CD MST Continus® (Napp)

Tablets, all m/r, f/c, morphine sulphate 5 mg (white), net price 60-tab pack = £4.50; 10 mg (brown), 60-tab pack = £7.51; 15 mg (green), 60-tab pack = £13.16; 30 mg (purple), 60-tab pack = £18.03; 60 mg (orange), 60-tab pack = £35.16; 100 mg (grey), 60-tab pack = £55.67; 200 mg (green), 60-tab pack = £111.35. Label: 2, 25

Suspension (= sachet of granules to mix with water), m/r, pink, morphine sulphate 20 mg/sachet, net price 30-sachet pack = £28.60; 30 mg/sachet, 30-sachet pack = £29.72; 60 mg/sachet, 30-sachet pack = £59.44; 100 mg/sachet, 30-sachet pack = £99.07; 200 mg/sachet pack, 30-sachet pack = £198.14. Label: 2, 13

Dose: (suspension or tablets) severe pain uncontrolled by weaker opioids, 30 mg every 12 hours, increased to 60 mg every 12 hours when required, then further increments of 25–50% if necessary. For lower initial doses in patients who have not received other opioids, see Prescribing in Terminal Care, p. 12

CHILD severe, intractable pain in cancer, initially 200–800 micrograms/kg every 12 hours, then further increments of 30–50% if necessary

Note. Brand name prescriptions for MST Continus must also specify 'tablets' or 'suspension' (i.e. 'MST Continus tablets' or 'MST Continus suspension').

CD Oramorph® SR (Boehringer Ingelheim)

Tablets, all m/r, f/c, morphine sulphate 10 mg (buff), net price 60-tab pack = £6.76; 30 mg (violet), 60-tab pack = £16.23; 60 mg (orange), 60-tab pack = £31.64; 100 mg (grey), 60-tab pack = £50.10. Label: 2, 25

Dose: severe pain uncontrolled by weaker opioids, 30 mg every 12 hours, increased to 60 mg every 12 hours when required, then further increments of 25-50% if necessary. For lower initial doses in patients who have not received other opioids, see Prescribing in Terminal Care, p. 12 CHILD not recommended

Note. Brand name prescriptions for Oramorph SR must also specify 'tablets' (i.e. 'Oramorph SR tablets')

Injections

CD Morphine Sulphate Injection, morphine sulphate 10, 15, 20, and 30 mg/mL, net price 1- and 2-mL amp (all) = 54–92p

CD Min-I-Jet® Morphine Sulphate (IMS)

Injection, morphine sulphate 10 mg/mL, net price 2-mL disposable syringe = £6.05

CD Morphine and Atropine Injection

See section 15.1.4.3

Injection with anti-emetic

CAUTION. In myocardial infarction cyclizine may aggravate severe heart failure and counteract the haemodynamic benefits of opioids, see section 4.6. **Not recommended** in terminal care, see p. 12

CD Cyclimorph® (Wellcome)

Cyclimorph-10® *Injection*, morphine tartrate 10 mg, cyclizine tartrate 50 mg/mL. Net price 1-mL amp = £1.28

Dose: by subcutaneous, intramuscular, or intravenous injection, 1 mL, repeated not more than every 4 hours, with not more than 3 doses in any 24-hour period; CHILD 1–5 years 0.25–0.5 mL as a single dose, 6–12 years 0.5–1 mL as a single dose

Cyclimorph-15® *Injection*, morphine tartrate 15 mg, cyclizine tartrate 50 mg/mL. Net price 1-mL amp = £1.33

Dose: by subcutaneous, intramuscular, or intravenous injection, 1 mL, repeated not more often than every 4 hours, with not more than 3 doses in any 24-hour period

Suppositories

CD Morphine Suppositories, morphine hydrochloride or sulphate 15 mg, net price 12 = £3.54; 30 mg, 12 = £5.51. Label: 2

Available from Evans, Martindale

Note. Both the strength of the suppositories and the morphine salt contained in them must be specified by the prescriber

Mixed opium alkaloids

Mixed opium alkaloids do not have any advantage over morphine alone; alcoholic solution of Nepenthe® was liable to evaporation and is **not** recommended—it has now been **discontinued**.

ALFENTANIL

See section 15.1.4.3

BUPRENORPHINE

Indications: moderate to severe pain; peri-operative analgesia, see section 15.1.4.3

Cautions; Contra-indications; Side-effects: see under Morphine Salts and notes above; can give rise to mild withdrawal symptoms in patients dependent on opioids; effects only partially reversed by naloxone; **interactions:** Appendix 1 (opioid analgesics)

Dose: by sublingual administration, initially 200–400 micrograms every 8 hours, increasing if necessary to 200–400 micrograms every 6–8 hours; CHILD over 6 months, 16–25 kg, 100 micrograms; 25–37.5 kg, 100–200 micrograms; 37.5–50 kg, 200–300 micrograms

By intramuscular or slow intravenous injection, 300–600 micrograms every 6–8 hours; CHILD over 6 months 3–6 micrograms/kg every 6–8 hours (max. 9 micrograms/kg)

CD Temgesic® (R&C)

Tablets (sublingual), buprenorphine (as hydrochloride), 200 micrograms, net price 50-tab pack = £6.00; 400 micrograms, 50-tab pack = £12.00. Label: 2, 26

Injection, buprenorphine 300 micrograms (as hydrochloride)/mL. Net price 1-mL amp = 55p

CODEINE PHOSPHATE

Indications: mild to moderate pain

Cautions; Contra-indications; Side-effects: see under Morphine Salts and notes above; use of cough suppressants containing codeine or similar opioid analgesics not generally recommended in children and should be avoided altogether in those under 1 year; **interactions:** Appendix 1 (opioid analgesics)

Dose: by mouth, 30–60 mg every 4 hours when necessary, to a max. of 240 mg daily; CHILD 1–12 years, 3 mg/kg daily in divided doses

By intramuscular injection, 30–60 mg every 4 hours when necessary

Codeine Phosphate (Non-proprietary)

PoM *Tablets,* codeine phosphate 15 mg, net price 20 = 35p; 30 mg, 20 = 37p; 60 mg, 20 = £1.11. Label: 2

Note. As for schedule 2 controlled drugs, travellers needing to take codeine phosphate preparations abroad may require a doctor's letter explaining why they are necessary

PoM *Syrup,* codeine phosphate 25 mg/5 mL. Net price 100 mL = 79p. Label: 2

CD *Injection,* codeine phosphate 60 mg/mL. Net price 1-mL amp = £1.48

Codeine Linctuses
See section 3.9.1

Note. Codeine is an ingredient of some compound analgesic preparations, see sections 4.7.1 and 10.1.1 (Codafen Continus®)

DEXTROMORAMIDE

Indications: severe pain

Cautions; Contra-indications; Side-effects: see under Morphine Salts and notes above; only short duration of action (2–3 hours); avoid in obstetric analgesia (increased risk of neonatal depression); **interactions:** Appendix 1 (opioid analgesics)

Dose: by mouth, 5 mg increasing to 20 mg, when required

By rectum in suppositories, 10 mg when required

CD Palfium® (Boehringer Mannheim)

Tablets, both scored, dextromoramide (as tartrate) 5 mg, net price 60-tab pack = £4.66; 10 mg (peach), 60-tab pack = £9.21. Label: 2

Suppositories, dextromoramide 10 mg (as tartrate). Net price 10 = £2.29. Label: 2

DEXTROPROPOXYPHENE HYDROCHLORIDE

Indications: mild to moderate pain

Cautions; Contra-indications; Side-effects: see under Morphine Salts and notes above; occasional hepatotoxicity; porphyria (see section 9.8.2); compound preparations special hazard in overdose, see notes above; convulsions reported in overdose; contra-indicated in those who are suicidal or addiction prone; **interactions:** Appendix 1 (opioid analgesics)

Dose: 65 mg every 6–8 hours when necessary; CHILD not recomended

Note. 65 mg dextropropoxyphene hydrochloride ≡ 100 mg dextropropoxyphene napsylate

PoM Dextropropoxyphene (Non-proprietary)

Capsules, the equivalent of dextropropoxyphene hydrochloride 65 mg (as napsylate). Net price 20 = £1.64. Label: 2

Available from Lilly (NHS Doloxene®)

Note. Dextropropoxyphene is an ingredient of some compound analgesic preparations, see section 4.7.1

DIAMORPHINE HYDROCHLORIDE
(Heroin Hydrochloride)

Indications: see notes above; acute pulmonary oedema

Cautions; Contra-indications; Side-effects: see under Morphine Salts and notes above; **interactions:** Appendix 1 (opioid analgesics)

Dose: acute pain, *by subcutaneous or intramuscular injection,* 5 mg repeated every 4 hours if necessary (up to 10 mg for heavier well-muscled patients)

By slow intravenous injection, quarter to half corresponding intramuscular dose

Myocardial infarction, *by slow intravenous injection* (1 mg/minute), 5 mg followed by a further 2.5–5 mg if necessary; elderly or frail patients, reduce dose by half

Acute pulmonary oedema, *by slow intravenous injection* (1 mg/minute) 2.5–5 mg

Chronic pain, *by mouth or by subcutaneous or intramuscular injection,* 5–10 mg regularly every 4 hours; dose may be increased according to needs; intramuscular dose should be approximately half corresponding oral dose, and quarter to third corresponding oral *morphine* dose; see also Terminal Care, p.12

CD Diamorphine (Non-proprietary)

Tablets, diamorphine hydrochloride 10 mg. Net price 20 = 91p. Label: 2

Available from Aurum

Injection, powder for reconstitution, diamorphine hydrochloride. Net price 5-mg amp = £1.16, 10 mg amp = £1.34, 30 mg amp = £1.60, 100-mg amp = £4.42, 500-mg amp = £20.68

Available from Berk (Diagesil®), CP, Evans, Hillcross, Napp (Diaphine®)

CD Diamorphine Linctus
See section 3.9.1

DIHYDROCODEINE TARTRATE

Indications: moderate to severe pain

Cautions; Contra-indications; Side-effects: see under Morphine Salts and notes above

Dose: by mouth, 30 mg every 4–6 hours when necessary (see also notes above); CHILD over 4 years 0.5–1 mg/kg every 4–6 hours

By deep subcutaneous or intramuscular injection, up to 50 mg every 4–6 hours

---

Cautionary label wordings, see inside back cover

Prices are **net**, see p.1

Dihydrocodeine (Non-proprietary)

PoM *Tablets*, dihydrocodeine tartrate 30 mg. Net price 20 = 47p. Label: 2, 21

Available from most generic manufacturers

PoM *Elixir*, dihydrocodeine tartrate 10 mg/5 mL. Net price 150 mL = £2.40. Label: 2, 21

Available from Napp

CD *Injection*, dihydrocodeine tartrate 50 mg/mL. Net price 1-mL amp = 87p

Available from Napp (DF 118®)

Note. The brand name DF118® was formerly used for tablets of dihydrocodeine tartrate 30 mg

PoM **DF 118 Forte®** (Napp)

Tablets, dihydrocodeine tartrate 40 mg. Net price 100-tab pack = £12.05. Label: 2, 21

Dose: severe pain and chronic severe pain, 40 mg 3–4 times daily or at discretion of physician

Modified release

PoM **DHC Continus®** (Napp)

Tablets, m/r, dihydrocodeine tartrate 60 mg, net price 56-tab pack = £6.58; 90 mg, 56-tab pack = £10.36; 120 mg, 56-tab pack = £13.83. Label: 2, 25

Dose: chronic severe pain, 60–120 mg every 12 hours; CHILD not recommended

Note. Dihydrocodeine is an ingredient of some compound analgesic preparations, see section 4.7.1

DIPHENOXYLATE

See Co-phenotrope, section 1.4.2

DIPIPANONE HYDROCHLORIDE

Indications: moderate to severe pain

Cautions; Contra-indications; Side-effects: see under Morphine Salts and notes above; **interactions:** Appendix 1 (opioid analgesics)

CD **Diconal®** (Wellcome)

Tablets, pink, scored, dipipanone hydrochloride 10 mg, cyclizine hydrochloride 30 mg. Net price 50-tab pack = £7.59. Label: 2

Dose: 1 tablet gradually increased to 3 tablets every 6 hours; CHILD not recommended

CAUTION. **Not recommended** in terminal care, see p. 12

FENTANYL

See section 15.1.4.3

MEPTAZINOL

Indications: moderate to severe pain, including postoperative and obstetric pain and renal colic; peri-operative analgesia, see section 15.1.4.3

Cautions; Contra-indications; Side-effects: see under Morphine Salts and notes above; effects only partially reversed by naloxone

Dose: by mouth, 200 mg every 3–6 hours as required; CHILD not recommended

By *intramuscular injection*, 75–100 mg every 2–4 hours if necessary; obstetric analgesia, 100–150 mg according to patient's weight (2 mg/kg); CHILD not recommended

By *slow intravenous injection*, 50–100 mg every 2–4 hours if necessary; CHILD not recommended

PoM **Meptid®** (Monmouth)

Tablets, orange, f/c, meptazinol 200 mg. Net price 20 = £4.39. Label: 2

Injection, meptazinol 100 mg (as hydrochloride)/mL. Net price 1-mL amp = £1.92

METHADONE HYDROCHLORIDE

Indications: severe pain, see notes above; adjunct in treatment of opioid dependence, section 4.10

Cautions; Contra-indications; Side-effects: see under Morphine Salts and notes above; **interactions:** Appendix 1 (opioid analgesics)

Dose: by mouth or by subcutaneous or intramuscular injection, 5–10 mg every 6–8 hours, adjusted according to response; CHILD not recommended

CD **Methadone** (Non-proprietary)

Tablets, scored, methadone hydrochloride 5 mg. Net price 50 = £3.11. Label: 2

Available from Wellcome (Physeptone®)

Injection, methadone hydrochloride, 10 mg/mL, net price 1-mL amp = 90p, 2-mL amp = £1.37, 3.5-mL amp = £1.58, 5-mL amp = £1.65

Available from Martindale, Wellcome (Physeptone®)

Linctus, see section 3.9.1

Mixture 1 mg/mL, section 4.10

NALBUPHINE HYDROCHLORIDE

Indications: moderate to severe pain; peri-operative analgesia, see section 15.1.4.3

Cautions; Contra-indications; Side-effects: see under Morphine Salts and notes above; **interactions:** Appendix 1 (opioid analgesics)

Dose: by subcutaneous, intramuscular, or intravenous injection, 10–20 mg for 70 kg patient every 3–6 hours, adjusted as required; CHILD up to 300 micrograms/kg repeated once or twice as necessary

Myocardial infarction, *by slow intravenous injection*, 10–20 mg repeated after 30 minutes if necessary

PoM **Nubain®** (Du Pont)

Injection, nalbuphine hydrochloride 10 mg/mL. Net price 1-mL amp = 73p; 2-mL amp = £1.13

PAPAVERETUM

See section 15.1.4.3

PENTAZOCINE

Indications: moderate to severe pain, but see notes above

Cautions; Contra-indications; Side-effects: see under Morphine Salts and notes above; occasional hallucinations; avoid in patients dependent on opioids and in arterial or pulmonary hypertension and heart failure; porphyria (see section 9.8.2); **interactions:** Appendix 1 (opioid analgesics)

Dose: by mouth, pentazocine hydrochloride 50 mg every 3–4 hours preferably after food (range 25–100 mg); CHILD 6–12 years 25 mg

By subcutaneous, intramuscular, or intravenous injection, moderate pain, pentazocine 30 mg, severe pain 45–60 mg every 3–4 hours when necessary; CHILD over 1 year, *by subcutaneous or intramuscular injection*, up to 1 mg/kg, *by intravenous injection* up to 500 micrograms/kg

By rectum in suppositories, pentazocine 50 mg up to 4 times daily; CHILD not recommended

CD Pentazocine (Non-proprietary)
Capsules, pentazocine hydrochloride 50 mg. Net price 20 = £3.55. Label: 2, 21
Tablets, pentazocine hydrochloride 25 mg. Net price 20 = £1.59. Label: 2, 21
Injection, pentazocine 30 mg (as lactate)/mL. Net price 1-mL amp = £1.04; 2-mL amp = £1.99
Suppositories, pentazocine 50 mg (as lactate). Net price 20 = £12.30. Label: 2
Note. The brand name NHS Fortral® (Sanofi Winthrop) is used for all the above preparations of pentazocine

PETHIDINE HYDROCHLORIDE

Indications: moderate to severe pain, obstetric analgesia; peri-operative analgesia, see section 15.1.4.3

Cautions; Contra-indications; Side-effects: see under Morphine Salts and notes above; avoid in severe renal impairment; not suitable for severe continuing pain; convulsions reported in overdosage; **interactions:** Appendix 1 (opioid analgesics)

Dose: by mouth, 50–150 mg every 4 hours; CHILD 0.5–2 mg/kg

By subcutaneous or intramuscular injection, 25–100 mg, repeated after 4 hours; CHILD, *by intramuscular injection,* 0.5–2 mg/kg

By slow intravenous injection, 25–50 mg, repeated after 4 hours

Obstetric analgesia, *by subcutaneous or intramuscular injection,* 50–100 mg, repeated 1–3 hours later if necessary; max. 400 mg in 24 hours

CD Pethidine (Non-proprietary)
Tablets, pethidine hydrochloride 50 mg, net price 20 = 39p. Label: 2
Available from Roche
Injection, pethidine hydrochloride 50 mg/mL. Net price 1-mL amp = 10p; 2-mL amp = 13p. 10 mg/mL see section 15.1.4.3
Various strengths available from Martindale, Roche

CD Pamergan P100® (Martindale)
Injection, pethidine hydrochloride 50 mg, promethazine hydrochloride 25 mg/mL. Net price 2-mL amp = 69p
Dose: by intramuscular injection, for obstetric analgesia, 1–2 mL every 4 hours if necessary; severe pain, 1–2 mL every 4–6 hours if necessary; premedication, see section 15.1.4.3
Note. Although usually given intramuscularly, may be given intravenously after dilution to at least 10 mL with water for injections

PHENAZOCINE HYDROBROMIDE

Indications: severe pain
Cautions; Contra-indications; Side-effects: see under Morphine Salts and notes above; **interactions:** Appendix 1 (opioid analgesics)

Dose: by mouth or sublingually, 5 mg every 4–6 hours when necessary; single doses may be increased to 20 mg; CHILD not recommended

CD Narphen® (Napp)
Tablets, scored, phenazocine hydrobromide 5 mg. Net price 100-tab pack = £28.51. Label: 2

PHENOPERIDINE
See section 15.1.4.3

TRAMADOL HYDROCHLORIDE

Indications: moderate to severe pain
Cautions; Contra-indications; Side-effects: see under Morphine Salts and notes above; in addition to hypotension, hypertension also occasionally reported, anaphylaxis reported; caution if history of epilepsy (convulsions reported, usually after rapid intravenous injection); avoid in pregnancy and breast-feeding; not suitable as substitute in opioid-dependent patients; **interactions:** Appendix 1 (opioid anagesics)
GENERAL ANAESTHESIA. Not recommended for analgesia during light planes of general anaesthesia (increased operative recall reported)

Dose: by mouth, 50–100 mg every 4–6 hours; usual max. 400 mg daily; CHILD not recommended

By intramuscular injection or by intravenous injection (over 2–3 minutes) *or infusion,* 50–100 mg every 4–6 hours

Postoperative pain, 100 mg initially then 50 mg every 10–20 minutes if necessary during first hour to total max. 250 mg (including initial dose) in first hour, *then* 50–100 mg every 4–6 hours; max. 600 mg daily; CHILD not recommended

▼ PoM Zydol® (Searle)
Capsules, green/yellow, tramadol hydrochloride 50 mg. Net price 100-cap pack = £17.71. Label: 2
Injection, tramadol hydrochloride 50 mg/mL. Net price 2-mL amp = £1.30

4.7.3 Trigeminal neuralgia

Carbamazepine (section 4.8.1), taken during the acute stages of trigeminal neuralgia, reduces the frequency and severity of attacks. It has no effect on other forms of headache. A dose of 100 mg once or twice a day should be given initially and the dose slowly increased until the best response is obtained; most patients require 200 mg 3–4 times daily but a few may require an increased total daily dosage of up to 1.6 g. Plasma concentrations should be monitored when high doses are given. Occasionally extreme dizziness is encountered which is a further reason for starting treatment with a small dose and increasing it slowly.

Some cases of trigeminal neuralgia respond to **phenytoin** (section 4.8.1) given alone or in conjunction with carbamazepine. A combination of phenytoin and carbamazepine is only required in very refractory cases or in those unable to tolerate high doses of carbamazepine.

Although **tricyclic antidepressants** are not indicated for true trigeminal neuralgia they are more effective than carbamazepine in *post-herpetic neuralgia* and may also be useful in *oral and facial pain*, particularly if it is associated with depression.

4.7.4   Antimigraine drugs

4.7.4.1 Treatment of the acute migraine attack
4.7.4.2 Prophylaxis of migraine

4.7.4.1 TREATMENT OF THE ACUTE MIGRAINE ATTACK

Most migraine headaches respond to analgesics such as **aspirin** or **paracetamol** (section 4.7.1) but as peristalsis is often reduced during migraine attacks the medication may not be sufficiently well absorbed to be effective; dispersible or effervescent preparations should therefore preferably be used.

Ergotamine is used in patients with migraine that does not respond to analgesics; it should not be given in hemiplegic migraine. It relieves migraine headache by constricting cranial arteries but visual and other prodromal symptoms are not affected; vomiting may be made worse (but can be relieved by the addition of an anti-emetic).

The value of ergotamine is limited by difficulties in absorption and by its side-effects, particularly *nausea, vomiting, abdominal pain*, and *muscular cramps*. The recommended doses of ergotamine preparations should **not** be exceeded and treatment should **not** be repeated at intervals of less than 4 days.

In some patients repeated administration of ergotamine may cause *habituation*, and headache *may be provoked* by chronic overdosage or by sudden withdrawal. To avoid habituation the frequency of administration should be limited to **no more than** twice a month. It should **never** be prescribed prophylactically but in the management of cluster headache a low dose is occasionally given daily for 1 to 2 weeks [unlicensed indication].

There are various ergotamine preparations designed to improve absorption and best results are obtained when the dose is given early in an attack. An aerosol form (Medihaler-Ergotamine®) is acceptable to some patients. Sublingual ergotamine (Lingraine®) probably has no advantage over oral treatment.

Sumatriptan is a new 5-HT$_1$ agonist. It appears to be of considerable value in the treatment of an acute attack but experience is relatively limited. Sumatriptan should not be taken until 24 hours after ergotamine has been stopped. Conversely ergotamine should not be taken until 6 hours after sumatriptan.

Anti-emetics (section 4.6), such as **metoclopramide** by mouth or, if vomiting is likely, by intramuscular injection, or the phenothiazine and antihistamine anti-emetics, relieve the nausea associated with migraine attacks. Domperidone or prochlorperazine may be given rectally if vomiting is a problem. Metoclopramide has the added advantage of promoting gastric emptying and normal peristalsis. A single dose should be given at the onset of symptoms. Oral analgesic preparations containing metoclopramide are available (**important:** for warnings relating to extrapyramidal effects particularly in children and young adults, see p. 177).

ANALGESICS
Section 4.7.1

ANALGESICS WITH ANTI-EMETICS

Migraleve® (Charwell)
Tablets, all f/c, *pink tablets*, buclizine hydrochloride 6.25 mg, paracetamol 500 mg, codeine phosphate 8 mg; *yellow tablets*, paracetamol 500 mg, codeine phosphate 8 mg. Net price 48-tab Duopack (32 pink + 16 yellow) = £5.10; 48 pink = £5.56; 48 yellow = £4.70. Label: 2, 17, 30

Dose: 2 pink tablets at onset of attack, or if it is imminent, then 2 yellow tablets every 4 hours if necessary; max. in 24 hours 2 pink and 6 yellow; CHILD 10–14 years, half adult dose

PoM Migravess® (Bayer)
Tablets, effervescent, scored, metoclopramide hydrochloride 5 mg, aspirin 325 mg. Net price 30-tab pack = £3.60. Label: 13, 17, 32

Forte tablets, effervescent, scored, metoclopramide hydrochloride 5 mg, aspirin 450 mg. Net price 30-tab pack = £4.94. Label: 13, 17, 32

Dose: tablets or Forte tablets, 2 dissolved in water at onset of attack every 4 hours when necessary; max. 6 tablets in 24 hours; CHILD 12–15 years, half adult dose
IMPORTANT. Ingredients include metoclopramide which can cause **severe extrapyramidal effects**, particularly in children and young adults (for further details, see p. 177)

PoM Paramax® (Lorex)
Tablets, scored, paracetamol 500 mg, metoclopramide hydrochloride 5 mg. Net price 42-tab pack = £3.99. Label: 17, 30

Sachets, effervescent powder, sugar-free, the contents of 1 sachet = 1 tablet; to be dissolved in ¼ tumblerful of liquid before administration. Net price 42-sachet pack = £5.27. Label: 13, 17, 30

Dose: (tablets or sachets): 2 at onset of attack then every 4 hours when necessary to max. of 6 in 24 hours (young adult 15–19 years, over 60 kg, max. of 5 in 24 hours); ADOLESCENT and YOUNG ADULT 12–19 years, 30–59 kg, 1 at onset of attack then 1 every 4 hours when necessary to max. of 3 in 24 hours
IMPORTANT. Ingredients include metoclopramide which can cause **severe extrapyramidal effects**, particularly in children and young adults (for further details, see p. 177)

ERGOTAMINE TARTRATE

Indications: acute attacks of migraine and migraine variants unresponsive to analgesics

Cautions: risk of peripheral vasospasm (see advice below); elderly; should not be used for migraine prophylaxis; **interactions:** Appendix 1

(ergotamine) and under sumatriptan (Cautions), below

PERIPHERAL VASOSPASM. Warn patient to stop treatment immediately if numbness or tingling of extremities develops and to contact doctor.

Contra-indications: peripheral vascular disease, coronary heart disease, obliterative vascular disease and Raynaud's syndrome, hepatic or renal impairment, sepsis, severe or inadequately controlled hypertension, hyperthyroidism, pregnancy and breast-feeding, porphyria (see section 9.8.2)

Side-effects: nausea, vomiting, abdominal pain, and occasionally increased headache (see also notes above); repeated high dosage may cause ergotism with gangrene and confusion; pleural and peritoneal fibrosis may occur with excessive use

Dose: see under preparations below

PoM **Cafergot®** (Sandoz)

Tablets, ergotamine tartrate 1 mg, caffeine 100 mg. Net price 2 × 50-tab pack = £4.46. Label: 18, counselling, dosage

Dose: 1–2 tablets at onset; max. 4 tablets in 24 hours; not to be repeated at intervals of less than 4 days; max. 8 tablets in one week (but see also notes above); CHILD not recommended

Suppositories, ergotamine tartrate 2 mg, caffeine 100 mg. Net price 30 = £4.87. Label: 18, counselling, dosage

Dose: 1 suppository at onset; max. 2 in 24 hours; not to be repeated at intervals of less than 4 days; max. 4 suppositories in one week (but see also notes above); CHILD not recommended

PoM **Lingraine®** (Sanofi Winthrop)

Tablets (for sublingual use), green, ergotamine tartrate 2 mg. Net price 12 = £7.43. Label: 18, 26, counselling, dosage

Dose: 1 tablet at onset repeated after 30–60 minutes if necessary; max. 3 tablets in 24 hours and 6 tablets in one week (but see also notes above); CHILD not recommended

PoM **Medihaler-Ergotamine®** (3M)

Aerosol inhalation (oral), ergotamine tartrate 360 micrograms/metered inhalation. Net price 75-dose unit = £3.06. Label: 18, counselling, dosage

Additives: include CFC propellants

Dose: 360 micrograms (1 puff) repeated if necessary after 5 minutes; max. 6 inhalations in 24 hours and 15 inhalations in one week (but see also notes above); CHILD not recommended

PoM **Migril®** (Wellcome)

Tablets, scored, ergotamine tartrate 2 mg, cyclizine hydrochloride 50 mg, caffeine hydrate 100 mg. Net price 20 = £11.67. Label: 2, 18, counselling, dosage

Dose: 1 tablet at onset, followed after 30 minutes by ½–1 tablet, repeated every 30 minutes if necessary; max. 4 tablets per attack and 6 tablets in one week (but see also notes above); CHILD not recommended

ISOMETHEPTENE MUCATE

Indications: migraine attack

Cautions: cardiovascular disease, hepatic and renal impairment, diabetes mellitus, hyperthyroidism; **interactions:** Appendix 1 (sympathomimetics)

Contra-indications: glaucoma, severe cardiac, hepatic and renal impairment, severe hypertension, pregnancy and breast-feeding; porphyria (see section 9.8.2)

Side-effects: dizziness, circulatory disturbances, rashes, blood disorders also reported

Midrid® (Shire)

Capsules, red, isometheptene mucate 65 mg, paracetamol 325 mg. Net price 20 = £2.38. Label: 17, 30

Dose: migraine, 2 capsules at onset of attack, followed by 1 capsule every hour if necessary; max. 5 capsules in 12 hours; CHILD not recommended

SUMATRIPTAN

Indications: acute treatment of migraine attacks; cluster headache (subcutaneous injection only)

Cautions: not for prophylaxis; conditions which predispose to coronary artery disease (exclude pre-existing cardiac disease); hepatic or renal impairment; pregnancy and breast-feeding; see also notes above; recommended as monotherapy and should **not** be taken with other acute migraine therapies—should **not** be taken until 24 hours after stopping an ergotamine-containing preparation (conversely, ergotamine-containing preparations should **not** be taken until 6 hours after sumatriptan); avoid concomitant use with MAOIs (including moclobemide), serotonin-uptake inhibitors or lithium; other **interactions:** Appendix 1 (sumatriptan)

DRIVING. Drowsiness may affect performance of skilled tasks (e.g. driving)

Contra-indications: ischaemic heart disease; previous myocardial infarction; Prinzmetal's angina, coronary vasospasm; uncontrolled hypertension

CSM advice. Following reports of chest pain and tightness (coronary vasoconstriction) CSM has emphasised that sumatriptan should **not** be used in ischaemic heart disease or Prinzmetal's angina, and that use with ergotamine should be **avoided** (see also Cautions).

Side-effects: chest pain and tightness (may be intense, involve throat, and mimic angina pectoris—vasospasm may result in arrhythmia, ischaemia or myocardial infarction, see also CSM advice above; sensations of tingling, heat, heaviness, pressure, or tightness in any part of body; flushing, dizziness, feeling of weakness, paraesthesia; fatigue, drowsiness, altered liver function tests, transient increase in blood pressure reported; nausea and vomiting also reported; transient pain at injection site

Dose: by mouth, 100 mg as soon as possible after onset (patient not responding should not take second dose for same attack); dose may be repeated if migraine recurs; max. 300 mg in 24 hours

By subcutaneous injection using auto-injector, 6 mg as soon as possible after onset (patient not responding should not take second dose for same attack); dose may be repeated once after not less than 1 hour if symptoms recur; max. 12 mg in 24 hours

ELDERLY over 65 years and CHILD not recommended

IMPORTANT. **Not** for intravenous injection which may cause coronary vasospasm and angina

▼ PoM **Imigran**® (Glaxo)

Tablets, f/c, sumatriptan (as succinate) 100 mg, net price 3-tab pack = £24.00, 6-tab pack = £48.00. Label: 3, 10 patient information leaflet

Injection, sumatriptan (as succinate) 12 mg/mL (= 6 mg/0.5-mL syringe), net price, treatment pack (2 × 0.5-mL pre-filled syringes and auto-injector) = £41.14; refill pack (2 × 0.5-mL pre-filled syringes) = £39.14. Label: 3, 10 patient information leaflet

4.7.4.2 PROPHYLAXIS OF MIGRAINE

Where migraine attacks are frequent, search should be made for provocative factors such as stress or diet (chocolate, cheese, alcohol, etc.). Benzodiazepines should be avoided because of the risk of dependence. In patients with more than one attack a month, one of three main prophylactic agents may be tried: pizotifen, beta-blockers, or tricyclic antidepressants (even when the patient is not obviously depressed). Long-term treatment with any of these prophylactic drugs is undesirable; the need for continuing therapy should be reviewed at intervals of about 6 months. Oral contraceptives may precipitate or worsen migraine; patients reporting a sharp increase in frequency of migraine or focal features should be recommended alternative contraceptive measures.

Pizotifen is an antihistamine and serotonin antagonist structurally related to the tricyclic antidepressants. It affords good prophylaxis but may cause weight gain. To avoid undue drowsiness treatment may be started at 500 micrograms at night and gradually increased to 3 mg; it is rarely necessary to exceed this dose.

The **beta-blockers** propranolol, metoprolol, nadolol, and timolol (see section 2.4) are all effective. Propranolol is the most commonly used in an initial dose of 40 mg 2 to 3 times daily by mouth. Beta-blockers may also be given as a single daily dose of a long-acting preparation. The value of beta-blockers is limited by their contra-indications (see section 2.4) and by interaction with ergotamine (see Appendix 1, beta-blockers).

Tricyclic antidepressants (section 4.3.1) may usefully be prescribed in a dose, for example, of amitriptyline 10 mg at night, increasing to a maintenance dose of 50 to 75 mg at night.

There is some evidence that the **calcium-channel blockers** (see section 2.6.2), e.g. verapamil and nifedipine may be useful in migraine prophylaxis.

Cyproheptadine (see section 3.4.1), an antihistamine with serotonin-antagonist and calcium channel-blocking properties, may also be tried in refractory cases.

Clonidine (Dixarit®) is probably little better than placebo and may aggravate depression or produce insomnia. **Methysergide** has dangerous side-effects (retroperitoneal fibrosis and fibrosis of the heart valves and pleura); **important:** it should only be administered under hospital supervision.

CLONIDINE HYDROCHLORIDE

Indications: prevention of recurrent migraine (but see notes above), vascular headache, menopausal flushing; hypertension, see section 2.5.2

Cautions: depressive illness, concurrent antihypertensive therapy; porphyria (see section 9.8.2); **interactions:** Appendix 1 (clonidine)

Side-effects: dry mouth, sedation, dizziness, nausea, nocturnal restlessness; occasionally rashes

Dose: 50 micrograms twice daily, increased after 2 weeks to 75 micrograms twice daily if necessary; CHILD not recommended

PoM **Dixarit**® (Boehringer Ingelheim)
Tablets, blue, s/c, clonidine hydrochloride 25 micrograms. Net price 112-tab pack = £6.68
PoM **Catapres**® (hypertension), see section 2.5.2

METHYSERGIDE

Indications: prevention of severe recurrent migraine and cluster headache in patients who are refractory to other treatment and whose lives are seriously disrupted (**important:** hospital supervision only, see notes above)

Cautions: history of peptic ulceration; avoid abrupt withdrawal of treatment; after 6 months withdraw (gradually over 2 to 3 weeks) for reassessment for at least 1 month (see also notes above)

Contra-indications: renal, hepatic, pulmonary, and cardiovascular disease, severe hypertension, collagen disease, cellulitis, urinary-tract disorders, cachectic or septic conditions, pregnancy, breast-feeding

Side-effects: nausea, vomiting, heartburn, abdominal discomfort, drowsiness, and dizziness occur frequently in initial treatment; mental and behavioural disturbances, insomnia, oedema, weight gain, rashes, loss of scalp hair, cramps, arterial spasm (including coronary artery spasm with angina and possible myocardial infarction), paraesthesias of extremities, postural hypotension, and tachycardia also occur. Retroperitoneal and other abnormal fibrotic reactions may occur on prolonged administration, requiring immediate withdrawal of treatment

Dose: 1 mg at bedtime, gradually increased to 1–2 mg 2–3 times daily with food (see notes above); CHILD not recommended
Carcinoid syndrome, usual range, 12–20 mg daily (hospital supervision); CHILD not recommended

PoM **Deseril**® (Sandoz)
Tablets, s/c, methysergide 1 mg (as maleate). Net price 50-tab pack = £4.47. Label: 2, 21

PIZOTIFEN

Indications: prevention of vascular headache including classical migraine, common migraine, and cluster headache

Cautions: urinary retention; closed-angle glaucoma, renal impairment; pregnancy and breast-feeding; **interactions:** Appendix 1 (pizotifen)
DRIVING. Drowsiness may affect performance of skilled tasks (e.g. driving); effects of alcohol enhanced

Side-effects: antimuscarinic effects, drowsiness, increased appetite and weight gain; occasionally nausea, dizziness; CNS stimulation may occur in children

Dose: 1.5 mg at night *or* 500 micrograms 3 times daily (but see also notes above), adjusted according to response within the usual range 0.5–3 mg daily; max. single dose 3 mg, max. daily dose 4.5 mg; CHILD up to 1.5 mg daily in divided doses; max. single dose at night 1 mg

---

Sanomigran® (Sandoz)

Tablets, both ivory-yellow, s/c, pizotifen (as hydrogen malate), 500 micrograms, net price 20 = £1.56; 1.5 mg, 28-tab pack = £7.78. Label: 2

Elixir, sugar-free, pizotifen 250 micrograms (as hydrogen malate)/5 mL. Net price 300-mL pack = £4.12. Label: 2

4.8 Antiepileptics

4.8.1 Control of epilepsy
4.8.2 Drugs used in status epilepticus
4.8.3 Febrile convulsions

4.8.1 Control of epilepsy

The object of treatment is to prevent the occurrence of seizures by maintaining an effective plasma concentration of the drug. Careful adjustment of doses is necessary, starting with low doses and increasing gradually until seizures are controlled or there are overdose effects.

The frequency of administration is determined by the plasma half-life, and should be kept as low as possible to encourage better patient compliance. Most antiepileptics, when used in average dosage, may be given twice daily. Phenobarbitone and sometimes phenytoin, which have long half-lives, may often be given as a daily dose at bedtime. However, with large doses, some antiepileptics may need to be administered 3 times daily to avoid adverse effects associated with high peak plasma concentrations. Young children metabolise antiepileptics more rapidly than adults and therefore require more frequent doses and a higher amount per kilogram body-weight.

COMBINATION THERAPY. Therapy with several antiepileptic drugs concurrently should generally be avoided. Patients are best controlled with one antiepileptic. Combinations of drugs have been used on the grounds that their therapeutic effects were additive while their individual toxicity was reduced but there is no evidence for this. In fact, toxicity may be enhanced with combination therapy. A second drug should only be added to the regimen if seizures continue despite high plasma concentrations or toxic effects. The use of more than two antiepileptics is rarely justified. Another disadvantage of multiple therapy is that drug interactions occur between the various antiepileptics (see below). Moreover, it is illogical to combine primidone and phenobarbitone as the former is largely metabolised to phenobarbitone in the liver, which is responsible for most, if not all, of its antiepileptic action.

INTERACTIONS. Interactions between antiepileptics are complex and may enhance toxicity without a corresponding increase in antiepileptic effect. Interactions may be caused by *hepatic enzyme induction* or *hepatic enzyme inhibition*; *displacement from protein binding sites* is not usually a problem. These interactions are highly variable and unpredictable. Plasma monitoring is therefore often advisable with combination therapy.

Important examples of interactions caused by *enzyme induction* include reduction in plasma-carbamazepine concentration by phenytoin, phenobarbitone and primidone. The plasma-phenytoin concentration is reduced by vigabatrin but the mechanism of the interaction is unclear. Plasma-clonazepam and plasma-lamotrigine concentrations are reduced by carbamazepine, phenytoin, phenobarbitone and primidone.

Valproate is responsible for important examples of *inhibition of hepatic metabolism*, notably causing a marked increase in the plasma concentration of lamotrigine. Lamotrigine in turn may increase the plasma concentration of an active metabolite of carbamazepine.

For other important interactions see **Appendix 1**, and for FPA guidelines on enzyme-inducing antiepileptics and **oral contraceptives**, see section 7.3.1.

WITHDRAWAL. Abrupt withdrawal of antiepileptics, particularly the barbiturates and benzodiazepines, should be avoided, as this may precipitate severe rebound seizures. Reduction in dosage should be carried out in stages and, in the case of the barbiturates, the withdrawal process may take months. The changeover from one antiepileptic drug regimen to another should be made cautiously, withdrawing the first drug only when the new regimen has been largely established.

The decision to withdraw all antiepileptics from a seizure-free patient, and its timing, is often difficult and may depend on individual patient factors. Even in patients who have been seizure-free for several years, there is a significant risk of seizure recurrence on drug withdrawal.

DRIVING. Patients suffering from epilepsy may drive a motor vehicle (but not a heavy goods or public service vehicle) provided that they have had a seizure-free period of one year or, if subject to attacks only while asleep, have established a three-year period of asleep attacks without awake attacks. Patients affected by drowsiness should not drive or operate machinery.

PREGNANCY AND BREAST-FEEDING. During pregnancy, plasma concentrations of antiepileptics should be frequently monitored as they may fall, particularly in the later stages. There is an increased risk of teratogenicity associated with the use of anticonvulsant drugs. **Important:** in view of the increased risk of neural tube defects associated with carbamazepine and valproate the **CSM** has advised that women taking these drugs who *may become pregnant* should be **informed of the possible consequences** and those who *wish to become pregnant* should be referred to an appropriate specialist for advice. Women who become pregnant should be **counselled** and offered **antenatal screening** (alpha-fetoprotein measurement and a second trimester ultrasound scan).

Breast-feeding is acceptable with all antiepileptic drugs, taken in normal doses, with the possible exception of the barbiturates see Prescribing during Breast-feeding (Appendix 5).

PARTIAL SEIZURES WITH OR WITHOUT SECONDARY GENERALISATION

Carbamazepine and **phenytoin** are the drugs of choice for secondary generalised tonic-clonic seizures and for partial (focal) seizures themselves; controlled trials with **sodium valproate** suggest similar efficacy but more evidence is awaited. Phenobarbitone and primidone are also effective but are likely to be more sedating. Second-line drugs include clonazepam, clobazam, and acetazolamide. The new drugs **gabapentin, lamotrigine,** and **vigabatrin** are now available where control is difficult to obtain. Partial epilepsy and secondarily generalised seizures are more difficult to control than tonic-clonic seizures as part of a syndrome of primary generalised epilepsy.

GENERALISED SEIZURES

TONIC-CLONIC SEIZURES (GRAND MAL). The drugs of choice for *tonic-clonic seizures* occurring as part of a syndrome of *primary generalised epilepsy* are **carbamazepine, phenytoin,** and **sodium valproate. Phenobarbitone** and **primidone** are also effective but may be more sedating. The new drugs **lamotrigine** and **vigabatrin** are now available where control is difficult to obtain.

ABSENCE SEIZURES (PETIT MAL). **Ethosuximide** and **sodium valproate** are the drugs of choice in simple absence seizures. Sodium valproate is also highly effective in treating the tonic-clonic seizures which may co-exist with absence seizures in primary generalised epilepsy.

MYOCLONIC SEIZURES. Myoclonic seizures (myoclonic jerks) occur in a variety of syndromes, and response to treatment varies considerably. **Sodium valproate** is the drug of choice and **clonazepam, ethosuximide,** and other antiepileptic drugs may be used. For reference to the adjunctive use of piracetam, see section 4.9.3.

ATYPICAL ABSENCE, ATONIC, AND TONIC SEIZURES. These seizure types are usually seen in childhood, in specific epileptic syndromes, or associated with cerebral damage or mental retardation. They may respond poorly to the traditional drugs. **Phenytoin, sodium valproate, clonazepam, ethosuximide,** and **phenobarbitone** may be tried. Second-line antiepileptic drugs that are occasionally helpful, include **acetazolamide** and **corticosteroids**.

CARBAMAZEPINE

Carbamazepine is a drug of choice for simple and complex partial seizures and for tonic-clonic seizures regardless of whether they are primary or secondary to a focal discharge. It has a wider therapeutic index than phenytoin and the relationship between dose and plasma concentration is linear, but monitoring of plasma concentrations may be helpful in determining optimum dosage. It has generally fewer side-effects than phenytoin or the barbiturates, but reversible blurring of vision, dizziness, and unsteadiness are dose-related, and may be dose-limiting. These side-effects may be reduced by altering the timing of medication. It is essential to initiate carbamazepine therapy at a low dose and build this up over one or two weeks.

CARBAMAZEPINE

Indications: all forms of epilepsy except absence seizures; trigeminal neuralgia (section 4.7.3); prophylaxis in manic-depressive illness (4.2.3)

Cautions: hepatic or renal impairment; cardiac disease (see also Contra-indications); skin reactions (see also Side-effects), history of haematological reactions to other drugs; manufacturer recommends blood counts and hepatic and renal function tests (but evidence of practical value unsatisfactory); glaucoma; pregnancy (**important:** see p.193 and Appendix 4 (neural tube screening)), breast-feeding (see p.193); avoid sudden withdrawal; **interactions:** see p.193 and Appendix 1 (carbamazepine)

BLOOD, HEPATIC or SKIN DISORDERS. Patients or their carers should be told how to recognise signs of blood, liver, or skin disorders, and advised to seek immediate medical attention if symptoms such as fever, sore throat, rash, mouth ulcers, bruising, or bleeding develop. Leucopenia which is severe, progressive or associated with clinical symptoms requires withdrawal (if necessary under cover of suitable alternative).

Contra-indications: AV conduction abnormalities (unless paced); history of bone marrow depression, porphyria (see section 9.8.2)

Side-effects: nausea and vomiting, dizziness, drowsiness, headache, ataxia, confusion and agitation (elderly), visual disturbances (especially double vision and often associated with peak plasma concentrations); constipation or diarrhoea, anorexia; mild transient generalised erythematous rash may occur in a large number of patients (withdraw if worsens or is accompanied by other symptoms); leucopenia and other blood disorders (including thrombocytopenia, agranulocytosis and aplastic anaemia); other side-effects include cholestatic jaundice, hepatitis and acute renal failure, Stevens-Johnson syndrome, toxic epidermal necrolysis, alopecia, thromboembolism, arthralgia, fever, proteinuria, lymph node enlargement, cardiac conduction disturbances (sometimes arrhythmias), dyskinesias, paraesthesia, depression, impotence (and impaired fertility), gynaecomastia, galactorrhoea, aggression, activation of psychosis; photosensitivity, hyponatraemia and oedema also reported; suppositories may cause occasional rectal irritation

Dose: by mouth, epilepsy, initially, 100–200 mg 1–2 times daily, increased slowly to usual dose of 0.8–1.2 g daily in divided doses; in some cases 1.6–2 g daily may be needed; ELDERLY reduce initial dose; CHILD daily in divided doses, up to 1 year 100–200 mg, 1–5 years 200–400 mg, 5–10 years 400–600 mg, 10–15 years 0.6–1 g

By rectum, as suppositories, see below

Note. Plasma concentration for optimum response 4–12 mg/litre (20–50 micromol/litre)

PoM **Carbamazepine** (Non-proprietary)

Tablets, carbamazepine 100 mg, net price 20 = 58p; 200 mg, 20 = £1.08; 400 mg, 20 = £2.34. Label: 3

Available from APS, Cox, Generics, Hillcross, K Pharm., Norton (Epimaz®)

PoM **Tegretol**® (Geigy)

Tablets, all scored, carbamazepine 100 mg, net price 20 = 62p; 200 mg, 20 = £1.15; 400 mg, 56-tab pack = £6.56. Label: 3

Chewtabs, orange, carbamazepine 100 mg, net price 20 = £1.05; 200 mg, 20 = £1.96. Label: 3, 21, 24

Liquid, sugar-free, carbamazepine 100 mg/5 mL. Net price 300-mL pack = £5.72. Label: 3

Suppositories, carbamazepine 125 mg, net price 5 = £7.50; 250 mg, 5 = £10.00. Label: 3

Dose: epilepsy, for short-term use (max. 7 days) when oral therapy temporarily not possible; suppositories of 125 mg may be considered to be approximately equivalent in therapeutic effect to tablets of 100 mg but final adjustment should always depend on clinical response (plasma concentration monitoring recommended); max. by rectum 1 g daily in 4 divided doses

PoM **Tegretol**® **Retard** (Geigy)

Tablets, m-r, both scored, carbamazepine 200 mg (beige-orange), net price 20 = £1.50; 400 mg (brown-orange), 20 = £2.94. Label: 3, 25

Dose: epilepsy (ADULT and CHILD over 5 years), as above; trigeminal neuralgia, as section 4.7.3; total daily dose given in 2 divided doses

ETHOSUXIMIDE

Ethosuximide is the drug of choice in simple absence seizures; it may also be used in myoclonic seizures and in atypical absence, atonic, and tonic seizures.

ETHOSUXIMIDE

Indications: absence seizures

Cautions: see notes above; hepatic and renal impairment; pregnancy and breast-feeding (see notes above); avoid sudden withdrawal; porphyria (see section 9.8.2); **interactions:** Appendix 1 (ethosuximide)

Side-effects: gastro-intestinal disturbances, drowsiness, dizziness, ataxia, dyskinesia, hiccup, photophobia, headache, depression, and mild euphoria. Psychotic states, rashes, liver changes, and haematological disorders such as leucopenia and agranulocytosis occur rarely; systemic lupus erythematosus and erythema multiforme reported

Dose: ADULT and CHILD over 6 years initially, 500 mg daily, increased by 250 mg at intervals of 4–7 days to usual dose of 1–1.5 g daily; occasionally up to 2 g daily may be needed; CHILD up to 6 years 250 mg daily, increased gradually to a max. of 1 g daily

Note. Plasma concentration for optimum response 40–100 mg/litre (300–700 micromol/litre)

PoM **Emeside**® (LAB)

Capsules, orange, ethosuximide 250 mg. Net price 112-cap pack = £9.64

Syrup, black currant or orange, ethosuximide 250 mg/5 mL. Net price 200-mL pack = £5.22

PoM **Zarontin**® (P-D)

Capsules, orange, ethosuximide 250 mg. Net price 50-cap pack = £3.82

Syrup, red, ethosuximide 250 mg/5 mL. Net price 300-mL pack = £5.60

LAMOTRIGINE

Lamotrigine is a new antiepileptic for the adjunctive treatment of partial seizures and secondarily generalised tonic-clonic seizures which are not satisfactorily controlled with other antiepileptics.

LAMOTRIGINE

Indications: adjunctive treatment of partial seizures and secondarily generalised tonic-clonic seizures not satisfactorily controlled with other antiepileptics

Cautions: closely monitor (including hepatic, renal and clotting parameters) and consider withdrawal if rash, fever, influenza-like symptoms, drowsiness, or worsening of seizure control develops, especially in first month of treatment (although causal relationship not established, lamotrigine given with other antiepileptics has been associated with rapidly progressive illness with status epilepticus, multi-organ dysfunction and disseminated intravascular coagulation); avoid abrupt withdrawal (taper off over 2 weeks or longer); pregnancy and breast-feeding; **interactions:** see p. 193 and Appendix 1 (lamotrigine)

Contra-indications: hepatic or renal impairment

Side-effects: commonly rashes (see also Cautions)—fever, malaise, influenza-like symptoms, drowsiness and rarely hepatic dysfunction, lymphadenopathy, leucopenia, and thrombocytopenia reported in conjunction with rash; angioedema, Stevens-Johnson syndrome, toxic epidermal necrolysis and photosensitivity also reported; diplopia, blurred vision, dizziness, drowsiness, headache, ataxia, tiredness, gastro-intestinal disturbances, irritability, aggression, tremor, agitation, confusion; headache, nausea, dizziness, diplopia and ataxia in patients also taking carbamazepine usually resolve when dose of either drug reduced

Dose: with *valproate*, initially 25 mg every other day for 14 days then 25 mg daily for further 14 days; usual maintenance with valproate, 100–200 mg daily in 1–2 divided doses; *without valproate*, initially 50 mg daily for 14 days then 50 mg twice daily for further 14 days; usual maintenance without valproate 200–400 mg daily in 2 divided doses; ELDERLY not recommended

CHILD 2–12 years, *with valproate*, initially 200 micrograms/kg daily for 14 days then 500 micrograms/kg daily for further 14 days (those weighing less than 25 kg may receive 5 mg on alternate days for first 14 days); usual maintenance with valproate 1–5mg/kg daily in 1–2 divided doses; *without valproate*, initially 2 mg/kg daily in 2 divided doses for 14 days then 5 mg/kg daily in 2 divided doses for further 14 days; usual maintenance without valproate 5–15 mg/kg daily in 2 divided doses

▼ PoM **Lamictal**® (Wellcome)
Tablets, all yellow, lamotrigine 25 mg, net price 56-tab pack = £19.97; 50 mg, 56-tab pack = £33.95; 100 mg, 56-tab pack = £58.57
Dispersible tablets, lamotrigine 5 mg (scored), net price 28-tab pack = £7.96; 25 mg, 56-tab pack = £19.97; 100 mg, 56-tab pack = £58.57. Label: 13

PHENOBARBITONE AND OTHER BARBITURATES

Phenobarbitone is effective for tonic and partial seizures but may be sedative in adults and cause behavioural disturbances and hyperkinesia in children. It may be tried for atypical absence, atonic, and tonic seizures. Rebound seizures may be a problem on withdrawal. Monitoring plasma concentrations is less useful than with other drugs because tolerance occurs. **Methylphenobarbitone** is largely converted to phenobarbitone in the liver and has no advantages. **Primidone** is largely converted to phenobarbitone and this is probably responsible for its antiepileptic action. A small starting dose of primidone (125 mg) is essential, and the drug should be introduced over several weeks.

PHENOBARBITONE
(Phenobarbital)
Indications: all forms of epilepsy except absence seizures; status epilepticus, section 4.8.2
Cautions: elderly, debilitated, children, impaired renal or hepatic function, respiratory depression (avoid if severe), pregnancy and breast-feeding (see notes above); avoid sudden withdrawal; see also notes above; avoid in porphyria (see section 9.8.2); **interactions:** see p.193 and Appendix 1 (barbiturates and primidone)
Side-effects: drowsiness, lethargy, mental depression, ataxia and allergic skin reactions; paradoxical excitement, restlessness and confusion in the elderly and hyperkinesia in children; megaloblastic anaemia (may be treated with folic acid); overdosage: see Emergency Treatment of Poisoning, p.22

Dose: by mouth, 60–180 mg at night; CHILD 5–8 mg/kg daily
By intramuscular or intravenous injection, 50–200 mg, repeated after 6 hours if necessary; max. 600 mg daily; dilute injection 1 in 10 with water for injections before intravenous administration; status epilepticus, section 4.8.2
Note. For therapeutic purposes phenobarbitone and phenobarbitone sodium may be considered equivalent in effect. Plasma concentration for optimum response 15–40 mg/litre (60–180 micromol/litre)

CD [1]**Phenobarbitone Tablets,** phenobarbitone 15 mg, net price 20 = 7p; 30 mg, 20 = 7p; 60 mg, 20 = 11p; 100 mg, 20 = 36p. Label: 2
CD [1]**Phenobarbitone Elixir,** phenobarbitone 15 mg/5 mL in a suitable flavoured vehicle, containing alcohol 38%. Net price 100 mL = 78p. Label: 2
Note. Some hospitals supply alcohol-free formulations
CD [1]**Phenobarbitone Injection,** phenobarbitone sodium 200 mg/mL in propylene glycol 90% and water for injections 10%. Net price 1-mL amp = 47p
Note. Must be diluted before intravenous administration (see under Dose)
Available from Rhône-Poulenc Rorer (**CD** [1]Gardenal Sodium®), Martindale; other strengths also available from Martindale.
1. See p.7 for prescribing requirements for phenobarbitone

METHYLPHENOBARBITONE
(Methyphenobarbital)
Indications; Cautions; Side-effects: see under Phenobarbitone
Dose: 100–600 mg daily

CD Prominal® (Sanofi Winthrop)
Tablets, methylphenobarbitone 30 mg, net price 20 = 78p; 60 mg, 20 = £1.03; 200 mg, 20 = £2.20. Label: 2

PRIMIDONE
Indications: all forms of epilepsy except absence seizures; essential tremor (section 4.9.3)
Cautions; Side-effects: see under Phenobarbitone. Drowsiness, ataxia, nausea, visual disturbances, and rashes, particularly at first, usually reversible on continued administration; **interactions:** see p.193 and Appendix 1 (barbiturates and primidone)
Dose: epilepsy, initially, 125 mg daily at bedtime, increased by 125 mg every 3 days to 500 mg daily in 2 divided doses then increased by 250 mg every 3 days to a max. of 1.5 g daily in divided doses; CHILD 20–30 mg/kg daily in 2 divided doses
Note. Monitor plasma concentrations of derived phenobarbitone. Optimum range as for phenobarbitone.

PoM Mysoline® (Zeneca)
Tablets, scored, primidone 250 mg. Net price 100-tab pack = £1.77. Label: 2
Oral suspension, primidone 250 mg/5 mL. Net price 250-mL pack = £1.01. Label: 2

PHENYTOIN

Phenytoin is effective in tonic-clonic and partial seizures. It has a narrow therapeutic index and the relationship between dose and plasma concentration is non-linear; small dosage increases in some patients may produce large rises in plasma concentrations with acute toxic side-effects. Monitoring of plasma concentration greatly assists dosage adjustment. A few missed doses or a small change in drug absorption may result in a marked change in plasma concentration.

Phenytoin may cause coarse facies, acne, hirsutism, and gingival hyperplasia and so may be particularly undesirable in adolescent patients.

PHENYTOIN

Indications: all forms of epilepsy except absence seizures; trigeminal neuralgia (see section 4.7.3)

Cautions: hepatic impairment (reduce dose); pregnancy and breast-feeding (see notes above); avoid sudden withdrawal; avoid in porphyria (see section 9.8.2); see also notes above; **interactions:** see p.193 and Appendix 1 (phenytoin)

Side-effects: nausea, vomiting, mental confusion, dizziness, headache, tremor, transient nervousness, insomnia occur commonly; rarely dyskinesias, peripheral neuropathy; ataxia, slurred speech, nystagmus and blurred vision are signs of overdosage; rashes (discontinue, if mild re-introduce cautiously but discontinue immediately if recurrence), coarse facies, acne and hirsutism, fever and hepatitis; lupus erythematosus, erythema multiforme (Stevens-Johnson syndrome), toxic epidermal necrolysis, polyarteritis nodosa; lymphadenopathy; gingival hypertrophy and tenderness; rarely haematological effects, including megaloblastic anaemia (may be treated with folic acid), leucopenia, thrombocytopenia, agranulocytosis, and aplastic anaemia; plasma calcium may be lowered (rickets and osteomalacia)

Dose: by mouth, initially 3–4 mg/kg daily *or* 150–300 mg daily (as a single dose or in two divided doses) increased gradually as necessary (plasma monitoring, see notes above); usual dose 300–400 mg daily; max. 600 mg daily; CHILD 5–8 mg/kg daily (in 1 or 2 doses)

By intravenous injection—section 4.8.2

Note. Plasma concentration for optimum response 10–20 mg/litre (40–80 micromol/litre)

COUNSELLING. Take preferably with or after food

PoM Phenytoin (Non proprietary)

Capsules, phenytoin sodium 50 mg, net price 20 = 40p; 100 mg, 20 = 56p. Label: 27, counselling, administration

Available from APS, Cox, K Pharm.

Tablets, coated, phenytoin sodium 50 mg, net price 20 = 21p; 100 mg, 20 = 32p. Label: 27, counselling, administration

Available from Berk (Pentran®), Cox, K Pharm.

Note. On the basis of single dose tests there are no clinically relevant differences in bioavailability between available phenytoin sodium tablets and capsules but some clinics prefer patients to remain on the same brand whenever possible

PoM Epanutin® (P-D)

Capsules, phenytoin sodium 25 mg (white/purple), net price 20 = 39p; 50 mg (white/pink), 20 = 40p; 100 mg (white/orange), 20 = 56p; 300 mg (white/green), 20 = £1.69. Label: 27, counselling, administration

Infatabs® (= tablets, chewable), yellow, scored, phenytoin 50 mg. Net price 20 = £1.10. Label: 24

Note. Contain phenytoin 50 mg (as against phenytoin sodium) therefore care is needed on changing to capsules or tablets containing phenytoin sodium

Suspension, red, phenytoin 30 mg/5 mL. Net price 100 mL = 71p. Counselling, administration

Note. Suspension of phenytoin 90 mg in 15 mL may be considered to be approximately equivalent in therapeutic effect to capsules or tablets containing phenytoin sodium 100 mg, but nevertheless care is needed in making changes

VALPROATE

Sodium valproate is effective in controlling tonic-clonic seizures, particularly in primary generalised epilepsy. It is the drug of choice in myoclonic seizures, and may be tried in atypical absence, atonic, and tonic seizures. Controlled trials in partial epilepsy suggest that it has similar efficacy to that of carbamazepine and phenytoin, but more evidence is awaited. Plasma concentrations are not a useful index of efficacy, therefore routine monitoring is unhelpful. The drug has widespread metabolic effects, and may have dose-related side-effects. There has been concern over severe hepatic or pancreatic toxicity, although these effects are rare.

SODIUM VALPROATE

Indications: all forms of epilepsy

Cautions: in patients most at risk (e.g. children and those with history of liver disease) monitor liver function in first 6 months; pregnancy (**important** see notes above and Appendix 4 (neural tube screening)); breast-feeding; systemic lupus erythematosus; monitor platelet function before major surgery; may give false positive urine tests for ketones; avoid sudden withdrawal; porphyria (see section 9.8.2); see also notes above; **interactions:** see p.193 and Appendix 1 (valproate)

Contra-indications: active liver disease, family history of severe hepatic dysfunction

Side-effects: gastric irritation, nausea, ataxia and tremor; hyperammonaemia, increased appetite and weight gain; transient hair loss (regrowth may be curly), oedema, thrombocytopenia, and inhibition of platelet aggregation; impaired hepatic function leading rarely to fatal hepatic failure (see Cautions—withdraw treatment immediately if vomiting, anorexia, jaundice, drowsiness, or loss of seizure control occurs); amenorrhoea, rashes; rarely pancreatitis (measure plasma amylase in acute abdominal pain), leucopenia, red cell hypoplasia; irregular periods and amenorrhoea also reported, also gynaecomastia

Dose: by mouth, initially, 600 mg daily in divided doses, preferably after food, increasing by 200 mg/day at 3-day intervals to a max. of 2.5 g daily in divided doses, usual maintenance 1–2 g daily (20–30 mg/kg daily); CHILD up to 20 kg, initially 20 mg/kg daily in divided doses, may be increased gradually providing plasma concentrations monitored to 40 mg/kg daily; over 20 kg, initially 400 mg daily in divided doses increased gradually to 20–30 mg/kg daily; max. 35 mg/kg daily

By intravenous injection (over 3–5 minutes) or *by intravenous infusion*, continuation of valproate treatment when oral therapy not possible, same as current dose by oral route

Initiation of valproate therapy (when oral valproate not possible), *by intravenous injection* (over 3–5 minutes), 400–800 mg (up to 10 mg/kg) followed by *intravenous infusion* up to max. 2.5 g daily; CHILD, usually 20–30 mg/kg daily

PoM **Sodium Valproate** (Non-proprietary)

Tablets, e/c, sodium valproate 200 mg, net price 20 = 78p; 500 mg, 20 = £3.13. Label: 5, 25

Available from Cox, CP (Orlept®), Hillcross, Norton

Oral solution, sodium valproate 200 mg/5 mL. Net price 100 mL = £1.96

Available from CP, (Orlept®, sugar-free), Hillcross, Norton (sugar-free)

PoM **Epilim®** (Sanofi Winthrop)

Tablets (crushable), scored, sodium valproate 100 mg. Net price 20 = 78p

Tablets, both e/c, lilac, sodium valproate 200 mg, net price 20 = £1.28; 500 mg, 20 = £3.21. Label: 5, 25

Liquid, red, sugar-free, sodium valproate 200 mg/ 5 mL. Net price 300-mL pack = £5.89

Syrup, red, sodium valproate 200 mg/5 mL. Net price 300-mL pack = £5.89

PoM **Epilim Chrono®** (Sanofi Winthrop)

Tablets, m/r, all lilac, sodium valproate 200 mg (as sodium valproate and valproic acid), net price 100-tab pack = £7.70; 300 mg, 100-tab pack = £11.55; 500 mg, 100-tab pack = £19.25. Label: 25

Dose: ADULT and CHILD over 20 kg, as above, total daily dose given in 2 divided doses

PoM **Epilim® Intravenous** (Sanofi Winthrop)

Injection, powder for reconstitution, sodium valproate. Net price 400-mg vial (with 4-mL amp water for injections) = £8.77

Valproic acid

PoM **Convulex®** (Pharmacia)

Capsules, e/c, valproic acid 150 mg, net price 100-cap pack = £3.85; 300 mg, 100-cap pack = £7.70; 500 mg, 100-cap pack = £12.83

Dose: ADULT and CHILD initially 15 mg/kg daily in 2–4 divided doses, gradually increasing in steps of 5–10 mg/ kg up to 30 mg/kg daily

EQUIVALENCE TO SODIUM VALPROATE. Manufacturer advises that Convulex® has a 1:1 dose relationship with products containing sodium valproate, but nevertheless care is needed in making changes.

BENZODIAZEPINES

Clonazepam is occasionally used in tonic-clonic or partial seizures, but its sedative side-effects may be prominent. **Clobazam** may be used as adjunctive therapy in the treatment of epilepsy (section 4.1.2), but the effectiveness of these and other **benzodiazepines** may wane considerably after weeks or months of continuous therapy.

CLOBAZAM
Section 4.1.2

CLONAZEPAM

Indications: all forms of epilepsy; myoclonus; status epilepticus, section 4.8.2

Cautions: see notes above; respiratory disease; hepatic and renal impairment; elderly and debilitated; pregnancy and breast-feeding (see notes above); avoid sudden withdrawal; porphyria (see section 9.8.2); **interactions:** see p.193 and Appendix 1 (clonazepam)

DRIVING. Drowsiness may affect the performance of skilled tasks (e.g. driving); effects of alcohol enhanced

Contra-indications: respiratory depression; acute pulmonary insufficiency

Side-effects: drowsiness, fatigue, dizziness, muscle hypotonia, coordination disturbances; hypersalivation in infants, paradoxical aggression, irritability and mental changes; rarely, blood disorders, abnormal liver-function tests; overdosage: see Emergency Treatment of Poisoning, p.22

Dose: 1 mg (elderly, 500 micrograms), initially at night for 4 nights, increased over 2–4 weeks to a usual maintenance dose of 4–8 mg daily in divided doses; CHILD up to 1 year 250 micrograms increased as above to 0.5–1 mg, 1–5 years 250 micrograms increased to 1–3 mg, 5–12 years 500 micrograms increased to 3–6 mg

PoM **Rivotril®** (Roche)

Tablets, both scored, clonazepam 500 micrograms (beige), net price 20 = 88p; 2 mg, 20 = £1.18. Label: 2

Injection, section 4.8.2

OTHER DRUGS

Acetazolamide, a carbonic anhydrase inhibitor, is a second-line drug for both tonic-clonic and partial seizures. It is occasionally helpful in atypical absence, atonic, and tonic seizures.

Vigabatrin is a new antiepileptic for use in chronic epilepsy not satisfactorily controlled by other antiepileptics. It is useful in tonic-clonic and partial seizures but has prominent behavioural side-effects in some patients.

Piracetam (section 4.9.3) has been introduced recently as adjunctive treatment for myoclonus.

Gabapentin is a new antiepileptic which can be given as adjunctive therapy in partial epilepsy with or without secondary generalisation.

ACETAZOLAMIDE

Indications: see notes above

Cautions; Side-effects: see section 11.6

Dose: 0.25–1 g daily in divided doses; CHILD 125–750 mg daily

Preparations

See section 11.6

GABAPENTIN

Indications: adjunctive treatment of partial seizures with or without secondary generalisation not satisfactorily controlled with other antiepileptics

Cautions: avoid sudden withdrawal (taper off over at least 1 week); mixed seizure disorders that include absence seizures (which may be exacerbated); elderly (may need to reduce dose), renal impairment (reduce dose), false positive readings with some urinary protein tests, pregnancy and breast-feeding; **interactions:** Appendix 1 (gabapentin)

Side-effects: somnolence, dizziness, ataxia, fatigue, nystagmus, headache, tremor, diplopia, nausea and vomiting, rhinitis, amblyopia; also convulsions, pharyngitis, dysarthria, weight gain, dyspepsia, amnesia, nervousness, coughing

Dose: 300 mg on first day, then 300 mg twice daily on second day, then 300 mg 3 times daily on third day, then increased according to response to 1.2 g daily (in 3 equally divided doses); if necessary may be further increased in steps of 300 mg daily (in 3 divided doses) to max. 2.4 g daily, usual range 0.9–1.2 g daily; max. period between doses should not exceed 12 hours; CHILD not recommended

▼ PoM **Neurontin®** (P-D)

Capsules, gabapentin 100 mg (white), net price 100-cap pack = £22.86; 300 mg (yellow), 100-cap pack = £53.00; 400 mg (orange), 100-cap pack = £61.33. Label: 3. 5

VIGABATRIN

Indications: epilepsy not satisfactorily controlled by other antiepileptics

Cautions: renal impairment; elderly; closely monitor neurological function; avoid sudden withdrawal (taper off over 2–4 weeks); history of psychosis or behavioural problems; **interactions:** see p. 193 and Appendix 1 (vigabatrin)

Contra-indications: pregnancy (high doses teratogenic in *animals*) and breast-feeding

Side-effects: drowsiness, fatigue, dizziness, nervousness, irritability, depression, headache; less commonly confusion, aggression, psychosis, memory disturbance, visual disturbance (e.g. diplopia); weight gain and gastro-intestinal disturbances reported; excitation and agitation in children; occasional increase in seizure frequency (especially if myoclonic), decrease in liver enzymes, slight decrease in haemoglobin

Dose: with current antiepileptic therapy, initially 2 g daily in single or 2 divided doses then increased or decreased according to response in steps of 0.5–1 g; usual max. 4 g daily; CHILD initially 40 mg/kg daily increased according to response to 80–100 mg/kg daily; *or* body-weight 10–15 kg, 0.5–1 g daily; body-weight 15–30 kg, 1–1.5 g daily; body-weight 30–50 kg, 1.5–3 g daily; body-weight over 50 kg, 2–4 g daily

Infants with West's syndrome may require 100 mg/kg daily or more

PoM **Sabril®** (Merrell)

Tablets, f/c, scored, vigabatrin 500 mg, net price 100-tab pack = £44.85. Label: 3

Powder, sugar-free, vigabatrin 500 mg/sachet. Net price 50-sachet pack = £24.33. Label: 3, 13

*Note.*The contents of a sachet should be dissolved in water or a soft drink immediately before taking

4.8.2 Drugs used in status epilepticus

Major status epilepticus should be *treated initially* with intravenous **diazepam**, used with caution because of the risk of respiratory depression; in situations where facilities for resuscitation are not immediately available, *small doses* of diazepam can be given intravenously or the drug can be administered as a rectal solution (Stesolid®). Absorption from intramuscular injection or from suppositories is too slow for treatment of status epilepticus. When diazepam is given intravenously there may be a high risk of venous thrombophlebitis which is minimised by using an emulsion (Diazemuls®). **Clonazepam** and **lorazepam** are also used; lorazepam has the advantage of a long duration of action.

To *prevent recurrence* **phenytoin sodium** may be given by slow intravenous injection, with ECG monitoring in a dose of 15 mg/kg at a rate of not more than 50 mg/minute (in adults) followed by the maintenance dosage. Intramuscular use of phenytoin is not recommended (absorption is slow and erratic) and intravenous infusion is not recommended (precipitates). Alternatively, **phenobarbitone sodium** (section 4.8.1) can be given by intravenous injection in a dose of 15 mg/kg at a rate of not more than 100 mg/minute. Other drugs which can be tried include **chlormethiazole edisylate**, given by intravenous infusion. Chlormethiazole has a short half-life, and the rate of infusion can be titrated against the patient's clinical condition (see **cautions** on next page).

Paraldehyde also remains a valuable drug. Given rectally (or occasionally by deep intramuscular injection) it causes little respiratory depression and is therefore useful where facilities for resuscitation are poor.

If the above measures fail to control seizures, anaesthesia with **thiopentone** or **a non-barbiturate anaesthetic** should be instituted with full intensive care support.

DIAZEPAM

Indications: status epilepticus; convulsions due to poisoning (see Emergency Treatment of Poisoning); other indications, see sections 4.1.2, 10.2.2, 15.1.4.1

Cautions; Contra-indications; Side-effects: see section 4.1.2; hypotension and apnoea may occur; when given intravenously facilities for reversing respiratory depression with mechanical ventilation must be at hand (but see also notes above)

Dose: by intravenous injection, 10–20 mg at a rate of 0.5 mL (2.5 mg) per 30 seconds, repeated if necessary after 30–60 minutes; may be followed by *intravenous infusion* to max. 3 mg/kg over 3 hours; CHILD 200–300 micrograms/kg *or* 1 mg per year of age

By rectum as rectal solution, ADULT and CHILD over 3 years 10 mg; CHILD 1–3 years and ELDERLY 5 mg; repeat after 5 minutes if necessary

PoM Diazepam (Non-proprietary)
Injection (solution), diazepam 5 mg/mL. See Appendix 6. Net price 2-mL amp = 31p
Available from CP, Roche (Valium®)
Injection (emulsion), diazepam 5 mg/mL (0.5%). See Appendix 6. Net price 2-mL amp = 76p
Available from Dumex (Diazemuls®)
Rectal tubes (= rectal solution), diazepam 2 mg/ mL. Net price 2.5-mL (5-mg) tube = £1.27; 4 mg / mL, 2.5-mL (10-mg) tube = £1.62
Available from CP (Diazepam Rectubes®), Dumex (Stesolid®), Lagap

Oral preparations, section 4.1.2

CLONAZEPAM

Indications: status epilepticus; other forms of epilepsy, and myoclonus, section 4.8.1
Cautions; Contra-indications; Side-effects: see section 4.8.1. Hypotension and apnoea may occur and resuscitation facilities must be available
Dose: by intravenous injection into a large vein (over 30 seconds) *or by intravenous infusion,* 1 mg, repeated if necessary; CHILD all ages, 500 micrograms

PoM Rivotril® (Roche)
Injection, clonazepam 1 mg/mL in solvent, for dilution with 1 mL water for injections immediately before injection or as described in Appendix 6. Net price 1-mL amp (with 1 mL water for injections) = 71p

Oral preparations, section 4.8.1

CHLORMETHIAZOLE

(Clomethiazole)
Indications: status epilepticus; other indications, see sections 4.1.1, 4.10, 15.1.4.1; eclampsia, see data sheet
Cautions: see section 4.10 for general cautions; resuscitation facilities must be available; maintain clear airway (risk of mechanical obstruction in deep sedation); *rapid infusion* to be given only

under direct medical supervision (risk of apnoea and hypotension—special care in those susceptible to cerebral or cardiac complications, e.g. the elderly); during *continuous infusion* sleep induced may lapse into deep unconsciousness and patient must be kept under close and constant observation; *prolonged infusion* may lead to accumulation and delay recovery, may also cause electrolyte imbalance (infusion contains only Na+ 32 mmol/litre and no other electrolytes); **interactions:** Appendix 1 (chlormethiazole)

Contra-indications: acute pulmonary insufficiency

Side-effects: nasal congestion and irritation (with sneezing), conjunctival irritation, headache; localised thrombophlebitis, tachycardia and transient fall in blood pressure (apnoea and hypotension on rapid infusion, see cautions); see also section 4.10

Dose: by intravenous infusion, as a 0.8% solution of chlormethiazole edisylate, initially 5–15 mL (40–120 mg)/minute up to a total of 40–100 mL (320–800 mg), then continued if necessary at a reduced rate according to response (see notes above); usual rate 0.5–1 mL (4–8 mg)/minute; CHILD initially 0.01 mL (80 micrograms)/kg/ minute, then dose increased every 2–4 hours if necessary until seizures controlled or drowsiness occurs; if no seizure for 2 days dose gradually reduced every 4–6 hours (if seizures recur dose increased to previous level)

IMPORTANT. See cautions for intravenous infusion under Cautions (above)

PoM Heminevrin® (Astra)
Intravenous infusion 0.8%, chlormethiazole edisylate 8 mg/mL. Net price 500-mL bottle = £5.25

Oral preparations, section 4.10

LORAZEPAM

Indications: status epilepticus; other indications, section 4.1.2
Cautions; Contra-indications; Side-effects: see section 4.1.2; hypotension and apnoea may occur and resuscitation facilities must be available
Dose: by intravenous injection (into large vein), 4 mg; CHILD 2 mg

Preparations
Section 4.1.2

PARALDEHYDE

Indications: status epilepticus
Cautions: bronchopulmonary disease, hepatic impairment; avoid intramuscular injection near sciatic nerve (causes severe causalgia); intravenous route, specialist centres only with intensive care facilities (see notes above)
Side-effects: rashes; pain and sterile abscess after intramuscular injection; rectal irritation after enema

Dose: by deep intramuscular injection, as a single dose, 5–10 mL; usual max. 20 mL daily with not more than 5 mL at any one site; CHILD up to 3 months 0.5 mL, 3–6 months 1 mL, 6–12 months 1.5 mL, 1–2 years 2 mL, 3–5 years 3–4 mL, 6–12 years 5–6 mL

By intravenous infusion, formerly given in a dose of up to 4–5 mL diluted to a 4% solution with sodium chloride intravenous infusion 0.9%, but no longer recommended

By rectum, 5–10 mL, administered as a 10% enema in physiological saline; CHILD as for intramuscular dose

Note. Do not use paraldehyde if it has a brownish colour or an odour of acetic acid. Avoid contact with rubber and plastics.

PoM **Paraldehyde** (Non-proprietary)

Injection, sterile paraldehyde 5 mL and 10 mL amp
Note. May temporarily be unavailable

PHENYTOIN SODIUM

Indications: status epilepticus; seizures in neurosurgery; arrhythmias, see section 2.3.2

Cautions: hypotension and heart failure; resuscitation facilities must be available; injection solutions alkaline (irritant to tissues); see also section 4.8.1; **interactions:** see p.193 and Appendix 1 (phenytoin)

Contra-indications: sinus bradycardia, sino-atrial block, and second- and third-degree heart block; Stokes-Adams syndrome; porphyria (see section 9.8.2)

Side-effects: intravenous injection may cause cardiovascular and CNS depression (particularly if injection too rapid) with arrhythmias, hypotension, and cardiovascular collapse; alterations in respiratory function (including respiratory arrest)

Dose: by slow intravenous injection (with blood pressure and ECG monitoring), status epilepticus, 15 mg/kg at a rate not exceeding 50 mg per minute, as a loading dose (see also notes above). Maintenance doses of about 100 mg should be given thereafter at intervals of every 6 hours, monitored by measurement of plasma concentrations; rate and dose reduced according to weight; CHILD 15 mg/kg as a loading dose (neonate 15–20 mg/kg)

By intramuscular injection, not recommended (see notes above)

PoM **Epanutin Ready Mixed Parenteral®** (P-D)

Injection, phenytoin sodium 50 mg/mL with propylene glycol 40% and alcohol 10% in water for injections. Net price 5-mL amp = £4.07

Oral preparations, section 4.8.1

4.8.3 Febrile convulsions

Brief febrile convulsions need only simple treatment such as tepid sponging or bathing, or antipyretic medication, e.g. **paracetamol** (section 4.7.1).

Prolonged febrile convulsions (those lasting 15 minutes or longer), *recurrent convulsions,* or those occurring in a child at known risk must be treated more actively, as there is the possibility of resulting brain damage. **Diazepam** is the drug of choice given either by slow intravenous injection in a dose of 250 micrograms/kg (as Diazemuls®, section 4.8.2) or preferably rectally in solution (e.g. Stesolid®, section 4.8.2) in a dose of 500 micrograms/kg (max. 10 mg), repeated if necessary (for full details of dose, see p.200). The rectal route is preferred as satisfactory absorption is achieved within minutes and administration is much easier. Suppositories are not suitable because absorption is too slow.

Intermittent prophylaxis (i.e. the anticonvulsant administered at the onset of fever) is possible in only a small proportion of children. Again **diazepam** is the treatment of choice, orally or rectally.

The exact role of continuous prophylaxis in children at risk from prolonged or complex febrile convulsions is controversial. It is probably indicated in only a small proportion of children, including those whose first seizure occurred at under 14 months or who have pre-existing neurological abnormalities or who have had previous prolonged or focal convulsions. Thus long-term anticonvulsant prophylaxis is rarely indicated.

4.9 Drugs used in parkinsonism and related disorders

4.9.1 Dopaminergic drugs used in parkinsonism

4.9.2 Antimuscarinic drugs used in parkinsonism

4.9.3 Drugs used in essential tremor, chorea, tics, and related disorders

In idiopathic Parkinson's disease, progressive degeneration of pigment-containing cells of the substantia nigra leads to deficiency of the neurotransmitter dopamine. This, in turn, results in a neurohumoral imbalance in the basal ganglia, causing the characteristic signs and symptoms of the illness to appear. The pathogenesis of this process is still obscure and current drug therapy aims simply to correct the imbalance. Although this approach fails to prevent the progression of the disease, it greatly improves the quality and expectancy of life of most patients.

The patient should be advised at the outset of the limitations of treatment and possible side-effects. About 10 to 20% of patients are unresponsive to treatment.

ELDERLY. Antiparkinsonian drugs carry a special risk of inducing confusion in the elderly. It is particularly important to initiate treatment with low doses and to use small increments.

4.9.1   Dopaminergic drugs used in parkinsonism

Levodopa, used with a **dopa-decarboxylase inhibitor**, is the treatment of choice for patients disabled by idiopathic Parkinson's disease. It is least valuable in elderly patients and in those with long-standing disease who may not tolerate a dose large enough to overcome their deficit. It is also less valuable in patients with post-encephalitic disease who are particularly susceptible to the side-effects. Parkinsonism caused by generalised degenerative brain disease does not normally respond to levodopa. It should not be used for neuroleptic-induced parkinsonism.

Levodopa, the amino-acid precursor of dopamine, acts mainly by replenishing depleted striatal dopamine. It improves bradykinesia and rigidity more than tremor. It is generally administered in conjunction with an extracerebral dopa-decarboxylase inhibitor which prevents the peripheral degradation of levodopa to dopamine but, unlike levodopa, does not cross the blood-brain barrier. Effective brain concentrations of dopamine can thereby be achieved with lower doses of levodopa. At the same time the reduced peripheral formation of dopamine decreases peripheral side-effects such as nausea and vomiting and cardiovascular effects. There is also less delay in onset of therapeutic effect and a smoother clinical response. A disadvantage is an increased incidence of abnormal involuntary movements.

The extracerebral dopa-decarboxylase inhibitors given with levodopa are benserazide (in **co-beneldopa**) and carbidopa (in **co-careldopa**).

When co-careldopa 10/100 (10 mg of carbidopa for each 100 mg of levodopa) is used the dose of carbidopa may be insufficient to achieve full inhibition of extracerebral dopa-decarboxylase; co-careldopa 25/100 (25 mg of carbidopa for each 100 mg of levodopa) should then be used so that the daily dose of carbidopa is at least 75 mg.

Levodopa therapy should be initiated with low doses and gradually increased, by small increments, at intervals of 2 to 3 days. The final dose is usually a compromise between increased mobility and dose-limiting side-effects. Intervals between doses may be critical and should be chosen to suit the needs of the individual patient. Nausea and vomiting are rarely dose-limiting but doses should be taken after meals. Domperidone (section 4.6) may be useful in controlling vomiting. The most frequent dose-limiting side-effects of levodopa are involuntary movements and psychiatric complications. As the patient ages, the maintenance dose may need to be reduced.

During the first 6 to 18 months of levodopa therapy there may be a slow improvement in the response of the patient which is maintained for 1½ to 2 years; thereafter a slow decline may occur. Particularly troublesome is the 'on-off' effect the incidence of which increases as the treatment progresses. This is characterised by fluctuations in performance with normal performance during the 'on' period and weakness and akinesia lasting for 2 to 4 hours during the 'off' period.

'End-of-dose' deterioration may also occur where the duration of benefit after each dose becomes progressively shorter. Modified-release preparations may help with 'end-of-dose' deterioration or nocturnal immobility and rigidity.

Selegiline is a monoamine-oxidase-B inhibitor used in severe parkinsonism in conjunction with levodopa to reduce 'end-of-dose' deterioration. It has been suggested that early treatment with selegiline may also delay the need for levodopa therapy and possibly slow the rate of progression of the disease but this remains to be confirmed.

Bromocriptine acts by direct stimulation of surviving dopamine receptors. Although effective, it has no advantages over levodopa. It should be reserved for patients for whom levodopa alone is no longer adequate or who despite careful titration cannot tolerate levodopa. Its use is often limited by its side-effects and when used with levodopa, abnormal involuntary movements and confusional states are common.

Lysuride is a newly introduced drug for parkinsonism; it is similar to bromocriptine in its action.

Pergolide is another newly introduced drug; it acts mainly on dopamine D_2 receptors. Like bromocriptine and lysuride it is sometimes useful in reducing 'off' periods and in ameliorating fluctuations in the later stage of Parkinson's disease. All these dopaminergic drugs may cause serious neuropsychiatric side-effects and occasionally may cause retroperitoneal fibrosis.

Amantadine has modest antiparkinsonian effects. It improves mild bradykinetic disabilities as well as tremor and rigidity. Unfortunately only a small proportion of patients derive much benefit from this drug and tolerance to its effects occurs. However it has the advantage of being relatively free from side-effects.

Apomorphine is a potent stimulator of D_1 and D_2 receptors, which is sometimes helpful in stabilising patients experiencing unpredictable 'off' periods with levodopa treatment. It is essential to establish patients on domperidone for three days before starting apomorphine. Long-term specialist supervision is advisable throughout apomorphine treatment.

LEVODOPA

Indications: parkinsonism (but not drug-induced extrapyramidal symptoms), see notes above

Cautions: pulmonary disease, peptic ulceration, cardiovascular disease, diabetes mellitus, osteomalacia, open-angle glaucoma, skin melanoma, psychiatric illness (avoid if severe). In prolonged therapy, psychiatric, hepatic, haematological, renal, and cardiovascular surveillance is advisable. Warn patients who benefit from therapy to resume normal activities gradually; avoid abrupt withdrawal; pregnancy (toxicity in *animals*) and breast-feeding; **interactions:** Appendix 1 (levodopa)

Contra-indications: closed-angle glaucoma

Side-effects: anorexia, nausea and vomiting, insomnia, agitation, postural hypotension (rarely labile hypertension), dizziness, tachycardia, arrhythmias, reddish discoloration of urine and other body fluids, rarely hypersensitivity; abnormal involuntary movements and psychiatric symptoms which include hypomania and psychosis may be dose-limiting; depression, drowsiness, headache, flushing, sweating, gastro-intestinal bleeding, peripheral neuropathy, and liver enzyme changes also reported

Dose: initially 125–500 mg daily in divided doses after meals, increased according to response (but rarely used alone, see notes above)

PoM Brocadopa® (Yamanouchi)

Capsules, levodopa 125 mg, net price 20 = 71p; 250 mg, 20 = 85p; 500 mg, 20 = £1.52. Label: 14, 21

PoM Larodopa® (Cambridge)

Tablets, scored, levodopa 500 mg. Net price 20 = £2.88. Label: 14, 21

CO-BENELDOPA

A mixture of benserazide hydrochloride and levodopa in mass proportions corresponding to 1 part of benserazide and 4 parts of levodopa

Indications; Cautions; Contra-indications; Side-effects: see under Levodopa and notes above

Dose: expressed as levodopa, initially 50–100 mg twice daily, adjusted according to response; usual maintenance dose 400–800 mg daily in divided doses after meals

Note. When transferring patients from levodopa, 3 capsules co-beneldopa 25/100 (Madopar 125®) should be substituted for 2 g levodopa; the levodopa should be discontinued 12 hours beforehand

PoM Madopar® (Roche)

Capsules 62.5, blue/grey, co-beneldopa 12.5/50 (benserazide 12.5 mg (as hydrochloride), levodopa 50 mg). Net price 100-cap pack = £7.76. Label: 14, 21

Capsules 125, blue/pink, co-beneldopa 25/100 (benserazide 25 mg (as hydrochloride), levodopa 100 mg). Net price 100-cap pack = £10.81. Label: 14, 21

Capsules 250, blue/caramel, co-beneldopa 50/200 (benserazide 50 mg (as hydrochloride), levodopa 200 mg). Net price 100-cap pack = £18.43. Label: 14, 21

Dispersible tablets 62.5, scored, co-beneldopa 12.5/50 (benserazide 12.5 mg (as hydrochloride), levodopa 50 mg). Net price 100-tab pack = £8.29. Label: 14, 21, counselling, administration, see below

Dispersible tablets 125, scored, co-beneldopa 25/100 (benserazide 25 mg (as hydrochloride) levodopa 100 mg). Net price 100-tab pack = £14.70. Label: 14, 21, counselling, administration, see below

Note. The tablets may be dispersed in water or orange squash or swallowed whole

PoM Madopar® CR (Roche)

Capsules 125, m/r, dark green/light blue, co-beneldopa 25/100 (benserazide 25 mg (as hydrochloride), levodopa 100 mg). Net price 100-cap pack = £17.97. Label: 5, 14, 25

Dose: fluctuations in response to conventional levodopa/decarboxylase inhibitor preparations, initially 1 capsule substituted for every 100 mg of levodopa and given at same dosage frequency, subsequently increased every 2–3 days according to response; average increase of 50% needed over previous levodopa dose and titration may take up to 4 weeks; supplementary dose of conventional Madopar® may be needed with first morning dose; if response still poor to total daily dose of Madopar® CR plus Madopar® corresponding to 1.2 g levodopa, consider alternative therapy

CO-CARELDOPA

A mixture of carbidopa and levodopa; the proportions are expressed in the form x/y where x and y are the strengths in milligrams of carbidopa and levodopa respectively

Indications; Cautions; Contra-indications; Side-effects: see under Levodopa and notes above

Dose: expressed as levodopa, initially 100–125 mg 3–4 times daily adjusted according to response; usual maintenance dose 0.75–1.5 g daily in divided doses after food. See also under Sinemet-Plus®

Note. When transferring patients from levodopa, 3 tablets co-careldopa 25/250 (Sinemet-275®) should be substituted for 4 g levodopa; the levodopa should be discontinued 12 hours beforehand

PoM Sinemet® (Du Pont)

Tablets (Sinemet-110), blue, scored, co-careldopa 10/100 (carbidopa 10 mg (as monohydrate), levodopa 100 mg). Net price 20 = £1.71. Label: 14, 21

Tablets (Sinemet-275), blue, scored, co-careldopa 25/250 (carbidopa 25 mg (as monohydrate), levodopa 250 mg). Net price 20 = £3.57. Label: 14, 21

PoM Sinemet LS® (Du Pont)

Tablets, yellow, scored, co-careldopa 12.5/50 (carbidopa 12.5 mg (as monohydrate), levodopa 50 mg). Net price 84-tab pack = £6.87. Label: 14, 21

Note. 2 tablets Sinemet LS® ≡ 1 tablet Sinemet Plus®

PoM Sinemet-Plus® (Du Pont)

Tablets, yellow, scored, co-careldopa 25/100 (carbidopa 25 mg (as monohydrate), levodopa 100 mg). Net price 20 = £2.52. Label: 14, 21

Dose: initially 1 tablet 3 times daily, adjusted according to response to 8 daily in divided doses; larger doses by gradual substitution of Sinemet® for Sinemet-Plus®

Note. The daily dose of carbidopa required to achieve full inhibition of extracerebral dopa-decarboxylase is 75 mg; co-careldopa 25/100 provides an adequate dose of carbidopa when low doses of levodopa are needed

Modified release

PoM Half Sinemet® CR (Du Pont)

Tablets, m/r, pink, co-careldopa 25/100 (carbidopa 25 mg (as monohydrate), levodopa 100 mg). Net price 56-tab pack = £18.56. Label: 14, 25

Dose: for fine adjustment of Sinemet® CR dose (see below)

PoM Sinemet® CR (Du Pont)

Tablets, m/r, peach, co-careldopa 50/200 (carbidopa 50 mg (as monohydrate), levodopa 200 mg). Net price 56-tab pack = £21.84. Label: 14, 25

Dose: initial treatment or fluctuations in response to conventional levodopa therapy, 1 Sinemet® CR tablet twice daily; both dose and interval then adjusted according to response at intervals of not less than 3 days; if transferring from existing levodopa therapy withdraw 8 hours beforehand; 1 tablet Sinemet® CR twice daily can be substituted for a daily dose of levodopa 300–400 mg in conventional Sinemet® tablets

AMANTADINE HYDROCHLORIDE

Indications: Parkinson's disease (but not drug-induced extrapyramidal symptoms); antiviral, see section 5.3

Cautions: hepatic, or renal impairment (avoid if severe), congestive heart disease (may exacerbate oedema), confused or hallucinatory states, elderly, pregnancy (toxicity in *animals*), breast-feeding. Avoid abrupt discontinuation in Parkinson's disease; **interactions:** Appendix 1 (amantadine)
DRIVING. May affect performance of skilled tasks (e.g. driving)

Contra-indications: epilepsy, history of gastric ulceration, severe renal impairment

Side-effects: anorexia, nausea, nervousness, inability to concentrate, insomnia, dizziness, convulsions, hallucinations or feelings of detachment, blurred vision, gastro-intestinal disturbances, livedo reticularis and peripheral oedema; rarely leucopenia, rashes

Dose: 100 mg daily increased after one week to 100 mg twice daily (not later than 4 p.m.), usually in conjunction with other treatment

PoM Symmetrel® (Geigy)

Capsules, red-brown, amantadine hydrochloride 100 mg. Net price 100-cap pack = £16.89. Counselling, driving

Syrup, amantadine hydrochloride 50 mg/5 mL. Net price 150-mL pack = £3.17. Counselling, driving

APOMORPHINE HYDROCHLORIDE

Indications: refractory motor fluctuations in Parkinson's disease ('off' episodes) inadequately controlled by levodopa or other dopaminergics (for capable and motivated patients under specialist supervision)

Cautions: tendency to nausea and vomiting; pulmonary, cardiovascular or endocrine disease, renal impairment; elderly and debilitated, history of postural hypotension (special care on initiation); hepatic, haemopoietic, renal, and cardiovascular monitoring; *on administration with levodopa* test initially and every 6 months for haemolytic anaemia (development calls for specialist haematological care with dose reduction and possible discontinuation); **interactions:** Appendix 1 (apomorphine)

Contra-indications: respiratory or CNS depression, hypersensitiviy to opioids; neuropsychiatric problems or dementia; not suitable if 'on' response to levodopa marred by severe dyskinesia, hypotonia or psychiatric effects; pregnancy and breast-feeding

Side-effects: dyskinesias during 'on' periods (may require discontinuation); postural instability and falls (impaired speech and balance may not improve), increasing cognitive impairment, personality change and disabling dyskinesias during 'on' phase; nausea and vomiting (see below under Dose); confusion and hallucinations (if continued, specialist observation required with possible gradual dose reduction), sedation, postural hypotension; also euphoria, light-headedness, restlessness, tremors; haemolytic anaemia with levodopa (see Cautions) and rarely eosinophilia; local reactions common (include nodule formation and possible ulceration)—rotate injection sites, dilute with sodium chloride 0.9%, consider ultrasound, ensure no infection

Dose: ADULT over 18 years, *by subcutaneous injection*, usual range (after initiation as below) 3–30 mg daily in divided doses; subcutaneous infusion may be preferable in those requiring division of injections into more than 10 doses daily; max. single dose 10 mg; ADOLESCENT (under 18 years) and CHILD not recommended
By continuous subcutaneous infusion (those requiring division into more than 10 injections daily) initially 1 mg/hour daily increased according to response (not more often than every 4 hours) in max. steps of 500 micrograms/hour to max. 4 mg/hour (15–60 micrograms/kg/hour); change infusion site every 12 hours and give during waking hours only (24-hour infusions not advised unless severe night-time symptoms)—intermittent bolus boosts also usually needed (in those with severe dyskinesias only when absolutely necessary)
Total daily dose by either route (or combined routes) max. 100 mg

REQUIREMENTS FOR INITIATION. *Hospital admission* and at least 3 days of pretreatment with domperidone, *after at least 3 days* withhold existing antiparkinsonian medication overnight to provoke 'off' episode, *determine* threshold dose, *re-establish* other antiparkinsonian drugs, *determine* effective apomorphine regimen, *teach* to administer by subcutaneous injection into lower abdomen or outer thigh at first sign of 'off' episode, *discharge* from hospital, *monitor* frequently and *adjust* dosage regimen as appropriate (domperidone may normally be withdrawn over several weeks or longer)—for full details of initiation requirements see data sheet

▼ **PoM Britaject®** (Britannia)

Injection, apomorphine hydrochloride 10 mg/mL, net price 2-mL amp = £7.95, 5-mL amp = £15.95

BROMOCRIPTINE

Indications: parkinsonism (but not drug-induced extrapyramidal symptoms); endocrine disorders, see section 6.7.1

Cautions; Side-effects: see section 6.7.1

HYPOTENSIVE REACTIONS. Hypotensive reactions may be disturbing in some patients during the first few days of treatment and particular care should be exercised when driving or operating machinery; tolerance may be reduced by alcohol

Dose: first week 1–1.25 mg at night, second week 2–2.5 mg at night, third week 2.5 mg twice daily, fourth week 2.5 mg 3 times daily then increasing by 2.5 mg every 3–14 days according to response to a usual range of 10–40 mg daily; taken with food

Preparations
See section 6.7.1

LYSURIDE MALEATE
(Lisuride Maleate)

Indications: Parkinson's disease

Cautions: history of pituitary tumour; history of psychotic disturbance; pregnancy; porphyria (see section 9.8.2); **interactions:** Appendix 1 (lysuride)

HYPOTENSIVE REACTIONS. Hypotensive reactions may be disturbing in some patients during the first few days of treatment and particular care should be exercised when driving or operating machinery

Contra-indications: severe disturbances of peripheral circulation; coronary insufficiency

Side-effects: nausea and vomiting; dizziness; headache, lethargy, malaise, drowsiness, psychotic reactions (including hallucinations); occasionally severe hypotension, rashes; rarely abdominal pain and constipation; Raynaud's phenomenon reported

Dose: initially 200 micrograms at bedtime with food increased as necessary at weekly intervals to 200 micrograms twice daily (midday and bedtime) then to 200 micrograms 3 times daily (morning, midday, and bedtime); further increases made by adding 200 micrograms each week first to the bedtime dose, then to the midday dose and finally to the morning dose; max. 5 mg daily in 3 divided doses after food

PoM **Revanil®** (Roche)
Tablets, scored, lysuride maleate 200 micrograms. Net price 100-tab pack = £24.00. Label: 21, counselling, hypotensive reactions

---

PERGOLIDE
Indications: adjunct to levodopa in Parkinson's disease

Cautions: arrhythmias or underlying cardiac disease, history of confusion or hallucinations, dyskinesia (may cause or exacerbate), pregnancy, breast-feeding; increase dose gradually and avoid abrupt withdrawal; porphyria (see section 9.8.2); **interactions:** Appendix 1 (pergolide)

HYPOTENSIVE REACTIONS. Hypotensive reactions may be disturbing in some patients during the first few days of treatment and particular care should be exercised when driving or operating machinery

Side-effects: hallucinations, confusion, dyskinesia, somnolence, abdominal pain, nausea, dyspepsia, diplopia, rhinitis, dyspnoea, insomnia, constipation or diarrhoea, hypotension, tachycardia and arrhythmias reported

Dose: 50 micrograms daily for 2 days, increased gradually by 100–150 micrograms every third day over next 12 days, usually given in 3 divided doses; further increases of 250 micrograms every third day; usual maintenance 3 mg daily (above 5 mg daily not evaluated); during pergolide titration levodopa dose may be reduced cautiously

PoM **Celance®** (Lilly)
Tablets, all scored, pergolide (as mesylate) 50 micrograms (ivory), net price 30-tab pack = £11.00; 250 micrograms (green), 20 = £9.14; 1 mg (pink), 20 = £33.00. Counselling, hypotensive reactions

---

SELEGILINE
Indications: Parkinson's disease or symptomatic parkinsonism (but not drug-induced extrapyramidal symptoms), either used alone (in early disease) or as an adjunct to levodopa therapy

Cautions: side-effects of levodopa may be increased, concurrent levodopa dosage may need to be reduced by 20–50%; **interactions:** Appendix 1 (selegiline)

Side-effects: hypotension, nausea and vomiting, confusion, agitation

Dose: 10 mg in the morning, or 5 mg at breakfast and midday

PoM **Eldepryl®** (Britannia)
Tablets, both scored, selegiline hydrochloride 5 mg, net price 20 = £9.36; 10 mg, 20 = £18.13

4.9.2 Antimuscarinic drugs used in parkinsonism

Antimuscarinic drugs (less correctly termed 'anticholinergics') are the other main class of drugs used in Parkinson's disease. They are less effective than levodopa in idiopathic Parkinson's disease although they often usefully supplement its action. Patients with mild symptoms, particularly where tremor predominates, may be treated initially with antimuscarinic drugs (alone or with selegiline, section 4.9.1), levodopa being added or substituted as symptoms progress. They have value in postencephalitic parkinsonism.

Antimuscarinic drugs exert their antiparkinsonian effect by correcting the relative central cholinergic excess thought to occur in parkinsonism as a result of dopamine deficiency. In most patients their effects are only moderate, reducing tremor and rigidity to some effect but without significant action on bradykinesia. They exert a synergistic effect when used with levodopa and are also useful in reducing sialorrhoea.

The antimuscarinic drugs also reduce the symptoms of drug-induced parkinsonism as seen, for example, with antipsychotic drugs (section 4.2.1) but there is no justification for giving them simultaneously with antipsychotics unless parkinsonian side-effects occur. Tardive dyskinesia is not improved by the antimuscarinic drugs and may be made worse.

No important differences exist between the many synthetic antimuscarinic drugs available but some patients appear to tolerate one better than another. They may be taken before food if dry mouth is troublesome, or after food if gastro-intestinal symptoms predominate. Those most commonly used are **orphenadrine** and **benzhexol; benztropine** and **procyclidine** are also used. Benztropine is similar to benzhexol but is excreted more slowly; changes in dose therefore need to be carried out very gradually. Both procyclidine and benztropine may be given parenterally and are effective emergency treatment for acute drug-induced dystonic reactions which may be severe.

BENZHEXOL HYDROCHLORIDE
(Trihexyphenidyl Hydrochloride)

Indications: parkinsonism; drug-induced extrapyramidal symptoms (but not tardive dyskinesia, see notes above)

Cautions: cardiovascular disease, hepatic or renal impairment; avoid abrupt discontinuation of treatment; liable to abuse; **interactions:** Appendix 1 (antimuscarinics)

DRIVING. May affect performance of skilled tasks (e.g. driving)

Contra-indications: untreated urinary retention, closed-angle glaucoma, gastro-intestinal obstruction

Side-effects: dry mouth, gastro-intestinal disturbances, dizziness, blurred vision; less commonly urinary retention, tachycardia, hypersensitivity, nervousness, and with high doses in susceptible patients, mental confusion, excitement, and psychiatric disturbances which may necessitate discontinuation of treatment

Dose: 1 mg daily, gradually increased; usual maintenance dose 5–15 mg daily in 3–4 divided doses

PoM **Artane®** (Lederle)
Tablets, both scored, benzhexol hydrochloride 2 mg, net price 20 = 31p; 5 mg, 20 = 63p. Counselling, before or after food (see notes above), driving

PoM **Broflex®** (Bioglan)
Syrup, pink, benzhexol hydrochloride 5 mg/5 mL. Net price 200-mL pack = £5.21. Counselling, before or after food (see notes above), driving

BENZTROPINE MESYLATE
(Benzatropine Mesilate)

Indications; Cautions; Contra-indications; Side-effects: see under Benzhexol Hydrochloride, but causes sedation rather than stimulation; avoid in children under 3 years

Dose: by mouth, 0.5–1 mg daily usually at bedtime, gradually increased; max. 6 mg daily; usual maintenance dose 1–4 mg daily in single or divided doses

By intramuscular or intravenous injection, 1–2 mg, repeated if symptoms reappear

PoM **Cogentin®** (MSD)
Tablets, scored, benztropine mesylate 2 mg. Net price 20 = 29p. Label: 2
Injection, benztropine mesylate 1 mg/mL. Net price 2-mL amp = 92p

BIPERIDEN
Indications; Cautions; Contra-indications; Side-effects: see under Benzhexol Hydrochloride, but may cause drowsiness; injection may cause hypotension

Dose: by mouth, biperiden hydrochloride 1 mg twice daily, gradually increased to 2 mg 3 times daily; usual maintenance dose 3–12 mg daily in divided doses

By intramuscular or slow intravenous injection, biperiden lactate 2.5–5 mg up to 4 times daily

PoM **Akineton®** (Knoll)
Tablets, scored, biperiden hydrochloride 2 mg. Net price 100-tab pack = £4.60. Label: 2
Injection, biperiden lactate 5 mg/mL. Net price 1-mL amp = 69p

ORPHENADRINE HYDROCHLORIDE
Indications; Cautions; Contra-indications; Side-effects: see under Benzhexol Hydrochloride, but more euphoric; may cause insomnia; porphyria (see section 9.8.2)

Dose: 150 mg daily in divided doses, gradually increased; max. 400 mg daily

PoM **Biorphen®** (Bioglan)
Elixir, sugar-free, orphenadrine hydrochloride 25 mg/5 mL. Net price 200-mL pack = £5.95. Counselling, driving
PoM **Disipal®** (Yamanouchi)
Tablets, yellow, s/c, orphenadrine hydrochloride 50 mg. Net price 20 = 30p. Counselling, driving
Additives: include tartrazine

PROCYCLIDINE HYDROCHLORIDE
Indications; Cautions; Contra-indications; Side-effects: see under Benzhexol Hydrochloride

Dose: by mouth, 2.5 mg 3 times daily, gradually increased if necessary; usual max. 30 mg daily (60 mg daily in exceptional circumstances)

Acute dystonia, by intramuscular injection, 5–10 mg repeated if necessary after 20 minutes; max. 20 mg daily; by intravenous injection, 5 mg (usually effective within 5 minutes); an occasional patient may need 10 mg or more and may require up to half an hour to obtain relief

PoM **Procyclidine** (Non-proprietary)
Tablets, procyclidine hydrochloride 5 mg. Net price 20 = £1.11. Counselling, driving
PoM **Arpicolin®** (RP Drugs)
Syrup, procyclidine hydrochloride 2.5 mg/5 mL, net price 200-mL pack = £4.30; 5 mg/5 mL, 200-mL pack = £7.60. Counselling, driving

---

PoM Kemadrin® (Wellcome)
Tablets, scored, procyclidine hydrochloride 5 mg. Net price 20 = £1.17. Counselling, driving
Injection, procyclidine hydrochloride 5 mg/mL. Net price 2-mL amp = £1.49

4.9.3 Drugs used in essential tremor, chorea, tics, and related disorders

Tetrabenazine is mainly used to control movement disorders in Huntington's chorea and related disorders. It may act by depleting nerve endings of dopamine. It has useful action in only a proportion of patients and its use may be limited by the development of depression.

Haloperidol may be useful in improving motor tics and symptoms of Gilles de la Tourette syndrome and related choreas. **Pimozide** (see section 4.2.1 for CSM warning) and more recently **clonidine** (section 4.7.4.2) and **sulpiride** (section 4.2.1), are also used in Gilles de la Tourette syndrome.**Benzhexol** (section 4.9.2) at high dosage may also improve some movement disorders. It is sometimes necessary to build the dose up over many weeks, to 20 to 30 mg daily or higher. **Chlorpromazine** and **haloperidol** are used to relieve intractable hiccup (section 4.2.1).

Propranolol or another beta-adrenoceptor blocking drug (see section 2.4) may be useful in treating essential tremor or tremors associated with anxiety or thyrotoxicosis. Propranolol is given in a dosage of 40 mg 2 or 3 times daily, increased if necessary; 80 to 160 mg daily is usually required for maintenance.

Primidone in some cases provides relief from benign essential tremor; the dose is increased slowly to reduce side-effects.

Piracetam has been introduced recently as adjunctive treatment for myoclonus of cortical origin.

HALOPERIDOL
Indications: motor tics, adjunctive treatment in choreas and Gilles de la Tourette syndrome; other indications, section 4.2.1
Cautions; Contra-indications; Side-effects: see section 4.2.1
Dose: by mouth, 0.5–1.5 mg 3 times daily adjusted according to the response; 10 mg daily or more may occasionally be necessary in Gilles de la Tourette syndrome; CHILD, Gilles de la Tourette syndrome up to 10 mg daily

Preparations
Section 4.2.1

PIRACETAM
Indications: adjunctive treatment of cortical myoclonus
Cautions: avoid abrupt withdrawal; renal impairment (avoid if severe)
Contra-indications: hepatic and severe renal impairment; pregnancy and breast-feeding
Side-effects: diarrhoea, weight gain; somnolence, insomnia, nervousness, depression; hyperkinesia; rash

Dose: initially 7.2 g daily in 2–3 divided doses, increased according to response by 4.8 g daily every 3–4 days to max. 20 g daily (subsequently, attempts should be made to reduce dose of concurrent therapy); CHILD under 16 years not recommended
ORAL SOLUTION. Follow the oral solution with a glass of water (or soft drink) to reduce bitter taste.

▼ **PoM Nootropil®** (UCB Pharma)
Tablets, f/c, scored, piracetam 800 mg, net price 90-tab pack = £15.80; 1.2 g, 56-tab pack = £14.74. Label: 3
Oral solution, piracetam, 333.3 mg/mL, net price 300-mL pack = £21.93. Label: 3

PRIMIDONE
Indications: essential tremor; epilepsy, see section 4.8.1
Cautions; Contra-indications; Side-effects: see section 4.8.1
Dose: essential tremor, initially 50 mg daily increased gradually over 2–3 weeks according to response; max. 750 mg daily

Preparations
Section 4.8.1

TETRABENAZINE
Indications: movement disorders due to Huntington's chorea, senile chorea, and related neurological conditions
Cautions: pregnancy; avoid in breast-feeding; **interactions:** Appendix 1 (tetrabenazine)
DRIVING. May affect performance of skilled tasks (e.g. driving)
Side-effects: drowsiness, gastro-intestinal disturbances, depression, extrapyramidal dysfunction, hypotension
Dose: initially 12.5 mg twice daily (elderly 12.5 mg daily) gradually increased to 12.5–25 mg 3 times daily; max. 200 mg daily

PoM Nitoman® (Roche)
Tablets, pale yellow-buff, scored, tetrabenazine 25 mg. Net price 120 tab pack = £5.59. Label: 2

TORSION DYSTONIAS AND OTHER INVOLUNTARY MOVEMENTS

BOTULINUM A TOXIN-HAEMAGGLUTININ COMPLEX
Indications: blepharospasm and hemifacial spasm
CSM warning. Botulinum A toxin-haemagglutinin complex is licensed **only** for blepharospasm and hemifacial spasm; injection into the neck is an **unlicensed** route, persistent dysphagia and sequelae (including death) may result
Cautions: avoid deep or misplaced injections - relevant anatomy (and any alterations due to previous surgery) must be understood before injecting; as a biological product bear in mind potential for anaphylaxis; reduced blinking can lead to corneal exposure, persistent epithelial defect and corneal

ulceration (especially in those with VIIth nerve disorders)—careful testing of corneal sensation in previously operated eyes, avoidance of injection in lower lid area and vigorous treatment of epithelial defect needed; do not give with (or before) aminoglycoside antibiotics or spectinomycin; other **interactions:** Appendix 1 (botulinum A toxin)

COUNSELLING. All patients should be alerted to possible side-effects

Contra-indications: generalised disorders of muscle activity (e.g. myasthenia gravis); pregnancy and breast-feeding

Side-effects: ptosis, lacrimation and irritation (including dry eye, lagophthalmos and photophobia); also ectropion, keratitis, diplopia and entropion; angle-closure glaucoma reported; increased electrophysiologic jitter in some distant muscles; misplaced injections may paralyse nearby muscle groups and excessive doses may paralyse distant muscles; bruising, ecchymosis and swelling of soft eyelid tissues minimised by applying gentle pressure at injection site immediately after injection

Dose: see under preparations below

IMPORTANT. The doses are specific to each individual preparation and are not interchangeable

▼ PoM **Botox®** (Allergan)

Injection, powder for reconstitution, botulinum A toxin-haemagglutinin complex, net price 100-unit vial = £135.00

Dose: Blepharospasm, into medial and lateral orbicularis oculi of upper lid and lateral orbicularis oculi of lower lid (additional sites in brow area, lateral orbicularis and upper facial area may also be injected if spasms interfere with vision), initially 1.25–2.5 units at each site (total of up to 25 units per eye) increased to max. 5 units per site, if response inadequate (e.g. not longer than 2 months); total dose should not exceed 100 units every 12 weeks; CHILD not recommended

Hemifacial spasm or VIIth nerve disorders, as for unilateral blepharospasm (other affected facial muscles being injected with initial doses of 1.25–2.5 units; electromyographic control may be needed to identify affected small circumoral muscles; CHILD not recommended

DURATION OF ACTION. Initial effect usually within 3 days with peak after 1–2 weeks. Injections need to be repeated approximately every 12 weeks.

PoM **Dysport®** (Porton)

Injection, powder for reconstitution, botulinum A toxin-haemagglutinin complex, net price 500-unit vial = £170.00

Dose: Blepharospasm, initially 20 units medially and 40 units laterally into junction between preseptal and orbital parts of both upper and lower orbicularis oculi of each eye (total of 120 units per eye)—see package insert for diagram to aid placement of injections; subsequently, dose may need to be reduced to 20 units medially and 20 units laterally as above (total of 80 units per eye); dose may be further reduced to total of 60 units per eye by omitting medial lower lid injection; CHILD not recommended

Hemifacial spasm, as for unilateral blepharospasm, above; CHILD not recommended

DURATION OF ACTION. Initial effect usually within 2–4 days with peak after 2 weeks. Injections need to be repeated approximately every 8 weeks.

4.10   Drugs used in substance dependence

This section includes drugs used in alcohol dependence, cigarette smoking, and opioid dependence.

The health departments of the UK have produced a report, *Drug Misuse and Dependence* which contains guidelines on clinical management.

Drug Misuse and Dependence, London, HMSO, 1991 can be obtained from:

    HMSO Publications Centre
    PO Box 276, London SW8 5DT
    Telephone orders, 071-873 9090

or from HMSO bookshops and through all good booksellers.

It is **important** to be aware that *people who misuse drugs* may be at risk not only from the intrinsic toxicity of the drug itself but also from the practice of injecting preparations intended for administration by mouth. Excipients used in the production of oral dose forms are usually insoluble and may lead to *abscess formation at the site of injection,* or even to *necrosis and gangrene*; moreover, deposits in the heart or lungs may lead to *severe cardiac or pulmonary toxicity.* Additional hazards include *infection* following the use of a dirty needle or an unsterilised diluent.

ALCOHOL DEPENDENCE

Disulfiram (Antabuse®) is used as an adjunct to the treatment of alcohol dependence. It gives rise to extremely unpleasant systemic reactions after the ingestion of even small amounts of alcohol because it leads to accumulation of acetaldehyde in the body. Reactions include flushing of the face, throbbing headache, palpitations, tachycardia, nausea, vomiting, and, with large doses of alcohol, arrhythmias, hypotension, and collapse. Even the small amounts of alcohol included in many oral medicines may be sufficient to precipitate a reaction (even toiletries containing alcohol should be avoided). It may be advisable for patients to carry a card warning of the danger of administration of alcohol.

Chlormethiazole is used to attenuate withdrawal symptoms but itself has a dependence potential. In order to minimise the risk of dependence, administration of chlormethiazole should be limited to 9 days under inpatient supervision.

Benzodiazepines are also used in the management of withdrawal, but again have dependence potential (see section 4.1).

BENZODIAZEPINES
Section 4.1.2

CHLORMETHIAZOLE
(Clomethiazole)

Indications: see under Dose; insomnia, restlessness and agitation in the elderly (section 4.1.1); status epilepticus (section 4.8.2); sedation during regional anaesthesia (section 15.1.4.1); eclampsia, see data sheet

Cautions: cardiac and respiratory disease (confusional state may indicate hypoxia); history of drug abuse; marked personality disorder; pregnancy and breast-feeding; elderly (excessive sedation with higher doses); hepatic impairment (especially if severe since sedation can mask hepatic coma); renal impairment; avoid prolonged use (and abrupt withdrawal thereafter); **interactions:** Appendix 1 (chlormethiazole)

SPECIAL CAUTIONS FOR INTRAVENOUS INFUSION. Resuscitation facilities must be available; maintain clear airway (risk of mechanical obstruction in deep sedation); *rapid infusion* to be given only under direct medical supervision (risk of apnoea and hypotension—special care in those susceptible to cerebral or cardiac complications, e.g. the elderly); during *continuous infusion* sleep induced may lapse into deep unconsciousness and patient must be kept under close and constant observation; *prolonged infusion* may lead to accumulation and delay recovery, may also cause electrolyte imbalance (infusion contains only Na^+ 32 mmol/litre and no other electrolytes)

DRIVING. Drowsiness may persist the next day and affect performance of skilled tasks (e.g. driving); effects of alcohol enhanced

Contra-indications: acute pulmonary insufficiency; alcohol-dependent patients who continue to drink

Side-effects: nasal congestion and irritation (with sneezing), conjunctival irritation, headache; rarely, paradoxical excitement, confusion, dependence; gastro-intestinal disturbances, rash, urticaria, bullous eruption, anaphylaxis, alterations in liver enzymes also reported; on *intravenous infusion*, localised thrombophlebitis, tachycardia and transient fall in blood pressure (apnoea and hypotension on rapid infusion, see Cautions)

Dose: by mouth, alcohol withdrawal, initially 2–4 capsules, if necessary repeated after some hours; day 1 (first 24 hours), 9–12 capsules in 3–4 divided doses; day 2, 6–8 capsules in 3–4 divided doses; day 3, 4–6 capsules in 3–4 divided doses; then gradually reduced over days 4–6, total treatment for not more than 9 days

Note. For an equivalent therapeutic effect 1 capsule $\equiv$ 5 mL syrup

By intravenous infusion, acute alcohol withdrawal, when oral administration not practicable, as a 0.8% solution of chlormethiazole edisylate, initially 3–7.5 mL (24–60 mg)/minute until shallow sleep induced (from which patient can be easily awakened) then reduced to 0.5–1 mL (4–8 mg)/minute to achieve lowest possible rate to maintain shallow sleep and adequate spontaneous respiration; urgent deep sedation (direct medical supervision only) 40–100 mL (320–800 mg) over 3–5 minutes then reduced to maintenance as indicated above

IMPORTANT. See special cautions for intravenous infusion under Cautions (above)

PoM Heminevrin® (Astra)

Capsules, grey-brown, chlormethiazole base 192 mg in an oily basis. Net price 60-cap pack = £4.45. Label: 19

Syrup, sugar-free, chlormethiazole edisylate 250 mg/5 mL. Net price 300-mL pack = £3.72. Label: 19

Intravenous infusion 0.8%, chlormethiazole edisylate 8 mg/mL. Net price 500-mL bottle = £5.25

DISULFIRAM

Indications: adjunct in the treatment of chronic alcohol dependence (under specialist supervision)

Cautions: ensure that alcohol not consumed for at least 24 hours before initiating treatment; see also notes above; alcohol challenge **not** recommended on routine basis (if considered essential—specialist units only with resuscitation facilities); hepatic or renal impairment, respiratory disease, diabetes mellitus, epilepsy; **interactions:** Appendix 1 (disulfiram)

ALCOHOL REACTION. Patients should be warned of unpredictable and occasionally severe nature of disulfiram-alcohol interactions. Reactions can occur in 10 minutes and last several hours (may require intensive supportive therapy). Patients should not ingest alcohol at all and should be warned of possible presence of alcohol in liquid medicines and even in toiletries (alcohol should also be avoided for at least 1 week after stopping)

Contra-indications: cardiac failure, coronary artery disease, hypertension, severe personality disorder, suicide risk, pregnancy

Side-effects: initially drowsiness and fatigue; nausea, vomiting, halitosis, reduced libido; rarely psychotic reactions (depression, paranoia, schizophrenia, mania), allergic dermatitis, peripheral neuritis, hepatic cell damage

Dose: 800 mg as a single dose on first day, reducing over 5 days to 100–200 mg daily; should not be continued for longer than 6 months without review

PoM Antabuse 200® (CP)

Tablets, scored, disulfiram 200 mg. Net price 50-tab pack = £23.45. Label: 2, counselling, alcohol reaction

CIGARETTE SMOKING

Nicotine chewing gum or patches may be used as an adjunct to counselling; they are not available on the NHS.

NICOTINE PRODUCTS

Indications: adjunct to smoking cessation

Cautions: cardiovascular disease (avoid if severe); hyperthyroidism; diabetes mellitus; phaeochromocytoma, renal and hepatic impairment; exacerbation of gastritis and peptic ulcers, skin disorders (patches); should not smoke or use other nicotine replacement products when wearing patches; **interactions:** Appendix 1 (nicotine and tobacco)

Contra-indications: pregnancy, breast-feeding

Side-effects: headache and cold and influenza-like symptoms, dizziness and nausea, insomnia and increased dreaming; myalgia, aphthous ulceration (sometimes with swelling of tongue), palpitations, dyspepsia, skin reactions also reported with patches (discontinue if severe)

Dose: see under preparations, below

Chewing gum

NHS Nicorette® (Pharmacia)

Chewing gum, sugar-free, nicotine (as resin) 2 mg, net price pack of 30 = £2.98; pack of 105 = £8.05

NHS Nicorette Plus® (Pharmacia)

Chewing gum, sugar-free, nicotine (as resin) 4 mg, net price pack of 105 = £10.80

Note. Nicorette Mint® (nicotine 2 mg) and Nicorette Mint Plus® (nicotine 4 mg) also on sale to the public

Dose: initially one 2-mg piece (**Nicorette®**) chewed slowly for approx. 30 minutes, when urge to smoke occurs; patients needing more than 15 pieces of 2 mg daily may need the 4-mg strength (**Nicorette Plus®**); max. 15 pieces of 4-mg strength daily; withdraw gradually after 3 months

Patches

NHS Nicabate® (Merrell)

Patches, self-adhesive, all pinkish-brown, nicotine, *'7 mg' patch* (releasing approx. 7 mg/24 hours), net price 7 = £8.20, 14 = £15.59; *'14 mg' patch* (releasing approx. 14 mg/24 hours), 7 = £8.63, 14 = £16.42; *'21 mg' patch* (releasing approx. 21 mg/24 hours), 7 = £9.05, 14 = £17.23

ADMINISTRATION: apply to dry, non-hairy skin on trunk or upper arm, removing after 24 hours and siting replacement patch on different area (avoid using same area for several days); individuals smoking more than 10 cigarettes daily, initially '21-mg' patch for 4–6 weeks, then '14-mg' patch for 2–4 weeks, then '7-mg' patch for 2–4 weeks; individuals smoking 10 cigarettes daily or fewer or who have cardiovascular disease or who weigh less than 45 kg, initially '14-mg' patch daily for 4–6 weeks, then '7-mg' patch for a further 2–4 weeks; review treatment if abstinence not achieved in 3 months

NHS Niconil® (Elan)

Patches, self-adhesive, nicotine, *'11 mg' patch* (releasing approx. 11 mg/24 hours), net price 7 = £7.40; *'22 mg' patch* (releasing approx. 22 mg/24 hours), starter pack = £7.40, 7 = £7.40

ADMINISTRATION: apply to dry, non-hairy skin on trunk or upper arm, removing after 24 hours and siting replacement patch on different area (avoid using the same area for several days); initially '22 mg' patch daily usually for 4 weeks; then '11 mg' patch for 2 weeks; review treatment if abstinence not achieved in 3 months

NHS Nicorette® (Pharmacia)

Patches, self-adhesive, all beige, nicotine, *'5 mg' patch* (releasing approx. 5 mg/16 hours), net price 7 = £7.20; *'10 mg' patch* (releasing approx. 10 mg/16 hours), 7 = £8.36; *'15 mg' patch* (releasing approx. 15 mg/16 hours), 3 = £4.55, 7 = £9.07, 28 = £31.77

ADMINISTRATION: apply on waking to dry, non-hairy skin on hip, chest or upper arm, removing after approx. 16 hours, usually when retiring; site next patch on different area (avoid using same area for several days); initially '15-mg' patch for 16 hours daily for 8 weeks then '10-mg' patch for 16 hours daily for 2 weeks then '5-mg' patch for 16 hours daily for 2 weeks; review treatment if abstinence not achieved in 3 months

NHS Nicotinell TTS® (Zyma)

Patches, self-adhesive, all yellowish-ochre, nicotine, *'10' patch* (releasing approx. 7 mg/24 hours), net price 7 = £8.21; *'20' patch* (releasing approx. 14 mg/24 hours), 7 = £8.64; *'30' patch* (releasing approx. 21 mg/24 hours), 7 = £9.07

ADMINISTRATION: apply to dry, non-hairy skin on trunk or upper arm, removing after 24 hours and siting replacement patch on a different area (avoid using the same area for several days); individuals smoking 20 cigarettes daily or fewer, initially '20' patch daily; individuals smoking more than 20 cigarettes daily, initially '30' patch daily; withdraw gradually, reducing dose every 3–4 weeks; review treatment if abstinence not achieved in 3 months

---

OPIOID DEPENDENCE

Methadone is an opioid *agonist*. It can be substituted for opioids such as diamorphine, preventing the onset of withdrawal symptoms; it is itself addictive and should only be prescribed for those who are physically dependent on opioids. It is administered in a single daily dose usually as methadone mixture 1 mg/mL. The dose is adjusted according to the degree of dependence with the aim of gradual reduction.

Naltrexone is an opioid *antagonist*. It blocks the action of opioids such as diamorphine and precipitates withdrawal symptoms in opioid-dependent subjects. Since the euphoric action of opioid agonists is blocked by naltrexone it is given to former addicts as an aid to relapse prevention.

Lofexidine has been recently introduced for the alleviation of symptoms in patients undergoing opioid withdrawal. Like clonidine it appears to act centrally to produce a reduction in sympathetic tone but reduction in blood pressure is less marked.

LOFEXIDINE HYDROCHLORIDE

Indications: management of symptoms of opioid withdrawal

Cautions: severe coronary insufficiency, recent myocardial infarction, cerebrovascular disease, marked bradycardia (monitor pulse rate frequently); renal impairment; history of depression (on longer treatment); pregnancy and breast-feeding; withdraw gradually over 2–4 days (or longer) to minimise risk of rebound hypertension and associated symptoms; **interactions:** Appendix 1 (lofexidine)

Side-effects: drowsiness, dry mucous membranes (particularly dry mouth, throat and nose), hypotension, bradycardia, rebound hypertension on withdrawal (see Cautions)

Dose: initially, 200 micrograms twice daily, increased as necessary in steps of 200–400 micrograms daily to max. 2.4 mg daily; recommended duration of treatment 7–10 days if no opioid use (but longer may be required); withdraw gradually over 2–4 days or longer; CHILD not recommended

---

▼ PoM **BritLofex**® (Britannia)
Tablets, peach, f/c, lofexidine hydrochloride
200 micrograms. Net price 60-tab pack = £77.95.
Label: 2

METHADONE HYDROCHLORIDE
Indications: adjunct in treatment of opioid dependence, see notes above; analgesia, section 4.7.2
Cautions; Contra-indications; Side-effects: section 4.7.2; overdosage: see Emergency Treatment
of Poisoning, p.21
IMPORTANT: Methadone, even in low doses is a **special
hazard** for children; non-dependent adults are also at
risk; dependent adults are at risk if tolerance is incor-
rectly assessed during induction
Dose: initially 10–20 mg daily, increased by 10–
20 mg daily until no signs of withdrawal or intoxication; usual dose 40–60 mg daily; CHILD not
recommended (see also important note above)

CD **Methadone** (Non-proprietary)
Mixture 1 mg/mL, methadone hydrochloride 1 mg/
mL, net price 30-mL = 44p, 50-mL = £1.33, 100-
mL = £1.48, 500-mL = £7.39. Label: 2
Available from Martindale
IMPORTANT. This preparation is 2½ times the strength of
Methadone Linctus and is intended only for drug dependent persons for whom treatment is normally ordered on
form FP10(HP)(ad) or FP10(MDA), or in Scotland on
forms HBP(A) or GP10. The title includes the strength and
prescriptions should be written accordingly
INCOMPATIBILITY. Syrup preserved with hydroxybenzoate
esters may be incompatible with methadone hydrochloride.
Injection and *Tablets*, section 4.7.2
Linctus, see section 3.9.1

NALTREXONE HYDROCHLORIDE
Indications: adjunct to prevent relapse in detoxified formerly opioid-dependent patients
Cautions: hepatic and renal impairment; liver
function tests needed before and during treatment; test for opioid dependence with naloxone;
avoid concomitant use of opioids but increased
dose of opioid analgesic may be required for pain
(monitor for opioid intoxication); pregnancy,
breast-feeding
WARNING FOR PATIENTS. Patients need to be warned that
an attempt to overcome the block could result in acute
opioid intoxication
Contra-indications: patients currently dependent
on opioids; acute hepatitis or liver failure
Side-effects: nausea, vomiting, abdominal pain;
anxiety, nervousness, sleeping difficulty, headache, reduced energy; joint and muscle pain; less
frequently, loss of appetite, diarrhoea, constipation, increased thirst; chest pain; increased sweating and lachrymation; increased energy, 'feeling
down', irritability, dizziness, chills; delayed ejaculation, decreased potency; rash; occasionally,
liver function abnormalities; reversible idiopathic
thrombocytopenia reported
Dose: (initiate in specialist clinics only) 25 mg initially then 50 mg daily; the total weekly dose may
be divided and given on 3 days of the week for
improved compliance (e.g. 100 mg on Monday
and Wednesday, and 150 mg on Friday); CHILD
not recommended

PoM **Nalorex**® (Du Pont)
Tablets, orange, scored, naltrexone hydrochloride
50 mg. Net price 50-tab pack = £79.49

5: Drugs used in the treatment of

INFECTIONS

In this chapter, drug treatment is discussed under the following headings:

5.1 Antibacterial drugs
5.2 Antifungal drugs
5.3 Antiviral drugs
5.4 Antiprotozoal drugs
5.5 Anthelmintics

5.1 Antibacterial drugs

5.1.1 Penicillins
5.1.2 Cephalosporins, cephamycins and other beta-lactam antibiotics
5.1.3 Tetracyclines
5.1.4 Aminoglycosides
5.1.5 Macrolides
5.1.6 Clindamycin
5.1.7 Some other antibiotics
5.1.8 Sulphonamides and trimethoprim
5.1.9 Antituberculous drugs
5.1.10 Antileprotic drugs
5.1.11 Metronidazole and tinidazole
5.1.12 4-Quinolones
5.1.13 Urinary-tract infections

CHOICE OF A SUITABLE DRUG. Before selecting an antibiotic the clinician must first consider two factors—the patient and the known or likely causative organism. Factors related to the patient which must be considered include history of allergy, renal and hepatic function, resistance to infection (i.e. whether immunocompromised), ability to tolerate drugs by mouth, severity of illness, ethnic origin, age and, if female, whether pregnant, breast-feeding or taking an oral contraceptive.

The known or likely organism and its antibiotic sensitivity, in association with the above factors, will suggest one or more antibiotics, the final choice depending on the microbiological, pharmacological, and toxicological properties.

An example of a rational approach to the selection of an antibiotic is treatment of a urinary-tract infection in a patient complaining of nausea in early pregnancy. The organism is reported as being resistant to ampicillin but sensitive to nitrofurantoin (can cause nausea), gentamicin (can only be given by injection and best avoided in pregnancy), tetracycline (causes dental discoloration) and co-trimoxazole (folate antagonist therefore theoretical teratogenic risk), and cephalexin. The safest antibiotics in pregnancy are the penicillins and cephalosporins; therefore, cephalexin would be indicated for this patient.

The principles involved in selection of an antibiotic must allow for a number of variables including changing renal and hepatic function, increasing bacterial resistance, and new information on side-effects. Duration of therapy, dosage, and route of administration depend on site, type and severity of infection.

ANTIBIOTIC POLICIES. Many health authorities now place limits on the antibiotics that may be used in their hospitals, to achieve reasonable economy consistent with adequate cover, and to reduce the development of resistant organisms. An authority may indicate a range of drugs for general use, and permit treatment with other drugs only on the advice of the microbiologist or physician responsible for the control of infectious diseases.

BEFORE STARTING THERAPY. The following precepts should be considered before starting:

Viral infections should not be treated with antibiotics.

Samples should be taken for culture and sensitivity testing; 'blind' prescribing of an antibiotic for a patient ill with unexplained pyrexia usually leads to further difficulty in establishing the diagnosis.

An up-to-date knowledge of prevalent organisms and their current sensitivity is of great help in choosing an antibiotic before bacteriological confirmation is available.

The dose of an antibiotic will vary according to a number of factors including age, weight, renal function, and severity of infection. The prescribing of the so-called 'standard' dose in serious infections may result in failure of treatment or even death of the patient therefore it is important to prescribe a dose appropriate to the condition. On the other hand, for an antibiotic with a narrow margin between the toxic and therapeutic dose (e.g. an aminoglycoside) it is also important to avoid an excessive dose and plasma concentration monitoring may be required.

The route of administration of an antibiotic will often depend on the severity of the infection. Life-threatening infections require intravenous therapy. Whenever possible painful intramuscular injections should be avoided in children.

Duration of therapy depends on the nature of the infection and the response to treatment. Courses should not be unduly prolonged as they are wasteful and may lead to side-effects. However, in certain infections such as tuberculosis or chronic osteomyelitis it is necessary to continue treatment for relatively long periods. Conversely a single dose of an antibiotic may cure uncomplicated urinary-tract infections.

SUPERINFECTION. In general, broad-spectrum antibacterial drugs such as the cephalosporins are more likely to be associated with adverse reactions related to the selection of resistant organisms e.g. *fungal infections* or *pseudomembranous colitis* (antibiotic-associated colitis).

THERAPY. Suggested treatment is shown in table 1. When the pathogen has been isolated treatment may be changed to a more appropriate antibiotic if necessary. If no bacterium is cultured the antibiotic can be continued or stopped on clinical grounds. Infections for which prophylaxis is useful are listed in table 2.

Table 1. Summary of antibacterial therapy

Infection	Suggested antibacterial	Comment
1: Gastro-intestinal system		
Gastro-enteritis	Antibiotic not usually indicated	Frequently nonbacterial aetiology
Campylobacter enteritis	Erythromycin *or* ciprofloxacin	
Invasive salmonellosis	Ciprofloxacin *or* trimethoprim	Includes severe infections which may be invasive
Shigellosis	Ciprofloxacin *or* trimethoprim	Antibiotic not indicated for mild cases. Ciprofloxacin should be used for trimethoprim-resistant strains
Typhoid fever	Chloramphenicol *or* ciprofloxacin	Infections from Indian subcontinent, Middle-East, and South-East Asia may be chloramphenicol-resistant and ciprofloxacin may be more appropriate
Biliary-tract infection	Gentamicin *or* a cephalosporin	
Peritonitis	Gentamicin (*or* a cephalosporin) + metronidazole (*or* clindamycin)	
Peritoneal dialysis-associated peritonitis	Vancomycin[3] + gentamicin added to dialysis fluid	Discontinue either gentamicin or vancomycin when sensitivity known; treat for 5–10 days
2: Cardiovascular system		
Endocarditis caused by:		
Penicillin-sensitive streptococci (e.g. viridans streptococci)	Benzylpenicillin (*or* vancomycin if penicillin-allergic) + low-dose gentamicin (i.e. 60–80mg twice daily)	Treat for up to 4 weeks; stop gentamicin after 2 weeks if organism fully sensitive to penicillin. Oral amoxycillin[1] may be substituted for benzylpenicillin after 2 weeks
Streptococci with reduced sensitivity to penicillin e.g. *Streptococcus faecalis*	Benzylpenicillin (*or* vancomycin[3] if penicillin-allergic) + low-dose gentamicin (i.e. 60–80 mg twice daily)	Treat for 4 weeks
Staphylococcus aureus (and *Staphylococcus epidermidis*)	Flucloxacillin[2] + *either* gentamicin *or* fusidic acid (*or* vancomycin[3] alone if penicillin-allergic)	Treat for at least 4 weeks; stop gentamicin after 2 weeks
3: Respiratory system		
Haemophilus epiglottitis	Chloramphenicol *or* cefotaxime	Give intravenously
Exacerbations of chronic bronchitis	Amoxycillin[1] *or* trimethoprim *or* tetracycline	Note that 20% of pneumococci and 15% of *Haemophilus influenzae* strains tetracycline-resistant; 15% *H. influenzae* strains amoxycillin-resistant
Chlamydial infections	Tetracycline *or* erythromycin[4]	Treat for at least 10–14 days
Pneumonia:		
Previously healthy chest	Benzylpenicillin *or* amoxycillin[1]	Add flucloxacillin[2] if *Staphylococcus* suspected e.g. in influenza or measles; add erythromycin[4] if *Mycoplasma pneumoniae* or Legionella infection suspected (severe Legionella infections may require addition of rifampicin); pneumococci with decreased penicillin sensitivity being isolated but not yet common in UK
Previously unhealthy chest	Flucloxacillin[2] + amoxycillin[1] *or* erythromycin[4] alone; *if hospital acquired*, a broad-spectrum cephalosporin or an aminoglycoside	Substitute erythromycin[4] (*or* rifampicin and erythromycin[4], see above) for flucloxacillin if Legionella infection suspected; use erythromycin[4] if *Mycoplasma pneumoniae* infection suspected
4: Central nervous system		
Meningitis caused by:		
Meningococci	Benzylpenicillin *or* cefotaxime	Give rifampicin for 2 days before hospital discharge
Pneumococci	Cefotaxime	Substitute benzylpenicillin if organism penicillin-sensitive
Haemophilus influenzae	Chloramphenicol *or* cefotaxime	For *H. influenzae* type b give rifampicin for 4 days before hospital discharge
Listeria	Amoxycillin[1] + gentamicin	

1. Where amoxycillin is suggested ampicillin or an ester of ampicillin (see section 5.1.1.3) may be used.
2. Where flucloxacillin is suggested cloxacillin may be used.
3. Where vancomycin is suggested teicoplanin may be used.
4. Where erythromycin is suggested another macrolide (e.g. azithromycin or clarithromycin) may be used.

Table 1. Summary of antibacterial therapy (*continued*)

Infection	Suggested antibacterial	Comment
7: Urinary tract		
Acute pyelonephritis or prostatitis	Trimethoprim *or* gentamicin *or* cephalosporin *or* a 4-quinolone	Treat prostatitis with trimethoprim or a 4-quinolone for 4 weeks
'Lower' UTI	Trimethoprim *or* amoxycillin[1] *or* nitrofurantoin *or* oral cephalosporin	
7: Genital system		
Syphilis	Procaine penicillin (*or* tetracycline *or* erythromycin if penicillin-allergic)	Treat for 10–21 days
Gonorrhoea	Amoxycillin[1] with probenecid (*or* spectinomycin *or* a 4-quinolone if penicillin-allergic)	Single-dose treatment in uncomplicated infection; choice depends on locality where infection acquired; contact-tracing advised; remember chlamydia
Non-gonococcal urethritis	Tetracycline *or* erythromycin	Treat for 7–21 days; contact-tracing advised
Pelvic inflammatory disease	Metronidazole + doxycycline (or erythromycin) *or* co-amoxiclav alone	Remember gonorrhoea; co-amoxiclav is not active against chlamydia; severely ill patients may require gentamicin (or a 'second-generation' cephalosporin) + a tetracycline
9: Blood		
Septicaemia Initial 'blind' therapy	Aminoglycoside + a penicillin *or* a cephalosporin alone *In immunocompromised*, aminoglycoside + a broad-spectrum penicillin *or* a 'third-generation' cephalosporin alone	Choice depends on local resistance patterns and clinical presentation; add metronidazole if anaerobic infection suspected; add flucloxacillin[2] *or* vancomycin[3] if Gram-positive infection suspected
10: Musculoskeletal system		
Osteomyelitis and septic arthritis	Clindamycin alone *or* flucloxacillin[2] + fusidic acid. If *Haemophilus influenzae* give amoxycillin[1] *or* cefuroxime	Under 5 years of age may be *H. influenzae*. Treat acute disease for at least 6 weeks and chronic infection for at least 12 weeks
11: Eye		
Purulent conjunctivitis	Chloramphenicol *or* gentamicin eye-drops	
12: Ear, nose, and oropharynx		
Dental infections	Phenoxymethylpenicillin (*or* amoxycillin[1]) *or* erythromycin *or* metronidazole	Tetracycline for chronic destructive forms of periodontal disease
Sinusitis	Amoxycillin[1] *or* doxycycline	
Otitis externa	Flucloxacillin[2]	
Otitis media	Amoxycillin[1] (*or* erythromycin[4] if penicillin-allergic)	Initial parenteral therapy (in severe infections) with benzylpenicillin, then oral therapy with phenoxymethylpenicillin. Under 5 years of age may be *Haemophilus influenzae*
Throat infections Avoid amoxycillin if possibility of glandular fever, see section 5.1.1.3	Phenoxymethylpenicillin (*or* erythromycin[4] if penicillin-allergic)	Initial parenteral therapy (in severe infection) with benzylpenicillin, then oral therapy with phenoxymethylpenicillin *or* amoxycillin[1]; treat beta-haemolytic streptococcal infections for at least 10 days. Most infections are caused by viruses
13: Skin		
Impetigo	Topical fusidic acid *or* mupirocin; oral flucloxacillin[2] *or* erythromycin if widespread	Topical treatment for 7 days usually adequate; max. duration of topical treatment 10 days
Erysipelas	Phenoxymethylpenicillin	
Cellulitis	Phenoxymethylpenicillin + flucloxacillin[2] (*or* erythromycin alone if penicillin-allergic) *or* co-amoxiclav alone	Severe cellulitis may require parenteral benzylpenicillin + flucloxacillin or co-amoxiclav alone
Acne—see section 13.6		

1. Where amoxycillin is suggested ampicillin or an ester of ampicillin (see section 5.1.1.3) may be used.
2. Where flucloxacillin is suggested cloxacillin may be used.
3. Where vancomycin is suggested teicoplanin may be used.
4. Where erythromycin is suggested another macrolide (e.g. azithromycin or clarithromycin) may be used.

Table 2. Summary of antibacterial prophylaxis

Infection	Antibacterial and dose
Prevention of recurrence of rheumatic fever	Phenoxymethylpenicillin 250 mg twice daily *or* sulphadiazine 1 g daily (500 mg daily for patients under 30 kg)
Prevention of secondary case of meningococcal meningitis[1]	Rifampicin 600 mg every 12 hours for 2 days; CHILD 10 mg/kg (3 months–1 year, 5 mg/kg) every 12 hours for 2 days *or* ciprofloxacin 500 mg as a single dose [not licensed for this indication]; CHILD obtain further advice[1] *or* i/m ceftriaxone 250 mg as a single dose; CHILD under 12 years 125 mg
Prevention of secondary case of *Haemophilus influenzae* type b disease[1]	Rifampicin 600 mg once daily for 4 days (optimum regimen for adults); CHILD over 3 months 20 mg/kg once daily for 4 days (max. 600 mg daily)
Prevention of secondary case of diphtheria in non-immune patient	Erythromycin 500 mg every 6 hours for 5 days; CHILD up to 2 years 125 mg every 6 hours, 2–8 years 250 mg every 6 hours
Prevention of whooping cough	ADULT and CHILD erythromycin 50 mg/kg daily in 4 divided doses for 7–10 days
Prevention of pneumococcal infection following splenectomy or in patients with sickle cell disease	Phenoxymethylpenicillin 500 mg every 12 hours; CHILD under 5 years 125 mg every 12 hours, 6–12 years 250 mg every 12 hours—if cover also needed for *H. influenzae* in CHILD give amoxycillin instead (under 5 years 125 mg every 12 hours, over 5 years 250 mg every 12 hours)

Infection	Antibacterial and dose

Prevention of endocarditis in patients with heart-valve lesion, septal defect, patent ductus, or prosthetic valve
 	
Dental procedures that require antibiotic prophylaxis are:
  extractions
  scaling
  surgery involving gingival tissues
Antibiotic prophylaxis for dental procedures may be supplemented with *chlorhexidine gluconate gel 1%* or *chlorhexidine gluconate mouthwash 0.2%*, used 5 minutes before procedure
 	
If **clindamycin** is used, periodontal or other multistage procedures should not be repeated at intervals of less than 2 weeks
	Dental procedures *under local or no anaesthesia*, patients who have not received a penicillin more than once in the previous month, including those with a prosthetic valve (but not those who have had endocarditis), oral amoxycillin 3 g 1 hour before procedure; CHILD under 5 years quarter adult dose; 5–10 years half adult dose
	patients who are penicillin-allergic or have received a penicillin more than once in the previous month,
	oral clindamycin 600 mg 1 hour before procedure; CHILD under 5 years quarter adult dose; 5–10 years half-adult dose
	patients who have had endocarditis, amoxycillin + gentamicin, as under general anaesthesia
	
	Dental procedures *under general anaesthesia, no special risk* (including patients who have not received a penicillin more than once in the previous month),
	either i/m or i/v amoxycillin 1 g at induction, then oral amoxycillin 500 mg 6 hours later; CHILD under 5 years quarter adult dose; 5–10 years half adult dose
	or oral amoxycillin 3 g 4 hours before induction then oral amoxycillin 3 g as soon as possible after procedure; CHILD under 5 years quarter adult dose; 5–10 years half adult dose
	or oral amoxycillin 3 g + oral probenecid 1 g 4 hours before procedure;
	special risk (patients with a prosthetic valve or who have had endocarditis), i/m or i/v amoxycillin 1 g + i/m or i/v gentamicin 120 mg at induction, then oral amoxycillin 500 mg 6 hours later; CHILD under 5 years amoxycillin quarter adult dose, gentamicin 2 mg/kg, 5–10 years amoxycillin half adult dose, gentamicin 2 mg/kg
	patients who are penicillin-allergic or who have received a penicillin more than once in the previous month,
	either i/v vancomycin 1 g over at least 100 minutes then i/v gentamicin 120 mg at induction or 15 minutes before procedure; CHILD under 10 years vancomycin 20 mg/kg, gentamicin 2 mg/kg
	or i/v teicoplanin 400 mg + gentamicin 120 mg at induction or 15 minutes before procedure; CHILD under 14 years teicoplanin 6 mg/kg, gentamicin 2 mg/kg
	or i/v clindamycin 300 mg over at least 10 minutes at induction or 15 minutes before procedure then oral or i/v clindamycin 150 mg 6 hours later; CHILD under 5 years quarter adult dose; 5–10 years half adult dose
	
	Upper respiratory-tract procedures, as for dental procedures; post-operative dose may be given parenterally if swallowing is painful
	
	Genito-urinary procedures, as for *special risk* patients undergoing dental procedures under general anaesthesia except that clindamycin is not given, see above; if urine infected, prophylaxis should also cover infective organism
	
	Obstetric, gynaecological and gastro-intestinal procedures (prophylaxis required for patients with prosthetic valves or those who have had endocarditis only), as for genito-urinary procedures

Prevention of gas-gangrene in high lower-limb amputations or following major trauma	Benzylpenicillin 300–600 mg every 6 hours for 5 days *or* if penicillin-allergic metronidazole 500 mg every 8 hours

1. For details of those who should receive chemoprophylaxis contact a consultant in communicable disease control (or a consultant in infectious diseases or the local public health laboratory). Unless there has been mouth to mouth contact, hospital workers do not generally require chemoprophylaxis.

Table 2. Summary of antibacterial prophylaxis (*continued*)

Infection	Antibacterial and dose
Prevention of tuberculosis in susceptible close contacts	Isoniazid 300 mg daily for 6 months; (CHILD, isoniazid 5–10 mg/kg daily) *or* isoniazid 300 mg daily + rifampicin 600 mg daily (450 mg if less than 50 kg) for 3 months; (CHILD isoniazid 5–10 mg/kg daily + rifampicin 10 mg/kg daily)
Prevention of infection in abdominal surgery	
Operations on stomach or oesophagus for carcinoma, or cholecystectomy in patients with possibly infected bile	Single dose of gentamicin *or* a cephalosporin given in 2 hours before operation
Resections of colon and rectum for carcinoma, and resections in inflammatory bowel disease	Single dose of *either* gentamicin + metronidazole *or* cefuroxime + metronidazole given in 2 hours before operation
Hysterectomy	Metronidazole as suppository *or* single i/v dose

Joint prostheses and dental treatment.
Advice of a Working Party of the British Society for Antimicrobial Chemotherapy is that patients with prosthetic joint implants (including total hip replacements) do not require antibiotic prophylaxis for dental treatment. The Working Party considers that it is unacceptable to expose patients to the adverse effects of antibiotics when there is no evidence that such prophylaxis is of any benefit, but that those who develop any intercurrent infection require prompt treatment with antibiotics to which the infecting organisms are sensitive.

The Working Party has commented that joint infections have rarely been shown to follow dental procedures and are even more rarely caused by oral streptococci.

Immunosuppression and indwelling intraperitoneal catheters
Advice of a Working Party of the British Society for Antimicrobial Chemotherapy is that patients who are immunosuppressed (including transplant patients) and patients with indwelling intraperitoneal catheters do not require antibiotic prophylaxis for dental treatment provided there is no other indication for prophylaxis.

The Working Party has commented that there is little evidence that dental treatment is followed by infection in immunosuppressed and immunodeficient patients nor is there evidence that dental treatment is followed by infection in patients with indwelling intraperitoneal catheters.

5.1.1   Penicillins

5.1.1.1   Benzylpenicillin and phenoxymethylpenicillin
5.1.1.2   Penicillinase-resistant penicillins
5.1.1.3   Broad-spectrum penicillins
5.1.1.4   Antipseudomonal penicillins

The penicillins are bactericidal and act by interfering with bacterial cell wall synthesis. They diffuse well into body tissues and fluids, but penetration into the cerebrospinal fluid is poor except when the meninges are inflamed. They are excreted in the urine in therapeutic concentrations. Probenecid (see section 10.1.4) blocks the renal tubular excretion of the penicillins, producing higher and more prolonged plasma concentrations; it is not recommended in children under 2 years of age.

The most important side-effect of the penicillins is hypersensitivity, which causes rashes and, occasionally, anaphylaxis, which can be fatal. Patients who are allergic to one penicillin will be allergic to all as the hypersensitivity is related to the basic penicillin structure. A rare but serious toxic effect of the penicillins is encephalopathy due to cerebral irritation. This may result from excessively high doses but can also develop with normal doses given to patients with renal failure. The penicillins should **not** be given by intrathecal injection as they can cause encephalopathy which may be fatal.

A second problem relating to high doses of penicillin, or normal doses given to patients with renal failure, is the accumulation of electrolyte since most injectable penicillins contain either sodium or potassium.

Diarrhoea frequently occurs during oral penicillin therapy. It is most common with ampicillin and its derivatives, which can also cause pseudomembranous colitis.

5.1.1.1 BENZYLPENICILLIN AND PHENOXYMETHYLPENICILLIN

Benzylpenicillin (Penicillin G), the first of the penicillins, remains an important and useful antibiotic but is inactivated by bacterial penicillinases (beta-lactamases). It is the drug of choice for streptococcal, pneumococcal, gonococcal, and meningococcal infections and also for anthrax, diphtheria, gas-gangrene, leptospirosis, syphilis, tetanus, yaws, and treatment of Lyme disease in children. Pneumococci, meningococci, and gonococci which have decreased sensitivity to penicillin have been isolated. Benzylpenicillin is inactivated by gastric acid and absorption from the gut is low; therefore it is best given by injection. Benzylpenicillin may cause convulsions after high doses by intravenous injection or in renal failure.

Procaine penicillin is a sparingly soluble salt of benzylpenicillin. It is used in intramuscular depot preparations which provide therapeutic tissue concentrations for up to 24 hours. It is the preferred choice for the treatment of syphilis; neurosyphilis requires special consideration.

Phenoxymethylpenicillin (Penicillin V) has a similar antibacterial spectrum to benzylpenicillin, but is less active. It is gastric acid-stable, so is suitable for oral administration. It should not be used for serious infections because absorption can be unpredictable and plasma concentrations variable. It is indicated principally for respiratory-tract infections in children, for streptococcal tonsillitis, and for continuing treatment after one or more injections of benzylpenicillin when clinical response has begun. It should not be used for meningococcal or gonococcal infections. Phenoxymethylpenicillin is used for prophylaxis against streptococcal infections following rheumatic fever and against pneumococcal infections following splenectomy or in sickle cell disease.

BENZYLPENICILLIN
(Penicillin G)

Indications: throat infections, otitis media, streptococcal endocarditis, meningococcal and pneumococcal meningitis, pneumonia (see table 1); prophylaxis in limb amputation
Cautions: history of allergy; renal impairment; **interactions:** Appendix 1 (penicillins)
Contra-indications: penicillin hypersensitivity
Side-effects: sensitivity reactions including urticaria, fever, joint pains; angioedema; transient leucopenia and thrombocytopenia; anaphylactic shock in hypersensitive patients; diarrhoea after administration by mouth
Dose: by intramuscular or by slow intravenous injection or by infusion, 1.2 g daily in 4 divided doses, increased if necessary to 2.4 g daily or more (see also below); PREMATURE INFANT and NEONATE, 50 mg/kg daily in 2 divided doses, INFANT 1–4 weeks, 75 mg/kg daily in 3 divided doses; CHILD 1 month–12 years, 100 mg/kg daily in 4 divided doses (higher doses may be required, see also below)
Bacterial endocarditis, *by slow intravenous injection or by infusion,* 7.2 g daily in 4–6 divided doses
Meningitis, *by slow intravenous injection or by infusion,* 2.4 g every 4–6 hours; PREMATURE INFANT and NEONATE, 100 mg/kg daily in 2 divided doses; INFANT 1–4 weeks, 150 mg/kg daily in 3 divided doses; CHILD 1 month–12 years, 180–300 mg/kg daily in 4–6 divided doses
Important. If meningococcal disease is suspected general practitioners are advised to give a single injection of benzylpenicillin by intramuscular or by intravenous injection before transporting the patient urgently to hospital. Suitable doses are: ADULT 1.2 g; INFANT 300 mg; CHILD 1–9 years 600 mg, 10 years and over as for adult
Prophylaxis in limb amputation, section 5.1, table 2
By intrathecal injection, **not** recommended
Note. Benzylpenicillin doses in BNF may differ from those in data sheet

PoM Crystapen® (Britannia)
Injection, powder for reconstitution, benzylpenicillin sodium (unbuffered). Net price 600-mg vial = 44p, 2-vial 'GP pack' = £1.99
Electrolytes: Na+ 1.68 mmol/600-mg vial

PHENOXYMETHYLPENICILLIN
(Penicillin V)

Indications: tonsillitis, otitis media, erysipelas; rheumatic fever and pneumococcal infection prophylaxis (see table 2)
Cautions; Contra-indications; Side-effects: see under Benzylpenicillin; **interactions:** Appendix 1 (penicillins)
Dose: 250–500 mg every 6 hours; CHILD, every 6 hours, up to 1 year 62.5 mg, 1–5 years 125 mg, 6–12 years 250 mg
Rheumatic fever and pneumococcal infection prophylaxis, section 5.1, table 2

PoM Phenoxymethylpenicillin (Non-proprietary)
Tablets, phenoxymethylpenicillin (as potassium salt) 250 mg, net price 20 = 27p. Label: 9, 23
Available from APS (Apsin®), Berk, Cox, CP, Evans, K Pharm., Lagap
Oral solution, phenoxymethylpenicillin (as potassium salt) for reconstitution with water, net price 125 mg/5 mL, 100 mL = 65p; 250 mg/5 mL, 100 mL = 87p. Label: 9, 23
Available from APS (Apsin®), Cox, Evans, K Pharm.

PROCAINE PENICILLIN

Indications: penicillin-sensitive infections
Cautions; Contra-indications; Side-effects: see under Benzylpenicillin; **not** for intravenous administration
Dose: see below

PoM Bicillin® (Yamanouchi)
Injection, powder for reconstitution, procaine penicillin 1.8 g, benzylpenicillin sodium 360 mg. Net price 6-mL multidose vial = £2.70
Electrolytes: Na+ 1 mmol/vial
Dose: when reconstituted with 4.6 mL water for injections, 1 mL (procaine penicillin 300 mg, benzylpenicillin sodium 60 mg) every 12–24 hours by intramuscular injection
Primary syphilis, by intramuscular injection, 3 mL (4 mL in patients over 80 kg) daily for 10 days (14 days for secondary or latent syphilis)
Note. Reconstitution with 4.6 mL water for injections produces 6 mL

5.1.1.2 PENICILLINASE-RESISTANT PENICILLINS

Most staphylococci are now resistant to benzylpenicillin because they produce penicillinases. **Cloxacillin** and **flucloxacillin**, however, are not inactivated by these enzymes and are thus effective in infections caused by penicillin-resistant staphylococci, which is the sole indication for their use. They are acid-stable and can, therefore, be given by mouth as well as by injection.

Flucloxacillin is better absorbed from the gut than cloxacillin and is, therefore, to be preferred for oral therapy. For CSM warning on cholestatic jaundice see under Flucloxacillin.

Staph. aureus strains resistant to methicillin [now discontinued] (methicillin-resistant *Staphylococcus aureus*, MRSA) and cloxacillin have emerged in some hospitals; some of these organisms are only sensitive to vancomycin (section 5.1.7). Other alternatives include rifampicin and teicoplanin.

Temocillin is a new penicillin with activity against penicillinase-producing Gram-negative bacteria (except *Pseudomonas aeruginosa*); it is not active against Gram-positive bacteria.

CLOXACILLIN

Indications: infections due to penicillinase-producing staphylococci

Cautions; Contra-indications; Side-effects: see under Benzylpenicillin (section 5.1.1.1)

Dose: by mouth, 500 mg every 6 hours, at least 30 minutes before food

By intramuscular injection, 250 mg every 4–6 hours

By slow intravenous injection or by infusion, 500 mg every 4–6 hours

Doses may be doubled in severe infections

CHILD, any route, under 2 years quarter adult dose; 2–10 years half adult dose

Note. Oral liquid preparation no longer marketed

PoM Cloxacillin (Non-proprietary)

Capsules, cloxacillin (as sodium salt) 250 mg, net price 20 = £3.55; 500 mg, 20 = £7.11. Label: 9, 23

Available from Forley (Orbenin®), SmithKline Beecham

Injection, powder for reconstitution, cloxacillin (as sodium salt). Net price 250-mg vial = 91p; 500-mg vial = £1.81

Electrolytes: Na+ 0.59 mmol/250-mg vial, 1.18 mmol/500-mg vial

Available from Forley (Orbenin®), SmithKline Beecham

FLUCLOXACILLIN

Indications: infections due to penicillinase-producing staphylococci including otitis externa; adjunct in pneumonia, impetigo, cellulitis and in staphylococcal endocarditis (section 5.1 table 1)

Cautions; Contra-indications; Side-effects: see under Benzylpenicillin (section 5.1.1.1); hepatitis and cholestatic jaundice reported (see also CSM advice below); caution in porphyria (see section 9.8.2)

CHOLESTATIC JAUNDICE. CSM has advised that cholestatic jaudice may occur up to several weeks after treatment with flucloxacillin has been stopped. Administration for more than 2 weeks and increasing age are risk factors

Dose: by mouth, 250 mg every 6 hours, at least 30 minutes before food

By intramuscular injection, 250 mg every 6 hours

By slow intravenous injection or by infusion, 0.25–1 g every 6 hours

Doses may be doubled in severe infections

CHILD, any route, under 2 years quarter adult dose; 2–10 years half adult dose

PoM Flucloxacillin (Non-proprietary)

Capsules, flucloxacillin (as sodium salt) 250 mg, net price 20 = 95p; 500 mg, 20 = £2.04. Label: 9, 23

Available from APS, Ashbourne (Fluclomix®), Berk (Ladropen®), Cox, CP, Galen (Galfloxin®), K Pharm., Lagap, Norton, Yamanouchi (Stafoxil®)

Oral solution (= elixir or syrup), flucloxacillin (as sodium salt) for reconstitution with water, 125 mg/5 mL. Net price 100 mL = £3.51. Label: 9, 23

Available from APS, Cox, CP, Norton

Oral suspension (= mixture), flucloxacillin (as magnesium salt) for reconstitution with water, 125 mg/5 mL, net price 100 mL = £3.32; 250 mg/ 5 mL, 100 mL = £6.64. Label: 9, 23

Available from Berk (Ladropen®)

Injection, powder for reconstitution, flucloxacillin (as sodium salt). Net price 250-mg vial = 75p; 500-mg vial = £1.71

Available from Berk (Ladropen®)

PoM Floxapen® (Beecham)

Capsules, both black/caramel, flucloxacillin (as sodium salt) 250 mg, net price 20-cap pack = £4.62, 28-cap pack = £6.47; 500 mg, 28-cap pack = £12.95. Label: 9, 23

Syrup, flucloxacillin (as magnesium salt) for reconstitution with water, 125 mg/5 mL, net price 100 mL = £3.32; 250 mg/5 mL, 100 mL = £6.64. Label: 9, 23

Injection, powder for reconstitution, flucloxacillin (as sodium salt). Net price 250-mg vial = 93p; 500-mg vial = £1.86; 1-g vial = £3.71

Electrolytes: Na+ 0.57 mmol/250-mg vial, 1.13 mmol/500-mg vial, 2.26 mmol/1-g vial

TEMOCILLIN

Indications: infections due to penicillinase-producing Gram-negative bacteria except pseudomonas

Cautions; Contra-indications; Side-effects: see under Benzylpenicillin (section 5.1.1.1)

Dose: by intramuscular injection or by intravenous injection (over 3–4 minutes) *or by intravenous infusion*, 1–2 g every 12 hours

Acute uncomplicated urinary-tract infections, 1 g daily as a single dose or in divided doses

PoM Temopen® (Bencard)

Injection, powder for reconstitution, temocillin (as sodium salt). Net price 1-g vial = £15.00

Electrolytes: Na+ 5 mmol/g

5.1.1.3 BROAD-SPECTRUM PENICILLINS

Ampicillin is active against certain Gram-positive and Gram-negative organisms but is inactivated by penicillinases including those produced by *Staphylococcus aureus* and by common Gram-negative bacilli such as *Escherichia coli*. Almost all staphylococci, 50% of *E. coli* strains and 15% of *Haemophilus influenzae* strains are now resistant. The likelihood of resistance should therefore be considered before using ampicillin for the 'blind' treatment of infections; in particular, it should not be used for hospital patients without checking sensitivity.

Ampicillin is well excreted in the bile and urine. It is principally indicated for the treatment of exacerbations of chronic bronchitis and middle ear infections, both of which are usually due to *Streptococcus pneumoniae* and *H. influenzae*, and for urinary-tract infections (section 5.1.13) and gonorrhoea.

Ampicillin can be given by mouth but less than half the dose is absorbed, and absorption is further decreased by the presence of food in the gut. Higher plasma concentrations are obtained with the ampicillin esters **bacampicillin** and **pivampicillin**; their absorption is little affected by the presence of food, and the incidence of diarrhoea is less than with ampicillin.

Maculopapular rashes commonly occur with ampicillin (and amoxycillin) but are not usually related to true penicillin allergy. They almost always occur in patients with glandular fever; broad-spectrum penicillins should not therefore be used for 'blind' treatment of a sore throat. Rashes are also common in patients with chronic lymphatic leukaemia and in patients infected with the human immunodeficiency virus (HIV).

Amoxycillin is a derivative of ampicillin which differs by only one hydroxyl group and has a similar antibacterial spectrum. It is better absorbed than ampicillin when given by mouth, producing higher plasma and tissue concentrations; unlike ampicillin, absorption is not affected by the presence of food in the stomach. Amoxycillin is used for endocarditis prophylaxis (section 5.1, table 2); it may also be used for the treatment of Lyme disease in children.

Co-amoxiclav consists of amoxycillin with the beta-lactamase inhibitor clavulanic acid. Clavulanic acid itself has no significant antibacterial activity but, by inactivating penicillinases, it makes the combination active against penicillinase-producing bacteria that are resistant to amoxycillin. These include most *Staph. aureus*, 50% of *E. coli* strains, and up to 15% of *H. influenzae* strains, as well as many *Bacteroides* and *Klebsiella* spp. Co-amoxiclav may be used for pelvic inflammatory disease and for cellulitis (see section 5.1, table 1). For CSM warning on cholestatic jaundice see under Co-amoxiclav.

Combinations of ampicillin with flucloxacillin (as co-fluampicil) and ampicillin with cloxacillin (Ampiclox®) are available.

AMOXYCILLIN
(Amoxicillin)

Indications: see under Ampicillin; also endocarditis prophylaxis; adjunct in listerial meningitis (section 5.1, table1)

Cautions; Contra-indications; Side-effects: see under Ampicillin

Dose: *by mouth*, 250 mg every 8 hours, doubled in severe infections; CHILD up to 10 years, 125 mg every 8 hours, doubled in severe infections
Severe or recurrent purulent respiratory infection, 3 g every 12 hours; CHILD 2–5 years 750 mg every 12 hours, 5–10 years 1.5 g every 12 hours
Endocarditis prophylaxis, section 5.1, table 2

Short-course oral therapy
Dental abscess, 3 g repeated after 8 hours
Urinary-tract infections, 3 g repeated after 10–12 hours
Gonorrhoea, single dose of 2–3 g with probenecid 1 g
Otitis media, CHILD 3–10 years, 750 mg twice daily for 2 days
By intramuscular injection, 500 mg every 8 hours; CHILD, 50–100 mg/kg daily in divided doses
By intravenous injection or infusion, 500 mg every 8 hours increased to 1 g every 6 hours; CHILD, 50–100 mg/kg daily in divided doses

PoM Amoxycillin (Non-proprietary)
Capsules, amoxycillin (as trihydrate) 250 mg, net price 20 = 76p; 500 mg, 20 = £1.67. Label: 9
Available from APS, Ashbourne (Amix®), Berk (Almodan®), BHR (Amrit®), Cox, CP, Eastern (Amoram®), Galen (Galenamox®), K Pharm., Lagap, Medipharma (Amoxymed®), Norton, Rima (Rimoxallin®)
Oral suspension, amoxycillin (as trihydrate) for reconstitution with water, 125 mg/5 mL, net price 100 mL = £1.20; 250 mg/5 mL, 100 mL = £2.05. Label: 9
Available from APS, Ashbourne (Amix®), Berk (Almodan®), BHR (Amrit®), Cox, CP, Eastern (Amoram®), Galen (Galenamox®), K Pharm., Lagap, Medipharma (Amoxymed®), Norton, Rima (Rimoxallin®)
Sachets, sugar-free, amoxycillin 3 g (as trihydrate)/sachet, net price 2-sachet pack = £4.49, 14-sachet pack = £31.45. Label: 9, 13
Available from Norton

PoM Amoxil® (Bencard)
Capsules, both maroon/gold, amoxycillin (as trihydrate), 250 mg, net price 21-cap pack = £3.67; 500 mg, 21-cap pack = £7.35. Label: 9
Dispersible tablets, sugar-free, amoxycillin 500 mg (as trihydrate). Net price 21-tab pack = £8.48. Label: 9, 13
Fiztab (= chewable tablets), sugar-free, amoxycillin (as trihydrate) 125 mg, net price 20-tab pack = £2.20; 250 mg, 20-tab pack = £4.40; 500 mg, 20-tab pack = £8.80. Label: 9, 10 patient information leaflet
Note. Dose form not suitable for children under 3 years
Syrup SF, both sugar-free, amoxycillin (as trihydrate) for reconstitution with water, 125 mg/5 mL, net price 100 mL = £2.20; 250 mg/5 mL, 100 mL = £4.40. Label: 9
Paediatric suspension, amoxycillin 125 mg (as trihydrate)/1.25 mL when reconstituted with water. Net price 20 mL = £3.30. Label: 9, counselling, use of pipette
Sachets SF, powder, sugar-free, amoxycillin 750 mg (as trihydrate)/sachet, net price 4-sachet pack = £2.86; 3 g/sachet, 2-sachet pack = £4.73; 14-sachet pack = £33.11. Label: 9, 13
Injection, powder for reconstitution, amoxycillin (as sodium salt). Net price 250-mg vial = 36p; 500-mg vial = 66p; 1-g vial = £1.31
Electrolytes: Na+ 3.2 mmol/g

PoM **Flemoxin Solutab®** (Yamanouchi)
Dispersible tablets, sugar-free, both scored, amoxycillin (as trihydrate) 375 mg, net price 10-tab pack = £2.62; 750 mg, 10-tab pack = £5.25. Label: 9, 13
Dose: 375 mg every 12 hours, doubled in severe infections; CHILD 5–10 years half usual adult dose
Severe or recurrent respiratory-tract infection, see under Dose on p. 219

AMPICILLIN

Indications: urinary-tract infections, otitis media, sinusitis, chronic bronchitis, invasive salmonellosis, gonorrhoea
Cautions: history of allergy; renal impairment; erythematous rashes common in glandular fever, chronic lymphatic leukaemia, and HIV infection; **interactions:** Appendix 1 (penicillins)
Contra-indications: penicillin hypersensitivity
Side-effects: nausea, diarrhoea; rashes (discontinue treatment); rarely, pseudomembranous colitis; see also under Benzylpenicillin (section 5.1.1.1)
Dose: by mouth, 0.25–1 g every 6 hours, at least 30 minutes before food
Gonorrhoea, 2–3.5 g as a single dose with probenecid 1 g
Urinary-tract infections, 500 mg every 8 hours
By intramuscular injection or intravenous injection or infusion, 500 mg every 4–6 hours; higher doses in meningitis
CHILD under 10 years, any route, half adult dose

PoM **Ampicillin** (Non-proprietary)
Capsules, ampicillin 250 mg, net price 20 = 61p; 500 mg, 20 = £1.13. Label: 9, 23
Available from APS, Berk (Vidopen®), Cox, CP, K Pharm., Lagap, Norton, Rima (Rimacillin®), Yamanouchi (Amfipen®)
Oral suspension, ampicillin 125 mg/5 mL when reconstituted with water, net price 100 mL = 88p; 250 mg/5 mL, 100 mL = £1.07. Label: 9, 23
Available from APS, Berk, Cox, K Pharm., Lagap, Norton, Rima (Rimacillin®), Yamanouchi (Amfipen®)
PoM **Penbritin®** (Beecham)
Capsules, both black/red, ampicillin (as trihydrate) 250 mg, net price 28-cap pack = £2.05; 500 mg, 28-cap pack = £4.10. Label: 9, 23
Syrup, ampicillin (as trihydrate) for reconstitution with water, 125 mg/5 mL, net price 100 mL = £1.09; 250 mg/5 mL, 100 mL = £2.17. Label: 9, 23
Paediatric suspension, ampicillin 125 mg (as trihydrate)/1.25 mL. Net price 25 mL = £2.03. Label: 9, 23, counselling, use of pipette
Injection, powder for reconstitution, ampicillin (as sodium salt). Net price 250-mg vial = 33p; 500-mg vial = 67p
Electrolytes: Na+ 0.73 mmol/250-mg vial, 1.47 mmol/500-mg vial

With cloxacillin
PoM **Ampiclox®** (Beecham)
Capsules, black/purple, ampicillin 250 mg (as trihydrate), cloxacillin 250 mg (as sodium salt). Net price 20-cap pack = £7.00. Label: 9, 23
Dose: 1–2 capsules every 4–6 hours
Syrup, ampicillin 125 mg (as trihydrate), cloxacillin 125 mg (as sodium salt)/5 mL when reconstituted with water. Net price 100 mL = £5.00. Label: 9, 23
Dose: 10–20 mL every 4–6 hours; CHILD 1 month–2 years, quarter adult dose; 2–12 years, half adult dose
Injection, ampicillin 250 mg (as sodium salt), cloxacillin 250 mg (as sodium salt). Net price per vial = £1.36
Electrolytes: Na+ 1.32 mmol/vial
Dose: by intramuscular injection or intravenous injection or infusion, 1–2 vials every 4–6 hours; CHILD up to 2 years quarter adult dose, 2–10 years half adult dose
PoM **Ampiclox Neonatal®** (Beecham)
Suspension, sugar-free, ampicillin 60 mg (as trihydrate), cloxacillin 30 mg (as sodium salt)/0.6 mL when reconstituted with water. Net price 10 mL = £2.06. Label: 9, counselling, use of pipette
Dose: 0.6 mL every 4 hours
Injection, ampicillin 50 mg (as sodium salt), cloxacillin 25 mg (as sodium salt). Net price per vial = 42p.
Electrolytes: Na+ <0.5 mmol/vial
Dose: NEONATE and PREMATURE INFANT, by intramuscular injection or by intravenous injection or infusion, 1 vial every 8 hours

With flucloxacillin
See Co-fluampicil

BACAMPICILLIN HYDROCHLORIDE
Indications; Cautions; Contra-indications; Side-effects: see under Ampicillin
Dose: 400 mg 2–3 times daily, doubled in severe infections; CHILD over 5 years, 200 mg 3 times daily
Uncomplicated gonorrhoea, 1.6 g as a single dose with probenecid 1 g

PoM **Ambaxin®** (Upjohn)
Tablets, scored, bacampicillin hydrochloride 400 mg. Net price 20 = £6.34. Label: 9

CO-AMOXICLAV
A mixture of amoxycillin (as the trihydrate or as the sodium salt) and clavulanic acid (as potassium clavulanate); the proportions are expressed in the form *x/y* where *x* and *y* are the strengths in milligrams of amoxycillin and clavulanic acid respectively
Indications; Cautions; Contra-indications; Side-effects: see under Ampicillin and notes above; also caution in severe hepatic impairment, pregnancy and breast-feeding; hepatitis, cholestatic jaundice (see also CSM advice below), and erythema multiforme (including Stevens-Johnson syndrome) reported; phlebitis at injection site

also reported; treatment not to exceed 14 days without review

CHOLESTATIC JAUNDICE. CSM has advised that cholestatic jaundice may occur up to 6 weeks after treatment with co-amoxiclav has been stopped. Clavulanic acid is likely to be responsible

Dose: by mouth, expressed as amoxycillin, 250 mg every 8 hours, dose doubled in severe infections; CHILD see under preparations below (under 6 years Augmentin® '125/31 SF' suspension; 6–12 years Augmentin® '250/62 SF' suspension)

By intravenous injection over 3–4 minutes *or by intravenous infusion,* expressed as amoxycillin, 1 g every 8 hours increased to 1 g every 6 hours in more serious infections; INFANTS up to 3 months 25 mg/kg every 8 hours (every 12 hours in the perinatal period and in premature infants); CHILD 3 months–12 years, 25 mg/kg every 8 hours increased to 25 mg/kg every 6 hours in more serious infections

Surgical prophylaxis, expressed as amoxycillin, 1 g at induction; for high risk procedures (e.g. colorectal surgery) a further 2–3 doses may be given every 8 hours in first 24 hours (longer if significantly increased risk of infection)

PoM Augmentin® (Beecham)

Tablets 375 mg, f/c, co-amoxiclav 250/125 (amoxycillin 250 mg as trihydrate, clavulanic acid 125 mg as potassium salt). Net price 21-tab pack = £7.35; 30-tab pack = £10.64. Label: 9

Tablets 625 mg, f/c, co-amoxiclav 500/125 (amoxycillin 500 mg as trihydrate, clavulanic acid 125 mg as potassium salt). Net price 21-tab pack = £13.00. Label: 9

Dispersible tablets, sugar-free, co-amoxiclav 250/125 (amoxycillin 250 mg as trihydrate, clavulanic acid 125 mg as potassium salt). Net price 21-tab pack = £8.25. Label: 9, 13

Suspension '125/31 SF', sugar-free, co-amoxiclav 125/31 (amoxycillin 125 mg as trihydrate, clavulanic acid 31 mg as potassium salt)/5 mL when reconstituted with water. Net price 100 mL = £3.43. Label: 9

Note. Suspension contains aspartame 12.5 mg/5 mL (see section 9.4.1)

Dose: CHILD under 1 year 0.8 mL/kg daily in 3 divided doses; 1–6 years (10–18 kg) 5 mL every 8 hours, doubled in severe infections

Suspension '250/62 SF', sugar-free, co-amoxiclav 250/62 (amoxycillin 250 mg as trihydrate, clavulanic acid 62 mg as potassium salt)/5 mL when reconstituted with water. Net price 100 mL = £4.83. Label: 9

Note. Suspension contains aspartame 12.5 mg/5 mL (see section 9.4.1)

Dose: CHILD 6–12 years 5 mL every 8 hours, doubled in severe infections

Injection 600 mg, powder for preparing intravenous injections, co-amoxiclav 500/100 (amoxycillin 500 mg as sodium salt, clavulanic acid 100 mg as potassium salt). Net price per vial = £1.35

Electrolytes: Na+ 1.6 mmol, K+ 0.5 mmol/600-mg vial

Injection 1.2 g, powder for preparing intravenous injections, co-amoxiclav 1000/200 (amoxycillin 1 g as sodium salt, clavulanic acid 200 mg as potassium salt). Net price per vial = £2.70

Electrolytes: Na+ 3.1 mmol, K+ 1 mmol/1.2-g vial

CO-FLUAMPICIL

A mixture of equal parts by mass of flucloxacillin and ampicillin

Indications: mixed infections involving penicillinase-producing staphylococci

Cautions; Contra-indications; Side-effects: see under Ampicillin and Flucloxacillin

Dose: by mouth, co-fluampicil, 250/250 every 6 hours, dose doubled in severe infections; CHILD under 10 years half adult dose, dose doubled in severe infections

By intramuscular or slow intravenous injection or by intravenous infusion, co-fluampicil 250/250 every 6 hours, dose doubled in severe infections; CHILD under 2 years quarter adult dose, 2–10 years half adult dose, dose doubled in severe infections

PoM Co-fluampicil (Non-proprietary)

Capsules, co-fluampicil 250/250 (flucloxacillin 250 mg as sodium salt, ampicillin 250 mg as trihydrate). Net price 20 = £4.00. Label: 9, 23

Available from Cox, Generics (Flu-Amp®), Norton

PoM Magnapen® (Beecham)

Capsules, black/turquoise, co-fluampicil 250/250 (flucloxacillin 250 mg as sodium salt, ampicillin 250 mg as trihydrate). Net price 20-cap pack = £5.08. Label: 9, 23

Syrup, co-fluampicil 125/125 (flucloxacillin 125 mg as magnesium salt, ampicillin 125 mg as trihydrate)/5 mL when reconstituted with water. Net price 100 mL = £4.13. Label: 9, 23

Injection 500 mg, powder for reconstitution, co-fluampicil 250/250 (flucloxacillin 250 mg as sodium salt, ampicillin 250 mg as sodium salt). Net price per vial = £1.10

Electrolytes: Na+ 1.3 mmol/vial

PIVAMPICILLIN

Indications: see under Ampicillin

Cautions; Contra-indications; Side-effects: see under Ampicillin; hepatic and renal function tests required in long-term use; avoid in porphyria (see section 9.8.2)

Dose: 500 mg every 12 hours, doubled in severe infections; CHILD up to 1 year 40–60 mg/kg daily in 2–3 divided doses; 1–5 years 350–525 mg daily; 6–10 years 525–700 mg daily; doses can be doubled in severe infections

PoM Pondocillin® (Leo)

Tablets, f/c, pivampicillin 500 mg. Net price 20 = £4.12. Label: 5, 9, 21

Suspension, sugar-free, pivampicillin 175 mg/5 mL when reconstituted with water. Net price 50 mL = £1.72; 100 mL = £2.77. Label: 5, 9, 21

Cautionary label wordings, see inside back cover

Prices are **net**, see p.1

With pivmecillinam

PoM Miraxid® (Fisons)

Tablets, f/c, pivampicillin 125 mg, pivmecillinam hydrochloride 100 mg. Net price 20 = £2.52. Label: 9, 21, 27, counselling, posture (see below)

Dose: 2 tablets twice daily, increased to 3 tablets twice daily for severe infections; CHILD 6–10 years 1 tablet twice daily

COUNSELLING. Swallow whole with plenty of fluid during meals while sitting or standing

Miraxid® 450 tablets, f/c, pivampicillin 250 mg, pivmecillinam hydrochloride 200 mg. Net price 20 = £4.93. Label: 9, 21, 27, counselling, posture (see below)

Dose: 1 tablet twice daily, increased to 2 tablets twice daily for severe infections

COUNSELLING. Swallow whole with plenty of fluid during meals while sitting or standing

Paediatric suspension, pivampicillin 62.5 mg, pivmecillinam 46.2 mg/unit-dose sachet. Net price 10-sachet pack = £2.30. Label: 9, 13, 21

Dose: under 6 years 1 sachet twice daily increased to 2 sachets twice daily for severe infections, 6–10 years 2 sachets twice daily increased to 3 sachets twice daily for severe infections

---

5.1.1.4 ANTIPSEUDOMONAL PENICILLINS

The carboxypenicillins, **carbenicillin** and **ticarcillin**, are principally indicated for the treatment of serious infections caused by *Pseudomonas aeruginosa* although they may also have activity against certain other Gram-negative bacilli including *Proteus* spp. and *Bacteroides fragilis*. Carbenicillin has been replaced by ticarcillin which is more active against these organisms.

Timentin® (ticarcillin with clavulanic acid, section 5.1.1.3), is active against penicillinase-producing bacteria resistant to ticarcillin.

The ureidopenicillins, **azlocillin** and **piperacillin**, have a broad spectrum and are both more active than ticarcillin against *Ps. aeruginosa*.

Tazocin® (piperacillin with the beta-lactamase inhibitor tazobactam) is active against beta-lactamase producing bacteria resistant to the ureidopenicillins.

For pseudomonas septicaemias (especially in neutropenia or endocarditis) these antipseudomonal penicillins should be given with an aminoglycoside (e.g. gentamicin or netilmicin, section 5.1.4) as there is a synergistic effect. Penicillins and aminoglycosides must not, however, be mixed in the same syringe or infusion.

Owing to the sodium content of many of these antibiotics, high doses may lead to hypernatraemia.

AZLOCILLIN

Indications: infections due to *Pseudomonas aeruginosa*, see notes above

Cautions; Contra-indications; Side-effects: see under Benzylpenicillin (section 5.1.1.1); **interactions:** Appendix 1 (penicillins)

Dose: by intravenous injection, 2 g every 8 hours Serious infections, *by intravenous infusion,* 5 g every 8 hours; PREMATURE INFANT 50 mg/kg every 12 hours; NEONATE 100 mg/kg every 12 hours; INFANT 7 days–1 year 100 mg/kg every 8 hours; CHILD 1–14 years 75 mg/kg every 8 hours

PoM Securopen® (Bayer)

Injection, powder for reconstitution, azlocillin (as sodium salt). Net price 500-mg vial = £1.03; 1-g vial = £2.36; 2-g vial = £2.94

Electrolytes: Na+ 1.08 mmol/500-mg vial, 2.17 mmol/1-g vial, 4.33 mmol/2-g vial

Infusion, powder for reconstitution, azlocillin (as sodium salt). Net price 5 g vial = £7.20 (also available with 50 mL water for injections, transfer needle, and infusion bag)

Electrolytes: Na+ 10.84 mmol/5-g vial

CARBENICILLIN

Indications: infections due to *Pseudomonas aeruginosa* and *Proteus* spp., see notes above

Cautions; Contra-indications: see under Benzylpenicillin (section 5.1.1.1)

Side-effects: see under Benzylpenicillin (section 5.1.1.1); also hypokalaemia, alteration in platelet function

Dose: by slow intravenous injection or rapid infusion, severe systemic infections, 5 g every 4–6 hours; CHILD 250–400 mg/kg daily in divided doses

By intramuscular injection, urinary-tract infections, 2 g every 6 hours; CHILD 50–100 mg/kg daily in divided doses

PoM Pyopen® (Link)

Injection, powder for reconstitution, carbenicillin (as sodium salt). Net price 1-g vial = £3.00; 5 g vial = £13.13

Electrolytes: Na+ 5.4 mmol/1-g vial, 27.1 mmol/5-g vial

Also available from SmithKline Beecham (1-g vials)

PIPERACILLIN

Indications: infections due to *Pseudomonas aeruginosa*, see notes above

Cautions; Contra-indications; Side-effects: see under Benzylpenicillin (section 5.1.1.1)

Dose: by intramuscular or by slow intravenous injection or by intravenous infusion, 100–150 mg/kg daily (in divided doses), increased to 200–300 mg/kg daily in severe infections, and to at least 16 g daily in life-threatening infections; single doses over 2 g intravenous route only

PoM Pipril® (Lederle)

Injection, powder for reconstitution, piperacillin (as sodium salt). Net price 1-g vial = £2.79; 2-g vial = £5.53

Infusion, powder for reconstitution, piperacillin 4 g (as sodium salt), with 50-mL bottle water for injections and transfer needle. Net price complete unit = £11.65

Electrolytes: Na+ 1.94 mmol/g

With tazobactam
▼ PoM **Tazocin®** (Lederle)

Injection 2.25 g, powder for reconstitution, piperacillin 2 g (as sodium salt), tazobactam 250 mg (as sodium salt). Net price per vial = £7.24
Electrolytes. Na⁺ 4.48 mmol/2.25-g vial

Injection 4.5 g, powder for reconstitution, piperacillin 4 g (as sodium salt), tazobactam 500 mg (as sodium salt). Net price per vial = £13.16; infusion pack (4.5-g infusion bottle, 50-mL bottle water for injections and transfer needle) = £14.48
Electrolytes: Na⁺ 8.96 mmol/4.5-g vial

Dose: lower respiratory-tract, urinary-tract, intra-abdominal and skin infections, and septicaemia, ADULT and CHILD over 12 years, *by intravenous injection* over 3–5 minutes *or by intravenous infusion*, 2.25–4.5 g every 6–8 hours, usually 4.5 g every 8 hours; CHILD under 12 years, not yet recommended

TICARCILLIN

Indications: infections due to *Pseudomonas* and *Proteus* spp, see notes above

Cautions; Contra-indications; Side-effects: see under Benzylpenicillin (section 5.1.1.1)

Dose: by slow intravenous injection over 3–4 minutes *or by intravenous infusion*, 15–20 g daily in divided doses; CHILD 200–300 mg/kg daily in divided doses

Urinary-tract infections, *by intramuscular or slow intravenous injection*, 3–4 g daily in divided doses; CHILD 50–100 mg/kg daily in divided doses

PoM **Ticar®** (Link)

Injection, powder for reconstitution, ticarcillin (as sodium salt). Net price 1-g vial = £4.20; 5-g vial = £17.09

Infusion, powder for reconstitution, ticarcillin 5 g (as sodium salt) in infusion bottle, with transfer needle and diluent. Net price complete unit = £17.09
Electrolytes: Na⁺ 5.3 mmol/1-g vial, 26.7 mmol/5-g vial

With clavulanic acid
Note. For a CSM warning on cholestatic jaundice possibly associated with clavulanic acid, see under Co-amoxiclav p. 221.

PoM **Timentin®** (Beecham)

Injection 1.6 g, powder for reconstitution, ticarcillin 1.5 g (as sodium salt), clavulanic acid 100 mg (as potassium salt). Net price per vial = £3.04

Injection 3.2 g, powder for reconstitution, ticarcillin 3 g (as sodium salt), clavulanic acid 200 mg (as potassium salt). Net price per vial = £6.08
Electrolytes: Na⁺ 16 mmol, K⁺ 1 mmol /3.2-g vial
Dose: by intravenous infusion, 3.2 g every 6–8 hours increased to every 4 hours in more severe infections; CHILD 80 mg/kg every 6–8 hours (every 12 hours in neonates)

5.1.2 Cephalosporins, cephamycins, and other beta-lactam antibiotics

Antibiotics discussed in this section include the **cephalosporins**, such as cefotaxime, ceftazidime, cefuroxime, cephalexin and cephradine, the **cephamycin**, cefoxitin, the **monobactam**, aztreonam, and the **carbapenem** imipenem (a thienamycin derivative).

CEPHALOSPORINS AND CEPHAMYCINS

The cephalosporins are broad-spectrum antibiotics which are used for the treatment of septicaemia, pneumonia, meningitis, biliary-tract infections, peritonitis, and urinary-tract infections. All have a similar antibacterial spectrum although individual agents have differing activity against certain organisms. The pharmacology of the cephalosporins is similar to that of the penicillins, excretion being principally renal and blocked by probenecid.

The principal side-effect of the cephalosporins is hypersensitivity and about 10% of penicillin-sensitive patients will also be allergic to the cephalosporins. Haemorrhage due to interference with blood clotting factors has been associated with several cephalosporins.

Cephradine and **cephazolin** have generally been replaced by the newer cephalosporins mentioned below.

Cefuroxime and **cephamandole** are 'second generation' cephalosporins and are less susceptible than the earlier cephalosporins to inactivation by penicillinases. They are, therefore, active against certain bacteria which are resistant to the other drugs and have greater activity against *Haemophilus influenzae* and *Neisseria gonorrhoeae*.

Cefotaxime, **ceftazidime**, **ceftizoxime**, and **cefodizime** are 'third generation' cephalosporins with greater activity than the 'second generation' cephalosporins against certain Gram-negative bacteria. However, they are less active than cefuroxime and cephamandole against Gram-positive bacteria, most notably *Staphylococcus aureus*. Their broad anti bacterial spectrum may encourage superinfection with resistant bacteria or fungi.

Cefsulodin and **ceftazidime** have good activity against pseudomonas. Ceftazidime is also active against other Gram-negative bacteria. Cefsulodin has a very much narrower spectrum and should be used only for pseudomonal infections.

Ceftriaxone, a recently introduced 'third generation' cephalosporin has a longer half-life than other cephalosporins and therefore only needs once daily administration. Indications include serious infections such as septicaemia, pneumonia, and meningitis. The calcium salt of ceftriaxone forms a precipitate in the gall bladder which may rarely cause symptoms but these usually resolve when the antibiotic is stopped.

Cefoxitin, a cephamycin antibiotic, is active against bowel flora including *Bacteroides fragilis* and because of this it has been recommended for abdominal sepsis such as peritonitis.

ORALLY ACTIVE CEPHALOSPORINS. The orally active 'first generation' cephalosporins, **cephalexin**, **cephradine**, and **cefadroxil** and the 'second generation' cephalosporin, **cefaclor** have a similar antimicrobial spectrum. They are useful for urinary-tract infections which do not respond to other drugs or which occur in pregnancy. Cefaclor has good activity against *H. influenzae*, but is associated with protracted skin reactions especially in children. Cefadroxil has a longer duration of action than the other cephalosporins but poor activity against *H. influenzae*. **Cefuroxime axetil**, an ester of the 'second generation' cephalosporin cefuroxime, has the same antibacterial spectrum as the parent compound.

Cefixime has a longer duration of action than the other cephalosporins that are active by mouth. It is presently only licensed for acute infections. **Ceftibuten** is similar to cefixime but is less active against pneumococci.

Cefpodoxime proxetil, a new oral cephalosporin, is more active than the other oral cephalosporins against respiratory bacterial pathogens and it is licensed for upper and lower respiratory-tract infections.

CEFACLOR

Indications: infections due to sensitive Gram-positive and Gram-negative bacteria, but see notes above

Cautions: penicillin sensitivity; renal impairment (see Appendix 3); pregnancy and breast-feeding (but appropriate to use); false positive urinary glucose (if tested for reducing substances) and false positive Coombs' test; **interactions:** Appendix 1 (cephalosporins)

Contra-indications: cephalosporin hypersensitivity; porphyria (see section 9.8.2)

Side-effects: diarrhoea and rarely pseudomembranous colitis (CSM has warned both more likely with higher doses), nausea and vomiting, headache; allergic reactions including rashes, pruritus, urticaria, serum sickness-like reactions with rashes, fever and arthralgia, and anaphylaxis; erythema multiforme, toxic epidermal necrolysis reported; disturbances in liver enzymes, transient hepatitis and cholestatic jaundice; other side-effects reported include eosinophilia and blood disorders (including thrombocytopenia, agranulocytosis and aplastic anaemia); reversible interstitial nephritis, hyperactivity, nervousness, sleep disturbances, confusion, hypertonia, and dizziness

Dose: 250 mg every 8 hours, doubled for severe infections; max. 4 g daily; CHILD over 1 month, 20 mg/kg daily in 3 divided doses, doubled for severe infections, max. 1 g daily; *or* 1 month–1 year, 62.5 mg every 8 hours; 1–5 years, 125 mg; over 5 years, 250 mg; doses doubled for severe infections

PoM **Distaclor**® (Dista)
Capsules, cefaclor (as monohydrate) 250 mg (violet/white), net price 21-cap pack = £11.37; 500 mg (violet/grey), 20 = £21.66. Label: 9

Suspension, both pink, cefaclor (as monohydrate) for reconstitution with water, 125 mg/5 mL, net price 100 mL = £5.16; 250 mg/5 mL, 100 mL = £10.32. Label: 9

PoM **Distaclor MR**® (Lilly)
Tablets, m/r, both blue, cefaclor (as monohydrate) 375 mg, net price 14-tab pack = £10.83; 500 mg, 7-tab pack = £5.95. Label: 9, 21, 25

Dose: 375 mg every 12 hours with food, dose doubled for pneumonia
Lower urinary-tract infections, 375 mg every 12 hours with food *or* 500 mg at night

CEFADROXIL

Indications: see under Cefaclor; see also notes above

Cautions; Contra-indications; Side-effects: see under Cefaclor

Dose: patients over 40 kg, 0.5–1 g twice daily; skin, soft tissue, and simple urinary-tract infections, 1 g daily; CHILD under 1 year, 25 mg/kg daily in divided doses; 1–6 years, 250 mg twice daily; over 6 years, 500 mg twice daily

PoM **Baxan**® (Bristol-Myers)
Capsules, cefadroxil 500 mg (as monohydrate). Net price 20 = £5.64. Label: 9
Suspension, cefadroxil (as monohydrate) for reconstitution with water, 125 mg/5 mL, net price 60 mL = £1.75; 250 mg/5 mL, 60 mL = £3.48; 500 mg/5 mL, 60 mL = £5.21. Label: 9

CEFIXIME

Indications: see under Cefaclor and notes above
Cautions; Contra-indications; Side-effects: see under Cefaclor

Dose: 200–400 mg daily as a single dose or in 2 divided doses; CHILD 8 mg/kg daily as a single dose or in 2 divided doses *or* 6 months–1 year 75 mg; 1–4 years 100 mg; 5–10 years 200 mg; 11–12 years 300 mg

PoM **Suprax**® (Lederle)
Tablets, f/c, scored, cefixime 200 mg. Net price 20 = £27.39. Label: 9
Paediatric oral suspension, cefixime 100 mg/5 mL when reconstituted with water. Net price 37.5 mL (with double-ended spoon for measuring 3.75 mL or 5 mL since dilution not recommended) = £6.53; 75 mL = £11.72. Label: 9

CEFODIZIME

Indications: see under Dose
Cautions; Contra-indications; Side-effects: see under Cefaclor

Dose: by intramuscular or intravenous injection or by intravenous infusion, lower respiratory-tract infection (including pneumonia and bronchopneumonia), 1 g every 12 hours
Upper and lower urinary-tract infections (including acute and chronic pyelonephritis and cystitis), 1 g every 12 hours *or* 2 g daily (as a single dose); single doses over 1 g intravenous route only

▼ PoM **Timecef**® (Roussel)
Injection, powder for reconstitution, cefodizime
(as sodium salt), net price 1-g vial = £11.04
Electrolytes: Na⁺ 3.18 mmol/g

CEFOTAXIME

Indications: see under Cefaclor; surgical prophylaxis; Haemophilus epiglottitis and meningitis
(see section 5.1 table 1); see also notes above
Cautions; Contra-indications; Side-effects: see
under Cefaclor
*Dose: by intramuscular or intravenous injection
or by intravenous infusion*, moderate to serious
infection, 1 g every 8 hours; life-threatening
infection, 2 g every 8 hours; exceptionally, for
life-threatening infections due to organisms less
sensitive to cefotaxime, up to 12 g daily;
NEONATE, 50 mg/kg daily in 2–4 divided doses
increased to 150–200 mg/kg daily in severe infections; CHILD, 100–150 mg/kg daily in 2–4 divided
doses; increased up to 200 mg/kg daily in severe
infections
Urinary-tract and mild to moderate infections, 1 g
every 12 hours
Gonorrhoea 1 g as a single dose

PoM **Claforan**® (Roussel)
Injection, powder for reconstitution, cefotaxime
(as sodium salt). Net price 500-mg vial = £2.41;
1-g vial = £4.85; 2-g vial = £9.65
Electrolytes: Na⁺ 2.09 mmol/g

CEFOXITIN

Indications: see under Cefaclor; surgical prophylaxis; more active against Gram-negative bacteria
Cautions; Contra-indications; Side-effects: see
under Cefaclor
*Dose: by intramuscular or by slow intravenous
injection or by infusion*, 1–2 g every 6–8 hours,
increased in severe infections; max. 12 g daily;
CHILD up to 1 week 20–40 mg/kg every 12 hours;
1–4 weeks 20–40 mg/kg every 8 hours; over 1
month 20–40 mg/kg every 6–8 hours

PoM **Mefoxin**® (MSD)
Injection, powder for reconstitution, cefoxitin (as
sodium salt). Net price 1-g vial = £4.92; 2-g vial
= £9.84
Electrolytes: Na⁺ 2.3 mmol/g

CEFPODOXIME

Indications: respiratory-tract infections but in
pharyngitis and tonsillitis reserved for infections
which are recurrent, chronic, or resistant to other
antibiotics
Cautions; Contra-indications; Side-effects: see
under Cefaclor
Dose: upper respiratory-tract infections, 100 mg
twice daily with food (200 mg twice daily in
sinusitis)
Lower respiratory-tract infections (including
bronchitis and pneumonia), 100–200 mg twice
daily with food

▼ PoM **Orelox**® (Roussel)
Tablets, f/c, cefpodoxime 100 mg (as cefpodoxime
proxetil). Net price 10-tab pack = £9.26. Label: 5,
9, 21

CEFSULODIN

Indications: infections due to sensitive strains of
Ps. aeruginosa
Cautions; Contra-indications; Side-effects: see
under Cefaclor
*Dose: by intramuscular injection, or by slow intra-
venous injection, or by intravenous infusion*, 1–
4 g daily in 2–4 divided doses increased in severe
infections (e.g. severe pneumonia, osteomyelitis)
to 6 g daily or more; CHILD 20–50 mg/kg daily
Urinary-tract infections and chronic bronchitis,
1–3 g daily in 2–4 divided doses

PoM **Monaspor**® (Ciba)
Injection, powder for reconstitution, cefsulodin (as
sodium salt). Net price 1-g vial = £11.30
Electrolytes: Na⁺ 1.8 mmol/g

CEFTAZIDIME

Indications: see under Cefaclor; see also notes
above
Cautions; Contra-indications; Side-effects: see
under Cefaclor
*Dose: by deep intramuscular injection or intra-
venous injection or infusion*, 1 g every 8 hours *or*
2 g every 12 hours; 2 g every 8–12 hours in severe
infections; single doses over 1 g intravenous route
only; elderly usual max. 3 g daily; CHILD, up to 2
months 25–60 mg/kg daily in 2 divided doses,
over 2 months 30–100 mg/kg daily in 2–3 divided
doses; up to 150 mg/kg daily (max. 6 g daily) in 3
divided doses if immunocompromised or meningitis; intravenous route recommended for children
Urinary-tract and less serious infections, 0.5–1 g
every 12 hours
Pseudomonal lung infection in cystic fibrosis,
ADULT with normal renal function 100–150 mg/
kg daily in 3 divided doses; CHILD up to 150 mg/
kg daily (max. 6 g daily) in 3 divided doses; intravenous route recommended for children
Surgical prophylaxis, prostatic surgery, 1 g at
induction of anaesthesia repeated if necessary
when catheter removed

PoM **Fortum**® (Glaxo)
Injection, powder for reconstitution, ceftazidime
(as pentahydrate), with sodium carbonate, net
price 250-mg vial = £2.48, 500-mg vial = £4.95,
1-g vial = £9.90, 2-g vial (for injection and for
infusion, both) = £19.80, 3-g vial (for injection or
infusion) = £29.00; *infusion kit*, 2-g vial, 50-mL
bag sodium chloride intravenous infusion, transfer needle, swab, sealing cap, and label, complete
kit = £20.82
Electrolytes: Na⁺ 2.3 mmol/g

PoM **Kefadim**® (Lilly)

Injection, powder for reconstitution, ceftazidime (as pentahydrate), with sodium carbonate, net price 500-mg vial = £4.95, 1-g vial = £9.90, 2-g vial (for injection and for infusion, both) = £19.80
Electrolytes: Na⁺ 2.3 mmol/g

CEFTIBUTEN

Indications: see under Cefaclor and notes above
Cautions; Contra-indications; Side-effects: see under Cefaclor
Dose: ADULT and CHILD over 10 years (over 45 kg) 400 mg daily as a single dose; CHILD over 6 months 9 mg/kg daily as a single dose

▼ PoM **Cedax**® (Schering-Plough)

Capsules, ceftibuten (as dihydrate) 400 mg, net price 5-cap pack = £13.03, 7-cap pack = £17.50. Label: 9
Oral suspension, ceftibuten (as dihydrate) for reconstitution with water, 90 mg/5 mL, net price 60 mL = £7.63; 180 mg/5 mL, 60 mL = £15.26. Label: 9

CEFTIZOXIME

Indications: see under Cefaclor; see also notes above
Cautions; Contra-indications; Side-effects: see under Cefaclor
Dose: by deep intramuscular or slow intravenous injection or by intravenous infusion, 1–2 g every 8–12 hours increased in severe infections up to 8 g daily, in 3 divided doses; CHILD over 3 months 30–60 mg/kg daily in 2–4 divided doses, increased to 100–150 mg/kg daily for severe infections
Gonorrhoea, *by intramuscular injection,* 1 g as a single dose
Urinary-tract infections, *by deep intramuscular or slow intravenous injection or by infusion,* 0.5–1 g every 12 hours

PoM **Cefizox**® (Wellcome)

Injection, powder for reconstitution, ceftizoxime (as sodium salt). Net price 500-mg vial = £2.76; 1-g vial = £5.50; 2-g vial = £11.00
Electrolytes: Na⁺ 2.6 mmol/g

CEFTRIAXONE

Indications: see under Cefaclor and notes above; surgical prophylaxis
Cautions; Contra-indications; Side-effects: see under Cefaclor; also caution in hepatic impairment if accompanied by renal impairment; may displace plasma bilirubin—contra-indicated in infants under 6 weeks; calcium ceftriaxone may appear as a precipitate in urine or as gallstones

Dose: by intramuscular injection, or by intravenous injection over 2–4 minutes, *or by intravenous infusion,* 1 g daily as a single dose; 2–4 g daily as a single dose in severe infections; intramuscular doses over 1 g divided between more than one site
CHILD over 6 weeks 20–50 mg/kg daily as a single dose; up to 80 mg/kg as a single dose in severe infections; doses over 50 mg/kg by intravenous infusion only
Uncomplicated gonorrhoea, *by intramuscular injection,* 250 mg
Surgical prophylaxis, *by intramuscular injection or by intravenous injection* over 2–4 minutes, 1 g as a single dose; colorectal surgery, *by intramuscular or by intravenous injection* over 2–4 minutes *or by intravenous infusion,* 2 g; intramuscular doses over 1 g divided between more than one site
Prophylaxis of meningococcal meningitis, section 5.1 (table 2)

▼ PoM **Rocephin**® (Roche)

Injection, powder for reconstitution, ceftriaxone (as sodium salt), net price 250-mg vial = £2.87; 1-g vial = £11.46; 2-g vial = £22.92
Electrolytes: Na⁺ 3.6 mmol/g

CEFUROXIME

Indications: see under Cefaclor; surgical prophylaxis; more active against *Haemophilus influenzae* and *Neisseria gonorrhoeae*
Cautions; Contra-indications; Side-effects: see under Cefaclor
Dose: by mouth (as cefuroxime axetil), 250 mg twice daily in most infections including mild to moderate lower respiratory-tract infections (e.g. bronchitis); doubled for more severe lower respiratory-tract infections or if pneumonia suspected
Urinary-tract infection, 125 mg twice daily, doubled in pyelonephritis
Gonorrhoea, 1 g as a single dose
CHILD over 3 months, 125 mg twice daily, if necessary doubled in child over 2 years with otitis media
By intramuscular injection or intravenous injection or infusion, 750 mg every 6–8 hours; 1.5 g every 6–8 hours in severe infections; single doses over 750 mg intravenous route only
CHILD usual dose 60 mg/kg daily (range 30–100 mg/kg daily) in 3–4 divided doses (2–3 divided doses in neonates)
Gonorrhoea, 1.5 g as a single dose by intramuscular injection (divided between 2 sites)
Surgical prophylaxis, 1.5 g by intravenous injection at induction; may be supplemented with 750 mg intramuscularly 8 and 16 hours later (abdominal, pelvic, and orthopaedic operations) *or* followed by 750 mg intramuscularly every 8 hours for further 24–48 hours (cardiac, pulmonary, oesophageal, and vascular operations)
Meningitis, 3 g intravenously every 8 hours; CHILD, 200–240 mg/kg daily (in 3–4 divided doses) reduced to 100 mg/kg daily after 3 days or on clinical improvement; NEONATE, 100 mg/kg daily reduced to 50 mg/kg daily

---

Abbreviations and symbols, see inside front cover

PoM **Zinacef**® (Glaxo)

Injection, powder for reconstitution, cefuroxime (as sodium salt). Net price 250-mg vial = 88p; 750-mg vial = £2.64; 1.5-g vial (for injection and for infusion) = £5.29; *infusion kit*, 750-mg vial, 50-mL bag sodium chloride intravenous infusion, transfer needle, swab, sealing cap, and label, complete kit = £3.67; *Zinacef/Metronidazole infusion kit*, 750-mg vial, 100-mL bag metronidazole 5 mg/mL, transfer needle, swab, sealing cap and label, complete kit = £3.77

Electrolytes: Na+ 1.8 mmol/750-mg vial

PoM **Zinnat**® (Glaxo)

Tablets, both f/c, cefuroxime 125 mg (as cefuroxime axetil), net price 14-tab pack = £4.73; 250 mg, 14-tab pack = £9.45. Label: 9, 21, 25

Suspension, cefuroxime (as cefuroxime axetil) 125 mg/5 mL when reconstituted with water. Net price 70 mL = £5.40. Label: 9, 21

Sachets, cefuroxime (as cefuroxime axetil) 125 mg/sachet, net price 14-sachet pack = £5.40. Label: 9, 13, 21

CEPHALEXIN
(Cefalexin)

Indications: see under Cefaclor

Cautions; Contra-indications; Side-effects: see under Cefaclor

Dose: 250 mg every 6 hours *or* 500 mg every 8–12 hours increased to 1–1.5 g every 6–8 hours for severe infections; CHILD, 25 mg/kg daily in divided doses, doubled for severe infections, max. 100 mg/kg daily; *or* under 1 year, 125 mg every 12 hours; 1–5 years, 125 mg every 8 hours; 6–12 years, 250 mg every 8 hours

PoM **Cephalexin** (Non-proprietary)

Capsules, cephalexin 250 mg, net price 20 = £2.34; 500 mg, 20 = £4.53. Label: 9

Available from APS, Berk, Hillcross

Tablets, cephalexin 250 mg, net price 20 = £2.44; 500 mg, 20 = £4.54. Label: 9

Available from APS, Berk, Hillcross, Norton

Oral suspension, cephalexin for reconstitution with water, 125 mg/5 mL, net price 100 mL = £1.27; 250 mg/5 mL, 100 mL = £2.55. Label: 9

Available from APS, Berk, Hillcross

PoM **Ceporex**® (Glaxo)

Capsules, both caramel/grey, cephalexin 250 mg, net price 28-cap pack = £4.47; 500 mg, 28-cap pack = £9.56. Label: 9

Tablets, all pink, f/c, cephalexin 250 mg, net price 28-tab pack = £4.47; 500 mg, 28-tab pack = £8.72; 1 g (scored), 14-tab pack = £8.72. Label: 9

Paediatric drops, orange, cephalexin 125 mg/1.25 mL when reconstituted with water. Net price 10 mL = £1.52. Label: 9, counselling, use of pipette

Syrup, all orange, cephalexin for reconstitution with water, 125 mg/5 mL, net price 100 mL = £1.59; 250 mg/5 mL, 100 mL = £3.19; 500 mg/5 mL, 100 mL = £6.19. Label: 9

PoM **Keflex**® (Lilly)

Capsules, cephalexin 250 mg (green/white), net price 28-cap pack = £3.57; 500 mg (pale green/dark green), 28-cap pack = £6.97. Label: 9

Tablets, both peach, cephalexin 250 mg, net price 28-tab pack = £3.57; 500 mg (scored), 28-tab pack = £6.97. Label: 9

Suspension, cephalexin for reconstitution with water, 125 mg/5 mL (pink), net price 100 mL = £1.27; 250 mg/5 mL (orange), 100 mL = £2.55. Label: 9

CEPHAMANDOLE
(Cefamandole)

Indications: see under Cefaclor; surgical prophylaxis

Cautions; Contra-indications; Side-effects: see under Cefaclor

Dose: by deep intramuscular injection or intravenous injection over 3–5 minutes or by intravenous infusion, 0.5–2 g every 4–8 hours; CHILD over 1 month, 50–100 mg/kg daily in 3–6 divided doses increased to 150 mg/kg daily for severe infections

Surgical prophylaxis, *by intramuscular or intravenous injection*, 1–2 g 30–60 minutes before surgery followed by 1–2 g every 6 hours for 24–48 hours (up to 72 hours for implantation of prostheses)

PoM **Kefadol**® (Dista)

Injection, powder for reconstitution, cephamandole (as nafate) with sodium carbonate. Net price 1-g vial = £3.91

Electrolytes: Na+ 1.19 mmol/1-g vial

CEPHAZOLIN
(Cefazolin)

Indications: see under Cefaclor; surgical prophylaxis

Cautions; Contra-indications; Side-effects: see under Cefaclor

Dose: by intramuscular injection or intravenous injection or infusion, 0.5–1 g every 6–12 hours; CHILD, 25–50 mg/kg daily (in divided doses), increased to 100 mg/kg daily in severe infections

PoM **Kefzol**® (Lilly)

Injection, powder for reconstitution, cephazolin (as sodium salt). Net price 500-mg vial = £2.45; 1-g vial = £4.63

Electrolytes: Na+ 2.1 mmol/g

CEPHRADINE
(Cefradine)

Indications: see under Cefaclor; surgical prophylaxis

Cautions; Contra-indications; Side-effects: see under Cefaclor

Dose: by mouth, 250–500 mg every 6 hours *or* 0.5–1 g every 12 hours; CHILD, 25–50 mg/kg daily in divided doses

By intramuscular injection or intravenous injection or infusion, 0.5–1 g every 6 hours, increased to 8 g daily in severe infections; CHILD 50–100 mg/kg daily in 4 divided doses

PoM Velosef® (Squibb)

Capsules, cephradine 250 mg (orange/blue), net price 20-cap pack = £3.55; 500 mg, 20-cap pack = £7.00. Label: 9

Syrup, cephradine 250 mg/5 mL when reconstituted with water. Net price 100 mL = £4.22. Label: 9

Injection, powder for reconstitution, cephradine. Net price 500-mg vial = 99p; 1-g vial = £1.95

OTHER BETA-LACTAM ANTIBIOTICS

Aztreonam is a monocyclic beta-lactam ('monobactam') antibiotic with an antibacterial spectrum limited to Gram-negative aerobic bacteria including *Pseudomonas aeruginosa*, *Neisseria meningitidis*, and *Haemophilus influenzae*; it should not be used alone for 'blind' treatment since it is not active against Gram-positive organisms. Aztreonam is also effective against *Neisseria gonorrhoeae* (but not against concurrent chlamydial infection). Side-effects are similar to those of the other beta-lactams although aztreonam may be less likely to cause hypersensitivity in penicillin-sensitive patients.

Imipenem, a carbapenem, is the first thienamycin beta-lactam antibiotic; it has a broad spectrum of activity which includes many aerobic and anaerobic Gram-positive and Gram-negative bacteria. Imipenem is partially inactivated in the kidney by enzymatic activity and is therefore administered in combination with **cilastatin**, a specific enzyme inhibitor, which blocks its renal metabolism. Side-effects are similar to those of other beta-lactam antibiotics; neurotoxicity has been observed at very high dosage or in renal failure.

AZTREONAM

Indications: Gram-negative infections including *Pseudomonas aeruginosa*, *Haemophilus influenzae*, and *Neisseria meningitidis*

Cautions: hypersensitivity to beta-lactam antibiotics; hepatic impairment; reduce dose in renal impairment; **interactions:** Appendix 1 (aztreonam)

Contra-indications: aztreonam hypersensitivity; pregnancy and breast-feeding

Side-effects: nausea, vomiting, diarrhoea, abdominal cramps; mouth ulcers, altered taste; jaundice and hepatitis; blood disorders (including thrombocytopenia and neutropenia); urticaria and rashes

Dose: by intramuscular injection or intravenous injection or infusion, 1 g every 8 hours *or* 2 g every 12 hours; 2 g every 6–8 hours for severe infections (including systemic *Pseudomonas aeruginosa* and lung infections in cystic fibrosis); single doses over 1 g intravenous route only

CHILD over 1 week, *by intravenous injection or infusion*, 30 mg/kg every 6–8 hours increased in severe infections for child of 2 years or older to 50 mg/kg every 6–8 hours; max. 8 g daily

Urinary-tract infections, 0.5–1 g every 8–12 hours

Gonorrhoea/cystitis, *by intramuscular injection*, 1 g as a single dose

PoM Azactam® (Squibb)

Injection, powder for reconstitution, aztreonam. Net price 500-mg vial = £4.48; 1-g vial = £8.95; 2-g vial = £17.90

IMIPENEM WITH CILASTATIN

Indications: aerobic and anaerobic Gram-positive and Gram-negative infections; surgical prophylaxis; not indicated for CNS infections

Cautions: hypersensitivity to penicillins, cephalosporins and other beta-lactam antibiotics; renal impairment; CNS disorders (e.g. epilepsy); pregnancy

Contra-indications: hypersensitivity to imipenem or cilastatin; breast-feeding

Side-effects: nausea, vomiting, diarrhoea (pseudomembranous colitis reported), taste disturbances; blood disorders, positive Coombs test; allergic reactions (with rash, pruritus, urticaria, fever, anaphylactic reactions, rarely toxic epidermal necrolysis); myoclonic activity, convulsions, confusion and mental disturbances reported; slight increases in liver enzymes and bilirubin reported; increases in serum creatinine and blood urea; red coloration of urine in children reported; local reactions: erythema, pain and induration, and thrombophlebitis

Dose: by deep intramuscular injection, mild to moderate infections, in terms of imipenem, 500–750 mg every 12 hours; gonococcal urethritis or cervicitis, 500 mg as a single dose

By intravenous infusion, in terms of imipenem, 1–2 g daily in 3–4 divided doses; less sensitive organisms, up to 50 mg/kg daily (to max. 4 g daily); CHILD 3 months and older, 60 mg/kg (up to max. of 2 g) daily in 4 divided doses

Surgical prophylaxis, *by intravenous infusion*, 1 g at induction of anaesthesia repeated after 3 hours, supplemented in high risk (e.g. colorectal) surgery by doses of 500 mg 8 and 16 hours after induction

PoM Primaxin® (MSD)

Intramuscular injection, powder for reconstitution, imipenem (as monohydrate) 500 mg with cilastatin (as sodium salt) 500 mg. Net price 15-mL vial = £15.00

Electrolytes: Na⁺ 1.47 mmol/vial

Intravenous infusion, powder for reconstitution, imipenem (as monohydrate) 250 mg with cilastatin (as sodium salt) 250 mg. Net price 60-mL vial = £9.00

Electrolytes: Na⁺ 0.86 mmol/vial

Intravenous infusion, powder for reconstitution, imipenem (as monohydrate) 500 mg with cilastatin (as sodium salt) 500 mg. Net price 120-mL vial = £15.00

Electrolytes: Na⁺ 1.72 mmol/vial

5.1.3   Tetracyclines

The tetracyclines are broad-spectrum antibiotics whose value has decreased owing to increasing bacterial resistance. They remain, however, the treatment of choice for infections caused by chlamydia (trachoma, psittacosis, salpingitis, urethritis, and lymphogranuloma venereum), rickettsia (including Q-fever), mycoplasma (respiratory and genital infections), brucella (doxycycline with rifampicin), and the spirochaete, *Borrelia burgdorferi* (Lyme disease). They are also used in acne, in destructive (refractory) periodontal disease, in exacerbations of chronic bronchitis (because of their activity against *Haemophilus influenzae*), and for leptospirosis in penicillin hypersensitivity (as an alternative to erythromycin).

Microbiologically, there is little to choose between the various tetracyclines, the only exception being **minocycline** which has a broader spectrum, is active against *Neisseria meningitidis* and has been used for meningococcal prophylaxis; however it may cause dizziness and vertigo.

The tetracyclines are deposited in growing bone and teeth (being bound to calcium) causing staining and occasionally dental hypoplasia, and should **not** be given to children under 12 years or to pregnant women. With the exception of **doxycycline** and **minocycline** the tetracyclines may exacerbate renal failure and should **not** be given to patients with kidney disease. Absorption of tetracyclines is decreased by milk (except doxycycline and minocycline), antacids, and calcium, iron and magnesium salts.

TETRACYCLINE

Indications: exacerbations of chronic bronchitis; brucellosis (see also notes above), chlamydia, mycoplasma, and rickettsia; pleural effusions due to malignancy or cirrhosis; acne vulgaris (see section 13.6)

Cautions: hepatic impairment (avoid intravenous administration); renal impairment (avoid if severe); rarely causes photosensitivity; **interactions:** Appendix 1 (tetracyclines)

Contra-indications: severe renal impairment, pregnancy and breast-feeding (see also Appendices 4 and 5), children under 12 years of age, systemic lupus erythematosus

Side-effects: nausea, vomiting, diarrhoea; erythema (discontinue treatment); headache and visual disturbances may indicate benign intracranial hypertension; pancreatitis and pseudomembranous colitis reported

Dose: by mouth, 250 mg every 6 hours, increased in severe infections to 500 mg every 6–8 hours
Acne, see section 13.6
Primary, secondary, or latent syphilis, 500 mg every 6 hours for 15 days
Non-gonococcal urethritis, 500 mg every 6 hours for 7–14 days (21 days if failure or relapse following the first course)

By intravenous infusion, 500 mg every 12 hours; max. 2 g daily
Pleural effusions, see under Achromycin® intravenous infusion

COUNSELLING. Tablets or capsules should be swallowed whole with plenty of fluid while sitting or standing

PoM Tetracycline (Non-proprietary)
Tablets, coated, tetracycline hydrochloride 250 mg. Net price 20 = 29p. Label: 7, 9, 23, counselling, posture, see above

PoM Achromycin® (Lederle)
Capsules, orange, tetracycline hydrochloride 250 mg. Net price 20 = 92p. Label: 7, 9, 23, counselling, posture, see above
Tablets, orange, f/c, tetracycline hydrochloride 250 mg. Net price 20 = 66p. Label: 7, 9, 23, counselling, posture, see above
Intravenous infusion, powder for reconstitution, tetracycline hydrochloride. Net price 250-mg vial = £1.24; 500-mg vial = £1.98
Dose: infections, see above
Recurrent pleural effusions, by intrapleural instillation, 500 mg in 30–50 mL sodium chloride intravenous infusion 0.9%

PoM Sustamycin® (Boehringer Mannheim)
Capsules, m/r, light blue/dark blue, tetracycline hydrochloride 250 mg. Net price 20 = £2.07. Label: 7, 9, 23, 25
Dose: 2 capsules initially, then 1 every 12 hours

PoM Tetrabid-Organon® (Organon)
Capsules, m/r, purple/yellow, tetracycline hydrochloride 250 mg. Net price 20 = £1.73. Label: 7, 9, 23, 25
Dose: 2 capsules initially, then 1 every 12 hours; acne, 1 daily

PoM Tetrachel® (Berk)
Capsules, orange, tetracycline hydrochloride 250 mg. Net price 20 = 49p. Label: 7, 9, 23, counselling, posture, see above
Tablets, orange, f/c, tetracycline hydrochloride 250 mg. Net price 20 = 34p. Label: 7, 9, 23, counselling, posture, see above

Compound preparations
PoM Deteclo® (Lederle)
Tablets, blue, f/c, tetracycline hydrochloride 115.4 mg, chlortetracycline hydrochloride 115.4 mg, demeclocycline hydrochloride 69.2 mg. Net price 20 = £2.48. Label: 7, 9, 11, 23, counselling, posture, see above
Dose: 1 tablet every 12 hours; 3–4 tablets daily in more severe infections

PoM Mysteclin® (Squibb)
Tablets, orange, s/c, tetracycline hydrochloride 250 mg, nystatin 250 000 units. Net price 20 = £1.34. Label: 7, 9, 23, counselling, posture, see above

DEMECLOCYCLINE HYDROCHLORIDE

Indications: see under Tetracycline; also inappropriate secretion of antidiuretic hormone, section 6.5.2

Cautions; Contra-indications; Side-effects: see under Tetracycline, but photosensitivity is more common

Dose: 150 mg every 6 hours *or* 300 mg every 12 hours

PoM Ledermycin® (Lederle)
Capsules, red, demeclocycline hydrochloride 150 mg. Net price 20 = £4.13. Label: 7, 9, 11, 23

DOXYCYCLINE

Indications: see under Tetracycline; brucellosis (with rifampicin); also chronic prostatitis and sinusitis; pelvic inflammatory disease (with metronidazole, section 5.1, table 1)

Cautions; Contra-indications; Side-effects: see under Tetracycline, but may be used in renal impairment; avoid in porphyria (see section 9.8.2)

Dose: 200 mg on first day, then 100 mg daily; severe infections (including chronic urinary-tract infections), 200 mg daily

Acne, 50 mg daily for 6–12 weeks or longer

COUNSELLING. Capsules should be swallowed whole with plenty of fluid during meals while sitting or standing

PoM **Doxycycline** (Non-proprietary)
Capsules, doxycycline 100 mg (as hydrochloride). Net price 20 = £7.24. Label: 6, 9, 11, 27, counselling, posture, see above
Available from APS, Ashbourne (Demix®), Berk (Cyclodox®), Hillcross, ISIS (Ramysis®), K Pharm., Lagap (Doxylar®), Norton

PoM **Nordox®** (Panpharma)
Capsules, green, doxycycline 100 mg (as hydrochloride). Net price 10-cap pack = £4.66. Label: 6, 9, 11, 27, counselling, posture, see above

PoM **Vibramycin®** (Invicta)
Capsules, doxycycline (as hydrochloride) 50 mg (green/ivory), net price 28-cap pack = £7.74; 100 mg (green), 8-cap pack = £4.18. Label: 6, 9, 11, 27, counselling, posture, see above

PoM **Vibramycin-D®** (Invicta)
Dispersible tablets, off-white, doxycycline 100 mg. Net price 8-tab pack = £4.91. Label: 6, 9, 11, 13

LYMECYCLINE

Indications; Cautions; Contra-indications; Side-effects: see under Tetracycline
Dose: 408 mg every 12 hours

PoM **Tetralysal 300®** (Pharmacia)
Capsules, lymecycline 408 mg (≡ tetracycline 300 mg). Net price 20-cap pack = £2.96. Label: 6, 9

MINOCYCLINE

Indications: see under Tetracycline; also meningococcal carrier state

Cautions; Contra-indications: see under Tetracycline, but may be used in renal impairment

Side-effects: see under Tetracycline; also dizziness and vertigo (more common in women); severe exfoliative rashes, pigmentation (sometimes irreversible), and liver damage reported

Dose: 100 mg twice daily

Acne, 50 mg twice daily for minimum course of 6 weeks

PoM **Minocycline** (Non-proprietary)
Capsules, minocycline (as hydrochloride) 50 mg, net price 56-cap pack = £17.20; 100 mg, 28-cap pack = £14.74. Label: 6, 9
Available from Merck (Aknemin®)

Tablets, minocycline (as hydrochloride) 50 mg, net price 84-tab pack = £26.34; 100 mg, 20 = £12.83. Label: 6, 9
Available from APS, Ashbourne (Blemix®), Hillcross, K Pharm., Lederle (Minocin®), Norton

PoM **Minocin MR®** (Lederle)
Capsules, m/r, yellow/brown (enclosing yellow and orange pellets), minocycline (as hydrochloride) 100 mg. Net price 49-cap pack = £26.99. Label: 6, 25
Dose: acne, 1 capsule daily

OXYTETRACYCLINE

Indications; Cautions; Contra-indications; Side-effects: see under Tetracycline; avoid in porphyria (see section 9.8.2)
Dose: 250–500 mg every 6 hours

PoM **Oxytetracycline** (Non-proprietary)
Tablets, coated, oxytetracycline dihydrate 250 mg, net price 20 = 25p. Label: 7, 9, 23
Available from APS, Ashbourne (Oxytetramix®), Berk (Berkmycen®, contain tartrazine), Cox, CP, DDSA (Oxymycin®), K Pharm., Norton

PoM **Terramycin®** (Pfizer)
Capsules, yellow, oxytetracycline 250 mg (as hydrochloride). Net price 28-cap pack = 96p. Label: 7, 9, 23
Tablets, yellow, s/c, oxytetracycline 250 mg (as dihydrate). Net price 28-tab pack = 96p. Label: 7, 9, 23

5.1.4 Aminoglycosides

These include amikacin, gentamicin, kanamycin, neomycin, netilmicin, streptomycin, and tobramycin. All are bactericidal and active against some Gram-positive and many Gram-negative organisms. Amikacin, gentamicin, and tobramycin are also active against *Pseudomonas aeruginosa*; streptomycin is active against *Mycobacterium tuberculosis* and is now almost entirely reserved for tuberculosis (section 5.1.9).

The aminoglycosides are not absorbed from the gut (although there is a risk of absorption in inflammatory bowel disease and liver failure) and must therefore be given by injection for systemic infections.

Excretion is principally via the kidney and accumulation occurs in renal impairment.

Most side-effects of this group of antibiotics are dose-related therefore care must be taken with dosage and whenever possible treatment should not exceed 7 days. The important side-effects are ototoxicity, and to a lesser degree nephrotoxicity; they occur most commonly in the elderly and in patients with renal failure.

If there is impairment of renal function (or high pre-dose plasma concentrations) the interval between doses must be increased; if the renal impairment is severe the dose itself should be reduced as well.

Aminoglycosides may impair neuromuscular transmission and should not be given to patients with myasthenia gravis; large doses given during surgery have been responsible for a transient myasthenic syndrome in patients with normal neuromuscular function.

Aminoglycosides should not be given with potentially ototoxic diuretics (e.g. frusemide and ethacrynic acid); if concurrent use is unavoidable administration of the aminoglycoside and of the diuretic should be separated by as long a period as practicable.

PLASMA CONCENTRATIONS. Plasma concentration monitoring avoids both excessive and subtherapeutic concentrations thus preventing toxicity and ensuring efficacy. Concentrations should be measured approximately 1 hour after intramuscular or intravenous administration and also just before the next dose.

If possible plasma aminoglycoside concentrations should be measured in all patients and **must** be determined in *infants*, in *elderly*, in *obesity*, and in *cystic fibrosis, or* if *high doses* are being given, *or* if there is *renal impairment, or* if treatment lasts *longer than 7 days.*

ONCE DAILY DOSAGE. Although aminoglycosides are generally given in 2–3 divided doses during the 24 hours, it has been suggested that *once daily administration* can reduce the risk of toxicity (while ensuring adequate plasma concentrations) but **expert advice** about dosage and plasma concentrations should be obtained.

Gentamicin is the most important of the aminoglycosides and is widely used for the treatment of serious infections. It is the aminoglycoside of choice in the UK. It has a broad spectrum but is inactive against anaerobes and has poor activity against haemolytic streptococci and pneumococci. When used for the 'blind' therapy of undiagnosed serious infections it is usually given in conjunction with a penicillin and/or metronidazole.

The daily dose is up to 5 mg/kg given in divided doses every 8 hours (if renal function is normal); whenever possible treatment should not exceed 7 days. Higher doses are occasionally indicated for serious infections, especially in the neonate or the compromised host. A lower dose of 80 mg twice daily (60 mg for lighter or elderly patients) in association with benzylpenicillin is sufficient for endocarditis due to oral streptococci (often termed *Streptococcus viridans*) and gut streptococci.

Amikacin is a derivative of kanamycin and has one important advantage over gentamicin in that it is stable to 8 of the 9 classified aminoglycoside-inactivating enzymes whereas gentamicin is inactivated by 5. It is principally indicated for the treatment of serious infections caused by Gram-negative bacilli resistant to gentamicin.

Kanamycin has been superseded by other aminoglycosides.

Netilmicin has similar activity to gentamicin, but may cause less ototoxicity in those needing treatment for longer than 10 days. Netilmicin is active against a number of gentamicin-resistant Gram-negative bacilli but is less active against *Ps. aeruginosa* than gentamicin or tobramycin.

Tobramycin is similar to gentamicin. It is slightly more active against *Ps. aeruginosa* but shows less activity against certain other Gram-negative bacteria.

Neomycin is too toxic for parenteral administration and can only be used for infections of the skin or mucous membranes or to reduce the bacterial population of the colon prior to bowel surgery or in hepatic failure. Oral administration may lead to malabsorption. Small amounts of neomycin may be absorbed from the gut in patients with hepatic failure and, as these patients may also be uraemic, cumulation may occur with resultant ototoxicity.

PREGNANCY. Where possible, the aminoglycosides should be avoided in pregnancy as they cross the placenta and can cause fetal eighth nerve damage.

GENTAMICIN

Indications: septicaemia and neonatal sepsis; meningitis and other CNS infections; biliary-tract infection, acute pyelonephritis or prostatitis, endocarditis caused by *Strep. viridans* or *Strep. faecalis* (with a penicillin); pneumonia in hospital patients, adjunct in listerial meningitis (section 5.1, table 1)

Cautions: renal impairment, infants and elderly (adjust dose and monitor renal, auditory and vestibular function together with plasma gentamicin concentrations); avoid prolonged use; see also notes above; **interactions:** Appendix 1 (aminoglycosides)

Contra-indications: pregnancy, myasthenia gravis

Side-effects: vestibular and auditory damage, nephrotoxicity; rarely, hypomagnesaemia on prolonged therapy, pseudomembranous colitis; see also notes above

Dose: by *intramuscular or by slow intravenous injection* over at least 3 minutes *or by intravenous infusion*, 2–5 mg/kg daily (in divided doses every 8 hours), see also notes above; reduce dose and measure plasma concentrations in renal impairment

CHILD up to 2 weeks, 3 mg/kg every 12 hours; 2 weeks–12 years, 2 mg/kg every 8 hours

By intrathecal injection, 1 mg daily (increased if necessary to 5 mg daily), with 2–4 mg/kg daily *by intramuscular injection* (in divided doses every 8 hours)

Endocarditis prophylaxis, section 5.1, table 2

Note. One-hour ('peak') concentration should not exceed 10 mg/litre; pre-dose ('trough') concentration should be less than 2 mg/litre

PoM Gentamicin (Non-proprietary)

Injection, gentamicin (as sulphate), net price 10 mg/mL, 1-mL amp = 50p; 40 mg/mL, 1-mL amp = £1.32, 2-mL amp = £1.81, 2-mL vial = £1.86
Available from David Bull

PoM **Cidomycin®** (Roussel)

Injection, gentamicin 40 mg (as sulphate)/mL. Net price 2-mL amp or vial = £1.55

Paediatric injection, gentamicin 10 mg (as sulphate)/mL. Net price 2-mL vial = 65p

Intrathecal injection, gentamicin 5 mg (as sulphate)/mL. Net price 1-mL amp = 77p

PoM **Genticin®** (Roche)

Injection, gentamicin 40 mg (as sulphate)/mL. Net price 2-mL amp = £1.58

PoM **Isotonic Gentamicin Injection** (Baxter)

Intravenous infusion, gentamicin 800 micrograms (as sulphate)/mL in sodium chloride intravenous infusion 0.9%. Net price 100-mL (80-mg) Viaflex® bag = £1.61

Electrolytes: Na⁺ 15.4 mmol/100-mL bag

AMIKACIN

Indications: serious Gram-negative infections resistant to gentamicin

Cautions; Contra-indications; Side-effects: see under Gentamicin

Dose: by intramuscular or by slow intravenous injection or by infusion, 15 mg/kg daily in 2 divided doses, see also notes above

Note. One-hour ('peak') concentration should not exceed 30 mg/litre; pre-dose ('trough') concentration should be less than 10 mg/litre

PoM **Amikin®** (Bristol-Myers)

Injection, amikacin 250 mg (as sulphate)/mL. Net price 2-mL vial = £10.14

Electrolytes: Na⁺ < 0.5 mmol/vial

Paediatric injection, amikacin 50 mg (as sulphate)/mL. Net price 2-mL vial = £2.36

Electrolytes: Na⁺ < 0.5 mmol/vial

KANAMYCIN

Indications: superseded by other aminoglycosides (see notes above)

Cautions; Contra-indications; Side-effects: see under Gentamicin

Dose: by intramuscular injection, 250 mg every 6 hours *or* 500 mg every 12 hours, see also notes above

By intravenous infusion, 15–30 mg/kg daily in divided doses every 8–12 hours, see also notes above

Note. One-hour ('peak') concentration should not exceed 30 mg/litre; pre-dose ('trough') concentration should be less than 10 mg/litre

PoM **Kannasyn®** (Sanofi Winthrop)

Powder (for preparing injections), kanamycin (as acid sulphate). Net price 1-g vial = £23.77

NEOMYCIN SULPHATE

Indications: bowel sterilisation prior to surgery, see also notes above

Cautions; Contra-indications; Side-effects: see under Gentamicin but too toxic for systemic use, see notes above; avoid in renal impairment

Dose: by mouth, bowel sterilisation, 1 g every 4 hours

PoM **Neomycin Elixir,** neomycin sulphate 100 mg/5 mL. Net price 100 mL = 69p

PoM **Mycifradin®** (Upjohn)

Tablets, neomycin sulphate 500 mg. Net price 20 = £3.60

PoM **Nivemycin®** (Boots)

Tablets, neomycin sulphate 500 mg. Net price 20 = £2.17

Elixir, neomycin sulphate 100 mg/5 mL. Net price 100 mL = 69p

NETILMICIN

Indications: serious Gram-negative infections resistant to gentamicin

Cautions; Contra-indications; Side-effects: see under Gentamicin

Dose: by intramuscular injection or by intravenous injection over 3–5 minutes or by intravenous infusion, 4–6 mg/kg daily, as a single daily dose or in divided doses every 8 or 12 hours; in severe infections, up to 7.5 mg/kg daily in divided doses every 8 hours (reduced as soon as clinically indicated, usually within 48 hours) NEONATE up to 1 · week, 3 mg/kg every 12 hours; INFANT over 1 week, 2.5–3 mg/kg every 8 hours; CHILD 2–2.5 mg/kg every 8 hours

Urinary-tract infection, 150 mg as a single daily dose for 5 days

Gonorrhoea, 300 mg as a single dose

Note. For divided daily dose regimens, one-hour ('peak') concentration should not exceed 12 mg/litre; pre-dose ('trough') concentration should be less than 2 mg/litre

PoM **Netillin®** (Schering-Plough)

Injection, netilmicin (as sulphate) 10 mg/mL, net price 1.5-mL (15-mg) amp = £1.49; 50 mg/mL, 1-mL (50-mg) amp = £2.21; 100 mg/mL, 1-mL (100-mg) amp = £2.88; 1.5-mL (150-mg) amp = £4.11, 2-mL (200-mg) amp = £5.33

TOBRAMYCIN

Indications: see under Gentamicin and notes above

Cautions; Contra-indications; Side-effects: see under Gentamicin

Dose: by intramuscular injection or by slow intravenous injection or by intravenous infusion, 3 mg/kg daily in divided doses every 8 hours, see also notes above; in severe infections up to 5 mg/kg daily in divided doses every 6–8 hours (reduced to 3 mg/kg as soon ,as clinically indicated); NEONATE 2 mg/kg every 12 hours; CHILD over 1 week 2–2.5 mg/kg every 8 hours

Urinary-tract infection, *by intramuscular injection,* 2–3 mg/kg daily as a single dose

Note. One-hour ('peak') concentration should not exceed 10 mg/litre; pre-dose ('trough') concentration should be less than 2 mg/litre

PoM **Nebcin®** (Lilly)

Injection, tobramycin (as sulphate) 10 mg/mL, net price 2-mL (20-mg) vial = £1.19; 40 mg/mL, 1-mL (40-mg) vial = £1.61, 2-mL (80-mg) vial = £2.89

5.1.5 Macrolides

Erythromycin has an antibacterial spectrum that is similar but not identical to that of penicillin; it is thus an alternative in penicillin-allergic patients.

Indications for erythromycin include respiratory infections, whooping-cough, legionnaires' disease, and campylobacter enteritis. It has activity against gut anaerobes and has been used with neomycin for prophylaxis before bowel surgery. It is active against many penicillin-resistant staphylococci but some are now also resistant to erythromycin. Erythromycin is also active against chlamydia and mycoplasmas.

Erythromycin causes nausea, vomiting, and diarrhoea in some patients; in mild to moderate infections this can be avoided by giving a lower dose (250 mg 4 times daily) but if a more serious infection, such as Legionella pneumonia, is suspected higher doses are needed.

Azithromycin is a new macrolide with slightly less activity than erythromycin against Gram-positive bacteria but enhanced activity against some Gram-negative organisms. Plasma concentrations are very low but tissue concentrations are much higher. It has a long tissue half-life and once daily dosage is recommended.

Clarithromycin is an erythromycin derivative with slightly greater activity than the parent compound. Tissue concentrations are higher than with erythromycin. It is given twice daily.

Azithromycin and clarithromycin cause fewer gastro-intestinal side-effects than erythromycin.

Spiramycin is also a macrolide (see section 5.4.7).

ERYTHROMYCIN

Indications: alternative to penicillin in hypersensitive patients; campylobacter enteritis, pneumonia, legionnaires' disease, syphilis, non-gonococcal urethritis, chronic prostatitis, acne vulgaris (see section 13.6); diphtheria and whooping cough prophylaxis

Cautions: hepatic and renal impairment; prolongation of QT interval (ventricular tachycardia reported); pregnancy and breast-feeding; **interactions:** Appendix 1 (erythromycin and other macrolides)

CSM Warning. Avoid concomitant administration with astemizole or terfenadine, see also p. 130 [other interactions, Appendix 1]

Contra-indications: porphyria (see section 9.8.2); estolate contra-indicated in liver disease

Side-effects: nausea, vomiting, abdominal discomfort, diarrhoea after large doses (pseudomembranous colitis reported); urticaria, rashes and other allergic reactions; reversible hearing loss also reported after large doses; if given for more than 14 days may occasionally cause cholestatic jaundice

Dose: by mouth, ADULT and CHILD over 8 years, 250–500 mg every 6 hours *or* 0.5–1 g every 12 hours (see notes above); up to 4 g daily in severe infections; CHILD up to 2 years 125 mg every 6 hours, 2–8 years 250 mg every 6 hours, doses doubled for severe infections

Acne, see section 13.6

Early syphilis, 500 mg 4 times daily for 14 days

By intravenous infusion, ADULT and CHILD severe infections, 50 mg/kg daily by continuous infusion *or* in divided doses every 6 hours; mild infections (oral treatment not possible), 25 mg/kg daily

PoM Erythromycin (Non-proprietary)
Tablets, e/c, erythromycin 250 mg, net price 20 = 79p; 500 mg, 20 = £1.66. Label: 5, 9, 25
Available from APS, Ashbourne (Rommix®), Berk (Erycen®), Cox, CP, K Pharm., Norton
Mixture, erythromycin (as ethyl succinate) 125 mg/5 mL, net price 100 mL = £1.14; 250 mg/5 mL, 100 mL = £1.73; 500 mg/5 mL, 100 mL = £3.88. Label: 9
Available from APS, Ashbourne (Rommix®), Berk, Cox, CP, K Pharm., Norton, RP Drugs (Arpimycin®)

PoM Erythromycin Lactobionate (Non-proprietary)
Intravenous infusion, powder for reconstitution, erythromycin (as lactobionate), net price 1-g vial = £9.98
Available from Abbott, David Bull

PoM Erymax® (Elan)
Capsules, opaque orange/clear orange, enclosing orange and white e/c pellets, erythromycin 250 mg. Net price 30-cap pack = £6.08. Label: 5, 9, 25
Dose: 1 every 6 hours *or* 2 every 12 hours; acne, 1 twice daily then 1 daily after 1 month

PoM Erythrocin® (Abbott)
Tablets, both f/c, erythromycin (as stearate), 250 mg, net price 20 = £2.60; 500 mg, 20 = £5.46. Label: 9

PoM Erythromid® (Abbott)
Tablets, both orange, e/c, f/c, erythromycin 250 mg, net price 20 = 84p; 500 mg (*Erythromid DS®*), 20 = £1.89. Label: 5, 9, 25

PoM Erythroped® (Abbott)
Suspension, erythromycin (as ethyl succinate) for reconstitution with water, 125 mg/5 mL (*Suspension PI*), net price 140 mL = £2.60; 250 mg/5 mL, 140 mL = £4.92; 500 mg/5 mL (*Suspension forte*), 140 mL = £8.73. Label: 9
Suspension SF, sugar-free, erythromycin (as ethyl succinate) for reconstitution with water, 125 mg/5 mL (*Suspension PI SF*), net price 140 mL = £2.68; 250 mg/5 mL, 140 mL = £5.22. Label: 9
Granules, erythromycin (as ethyl succinate), 125 mg/sachet (*Granules PI*), net price 28-sachet pack = £3.65; 250 mg/sachet, 28-sachet pack = £6.15; 500 mg/sachet (*Granules forte*), 28-sachet pack = £9.95. Label: 9, 13

PoM Erythroped A® (Abbott)
Tablets, yellow, f/c, erythromycin 500 mg (as ethyl succinate). Net price 28-tab pack = £7.88. Label: 9
Granules, erythromycin 1 g (as ethyl succinate)/sachet. Net price 14-sachet pack = £9.15. Label: 9, 13

PoM Ilosone® (Dista)

Capsules, ivory/red, erythromycin 250 mg (as estolate). Net price 20 = £5.71. Label: 9

Tablets, pink, erythromycin 500 mg (as estolate). Net price 12-tab pack = £6.82. Label: 9

Suspension, both orange, erythromycin (as estolate) 125 mg/5 mL, net price 100 mL = £3.45; 250 mg/5 mL (*Suspension forte*), 100 mL = £6.72. Label: 9

AZITHROMYCIN

Indications: respiratory-tract infections; otitis media; skin and soft-tissue infections; uncomplicated genital chlamydial infections

Cautions; Side-effects: see under Erythromycin; caution in pregnancy and breast-feeding; mild neutropenia reported; **interactions:** Appendix 1 (erythromycin and other macrolides)

CSM Warning. Avoid concomitant administration with astemizole or terfenadine, see also p. 130 [other interactions, Appendix 1]

Contra-indications: hepatic impairment

Dose: 500 mg once daily for 3 days; CHILD over 6 months 10 mg/kg once daily for 3 days; *or* bodyweight 15–25 kg, 200 mg once daily for 3 days; body-weight 26–35 kg, 300 mg once daily for 3 days; body-weight 36–45 kg, 400 mg once daily for 3 days

Genital chlamydial infections, 1 g as a single dose

PoM Zithromax® (Richborough)

Capsules, azithromycin (as dihydrate) 250 mg. Net price 4-cap pack = £8.95, 6-cap pack = £13.43. Label: 5, 9, 23

Oral suspension, azithromycin (as dihydrate) 200 mg/5 mL when reconstituted with water. Net price 15-mL pack = £5.08, 22.5-mL pack = £7.62, 30-mL pack = £13.80. Label: 5, 9, 23

CLARITHROMYCIN

Indications: respiratory-tract infections, mild to moderate skin and soft tissue infections

Cautions; Side-effects: see under Erythromycin; reduce dose in renal impairment; caution in pregnancy and breast-feeding; also reported, headache, taste disturbances, stomatitis, glossitis, and raised liver enzymes; on intravenous infusion, local tenderness, phlebitis; **interactions:** Appendix 1 (erythromycin and other macrolides)

CSM Warning. Avoid concomitant administration with astemizole or terfenadine, see also p. 130 [other interactions, Appendix 1]

Dose: by mouth, 250 mg every 12 hours for 7 days, increased in severe infections to 500 mg every 12 hours for up to 14 days; CHILD body-weight under 8 kg, 7.5 mg/kg twice daily; 8–11 kg (1–2 years), 62.5 mg twice daily; 12–19 kg (3–6 years), 125 mg twice daily; 20–29 kg (7–9 years), 187.5 mg twice daily; 30–40 kg (10–12 years), 250 mg twice daily

By intravenous infusion into larger proximal vein, 500 mg twice daily; CHILD not recommended

PoM Klaricid® (Abbott)

Tablets, yellow, f/c, clarithromycin 250 mg. Net price 14-tab pack = £10.71. Label: 9

Paediatric suspension, clarithromycin 125 mg/5 mL when reconstituted with water. Net price 70 mL = £6.00, 100 mL = £9.08. Label: 9

Intravenous infusion, powder for reconstitution, clarithromycin. Net price 500-mg vial = £12.14

Electrolytes: Na⁺ < 0.5 mmol/500-mg vial

5.1.6   Clindamycin

Clindamycin has only a limited use because of serious side-effects. Its most serious toxic effect is pseudomembranous colitis (see section 1.5) which may be fatal and is most common in middle-aged and elderly women, especially following operation. Although it can occur with most antibiotics it is more frequently seen with clindamycin. Patients should therefore discontinue treatment immediately if diarrhoea develops.

Clindamycin is active against Gram-positive cocci, including penicillin-resistant staphylococci and also against many anaerobes, especially *Bacteroides fragilis.* It is well concentrated in bone and excreted in bile and urine.

Clindamycin is recommended for staphylococcal joint and bone infections such as osteomyelitis, and intra-abdominal sepsis. Clindamycin is also used for endocarditis prophylaxis (section 5.1, table 2).

CLINDAMYCIN

Indications: staphylococcal bone and joint infections, peritonitis; endocarditis prophylaxis, section 5.1, Table 2

Cautions: discontinue immediately if diarrhoea or colitis develops; hepatic or renal impairment; monitor liver function and blood counts on prolonged therapy and in neonates and infants; pregnancy; breast-feeding (see Appendix 5); **interactions:** Appendix 1 (clindamycin)

Contra-indications: diarrhoeal states

Side-effects: diarrhoea (discontinue treatment), abdominal discomfort, nausea, vomiting, pseudomembranous colitis; rash; jaundice and altered liver function tests; neutropenia, eosinophilia, agranulocytosis and thrombocytopenia reported; pain, induration, and abscess after intramuscular injection; thrombophlebitis after intravenous injection

Dose: by mouth, 150–300 mg every 6 hours; up to 450 mg every 6 hours in severe infections; CHILD, 3–6 mg/kg every 6 hours

COUNSELLING. Patients should discontinue immediately and contact doctor if diarrhoea develops; capsules should be swallowed with a glass of water.

By deep intramuscular injection or by intravenous infusion, 0.6–2.7 g daily in 2–4 divided doses; life-threatening infection, up to 4.8 g daily; single doses above 600 mg by intravenous infusion only; single doses by intravenous infusion not to exceed 1.2 g

CHILD over 1 month, 15–40 mg/kg daily in 3–4 divided doses; severe infections, at least 300 mg daily regardless of weight

Endocarditis prophylaxis, section 5.1, Table 2

PoM Dalacin C® (Upjohn)

Capsules, clindamycin (as hydrochloride) 75 mg (lavender), net price 16-cap pack = £4.14; 150 mg, (lavender/maroon), 16-cap pack = £7.62. Label: 9, 27, counselling, see above (diarrhoea)

Paediatric suspension, pink, clindamycin 75 mg (as palmitate hydrochloride)/5 mL when reconstituted with purified water (freshly boiled and cooled). Net price 100 mL = £6.62. Label: 9, 27, counselling, see above (diarrhoea)

Injection, clindamycin 150 mg (as phosphate)/mL. Net price 2-mL amp = £5.17; 4-mL amp = £10.29

5.1.7 Some other antibiotics

Antibacterials discussed in this section include chloramphenicol, fusidic acid, spectinomycin, glycopeptide antibiotics (vancomycin and teicoplanin), and the polymyxin, colistin.

CHLORAMPHENICOL

Chloramphenicol is a potent, potentially toxic, broad-spectrum antibiotic which should be reserved for the treatment of life-threatening infections, particularly those caused by *Haemophilus influenzae*, and also for typhoid fever.

Its toxicity renders it unsuitable for systemic use except in the circumstances indicated above.

Eye-drops of chloramphenicol (see section 11.3.1) are useful for bacterial conjunctivitis.

CHLORAMPHENICOL

Indications: see notes above

Cautions: avoid repeated courses and prolonged treatment; reduce doses in hepatic or renal impairment; blood counts required before and periodically during treatment; may cause 'grey syndrome' in neonates (monitor plasma concentrations); **interactions:** Appendix 1 (chloramphenicol)

Contra-indications: pregnancy (see also Appendix 4), breast-feeding, porphyria (see section 9.8.2)

Side-effects: blood disorders including irreversible aplastic anaemia (aplastic anaemia attributed to chloramphenicol has terminated in leukaemia), peripheral neuritis, optic neuritis, erythema multiforme, nausea, vomiting, diarrhoea; nocturnal haemoglobinuria reported

Dose: by mouth or by intravenous injection or infusion, 50 mg/kg daily in 4 divided doses (exceptionally, can be doubled for severe infections such as septicaemia and meningitis, providing high doses reduced as soon as clinically indicated); CHILD, haemophilus epiglottitis and pyogenic meningitis, 50–100 mg/kg daily in divided doses (high dosages decreased as soon as clinically indicated); INFANTS under 2 weeks 25 mg/kg daily (in 4 divided doses), 2 weeks–1 year 50 mg/kg daily (in 4 divided doses)

Note. Plasma concentration monitoring required in neonates and preferred in those under 4 years of age; recommended peak plasma concentration (measured approx. 1 hour after intravenous injection or infusion) 15–25 mg/litre; pre-dose ('trough') concentration should not exceed 15 mg/litre

PoM Chloromycetin® (P-D)

Capsules, white/grey, chloramphenicol 250 mg. Net price 20 = £1.64

Suspension, chloramphenicol 125 mg (as palmitate)/5 mL. Net price 100 mL = £3.85

Injection, powder for reconstitution, chloramphenicol (as sodium succinate). Net price 300-mg vial = £5.16; 1.2-g vial = £5.03

Electrolytes: Na⁺ 0.94 mmol/300-mg vial, 3.75 mmol/1.2-g vial

PoM Kemicetine® (Pharmacia)

Injection, powder for reconstitution, chloramphenicol (as sodium succinate). Net price 1-g vial = £1.21

Electrolytes: Na⁺ 3.14 mmol/g

FUSIDIC ACID

Fusidic acid and its salts are narrow-spectrum antibiotics. The only indication for their use is in infections caused by penicillin-resistant staphylococci, especially osteomyelitis, as they are well concentrated in bone; they are also used for staphylococcal endocarditis (section 5.1, table 1). A second antistaphylococcal antibiotic is usually required to prevent emergence of resistance.

SODIUM FUSIDATE

Indications: see notes above

Cautions: liver-function tests required

Side-effects: nausea, vomiting, rashes, reversible jaundice, especially after high dosage or rapid infusion (withdraw therapy if persistent)

Dose: see under Preparations, below

PoM Fucidin® (Leo)

Tablets, f/c, sodium fusidate 250 mg. Net price 20 = £13.54. Label: 9

Dose: 500 mg every 8 hours, doubled for severe infections

Suspension, orange, fusidic acid 250 mg/5 mL. Net price 50 mL = £7.58. Label: 9, 21

Dose: as fusidic acid, ADULT 750 mg every 8 hours; CHILD up to 1 year 50 mg/kg daily (in 3 divided doses), 1–5 years 250 mg every 8 hours, 5–12 years 500 mg every 8 hours

Note. Fusidic acid is incompletely absorbed and doses recommended for suspension are proportionately higher than those for sodium fusidate tablets

Intravenous infusion, powder for reconstitution, diethanolamine fusidate 580 mg (≡ sodium fusidate 500 mg), with buffer. Net price per vial (with diluent) = £4.53

Electrolytes: Na⁺ 14 mmol/vial when reconstituted with buffer

Dose: as diethanolamine fusidate, by intravenous infusion, ADULT over 50 kg, 580 mg 3 times daily; ADULT under 50 kg and CHILD, 6–7 mg/kg 3 times daily

SPECTINOMYCIN

Spectinomycin is active against Gram-negative organisms, including *N. gonorrhoeae.* Its only indication is the treatment of gonorrhoea caused by penicillin-resistant organisms or in a penicillin-allergic patient.

SPECTINOMYCIN

Indications: see notes above

Cautions: pregnancy and breast-feeding; **interactions:** Appendix 1 (spectinomycin)

Side-effects: nausea, dizziness, urticaria, fever

Dose: by deep intramuscular injection, 2 g; up to 4 g in difficult-to-treat cases and in geographical areas of resistance; CHILD over 2 years, if no alternative treatment, 40 mg/kg

PoM Trobicin® (Upjohn)

Injection, powder for reconstitution, spectinomycin (as hydrochloride). Net price 2-g vial (with diluent) = £8.16

VANCOMYCIN AND TEICOPLANIN

The glycopeptide antibiotics vancomycin and teicoplanin have bactericidal activity against aerobic and anaerobic Gram-positive bacteria.

Vancomycin is the drug of choice for antibiotic-associated pseudomembranous colitis, for which it is given by mouth; a dose of 125 mg every 6 hours for 7 to 10 days is considered to be adequate; it is not significantly absorbed by mouth. It has a limited use by the intravenous route in the prophylaxis and treatment of endocarditis and other serious infections caused by Gram-positive cocci including multi-resistant staphylococci. It has a relatively long duration of action and can therefore be given every 12 hours; plasma concentrations should be monitored (especially in patients with renal impairment in whom the dose may need marked reduction). It is ototoxic and nephrotoxic.

Teicoplanin is very similar to vancomycin but has a significantly longer duration of action allowing once daily administration. Unlike vancomycin, teicoplanin can be given by intramuscular as well as by intravenous injection.

VANCOMYCIN

Indications: see notes above

Cautions: avoid rapid infusion (risk of anaphylactoid reactions, see Side-effects); rotate infusion sites; renal impairment; elderly; avoid if history of deafness; blood counts, urinalysis and renal function tests required in all patients; monitor auditory function and plasma-vancomycin concentration in elderly or if renal impairment; pregnancy and breast-feeding; systemic absorption may follow oral administration especially in inflammatory bowel disorders or following multiple doses; **interactions:** Appendix 1 (vancomycin)

Side-effects: after parenteral administration: nephrotoxicity including renal failure and interstitial nephritis; ototoxicity (discontinue if tinnitus occurs); blood disorders including neutropenia (usually after 1 week or cumulative dose of 25 g), rarely agranulocytosis and thrombocytopenia; nausea; chills; fever; eosinophilia, anaphylaxis, rashes (including exfoliative dermatitis, Stevens-Johnson syndrome and vasculitis); phlebitis (irritant to tissue); on rapid infusion, severe hypotension (including shock and cardiac arrest), wheezing, dyspnoea, urticaria, pruritus, flushing of the upper body ('red man' syndrome), pain and muscle spasm of back and chest

Dose: by mouth, 125 mg every 6 hours for 7–10 days, see notes above; CHILD 5 mg/kg every 6 hours, over 5 years, half adult dose

Note. Oral paediatric dose is lower than that on data sheet but is adequate

By intravenous infusion, 500 mg over at least 60 minutes every 6 hours *or* 1 g over at least 100 minutes every 12 hours; NEONATE up to 1 week, 15 mg/kg initially then 10 mg/kg every 12 hours; INFANT 1–4 weeks, 15 mg/kg initially then 10 mg/kg every 8 hours; CHILD over 1 month, 10 mg/kg every 6 hours

Endocarditis prophylaxis, section 5.1, table 2

Note. Plasma concentration monitoring required; peak plasma concentration (measured approx. 1 hour after intravenous infusion) should not exceed 30 mg/litre; predose ('trough') concentration should not exceed 10 mg/litre

PoM Vancocin® (Lilly)

Matrigel capsules, vancomycin (as hydrochloride) 125 mg (blue/peach), net price 20-cap pack = £63.08; 250 mg (blue/grey), 20-cap pack = £126.16

Injection, powder for reconstitution, vancomycin (as hydrochloride). Net price 250-mg vial = £4.76; 500-mg vial = £8.66; 1-g vial = £17.32

Note. Can be used to prepare solution for oral administration

---

TEICOPLANIN

Indications: potentially serious Gram-positive infections including endocarditis, dialysis-associated peritonitis, and serious infections due to *Staphylococcus aureus*

Cautions: vancomycin sensitivity; blood counts and liver and kidney function tests required; reduce dose in renal impairment (and monitor renal and auditory function on prolonged administration or if other nephrotoxic drugs given); reduce dose in elderly; pregnancy and breast-feeding

Side-effects: nausea, vomiting, diarrhoea; rash, fever, bronchospasm, anaphylactic reactions; dizziness, headache; blood disorders including eosinophilia, leucopenia, and thrombocytopenia; disturbances in liver enzymes, transient increase of serum creatinine; tinnitus, mild hearing loss, and vestibular disorders also reported; local reactions include erythema, pain, and thrombophlebitis

Dose: by intravenous injection or infusion, 400 mg initially, subsequently 200 mg daily; severe infections, 400 mg every 12 hours for 3 doses initially, subsequently 400 mg daily; the subsequent doses can alternatively be given *by intramuscular injection*; higher doses may be required in patients of over 85 kg and in severe burns or endocarditis (see data sheet)

CHILD over 2 months *by intravenous injection or infusion*, initially 10 mg/kg every 12 hours for 3 doses, subsequently 6 mg/kg daily (severe infections or in neutropenia, 10 mg/kg daily); NEONATE *by intravenous infusion*, initially a single dose of 16 mg/kg, subsequently 8 mg/kg daily
Endocarditis prophylaxis, section 5.1, table 2

PoM **Targocid**® (Merrell)
Injection, powder for reconstitution, teicoplanin, net price 200-mg vial (with diluent) = £26.05; 400-mg vial (with diluent) = £52.10
Electrolytes: Na⁺ < 0.5 mmol/200- and 400-mg vial

POLYMYXINS

The polymyxin antibiotic, colistin, is active against Gram-negative organisms, including *Pseudomonas aeruginosa*. It is **not** absorbed by mouth and thus needs to be given by injection to obtain a systemic effect; however, it is toxic and has few, if any, indications for systemic use.

Colistin is used by mouth in bowel sterilisation regimens in neutropenic patients (usually with nystatin); it is **not** recommended for gastro-intestinal infections. It is also given by inhalation of a nebulised solution as an adjunct to standard antibiotic therapy.

Both colistin and polymyxin B are included in some preparations for topical application.

COLISTIN

Indications: see notes above
Cautions: renal impairment; porphyria (see section 9.8.2); **interactions:** Appendix 1 (colistin)
Contra-indications: myasthenia gravis; pregnancy; breast-feeding
Side-effects: perioral and peripheral paraesthesia, vertigo, muscle weakness, apnoea, nephrotoxicity; rarely vasomotor instability, slurred speech, visual disturbance, confusion and psychosis, neurotoxicity reported with excessive doses; bronchospasm on inhalation
Dose: by mouth, bowel sterilisation, 1.5–3 million units every 8 hours
By intramuscular injection or intravenous injection or infusion, 2 million units every 8 hours (but see notes above)
By inhalation of nebulised solution, patients over 40 kg, 1 million units every 12 hours; patients under 40 kg, 500 000 units every 12 hours
Note. Colistin doses in BNF may differ from those in data sheet

PoM **Colomycin**® (Pharmax)
Tablets, scored, colistin sulphate 1.5 million units. Net price 50 = £65.11
Syrup, pink, colistin sulphate 250 000 units/5 mL when reconstituted with water. Net price 80 mL = £3.88
Injection, powder for reconstitution, colistin sulphomethate sodium. Net price 500 000-unit vial = £1.27; 1 million-unit vial = £1.88
Electrolytes: (before reconstitution) Na⁺ < 0.5 mmol/500 000- and 1 million-unit vial

5.1.8 Sulphonamides and trimethoprim

The importance of the sulphonamides has decreased as a result of increasing bacterial resistance and their replacement by antibiotics which are generally more active and less toxic.

Sulphamethoxazole and trimethoprim have been used in combination (as co-trimoxazole) because of their synergistic activity. Increasing bacterial resistance to sulphonamides and the high incidence of sulphonamide-related side-effects have however diminished the value of co-trimoxazole.

Indications for **co-trimoxazole** include urinary-tract infections, prostatitis, exacerbations of chronic bronchitis, and invasive salmonella infections, but trimethoprim alone is now preferred. High doses of co-trimoxazole are used for *Pneumocystis carinii* infections. Co-trimoxazole is no longer recommended for gonorrhoea.

Trimethoprim can be used alone for urinary- and respiratory-tract infections and for prostatitis, shigellosis, and invasive salmonella infections. Side-effects are less than with co-trimoxazole especially in older patients; therefore it should be used in place of co-trimoxazole for most infections (except pneumocystis).

Side-effects of the sulphonamides include rashes, which are common, the Stevens-Johnson syndrome (erythema multiforme), renal failure (especially with the less soluble preparations), and blood dyscrasias, notably marrow depression and agranulocytosis.

Side-effects of co-trimoxazole are similar to those of the sulphonamides but a particular watch should be kept for haematological effects and special care should be taken in patients who may be folate deficient such as the elderly and chronic sick, and in those receiving prolonged treatment or high doses. There have been reports of deaths in patients over the age of 65 years being treated with co-trimoxazole and almost certainly associated with the sulphonamide component. For this reason co-trimoxazole should be used with care in the elderly and preferably only if there is no acceptable alternative.

The **longer-acting sulphonamide**, sulfametopyrazine which is highly bound to plasma proteins, has the advantage of requiring less frequent administration, but toxic effects due to accumulation are more likely to occur.

For *topical preparations* of sulphonamides used in the treatment of burns see section 13.10.1.1.

CO-TRIMOXAZOLE

A mixture of trimethoprim and sulphamethoxazole in the proportions of 1 part to 5 parts
Indications: see notes above
Cautions: blood counts in prolonged treatment, maintain adequate fluid intake, renal impairment, breast-feeding; photosensitivity; elderly patients (**important:** see notes above); G6PD deficiency

---

(see section 9.1.5); **interactions:** Appendix 1 (co-trimoxazole)

BLOOD DISORDERS AND RASHES. A reminder that treatment should be stopped immediately if blood disorders or rashes develop (see notes above)

Contra-indications: pregnancy (see Appendix 4), infants under 6 weeks (risk of kernicterus), renal or hepatic failure, jaundice, blood disorders; porphyria (see section 9.8.2)

Side-effects: nausea, vomiting, diarrhoea, glossitis, rashes, erythema multiforme (includes Stevens-Johnson syndrome), epidermal necrolysis, pancreatitis, eosinophilia, agranulocytosis, granulocytopenia, purpura, leucopenia, thrombocytopenia; megaloblastic anaemia due to trimethoprim; pseudomembranous colitis, jaundice and hepatic necrosis reported

Dose: by mouth, 960 mg every 12 hours, increased to 1.44 g in severe infections; 480 mg every 12 hours if treated for more than 14 days; CHILD, every 12 hours, 6 weeks to 5 months, 120 mg; 6 months to 5 years, 240 mg; 6–12 years, 480 mg
Prophylaxis of recurrent urinary-tract infection, 480 mg at night; CHILD 6–12 mg/kg at night
Gonorrhoea, 1.92 g every 12 hours for 2 days, or 2.4 g followed by a further dose of 2.4 g after 8 hours but see notes above
High-dose therapy for *Pneumocystis carinii* infections, 120 mg/kg daily in divided doses for 14 days
By intramuscular injection or intravenous infusion, 960 mg every 12 hours increased to 1.44 g every 12 hours in severe infections; CHILD *by intravenous infusion*, 36 mg/kg daily in 2 divided doses increased to 54 mg/kg daily in severe infections
Note. 480 mg of co-trimoxazole consists of sulphamethoxazole 400 mg and trimethoprim 80 mg

PoM **Co-trimoxazole** (Non-proprietary)
Tablets, co-trimoxazole 480 mg, net price 20 = 61p; 960 mg, 20 = £2.59. Label: 9
Available from APS, Ashbourne (Comixco®), Cox (480 mg), CP, DDSA (Fectrim®, Fectrim® Forte), K Pharm., Norton
Dispersible tablets, co-trimoxazole 480 mg. Net price 20 = £1.72. Label: 9, 13
Available from APS, Norton (Comox®)
Paediatric oral suspension, co-trimoxazole 240 mg/5 mL. Net price 100 mL = £1.75. Label: 9
Available from APS, Ashbourne (Comixco®), CP, Lagap (Laratrim®), Norton, RP Drugs (Chemotrim®)
Oral suspension, co-trimoxazole 480 mg/5 mL. Net price 100 mL = £3.00. Label: 9
Available from CP, Lagap (Laratrim®)
Strong sterile solution, co-trimoxazole 96 mg/mL. For dilution and use as an intravenous infusion. Net price 5-mL amp = £1.59, 10-mL amp = £2.97
Available from David Bull

PoM **Bactrim®** (Roche)
Drapsules® (= tablets), orange, f/c, co-trimoxazole 480 mg. Net price 20 = £2.49. Label: 9
Double-strength tablets, scored, co-trimoxazole 960 mg. Net price 20 = £3.54. Label: 9
Paediatric syrup, sugar-free, yellow, co-trimoxazole 240 mg/5 mL. Net price 100 mL = £2.09. Label: 9

PoM **Septrin®** (Wellcome)
Tablets, co-trimoxazole 480 mg. Net price 20 = £3.03. Label: 9
Dispersible tablets, orange, sugar-free, co-trimoxazole 480 mg. Net price 20 = £3.55. Label: 9, 13
Forte tablets, scored, co-trimoxazole 960 mg. Net price 20 = £5.05. Label: 9
Adult suspension, co-trimoxazole 480 mg/5 mL. Net price 100 mL = £4.74. Label: 9
Paediatric suspension, sugar-free, co-trimoxazole 240 mg/5 mL. Net price 100 mL = £2.63. Label: 9
Intravenous infusion, co-trimoxazole 96 mg/mL. To be diluted before use. Net price 5-mL amp = £1.59

SULFAMETOPYRAZINE

Indications: urinary-tract infections, chronic bronchitis
Cautions; Contra-indications; Side-effects: see under Co-trimoxazole
Dose: 2 g once weekly

PoM **Kelfizine W®** (Pharmacia)
Tablets, sulfametopyrazine 2 g. Tablets to be taken in water. Net price 5-tab pack = £6.68. Label: 9, 13

SULPHADIAZINE
(Sulfadiazine)

Indications: meningococcal meningitis, prevention of rheumatic fever recurrence
Cautions; Contra-indications; Side-effects: see under Co-trimoxazole; avoid in severe renal impairment
Dose: by deep intramuscular injection or intravenous infusion, 2 g initially then 1 g every 6 hours for 2 days, followed by oral treatment for a further 5 days

PoM **Sulphadiazine** (Non-proprietary)
Tablets, sulphadiazine 500 mg. Net price 20 = £5.10. Label: 9, 27
Available from CP
Injection, sulphadiazine 250 mg (as sodium salt)/mL. Net price 4-mL amp = 94p
Available from Rhône-Poulenc Rorer

SULPHADIMIDINE

Indications: urinary-tract infections; meningococcal meningitis
Cautions; Contra-indications; Side-effects: see under Co-trimoxazole
Dose: by mouth, 2 g initially, then 0.5–1 g every 6–8 hours

PoM **Sulphadimidine** (Non-proprietary)
Tablets, sulphadimidine 500 mg. Net price 20 = £3.00. Label: 9, 27
Available from CP

TRIMETHOPRIM

Indications: urinary-tract infections, acute and chronic bronchitis

Cautions: renal impairment, breast-feeding, predisposition to folate deficiency, blood counts required on long-term therapy; **interactions:** Appendix 1 (trimethoprim)

Contra-indications: severe renal impairment, pregnancy, neonates; porphyria (see section 9.8.2)

Side-effects: gastro-intestinal disturbances including nausea and vomiting, pruritus, rashes, depression of haemopoiesis

Dose: by mouth, acute infections, 200 mg every 12 hours; CHILD, twice daily, 2–5 months 25 mg, 6 months–5 years 50 mg, 6–12 years 100 mg

Chronic infections and prophylaxis, 100 mg at night; CHILD 1–2 mg/kg at night

By slow intravenous injection or infusion, 150–250 mg every 12 hours; CHILD under 12 years, 6–9 mg/kg daily in 2–3 divided doses

PoM Trimethoprim (Non-proprietary)

Tablets, trimethoprim 100 mg, net price 20 = 42p; 200 mg, 20 = 71p. Label: 9

Available from APS, Ashbourne (Triprimix®), Berk (Trimopan®), Cox, CP, K Pharm., Lagap (Trimogal®), Norton

PoM Ipral® (Squibb)

Tablets, trimethoprim 100 mg, net price 20 = 80p; 200 mg, 20 = £1.71. Label: 9

PoM Monotrim® (Duphar)

Tablets, both scored, trimethoprim 100 mg, net price 20 = 82p; 200 mg, 20 = £1.44. Label: 9

Suspension, sugar-free, trimethoprim 50 mg/5 mL. Net price 100 mL = £1.77. Label: 9

Injection, trimethoprim 20 mg (as lactate)/mL. Net price 5-mL amp = £1.11

PoM Trimopan® (Berk)

Suspension, sugar-free, trimethoprim 50 mg/5 mL. Net price 100 mL = £2.34. Label: 9

5.1.9 Antituberculous drugs

Tuberculosis is treated in two phases—an *initial phase* using at least three drugs and a *continuation phase* using two drugs. Treatment requires specialised knowledge, particularly where the disease involves resistant organisms or non-respiratory organs.

The regimens given below are recommended by the Joint Tuberculosis Committee of the British Thoracic Society for the treatment of tuberculosis in the UK; variations occur in other countries.

INITIAL PHASE. The concurrent use of at least three drugs during the initial phase is designed to reduce the population of viable bacteria as rapidly as possible and to prevent the emergence of drug-resistant bacteria. Treatment of choice for the initial phase is the daily use of isoniazid, rifampicin, and pyrazinamide; ethambutol is added if drug resistance is thought likely. Streptomycin is now rarely used in the UK but it may be added if the organism is resistant to isoniazid. The initial phase drugs should be continued for 2 months.

CONTINUATION PHASE. After the initial phase, treatment is continued for a further 4 months with isoniazid and rifampicin; longer treatment may be necessary for bone and joint infections, for meningitis, or for resistant organisms.

Recommended dosage for standard unsupervised 6-month regimen

Isoniazid (for 6 months)	ADULT 300 mg daily; CHILD 10 mg/kg (max. 300 mg) daily
Rifampicin (for 6 months)	ADULT under 50 kg 450 mg daily, 50 kg and over 600 mg daily: CHILD 10 mg/kg daily
Pyrazinamide (for first 2 months only)	ADULT under 50 kg 1.5 g, 50 kg and over 2 g daily; CHILD 35 mg/kg daily

Note. Ethambutol and streptomycin are included in treatment regimens if resistance is suspected; see notes below for doses

PREGNANCY AND BREAST-FEEDING. The standard regimen (above) may be used during pregnancy and breast-feeding; pyridoxine supplements are advisable. Streptomycin should not be given in pregnancy.

CHILDREN. As for adults, children are given isoniazid, rifampicin, and pyrazinamide for the first 2 months followed by isoniazid and rifampicin during the next 4 months. If pyrazinamide is omitted from the initial phase, then treatment with isoniazid and rifampicin should be given for 9 months. Except in exceptional circumstances (e.g. drug resistance) ethambutol should be **avoided** in young children because of the difficulty in testing eyesight and in obtaining reports of visual symptoms (see below).

SUPERVISED TREATMENT. Treatment needs to be fully supervised in patients who cannot be relied upon to comply with the treatment regimen. These patients are given isoniazid, rifampicin, and pyrazinamide 3 times a week under supervision for the first 2 months followed by isoniazid and rifampicin three times a week for a further 4 months.

Recommended dosage for intermittent supervised treatment

Isoniazid (for 6 months)	ADULT and CHILD 15 mg/kg 3 times a week
Rifampicin (for 6 months)	ADULT 600–900 mg 3 times a week; CHILD 15 mg/kg 3 times a week
Pyrazinamide (for first 2 months only)	ADULT under 50 kg 2 g 3 times a week, 50 kg and over 2.5 g; CHILD 50 mg/kg 3 times a week
	or
	ADULT under 50 kg 3 g twice a week, 50 kg and over 3.5 g; CHILD 75 mg/kg twice a week

Note. Ethambutol and streptomycin are included in treatment regimens if resistance is suspected; see notes below for doses

IMMUNOCOMPROMISED PATIENTS. Immunocompromised patients may develop tuberculosis owing to reactivation of previously latent disease or to new infection. Multi-resistant *Mycobacterium tuberculosis* may be present or the infection may be caused by other mycobacteria e.g. *M. avium* complex in which case specialist advice is needed. Culture should always be carried out and the type of organism and its sensitivity confirmed. A minimum duration of treatment of 9 months is currently recommended for *M. tuberculosis* infection.

> Major causes of treatment failure are incorrect prescribing by the physician and inadequate compliance by the patient. Avoid both excessive and inadequate dosage. Treatment should be supervised by a specialist physician.

Isoniazid is cheap and highly effective. Like rifampicin it should always be included in any antituberculous regimen unless there is a specific contra-indication. Its only common side-effect is peripheral neuropathy which is more likely to occur where there are pre-existing risk factors such as diabetes and alcoholism and in chronic renal failure and malnutrition. In these circumstances pyridoxine 10 mg daily should be given prophylactically from the start of treatment. Other side-effects such as hepatitis and psychosis are rare.

Rifampicin is a key component of any antituberculous regimen. Like isoniazid it should always be included unless there is a specific contra-indication.

During the first two months of rifampicin administration transient disturbance of liver function with elevated serum transaminases is common but generally does not require interruption of treatment. Occasionally more serious liver toxicity requires a change of treatment particularly in those with pre-existing liver disease.

On intermittent treatment six toxicity syndromes have been recognised—influenzal, abdominal, and respiratory symptoms, shock, renal failure, and thrombocytopenic purpura—and can occur in 20 to 30% of patients.

Rifampicin induces hepatic enzymes which accelerate the metabolism of several drugs including oestrogens, corticosteroids, phenytoin, sulphonylureas, and anticoagulants. **Important:** the effectiveness of oral contraceptives is reduced and alternative family planning advice should be offered (see section 7.3.1).

Rifabutin, a newly introduced rifamycin, is indicated for *prophylaxis* against *M. avium* complex infections in patients with a low CD4 count; it is also licensed for the *treatment* of non-tuberculous mycobacterial disease and pulmonary tuberculosis. As with rifampicin it induces hepatic enzymes and the effectiveness of oral contraceptives is reduced requiring alternative family planning methods.

Pyrazinamide is a bactericidal drug only active against intracellular dividing forms of *Mycobacterium tuberculosis*; it exerts its main effect only in the first two or three months. It is particularly useful in tuberculous meningitis because of good meningeal penetration. It is not active against *M. bovis*.

Ethambutol is included in a treatment regimen if resistance is suspected; it can be omitted if the risk of resistance is low. For unsupervised treatment

ethambutol is given in a dose of 25 mg/kg daily in the initial phase followed by 15 mg/kg daily in the continuation phase (*or* 15 mg/kg daily throughout); in fully supervised intermittent treatment ethambutol is given in a dose of 30 mg/kg 3 times a week *or* 45 mg/kg twice a week.

Side-effects of ethambutol are largely confined to visual disturbances in the form of loss of acuity, colour blindness, and restriction of visual fields. These toxic effects are more common where excessive dosage is used or the patient's renal function is impaired, in which case the drug should be **avoided**. The earliest features of ocular toxicity are subjective and patients should be advised to discontinue therapy immediately if they develop deterioration in vision and promptly seek further advice. Early discontinuation of the drug is almost always followed by recovery of eyesight. Patients who cannot understand warnings about visual side-effects should, if possible, be given an alternative drug. In particular, ethambutol should be **avoided** in children until they are at least 6 years old and capable of reporting symptomatic visual changes accurately.

Ophthalmic examination should be performed before, and at intervals during, treatment.

Streptomycin is now rarely used in the UK except for resistant organisms. It is given intramuscularly in a standard dose of 1 g daily, reduced to 500–750 mg in patients under 50 kg or those over 40 years of age. For fully supervised intermittent treatment streptomycin is given in a dose of 1 g 3 times a week, reduced to 750 mg 3 times a week in patients under 50 kg. Children are given streptomycin in a dose of 15–20 mg/kg daily or for fully supervised intermittent treatment, 15–20 mg/kg 3 times a week. Plasma drug concentrations should be measured, particularly in patients with impaired renal function in whom streptomycin must be used with great care. Side-effects increase after a cumulative dose of 100 g, which should only be exceeded in exceptional circumstances.

Second-line drugs available for infections caused by resistant organisms, or when first-line drugs cause unacceptable side-effects, include capreomycin, cycloserine, and prothionamide (no longer on UK market). Advice on the availability of second-line antituberculous drugs can be obtained from Regional Drug Information Services

CAPREOMYCIN

Indications: in combination with other drugs, tuberculosis resistant to first-line drugs

Cautions: renal, hepatic, or auditory impairment; monitor renal, hepatic, auditory, and vestibular function and electrolytes; pregnancy (teratogenic in *animals*) and breast-feeding; **interactions:** Appendix 1 (capreomycin)

Side-effects: hypersensitivity reactions including urticaria and rashes; leucocytosis or leucopenia, rarely thrombocytopenia; changes in liver function tests; nephrotoxicity; electrolyte disturbances; hearing loss with tinnitus and vertigo;

neuromuscular block after large doses, pain and induration at injection site

Dose: by deep intramuscular injection, 1 g daily (not more than 20 mg/kg) for 2–4 months, then 1 g 2–3 times each week

PoM **Capastat®** (Dista)
Injection, powder for reconstitution, capreomycin sulphate 1 million units ($\equiv$ capreomycin approx. 1 g). Net price per vial = £3.45

CYCLOSERINE

Indications: in combination with other drugs, tuberculosis resistant to first-line drugs
Cautions: discontinue (or reduce dose) if allergic dermatitis or symptoms of CNS toxicity; reduce dose in renal impairment (avoid if severe); monitor haematological, renal, and hepatic function; pregnancy and breast-feeding; **interactions:** Appendix 1 (cycloserine)
Contra-indications: severe renal impairment, epilepsy, depression, severe anxiety, psychotic states, alcohol dependence, porphyria (see section 9.8.2)
Side-effects: mainly neurological, including headache, dizziness, vertigo, drowsiness, tremor, convulsions; psychosis, depression; rashes; megaloblastic anaemia; changes in liver function tests
Dose: initially 250 mg every 12 hours for 2 weeks increased according to blood concentration and response to max. 500 mg every 12 hours; CHILD initially 10 mg/kg daily adjusted according to blood concentration and response
Note. Blood concentration monitoring required especially in renal impairment or if dose exceeds 500 mg daily or if signs of toxicity; blood concentration should not exceed 30 mg/litre

PoM **Cycloserine** (Lilly)
Capsules, red/grey cycloserine 250 mg, net price 20 = £17.16. Label: 2, 8

ETHAMBUTOL HYDROCHLORIDE

Indications: tuberculosis, in combination with other drugs
Cautions: reduce dose in renal impairment; elderly; pregnancy; warn patients to report visual changes—see notes above
Contra-indications: young children (see notes), optic neuritis, poor vision
Side-effects: optic neuritis, red/green colour blindness, peripheral neuritis
Dose: ADULT and CHILD over 6 years, see notes above

PoM **Myambutol®** (Lederle)
Tablets, ethambutol hydrochloride 100 mg (yellow), net price 100-tab pack = £7.22; 400 mg (grey), 100-tab pack = £25.84. Label: 8
PoM **Mynah®** (Lederle)
Mynah 250 tablets, yellow, ethambutol hydrochloride 250 mg, isoniazid 100 mg. Net price 84-tab pack = £16.04. Label: 8, 23
Mynah 300 tablets, orange, ethambutol hydrochloride 300 mg, isoniazid 100 mg. Net price 84-tab pack = £19.17. Label: 8, 23

ISONIAZID

Indications: tuberculosis, in combination with other drugs; prophylaxis—section 5.1, Table 2
Cautions: hepatic and renal impairment; slow acetylator status (increased risk of side-effects); epilepsy; history of psychosis; alcoholism; pregnancy and breast-feeding; porphyria (see section 9.8.2); **interactions:** Appendix 1 (isoniazid)
Contra-indications: drug-induced liver disease
Side-effects: nausea, vomiting; peripheral neuritis with high doses (pyridoxine prophylaxis, see notes above), optic neuritis, convulsions, psychotic episodes; hypersensitivity reactions including fever, erythema multiforme, purpura, agranulocytosis; hepatitis (especially over age of 35); systemic lupus erythematosus-like syndrome, pellagra, hyperglycaemia, and gynaecomastia reported
Dose: by mouth or by intramuscular or intravenous injection, see notes above

PoM **Isoniazid** (Non-proprietary)
Tablets, isoniazid 50 mg, net price 20 = £1.38; 100 mg, 20 = 39p. Label: 8, 22
Elixir (BPC), isoniazid 50 mg, citric acid monohydrate 12.5 mg, sodium citrate 60 mg, concentrated anise water 0.05 mL, compound tartrazine solution 0.05 mL, glycerol 1 mL, double-strength chloroform water 2 mL, water to 5 mL. Label: 8, 22
'Special order' [unlicensed] product; contact Penn, RP Drugs or regional hospital manufacturing unit
PoM **Rimifon®** (Cambridge)
Injection, isoniazid 25 mg/mL. Net price 2-mL amp = £1.32

PYRAZINAMIDE

Indications: tuberculosis in combination with other drugs
Cautions: impaired renal function, diabetes, gout; **interactions:** Appendix 1 (pyrazinamide)
Contra-indications: liver damage, porphyria (see section 9.8.2)
Side-effects: hepatotoxicity including fever, anorexia, hepatomegaly, jaundice, liver failure; nausea, vomiting, arthralgia, sideroblastic anaemia, urticaria
Dose: see notes above

PoM **Zinamide®** (MSD)
Tablets, scored, pyrazinamide 500 mg. Net price 20 = £1.44. Label: 8

RIFABUTIN

Indications: see under Dose
Cautions: see under Rifampicin; reduce dose in severe renal impairment
Side-effects: nausea, vomiting; leucopenia, thrombocytopenia, anaemia; raised liver enzymes, jaundice; uveitis following high doses or administration with drugs which raise plasma concentration—see also interactions: Appendix 1 (rifamycins); also hypersensitivity reactions

including fever, rash, eosinophilia, broncho-spasm, shock; urine, saliva and other body secretions coloured orange-red

Dose: prophylaxis of *Mycobacterium avium* complex infections in immunosuppressed patients with low CD4 count (see data sheet), 300 mg daily as a single dose

Treatment of non-tuberculous mycobacterial disease, in combination with other drugs, 450–600 mg daily as a single dose for up to 6 months after cultures negative

Treatment of pulmonary tuberculosis, in combination with other drugs, 150–450 mg daily as a single dose for at least 6 months

CHILD not recommended

▼ PoM **Mycobutin®** (Pharmacia)

Capsules, red-brown, rifabutin 150 mg. Net price 30-cap pack = £82.29. Label: 8, 14, counselling, lenses, see under Rifampicin

RIFAMPICIN

Indications: see under Dose

Cautions: reduce dose in hepatic impairment (see Appendix 2; liver function tests and blood counts in hepatic disorders and on prolonged therapy); renal impairment (if above 600 mg daily); pregnancy and breast-feeding (see notes above and Appendixes 4 and 5); **important:** advise patients on oral contraceptives to use additional means (see also section 7.3.1); discolours soft contact lenses; see also notes above; **interactions:** Appendix 1 (rifamycins)

Note. If treatment interrupted re-introduce with low dosage and increase gradually; discontinue permanently if serious side-effects develop

Contra-indications: jaundice, porphyria (see section 9.8.2)

Side-effects: gastro-intestinal symptoms including anorexia, nausea, vomiting, diarrhoea (pseudomembranous colitis reported); those occurring mainly on intermittent therapy include influenzal syndrome (with chills, fever, dizziness, bone pain), respiratory symptoms (including shortness of breath), collapse and shock, haemolytic anaemia, acute renal failure, and thrombocytopenic purpura; alterations of liver function, jaundice; flushing, urticaria, and rashes; other side-effects reported include oedema, muscular weakness and myopathy, leucopenia, eosinophilia, menstrual disturbances; urine, saliva, and other body secretions coloured orange-red; thrombophlebitis reported if infusion used for prolonged period

Dose: brucellosis, legionnaires' disease and serious staphylococcal infections, in combination with other drugs, *by mouth or by intravenous infusion,* 0.6–1.2 g daily in 2–4 divided doses

Tuberculosis, in combination with other drugs, see notes above

Leprosy, section 5.1.10

Prophylaxis of meningococcal meningitis and *Haemophilus influenzae* (type b) infection, section 5.1, Table 2

PoM **Rifampicin** (Non-proprietary)

Capsules, rifampicin 150 mg, net price 20 = £3.44; 300 mg, 20 = £6.88. Label: 8, 14, 22, counselling, see lenses above

Available from APS, Generics

PoM **Rifadin®** (Merrell)

Capsules, rifampicin 150 mg (blue/red), net price 20 = £3.73; 300 mg (red), 20 = £7.45. Label: 8, 14, 22, counselling, see lenses above

Syrup, red, rifampicin 100 mg/5 mL. Net price 120 mL = £3.62. Label: 8, 14, 22, counselling, see lenses above

Intravenous infusion, powder for reconstitution, rifampicin. Net price 600-mg vial (with solvent) = £7.80

Electrolytes: Na⁺ < 0.5 mmol/vial

PoM **Rimactane®** (Ciba)

Capsules, rifampicin 150 mg (red), net price 56-tab pack = £9.63; 300 mg (red/brown), 56-tab pack = £19.26. Label: 8, 14, 22, counselling, see lenses above

Syrup, red, rifampicin 100 mg/5 mL. Net price 100 mL = £2.78. Label: 8, 14, 22, counselling, see lenses above

Intravenous infusion, powder for reconstitution, rifampicin (as sodium salt). Net price 300-mg vial (with diluent) = £7.28

Electrolytes: Na⁺ < 0.5 mmol/vial

Note. Owing to risk of contact sensitisation care must be taken to avoid contact during preparation and infusion

Combined preparations

PoM **Rifater®** (Merrell)

Tablets, pink-beige, s/c, rifampicin 120 mg, isoniazid 50 mg, pyrazinamide 300 mg. Net price 20 = £4.29. Label: 8, 14, 22, counselling, see lenses above

Dose: initial treatment of pulmonary tuberculosis, patients up to 40 kg 3 tablets daily preferably before breakfast, 40–49 kg 4 tablets daily, 50–64 kg 5 tablets daily, 65 kg or more, 6 tablets daily; not suitable for use in children

PoM **Rifinah 150®** (Merrell)

Tablets, pink, rifampicin 150 mg, isoniazid 100 mg. Net price 84-tab pack = £16.18. Label: 8, 14, 22, counselling, see lenses above

Dose: ADULT under 50 kg, 3 tablets daily, preferably before breakfast

PoM **Rifinah 300®** (Merrell)

Tablets, orange, rifampicin 300 mg, isoniazid 150 mg. Net price 56-tab pack = £21.38. Label: 8, 14, 22, counselling, see lenses above

Dose: ADULT 50 kg and over, 2 tablets daily, preferably before breakfast

PoM **Rimactazid 150®** (Ciba)

Tablets, pink, s/c, rifampicin 150 mg, isoniazid 100 mg. Net price 84-tab pack = £14.93. Label: 8, 14, 22, counselling, see lenses above

Additives: include gluten

Dose: ADULT under 50 kg, 3 tablets daily, preferably before breakfast

PoM Rimactazid 300® (Ciba)

Tablets, orange, s/c, rifampicin 300 mg, isoniazid 150 mg. Net price 56-tab pack = £18.06. Label: 8, 14, 22, counselling, see lenses above

Additives: include gluten

Dose: ADULT 50 kg and over, 2 tablets daily, preferably before breakfast

STREPTOMYCIN

Indications: tuberculosis, in combination with other drugs

Cautions; Contra-indications; Side-effects: see under Aminoglycosides, section 5.1.4; also hypersensitivity reactions, paraesthesia of mouth

Dose: by deep intramuscular injection, see notes above

PoM Streptomycin Sulphate (Evans)

Injection, powder for reconstitution, streptomycin (as sulphate). Net price 1-g vial = £5.62

5.1.10 Antileprotic drugs

Advice from a member of the Panel of Leprosy Opinion is essential for the treatment of leprosy (Hansen's disease). Details of the Panel can be obtained from the Department of Health telephone 071-972 4480.

For over twenty years the mainstay of leprosy treatment was dapsone monotherapy but resistance to dapsone became an increasing concern. The World Health Organization has made recommendations to overcome this problem of dapsone resistance and to prevent the emergence of resistance to other antileprotic drugs. These recommendations are based on the same principles as for the chemotherapy of tuberculosis. Drugs recommended are **dapsone**, **rifampicin**, and **clofazimine**; ethionamide or prothionamide (which are not marketed in the UK) are no longer recommended unless absolutely necessary.

A three-drug regimen is recommended for *multi bacillary leprosy* (lepromatous, borderline-lepromatous, and borderline leprosy) and a two-drug regimen for those suffering from *paucibacillary leprosy* (borderline-tuberculoid, tuberculoid, and indeterminate). These regimens, which are widely applicable throughout the world (with minor local variations), are as follows:

Multibacillary leprosy (3-drug regimen)

Rifampicin	600 mg once-monthly, supervised (450 mg for those weighing less than 35 kg)
Dapsone	100 mg daily, self-administered
Clofazimine	300 mg once-monthly, supervised, *and* 50 mg daily, self-administered

Note. Substitution of clofazimine with ethionamide or prothionamide is no longer recommended unless absolutely necessary; administration (in a dose of 250–375 mg daily) should be under medical supervision, with periodic checks for hepatotoxicity

Treatment should be given for at least 2 years and be continued, wherever possible, up to smear negativity. It should be continued unchanged during both type I (reversal) or type II (erythema nodosum leprosum) reactions which, if severe, should receive their own specific treatment (e.g. prednisolone or increased clofazimine dosage).

Paucibacillary leprosy (2-drug regimen)

Rifampicin	600 mg once-monthly, supervised (450 mg for those weighing less than 35 kg)
Dapsone	100 mg daily, self-administered

Treatment should be given for 6 months. If treatment is interrupted the regimen should be recommenced where it was left off to complete the full course.

Neither the multibacillary nor the paucibacillary antileprosy regimen is sufficient to treat tuberculosis, therefore patients who also have tuberculosis should be given appropriate antituberculous drugs in addition to the antileprosy regimen.

DAPSONE

Indications: leprosy, dermatitis herpetiformis

Cautions: cardiac or pulmonary disease; anaemia (treat severe anaemia before starting); G6PD-deficiency (including breast-feeding of affected children, see section 9.1.5); pregnancy; avoid in porphyria (see section 9.8.2); **interactions:** Appendix 1 (dapsone)

Side-effects: (dose-related and uncommon at doses used for leprosy), neuropathy, allergic dermatitis, anorexia, nausea, vomiting, headache, insomnia, tachycardia, anaemia, hepatitis, agranulocytosis

Dose: leprosy, 1–2 mg/kg daily, see notes above
Dermatitis herpetiformis, see specialist literature

PoM Dapsone (Non-proprietary)

Tablets, dapsone 50 mg, net price 20 = 54p; 100 mg, 20 = 73p. Label: 8

Available from Cox

CLOFAZIMINE

Indications: leprosy

Cautions: hepatic and renal impairment—function tests required

Side-effects: nausea, giddiness, headache, and diarrhoea with high doses, skin and urine coloured (red), lesions discoloured (blue-black)

Dose: leprosy, see notes above
Lepromatous lepra reactions, dosage increased to 300 mg daily for max. of 3 months

PoM Lamprene® (Geigy)

Capsules, brown, clofazimine 100 mg. Net price 20 = £1.65. Label: 8, 14, 21

RIFAMPICIN

Section 5.1.9

5.1.11   Metronidazole and tinidazole

Metronidazole is an antimicrobial drug with high activity against anaerobic bacteria and protozoa; indications include trichomonal vaginitis (section 5.4.3), bacterial vaginosis (notably *Gardnerella vaginalis* infections), and *Entamoeba histolytica* and *Giardia lamblia* infections (section 5.4.2). It is also used for surgical and gynaecological sepsis in which its activity against colonic anaerobes, especially *Bacteroides fragilis*, is important. Metronidazole is also effective in the treatment of pseudomembranous colitis (in a dose of 400 mg by mouth three times daily). Topical metronidazole (see section 13.10.1.2) reduces the odour produced by anaerobic bacteria in fungating tumours; it is also used in the management of rosacea.

Tinidazole is similar to metronidazole but has a longer duration of action.

METRONIDAZOLE

Indications: anaerobic infections (including dental), see under Dose below; protozoal infections, section 5.4.2

Cautions: disulfiram-like reaction with alcohol, hepatic impairment; pregnancy and breast-feeding (manufacturer advises avoidance of high-dose regimens); **interactions:** Appendix 1 (metronidazole)

Side-effects: nausea, vomiting, unpleasant taste, and gastro-intestinal disturbances; rashes, urticaria and angioedema; rarely drowsiness, headache, dizziness, ataxia, and darkening of urine; on prolonged or intensive therapy peripheral neuropathy, transient epileptiform seizures, and leucopenia

Dose: anaerobic infections (usually treated for 7 days), *by mouth*, 800 mg initially then 400 mg every 8 hours; *by rectum*, 1 g every 8 hours for 3 days, then 1 g every 12 hours; *by intravenous infusion*, 500 mg every 8 hours; CHILD, any route, 7.5 mg/kg every 8 hours

Leg ulcers and pressure sores, *by mouth*, 400 mg every 8 hours for 7 days

Bacterial vaginosis, *by mouth*, 400 mg twice daily for 7 days *or* 2 g as a single dose

Acute ulcerative gingivitis, *by mouth*, 200 mg every 8 hours for 3 days; CHILD 1–3 years 50 mg every 8 hours for 3 days; 3–7 years 100 mg every 12 hours; 7–10 years 100 mg every 8 hours

Acute dental infections, *by mouth*, 200 mg every 8 hours for 3–7 days

Surgical prophylaxis, *by mouth*, 400 mg every 8 hours started 24 hours before surgery, then continued postoperatively *by intravenous infusion* or *by rectum* (see below) until oral administration can be resumed; CHILD 7.5 mg/kg every 8 hours

By rectum, 1 g every 8 hours; CHILD 125–250 mg every 8 hours

By intravenous infusion, 500 mg shortly before surgery then every 8 hours until oral administration can be started; CHILD, 7.5 mg/kg every 8 hours

PoM Metronidazole (Non-proprietary)

Tablets, metronidazole 200 mg, net price 20 = 47p; 400 mg, 20 = £1.00. Label: 4, 9, 21, 25, 27

Available from APS, Cox, CP, DDSA (Vaginyl®), K Pharm., Lagap (Metrolyl®), Lederle (Zadstat®), Norton

Suspension, metronidazole (as benzoate) 200 mg/ 5 mL. Net price 100 mL = £4.41. Label: 4, 9, 23

Available from RP Drugs

Intravenous infusion, metronidazole 5 mg/mL. Net price 20-mL amp = £1.80

Available from David Bull

PoM Flagyl® (Rhône-Poulenc Rorer)

Tablets, both f/c, ivory, metronidazole 200 mg, net price 21-tab pack = £2.14; 400 mg, 14-tab pack = £3.03. Label: 4, 9, 21, 25, 27

Intravenous infusion, metronidazole 5 mg/mL. Net price 100-mL Viaflex® bag = £3.41

Electrolytes: Na⁺ 13.6 mmol/100-mL bottle or bag

Suppositories, metronidazole 500 mg, net price 10 = £6.60; 1 g, 10 = £10.02. Label: 4, 9

PoM Flagyl S® (Rhône-Poulenc Rorer)

Suspension, metronidazole 200 mg (as benzoate)/ 5 mL. Net price 100 mL = £4.41. Label: 4, 9, 23

PoM Metrogel®: see section 13.10.1.2

PoM Metrolyl® (Lagap)

Intravenous infusion, metronidazole 5 mg/mL. Net price 100-mL Steriflex® bag = £4.05

Electrolytes: Na⁺ 14.53 mmol/100-mL bag

Suppositories, metronidazole 500 mg, net price 10 = £4.25; 1 g, 10 = £6.80. Label: 4, 9

PoM Metrotop®: see section 13.10.1.2

PoM Zadstat® (Lederle)

Suppositories, metronidazole 500 mg, net price 10 = £4.14; 1 g, 10 = £6.63. Label: 4, 9

With antifungal

PoM Flagyl Compak® (Rhône-Poulenc Rorer)

Treatment pack, tablets, off-white, f/c, metronidazole 400 mg), with pessaries, yellow, nystatin 100 000 units. Net price 14 tablets and 14 pessaries (with applicator) = £4.13

Dose: for mixed trichomonal and candidal infections, 1 tablet twice daily for 7 days and 1 pessary inserted twice daily for 7 days *or* 1 pessary at night for 14 nights

---

TINIDAZOLE

Indications: anaerobic infections, see under Dose below; protozoal infections, section 5.4.2

Cautions; Side-effects: see under Metronidazole; pregnancy (manufacturer advises avoidance in first trimester)

Dose: anaerobic infections *by mouth*, 2 g initially, followed by 1 g daily *or* 500 mg twice daily, usually for 5–6 days

Bacterial vaginosis and acute ulcerative gingivitis, a single 2-g dose

Abdominal surgery prophylaxis, a single 2-g dose approximately 12 hours before surgery

PoM Fasigyn® (Pfizer)

Tablets, f/c, tinidazole 500 mg. Net price 20-tab pack = £11.50. Label: 4, 9, 21, 25

5.1.12   4-Quinolones

Antibacterials discussed in this section include acrosoxacin, ciprofloxacin, ofloxacin, and the urinary antiseptics cinoxacin, nalidixic acid, and norfloxacin.

Acrosoxacin is used only in the treatment of gonorrhoea in patients allergic to penicillins or who have strains resistant to penicillins and other antibiotics.

Nalidixic acid, **cinoxacin**, and **norfloxacin** are effective in uncomplicated urinary-tract infections.

Ciprofloxacin is active against both Gram-positive and Gram-negative bacteria. It is particularly active against Gram-negative bacteria, including salmonella, shigella, campylobacter, neisseria, and pseudomonas. Ciprofloxacin only has moderate activity against Gram-positive bacteria such as *Streptococcus pneumoniae* and *Strep. faecalis*; it is not the drug of first choice for pneumococcal pneumonia. It is active against chlamydia and some mycobacteria. Most anaerobic organisms are not susceptible. Uses for ciprofloxacin include infections of the respiratory (but not for pneumococcal pneumonia, see above) and urinary tracts, and of the gastro-intestinal system (including typhoid fever), and gonorrhoea and septicaemia caused by sensitive organisms. Although licensed for skin and soft tissue infections there is a high incidence of staphylococcal resistance and it should be avoided in methicillin-resistant Staphylococcus aureus (MRSA) infections.

Ofloxacin is used for urinary-tract infections, lower respiratory-tract infections, gonorrhoea, and non-gonococcal urethritis and cervicitis.

CAUTIONS. 4-Quinolones should be used with caution in patients with epilepsy or a history of epilepsy, in hepatic or renal impairment, in pregnancy, during breast-feeding, and in children or adolescents (arthropathy has developed in weight-bearing joints in young *animals*). The CSM has warned that 4-quinolones may induce **convulsions** in patients with or without a history of convulsions; taking NSAIDs at the same time may also induce them. Other **interactions**: Appendix 1 (4-quinolones).

SIDE-EFFECTS. Common side-effects of the 4-quinolones include nausea, vomiting, abdominal pain, diarrhoea (rarely pseudomembranous colitis), headache, dizziness, sleep disorders, rash, pruritus, fever, anaphylaxis, photosensitivity, increase in blood urea and creatinine, transient disturbances in liver enzymes and bilirubin, arthralgia and myalgia, blood disorders (including eosinophilia, leucopenia, thrombocytopenia, and altered prothrombin concentration). Less frequent side-effects include anorexia, restlessness, depression, hallucinations, confusion, and disturbances in vision, taste and smell; also isolated reports of intracranial hypertension and tendon damage. Side-effects that have been reported to the CSM also include haemolytic anaemia, renal impairment, hepatic dysfunction, anaphylaxis, and hypoglycaemia. The drug should be **discontinued** if mental, neurological or hypersensitivity reactions occur with the first dose.

CIPROFLOXACIN

Indications: Gram-negative and Gram-positive infections, see notes above; surgical prophylaxis in upper gastro-intestinal procedures

Cautions; Side-effects: see notes above; avoid excessive alkalinity of urine and ensure adequate fluid intake (risk of crystalluria); not recommended in children or growing adolescents; caution in G6PD deficiency (see section 9.1.5); anaphylaxis reported, also reported dyspepsia, flatulence, dysphagia, tremor, convulsions, jaundice and hepatitis with necrosis, renal failure, nephritis, vasculitis, Stevens-Johnson syndrome, Lyell syndrome, petechiae, haemorrhagic bullae, tenosynovitis and tachycardia; pain and phlebitis at injection site; **interactions:** Appendix 1 (4-quinolones)

DRIVING. May impair performance of skilled tasks (e.g. driving); effects of alcohol enhanced

Dose: *by mouth*, respiratory-tract infections, 250–750 mg twice daily

Urinary-tract infections, 250–500 mg twice daily (250 mg twice daily for 3 days in acute uncomplicated cystitis)

Gonorrhoea, 250 mg as a single dose; 500 mg may be required in resistant cases

Most other infections, 500–750 mg twice daily

Surgical prophylaxis, 750 mg 60–90 minutes before procedure

Prophylaxis of meningococcal meningitis [not licensed], section 5.1, table 2

By intravenous infusion (over 30–60 minutes), 200 mg twice daily

Urinary-tract infections, 100 mg twice daily

Gonorrhoea, 100 mg as a single dose

CHILD not recommended (see above) but where benefit outweighs risk, *by mouth*, 7.5–15 mg/kg daily in 2 divided doses *or by intravenous infusion*, 5–10 mg/kg daily in 2 divided doses

PoM Ciproxin® (Baypharm)

Tablets, all f/c, ciprofloxacin (as hydrochloride) 250 mg (scored), net price 10-tab pack = £7.30, 20-tab pack = £15.00; 500 mg (scored), 10-tab pack = £13.75, 20-tab pack = £27.50; 750 mg, 10-tab pack = £20.00. Label: 6, 9, 25, counselling, driving

Intravenous infusion, ciprofloxacin 2 mg (as lactate)/mL, net price 50 mL bottle = £10.18; 100-mL bottle = £19.85

Electrolytes: Na+ 15.4 mmol/100-mL bottle

ACROSOXACIN

(Rosoxacin)

Indications: gonorrhoea

Cautions; Side-effects: see notes above; avoid frequent repeat doses in patients under 18 years; **interactions:** Appendix 1 (4-quinolones)

DRIVING. May impair performance of skilled tasks (e.g. driving)

Dose: 300 mg as a single dose on an empty stomach

PoM Eradacin® (Sanofi Winthrop)

Capsules, red/yellow, acrosoxacin 150 mg. Net price 20-cap pack = £31.15. Label: 2, 23

CINOXACIN

Indications: urinary-tract infections

Cautions; Side-effects: see notes above; avoid in severe renal impairment; also reported, peripheral and oral oedema, tinnitus, perineal burning; **interactions:** Appendix 1 (4-quinolones)

Dose: 500 mg every 12 hours; prophylaxis, 500 mg at night

PoM Cinobac® (Lilly)

Capsules, green/orange, cinoxacin 500 mg. Net price 14-cap pack = £10.41. Label: 9

NALIDIXIC ACID

Indications: urinary-tract infections

Cautions; Side-effects: see notes above; avoid in porphyria (see section 9.8.2) and if history of convulsive disorders, avoid strong sunlight, false positive urinary glucose (if tested for reducing substances); caution in G6PD deficiency (see section 9.1.5); also reported toxic psychosis and convulsions, weakness, increased intracranial pressure, paraesthesia, cranial nerve palsy, cholestasis, metabolic acidosis; **interactions:** Appendix 1 (4-quinolones)

Dose: 1 g every 6 hours for 7 days, reduced in chronic infections to 500 mg every 6 hours; CHILD over 3 months max. 50 mg/kg daily in divided doses; reduced in prolonged therapy to 30 mg/kg daily

PoM Nalidixic Acid (Non-proprietary)

Tablets, nalidixic acid 500 mg. Net price 56-tab pack = £10.80. Label: 9, 11
Available from Norton

PoM Mictral® (Sanofi Winthrop)

Granules, effervescent, nalidixic acid 660 mg, sodium citrate (as sodium citrate and citric acid) 4.1 g/sachet (Na⁺ 41 mmol/sachet). Net price 9-sachet pack = £5.48. Label: 9, 11, 13
Dose: 1 sachet in water 3 times daily for 3 days

PoM Negram® (Sanofi Winthrop)

Tablets, beige, nalidixic acid 500 mg. Net price 56-tab pack = £12.83. Label: 9, 11

Suspension, pink, sugar-free, nalidixic acid 300 mg/5 mL. Net price 150 mL = £12.85. Label: 9, 11

PoM Uriben® (RP Drugs)

Suspension, pink, nalidixic acid 300 mg/5 mL. Net price 200 mL = £16.25; 500 mL = £34.65. Label: 9, 11

NORFLOXACIN

Indications: see under Dose

Cautions; Side-effects: see notes above; avoid in prepubertal children and growing adolescents; also reported, anorexia, depression, anxiety, tinnitus, toxic epidermal necrolysis, erythema multiforme (Stevens-Johnson syndrome); **interactions:** Appendix 1 (4-quinolones)

Dose: urinary-tract infections, 400 mg twice daily for 7–10 days (for 3 days in uncomplicated lower urinary-tract infections)
Chronic relapsing urinary-tract infections, 400 mg twice daily for 12 weeks; may be reduced to 400 mg once daily if adequate suppression within first 4 weeks

PoM Utinor® (MSD)

Tablets, norfloxacin 400mg. Net price 6-tab pack = £2.88, 14-tab pack = £6.72. Label: 6, 9

OFLOXACIN

Indications: see under Dose

Cautions; Side-effects: see notes above; caution in history of psychiatric illness and in G6PD deficiency; avoid strong sunlight; avoid in epilepsy or history of epilepsy and in children and adolescents; also reported, inflammation and rupture of tendons, erythema mutiforme, vasculitic reactions, angioedema, anxiety, unsteady gait and tremor, paraesthesia, neuropathy, psychotic reactions (discontinue treatment—see notes above); tachycardia, anaemia, agranulocytosis and pancytopenia; on intravenous infusion, hypotension and local reactions (including thrombophlebitis); **interactions:** Appendix 1 (4-quinolones)
DRIVING. May affect performance of skilled tasks (e.g. driving); effects enhanced by alcohol

Dose: by mouth, urinary-tract infections, 200–400 mg daily preferably in the morning, increased if necessary in upper urinary-tract infections to 400 mg twice daily
Lower respiratory-tract infections, 400 mg daily preferably in the morning, increased if necessary to 400 mg twice daily
Uncomplicated gonorrhoea, 400 mg as a single dose
Non-gonococcal urethritis and cervicitis, 400 mg daily in single or divided doses
By intravenous infusion (over at least 30 minutes), complicated urinary-tract infection, 200 mg daily
Lower respiratory-tract infection, 200 mg twice daily
Septicaemia, 200 mg twice daily
Severe or complicated infections, dose may be increased to 400 mg twice daily

PoM Tarivid® (Hoechst, Roussel)

Tablets, f/c, scored, ofloxacin 200 mg, net price 10-tab pack = £10.26, 20-tab pack = £20.50; 400 mg (yellow), 5-tab pack = £10.24, 10-tab pack = £20.43. Label: 6, 9, 11, counselling, driving

▼*Intravenous infusion,* ofloxacin (as hydrochloride) 2 mg/mL, net price 50-mL bottle = £15.41; 100-mL bottle = £22.01 (both hosp. only)

5.1.13   Urinary-tract infections

Urinary-tract infection is more common in women than in men; when it occurs in men there is frequently an underlying abnormality of the renal tract. Recurrent episodes of infection are an indication for radiological investigation especially in children in whom untreated pyelonephritis may lead to permanent kidney damage.

Escherichia coli is the most common cause of urinary-tract infection. Less common causes include Proteus and Klebsiella spp. *Pseudomonas aeruginosa* infections are almost invariably associated with functional or anatomical abnormalities of the renal tract. *Staphylococcus epidermidis* and *Enterococcus faecalis* infection may complicate catheterisation or instrumentation. Whenever possible a specimen of urine should be collected for culture and sensitivity testing before starting antibiotic therapy.

Uncomplicated lower urinary-tract infections often respond to ampicillin, nalidixic acid, nitrofurantoin, or trimethoprim given for 5–7 days; those caused by fully sensitive bacteria respond to two 3-g doses of amoxycillin (section 5.1.1.3). Bacterial resistance, however, especially to ampicillin (to which approximately 50% of *E. coli* are now resistant), has increased the importance of urine culture prior to therapy. Alternatives for resistant organisms include co-amoxiclav (amoxycillin with clavulanic acid), an oral cephalosporin, ciprofloxacin, and fosfomycin. Hexamine should **not** be used as it is only bacteriostatic, requires acid urine, and frequently causes side-effects.

Long-term low dose therapy may be required in selected patients to prevent *recurrence of infection*; indications include frequent relapses and significant kidney damage. Trimethoprim and nitrofurantoin have been recommended for long-term therapy.

Acute pyelonephritis can be associated with septicaemia and is best treated initially by injection of a broad-spectrum antibiotic such as aztreonam, cefuroxime, ciprofloxacin, or gentamicin especially if the patient is vomiting or severely ill.

Prostatitis can be difficult to cure and requires treatment for several weeks with an antibiotic which penetrates prostatic tissue such as trimethoprim, erythromycin, or ciprofloxacin.

Where infection is localised and associated with an indwelling *catheter* a bladder instillation is often effective (see section 1.4.4).

Patients with *heart-valve lesions* undergoing instrumentation of the urinary tract should be given a parenteral antibiotic to prevent bacteraemia and endocarditis (section 5.1, Table 2).

Urinary-tract infection in *pregnancy* may be asymptomatic and requires prompt treatment to prevent progression to acute pyelonephritis. Penicillins and cephalosporins can be given in pregnancy but trimethoprim, sulphonamides, 4-quinolones, and tetracyclines should be avoided.

In *renal failure* antibiotics normally excreted by the kidney accumulate with resultant toxicity unless the dose is reduced. This applies especially to the aminoglycosides which should be used with great caution; tetracyclines, hexamine, and nitrofurantoin should be avoided altogether.

FOSFOMYCIN

Indications: acute uncomplicated lower urinary-tract infection; prophylaxis in transurethral procedures

Cautions: pregnancy and breast-feeding; not recommended in patients over 75 years or in severe renal impairment (inadequate urinary concentrations); **interactions:** Appendix 1 (fosfomycin)

Side-effects: nausea, diarrhoea, heartburn; rash

Dose: urinary-tract infection, 3 g as a single dose at bedtime after emptying bladder; CHILD over 5 years 2 g as a single dose

Prophylaxis in transurethral procedures, 3 g as a single dose 3 hours before procedure followed by 3 g 24 hours after procedure

▼ PoM **Monuril**® (Pharmax)

Granules, fosfomycin (as trometamol) 3 g/sachet, net price 1-sachet pack = £5.95. Label: 13, 23

Paediatric granules, fosfomycin (as trometamol) 2 g/sachet, net price 1-sachet pack = £4.75. Label: 13, 23

NITROFURANTOIN

Indications: urinary-tract infections

Cautions: anaemia; diabetes mellitus; electrolyte imbalance; vitamin B and folate deficiency; pulmonary disease; hepatic impairment; monitor lung and liver function on long-term therapy, especially in the elderly; susceptibility to peripheral neuropathy; false positive urinary glucose (if tested for reducing substances); urine may be coloured yellow or brown; **interactions:** Appendix 1 (nitrofurantoin)

Contra-indications: impaired renal function, infants less than 3 months old, G6PD deficiency (including pregnancy at term, and breast-feeding of affected infants, see section 9.1.5 and Appendixes 4 and 5), porphyria (see section 9.8.2)

Side-effects: anorexia, nausea, vomiting, and diarrhoea; acute and chronic pulmonary reactions; peripheral neuropathy; also reported, angioedema, urticaria, rash and pruritus; rarely, cholestatic jaundice, hepatitis, exfoliative dermatitis, erythema multiforme, pancreatitis, arthralgia, blood disorders (including agranulocytosis, thrombocytopenia, and aplastic anaemia), and transient alopecia

Dose: acute uncomplicated infection, 50 mg every 6 hours with food for 7 days; CHILD over 3 months, 3 mg/kg daily in 4 divided doses

Severe chronic recurrent infection, 100 mg every 6 hours with food for 7 days (dose reduced or discontinued if severe nausea)

Prophylaxis (but see Cautions), 50–100 mg at night; CHILD over 3 months, 1 mg/kg at night

PoM **Nitrofurantoin** (Non-proprietary)

Tablets, nitrofurantoin 50 mg and 100 mg. Label: 9, 14, 21

Available from Biorex

PoM **Furadantin**® (Procter & Gamble Pharm.)

Tablets, all yellow, scored, nitrofurantoin 50 mg, net price 20 = £1.96; 100 mg, 20 = £3.62. Label: 9, 14, 21

Suspension, yellow, sugar-free, nitrofurantoin 25 mg/5 mL. Net price 300 mL = £4.95. Label: 9, 14, 21

PoM **Macrobid**® (Procter & Gamble Pharm.)
Capsules, m/r, blue/yellow, nitrofurantoin 100 mg
(as nitrofurantoin macrocrystals and nitrofurantoin monohydrate). Net price 14-cap pack =
£4.89. Label: 9, 14, 21, 25
> *Dose:* uncomplicated urinary-tract infection, 1 capsule
> twice daily with food
> Genito-urinary surgical prophylaxis, 1 capsule twice
> daily on day of procedure and for 3 days after

PoM **Macrodantin**® (Procter & Gamble Pharm.)
Capsules, nitrofurantoin 50 mg (yellow/white), net
price 28-cap pack = £3.05; 100 mg (yellow), 20 =
£3.84. Label: 9, 14, 21

HEXAMINE HIPPURATE
(Methenamine hippurate)
> *Indications:* prophylaxis and long-term treatment of
> recurrent urinary-tract infections
> *Cautions:* pregnancy; **interactions:** Appendix 1 (hex-
> amine)
> *Contra-indications:* severe renal impairment, dehydra-
> tion, metabolic acidosis
> *Side-effects:* gastro-intestinal disturbances, bladder irrita-
> tion, rash
> *Dose:* 1 g every 12 hours (may be increased in patients
> with catheters to 1 g every 8 hours); CHILD 6–12 years
> 500 mg every 12 hours

Hiprex® (3M)
Tablets, scored, hexamine hippurate 1 g. Net price 60-tab
pack = £7.40. Label: 9

5.2   Antifungal drugs

Fungal infections are frequently associated with a
defect in host resistance which should, if possible,
be corrected otherwise drug therapy may fail. Similarly, treatment of dermatophyte infection may be
unsuccessful until the animal source has been
removed or controlled.

For local treatment of fungal infections see also
sections 7.2.2 (genital), 7.4.4 (bladder), 11.3.2
(eye), 12.1.1 (ear), 12.3.3 (oropharynx), and
13.10.2 (skin).

POLYENE ANTIFUNGALS. The polyene antifungals
include amphotericin and nystatin.

Amphotericin is not absorbed from the gut and is
the only polyene antibiotic which can be given
parenterally. It is used for the treatment of systemic
fungal infections and is active against most fungi
and yeasts. It is highly protein bound and penetrates
poorly into body fluids and tissues. When given
parenterally amphotericin is toxic and side-effects
are common.

A formulation of amphotericin encapsulated in
liposomes (AmBisome®) is now available and is
apparently significantly less toxic than the parent
compound. A colloidal dispersion of amphotericin
and sodium cholesteryl sulphate (Amphocil®) has
also recently been made available. Both are recommended for systemic mycoses when amphotericin
alone is contra-indicated because of toxicity, especially nephrotoxicity.

Nystatin is not absorbed when given by mouth
and is too toxic for parenteral use. It is active

against a number of yeasts and fungi but is principally used for *Candida albicans* infections of skin
and mucous membranes. It is also used in the treatment of intestinal candidiasis.

IMIDAZOLE ANTIFUNGALS. The imidazole antifungals include clotrimazole, econazole, isoconazole,
ketoconazole, miconazole, sulconazole, and tioconazole; they are active against a wide range of fungi
and yeasts. Their main indications are vaginal
candidiasis and dermatophyte infections. Clotrimazole, econazole, isoconazole, sulconazole, and tioconazole are used for local treatment.

Miconazole is used for local treatment and can be
given by mouth for oral and intestinal infection; it
can also be given parenterally for systemic infections including aspergillosis, candidiasis, and
cryptococcosis but the injection contains polyethoxylated castor oil which may give rise to hypersensitivity reactions.

Ketoconazole is significantly better absorbed after
oral administration than the other imidazoles, but has
been associated with fatal hepatotoxicity. The CSM
has advised that prescribers should weigh the potential
benefits of ketoconazole treatment against the liver
damage risk and should carefully monitor patients
both clinically and biochemically. It should **not** be
given for superficial fungal infections.

TRIAZOLE ANTIFUNGALS. The triazole antifungals
include fluconazole and itraconazole which are
absorbed by mouth.

Fluconazole is an oral triazole antifungal indicated for local and systemic candidiasis and cryptococcal infections.

Itraconazole is indicated for oropharyngeal and
vulvovaginal candidiasis, pityriasis versicolor, and
tinea corporis and pedis; it is metabolised in the
liver and should not be given to patients with a history of liver disease.

OTHER ANTIFUNGALS. **Flucytosine** is a synthetic
antifungal drug which is only active against yeasts
and has been used for the treatment of systemic
candidiasis, cryptococcosis, and torulopsosis. It is
well absorbed from the gut and distributed widely
in the body. Side-effects are uncommon but bone-
marrow depression can occur and weekly blood
counts are necessary during prolonged therapy.
Synergy has been demonstrated with amphotericin.
Resistance to flucytosine is not uncommon and can
develop during therapy; sensitivity testing is, therefore, essential before and during treatment.

Griseofulvin is selectively concentrated in keratin and is the drug of choice for widespread or
intractable dermatophyte infections. It is well
absorbed from the gut but is inactive when applied
topically. It is more effective in skin than in nail
infections and treatment must be continued for several weeks or even months. Side-effects are uncommon.

Terbinafine, an allylamine antifungal, has
recently been introduced for ringworm infections
where oral treatment is considered appropriate.

> **Oral versus topical antifungal preparations.** Oral antifungal preparations should preferably be reserved for those who are resistant to (or intolerant of) topical preparations

AMPHOTERICIN
(Amphotericin B)

Indications: See under Dose

Cautions: when given parenterally, toxicity common (close supervision necessary); hepatic and renal-function tests, blood counts, and plasma electrolyte monitoring required; other nephrotoxic drugs, corticosteroids (avoid except to control reactions), antineoplastics; pregnancy and breast-feeding; frequent change of injection site (irritant); **interactions:** Appendix 1 (amphotericin)

Side-effects: when given parenterally, anorexia, nausea and vomiting, diarrhoea, epigastric pain; febrile reactions, headache, muscle and joint pain; anaemia; disturbances in renal function (including hypokalaemia and hypomagnesaemia) and renal toxicity; also cardiovascular toxicity (including arrhythmias), blood disorders, neurological disorders (including hearing loss, diplopia, convulsions, peripheral neuropathy), abnormal liver function (discontinue treatment), rash, anaphylactoid reactions

Dose: by mouth, intestinal candidiasis, 100–200 mg every 6 hours

Oral and perioral infections, see section 12.3.2

By intravenous infusion, see under preparations, below

PoM Fungilin® (Squibb)
Tablets, yellow, scored, amphotericin 100 mg. Net price 56-tab pack = £8.32. Label: 9

Lozenges—see section 12.3.2

Suspension, yellow, sugar-free, amphotericin 100 mg/mL. Net price 12 mL = £2.31. Label: 9, counselling, use of pipette

PoM Fungizone® (Squibb)
Intravenous infusion, powder for reconstitution, amphotericin (as sodium deoxycholate complex). Net price 50 mg vial = £3.70

Electrolytes: Na+ < 0.5 mmol/vial

Dose: by intravenous infusion, systemic fungal infections, 250 micrograms/kg daily, gradually increased if tolerated to 1 mg/kg daily; max. (severe infection) 1.5 mg/kg daily or on alternate days

Note. Prolonged treatment usually necessary; if interrupted for longer than 7 days recommence at 250 micrograms/kg daily and increase gradually

Lipid formulations
PoM AmBisome® (Vestar)
Intravenous infusion, powder for reconstitution, amphotericin 50 mg encapsulated in liposomes. Net price 50-mg vial = £145.00

Electrolytes: Na+ < 0.5 mmol/vial

Dose: severe systemic or deep mycoses where toxicity (particularly nephrotoxicity) precludes use of conventional amphotericin, by intravenous infusion, ADULT and CHILD initially 1 mg/kg daily as a single dose increased gradually if necessary to 3 mg/kg daily as a single dose

▼ PoM Amphocil® (Zeneca)
Intravenous infusion, powder for reconstitution, amphotericin as a complex with sodium cholesteryl sulphate. Net price 50-mg vial = £109.00, 100-mg vial = £199.00

Electrolytes: Na+ < 0.5 mmol/vial

Dose: severe systemic or deep mycoses where toxicity or renal failure preclude use of conventional amphotericin, by intravenous infusion, ADULT and CHILD initially 1 mg/kg daily as a single dose increased gradually if necessary to 3–4 mg/kg daily as a single dose

FLUCONAZOLE

Indications: see under Dose

Cautions: renal impairment; pregnancy (toxicity at high doses in *animal* studies) and breast-feeding; children (use only if imperative and if no alternative treatment; not recommended under 1 year); raised liver enzymes; **interactions:** Appendix 1 (antifungals, imidazole and triazole)

CSM Warning. Avoid concomitant administration with astemizole or terfenadine, see also p. 130 [other interactions, Appendix 1]

Side-effects: nausea, abdominal discomfort, diarrhoea, and flatulence; occasionally abnormalities of liver enzymes; rarely rash (discontinue treatment); angioedema, anaphylaxis and Stevens-Johnson syndrome reported; fixed drug eruption also reported

Dose: acute or recurrent vaginal candidiasis, *by mouth,* a single dose of 150 mg

Mucosal candidiasis (except vaginal), *by mouth,* 50 mg daily (100 mg daily in unusually difficult infections) given for 7–14 days in oropharyngeal candidiasis (max. 14 days except in severely immunocompromised patients); for 14 days in atrophic oral candidiasis associated with dentures; for 14–30 days in other mucosal infections (e.g. oesophagitis, candiduria)

Tinea pedis, corporis, cruris, versicolor, and dermal candidiasis, *by mouth,* 50 mg daily for 2–4 weeks (for up to 6 weeks in tinea pedis); max. duration of treatment 6 weeks

Systemic candidiasis and cryptococcal infections (including meningitis), *by mouth or intravenous infusion,* 400 mg initially then 200 mg daily, increased if necessary to 400 mg daily; treatment continued according to response (at least 6–8 weeks for cryptococcal meningitis)

Prevention of relapse of cryptococcal meningitis in AIDS patients after completion of primary therapy, 100–200 mg daily

Prevention of fungal infections in immunocompromised patients following cytotoxic chemotherapy or radiotherapy, 50 mg daily; 100 mg daily if risk of severe recurrent infections

CHILD over 1 year (see Cautions), *by mouth or by intravenous infusion,* superficial candidal infections, 1–2 mg/kg daily; systemic candidiasis and cryptococcal infections, 3–6 mg/kg daily (in serious life-threatening infections up to 12 mg/kg daily has been given to children aged 5–13 years—max. 400 mg daily)

PoM **Diflucan®** (Pfizer)
Capsules, fluconazole 50 mg (blue/white), net price 7-cap pack = £16.61; 150 mg (blue), single-capsule pack = £7.12; 200 mg (purple/white), 7-cap pack = £66.42. Label: 50 and 200 mg, 9
Oral suspension, fluconazole for reconstitution with water, 50 mg/5 mL, net price 35 mL = £16.61; 200 mg/5 mL, 35 mL = £66.42. Label: 9
Intravenous infusion, fluconazole 2 mg/mL in sodium chloride intravenous infusion 0.9%, net price 25-mL bottle = £7.32; 100-mL bottle = £29.28
Electrolytes: Na+ 15 mmol/100-mL bottle

FLUCYTOSINE

Indications: systemic yeast and fungal infections; adjunct to amphotericin in cryptococcal meningitis, in severe systemic candidiasis and in other severe or long-standing infections
Cautions: hepatic impairment, renal impairment (reduce dose and monitor plasma concentrations), elderly, blood disorders, liver- and kidney-function tests and blood counts required (weekly in renal impairment or blood disorders); pregnancy, breast-feeding
Side-effects: nausea, vomiting, diarrhoea, rashes; less frequently confusion, hallucinations, convulsions, headache, sedation, vertigo, alterations in liver function tests (hepatitis and hepatic necrosis reported); blood disorders including thrombocytopenia, leucopenia, and aplastic anaemia reported
Dose: by mouth or by intravenous infusion over 20–40 minutes, 200 mg/kg daily in 4 divided doses; extremely sensitive organisms, 100–150 mg/kg daily may be sufficient
Note. Plasma concentration for optimum response 25–50 mg/litre (200–400 micromol/litre)—should not be allowed to exceed 80 mg/litre (620 micromol/litre)

PoM **Alcobon®** (Roche)
Tablets, scored, flucytosine 500 mg. Net price 20 = £10.37 (hosp. only)
Intravenous infusion, flucytosine 10 mg/mL. Net price 250-mL infusion bottle = £18.21 (hosp. only)
Electrolytes: Na+ 34.44 mmol/250-mL bottle

GRISEOFULVIN

Indications: dermatophyte infections of the skin, scalp, hair and nails, where topical therapy has failed or is inappropriate
Cautions: rarely aggravation or precipitation of systemic lupus erythematosus; breast-feeding; interactions: Appendix 1 (griseofulvin)
DRIVING. May impair performance of skilled tasks (e.g. driving); effects of alcohol enhanced
Contra-indications: liver failure, porphyria (see section 9.8.2); pregnancy
Side-effects: headache, nausea, vomiting, rashes, photosensitivity; dizziness, fatigue, agranulocytopenia and leucopenia reported; lupus erythematosus, erythema multiforme, toxic epidermal necrolysis, peripheral neuropathy, confusion and impaired co-ordination also reported

Dose: 500 mg daily, in divided doses or as a single dose, in severe infection dose may be doubled, reducing when response occurs; CHILD, 10 mg/kg daily in divided doses or as a single dose

PoM **Fulcin®** (Zeneca)
Tablets, griseofulvin 125 mg (scored), net price 20 = 61p; 500 mg (f/c), 20 = £2.29. Label: 9, 21, counselling, driving
Oral suspension, brown, griseofulvin 125 mg/5 mL. Net price 100 mL = £1.10. Label: 9, 21, counselling, driving
PoM **Grisovin®** (Glaxo)
Tablets, both f/c, griseofulvin 125 mg, net price 20 = 47p; 500 mg, 20 = £1.75. Label: 9, 21, counselling, driving

ITRACONAZOLE

Indications: oropharyngeal and vulvovaginal candidiasis; pityriasis versicolor and other dermatophyte infections
Cautions: avoid if history of liver disease; liver function tests required if anorexia, nausea, vomiting, fatigue, abdominal pain or dark urine (discontinue if test abnormal); renal impairment (bioavailability may be reduced); discontinue treatment if peripheral neuropathy; pregnancy (toxicity in *animal* studies) and breast-feeding; interactions: Appendix 1 (antifungals, imidazole and triazole)
CSM Warning. Avoid concomitant administration with astemizole or terfenadine, see also p. 130 [other interactions, Appendix 1]
Side-effects: nausea, abdominal pain, dyspepsia, headache, dizziness; allergic reactions (including pruritus, rash, urticaria and angioedema), liver damage, and Stevens-Johnson syndrome reported
Dose: oropharyngeal candidiasis, 100 mg daily (200 mg daily in AIDS or neutropenia) for 15 days
Vulvovaginal candidiasis, 200 mg twice daily for 1 day
Pityriasis versicolor, 200 mg daily for 7 days
Tinea corporis and tinea cruris, 100 mg daily for 15 days
Tinea pedis and tinea manuum, 100 mg daily for 30 days
CHILD and ELDERLY not recommended

PoM **Sporanox®** (Janssen)
Capsules, blue/pink, enclosing coated beads, itraconazole 100 mg. Net price 4-cap pack = £5.99; 15-cap pack = £22.46. Label: 5, 9, 21, 25

KETOCONAZOLE

Indications: systemic mycoses, serious chronic resistant mucocutaneous candidiasis, serious resistant gastro-intestinal mycoses, chronic resistant vaginal candidiasis, resistant dermatophyte infections of skin or finger nails (not toe nails); prophylaxis of mycoses in immunosuppressed patients
Cautions: **important:** monitor liver function clinically and biochemically—for treatment lasting

---

longer than 14 days perform liver function tests before starting, 14 days after starting, then at monthly intervals (for details see data sheet); pregnancy (teratogenicity in *animal* studies, packs carry a warning to avoid in pregnancy); avoid in porphyria (see section 9.8.2); **interactions:** Appendix 1 (antifungals, imidazole and triazole)

CSM Warning. Avoid concomitant administration with astemizole or terfenadine, see also p. 130 [other interactions, Appendix 1]

Contra-indications: hepatic impairment

Side-effects: nausea, vomiting, abdominal pain; headache; rashes, urticaria, pruritus; rarely thrombocytopenia, gynaecomastia; fatal liver damage—for CSM advice see notes above, risk of developing hepatitis greater if given for longer than 14 days

Dose: 200 mg once daily with food, usually for 14 days; if response inadequate after 14 days continue until at least 1 week after symptoms have cleared and cultures become negative; max. 400 mg daily.

CHILD, 3 mg/kg daily

Chronic resistant vaginal candidiasis, 400 mg daily with food for 5 days

PoM Nizoral® (Janssen)

Tablets, scored, ketoconazole 200 mg. Net price 30-tab pack = £15.69. Label: 5, 9, 21

Suspension, pink, ketoconazole 100 mg/5 mL. Net price 100 mL with pipette = £7.16. Label: 5, 9, 21, counselling, use of pipette

MICONAZOLE

Indications: see under Dose

Cautions: change infusion site to avoid phlebitis; pregnancy; avoid in porphyria (see section 9.8.2); **interactions:** Appendix 1 (antifungals, imidazole and triazole)

CSM Warning. Avoid concomitant administration with astemizole or terfenadine, see also p. 130 [other interactions, Appendix 1]

Side-effects: nausea and vomiting, pruritus, rashes

Dose: by mouth as tablets, oral and intestinal fungal infections, 250 mg every 6 hours for 10 days or up to 2 days after symptoms clear; as oral gel, see under Daktarin® oral gel

By intravenous infusion, systemic fungal infections, initially, 600 mg every 8 hours; CHILD, max. 15 mg/kg every 8 hours up to 40 mg/kg/day

Daktarin® (Janssen)

PoM *Tablets,* scored, miconazole 250 mg. Net price 20-tab pack = £14.89. Label: 9, 21

Note. Can be sucked for oral treatment

PoM[1] *Oral gel,* sugar-free, miconazole 25 mg/mL. Net price 80 g = £5.00. Label: 9, counselling advised, hold in mouth, after food

Dose: oral and intestinal fungal infections, 5–10 mL in the mouth after food 4 times daily; retain near lesions before swallowing; CHILD under 2 years, 2.5 mL twice daily, 2–6 years, 5 mL twice daily, over 6 years, 5 mL 4 times daily

Localised lesions, smear affected area with clean finger; a 15-g tube (net price £1.95) also available

1. 15-g tube can be sold to public

PoM *Intravenous solution,* miconazole 10 mg/mL. For dilution and use as an infusion. Net price 20-mL amp = £1.47 (hosp. only)

Note. Contains polyethoxylated castor oil which has been associated with anaphylaxis

NYSTATIN

Indications: candidiasis

Side-effects: nausea, vomiting, diarrhoea at high doses; oral irritation and sensitisation; rash (including urticaria) and rarely Stevens-Johnson syndrome reported

Dose: by mouth, intestinal candidiasis 500 000 units every 6 hours, doubled in severe infections; CHILD 100 000 units 4 times daily

Prophylaxis, 1 million units daily; NEONATE 100 000 units daily as a single dose

For use as a mouthwash in oral candidiasis, see section 12.3.2

PoM Nystan® (Squibb)

Tablets, brown, s/c, nystatin 500 000 units. Net price 56-tab pack = £4.70. Label: 9

Pastilles—see section 12.3.2

Suspension, yellow, nystatin 100 000 units/mL. Net price 30 mL with pipette = £2.05. Label: 9, counselling, use of pipette

Suspension, gluten-, lactose-, and sugar-free, nystatin 100 000 units/mL when reconstituted with water. Net price 24 mL with pipette = £1.67. Label: 9, counselling, use of pipette

PoM Nystatin-Dome® (Lagap)

Suspension, yellow, nystatin 100 000 units/mL. Net price 30 mL with 1-mL spoon = £2.50. Label: 9, counselling, use of 1-mL spoon

TERBINAFINE

Indications: dermatophyte infections of the nails, ringworm infections (including tinea pedis, cruris, and corporis) where oral therapy appropriate (due to site, severity or extent)

Cautions: hepatic and renal impairment; pregnancy, breast-feeding; **interactions:** Appendix 1 (terbinafine)

Side-effects: abdominal discomfort, loss of appetite, nausea, diarrhoea; headache; rash and urticaria occasionally with arthralgia or myalgia; serious skin reactions including Stevens-Johnson syndrome and toxic epidermal necrolysis reported (discontinue treatment if progressive skin rash); also reported, taste disturbance, photosensitivity, and rarely liver toxicity including jaundice, cholestasis and hepatitis

Dose: 250 mg daily usually for 2–6 weeks in tinea pedis, 2–4 weeks in tinea cruris, 4 weeks in tinea corporis, 6 weeks–3 months or longer in nail infections; CHILD not recommended

▼ **PoM Lamisil®** (Sandoz)

Tablets, off-white, scored, terbinafine 250 mg (as hydrochloride), net price 14-tab pack = £23.16, 28-tab pack = £44.66. Label: 9

5.3   Antiviral drugs

The specific therapy of virus infections is generally unsatisfactory and treatment is, therefore, primarily symptomatic. Fortunately, the majority of infections resolve spontaneously. For **interferon** preparations used in hepatitis B infections, see section 8.2.4.

HERPES SIMPLEX AND VARICELLA–ZOSTER

Acyclovir is active against herpes viruses but does not eradicate them. It is effective only if started at the onset of infection. Uses of acyclovir include the systemic treatment of varicella–zoster (chickenpox–shingles) and the systemic and topical treatment of herpes simplex infections of the skin and mucous membranes (including initial and recurrent genital herpes); it is also used topically in the eye. It can be life-saving in herpes simplex and varicella–zoster infections in the immunocompromised, and is also used in the immunocompromised for prevention of recurrence and prophylaxis. Acyclovir may also be given by mouth to immunocompetent adults and older adolescents with chickenpox; it is not generally indicated for immunocompetent children in whom the disease is milder. See also section 11.3.3 (eye) and section 13.10.3 (skin, including herpes labialis).

Famciclovir is similar to acyclovir but need only be given 3 times daily; it is recommended for herpes zoster only.

Idoxuridine is also only effective if started at the onset of infection; it is too toxic for systemic use. It has been used topically in the treatment of herpes simplex lesions of the skin and external genitalia with variable results; it has also been used topically in the treatment of zoster, but evidence of its value is dubious. See also section 11.3.3 (eye) and section 13.10.3 (skin, including herpes labialis).

Inosine pranobex has been used by mouth for herpes simplex infections; its effectiveness has not been established.

Amantadine has been used by mouth for herpes zoster but, again, its effectiveness has not been established. Amantadine may be used for prophylaxis during an outbreak of influenza A in:

unimmunised patients in 'at risk' groups (see p. 474), for 2 weeks while the vaccine takes effect

patients in 'at risk' groups for whom immunisation is contra-indicated, for the duration of the outbreak

health care workers and other key personnel (to prevent disruption of service), during an epidemic.

ACYCLOVIR

(Aciclovir)

Indications: herpes simplex and varicella–zoster (see also under Dose)

Cautions: maintain adequate hydration; renal impairment (see Appendix 3); pregnancy and breast-feeding; **interactions:** Appendix 1 (acyclovir and famciclovir)

Side-effects: rashes; gastro-intestinal disturbances; rises in bilirubin and liver enzymes, increases in blood urea and creatinine, decreases in haematological indices, headache, neurological reactions (including dizziness), fatigue; on intravenous infusion, severe local inflammation (sometimes leading to ulceration), also confusion, hallucinations, agitation, tremors, somnolence, psychosis, convulsions and coma

Dose: by mouth,

Herpes simplex, treatment, 200 mg (400 mg in the immunocompromised or if absorption impaired) 5 times daily, usually for 5 days; CHILD under 2 years, half adult dose, over 2 years, adult dose

Herpes simplex, prevention of recurrence, 200 mg 4 times daily *or* 400 mg twice daily possibly reduced to 200 mg 2 or 3 times daily and interrupted every 6–12 months

Herpes simplex, prophylaxis in the immunocompromised, 200–400 mg 4 times daily; CHILD under 2 years, half adult dose, over 2 years, adult dose

Varicella and herpes zoster, treatment, 800 mg 5 times daily for 7 days; CHILD, varicella, 20 mg/kg (max. 800 mg) 4 times daily for 5 days *or* under 2 years 200 mg 4 times daily, 2–5 years 400 mg 4 times daily, over 6 years 800 mg 4 times daily

By intravenous infusion over 1 hour, herpes simplex or recurrent varicella–zoster 5 mg/kg every 8 hours; doubled in primary and recurrent varicella–zoster in the immunocompromised, and in simplex encephalitis; CHILD up to 3 months 10 mg/kg every 8 hours; 3 months–12 years, 250 mg/m² every 8 hours, dose doubled in the immunocompromised and in simplex encephalitis

By topical application, herpes simplex (*cream or eye ointment* as appropriate) every 4 hours (5 times daily), see sections 13.10.3 and 11.3.3

Note. Cream should not be used on mucous membranes

PoM Zovirax® (Wellcome)

Tablets, acyclovir 200 mg (blue), net price 25-tab pack = £28.89; 400 mg (pink), 56-tab pack = £105.95; 800 mg (dispersible, scored, *Shingles Treatment Pack*), 35-tab pack = £107.30. Label: 9

Suspension, both off-white, sugar-free, acyclovir 200 mg/5 mL, net price 125 mL = £28.89; 400 mg/5 mL (*Chickenpox Treatment*) 50 mL = £16.14. Label: 9

Intravenous infusion, powder for reconstitution, acyclovir (as sodium salt). Net price 250-mg vial = £10.91; 500-mg vial = £20.22

Electrolytes: Na⁺ 1.1 mmol/250-mg vial

Cream, see section 13.10.3

Eye ointment, see section 11.3.3

AMANTADINE HYDROCHLORIDE

Indications: see under Dose; parkinsonism, see section 4.9.1

Cautions; Contra-indications; Side-effects: see section 4.9.1

Dose: herpes zoster, 100 mg twice daily for 14 days, if necessary extended for a further 14 days for post-herpetic neuralgia

Influenza A₂, treatment, 100 mg twice daily for 5–7 days; prophylaxis, 100 mg twice daily (but see below) for as long as required (usually 7–10 days); CHILD 10–15 years, 100 mg daily

Department of Health guidelines. For prophylaxis of influenza A the Department of Health has advised that the recommended dose of amantadine should be reduced to 100 mg daily since higher doses are associated with more adverse effects (notably insomnia, restlessness, anxiety, nausea, anorexia, and occasionally, convulsions—mainly in the elderly taking doses higher than 100 mg daily)

Preparations
See section 4.9.1

FAMCICLOVIR

Indications: treatment of herpes zoster

Cautions: renal impairment; pregnancy and breast-feeding; **interactions:** Appendix 1 (acyclovir and famciclovir)

Side-effects: nausea; headache

Dose: 250 mg 3 times daily for 7 days; CHILD not recommended

▼ PoM **Famvir**® (SmithKline Beecham)
Tablets, f/c, famciclovir 250 mg. Net price 21-tab pack = £107.35. Label: 9

INOSINE PRANOBEX

Indications: see under Dose

Cautions: avoid in renal impairment; history of gout or hyperuricaemia

Side-effects: reversible increases in serum and urinary uric acid

Dose: mucocutaneous herpes simplex, 1 g 4 times daily for 7–14 days

Adjunctive treatment of genital warts, 1 g 3 times daily for 14–28 days

PoM **Imunovir**® (Leo)
Tablets, inosine pranobex 500 mg. Net price 100 = £36.31. Label: 9

HUMAN IMMUNODEFICIENCY VIRUS

Zidovudine inhibits the human immunodeficiency virus (HIV) but does not eradicate it from the body; it is not therefore a cure for AIDS but may delay progression of the disease. It is now also being recommended for asymptomatic HIV antibody positive individuals. Zidovudine is toxic and expensive and should only be prescribed by those experienced in its use.

Didanosine also inhibits the human immunodeficiency virus but does not eradicate it from the body. It is indicated for the treatment of symptomatic HIV infection in adult patients who are intolerant of zidovudine *or* who have shown significant clinical or immunological deterioration during zidovudine therapy *or* when zidovudine is inappropriate.

ZIDOVUDINE
(Azidothymidine, AZT)

Indications: management of advanced human immunodeficiency virus (HIV) disease such as acquired immunodeficiency syndrome (AIDS) or AIDS-related complex; early symptomatic or asymptomatic HIV infection with markers indicating risk of disease progression

Cautions: haematological toxicity (blood tests at least every 2 weeks for first 3 months then at least once a month, early disease with good bone marrow reserves may require less frequent tests e.g. every 1–3 months); vitamin B₁₂ deficiency (increased risk of neutropenia); adjust dose according to data sheet if anaemia or myelosuppression; renal impairment; hepatic impairment, monitor closely patients at risk of liver disease (especially obese women) including those with hepatomegaly and hepatitis; risk of lactic acidosis, see Side-effects; elderly; pregnancy; avoid in breast-feeding; **interactions:** Appendix 1 (zidovudine)

DRIVING. May impair performance of skilled tasks (e.g. driving); effects of alcohol may be enhanced

Contra-indications: abnormally low neutrophil counts or haemoglobin values (see data sheet)

Side-effects: anaemia (may require transfusion), neutropenia, and leucopenia (all more frequent with high dose and advanced disease); also include, nausea and vomiting, anorexia, abdominal pain, dyspepsia, headache, rash, fever, myalgia, paraesthesia, insomnia, malaise, and asthenia; also reported, convulsions (and other cerebral effects), myopathy, nail pigmentation, pancytopenia (with bone marrow hypoplasia and rarely thrombocytopenia), liver disorders including fatty change and raised bilirubin (suspend treatment if progressive hepatomegaly or rapidly elevating plasma aminotransferase), lactic acidosis (with tachypnoea, dyspnoea, and reduced plasma bicarbonate—suspend treatment)

Dose: by mouth symptomatic disease, 200 mg every 4 hours (total 1.2 g daily) for 70-kg patient; for advanced disease with poorer tolerance dose may be reduced to maintenance of 100 mg every 4 hours (total 600 mg daily); daily dosage can be given in 4–5 divided doses

Asymptomatic disease, initially 500 mg daily increased if disease progresses to 1.5 g daily CHILD over 3 months initially 180 mg/m² every 6 hours

By intravenous infusion, patients temporarily unable to take oral zidovudine, 2.5 mg/kg every 4 hours; not to be given for more than 2 weeks

PoM **Retrovir**® (Wellcome)
Capsules, zidovudine 100 mg (white/blue band), net price 100 = £124.95; 250 mg (blue/white), 40-cap pack = £124.95
Syrup, zidovudine 50 mg/5 mL. Net price 200-mL pack with 10-mL oral syringe = £24.99
Injection, zidovudine 10 mg/mL. For dilution and use as an intravenous infusion. Net price 20-mL vial = £11.94

DIDANOSINE
(DDI)

Indications: symptomatic HIV infection in patients who are intolerant of zidovudine *or* who have shown significant clinical or immunological deterioration during zidovudine therapy *or* when zidovudine is inappropriate

Cautions: history of pancreatitis (extreme caution, see also below); peripheral neuropathy or hyperuricaemia (see under Side-effects); monitor liver enzymes (suspend if significant elevation)—see also Contra-indications; hepatic and renal impairment (see Appendixes 2 and 3); pregnancy; avoid tetracyclines at same time of day (didanosine tablets contain aluminium and magnesium antacids) PANCREATITIS. If raised serum amylase suspend treatment (even if asymptomatic) until diagnosis of pancreatitis excluded; on return to normal values re-initiate treatment only if essential (using low dose increased gradually if appropriate). Whenever possible avoid concomitant treatment with other drugs known to cause pancreatic toxicity (e.g. intravenous pentamidine isethionate); monitor closely if concomitant therapy unavoidable. Since significant elevations of triglycerides cause pancreatitis monitor closely if elevated

Contra-indications: hepatic abnormalities due to previous didanosine treatment; breast-feeding

Side-effects: pancreatitis (see also under Cautions); peripheral neuropathy especially in advanced HIV infection—suspend (reduced dose may be tolerated when symptoms resolve); asymptomatic hyperuricaemia (suspend treatment if measures to reduce uric acid concentration fail); diarrhoea (occasionally serious); also reported, nausea, vomiting, confusion, insomnia, chills, fever, headache, pain, rash, pruritus, asthenia, convulsions, pneumonia

Dose: ADULT under 60 kg 125 mg every 12 hours, 60 kg and over 200 mg every 12 hours; CHILD safety and efficacy not established, see data sheet for details

COUNSELLING. Each dose to be taken as 2 tablets (total 4 tablets daily) chewed thoroughly, crushed or dispersed in water; clear apple juice may be added for flavouring

▼ PoM **Videx®** (Bristol-Myers)

Tablets, both with aluminium and magnesium antacids, didanosine 25 mg, net price 60-tab pack = £28.60; 100 mg, 60-tab pack = £88.00. Each tablet contains Al^{3+} 8.4 mmol, Mg^{2+} 7.9 mmol, Na^+ 11.5 mmol. Label: 23, counselling, administration, see above

Additives: include aspartame

CYTOMEGALOVIRUS (CMV)

Ganciclovir is related to acyclovir but is more active against cytomegalovirus; it is also much more toxic than acyclovir. It should therefore only be prescribed when the potential benefit outweighs the risks. Ganciclovir causes profound myelosuppression when given with zidovudine; the two should not normally be given together particularly during initial ganciclovir therapy.

Foscarnet is also active against cytomegalovirus but is recommended only for retinitis in AIDS patients in whom ganciclovir is contra-indicated or is inappropriate; it is toxic and can cause renal impairment in up to 50% of patients.

GANCICLOVIR

Indications: life-threatening or sight-threatening cytomegalovirus infections in immunocompromised patients only; prevention of cytomegalovirus disease during immunosuppressive therapy following organ transplantation

Cautions: close monitoring of blood counts (see data sheet); history of cytopenia; low platelet count; concomitant use of myelosuppressants or drugs which inhibit rapid cell replication; potential carcinogen; renal impairment; ensure adequate hydration during administration; vesicant—infuse into vein with adequate flow preferably via a plastic cannula; not for neonatal or congenital cytomegalovirus disease; **interactions:** see notes above and Appendix 1 (ganciclovir)

Contra-indications: pregnancy (includes effective contraception during treatment and barrier contraception for men for 90 days after treatment); breast-feeding (until 72 hours after last dose); hypersensitivity to ganciclovir or acyclovir; abnormally low neutrophil counts (see data sheet)

Side-effects: most frequent, leucopenia and thrombocytopenia; less frequent, anaemia, fever, rash, abnormal liver function tests; also chills, oedema, infections, malaise; nausea, vomiting, anorexia, gastro-intestinal haemorrhage, abdominal pain; arrhythmias, hypertension, hypotension; dyspnoea; psychosis, confusion, nervousness, drowsiness, dizziness, ataxia, paraesthesia, tremor, headache, coma; eosinphilia; decrease in blood glucose; haematuria, raised serum creatinine and blood urea nitrogen; aspermatogenesis; retinal detachment in AIDS patients with retinitis; alopecia, pruritus, urticaria; local inflammation, pain and phlebitis at injection site

Dose: by intravenous infusion over 1 hour, initially 5 mg/kg every 12 hours given for 14–21 days for treatment or for 7–14 days for prevention; maintenance (for patients at risk of relapse of retinitis) 6 mg/kg daily on 5 days per week *or* 5 mg/kg daily every day

In renal impairment, consult data sheet

PoM **Cymevene®** (Syntex)

Intravenous infusion, powder for reconstitution, ganciclovir (as sodium salt). Net price 500-mg vial (with in-line filter) = £35.58

Electrolytes: Na+ 2 mmol/500-mg vial

CAUTION IN HANDLING. Wear polythene gloves and safety glasses when reconstituting; if solution contacts skin or mucosa immediately wash with soap and water

---

FOSCARNET SODIUM

Indications: cytomegalovirus retinitis in patients with AIDS in whom ganciclovir is inappropriate

Cautions: renal impairment (avoid if severe), hypocalcaemia, monitor serum creatinine and serum calcium concentrations every second day; ensure adequate hydration

Contra-indications: pregnancy, breast-feeding

Side-effects: nausea, vomiting, headache, fatigue, rash; impairment of renal function including acute renal failure, symptomatic hypocalcaemia; decreased haemoglobin concentration; rarely hypoglycaemia, convulsions; thrombophlebitis if given undiluted by peripheral vein

Dose: by intravenous infusion, 20 mg/kg over 30 minutes then 21–200 mg/kg daily according to renal function for 2–3 weeks

PoM **Foscavir**® (Astra)

Intravenous infusion, foscarnet sodium hexahydrate 24 mg/mL, net price 250-mL bottle = £31.35, 500-mL bottle = £53.58

RESPIRATORY SYNCYTIAL VIRUS

Tribavirin inhibits a wide range of DNA and RNA viruses. It is given by inhalation for the treatment of severe bronchiolitis caused by the respiratory syncytial virus in infants, especially when they have other serious diseases. It is also effective in lassa fever.

TRIBAVIRIN
(Ribavirin)

Indications: severe respiratory syncytial virus bronchiolitis in infants and children

Cautions: maintain standard supportive respiratory and fluid management therapy; monitor equipment for precipitation

Contra-indications: pregnancy

Side-effects: reticulocytosis; also worsening respiration, bacterial pneumonia, and pneumothorax reported

Dose: by aerosol inhalation or nebulisation (via small particle aerosol generator) of solution containing 20 mg/mL for 12–18 hours for at least 3 days; max. 7 days

PoM **Virazid**® (Britannia)

Inhalation, tribavirin 6 g for reconstitution with 300 mL water for injections. Net price 3 × 6-g vials = £585.00

5.4   Antiprotozoal drugs

Cautionary label wordings, see inside back cover

Advice on specific problems available from:

Malaria Reference
Laboratory	071-636 8636 (prophylaxis only)
Birmingham	021-766 6611
Glasgow	041-946 7120
Liverpool	051-708 9393
London	071-387 4411 (treatment)
	071-388 9600 (travel prophylaxis)
Oxford	(0865) 225217
Recorded advice for Travellers	0891 600350

(48p/minute standard rate, 36p/minute cheap rate)

5.4.1   Antimalarials

Recommendations on the prophylaxis and treatment of malaria reflect guidelines agreed by UK malaria specialists.

The centres listed above should be consulted for advice on special problems.

TREATMENT OF MALARIA

If the infective species is **not known** or if the infection is **mixed** initial treatment should be with quinine, mefloquine, or halofantrine as for *falciparum malaria.*

FALCIPARUM MALARIA (TREATMENT)

Falciparum malaria (malignant malaria) is caused by *Plasmodium falciparum.* In most parts of the world *P. falciparum* is now resistant to chloroquine which should not therefore be given for treatment[1].

Quinine, mefloquine, or **halofantrine** can be given *by mouth* if the patient can swallow tablets and there are no serious manifestations (e.g. impaired consciousness); quinine should be given *by intravenous infusion* (see below) if the patient is seriously ill or unable to take tablets.

The adult dosage regimen for **quinine** *by mouth* is:

600 mg (of quinine salt[2]) every 8 hours for 7 days *and* (if quinine resistance known or suspected)

either followed by **Fansidar**® 3 tablets as a single dose

or (if Fansidar®-resistant) *followed by* **tetracycline** 250 mg every 6 hours for 7 days when renal function has returned to normal.

1. For chloroquine-sensitive strains of falciparum malaria chloroquine is effective by mouth in the dosage schedule outlined under benign malarias but it should **not** be used unless there is an **unambiguous exposure history** in one of the few remaining areas of chloroquine sensitivity.
   If the patient with a chloroquine-sensitive infection is seriously ill, chloroquine is given by continuous intravenous infusion. The dosage (for adults and children) is chloroquine 10 mg/kg (of base) infused over 8 hours, followed by three 8-hour infusions of 5 mg/kg (of base) each. Oral therapy is started as soon as possible to complete the course; the total cumulative dose for the course should be 25 mg/kg of base.
2. Valid for quinine hydrochloride, dihydrochloride, and sulphate; not valid for quinine bisulphate which contains a correspondingly smaller amount of quinine.

Prices are **net**, see p.1

Alternatively **mefloquine** or **halofantrine** (**important:** see CSM warning below) may be given instead of quinine but resistance has been reported in several countries.

The adult dosage regimen for **mefloquine** *by mouth* is:

20 mg/kg (of mefloquine base) as a single dose (up to maximum 1.5 g) *or preferably* as 2 divided doses 6–8 hours apart.

The adult dosage regimen for **halofantrine** (**important:** see CSM warning below) *by mouth* is:

1.5 g of halofantrine hydrochloride divided into three doses of 500 mg given at intervals of 6 hours (on an empty stomach); this course should be repeated after an interval of 1 week.

It is not necessary to give Fansidar® or tetracycline after mefloquine or halofantrine treatment.

Halofantrine—arrhythmias

The CSM has recommended that in order to reduce the likelihood of arrhythmias, halofantrine:

1. Should **not** be taken with meals;

2. Should **not** be taken with other drugs which may induce arrhythmias (e.g. chloroquine, mefloquine, quinine, tricyclic antidepressants, antipsychotics, certain anti-arrhythmics, and antihistamines such as astemizole and terfenadine);

3. Should **not** be taken with drugs causing electrolyte disturbances;

4. Should **not** be administered to those with known prolongation of the QT interval;

5. Should **not** be administered to those with any form of cardiac disease associated with QT interval prolongation or ventricular arrhythmias (e.g. coronary heart disease, cardiomyopathy, and congenital heart disease).

If the patient is seriously ill, **quinine** should be given *by intravenous infusion*. The adult dosage regimen for quinine *by infusion* is:

loading dose[3] of 20 mg/kg[4] (up to maximum 1.4 g) of quinine salt[2] infused over 4 hours *then after 8–12 hours* maintenance dose of 10 mg/kg[5] (up to maximum 700 mg) of quinine salt[2] infused over 4 hours every 8–12 hours (until patient can swallow tablets to complete the 7-day course) *either followed by* Fansidar® *or* (when renal function has returned to normal) tetracycline as above.

CHILDREN.

Oral. Quinine is well tolerated by children although the salts are bitter. The dosage regimen for quinine *by mouth* for children is:

10 mg/kg (of quinine salt[2]) every 8 hours for 7 days *then* (if quinine resistance known or suspected)
Fansidar® as a single dose: up to 4 years ½ tablet, 5–6 years 1 tablet, 7–9 years 1½ tablets, 10–14 years 2 tablets.

Alternatively mefloquine or halofantrine may be given instead of quinine; it is not necessary to give Fansidar® after mefloquine or halofantrine treat-

ment. The dosage regimen for mefloquine *by mouth* for children is calculated on a mg/kg basis as for adults (see above). The dosage regimen for halofantrine *by mouth* (**important:** see CSM warning above) for children over 37 kg is the same as for adults (see above); the dosage regimen for halofantrine for smaller children is reduced as follows:
weight under 23 kg, no suitable dose form;
weight 23–31 kg, 3 doses of 250 mg at intervals of 6 hours;
weight 32–37 kg, 3 doses of 375 mg at intervals of 6 hours.

This course of halofantrine should be repeated after an interval of 1 week.

Parenteral. The dosage regimen for quinine *by intravenous infusion* for children is calculated on a mg/kg basis as for adults (see above).

PREGNANCY. Falciparum malaria is particularly dangerous in pregnancy, especially in the last trimester. The adult treatment doses of oral and intravenous quinine given above (including the loading dose) can safely be given to pregnant women. Halofantrine is contra-indicated in pregnancy and tetracycline should be avoided (causes dental discoloration); Fansidar® and mefloquine are also best avoided until more information is available.

BENIGN MALARIAS (TREATMENT)

Benign malaria is usually caused by *Plasmodium vivax* and less commonly by *P. ovale* and *P. malariae*. **Chloroquine**[6] is the drug of choice for the treatment of benign malarias (but chloroquine-resistant *P. vivax* infection has been reported from New Guinea).

The adult dosage regimen for **chloroquine** *by mouth* is:

initial dose of 600 mg (of base) *then*
a single dose of 300 mg after 6 to 8 hours *then*
a single dose of 300 mg daily for 2 days
(approximate total cumulative dose of 25 mg/kg of base)

---

2. Valid for quinine hydrochloride, dihydrochloride, and sulphate; not valid for quinine bisulphate which contains a correspondingly smaller amount of quinine.

3. In intensive care units the loading dose can alternatively be given as quinine salt[2] 7 mg/kg infused over 30 minutes followed immediately by 10 mg/kg over 4 hours then (after 8 hours) maintenance dose as described.

4. **Important:** the loading dose of 20 mg/kg should not be used if the patient has received quinine (or quinidine) or mefloquine during the previous 24 hours—for **additional warnings** relating to halofantrine, see above

5. Maintenance dose should be reduced to 5–7 mg/kg of salt if parenteral treatment is required for more than 48 hours.

6. Halofantrine and mefloquine are also active in benign malarias but are not required since chloroquine is usually effective; as with chloroquine a radical cure with primaquine is required for *P. vivax* and *P. ovale* infections.

Chloroquine alone is adequate for *P. malariae* infections but in the case of *P. vivax* and *P. ovale*, a *radical cure* (to destroy parasites in the liver and thus prevent relapses) is required. This is achieved with **primaquine**[7] in an adult dosage of 15 mg daily for 14 to 21 days given after the chloroquine; a 21-day (or even longer) course may be needed for Chesson-type strains of *P. vivax* from south-east Asia and western Pacific.

CHILDREN. The dosage regimen of chloroquine for benign malaria in children is:
 initial dose of 10 mg/kg (of base) *then*
 a single dose of 5 mg/kg after 6–8 hours *then*
 a single dose of 5 mg/kg daily for 2 days
For a *radical cure* children are then given primaquine[7] in a dose of 250 micrograms/kg daily.

PREGNANCY. The adult treatment doses of chloroquine can be given for benign malaria. In the case of *P. vivax* or *P. ovale*, however, the radical cure with primaquine should be **postponed** until the pregnancy is over; instead chloroquine should be continued at a dose of 600 mg each week during the pregnancy

PROPHYLAXIS AGAINST MALARIA

The recommendations on prophylaxis reflect guidelines agreed by UK malaria specialists; the advice is aimed at residents of the UK who travel to endemic areas for short stays. The choice of drug (see next page) takes account of:

 risk of exposure to malaria;
 extent of drug resistance;
 efficacy of the recommended drugs;
 side-effects of the drugs;
 patient-related criteria (e.g. age, pregnancy, renal or hepatic impairment).

NETS AND REPELLENTS. The most important point to remember is that **prophylaxis is relative and not absolute**, and that breakthrough can occur with any of the drugs recommended anywhere in the world. Travellers should be warned that **personal protection** against being bitten (e.g. keep well covered, use mosquito nets, repellents etc.) is **very important**.

7. Before starting primaquine the blood should be tested for glucose-6-phosphate dehydrogenase (G6PD) activity as the drug can cause haemolysis in patients who are deficient in the enzyme. If the patient is G6PD deficient primaquine, in a dose for adults of 30 mg once a week (children 500–750 micrograms/kg once a week) for 8 weeks, has been found useful and without undue harmful effects.

LENGTH OF PROPHYLAXIS. In order to determine tolerance and to establish habit, prophylaxis should be started one week (preferably two weeks in the case of mefloquine) before travel into an endemic area (or if not possible at earliest opportunity up to 1 or 2 days before travel); it should be continued for **at least 4 weeks after leaving**. Mefloquine prophylaxis is appropriate for up to 3 months; longer prophylaxis requires individual assessment (and specialist advice may need to be sought).

RETURN FROM MALARIAL REGION. It is important to be aware that **any illness** that occurs within 1 year and **especially within 3 months of return might be malaria**. Travellers should be warned of this and told that if they develop any illness **particularly within 3 months** of their return they should go **immediately** to a doctor and specifically mention their exposure to malaria.

CHILDREN. The following prophylactic doses are based on guidelines agreed by UK malaria experts and may differ from advice in data sheets. If in doubt telephone centres listed on p. 255.

Age	Weight (kg)	Fraction of adult dose	
		Chloroquine Proguanil	Maloprim®
0–5 weeks		⅛	—
6 weeks–11 months		¼	—
1–5 years	10–19	½	¼
6–11 years	20–39	¾	½
12 years	40	adult dose	adult dose

Note. Weight is a better guide than age for children over 6 months old. Specialist advice should be obtained for use of Maloprim® in children under 1 year of age.

For children's doses of mefloquine see p. 260.

Prophylaxis is required in **breast-fed infants**; although antimalarials are excreted in milk, the amounts are too variable to give reliable protection.

PREGNANCY. Chloroquine and proguanil may be given in usual doses in areas where *P. falciparum* strains are sensitive; in the case of proguanil, folate supplements (folic acid 5 mg daily) should be given. Maloprim® is contra-indicated in the first trimester; folate supplements should be given if Maloprim® is prescribed in the second and third trimester. Mefloquine should also be avoided (see p. 260). The centres listed on p. 255 should be consulted for advice on prophylaxis in resistant areas.

SPECIFIC RECOMMENDATIONS

North Africa and the Middle East

Risk *extremely low* in Algeria, tourist areas of Egypt, Libya, Morocco, Tunisia, most tourist areas of Turkey:

> no prophylaxis recommended but consider malaria if fever presents

Risk *very low* in major cities (therefore no prophylaxis recommended but consider malaria if fever presents) and *present but usually low* in rural (delta) areas of Egypt (June–October), North Iraq (May–November), Syria (May–October), south coast of Turkey (Anatolia, Side) and border with Syria (March–November), United Arab Emirates; also rural Mauritius:

> chloroquine 300 mg (as base) once weekly
>
> **or**
>
> proguanil hydrochloride 200 mg once daily

Risk *present* in Afghanistan, Iran, Oman, rural Saudi Arabia, Yemen:

> **both**
> chloroquine 300 mg (as base) once weekly
> **and**
> proguanil hydrochloride 200 mg once daily

Sub-Saharan Africa

Risk *very high* in Kenya, Malawi, Tanzania, Uganda, Zambia (**important:** mefloquine particularly recommended in these countries, see below) and *sometimes very high* in rest of sub-Saharan African countries (including the Gambia), in game parks of South Africa and rural Natal and Transvaal, and in Comoros, Madagascar, Principe, and São Tomé:

> **preferably**
> mefloquine 250 mg once weekly
>
> **or**
> (if mefloquine not appropriate)
>
> **both**
> chloroquine 300 mg (as base) once weekly
> **and**
> proguanil hydrochloride 200 mg once daily

Important: mefloquine particularly recommended in Kenya, Malawi, Tanzania, Uganda, and Zambia (except for long-term travellers, women who are pregnant or likely to become pregnant, or others in whom mefloquine contraindicated).
In Zimbabwe and neighbouring countries, Maloprim® (also known as Deltaprim®) prophylaxis is widely used by local residents (sometimes with chloroquine), but it is not advised by UK malaria experts in order to simplify UK guidelines especially for those travelling to more than one country.

South Asia

Risk *variable* in Bangladesh, Bhutan, India, Nepal, Pakistan, Sri Lanka:

> **both**
> chloroquine 300 mg (as base) once weekly
> **and**
> proguanil hydrochloride 200 mg once daily

South-East Asia

Risk *very low* in tourist areas and cities of Bali, Brunei, China, Hong Kong, peninsular Malaysia, Philippines, Sarawak, Singapore, Thailand (Bangkok and main tourist areas only):

> no prophylaxis recommended but consider malaria if fever presents

Risk *substantial* in Cambodia (**important:** specialist advice needed for western Cambodia, see below), some rural areas of China, Indonesia (except Bali), Laos, some rural areas of peninsular Malaysia, Myanmar (Burma), some rural areas of Philippines, Sabah, rural Thailand (**important:** specialist advice needed for border areas, see below), Vietnam:

> mefloquine 250 mg once weekly
>
> **or**
>
> **both**
> chloroquine 300 mg (as base) once weekly
> **and**
> proguanil hydrochloride 200 mg once daily

Mefloquine preferred (except for long-term travellers, women who are pregnant or likely to become pregnant, or others in whom mefloquine contra-indicated)
Important: above regimes may not be appropriate for border areas of Thailand and western Cambodia—specialist advice needed

Oceania

Risk *high* in Papua New Guinea, Solomon Islands, Vanuatu:

> mefloquine 250 mg once weekly
>
> **or**
>
> **both**
> Maloprim® 1 tablet once weekly
> **and**
> chloroquine 300 mg (as base) once weekly

Latin America

Risk *variable* in Belize, rural Costa Rica, Dominican Republic, El Salvador, Guatemala, Haiti, Honduras, rural and little visited areas of Mexico, Nicaragua, rural Paraguay (October–May), Peru (below 1500 m), a few areas of Argentina:

> chloroquine 300 mg (as base) once weekly

Latin America *continued on next page*

Latin America *(continued)*

Risk *variable to high* in Bolivia (below 2500 m), some rural areas of Brazil, Colombia, Ecuador, French Guiana, Guyana, Panama, Suriname, rural Venezuela:

> **both**
> chloroquine 300 mg (as base) once weekly
> **and**
> proguanil hydrochloride 200 mg once daily

In Amazonia region of Brazil, mefloquine 250 mg once weekly recommended for short-term travellers (where not contra-indicated).

STANDBY TREATMENT. Adults travelling for prolonged periods to areas of chloroquine-resistance who are unlikely to have easy access to medical care should carry a standby treatment course. Self-medication should be **avoided** if medical help is accessible; prophylaxis should be continued during and after the attack.

In order to avoid excessive self-medication, the traveller should be provided with **written instructions** that urgent medical attention should be sought if fever (38°C or more) develops 7 days (or more) after arriving in a malarious area and that self treatment is indicated if medical help is not immediately available or the condition is worsening.

In view of the continuing emergence of resistant strains and of the different regimens required for different areas expert advice should be sought on the best treatment course for an individual traveller.

CHLOROQUINE

Indications: chemoprophylaxis and treatment of malaria; rheumatoid arthritis and lupus erythematosus—see section 10.1.3

Cautions: hepatic and renal impairment, pregnancy (but for malaria benefit outweighs risk, see Appendix 4, Antimalarials), may exacerbate psoriasis, neurological disorders (especially history of epilepsy), may aggravate myasthenia gravis, severe gastro-intestinal disorders, G6PD deficiency (see section 9.1.5); ophthalmic examination and long-term therapy, see p. 390; avoid concurrent therapy with hepatotoxic drugs and with halofantrine (see CSM advice under Halofantrine)—other **interactions**: Appendix 1 (chloroquine)

Side-effects: gastro-intestinal disturbances, headache, visual disturbances, irreversible retinal damage, corneal opacities, depigmentation or loss of hair, skin reactions; ECG changes; rarely blood disorders (thrombocytopenia, agranulocytosis, and aplastic anaemia), psychosis; **important:** very toxic in overdosage—immediate advice from poisons centres essential (see also p. 22)

Dose: see notes above

COUNSELLING. Warn travellers about **importance** of avoiding mosquito bites, **importance** of taking prophylaxis regularly, and **importance** of immediate visit to doctor if ill within 1 year and **especially** within 3 months of return. For details, see notes above

PoM ***Avloclor®** (Zeneca)

Tablets, scored, chloroquine phosphate 250 mg (≡chloroquine base 155 mg). Net price 20-tab pack = £1.11. Label: 5, counselling, prophylaxis, see above

* Can be sold to the public provided it is licensed and labelled for the prophylaxis of malaria

Nivaquine® (Rhône-Poulenc Rorer)

PoM* *Tablets*, f/c, yellow, chloroquine sulphate 200 mg (≡chloroquine base 150 mg). Net price 28-tab pack = £1.01. Label: 5, counselling, prophylaxis, see above

PoM* *Syrup*, golden, chloroquine sulphate 68 mg/5 mL (≡chloroquine base 50 mg/5 mL). Net price 100 mL = £2.12. Label: 5, counselling, prophylaxis, see above

* Can be sold to the public provided it is licensed and labelled for the prophylaxis of malaria

PoM *Injection*, chloroquine sulphate 54.5 mg/mL (≡chloroquine base 40 mg/mL). Net price 5-mL amp = 50p

HALOFANTRINE HYDROCHLORIDE

Indications: treatment of uncomplicated chloroquine-resistant falciparum malaria or of chloroquine-resistant vivax malaria, see notes above

Cautions: no experience of use in cerebral or complicated malaria; cardiac disease (see below); **interactions:** see below and Appendix 1 (halofantrine)

ARRHYTHMIAS. Halofantrine prolongs QT interval and has a potential for inducing hazardous arrhythmias in susceptible individuals, especially if dose excessive or if taken with food (which enhances absorption). Recommendations of the **CSM** are that halofantrine

should **not** be taken with meals;

should **not** be taken with other drugs which may induce arrhythmias (e.g. *chloroquine, mefloquine, quinine, tricyclic antidepressants, antipsychotics, certain antiarrhythmias, and antihistamines such as astemizole and terfenadine*);

should **not** be taken with drugs causing electrolyte disturbances;

should **not** be administered to those with known prolongation of the QT interval;

should **not** be administered to those with any form of cardiac disease associated with QT interval prolongation or ventricular arrhythmias (e.g. coronary heart disease, cardiomyopathy, and congenital heart disease).

Contra-indications: cardiac disorders including family history of congenital QT interval prolongation (**important:** see also above); other conditions associated with prolonged QT interval (e.g. hypokalaemia, hypomagnesaemia or other electrolyte disorders, thiamine deficiency); unexplained syncopal attacks; pregnancy and breast-feeding (avoid during treatment)

Side-effects: diarrhoea, abdominal pain, nausea, vomiting; transient elevation of serum transaminases; pruritus, rash, intravascular haemolysis, and hypersensitivity reactions also reported; **important**: ventricular arrhythmias (see also above)

Dose: see notes above

▼ PoM **Halfan®** (SK&F)

Tablets, scored, halofantrine hydrochloride 250 mg. Net price 12-tab pack = £13.96. Label: 23

MEFLOQUINE

Indications: chemoprophylaxis of malaria, treatment of uncomplicated falciparum malaria and chloroquine-resistant vivax malaria, see notes above

Cautions: exclude pregnancy before starting chemoprophylaxis (**important teratogenic risk**); avoid for chemoprophylaxis in severe hepatic and in renal impairment; cardiac conduction disorders; epilepsy (avoid for prophylaxis); not recommended in young children (under 15 kg); halofantrine must not be given with or after mefloquine (danger of fatal arrhythmias—see also under Halofantrine); other **interactions:** Appendix 1 (mefloquine)

DRIVING. May affect performance of skilled tasks (e.g. driving); effects may persist for up to 3 weeks

Contra-indications: chemoprophylaxis in pregnancy (teratogenic in *animals*, **avoid** pregnancy **during** and for **3 months after**), breast-feeding, and history of psychiatric disturbances or convulsions; hypersensitivity to quinine

Side-effects: nausea, vomiting, diarrhoea, abdominal pain; dizziness and loss of balance; rarely headache, visual disturbances, neuropsychiatric disturbances (discontinue prophylaxis), weakness, paraesthesia, rash, pruritus, and disturbances in liver function tests; very rarely cardiac conduction alterations, bradycardia, myalgia, loss of appetite, urticaria, thrombocytopenia, leucopenia; erythema multiforme (and Stevens-Johnson syndrome) reported

Dose: short-term chemoprophylaxis (up to 3 months), 250 mg each week starting 1–2 weeks before departure (see p. 257) and continued for 4 weeks after leaving malarious area; CHILD 15–19 kg (2–5 years) quarter adult dose, 20–30 kg (6–8 years) half adult dose, 31–45 kg (9–11 years) three-quarters adult dose

Longer chemoprophylaxis (more than 3 months), on individual assessment (not licensed, specialist advice may need to be sought)

Treatment, see notes above

COUNSELLING. Warn travellers about **importance** of avoiding mosquito bites, **importance** of taking prophylaxis regularly, and **importance** of immediate visit to doctor if ill within 1 year and **especially** within 3 months of return. For details, see notes above

PoM **Lariam®** (Roche)

Tablets, scored, mefloquine (as hydrochloride) 250 mg. Net price 8-tab pack = £14.53. Label: 21, 25, 27, counselling, driving, prophylaxis, see above

PRIMAQUINE

Indications: adjunct in the treatment of *Plasmodium vivax* and *P. ovale* malaria (eradication of liver stages)

Cautions: G6PD deficiency (see notes above); systemic diseases associated with granulocytopenia (e.g. rheumatoid arthritis, lupus erythematosus); pregnancy and breast-feeding; **interactions:** Appendix 1 (primaquine)

Side-effects: nausea, vomiting, abdominal pain; less commonly methaemoglobinaemia, haemolytic anaemia especially in G6PD deficiency

Dose: see notes above

Primaquine (Non-proprietary)

Tablets, primaquine (as phosphate) 7.5 mg

Available from Durbin [unlicensed—special order]

PROGUANIL HYDROCHLORIDE

Indications: chemoprophylaxis of malaria

Cautions: severe renal impairment; pregnancy (folate supplements needed); **interactions:** Appendix 1 (proguanil)

Side-effects: mild gastric intolerance and diarrhoea; occasionally mouth ulcers and stomatitis; skin reaction and hair loss reported

Dose: see notes above

COUNSELLING. Warn travellers about **importance** of avoiding mosquito bites, **importance** of taking prophylaxis regularly, and **importance** of immediate visit to doctor if ill within 1 year and **especially** within 3 months of return. For details, see notes above

Paludrine® (Zeneca)

Tablets, scored, proguanil hydrochloride 100 mg. Net price 20 = 91p. Label: 21, counselling, prophylaxis, see above

PYRIMETHAMINE

Indications: malaria (but used only in combined preparations incorporating dapsone or sulphadoxine); toxoplasmosis (section 5.4.7)

Cautions: hepatic or renal impairment; folate supplements in pregnancy, blood counts required with prolonged treatment; **interactions:** Appendix 1 (pyrimethamine)

Side-effects: depression of haematopoiesis with high doses, rashes, insomnia

Daraprim® (Wellcome)

Tablets, scored, pyrimethamine 25 mg. Net price 30-tab pack = £2.22

Dose: malaria, no dose stated because not recommended

With sulfadoxine

ADDITIONAL CAUTIONS: Severe adverse reactions on long-term use therefore not for prophylaxis; pregnancy (see also Appendix 4) and breast-feeding (see also Appendix 5); **interactions**: Appendix 1

PoM **Fansidar®** (Roche)

Tablets, scored, pyrimethamine 25 mg, sulfadoxine 500 mg. Net price 10-tab pack = £2.77

Dose: treatment, see notes above

Chemoprophylaxis, not recommended by UK experts

With dapsone
ADDITIONAL CAUTIONS: G6PD deficiency (see section
9.1.5); pregnancy (see also Appendix 4) and breast-feeding (see also Appendix 5); **interactions**: Appendix 1

PoM Maloprim® (Wellcome)

Tablets, scored, pyrimethamine 12.5 mg, dapsone
100 mg. Net price 30-tab pack = £2.76. Counselling, prophylaxis, see above
Dose: limited use, see Chemoprophylaxis
COUNSELLING. Warn travellers about **importance** of
avoiding mosquito bites, **importance** of taking prophylaxis regularly, and **importance** of immediate visit to
doctor if ill within 1 year and **especially** within 3
months of return. For details, see notes above

QUININE

Indications: falciparum malaria; nocturnal leg
cramps, see section 10.2.2
Cautions: atrial fibrillation, conduction defects,
heart block, pregnancy; monitor blood glucose
concentration during parenteral treatment; G6PD
deficiency (see section 9.1.5); avoid concurrent
administration with halofantrine (see CSM advice
under Halofantrine), other **interactions**: Appendix 1 (quinine)
Contra-indications: haemoglobinuria, optic neuritis
Side-effects: cinchonism, including tinnitus, headache, hot and flushed skin, nausea, abdominal
pain, rashes, visual disturbances (including temporary blindness), confusion; hypersensitivity
reactions including angioedema, blood disorders
(including thrombocytopenia and intravascular
coagulation), and acute renal failure; hypoglycaemia (especially after parenteral administration);
cardiovascular effects (see Cautions); **important:**
very toxic in overdosage—immediate advice
from poisons centres essential (see also p. 22)
Dose: see notes above
Note. Quinine (anhydrous base) 100 mg ≡ quinine bisulphate 169 mg ≡ quinine dihydrochloride 122 mg ≡ quinine hydrochloride 122 mg ≡ quinine sulphate 121 mg.
Quinine bisulphate 300-mg tablets are available but provide smaller amounts of quinine than the dihydrochloride, hydrochloride, or sulphate

PoM Quinine Sulphate (Non-proprietary)
Tablets, coated, quinine sulphate 200 mg, net price
20 = 77p; 300 mg, 20 = 61p
PoM Quinine Dihydrochloride
Injection, quinine dihydrochloride 300 mg/mL.
For dilution and use as an infusion. 1- and 2-mL
amps
Injection available from Martindale and Penn (both spe-
cial order) or from specialist centres (see p. 255)
Note. Intravenous injection of quinine is so hazardous that
it has been superseded by infusion

5.4.2 Amoebicides

Metronidazole is the drug of choice for *acute invasive amoebic dysentery* since it is very effective
against vegetative forms of *Entamoeba histolytica*
in ulcers; it is given in an adult dose of 800 mg three
times daily for 5 days. **Tinidazole** is also effective.
Metronidazole and tinidazole are also active against
amoebae which may have migrated to the liver.

Treatment with metronidazole (or tinidazole) is followed by a 10-day course of diloxanide furoate.

Diloxanide furoate is the drug of choice for
asymtomatic patients with *E. histolytica* cysts in the
faeces; metronidazole and tinidazole are relatively
ineffective. Diloxanide furoate is relatively free
from toxic effects and the usual course is of 10
days, given alone for chronic infections or following metronidazole or tinidazole treatment.

For *amoebic abscesses* of the liver **metronidazole** is effective in doses of 400 mg 3 times daily
for 5–10 days; tinidazole is an alternative. The
course may be repeated after 2 weeks if necessary.
Aspiration of the abscess is indicated where it is
suspected that it may rupture or where there is no
improvement after 72 hours of metronidazole; the
aspiration may need to be repeated. Aspiration aids
penetration of metronidazole and, for abscesses
with more than 100 mL of pus, if carried out in conjunction with drug therapy, may reduce the period
of disability.

Rarely, where metronidazole and tinidazole
appear to be ineffective, dehydroemetine may be
used (but the risk of side-effects is much greater).
Diloxanide furoate is not effective against hepatic
amoebiasis, but a 10-day course should be given at
the completion of metronidazole or tinidazole treatment to destroy any amoebae in the gut.

DILOXANIDE FUROATE

Indications: chronic amoebiasis—see notes
Side-effects: flatulence, vomiting, urticaria, pru-
ritus
Dose: 500 mg every 8 hours for 10 days; CHILD
20 mg/kg daily in 3 divided doses.
See also notes above

PoM Furamide® (Boots)
Tablets, scored, diloxanide furoate 500 mg. Label: 9
Available only on direct order from Boots
PoM Entamizole® (Boots)
Tablets, off-white, diloxanide furoate 250 mg, metronid-
azole 200 mg. Label: 4, 9, 21, 25
Available only on direct order from Boots
Dose: amoebiasis, 2 tablets 3 times daily for 5 days;
CHILD 5–12 years ½–1 tablet, according to age, for 5
days
Treatment may be extended to 10 days in refractory
cases; not suitable for prolonged (e.g. prophylactic) use

METRONIDAZOLE

Indications: see under Dose below; anaerobic
infections, section 5.1.11
Cautions; Side-effects: section 5.1.11
Dose: by mouth, invasive intestinal amoebiasis,
800 mg every 8 hours for 5 days; CHILD 1–3 years
200 mg every 8 hours; 3–7 years 200 mg every 6
hours; 7–10 years 400 mg every 8 hours
Extra-intestinal amoebiasis (including liver
abscess) and symptomatic amoebic cyst passers,
400–800 mg every 8 hours for 5–10 days; CHILD
1–3 years 100–200 mg every 8 hours; 3–7 years
100–200 mg every 6 hours; 7–10 years 200–
400 mg every 8 hours

Urogenital trichomoniasis, 200 mg every 8 hours for 7 days *or* 400 mg every 12 hours for 7 days, *or* 800 mg in the morning and 1.2 g at night for 2 days, *or* 2 g as a single dose; CHILD 1–3 years 50 mg every 8 hours for 7 days; 3–7 years 100 mg every 12 hours; 7–10 years 100 mg every 8 hours
Giardiasis, 2 g daily for 3 days; CHILD 1–3 years 500 mg daily; 3–7 years 600–800 mg daily; 7–10 years 1 g daily

Preparations
Section 5.1.11

TINIDAZOLE
Indications: see under Dose below; anaerobic infections, section 5.1.11
Cautions; Side-effects: section 5.1.11
Dose: intestinal amoebiasis, 2 g daily for 2–3 days; CHILD 50–60 mg/kg daily for 3 days
Amoebic involvement of liver, 1.5–2 g daily for 3–5 days; CHILD 50–60 mg/kg daily for 5 days
Urogenital trichomoniasis and giardiasis, single 2-g dose (repeated once if necessary); CHILD single dose of 50–75 mg/kg

Preparations
Section 5.1.11

5.4.3   Trichomonacides
Metronidazole (section 5.4.2) is the treatment of choice for *Trichomonas vaginalis* infection.
If metronidazole is ineffective, **tinidazole** may be tried; it is usually given as a single 2-g dose, with food. A further 2-g dose may be given if there is no clinical improvement.
Alcohol should be avoided during treatment with both metronidazole and tinidazole.

5.4.4   Antigiardial drugs
Metronidazole (section 5.4.2) is the treatment of choice for *Giardia lamblia* infections, given by mouth in a dosage of 2 g daily for 3 days or 400 mg every 8 hours for 5 days.
Alternative treatments are **tinidazole** (section 5.4.2) 2 g as a single dose or **mepacrine hydrochloride** 100 mg every 8 hours for 5–7 days.

MEPACRINE HYDROCHLORIDE
Indications: giardiasis
Cautions: hepatic impairment, elderly, history of psychosis; avoid in psoriasis; **interactions:** Appendix 1 (mepacrine)
Side-effects: gastro-intestinal disturbances; dizziness, headache; with large doses nausea, vomiting and occasionally transient acute toxic psychosis and CNS stimulation; on prolonged treatment yellow discoloration of skin and urine, chronic dermatoses (including severe exfoliative dermatitis), hepatitis, aplastic anaemia; also reported blue/black discoloration of palate and nails and corneal deposits with visual disturbances
Dose: 100 mg every 8 hours for 5–7 days; CHILD 2 mg/kg every 8 hours

Mepacrine Hydrochloride
Tablets, mepacrine hydrochloride 100 mg. Label: 4, 9, 14, 21
Available from Boots [unlicensed—special order]

5.4.5   Leishmaniacides
Cutaneous leishmaniasis frequently heals spontaneously but if skin lesions are extensive or unsightly, treatment is indicated, as it is in visceral leishmaniasis (kala-azar).
Sodium stibogluconate, an organic pentavalent antimony compound, is the treatment of choice for visceral leishmaniasis. The dose is 20 mg/kg daily (max. 850 mg) for at least 20 days by intramuscular or intravenous injection; the dosage varies with different geographical regions and expert advice should be obtained. Skin lesions are treated for 10 days.
Pentamidine isethionate (section 5.4.8) has been used in antimony-resistant visceral leishmaniasis, but although the initial response is often good, the relapse rate is high; it is associated with serious side-effects. Other treatments include paromomycin (*Farmitalia Carlo Erba*, not on UK Market) or liposomal amphotericin [section 5.2 but not licensed for leishmaniasis].

SODIUM STIBOGLUCONATE
Indications: leishmaniasis
Cautions: intravenous injections must be given slowly and stopped if coughing or substernal pain develops; intramuscular injection painful
Contra-indications: pneumonia, myocarditis, nephritis, hepatitis
Side-effects: anorexia, vomiting, coughing, substernal pain
Dose: see notes above

PoM **Pentostam®** (Wellcome)
Injection, sodium stibogluconate equivalent to pentavalent antimony 100 mg/mL. Net price 100-mL bottle = £68.01

5.4.6   Trypanocides
The prophylaxis and treatment of trypanosomiasis is difficult and differs according to the strain of organism. Expert advice should therefore be obtained.

5.4.7   Drugs for toxoplasmosis
Most infections caused by *Toxoplasma gondii* are self-limiting, and treatment is not necessary. Exceptions are patients with eye involvement (toxoplasma choroidoretinitis), and those who are immunosuppressed. The treatment of choice is a combination of pyrimethamine and sulphadiazine, given for several weeks (expert advice **essential**). Pyrimethamine is a folate antagonist, and adverse reactions to this combination are relatively common (folinic acid supplements and weekly blood counts needed).
If toxoplasmosis is acquired in pregnancy, transplacental infection may lead to severe disease in the

fetus. The pyrimethamine and sulphadiazine combination is best avoided in pregnancy but there are encouraging reports with spiramycin (not on UK market).

5.4.8 Drugs for Pneumocystis pneumonia

Pneumonia caused by *Pneumocystis carinii* occurs in immunosuppressed or severely debilitated patients. It is the commonest cause of pneumonia in AIDS. **Co-trimoxazole** (section 5.1.8) in high dosage is the drug of choice for the treatment of pneumocystis pneumonia. **Pentamidine isethionate** is an alternative to co-trimoxazole and is particularly indicated for patients with a history of adverse reactions to, or who have not responded to, co-trimoxazole. Pentamidine isethionate is a potentially toxic drug that can cause severe hypotension during or immediately after administration; it should only be administered by those experienced in its use. Pentamidine isethionate is given by intravenous infusion but can also be administered by inhalation which reduces side-effects (although systemic absorption may still occur); intermittent prophylactic inhalation may prevent relapse.

PENTAMIDINE ISETHIONATE
(Pentamidine isetionate)

Indications: see under Dose (should only be given by specialists)

Cautions: risk of severe hypotension following administration (establish baseline blood pressure and administer with patient lying down); monitor blood pressure closely during administration, and at regular intervals, until treatment concluded); hepatic and renal impairment; hypertension or hypotension; hyperglycaemia or hypoglycaemia; leucopenia, thrombocytopenia, or anaemia; carry out laboratory monitoring for all functions according to data sheet

Side-effects: severe reactions, sometimes fatal, due to hypotension, hypoglycaemia, pancreatitis, and arrhythmias; also leucopenia, thrombocytopenia, acute renal failure, hypocalcaemia; also reported: azotaemia, abnormal liver-function tests, leucopenia, anaemia, hyperkalaemia, nausea and vomiting, dizziness, syncope, flushing, hyperglycaemia, rash, and taste disturbances; bronchoconstriction reported on inhalation; discomfort, pain, induration, abscess formation, and muscle necrosis at injection site

Dose: Pneumocystis carinii pneumonia, *by intravenous infusion*, 4 mg/kg daily for at least 14 days (reduced according to data sheet in renal impairment)

By inhalation of nebulised solution (using suitable equipment—see data sheet) 600 mg pentamidine isethionate daily for 3 weeks; secondary prevention, 300 mg every 4 weeks *or* 150 mg every 2 weeks

Visceral leishmaniasis (Kala-azar), *by deep intramuscular injection*, 3–4 mg/kg on alternate days to max. total of 10 injections; course may be repeated if necessary

Cutaneous leishmaniasis, *by deep intramuscular injection*, 3–4 mg/kg once or twice weekly until condition resolves (but see also section 5.4.5)

Trypanosomiasis, *by deep intramuscular injection or intravenous infusion*, 4 mg/kg daily or on alternate days to total of 7–10 injections

Note. Direct bolus intravenous injection should be avoided whenever possible and **never** given rapidly; intramuscular injections should be deep and preferably given into the buttock

PoM **Pentacarinat®** (Rhône-Poulenc Rorer)
Injection, powder for reconstitution, pentamidine isethionate. Net price 300-mg vial = £15.58
Nebuliser solution, pentamidine isethionate. Net price 300-mg bottle = £16.45

5.5   Anthelmintics

5.5.1   Drugs for threadworms
5.5.2   Ascaricides
5.5.3   Drugs for tapeworm infections
5.5.4   Drugs for hookworms
5.5.5   Schistosomicides
5.5.6   Filaricides
5.5.7   Drugs for guinea worms
5.5.8   Drugs for strongyloidiasis

Advice on prophylaxis and treatment of helminth infections is available from:

Birmingham	021-766 6611
Glasgow	041-946 7120
Liverpool	051-708 9393
London	071-387 4411 (treatment)

5.5.1   Drugs for threadworms
(pinworms, *Enterobius vermicularis*)

Anthelmintics are effective in threadworm infections, but their use needs to be combined with hygienic measures to break the cycle of auto-infection. All members of the family require treatment.

Adult threadworms do not live for longer than 6 weeks and for development of fresh worms, ova must be swallowed and exposed to the action of digestive juices in the upper intestinal tract. Direct multiplication of worms does not take place in the large bowel. Adult female worms lay ova on the peri-anal skin which causes pruritus; scratching the area then leads to ova being transmitted on fingers to the mouth, often via food eaten with unwashed hands. Washing hands and scrubbing nails before each meal and after each visit to the toilet is essential. A bath taken immediately after rising will remove ova laid during the night.

Mebendazole is the drug of choice for patients of all ages over 2 years. It is given as a single dose; as reinfection is very common, a second dose may be given after 2–3 weeks.

Piperazine salts are preferably given daily for 7 days (followed by a second course if necessary 7 days later); single-dose preparations are also available.

Pyrantel is equally effective. It is given as a single dose of 10 mg/kg (max. 1 g); cure-rates are improved if one or two further doses are given at intervals of 2 weeks.

MEBENDAZOLE

Indications: threadworm, roundworm, whipworm, and hookworm infections

Cautions: pregnancy (toxicity in *rats*), breast-feeding; **interactions:** Appendix 1 (mebendazole)

Note. The package insert in the Vermox® pack includes the statement that it is not suitable for women known to be pregnant or children under 2 years

Side-effects: rarely abdominal pain, diarrhoea; hypersensitivity reactions (including exanthema, rash, urticaria, and angioedema) reported

Dose: threadworms, ADULT and CHILD over 2 years, 100 mg as a single dose; if reinfection occurs second dose may be needed after 2–3 weeks; CHILD under 2 years, not yet recommended

Roundworms—section 5.5.2

Hookworms—section 5.5.4

PoM ¹**Vermox®** (Janssen)

Tablets, orange, scored, chewable, mebendazole 100 mg. Net price 6-tab pack = £1.53

Suspension mebendazole 100 mg/5 mL. Net price 30 mL = £1.77

1. Can be sold to the public if supplied for oral use in the treatment of enterobiasis in adults and children over 2 years provided its container or package is labelled to show a max. single dose of 100 mg and it is supplied in a container or package containing not more than 400 mg; a proprietary brand (Ovex®) is also on sale to the public.

PIPERAZINE

Indications: threadworm and roundworm infections

Cautions: renal impairment (avoid if severe), liver disease, neurological disease; epilepsy, pregnancy (see also Appendix 4—packs on sale to the general public carry a warning to avoid in epilepsy and pregnancy); **interactions:** Appendix 1 (piperazine)

Side-effects: nausea, vomiting, colic, diarrhoea; allergic reactions including urticaria, broncho-spasm, and rare reports of Stevens-Johnson syndrome and angioedema; rarely dizziness, muscular incoordination ('worm wobble'); drowsiness, confusion and clonic contractions in patients with neurological or renal abnormalities

Dose: see under Preparations, below

Piperazine Citrate (Non-proprietary)

Elixir, piperazine hydrate 750 mg/5 mL (as citrate) Available from Cupal (Expelix®), De Witt (De Witt's Worm Syrup)

Dose: threadworms, 15 mL once daily for 7 days; CHILD under 2 years (on doctor's advice only) 0.3–0.5 mL/kg once daily for 7 days, 2–3 years 5 mL once daily for 7 days, 4–6 years 7.5 mL once daily for 7 days, 7–12 years 10 mL once daily for 7 days; repeat course after 1 week if necessary

Roundworms, 30 mL as a single dose; CHILD under 1 year (on doctor's advice only) 0.8 mL/kg as a single dose, 1–3 years 10 mL as a single dose, 4–5 years 15 mL as a single dose, 6–8 years 20 mL as a single dose, 9–12 years 25 mL as a single dose; repeat dose after 2 weeks

Pripsen® (R&C)

Oral powder, cream, piperazine phosphate 4 g and sennosides 15.3 mg/sachet. Net price two-dose sachet pack = £1.31. Label: 13

Dose: threadworms, stirred into a small glass of milk or water and drunk immediately, ADULT and CHILD over 6 years, 1 sachet, repeat after 14 days; INFANT 3 months–1 year, one-third sachet (2.5 mL powder), repeat after 14 days; CHILD 1–6 years, two-thirds sachet (5 mL powder), repeat after 14 days

Roundworms, first dose as for threadworms; repeat at monthly intervals for up to 3 months if reinfection risk

5.5.2   Ascaricides

(common roundworm infections)

Levamisole (not on UK market) is very effective against *Ascaris lumbricoides* and is generally considered to be the drug of choice. It is very well tolerated; mild nausea or vomiting has been reported in about 1% of treated patients; it is given as a single dose of 120–150 mg in adults.

Mebendazole (section 5.5.1) is also active against ascaris; the usual dose is 100 mg twice daily for 3 days. **Pyrantel** is also an effective broad-spectrum anthelmintic and a single dose of 10 mg/kg (max. 1 g) is usually sufficient to eradicate ascaris; it may occasionally produce mild nausea but experience shows it to be a very safe drug. **Piperazine** may also be given in a single adult dose equivalent to 4–4.5 g of piperazine hydrate see Piperazine, above.

PYRANTEL

Indications: roundworm, threadworm, and hook-worm infections

Cautions: liver disease, pregnancy; **interactions:** Appendix 1 (pyrantel)

Side-effects: anorexia, abdominal cramps, nausea, vomiting, diarrhoea; headache, dizziness, sleep disturbance; rash

Dose: ADULT and CHILD over 6 months, *Ascaris lumbricoides* alone, a single dose of 5 mg/kg; mixed infections involving *Ascaris lumbricoides*, single dose of 10 mg/kg

Hookworm—section 5.5.4

Threadworm—section 5.5.1

PoM **Combantrin®** (Pfizer)
Tablets, orange, pyrantel 125 mg (as embonate).
  Net price 6-tab pack = 64p

5.5.3   Drugs for tapeworm infections

TAENICIDES

Niclosamide is the most widely used drug for tapeworm infections and side-effects are limited to occasional gastro-intestinal upset, lightheadedness, and pruritus; it is not effective against larval worms. Fears of developing cysticercosis in *Taenia solium* infections have proved unfounded. All the same, it is wise to anticipate this possibility by using an anti-emetic on wakening.

Praziquantel (Biltricide®, not on UK market) is as effective as niclosamide and is given as a single dose of 10–20 mg/kg after a light breakfast (a single dose of 25 mg/kg for *Hymenolepis nana*).

NICLOSAMIDE

Indications: tapeworm infections—see notes above and under Dose
Side-effects: nausea, retching, abdominal pain; lightheadedness; pruritus
Dose: Taenia solium, ADULT and CHILD over 6 years 2 g as a single dose after a light breakfast followed by a purgative after 2 hours; CHILD under 2 years 500 mg, 2–6 years 1 g
T. saginata and *Diphyllobothrium latum*, as for *T. solium* but half the dose may be taken after breakfast and the remainder 1 hour later followed by a purgative 2 hours after last dose
Hymenolepis nana, ADULT and CHILD over 6 years 2 g as a single dose on first day then 1 g daily for 6 days; CHILD under 2 years 500 mg on first day then 250 mg daily for 6 days, 2–6 years 1 g on first day then 500 mg daily for 6 days
COUNSELLING. Tablets should be chewed thoroughly (or crushed) before washing down with water

Yomesan® (Bayer)
Tablets, yellow, chewable, niclosamide 500 mg.
  Net price 4-tab pack = £1.41. Label: 4, 24, counselling, administration

HYDATID DISEASE

Cysts caused by *Echinococcus granulosus* grow slowly and asymptomatic patients do not always require treatment. Surgical treatment remains the method of choice in many situations. **Albendazole** is used in conjunction with surgery to reduce the risk of recurrence or as primary treatment in inoperable cases. Alveolar echinococcosis due to *E. multilocularis* is usually fatal if untreated. Surgical removal with albendazole cover is the treatment of choice, but where effective surgery is impossible, repeated cycles of albendazole (for a year or more) may help. Careful monitoring of liver function is particularly important during drug treatment.

ALBENDAZOLE
Indications: adjunct to surgery in hydatid cysts caused by *Echinococcus granulosus* or *E. multilocularis*, or primary treatment if surgery not possible; strongyloidiasis (section 5.5.8)
Cautions: blood counts and liver function tests before treatment and twice during each cycle; breast-feeding; exclude pregnancy before starting treatment (non-hormonal contraception during and for 1 month after treatment)
Contra-indications: pregnancy (see also Cautions)
Side-effects: gastro-intestinal disturbances, headache, dizziness, changes in liver enzymes; rarely reversible alopecia; rash, fever, blood disorders including leucopenia and pancytopenia reported; allergic shock if cyst leakage; convulsions and meningism in cerebral disease
Dose: E. granulosus, ADULT over 60 kg, medical treatment, 800 mg daily in divided doses for 28 days followed by 14 tablet-free days; up to 3 cycles of treatment may be given
Adjunct in surgical treatment, *pre-surgery*, 800 mg daily in divided doses for 28 days followed by 14 tablet-free days, repeat cycle once before surgery; *post-surgery* (if viable cysts after pre-surgery treatment, or if no pre-surgery treatment, or if only short pre-surgery course), 800 mg daily in divided doses for 28 days followed by 14 tablet-free days, repeat cycle once
E. multilocularis, ADULT over 60 kg, 800 mg daily in divided doses for 28 days followed by 14 tablet-free days; prolonged treatment may be required, see notes above

▼ PoM **Eskazole®** (SmithKline Beecham)
Tablets, orange, scored, chewable, albendazole 400 mg. Net price 60-tab pack = £72.00. Label: 9

5.5.4   Drugs for hookworms
(ancylostomiasis, necatoriasis)

Hookworms live in the upper small intestine and draw blood from the point of their attachment to their host. An iron-deficiency anaemia may thereby be produced and, if present, effective treatment of the infection requires not only expulsion of the worms but treatment of the anaemia.

Mebendazole (section 5.5.1) has a useful broad-spectrum activity, and is effective against hookworms; the usual dose is 100 mg twice daily for 3 days.

Pyrantel (section 5.5.2) is also very effective against hookworms; its side-effects are limited to occasional nausea and vomiting. The usual dose is 10 mg/kg (max. 1 g) given as a single dose for light infections; heavy infections may need single daily doses for 3 days

5.5.5   Schistosomicides
(bilharziasis)

Adult *Schistosoma haematobium* worms live in the genito-urinary veins and adult *S. mansoni* in those of the colon and mesentery. *S. japonicum* is more widely distributed in veins of the alimentary tract and portal system.

Praziquantel (Biltricide®, not on UK market) is effective against all human schistosomes. The dose is 40 mg/kg in 2 divided doses 4–6 hours apart on one day (60 mg/kg in 3 divided doses on one day for *S. japonicum* infections). No serious toxic effects have been reported. Of all the available schistosomicides, it has the most attractive combination of effectiveness, broad-spectrum activity, and low toxicity.

Oxamniquine (may no longer be available) is effective against *S. mansoni* infections only. It is a quinoline compound given by mouth; the dosage ranges from 15 mg/kg as a single dose to a total of 60 mg/kg over 2 to 3 days according to the geographical region. It can occasionally cause convulsions.

Metriphonate (Bilarcil®, not on UK market) is effective against *S. haematobium* infections only; it may be used if praziquantel is not available.

Hycanthone, lucanthone, niridazole, and stibocaptate have now been superseded.

5.5.6   Filaricides

Diethylcarbamazine (Hetrazan®, *Lederle*) is effective against microfilariae and adults of *Loa loa*, *Wuchereria bancrofti*, and *Brugia malayi*. To minimise reactions treatment is commenced with a dose of diethylcarbamazine citrate 1 mg/kg and increased gradually over 3 days to 6 mg/kg daily in divided doses; this dosage is maintained for 21 days and usually gives a radical cure for these infections. Close medical supervision is necessary particularly in the early phase of treatment.

In heavy infections there may be a febrile reaction, and in heavy *Loa loa* infection there is a small risk of encephalopathy. In such cases treatment must be given under careful in-patient supervision and stopped at the first sign of cerebral involvement (and specialist advice sought).

Ivermectin (Mectizan®, *MSD*, not on UK market) is very effective in *onchocerciasis* and it is now the drug of choice. A single dose of 150 micrograms/kg by mouth produces a prolonged reduction in microfilarial levels. Retreatment at intervals of 6 to 12 months depending on symptoms must be given until the adult worms die out. Reactions are usually slight and most commonly take the form of temporary aggravation of itching and rash. Diethylcarbamazine or suramin should no longer be used for onchocerciasis because of their toxicity.

5.5.7   Drugs for guinea worms
(dracontiasis)

Metronidazole has been reported to be effective against *Dracunculus medinensis* in a dose of 400 mg three times daily for 5 days. In India, **mebendazole** has been reported as effective at a dosage of 200 mg twice daily for 7 days.

5.5.8   Drugs for strongyloidiasis

Adult *Strongyloides stercoralis* live in the gut and produce larvae which penetrate the gut wall and invade the tissues, setting up a cycle of auto-infection. **Thiabendazole** is the drug of choice, at a dosage of 25 mg/kg (max. 1.5 g) every 12 hours for 3 days. **Albendazole** (section 5.5.3) is an alternative with fewer side-effects; it is given in a dose of 400 mg daily for 3 days, repeated after 3 weeks if necessary.

THIABENDAZOLE
(Tiabendazole)

Indications: strongyloidiasis, cutaneous and visceral larva migrans, dracontiasis, symptoms of trichinosis; secondary treatment for threadworm when mixed with above infestations; adjunct in hookworm, whipworm, or roundworm

Cautions: hepatic or renal impairment, discontinue if hypersensitivity reactions occur; **interactions:** Appendix 1 (thiabendazole)

DRIVING. May impair performance of skilled tasks (e.g. driving)

Contra-indications: pregnancy (teratogenesis in *animal* studies)

Side-effects: anorexia, nausea, vomiting, dizziness, diarrhoea, headache, pruritus, drowsiness; hypersensitivity reactions including fever, chills, angioedema, rashes, erythema multiforme; rarely tinnitus, collapse, parenchymal liver damage

Dose: see notes above

PoM Mintezol® (MSD)
Tablets, orange, chewable, thiabendazole 500 mg.
Net price 6-tab pack = 62p. Label: 3, 21, 24

6: Drugs used in the treatment of disorders of the
ENDOCRINE SYSTEM

In this chapter, drug treatment is discussed under the following headings:

6.1	Drugs used in diabetes
6.2	Thyroid and antithyroid drugs
6.3	Corticosteroids
6.4	Sex hormones
6.5	Hypothalamic and pituitary hormones
6.6	Drugs affecting bone metabolism
6.7	Other endocrine drugs

6.1 Drugs used in diabetes

6.1.1	Insulin
6.1.2	Oral antidiabetic drugs
6.1.3	Diabetic ketoacidosis
6.1.4	Treatment of hypoglycaemia
6.1.5	Treatment of diabetic neuropathy
6.1.6	Diagnostic and monitoring agents for diabetes mellitus

6.1.1 Insulin

6.1.1.1	Short-acting insulin
6.1.1.2	Intermediate- and long-acting insulins
6.1.1.3	Hypodermic equipment

Insulin plays a key role in the body's regulation of carbohydrate, fat, and protein metabolism. Diabetes mellitus is due to a deficiency in insulin synthesis and secretion. Patients are generally described as insulin-dependent diabetics (type 1) or non-insulin-dependent diabetics (type 2), although many of the latter need insulin to maintain satisfactory control.

Insulin is a polypeptide hormone of complex structure. It is extracted mainly from pork pancreas and purified by crystallisation; it can also be made biosynthetically by recombinant DNA technology using *Escherichia coli* or semisynthetically by enzymatic modification of porcine material (see under Human Insulins, below). All insulin preparations are to a greater or lesser extent immunogenic in man but immunological resistance to insulin action is uncommon.

Insulin is inactivated by gastro-intestinal enzymes, and must therefore be given by injection; the subcutaneous route is ideal for most circumstances. It is usually injected into the upper arms, thighs, buttocks, or abdomen; there may be increased absorption from a limb site if the limb is used in strenuous exercise. Insulin is most readily administered by injection devices ('pens') (section 6.1.1.3) which hold insulin in cartridge form and meter the required dose. The more conventional syringe and needle is still preferred by many and is also required for insulins not available in cartridge form. Subcutaneous insulin injections generally cause no problems although fat hypertrophy is not rare; to some extent it can be avoided by rotating the injection sites. Local allergic reactions are now scarcely ever seen.

Insulin can also be given by continuous subcutaneous infusion using soluble insulin in an infusion pump. This technique has a limited place in the treatment of diabetes, and provides for continuous basal insulin infusion with prandial boosts. There are many disadvantages to the technique. Patients using it must be well-motivated, reliable, and able to monitor their own blood glucose, and must have access to expert advice both day and night.

CHOICE OF TREATMENT. About 25% of diabetics require insulin treatment; apart from those presenting in ketoacidosis, insulin is needed by most of those with a rapid onset of symptoms, weight loss, weakness, and sometimes vomiting, often associated with ketonuria. The majority of those who are obese can be managed by restriction of carbohydrate or energy intake alone or with the subsequent administration of oral hypoglycaemic drugs. Most children require insulin from the outset.

MANAGEMENT OF DIABETIC PATIENTS. The aim of treatment is to achieve the best possible control of plasma glucose without making the patient obsessional, and avoiding disabling hypoglycaemia; close co-operation is needed between the patient and the medical team since good control of insulin dependent patients reduces the incidence of complications. Mixtures of available insulin preparations may be required and these combinations have to be worked out for the individual patient. Insulin requirements may be affected by variations in lifestyle, infection, and corticosteroids, and sometimes by a very small amount when the oral contraceptive pill is taken. In pregnancy insulin requirements should be assessed frequently by an experienced diabetic physician.

Many patients now monitor their own blood glucose concentrations using blood glucose strips (with or without electronic meters). Since blood glucose concentrations oscillate substantially throughout the day, 'normoglycaemia' cannot always be achieved throughout a 24-hour period without causing damaging hypoglycaemia. It is therefore best to recommend that patients should maintain blood glucose concentrations of between 4 and 10 mmol/litre for most of the time, while accepting that on occasions, for brief periods, they will be above or below these values. Patients should be advised to look for 'peaks' and 'troughs' of blood glucose, and to adjust their insulin dosage only once or twice weekly. Overall it is ideal to aim for an HbA_{1c} level of less than 7% (normal range 4–6%) or an HbA_1 of less than 8.8% (normal range 5.0–7.5%) although this is not always possible without causing disabling hypoglycaemia. Fructosamine can also be used for assessment of control: this is a simpler and cheaper but less reliable measurement of glycated serum proteins.

The energy and carbohydrate intake must be adequate to allow normal growth and development but obesity must be avoided. The carbohydrate intake must be regulated and should be distributed throughout the day. Fine control of plasma glucose can be achieved by moving portions of carbohydrate from one meal to another without altering the total intake.

Insulin doses are determined on an individual basis, by gradually increasing the dose but avoiding troublesome hypoglycaemic reactions.

There are 3 main types of insulin preparations:

1. those of **short** duration which have a relatively rapid onset of action, namely soluble forms of insulin;
2. those with an **intermediate** action, e.g. Isophane Insulin Injection and Insulin Zinc Suspension; and
3. those whose action is slower in onset and lasts for **long** periods, e.g. Human Ultratard®.

The *duration of action* of different insulin preparations varies considerably from one patient to another, and needs to be assessed for every individual; those indicated below are only approximations. The type of insulin used and its dose and frequency of administration depend on the particular needs of the patient. Most patients are best started on insulins of intermediate action twice daily and a short-acting insulin can later be added to cover any hyperglycaemia which may follow breakfast or evening meal.

Some recommended insulin regimens

Insulin	Regimen
1. Short-acting insulin mixed with Intermediate-acting insulin	twice daily (before meals)
2. Short-acting insulin mixed with Intermediate-acting insulin	before breakfast
Short-acting insulin	before evening meal
Intermediate-acting insulin	bedtime
3. Short-acting insulin	three times daily (before breakfast, midday and evening meal)
Intermediate-acting insulin	bedtime
4. Short-acting insulin mixed with Intermediate-acting insulin	before breakfast (sufficient in some cases)

HUMAN INSULINS. There are differences in the amino-acid sequence in animal and human insulins; most available insulins are either porcine in origin or of human sequence prepared by modification of porcine material (emp) or biosynthetically (crb, prb, or pyr). Preparations of human sequence insulin should theoretically be less immunogenic, but in trials no real advantage has been shown.

HYPOGLYCAEMIA. This is a potential hazard when the type of insulin is changed, especially when converting from beef to human insulin. The conversion from beef to human sequence insulin should always be undertaken with specialist advice; it is usual to reduce the total dose by about 10%, with careful monitoring for the first few days. When changing from porcine to human sequence insulin, a dose change is not usually needed, but careful monitoring is advised. Loss of warning of hypoglycaemia is a common problem among insulin-treated patients and can be a serious hazard, especially for drivers. The cause is not known, but very tight control of diabetes appears to lower the blood glucose concentration needed to trigger hypoglycaemic symptoms. Beta-blockers can also blunt hypoglycaemic awareness (and can delay recovery).

Some patients have reported loss of warning of hypoglycaemia after transfer to human insulin. Patients should be warned of this possibility and if they believe that human insulin is responsible for their loss of warning it is reasonable to transfer them back to porcine insulin. When prescribing insulin great care should be taken to specify whether a human or an animal preparation is required. Indications for changing from animal to human preparations must be very carefully considered in the light of these reported problems.

DRIVING. Car drivers need to be particularly careful to avoid hypoglycaemia (see above) and should be warned of the problems. They should normally check their blood glucose concentration before driving and, on long journeys, at intervals of approximately two hours. If hypoglycaemia occurs a car driver should switch off the ignition until recovery is complete, which may take up to 15 minutes or longer. Driving is not permitted when hypoglycaemic awareness has been lost.

UNITS. The word 'unit' should **not** be abbreviated.

6.1.1.1 SHORT-ACTING INSULIN

Soluble Insulin is a short-acting form of insulin. For maintenance regimens it is usual to inject it 15 to 30 minutes before meals.

Soluble insulin is the only appropriate form of insulin for use in diabetic emergencies and at the time of surgical operations. It has the great advantage that it can be given intravenously and intramuscularly, as well as subcutaneously.

When injected subcutaneously, soluble insulin has a rapid onset of action (after 30 to 60 minutes), a peak action between 2 and 4 hours, and a duration of action of up to 8 hours. Human sequence preparations tend to have a more rapid onset and a shorter overall duration.

When injected intravenously, soluble insulin has a very short half-life of only about 5 minutes and its effect disappears within 30 minutes.

SOLUBLE INSULIN

(Insulin Injection; Neutral Insulin)

A sterile solution of insulin (i.e. bovine or porcine) or of human insulin; pH 6.6–8.0

Indications: diabetes mellitus; diabetic ketoacidosis (section 6.1.3)

Cautions: see notes above; reduce dose in renal impairment; **interactions:** Appendix 1 (antidiabetics)

Side-effects: see notes above; local reactions and fat hypertrophy at injection site; overdose causes hypoglycaemia

Dose: by subcutaneous, intramuscular, or intravenous injection or intravenous infusion, according to patient's requirements

COUNSELLING. Show bottle to patient and confirm that patient is expecting the version dispensed

Highly purified animal
Hypurin Neutral® (CP)
Injection, soluble insulin (bovine, highly purified) 100 units/mL. Net price 10-mL vial = £10.97
Velosulin® (Novo Nordisk, Wellcome)
Injection, soluble insulin (porcine, highly purified) 100 units/mL. Net price 10-mL vial = £6.58

Human sequence
Human Actrapid® (Novo Nordisk)
Injection, soluble insulin (human, pyr) 100 units/mL. Net price 10-mL vial = £9.42; 5 × 1.5-mL Penfill® cartridge (for NHS NovoPen® devices) = £7.50; 5 × 3-mL Actrapid® prefilled disposable injection devices (range 2–78 units allowing 2-unit dosage adjustments) = £26.33
Human Velosulin® (Novo Nordisk, Wellcome)
Injection, soluble insulin (human, emp) 100 units/mL. Net price 10-mL vial = £9.42
Humulin S® (Lilly)
Injection, soluble insulin (human, prb) 100 units/mL. Net price 10-mL vial = £9.98; 5 × 1.5-mL cartridge (for NHS B-D pen®) = £8.30
Pur-In® Neutral (CP)
Injection, soluble insulin (human, emp) 100 units/mL. Net price 10-mL vial = £8.45; 5 × 3-mL cartridge (for NHS Pur-In Pen® device) − £15.38

Mixed preparations, see Biphasic Insulin and Biphasic Isophane Insulin (section 6.1.1.2)

6.1.1.2 INTERMEDIATE- AND LONG-ACTING INSULINS

When given by subcutaneous injection intermediate- and long-acting insulins have an onset of action of approximately 1–2 hours, a maximal effect at 4–12 hours, and a duration of 16–35 hours. Some are given twice daily in conjunction with short-acting (soluble) insulin, and others are given once daily, particularly in elderly patients. They can be mixed with soluble insulin in the syringe, essentially retaining the properties of the two components, although there may be some blunting of the initial effect of the soluble insulin component (especially on mixing with protamine zinc insulin, see below).

Isophane Insulin is a suspension of insulin with protamine which is of particular value for initiation of twice-daily insulin regimens. Patients usually mix isophane with soluble insulin but ready-mixed preparations may be appropriate (**Biphasic Isophane Insulin**).

Biphasic Insulin is another ready-mixed insulin suitable for twice-daily injection.

Insulin Zinc Suspension (Amorphous) has an intermediate duration of action and **Insulin Zinc Suspension (Crystalline)** a more prolonged duration of action. These preparations may be used independently or in **Insulin Zinc Suspension** (30% amorphous, 70% crystalline).

Protamine Zinc Insulin is usually given once daily in conjunction with short-acting (soluble) insulin. It has the drawback of binding with the soluble insulin when mixed in the same syringe, and is now rarely used.

INSULIN ZINC SUSPENSION
(Insulin Zinc Suspension (Mixed); I. Z. S.)
A sterile neutral suspension of bovine and/or porcine insulin or of human insulin in the form of a complex obtained by the addition of a suitable zinc salt; consists of rhombohedral crystals (10–40 microns) and of particles of no uniform shape (not exceeding 2 microns)
Indications: diabetes mellitus (long acting)
Cautions; Side-effects: see under Soluble Insulin (section 6.1.1.1)
Dose: by subcutaneous injection, according to patient's requirements
COUNSELLING. Show bottle to patient and confirm that patient is expecting the version dispensed

Highly purified animal
Hypurin Lente® (CP)
Injection, insulin zinc suspension (bovine, highly purified) 100 units/mL. Net price 10-mL vial = £10.97
Lentard MC® (Novo Nordisk)
Injection, insulin zinc suspension (bovine and porcine, highly purified) 100 units/mL. Net price 10-mL vial = £5.78

Human sequence
Human Monotard® (Novo Nordisk)
Injection, insulin zinc suspension (human, pyr) 100 units/mL. Net price 10-mL vial = £9.42
Humulin Lente® (Lilly)
Injection, insulin zinc suspension (human, prb) 100 units/mL. Net price 10-mL vial = £9.98

INSULIN ZINC SUSPENSION (AMORPHOUS)
(Amorph. I. Z. S.)
A sterile neutral suspension of bovine or porcine insulin in the form of a complex obtained by the addition of a suitable zinc salt; consists of particles of no uniform shape (not exceeding 2 microns)
Indications: diabetes mellitus (intermediate acting)
Cautions; Side-effects: see under Soluble Insulin (section 6.1.1.1)
Dose: by subcutaneous injection, according to patient's requirements
COUNSELLING. Show bottle to patient and confirm that patient is expecting the version dispensed

Semitard MC® (Novo Nordisk)

Injection, insulin zinc suspension (amorphous) (porcine, highly purified) 100 units/mL. Net price 10-mL vial = £6.28

INSULIN ZINC SUSPENSION (CRYSTALLINE)

(Cryst. I. Z. S.)

A sterile neutral suspension of bovine insulin or of human insulin in the form of a complex obtained by the addition of a suitable zinc salt; consists of rhombohedral crystals (10–40 microns)

Indications: diabetes mellitus (duration of action, see below)

Cautions; Side-effects: see under Soluble Insulin (section 6.1.1.1)

Dose: by subcutaneous injection, according to patient's requirements

COUNSELLING. Show bottle to patient and confirm that patient is expecting the version dispensed

Human sequence
Human Ultratard® (Novo Nordisk)

(long acting)

Injection, insulin zinc suspension, crystalline (human, pyr) 100 units/mL. Net price 10-mL vial = £9.42

Humulin Zn® (Lilly)

(intermediate acting)

Injection, insulin zinc suspension, crystalline (human, prb) 100 units/mL. Net price 10-mL vial = £9.98

ISOPHANE INSULIN

(Isophane Insulin Injection; Isophane Protamine Insulin Injection; Isophane Insulin (NPH))

A sterile suspension of bovine or porcine insulin or of human insulin in the form of a complex obtained by the addition of protamine sulphate or another suitable protamine

Indications: diabetes mellitus (intermediate acting)

Cautions; Side-effects: see under Soluble Insulin (section 6.1.1.1); protamine may cause allergic reactions

Dose: by subcutaneous injection, according to patient's requirements

COUNSELLING. Show bottle to patient and confirm that patient is expecting the version dispensed

Highly purified animal
Hypurin Isophane® (CP)

Injection, isophane insulin (bovine, highly purified) 100 units/mL. Net price 10-mL vial = £10.97

Insulatard® (Novo Nordisk, Wellcome)

Injection, isophane insulin (porcine, highly purified) 100 units/mL. Net price 10-mL vial = £6.58

Human sequence
Human Insulatard® (Novo Nordisk, Wellcome)

Injection, isophane insulin (human, emp) 100 units/mL. Net price 10-mL vial = £9.42; 5 ×

3-mL prefilled disposable injection devices (range 2–78 units allowing 2-unit dosage adjustment) = £26.33

Human Protaphane® (Novo Nordisk)

Injection, isophane insulin (human, pyr) 100 units/mL. Net price 10-mL vial = £9.42; 5 × 1.5-mL Penfill® cartridge (for NHS Novopen® devices) = £7.90

Humulin I® (Lilly)

Injection, isophane insulin (human, prb) 100 units/mL. Net price 10-mL vial = £9.98; 5 × 1.5-mL cartridge (for NHS B-D pen®) = £8.30

Pur-In® Isophane (CP)

Injection, isophane insulin (human, emp) 100 units/mL. Net price 10-mL vial = £8.45; 5 × 3-mL cartridge (for NHS Pur-In Pen® device) = £16.20

Mixed preparations, see Biphasic Isophane Insulin (below)

PROTAMINE ZINC INSULIN

(Protamine Zinc Insulin Injection)

A sterile suspension of insulin in the form of a complex obtained by the addition of a suitable protamine and zinc chloride; this preparation was included in BP 1980 but is not included in BP 1988

Indications: diabetes mellitus (long acting)

Cautions; Side-effects: see under Soluble Insulin (section 6.1.1.1); protamine may cause allergic reactions; see also notes above

Dose: by subcutaneous injection, according to patient's requirements

COUNSELLING. Show bottle to patient and confirm that patient is expecting the version dispensed

Hypurin Protamine Zinc® (CP)

Injection, protamine zinc insulin (bovine, highly purified) 100 units/mL. Net price 10-mL vial = £11.76

BIPHASIC INSULINS

BIPHASIC INSULIN

(Biphasic Insulin Injection)

A sterile suspension of crystals containing bovine insulin in a solution of porcine insulin

Indications: diabetes mellitus (intermediate acting)

Cautions; Side-effects: see under Soluble Insulin (section 6.1.1.1)

Dose: by subcutaneous injection, according to patient's requirements

COUNSELLING. Show bottle to patient and confirm that patient is expecting the version dispensed

Rapitard MC® (Novo Nordisk)

Injection, biphasic insulin (highly purified) 100 units/mL. Net price 10-mL vial = £5.78

BIPHASIC ISOPHANE INSULIN
(Biphasic Isophane Insulin Injection)

A sterile buffered suspension of porcine insulin complexed with protamine sulphate (or another suitable protamine) in a solution of porcine insulin *or* a sterile buffered suspension of human insulin complexed with protamine sulphate (or another suitable protamine) in a solution of human insulin

Indications: diabetes mellitus (intermediate acting)

Cautions; Side-effects: see under Soluble Insulin (section 6.1.1.1); protamine may cause allergic reactions

Dose: by subcutaneous injection, according to the patient's requirements

COUNSELLING. Show bottle to patient and confirm that patient is expecting the version dispensed

Highly purified animal

Initard 50/50® (Novo Nordisk, Wellcome)

Injection, biphasic isophane insulin (porcine, highly purified), 50% soluble, 50% isophane. 100 units/mL. Net price 10-mL vial = £6.58

Mixtard 30/70® (Novo Nordisk, Wellcome)

Injection, biphasic isophane insulin (porcine, highly purified), 30% soluble, 70% isophane, 100 units/mL. Net price 10-mL vial = £6.58

Human sequence

Human Actraphane 30/70® (Novo Nordisk)

Injection, biphasic isophane insulin (human, pyr), 30% soluble, 70% isophane, 100 units/mL. Net price 10-mL vial = £9.42

Human Initard 50/50® (Novo Nordisk Wellcome)

Injection, biphasic isophane insulin (human, emp), 50% soluble, 50% isophane, 100 units/mL. Net price 10-mL vial = £9.42

Human Mixtard 30/70® (Novo Nordisk Wellcome)

Injection, biphasic isophane insulin (human, emp), 30% soluble, 70% isophane, 100 units/mL. Net price 10-mL vial = £9.42

Humulin M1® (Lilly)

Injection, biphasic isophane insulin (human, prb), 10% soluble, 90% isophane, 100 units/mL. Net price 10-mL vial = £9.98; 5 × 1.5-mL cartridge (for NHS B-D pen®) = £8.30

Humulin M2® (Lilly)

Injection, biphasic isophane insulin (human, prb), 20% soluble, 80% isophane, 100 units/mL. Net price 10-mL vial = £9.98; 5 × 1.5-mL cartridge (for NHS B-D pen®) = £8.30

Humulin M3® (Lilly)

Injection, biphasic isophane insulin (human, prb), 30% soluble, 70% isophane, 100 units/mL. Net price 10-mL vial =£9.98; 5 × 1.5-mL cartridge (for NHS B-D pen®) = £8.30

Humulin M4® (Lilly)

Injection, biphasic isophane insulin (human, prb), 40% soluble, 60% isophane, 100 units/mL. Net price 10-mL vial = £9.98; 5 × 1.5-mL cartridge (for NHS B-D pen®) = £8.30

PenMix 10/90® (Novo Nordisk)

Injection, biphasic isophane insulin (human, pyr), 10% soluble, 90% isophane, 100 units/mL. Net price 5 × 1.5-mL Penfill® cartridge (for NHS Novopen® devices) = £7.90; 5 × 3-mL pre-filled disposable injection devices (range 2–78 units, allowing 2-unit dosage adjustment) = £26.33

PenMix 20/80® (Novo Nordisk)

Injection, biphasic isophane insulin (human, pyr), 20% soluble, 80% isophane, 100 units/mL. Net price 5 × 1.5-mL Penfill® cartridge (for NHS Novopen® devices) = £7.90; 5 × 3-mL pre-filled disposable injection devices (range 2–78 units, allowing 2-unit dosage adjustment) = £26.33

PenMix 30/70® (Novo Nordisk)

Injection, biphasic isophane insulin (human, pyr), 30% soluble, 70% isophane, 100 units/mL. Net price 5 × 1.5-mL Penfill® cartridge (for NHS Novopen® devices) = £7.90; 5 × 3-mL pre-filled disposable injection devices (range 2–78 units, allowing 2-unit dosage adjustment) = £26.33

PenMix 40/60® (Novo Nordisk)

Injection, biphasic isophane insulin (human, pyr), 40% soluble, 60% isophane, 100 units/mL. Net price 5 × 1.5-mL Penfill® cartridge (for NHS Novopen® devices) = £7.90; 5 × 3-mL pre-filled disposable injection devices (range 2–78 units, allowing 2-unit dosage adjustments) = £26.33

PenMix 50/50® (Novo Nordisk)

Injection, biphasic isophane insulin (human, pyr), 50% soluble, 50% isophane, 100 units/mL. Net price 5 × 1.5-mL Penfill® cartridge (for NHS Novopen® devices) = £7.90; 5 × 3-mL pre-filled disposable injection devices (range 2–78 units, allowing 2-unit dosage adjustment) = £26.33

Pur-In® Mix 15/85 (CP)

Injection, biphasic isophane insulin (human, emp) 15% soluble, 85% isophane, 100 units/mL. Net price 10-mL vial = £8.45; 5 × 3-mL cartridge (for NHS Pur-In Pen® device) = £16.20

Pur-In® Mix 25/75 (CP)

Injection, biphasic isophane insulin (human, emp), 25% soluble, 75% isophane, 100 units/mL. Net price 10-mL vial = £8.45; 5 × 3-mL cartridge (for NHS Pur-In Pen® device) = £16.20

Pur-In® Mix 50/50 (CP)

Injection, biphasic isophane insulin (human, emp), 50% soluble, 50% isophane, 100 units/mL. Net price 10-mL vial = £8.45; 5 × 3-mL cartridge (for NHS Pur-In Pen® device) = £16.20

6.1.1.3 HYPODERMIC EQUIPMENT

Patients should be advised on the safe disposal of lancets, single-use syringes, and needles. Suitable arrangements for the safe disposal of contaminated waste must be made before these products are prescribed for patients who are carriers of infectious diseases.

Injection devices

NHS Autopen® (Owen Mumford)

Injection device, for use with Lilly and Novo Nordisk 1.5-mL insulin cartridges; allows adjustment of dosage in multiples of one unit, max. 16 units (single unit version); two units, max. 32 units (two unit version). Net price (both) = £13.96

NHS B-D Pen® (Becton Dickinson)

Injection device, for use with Lilly 1.5-mL insulin cartridges; allows adjustment of dosage in multiples of one unit, max. 30 units. Net price = £23.86. Also available from clinics

NHS NovoPen II® (Novo Nordisk)

Injection device, for use with Penfill® insulin cartridges; allows adjustment of dosage in multiples of two units, max. 36 units. Available only from clinics

NHS Penject® (Hypoguard)

Injection device, for use with B-D U100 1mL syringe; allows adjustment of dosage in multiples of two units. Net price = £18.40

NHS Pur-In Pen® (CP)

Injection devices, for use with Pur-In® insulin cartridges; allows adjustment of dosage in multiples of one unit (Pur-In Pen® 1), two units (Pur-In Pen® 2), and four units (Pur-In Pen® 4); max. 40 units. Available only from clinics

Lancets— sterile, single use

Type A (Drug Tariff). Mount fluted longitudinally; compatible with **NHS** Autoclix® (BM Diagnostics), **NHS** Monojector® (Sherwood), and **NHS** Soft Touch® (BM Diagnostics) finger-pricking devices

Available from Owen Mumford (Unilet G®, net price 100-lancet pack = £3.17; 200-lancet pack = £6.01), Sherwood (Monolet®, net price 100-lancet pack = £3.15; 200-lancet pack = £6.00; Monolet Extra®, net price 100-lancet pack = £3.15)

Type B (Drug Tariff). Mount with concentric ribs; compatible with **NHS** Autolet® (Owen Mumford) and **NHS** Glucolet® (Bayer Diagnostics) finger-pricking devices

Available from Bayer Diagnostics (Ames®, net price 200-lancet pack = £6.24), Owen Mumford (Unilet®, net price 100-lancet pack = £3.17; 200-lancet pack = £6.01)

Type C (Drug Tariff). Mount flat and oblong; compatible with **NHS** Autolance® (Becton Dickinson) finger-pricking device

Available from Becton Dickinson (B-D Microfine®, net price 100-lancet pack = £3.02)

Needles

Hypodermic Needle , Sterile single use (Drug Tariff). For use with re-usable glass syringe, sizes 0.5 mm (25G), 0.45 mm (26G), 0.4 mm (27G). Net price 100-needle pack = £2.20

Available from Becton Dickinson (Microlance®), Sherwood (Monoject®), Sabre (Sabre Gillette®)

Needle Clipping Device (Drug Tariff). Consisting of a clipper to remove needle from its hub and container from which cut-off needles cannot be retrieved; designed to hold 1200 needles, not suitable for use with lancets. Net price = £1.08

Available from Becton Dickinson (B-D Safe-clip®)

Subcutaneous infusion pumps

NHS MS36® (Graseby Medical)

Infusion pump, for use with any brand of U100 soluble insulin. Net price = £782.00

Syringes

Clickcount® (Hypoguard). Calibrated glass with Luer taper conical fitting, supplied with dosage chart and strong box for blind patients for whom the Pre-Set syringe is unsuitable. Net price 1 mL = £17.42

Hypodermic Syringe (Drug Tariff). Calibrated glass with Luer taper conical fitting, for use with U100 insulin. Net price 0.5 mL and 1 mL = £10.71

Available from Rand Rocket (Abcare®)

Pre-Set U100 Insulin Syringe (Drug Tariff). Calibrated glass with Luer taper conical fitting, supplied with dosage chart and strong box, for blind patients. Net price 1 mL = £17.43

Available from Rand Rocket

U100 Insulin Syringe with Needle (Drug Tariff). Disposable with fixed or separate needle for single use or single patient-use, colour coded orange, 0.45 mm (26G), 0.4 mm (27G), 0.36 mm (28G), 0.33 mm (29G). Net price, 0.3 mL, 0.5 mL and 1 mL (with needle), 10 = £1.11

Available from Becton Dickinson (B-D Micro-Fine®+, Plastipak®), Braun (Omnikan®), Rand Rocket (Clinipak®), Sabre (Sabre Gillette®), Sherwood (Monoject® Ultra), Steriseal (Insupak®), Terumo (Myjector®)

Syringe carrying case (Drug Tariff). For use with Clickcount® and Hypodermic insulin syringe. Net price 1 = £2.64; screw cap (to convert for use with Pre-Set U 100 insulin syringe) = 71p

6.1.2   Oral antidiabetic drugs

6.1.2.1   Sulphonylureas
6.1.2.2   Biguanides
6.1.2.3   Other antidiabetics

Oral antidiabetic drugs are used for non-insulin-dependent (type 2) diabetes; they should not be prescribed until patients have been shown not to respond adequately to at least three months' restriction of energy and carbohydrate intake. They should be used to augment the effect of diet, and not to replace it.

6.1.2.1 SULPHONYLUREAS

The sulphonylureas act mainly by augmenting insulin secretion and consequently are effective only when some residual pancreatic beta-cell activity is present; during long-term administration they also have an extrapancreatic action. All may lead to hypoglycaemia 4 hours or more after food but this is usually an indication of overdose, and is relatively uncommon.

There are several sulphonylureas but there is no evidence for any difference in their effectiveness. Only **chlorpropamide** has appreciably more side-effects, mainly because of its very prolonged duration of action and the consequent hazard of hypoglycaemia (but also as a result of the common and unpleasant chlorpropamide-alcohol flush phenomenon). Selection of an individual sulphonylurea depends otherwise on the age of the patient and renal function (see below), or more generally just on personal preference.

Elderly patients are particularly prone to the dangers of hypoglycaemia when long-acting sulphonylureas are used; **chlorpropamide**, and also preferably **glibenclamide**, should be avoided in these patients and replaced by others, such as **gliclazide** or **tolbutamide**.

CAUTIONS AND CONTRA-INDICATIONS. These drugs tend to encourage weight gain and should only be prescribed if poor control and symptoms persist despite adequate attempts at dieting. They should not be used during breast-feeding, and caution is needed in the elderly and those with hepatic and renal insufficiency because of the hazard of hypoglycaemia. The short-acting tolbutamide may be used in renal impairment, as may gliquidone and gliclazide which are principally metabolised and inactivated in the liver. Sulphonylureas should be avoided in porphyria (see section 9.8.2).

Insulin therapy should be instituted temporarily during intercurrent illness (such as myocardial infarction, coma, infection, and trauma) and during surgery since control of diabetes with the sulphonylureas is often inadequate in such circumstances. Insulin therapy is also usually substituted during pregnancy (see also Appendix 4). Sulphonylureas are contra-indicated in the presence of ketoacidosis.

SIDE-EFFECTS. These are generally mild and infrequent and include gastro-intestinal disturbances and headache.

Chlorpropamide may cause facial flushing after drinking alcohol; this effect is not normally witnessed with other sulphonylureas. Chlorpropamide may also enhance antidiuretic hormone and very rarely cause hyponatraemia.

Sensitivity reactions (usually in first 6–8 weeks of therapy) include transient rashes which rarely progress to erythema multiforme and exfoliative dermatitis, fever, and jaundice; photosensitivity has also rarely been reported with chlorpropamide. Blood disorders are rare too but include thrombocytopenia, agranulocytosis, and aplastic anaemia. All these phenomena are very rare.

CHLORPROPAMIDE

Indications: diabetes mellitus (for use in diabetes insipidus, see section 6.5.2)

Cautions; Contra-indications; Side-effects: see notes above; **interactions:** Appendix 1 (antidiabetics)

Dose: initially 250 mg daily (elderly patients 100–125 mg but avoid—see notes above), adjusted according to response; max. 500 mg daily; taken with breakfast

PoM **Chlorpropamide** (Non-proprietary)
Tablets, chlorpropamide 100 mg, net price 20 = 18p; 250 mg, 20 = 27p. Label:4
Available from APS, Cox, CP
PoM **Diabinese**® (Pfizer)
Tablets, scored, chlorpropamide 100 mg, net price 28-tab pack = 56p; 250 mg, 28-tab pack = £1.23. Label: 4

GLIBENCLAMIDE

Indications: diabetes mellitus

Cautions; Contra-indications; Side-effects: see notes above; **interactions:** Appendix 1 (antidiabetics)

Dose: initially 5 mg daily (elderly patients 2.5 mg (but see also notes above)), adjusted according to response; max. 15 mg daily; taken with breakfast

PoM **Glibenclamide** (Non-proprietary)
Tablets, glibenclamide 2.5 mg, net price 20 = 44p; 5 mg, 20 = 41p
Available from APS (Libanil®), Ashbourne (Diabetamide®), Berk (Calabren®), Cox, CP, Generics, Hillcross, K Pharm., Lagap (Malix®)
PoM **Daonil**® (Hoechst)
Tablets, scored, glibenclamide 5 mg. Net price 28-tab pack = £2.63
PoM **Semi-Daonil**® (Hoechst)
Tablets, scored, glibenclamide 2.5 mg. Net price 28-tab pack = £1.58
PoM **Euglucon**® (Roussel)
Tablets, glibenclamide 2.5 mg, net price 28-tab pack = £1.58; 5 mg (scored), 28-tab pack = £2.63

GLICLAZIDE

Indications: diabetes mellitus

Cautions; Contra-indications; Side-effects: see notes above; **interactions:** Appendix 1 (antidiabetics)

Dose: initially, 40–80 mg daily, adjusted according to response; up to 160 mg as a single dose, with breakfast; higher doses divided; max. 320 mg daily

PoM **Diamicron**® (Servier)
Tablets, scored, gliclazide 80 mg. Net price 60 = £7.00

GLIPIZIDE

Indications: diabetes mellitus

Cautions; Contra-indications; Side-effects: see notes above; **interactions:** Appendix 1 (antidiabetics)

Dose: initially 2.5–5 mg daily, adjusted according to response; max. 40 mg daily; up to 15 mg may be given as a single dose before breakfast; higher doses divided

PoM **Glibenese**® (Pfizer)
Tablets, scored, glipizide 5 mg. Net price 56-tab pack = £3.63
PoM **Minodiab**® (Pharmacia)
Tablets, glipizide 2.5 mg, net price 60 = £3.31; 5 mg (scored), 60 = £3.54

GLIQUIDONE

Indications: diabetes mellitus

Cautions; Contra-indications; Side-effects: see notes above; **interactions:** Appendix 1 (antidiabetics)

Dose: initially 15 mg daily before breakfast, adjusted to 45–60 mg daily in 2 or 3 divided doses; max. single dose 60 mg, max. daily dose 180 mg

PoM **Glurenorm®** (Sanofi Winthrop)

Tablets, scored, gliquidone 30 mg. Net price 100 = £17.54

TOLAZAMIDE

Indications: diabetes mellitus

Cautions; Contra-indications; Side-effects: see notes above; **interactions:** Appendix 1 (antidiabetics)

Dose: initially 100–250 mg daily with breakfast adjusted according to response; max. 1 g daily; higher doses divided

PoM **Tolanase®** (Upjohn)

Tablets, both scored, tolazamide 100 mg, net price 20 = £1.13; 250 mg, 20 = £2.46

TOLBUTAMIDE

Indications: diabetes mellitus

Cautions; Contra-indications; Side-effects: see notes above; **interactions:** Appendix 1 (antidiabetics)

Dose: 0.5–1.5 g (max. 2 g) daily in divided doses (see notes above)

PoM **Tolbutamide** (Non-proprietary)

Tablets, tolbutamide 500 mg. Net price 20 = 29p

Available from APS, Cox, CP, Evans, Hillcross, K Pharm.

PoM **Rastinon®** (Hoechst)

Tablets, scored, tolbutamide 500 mg. Net price 20 = 67p

6.1.2.2 BIGUANIDES

Metformin, the only available biguanide, has a different mode of action from the sulphonylureas, and is not interchangeable with them. It exerts its effect mainly by decreasing gluconeogenesis and by increasing peripheral utilisation of glucose; since it only acts in the presence of endogenous insulin it is only effective in diabetics with some residual functioning pancreatic islet cells. Metformin is used in the treatment of non-insulin-dependent diabetics when strict dieting and sulphonylurea treatment have failed to control diabetes, especially in overweight patients, in whom it may, if necessary, be used first. It can be used alone or with a sulphonylurea. It does not exert a hypoglycaemic action in non-diabetic subjects unless given in overdose. Gastro-intestinal side-effects are initially common, and may persist in some patients, particularly when very high doses such as 3 g daily are given

Metformin is not free from the hazard of lactic acidosis but this occurs almost exclusively in renal failure patients, in whom it should not be used.

METFORMIN HYDROCHLORIDE

Indications: diabetes mellitus (see notes above)

Cautions: see notes above; **interactions:** Appendix 1 (antidiabetics)

Contra-indications: hepatic or renal impairment (withdraw if renal impairment suspected), predisposition to lactic acidosis, heart failure, severe infection or trauma, dehydration, alcohol dependence; pregnancy, breast-feeding

Side-effects: anorexia, nausea, vomiting, diarrhoea (usually transient), lactic acidosis (withdraw treatment), decreased vitamin-B_{12} absorption

Dose: 500 mg every 8 hours *or* 850 mg every 12 hours with or after food; max. 3 g daily in divided doses though most physicians limit this to 2 g daily (see notes above)

PoM **Metformin** (Non-proprietary)

Tablets, coated, metformin hydrochloride 500 mg, net price 20 = 33p; 850 mg, 20 = 58p. Label: 21

Available from APS, Berk, Cox, Evans, Hillcross, K Pharm., Lagap (Orabet®), Norton

PoM **Glucophage®** (Lipha)

Tablets, f/c, metformin hydrochloride 500 mg, net price 84-tab pack = £2.00; 850 mg, 56-tab pack = £2.22. Label: 21

6.1.2.3 OTHER ANTIDIABETICS

Acarbose, an inhibitor of intestinal alpha glucosidases, delays the digestion of starch and sucrose and hence the increase in blood glucose levels which follow a carbohydrate-containing meal. It has been recently introduced for the treatment of non-insulin-dependent (type 2) diabetes.

Guar gum, if taken in adequate quantities, results in some reduction of postprandial plasma-glucose concentrations in diabetes mellitus, probably by retarding carbohydrate absorption. It is also used to relieve symptoms of the dumping syndrome.

ACARBOSE

Indications: diabetes mellitus inadequately controlled by diet or by diet with oral hypoglycaemic agents

Cautions: monitor hepatic transaminase levels (higher doses); may enhance hypoglycaemic effects of insulin and sulphonylureas (hypoglycaemic episodes may be treated with oral glucose but not with sucrose); **interactions:** Appendix 1 (acarbose)

Contra-indications: pregnancy and breast-feeding; inflammatory bowel disease (e.g. ulcerative colitis, Crohn's disease), partial intestinal obstruction (or predisposition); hepatic impairment, severe renal impairment; hernia, history of abdominal surgery

Side-effects: flatulence, soft stools, diarrhoea (may need to reduce dose or withdraw), abdominal distention and pain

Note. Antacids not recommended for treating side-effects (unlikely to be benificial)

Dose: 50 mg 3 times daily, increased if necessary after 6–8 weeks to 100 mg 3 times daily; max. 200 mg 3 times daily; CHILD not recommended

COUNSELLING. The tablets should either be chewed with first mouthful of food or swallowed whole with a little liquid immediately before food. In order to counteract possible hypoglycaemia, patients receiving insulin or a sulphonylurea as well as acarbose need to carry glucose (not sucrose—acarbose interferes with sucrose absorption)

▼ PoM **Glucobay**® (Bayer)

Tablets, acarbose 50 mg, net price 90-tab pack = £14.10; 100 mg (scored). 90-tab pack = £17.70. Counselling, administration

GUAR GUM

Indications: see notes above

Cautions: maintain adequate fluid intake; **interactions:** Appendix 1 (guar gum)

COUNSELLING. Preparations that swell in contact with liquid should always be carefully swallowed with water and should not be taken imediately before going to bed.

Contra-indications: gastro-intestinal obstruction

Side-effects: flatulence, abdominal distension, intestinal obstruction

Guarem® (Rybar)

Granules, ivory, sugar-free, guar gum 5 g/sachet, net price 50 sachets = £9.72; 100 sachets = £15.67. Label: 13, counselling, administration

Dose: 5 g stirred into 200 mL fluid 3 times daily immediately before main meals (or sprinkled on food and eaten accompanied by 200 mL fluid)

Guarina® (Norgine)

Granules, dispersible, guar gum 5 g/sachet. Net price 60 sachets = £8.73. Label: 13, counselling, administration

Dose: 5 g stirred into 150 mL fluid immediately before main meals up to 3 times daily (or sprinkled on food and eaten accompanied by 150 mL of fluid)

6.1.3 Diabetic ketoacidosis

Soluble insulin, the only form of insulin that may be given intravenously, is used in the management of diabetic ketoacidotic and hyperosmolar non-ketotic coma. It is preferable to use the type of soluble insulin that the patient has been using previously. It is necessary to achieve and to maintain an adequate plasma-insulin concentration until the metabolic disturbance is brought under control.

Insulin is best given by *intravenous infusion*, using an infusion pump, and diluted to 1 unit/mL (care in mixing, see Appendix 6). Adequate plasma concentrations can usually be maintained with infusion rates of 6 units/hour for adults and 0.1 units/kg/hour for children. Blood glucose is expected to decrease by about 5 mmol/hour; if the response is inadequate the infusion rate can be doubled or quadrupled. When the plasma glucose has fallen to 10 mmol/litre the infusion rate can be reduced to 1 to 2 units/hour for adults (about 0.02 units/kg/hour for children) and continued until the patient is ready to take food by mouth. The insulin infusion should

not be stopped before subcutaneous insulin has been started.

No matter how large, a bolus intravenous injection of insulin can only provide an adequate plasma concentration for a short time, therefore if facilities for intravenous infusion are not available the insulin is given by *intramuscular injection.* An initial loading dose of 20 units intramuscularly is followed by 6 units intramuscularly every hour until the plasma glucose concentration has fallen to 10 mmol/litre; intramuscular injections are then given every 2 hours. Although absorption of insulin is usually rapid after intramuscular injection, it may be impaired in the presence of hypotension and poor tissue perfusion; moreover depots of insulin may build up during treatment therefore late hypoglycaemia should be watched for and treated appropriately.

Intravenous replacement of fluid and electrolytes with **sodium chloride** intravenous infusion is an essential part of the management of ketoacidosis; **potassium chloride** is included in the infusion as appropriate to prevent the hypokalaemia induced by the insulin. **Sodium bicarbonate** infusion (1.26% or 2.74%) is only used in cases of extreme acidosis and shock since the acid-base disturbance is normally corrected by the insulin. **Glucose** solution (10%) is infused once the blood glucose has decreased below 10 mmol/litre but insulin infusion must continue. For glucose, see section 9.2.2.

6.1.4 Treatment of hypoglycaemia

Initially, glucose or 3 or 4 lumps of sugar should be taken with a little water. If necessary, this may be repeated in 10 to 15 minutes.

If hypoglycaemia causes unconsciousness, up to 50 mL of **50% glucose intravenous infusion** should be given intravenously (see section 9.2.2).

Glucagon can be given as an alternative to parenteral glucose in hypoglycaemia. It is a polypeptide hormone produced by the alpha cells of the islets of Langerhans. Its action is to increase plasma glucose concentration by mobilising glycogen stored in the liver. It has the advantage that it can be injected by any route (intramuscular, subcutaneous, or intravenous) in a dose of 1 mg (1 unit) in circumstances when an intravenous injection of glucose would be difficult or impossible to administer. It may be issued to close relatives of insulin-treated patients for emergency use in hypoglycaemic attacks. It is often advisable to prescribe on an 'if necessary' basis to hospitalised insulin-treated patients, so that it may be given rapidly by the nurses during an hypoglycaemic emergency. If not effective in 15 minutes intravenous glucose should be given.

GLUCAGON

Indications: see under Dose

Cautions: see notes above. Ineffective in chronic hypoglycaemia, starvation, and adrenal insufficiency

Contra-indications: insulinoma, phaeochromocytoma, glucagonoma

Side-effects: nausea, vomiting, diarrhoea, hypokalaemia, rarely hypersensitivity reactions

Dose: by subcutaneous, intramuscular, or intravenous injection, adults and children 0.5–1 unit; if no response after 15 minutes intravenous glucose should be given

Diagnostic aid, see data sheet

Beta-blocker poisoning, see p. 22

*Note.*1 unit of glucagon = 1 mg of glucagon or glucagon hydrochloride

PoM **Glucagon Injection,** powder for reconstitution, glucagon (as hydrochloride, with lactose). Net price 1-unit (1-mg) vial (Lilly) = £7.10; 1-mg vial (Novo Nordisk) = £6.83; 10-mg vial (Novo Nordisk) = £39.98 (all with diluent)

Note. If given in doses higher than 2 units (as in betablocker poisoning p. 22) reconstitute with water for injection instead of diluent

---

CHRONIC HYPOGLYCAEMIA

Diazoxide, administered by mouth, is useful in the management of patients with chronic hypoglycaemia from excess endogenous insulin secretion, either from an islet cell tumour or islet cell hyperplasia. It has no place in the management of acute hypoglycaemia.

DIAZOXIDE

Indications: chronic intractable hypoglycaemia (for use in hypertensive crisis see section 2.5.1)

Cautions: ischaemic heart disease, pregnancy, labour, impaired renal function; haematological examinations and blood pressure monitoring required during prolonged treatment; growth, bone, and developmental checks in children; **interactions:** Appendix 1 (diazoxide)

Side-effects: anorexia, nausea, vomiting, hyperuricaemia, hypotension, oedema, tachycardia, arrhythmias, extrapyramidal effects; hypertrichosis on prolonged treatment

Dose: by mouth, adults and children, initially 5 mg/kg daily in 2–3 divided doses

PoM **Eudemine®** (Evans)

Tablets, diazoxide 50 mg. Net price 20 = £7.68

6.1.5   Treatment of diabetic neuropathy

*Note.*Several recommendations in this section involve non-licensed indications

Optimal diabetic control is beneficial for the management of *painful neuropathy.* Most patients should be treated with insulin, and relief can probably be accelerated by continuous insulin infusion. **Non-opioid analgesics** such as aspirin and paracetamol (see section 4.7.1) are indicated. Relief may also be obtained with the **tricyclic antidepressants,** amitriptyline, imipramine, and nortriptyline (see section 4.3.1) with or without a low dose of a **phenothiazine** (see section 4.2). **Carbamazepine**

(see section 4.8.1) or mexiletine may be useful; lignocaine has also been used but needs further evaluation.

In *autonomic neuropathy* diabetic diarrhoea can often be aborted by two or three doses of **tetracycline** 250 mg (see section 5.1.3). Otherwise **codeine phosphate** (see section 1.4.2) is the best drug, but all other antidiarrhoeal preparations can be tried. **Anti-emetics** or **cisapride** may control vomiting in gastroparesis. In the rare cases where they do not, erythromycin (especially when given intravenously) has been shown to be of benefit but further studies are needed.

In *neuropathic postural hypotension* an increased salt intake and the use of the **mineralocorticoid** fludrocortisone 100 to 400 micrograms daily (see section 6.3.1) help by increasing plasma volume but uncomfortable oedema is a common side-effect. Fludrocortisone can also be combined with **flurbiprofen** (see section 10.1.1) and **ephedrine hydrochloride** (see section 3.1.1.2).

Gustatory sweating can be treated with **antimuscarinics** (see section 1.2), poldine methylsulphate is the best but propantheline bromide may also be used; side-effects are common. In some patients with *neuropathic oedema*, **ephedrine hydrochloride** 30 to 60 mg three times daily offers impressive relief.

6.1.6   Diagnostic and monitoring agents for diabetes mellitus

---

BLOOD GLUCOSE MONITORING

Blood glucose monitoring gives a direct measure of the glucose concentration at the time of the test and can detect hypoglycaemia as well as hyperglycaemia. It is a method of assessing diabetic control, especially where tight control is essential e.g. in pregnancy. Patients should be properly trained in the use of blood glucose monitoring systems and to take appropriate action on the results obtained. Inadequate understanding of the normal fluctuations in blood glucose may lead to confusion and inappropriate action. It is ideal for patients to observe the 'peaks' and 'troughs' of blood glucose over 24 hours and make adjustments of their insulin no more than once or twice weekly. Daily alterations to the insulin dose are highly undesirable (except during illness).

Blood glucose concentration evaluation may be carried out visually (using a colour comparison chart) or by means of a meter. Meters give a more precise reading and are useful for patients with poor eyesight or who are colour blind.

Note. In the U. K. blood glucose concentration is expressed in mmol/litre and the British Diabetic Association advises its members that these units should be used for self blood glucose monitoring. In other European countries units of mg/100 mL (or mg/dL) are commonly used.

It is advisable to check that the meter is pre-set in the correct units.

Test strips

Biocare Glucose VT® (Biocare)

Reagent strips, for blood glucose monitoring, visual range (1.1–44.4 mmol/litre). Net price 50-strip pack = £8.50

BM-Accutest® (BM Diagnostics)

Reagent strips, for blood glucose monitoring, range (1.1–33.3 mmol/litre), for use with **NHS** Accutrend® meter only. Net price 50-strip pack = £12.79

BM-Test 1–44® (BM Diagnostics)

Reagent strips, for blood glucose monitoring, visual range (1–44 mmol/litre) meter range (0.5–27.7 mmol/litre), suitable for use with **NHS** Reflolux® S. Net price 50-strip pack = £14.01

Dextrostix® (Bayer Diagnostics)

Reagent strips, for blood glucose monitoring, visual range (1.4–14 mmol/litre). Net price 50-strip pack = £13.99

ExacTech® (MediSense)

Biosensor strips, for blood glucose monitoring, range (2.2–25 mmol/litre), for use with **NHS** ExacTech® meter only. Net price 50-strip pack = £12.93

Glucostix® (Bayer Diagnostics)

Reagent strips, for blood glucose monitoring, visual range (1–44 mmol/litre), meter range (2–22 mmol/litre), suitable for use with **NHS** Glucometer® GX. Net price 50-strip pack = £13.99

Hypoguard® GA (Hypoguard)

Reagent strips, for blood glucose monitoring, visual range (1–22 mmol/litre), meter range (0–22 mmol/litre), suitable for use with **NHS** Hypocount® GA. Net price 50-strip pack = £12.21

Hypoguard® Supreme (Hypoguard)

Reagent strips, for blood glucose monitoring, visual range 1–22 mmol/litre, meter range (2–22 mmol/litre), suitable for use with **NHS** Hypocount® Supreme meter. Net price 50-strip pack = £12.73

Medisense G2® (MediSense)

Sensor strips, for blood glucose monitoring, range (1.1–33.3 mmol/litre) for use with **NHS** Medisense Companion® 2 or **NHS** Medisense Pen® 2 meter only. Net price 50-strip pack = £12.93

Medi-Test® Glycaemic C (BHR)

Reagent strips, for blood glucose monitoring, visual range (1.1–44.4 mmol/litre), meter range (1.1–33.3 mmol/litre), suitable for use with **NHS** Glycotronic® C meter. Net price 50-strip pack = £12.95

One Touch® (LifeScan)

Reagent strips, for blood glucose monitoring, range (0–33.3 mmol/litre), for use with **NHS** One Touch® meter. Net price 50-strip pack = £12.43

Meters

NHS Accutrend® (BM Diagnostics)

Meter for blood glucose monitoring (for use with BM-Accutest® test strips) = £49.00

NHS ExacTech® (MediSense)

Meters (Sensor) for blood glucose monitoring for use with ExacTech® test strips. ExacTech Companion = £29.00, ExacTech Companion starter pack = £39.00, ExacTech Pen = £29.00, ExacTech Pen starter pack = £39.00

NHS Glucometer GX® (Bayer Diagnostics)

Meter for blood glucose monitoring (for use with Glucostix® test strips) = £25.00

NHS Glycotronic® C (BHR)

Meter for blood glucose monitoring (for use with Medi-Test® Glycaemic C test strips) = £31.00

NHS Hypocount® (Hypoguard)

Meters for blood glucose monitoring, Hypocount GA (for use with Hypoguard GA® test strips) = £24.95, Hypocount® Supreme (for use with Hypoguard® Supreme test strips) = £34.95

NHS Medisense® (MediSense)

Meters (Sensor) for blood glucose monitoring for use with Medisense G2® test strips. Medisense Companion 2 = £45.00, Medisense Pen 2 = £45.00

NHS One Touch® (LifeScan)

Meters for blood glucose monitoring for use with One Touch® test strips. One Touch Basic system pack = £39.00, One Touch II system pack = £59.00

NHS Reflolux® S (BM Diagnostics)

Meter for blood glucose monitoring (for use with BM-Test 1–44® test strips) = £29.00

URINALYSIS

Urine testing for glucose is useful in patients who find blood glucose monitoring difficult. Tests for glucose range from reagent strips specific to glucose to reagent tablets which detect all reducing sugars. Few patients still use *Clinitest*; *Clinistix* is suitable for screening purposes only. Tests for ketones and proteins are usually performed in clinics and patients are rarely required to do these tests for themselves.

Microalbuminuria can be detected with **NHS** Micral-Test® but this should be followed by confirmation with a 24-hour sample, since false positive results are common.

Glucose

Clinistix® (Bayer Diagnostics)

Reagent strips, for detection of glucose in urine. Net price 50-strip pack = £2.75

Clinitest® (Bayer Diagnostics)

Reagent tablets, for detection of glucose and other reducing substances in urine. Pocket set (test tube, dropper and 36 tablets), net price = £3.35, 36-tab pack = £1.69, 6-test tube pack = £1.93, 6-dropper pack = £1.93, **NHS** test tube rack set (6 tubes and 2 droppers) = £5.30

Diabur Test 5000® (BM Diagnostics)

Reagent strips, for detection of glucose in urine. Net price 50-strip pack = £2.28

Diastix® (Bayer Diagnostics)

Reagent strips, for detection of glucose in urine. Net price 50-strip pack = £2.34

Medi-Test® Glucose (BHR)

Reagent strips, for detection of glucose in urine. Net price 50-strip pack = £1.99

Ketones

Acetest® (Bayer Diagnostics)

Reagent tablets, for detection of ketones in urine. Net price 100-tab pack = £2.99

Ketostix® (Bayer Diagnostics)

Reagent strips, for detection of ketones in urine. Net price 50-strip pack = £2.34

Ketur Test® (BM Diagnostics)

Reagent strips, for detection of ketones in urine. Net price 50-strip pack = £2.18

Protein

Albustix® (Bayer Diagnostics)

Reagent strips, for detection of protein in urine. Net price 50-strip pack = £3.22

Albym Test® (BM Diagnostics)
Reagent strips, for detection of protein in urine. Net price 50-strip pack = £2.94

Other reagent strips available for urinalysis include NHS BM-Test-GP® (glucose and protein—BM Diagnostics), NHS Ketodiastix® (glucose and ketones— Bayer Diagnostics, NHS Medi-Test Combi 2® (glucose and protein—BHR), NHS Micral-Test® (albumin—BM Diagnostics), NHS Microbumintest® (albumin—Bayer Diagnostics), NHS Uristix® (glucose and protein— Bayer Diagnostics)

GLUCOSE TOLERANCE TEST

The **glucose** tolerance test is used in the diagnosis of diabetes mellitus. In the UK this generally involves giving 75 g of glucose BP (= dextrose monohydrate) by mouth to the fasting patient, and measuring plasma concentrations at intervals. At an international level, however, confusion has arisen because in different pharmacopoeias the title 'glucose' can mean the anhydrous form or the monohydrate. Sources at the World Health Organisation have therefore suggested that the form of dextrose should be standardised as anhydrous, and that the standard amount should be 75 g. The equivalent value (and titles) in the UK are:

Anhydrous glucose BP (anhydrous dextrose) 75 g = Glucose BP (dextrose monohydrate) 82.5 g

6.2   Thyroid and antithyroid drugs

6.2.1   Thyroid hormones
6.2.2   Antithyroid drugs

6.2.1   Thyroid hormones

Thyroid hormones are used in hypothyroidism (myxoedema), and also in diffuse non-toxic goitre, Hashimoto's thyroiditis (lymphadenoid goitre), and thyroid carcinoma. Neonatal hypothyroidism requires prompt treatment for normal development.

Thyroxine sodium is the treatment of choice for *maintenance* therapy. The initial dose should not exceed 100 micrograms daily, preferably before breakfast, or 25 to 50 micrograms in elderly patients or those with cardiac disease, increased by 25 to 50 micrograms at intervals of at least 4 weeks. The usual maintenance dose to relieve hypothyroidism is 100 to 200 micrograms daily which can be administered as a single dose.

In infants a daily dose of 10 micrograms/kg up to a maximum of 50 micrograms daily should be given; subsequent therapy should reach 100 micrograms daily by 5 years and adult doses by 12 years, guided by clinical response, growth assessment, and measurements of plasma thyroxine and thyroid-stimulating hormone.

Liothyronine sodium has a similar action to thyroxine but is more rapidly metabolised; 20 micrograms is equivalent to 100 micrograms of thyroxine. Its effects develop after a few hours and disappear within 24 to 48 hours of discontinuing

treatment. It may be used in *severe hypothyroid states* when a rapid response is desired.

Liothyronine by intravenous injection is the treatment of choice in *hypothyroid coma*. Adjunctive therapy includes intravenous fluids, hydrocortisone, and antibiotics; assisted ventilation is often required.

Dried **thyroid** should **not** be used as its effects are unpredictable.

THYROXINE SODIUM
Indications: hypothyroidism
Cautions: cardiovascular disorders, prolonged myxoedema, adrenal insufficiency; **interactions:** Appendix 1 (thyroxine)
Side-effects: arrhythmias, anginal pain, tachycardia, cramps in skeletal muscles, headache, restlessness, excitability, flushing, sweating, diarrhoea, excessive weight loss
Dose: see notes above

PoM Thyroxine (Non-proprietary)
Tablets, thyroxine sodium 25 micrograms, net price 20 = 13p; 50 micrograms, 20 = 16p; 100 micrograms, 20 = 5p
Various strengths available from APS, Cox, CP, Evans, Goldshield (including Eltroxin®), K Pharm.

LIOTHYRONINE SODIUM
(L-Tri-iodothyronine sodium)
Indications: see notes above
Cautions; Contra-indications; Side-effects: see under Thyroxine Sodium; has a more rapid effect
Dose: by mouth, initially 20 micrograms daily gradually increased to 60 micrograms daily in 2–3 divided doses; elderly patients should receive smaller initial doses, gradually increased; CHILD, adult dose reduced in proportion to body-weight
By slow intravenous injection, hypothyroid coma, 5–20 micrograms repeated every 12 hours or more frequently (every 4 hours if necessary); alternatively 50 micrograms initially then 25 micrograms every 8 hours reducing to 25 micrograms twice daily

PoM Tertroxin® (Link)
Tablets, scored, liothyronine sodium 20 micrograms. Net price 100-tab pack = £14.92
PoM Triiodothyronine (Link)
Injection, powder for reconstitution, liothyronine sodium (with dextran). Net price 20-microgram amp = £31.63

6.2.2   Antithyroid drugs
Antithyroid drugs are used to prepare patients for thyroidectomy. They are also used for prolonged periods in the hope of inducing life-long remission. In the UK the carbimazole is the most commonly used drug. Propylthiouracil may be used in patients who suffer sensitivity reactions to carbimazole as sensitivity is not necessarily displayed to both drugs. Both drugs act primarily by interfering with the synthesis of thyroid hormones.

Carbimazole is given in a daily dose of 20 to 60 mg and maintained at this dose until the patient becomes euthyroid, usually after 4 to 8 weeks; the dose may then be progressively reduced to a maintenance of between 5 and 15 mg daily; therapy is usually given for 18 months. Children may be given an initial dose of 15 mg daily, adjusted according to response. Rashes are common, and propylthiouracil may then be substituted. Pruritus and rashes can also be treated with antihistamines without discontinuing therapy, however patients should be advised to report any sore throat immediately because of the rare complication of agranulocytosis (see CSM warning, above).

Propylthiouracil is given in a daily dose of 300 to 600 mg and maintained on this dose until the patient becomes euthyroid; the dose may then be progressively reduced to a maintenance of between 50 and 150 mg daily.

Although antithyroid drugs have a short half-life they need only be given once daily because of their prolonged effect on the thyroid. Over-treatment with the rapid development of hypothyroidism is not uncommon and should be avoided particularly during pregnancy since it can cause fetal goitre.

A combination of carbimazole, 20 to 60 mg daily with thyroxine, 50 to 150 micrograms daily, may be used in a *blocking replacement regimen*; therapy is again usually given for 18 months. The blocking-replacement regimen is not suitable during pregnancy.

Unless operation or use of radioactive iodine is planned, treatment should be for at least a year.

Before partial thyroidectomy **iodine** may be given for 10 to 14 days in addition to carbimazole or propylthiouracil to assist control and reduce vascularity of the thyroid. Iodine should not be used for long-term treatment since its antithyroid action tends to diminish.

Radioactive sodium iodide (^{131}I) solution is used increasingly for the treatment of thyrotoxicosis at all ages, particularly where medical therapy or compliance is a problem, in patients with cardiac disease, and in patients who relapse after thyroidectomy.

Propranolol is useful for rapid relief of thyrotoxic symptoms and may be used in conjunction with antithyroid drugs or as an adjunct to radioactive iodine. Beta-blockers are also useful in neonatal thyrotoxicosis and in supraventricular arrhythmias due to hyperthyroidism. Propranolol may be used in conjunction with iodine to prepare mildly thyrotoxic patients for surgery but it is still preferable to make the patient euthyroid with carbimazole before surgery. Laboratory tests of thyroid function are not altered by beta-blockers. Most experience in treating thyrotoxicosis has been gained with propranolol but **nadolol** and **sotalol** are also used. For doses and preparations of beta-blockers see section 2.4.

Thyrotoxic crisis ('thyroid storm') requires emergency treatment with intravenous administration of fluids, propranolol (5 mg) and hydrocortisone (100 mg every 6 hours, as sodium succinate), as well as oral iodine solution and carbimazole or propylthiouracil which may need to be administered by nasogastric tube.

PREGNANCY AND BREAST-FEEDING. Radioactive iodine therapy is contra-indicated during pregnancy. Propylthiouracil and carbimazole can be given. Both drugs cross the placenta and in high doses may cause fetal goitre and hypothyroidism. Rarely, carbimazole has been associated with aplasia cutis of the neonate.

Carbimazole and propylthiouracil transfer to breast milk but this does not preclude breast-feeding as long as neonatal development is closely monitored and the lowest effective dose is used.

CARBIMAZOLE

Indications: hyperthyroidism

Cautions: large goitre; pregnancy, breast-feeding (see notes)

Side-effects: nausea, headache, rashes and pruritus, arthralgia; rarely alopecia, agranulocytosis **(see CSM warning above)**, jaundice

Dose: see notes above

COUNSELLING. Warn patient to tell doctor immediately if sore throat, mouth ulcers, bruising, fever, malaise, or non-specific illness develops

PoM Neo-Mercazole® (Roche)

Tablets, both pink, carbimazole 5 mg, net price 100-tab pack = £2.74; 20 mg, 100-tab pack = £10.14

IODINE AND IODIDE

Indications: thyrotoxicosis (pre-operative)

Cautions: pregnancy, children; not for long-term treatment

Contra-indications: breast-feeding

Side-effects: hypersensitivity reactions including coryza-like symptoms, headache, lachrymation, conjunctivitis, pain in salivary glands, laryngitis, bronchitis, rashes; on prolonged treatment depression, insomnia, impotence; goitre in infants of mothers taking iodides

Aqueous Iodine Oral Solution (Lugol's Solution), iodine 5%, potassium iodide 10% in purified water, freshly boiled and cooled, total iodine 130 mg/mL. Net price 100 mL = £1.15. Label: 27
Dose: 0.1–0.3 mL 3 times daily well diluted with milk or water

PROPYLTHIOURACIL
Indications: hyperthyroidism
Cautions; Side-effects: see under Carbimazole; also rarely tendency to haemorrhage; reduce dose in renal impairment; systemic lupus erythematosus reported
Dose: see notes above

PoM **Propylthiouracil** (Non-proprietary)
Tablets, propylthiouracil 50 mg. Net price 20 = £8.00
Available from CP, Evans

6.3   Corticosteroids

6.3.1   Replacement therapy
6.3.2   Comparisons of corticosteroids
6.3.3   Disadvantages of corticosteroids
6.3.4   Clinical management

6.3.1   Replacement therapy

The adrenal cortex normally secretes hydrocortisone (cortisol) which has glucocorticoid activity and weak mineralocorticoid activity. It also secretes the mineralocorticoid aldosterone.

In deficiency states, physiological replacement is best achieved with a combination of **hydrocortisone**[1] and the mineralocorticoid **fludrocortisone**; hydrocortisone alone does not usually provide sufficient mineralocorticoid activity for complete replacement.

In *Addison's disease* or following adrenalectomy, **hydrocortisone** 20 to 30 mg daily by mouth is usually required. This is given in 2 doses, the larger in the morning and the smaller in the evening, mimicking the normal diurnal rhythm of cortisol secretion. The optimum daily dose is determined on the basis of clinical response. Glucocorticoid therapy is supplemented by fludrocortisone 50 to 300 micrograms daily.

In *acute adrenocortical insufficiency,* **hydrocortisone** is given intravenously (preferably as sodium succinate) in doses of 100 mg every 6 to 8 hours in sodium chloride intravenous infusion 0.9%.

In *hypopituitarism* glucocorticoids should be given as in adrenocortical insufficiency, but since the production of aldosterone is also regulated by the renin-angiotensin system a mineralocorticoid is not usually required. Additional replacement ther-

1. Cortisone has generally been superseded by hydrocortisone; management with the more potent synthetic glucocorticoids such as prednisolone (with fludrocortisone) though practicable, offers no advantage. They tend to have less mineralocorticoid activity than hydrocortisone and their greater glucocorticoid activity is only of advantage in the treatment of inflammatory and neoplastic disease.

apy with thyroxine (section 6.2.1) and sex hormones (section 6.4) should be given as indicated by the pattern of hormone deficiency.

Corticosteroid cover for *adrenalectomy,* for *hypophysectomy* or for operations on patients on long-term treatment with corticosteroids is determined logically from the knowledge that in a normal person major stress will not lead to the secretion of more than 300 mg of cortisol in 24 hours; once the stress is over, cortisol production rapidly returns to its usual level of approximately 20 mg per 24 hours. A simple way of mimicking this is to administer hydrocortisone. On the day of operation hydrocortisone 100 mg (usually as the succinate) is given by intramuscular or intravenous injection with the premedication, and repeated every 8 hours. In the absence of complications, the dose can be halved every 24 hours until a normal maintenance dose of 20 to 30 mg per 24 hours is reached on the 5th post-operative day.

CORTISONE ACETATE
Section 6.3.4

FLUDROCORTISONE ACETATE
Indications: mineralocorticoid replacement in adrenocortical insufficiency
Cautions; Contra-indications; Side-effects: section 6.3.3
Dose: adrenocortical insufficiency, 50–300 micrograms daily; CHILD 5 micrograms/kg daily

PoM **Florinef®** (Squibb)
Tablets, pink, scored, fludrocortisone acetate 100 micrograms. Net price 20 = 96p. Label: 10 steroid card

HYDROCORTISONE
Section 6.3.4

6.3.2   Comparisons of corticosteroids

Betamethasone, dexamethasone, hydrocortisone, prednisolone, and prednisone are used for their anti-inflammatory effect; the following table shows equivalent anti-inflammatory doses.

Equivalent Anti-inflammatory Doses of Glucocorticoids

Drug	Equivalent anti-inflammatory dose (mg)
Betamethasone	0.75
Cortisone acetate	25
Dexamethasone	0.75
Hydrocortisone	20
Methylprednisolone	4
Prednisolone	5
Prednisone	5
Triamcinolone	4

Note. This table takes no account of mineralocorticoid effects (see text below), nor does it take account of variations in duration of action.

In comparing the relative potencies of corticosteroids in terms of their anti-inflammatory (glucocorticoid) effects it should be borne in mind that high anti-inflammatory (glucocorticoid) activity in itself is of no advantage unless it occurs in conjunction with relatively low mineralocorticoid activity so that the mineralocorticoid effect on water and electrolytes is not also increased.

The mineralocorticoid activity of **fludrocortisone** is so high that its anti-inflammatory activity is of no clinical relevance.

The mineralocorticoid effects of **cortisone** and **hydrocortisone** are too high for them to be used on a long-term basis for inflammatory disease suppression since fluid retention would be too great, but they are suitable for adrenal replacement therapy (section 6.3.1); hydrocortisone is preferred because cortisone is only active after conversion in the liver to hydrocortisone. Hydrocortisone is also used by intravenous injection for the emergency management of some conditions (section 6.3.4). The relatively moderate anti-inflammatory potency of hydrocortisone makes it a first-choice topical corticosteroid for the management of inflammatory skin conditions because side-effects (both topical and caused by absorption) are less marked (see section 13.4); cortisone is not active topically.

Prednisolone has predominantly glucocorticoid activity and is the corticosteroid most commonly used by mouth for long-term administration. **Prednisone** has a similar level of glucocorticoid activity but is only active after conversion in the liver to prednisolone; it is therefore not recommended.

Betamethasone and **dexamethasone** have very high glucocorticoid activity in conjunction with insignificant mineralocorticoid activity. This makes them particularly suitable for high-dose therapy in conditions where water retention would be a disadvantage (see *cerebral oedema*, section 6.3.4).

They also have a long duration of action and this, coupled with their lack of mineralocorticoid action makes them particularly suitable for conditions which require suppression of corticotrophin secretion (see *congenital adrenal hyperplasia*, section 6.3.4). Some esters of betamethasone and of **beclomethasone** exert a considerably more marked topical effect (e.g. on the skin or the lungs) than when given by mouth; use is made of this to obtain topical effects without corresponding systemic activity (e.g. for skin applications and asthma inhalations).

6.3.3   Disadvantages of corticosteroids

Overdosage or prolonged use may exaggerate some of the normal physiological actions of corticosteroids.

Mineralocorticoid effects include *hypertension*, *sodium and water retention and potassium loss*. They are most marked with fludrocortisone, but are significant with cortisone, hydrocortisone, corticotrophin, and tetracosactrin. Mineralocorticoid actions are negligible with the high potency glucocorticoids, betamethasone and dexamethasone, and

occur only slightly with methylprednisolone, prednisolone, prednisone, and triamcinolone.

Glucocorticoid effects include *diabetes* and *osteoporosis* which is a danger, particularly in the elderly, as it may result in osteoporotic fractures for example of the hip or vertebrae; in addition administration of high doses is associated with *avascular necrosis* of the femoral head. *Mental disturbances* may occur; a serious paranoid state or depression with risk of suicide may be induced, particularly in patients with a history of mental disorder. *Euphoria* is frequently observed. *Muscle wasting* (proximal myopathy) may also occur. Corticosteroid therapy is also weakly linked with *peptic ulceration* (the use of soluble or enteric-coated preparations to reduce the risk is speculative only).

High doses of corticosteroids may cause *Cushing's syndrome*, with moon face, striae, and acne; it is usually reversible on withdrawal of treatment, but this must always be gradually tapered to avoid symptoms of acute adrenal insufficiency (see Adrenal Suppression).

In children, administration of corticosteroids may result in *suppression of growth*. Corticosteroids given in high dosage during *pregnancy* may affect adrenal development in the child (but see also Appendix 4).

Modification of tissue reactions may result in spread of *infection*; suppression of clinical signs may allow diseases such as septicaemia or tuberculosis to reach an advanced stage before being recognised – **important:** for advice relating to measles and chickenpox (varicella) exposure, see p. 481 (measles) and p. 482 (varicella-zoster); see also CSM warning below.

CSM warning (severe chickenpox associated with systemic corticosteroids)
Unless they have had chickenpox, all patients receiving oral or parenteral corticosteroids for purposes other than replacement should be regarded as being *at risk of severe chickenpox*. Manifestations of fulminant illness include pneumonia, hepatitis and disseminated intravascular coagulation; rash is not necessarily a prominent feature. Patients (or parents of children) at risk who use systemic corticosteroids should be advised to take reasonable steps *to avoid close personal contact* with chickenpox or herpes zoster and *to seek urgent medical attention* if exposed to chickenpox. Passive immunisation with varicella-zoster immunoglobulin is needed by non-immune exposed patients receiving systemic corticosteroids or who have used them within the previous 3 months; it should preferably be given within 3 days of exposure (not later than 10 days). For further details see p. 482 and *Immunisation against Infectious Disease 1994*.

Currently there is no good evidence that topical, inhaled or rectal corticosteroids are associated with an increased risk of severe chickenpox.

For other references to the adverse effects of corticosteroids see section 11.4 (eye) and section 13.4 (skin).

ADRENAL SUPPRESSION. Administration of corticosteroids suppresses the secretion of corticotrophin and may lead to adrenal atrophy; withdrawal of treatment must therefore be gradual to avoid symptoms of *acute adrenal insufficiency*. When long-term treatment is to be discontinued, the dose should be reduced gradually over a period of several weeks or months depending on the dosage and duration of the therapy. Too rapid a reduction of corticosteroid dosage can lead to *acute adrenal insufficiency*, *hypotension*, and *death*. A number of minor withdrawal symptoms may also result such as *rhinitis*, *conjunctivitis*, *loss of weight*, *arthralgia*, and *painful itchy skin nodules*.

Adrenal atrophy can persist for years after stopping prolonged corticosteroid therapy, therefore any illness or surgical emergency may require temporary reintroduction of corticosteroid therapy to compensate for lack of sufficient adrenocortical response. Anaesthetists **must** therefore know whether a patient is taking or has been taking corticosteroids to avoid a precipitous fall in blood pressure during anaesthesia or in the immediate postoperative period. Patients should therefore carry cards giving details of their dosage and possible complications. These 'steroid cards' can be obtained from local Family Health Services Authority (FHSA).

In Scotland 'steroid cards' are available from Health Boards. In Northern Ireland they may be obtained from Central Services Agency, 27 Adelaide St, Belfast BT2 8FH.

Pharmacists may also obtain 'steroid cards' from the Royal Pharmaceutical Society of Great Britain.

Interactions: see Appendix 1 (corticosteroids).

6.3.4   Clinical management

Corticosteroids should not be used unless the benefits justify the hazards; the lowest dose that will produce an acceptable response should be used (see also under Administration, below). Dosage varies widely in different diseases and in different patients.

If the use of a corticosteroid can save or prolong life, as in *exfoliative dermatitis*, *pemphigus*, *acute leukaemia* or *acute transplant rejection*, high doses may need to be given, as the complications of therapy are likely to be less serious than the effects of the disease itself.

When long-term corticosteroid therapy is used in relatively benign chronic diseases such as *rheumatoid arthritis* the danger of treatment may become greater than the disabilities produced by the disease. To minimise side-effects the maintenance dose should be kept as low as possible (see also section 10.1.2.1).

When potentially less harmful measures are ineffective corticosteroids are used topically for the treatment of *inflammatory conditions of the skin* (see section 13.4). Corticosteroids should be avoided or used only under specialist supervision in *psoriasis* (see section 13.5).

I am a patient on—

STEROID TREATMENT

which must not be stopped abruptly

and in the case of intercurrrent illness may have to be increased

full details are available from the hospital or general ⟶ practitioners shown overleaf

STC1

INSTRUCTIONS

1   *DO NOT STOP taking the steroid drug except on medical advice. Always have a supply in reserve.*

2   *In case of feverish illness, accident, operation (emergency or otherwise), diarrhoea or vomiting the steroid treatment MUST be continued. Your doctor may wish you to have a LARGER DOSE or an INJECTION at such times.*

3   *If the tablets cause indigestion consult your doctor AT ONCE.*

4   *Always carry this card while receiving steroid treatment and show it to any doctor, dentist, nurse or midwife or anyone else who is giving you treatment.*

5   *After your treatment has finished you must still tell any doctor, dentist, nurse or midwife or anyone else who is giving you treatment that you have had steroid treatment.*

Corticosteroids are used both topically (by rectum) and systemically (by mouth or intravenously) in the management of *ulcerative colitis* and *Crohn's disease* (see sections 1.5 and 1.7.2).

Use can be made of the mineralocorticoid activity of fludrocortisone to treat *postural hypotension* in autonomic neuropathy (see section 6.1.5).

Very high doses of corticosteroids have been given by intravenous injection in *septic shock*. However a recent study (using methylprednisolone sodium succinate) did not demonstrate efficacy and, moreover, suggested a higher mortality in some subsets of patients given the high-dose corticosteroid therapy.

Dexamethasone and betamethasone have little if any mineralocorticoid action and their long duration of action makes them particularly suitable for suppressing corticotrophin secretion in *congenital adrenal hyperplasia* where the dose should be tailored to the individual on clinical grounds and by measurement of adrenal androgens and 17-hydroxyprogesterone. In common with all glucocorticoids their suppressive action on the hypothalamic-pituitary-adrenal axis is greatest and most prolonged when they are given at night. In most normal subjects a single dose of 1 mg of dexamethasone at night, depending on weight, is sufficient to inhibit corticotrophin secretion for 24 hours. This is the basis of the 'overnight dexamethasone suppression test' for diagnosing Cushing's syndrome.

Betamethasone and dexamethasone are also appropriate for conditions where water retention would be a disadvantage, as for example in treating traumatic *cerebral oedema* with doses of 12 to 20 mg daily.

In acute hypersensitivity reactions such as *angioedema* of the upper respiratory tract and *anaphylactic shock*, corticosteroids are indicated as an adjunct to emergency treatment with adrenaline (see section 3.4.3). In such cases hydrocortisone (as sodium succinate) by intravenous injection in a dose of 100 to 300 mg may be required.

Corticosteroids are preferably used by inhalation in the management of *asthma* (see section 3.2) but systemic therapy in association with bronchodilators is required for the emergency treatment of severe acute asthma (see section 3.1.1).

Corticosteroids may also be useful in conditions such as *rheumatic fever*, *chronic active hepatitis*, and *sarcoidosis*; they may also lead to remissions of acquired *haemolytic anaemia*, and some cases of the *nephrotic syndrome* (particularly in children) and *thrombocytopenic purpura*.

Corticosteroids can improve the prognosis of serious conditions such as *systemic lupus erythematosus*, *temporal arteritis*, and *polyarteritis nodosa*; the effects of the disease process may be suppressed and symptoms relieved, but the underlying condition is not cured, although it may ultimately burn itself out. It is usual to begin therapy in these conditions at fairly high dose, such as 40 to 60 mg prednisolone daily, and then to reduce the dose to the lowest commensurate with disease control.

For other reference to the use of corticosteroids see section 11.4 (eye), 12.1.1 (otitis externa), 12.2.1 (allergic rhinitis), and 12.3.1 (aphthous ulcers).

ADMINISTRATION. Whenever possible *local treatment* with creams, intra-articular injections, inhalations, eye-drops, or enemas should be used in preference to *systemic treatment*. The suppressive action of a corticosteroid on cortisol secretion is least when it is given in the morning, therefore in an attempt to reduce pituitary-adrenal suppression a corticosteroid (usually prednisolone) should normally be taken as a single dose in the morning. In an attempt to reduce pituitary-adrenal suppression further, the total dose for two days can sometimes be taken as a single dose on alternate days; alternate-day administration has not been very successful in the management of asthma (see section 3.2) but it can be suitable for rheumatoid arthritis (see section 10.1.2). Pituitary-adrenal suppression can also be reduced by means of intermittent therapy with short courses. In some conditions it may be possible to reduce the dose of corticosteroid by adding a small dose of an immunosuppressive drug (see section 8.2.1).

CHILDREN. In children the indications for corticosteroids are the same as for adults but risks are greater (see **Side-effects** and CSM warning relating to chickenpox, p. 281). The implications of starting these drugs are serious, and they should be used only when specifically indicated, in a minimal dosage, and for the shortest possible time. Prolonged or continuous treatment is rarely justified.

PREDNISOLONE

Indications: suppression of inflammatory and allergic disorders; see also notes above; inflammatory bowel disease, section 1.5; asthma, section 3.2; immunosuppression, section 8.2.2; rheumatic disease, section 10.1.2

Cautions; Contra-indications; Side-effects: section 6.3.3

Dose: by mouth, initially, up to 10–20 mg daily (severe disease, up to 60 mg daily), preferably taken in the morning after breakfast; can often be reduced within a few days but may need to be continued for several weeks or months

Maintenance, usual range, 2.5–15 mg daily, but higher doses may be needed; cushingoid side-effects increasingly likely with doses above 7.5 mg daily

By intramuscular injection, prednisolone acetate, 25–100 mg once or twice weekly (for preparation see section 10.1.2.2)

PoM **Prednisolone** (Non-proprietary)

Tablets, prednisolone 1 mg, net price 20 = 7p; 5 mg, 20 = 15p. Label: 10 steroid card, 21

Available from APS, Boots (Deltastab®), Cox, CP, Evans, Hillcross, K Pharm., Roussel (Precortisyl®)

Tablets, both e/c, prednisolone 2.5 mg (brown), net price 20 = 11p; 5 mg (red), 20 = 20p. Label: 5, 10 steroid card, 25

Available from APS, Biorex, Cox, Hillcross, K.Pharm. (2.5 mg), Lagap, Pfizer (Deltacortril Enteric®)

Injection, see section 10.1.2.2

PoM Precortisyl Forte® (Roussel)

Tablets, scored, prednisolone 25 mg. Net price 20 = £1.52. Label: 10 steroid card, 21

PoM Prednesol® (Glaxo)

Tablets, pink, scored, soluble, prednisolone 5 mg (as sodium phosphate). Net price 20 = £1.15. Label: 10 steroid card,13, 21

BETAMETHASONE

Indications: suppression of inflammatory and allergic disorders; congenital adrenal hyperplasia; cerebral oedema; see also notes above; ear, section 12.1.1; eye, section 11.4.1; nose, section 12.2.1

Cautions; Contra-indications; Side-effects: section 6.3.3

Dose: by mouth, usual range 0.5–5 mg daily. See also Administration (above)

By intramuscular injection or slow intravenous injection or infusion, 4–20 mg, repeated up to 4 times in 24 hours; CHILD, *by slow intravenous injection*, up to 1 year 1 mg, 1–5 years 2 mg, 6–12 years 4 mg

PoM Betnelan® (Evans)

Tablets, scored, betamethasone 500 micrograms. Net price 100-tab pack = £3.63. Label: 10 steroid card, 21

PoM Betnesol® (Evans)

Tablets, pink, scored, soluble, betamethasone 500 micrograms (as sodium phosphate). Net price 100-tab pack = £3.20. Label: 10 steroid card, 13, 21

Injection, betamethasone 4 mg (as sodium phosphate)/mL. Net price 1-mL amp = 65p. Label: 10 steroid card

---

CORTISONE ACETATE

Indications: section 6.3.1

Cautions; Contra-indications; Side-effects: section 6.3.3

Dose: by mouth, for replacement therapy, 25–37.5 mg daily in divided doses

PoM Cortistab® (Boots)

Tablets, both scored, cortisone acetate 5 mg, net price 20 = 16p; 25 mg, 20 = 66p. Label: 10 steroid card, 21

PoM Cortisyl® (Roussel)

Tablets, scored, cortisone acetate 25 mg. Net price 20 = £1.16. Label: 10 steroid card, 21

DEXAMETHASONE

Indications: suppression of inflammatory and allergic disorders; shock; diagnosis of Cushing's disease, congenital adrenal hyperplasia; cerebral oedema; see also notes above; rheumatic disease, section 10.1.2; eye, section 11.4.1

Cautions; Contra-indications; Side-effects: section 6.3.3; perineal irritation may follow intravenous administration of the phosphate ester

Dose: by mouth, usual range 0.5–9 mg daily. See also Administration (above)

See also section 8.1 (chemotherapy emesis)

By intramuscular injection or slow intravenous injection or infusion (as dexamethasone phosphate), initially 0.5–20 mg; CHILD 200–500 micrograms/kg daily

Cerebral oedema (as dexamethasone phosphate), *by intravenous injection*, 10 mg initially, then 4 mg *by intramuscular injection* every 6 hours as required for 2–10 days

PoM Dexamethasone (Organon)

Tablets, dexamethasone 500 micrograms, net price 20 = 64p; 2 mg, 20 = £2.19. Label: 10 steroid card, 21

Injection, dexamethasone sodium phosphate 5 mg/mL (≡ dexamethasone 4 mg/mL ≡ dexamethasone phosphate 4.8 mg/mL). Net price 1-mL amp = 83p; 2-mL vial = £1.27. Label: 10 steroid card

PoM Decadron® (MSD)

Tablets, scored, dexamethasone 500 micrograms. Net price 20 = 64p. Label: 10 steroid card, 21

Injection, dexamethasone phosphate 4 mg/mL (≡ dexamethasone 3.33 mg/mL ≡ dexamethasone sodium phosphate 4.17 mg/mL). Net price 2-mL vial = £1.76. Label: 10 steroid card

Note. Injection containing Dexamethasone phosphate 4 mg/mL (as sodium phosphate) is also available from David Bull

PoM Decadron Shock-Pak® (MSD)

Injection, dexamethasone 20 mg/mL (≡ dexamethasone sodium phosphate 25 mg/mL). Net price 5-mL vial = £15.13. Label: 10 steroid card

Dose: shock, *by intravenous injection or infusion*, 2–6 mg/kg, repeated if necessary after 2–6 hours (but see section 6.3.2)

FLUDROCORTISONE

See section 6.3.1

HYDROCORTISONE

Indications: adrenocortical insufficiency (section 6.3.1); shock; see also notes above; hypersensitivity reactions (such as anaphylactic shock and angioedema), section 3.4.5; inflammatory bowel disease, section 1.5; haemorrhoids, section 1.7.2; rheumatic disease, section 10.1.2; eye, 11.4.1; skin, section 13.4

Cautions; Contra-indications; Side-effects: section 6.3.3; perineal irritation may follow intravenous administration of the phosphate ester

Dose: by mouth, replacement therapy, 20–30 mg daily in divided doses—see section 6.3.1

By intramuscular injection or slow intravenous injection or infusion, 100–500 mg, 3–4 times in 24 hours or as required; CHILD *by slow intravenous injection* up to 1 year 25 mg, 1–5 years 50 mg, 6–12 years 100 mg

---

Oral preparations

PoM Hydrocortistab® (Boots)

Tablets, scored, hydrocortisone 20 mg. Net price 20 = 65p. Label: 10 steroid card, 21

PoM Hydrocortone® (MSD)

Tablets, scored, hydrocortisone 10 mg, net price 20 = 46p; 20 mg, 20 = 71p. Label: 10 steroid card, 21

Parenteral preparations

PoM Efcortelan Soluble® (Glaxo)

Injection, powder for reconstitution, hydrocortisone (as sodium succinate). Net price 100-mg vial (with 2-mL amp water for injections) = 67p. Label: 10 steroid card

PoM Efcortesol® (Glaxo)

Injection, hydrocortisone 100 mg (as sodium phosphate)/mL. Net price 1-mL amp = 75p; 5-mL amp = £3.40. Label: 10 steroid card

PoM Solu-Cortef® (Upjohn)

Injection, powder for reconstitution, hydrocortisone (as sodium succinate). Net price 100-mg vial (with 2-mL amp water for injections) = £1.02; without water for injections = 96p. Label: 10 steroid card

METHYLPREDNISOLONE

Indications: suppression of inflammatory and allergic disorders; cerebral oedema; see also notes above; rheumatic disease, section 10.1.2; skin, section 13.4

Cautions; Contra-indications; Side-effects: section 6.3.3; rapid intravenous administration of large doses has been associated with cardiovascular collapse

Dose: by mouth, usual range 2–40 mg daily. See also Administration (above)

By intramuscular injection or slow intravenous injection or infusion, initially 10–500 mg; graft rejection, up to 1 g daily *by intravenous infusion* for up to 3 days

Oral preparations

PoM Medrone® (Upjohn)

Tablets, scored, methylprednisolone 2 mg (pink), net price 30-tab pack = £2.69; 4 mg, 30-tab pack = £5.16; 16 mg, 14-tab pack = £6.68; 100 mg (blue), 20-tab pack = £40.27. Label: 10 steroid card, 21

Parenteral preparations

PoM Solu-Medrone® (Upjohn)

Injection, powder for reconstitution, methylprednisolone (as sodium succinate) (all with solvent). Net price 40-mg vial = £1.32; 125-mg vial = £3.96; 500-mg vial = £8.00; 1-g vial = £14.42; 2-g vial = £27.38. Label: 10 steroid card

Various strengths of methylprednisolone sodium succinate injection also available from David Bull

Intramuscular depot

PoM Depo-Medrone® (Upjohn)

Injection (aqueous suspension), methylprednisolone acetate 40 mg/mL. Net price 1-mL vial = £2.73; 2-mL vial = £4.90; 3-mL vial = £7.11. Label: 10 steroid card

Dose: by deep intramuscular injection into gluteal muscle, 40–120 mg, repeated every 2–3 weeks if required

PREDNISONE

Indications: suppression of inflammatory and allergic disorders; see also notes above

Cautions; Contra-indications; Side-effects: section 6.3.3. Avoid in liver disease

Dose: see Prednisolone

PoM Prednisone (Non-proprietary)

Tablets, prednisone 5 mg, net price 20 = 15p. Label: 10 steroid card, 21

PoM Decortisyl® (Roussel)

Tablets, scored, prednisone 5 mg. Net price 20 = 15p. Label: 10 steroid card, 21

TRIAMCINOLONE

Indications: suppression of inflammatory and allergic disorders; see also notes above; rheumatic disease, section 10.1.2; mouth, section 12.3.1; skin, section 13.4

Cautions; Contra-indications; Side-effects: section 6.3.3. Triamcinolone in high dosage has a greater tendency to cause proximal myopathy and should be avoided in chronic therapy

Dose: by mouth, 2–24 mg daily. See also Administration (above)

By deep intramuscular injection, into gluteal muscle, 40 mg of acetonide for depot effect, repeated at intervals according to the patient's response; max. single dose 100 mg

PoM Kenalog® (Squibb)

Injection (aqueous suspension), triamcinolone acetonide 40 mg/mL. Net price 1-mL vial (intramuscular/intra-articular) = £1.70; 1-mL syringe (intramuscular only) = £2.11; 2-mL syringe (intramuscular only) = £3.66. Label: 10 steroid card

PoM Ledercort® (Lederle)

Tablets, triamcinolone 2 mg (blue), net price 20 = £1.90; 4 mg, 20 = £3.78. Label: 10 steroid card, 21

Cautionary label wordings, see inside back cover

Prices are **net**, see p.1

6.4   Sex hormones

Sex hormones are described under the following section headings:

6.4.1   Female sex hormones
6.4.2   Male sex hormones and antagonists
6.4.3   Anabolic steroids

6.4.1   Female sex hormones

6.4.1.1   Oestrogens and HRT
6.4.1.2   Progestogens

6.4.1.1 OESTROGENS AND HRT

Oestrogens are necessary for the development of female secondary sexual characteristics; they also stimulate myometrial hypertrophy with endometrial hyperplasia.

In terms of oestrogenic activity *natural oestrogens* (oestradiol, oestrone, and oestriol) have a more appropriate profile for hormone replacement therapy (HRT) than *synthetic oestrogens* (ethinyl-oestradiol, mestranol, and stilboestrol); the profile of *conjugated oestrogens* resembles that of natural oestrogens.

Oestrogen therapy is given cyclically or continuously for a number of gynaecological conditions. If long-term therapy is required a progestogen should be added cyclically to prevent cystic hyperplasia of the endometrium and possible transformation to cancer (suitable preparations are available incorporating a progestogen, see below). This cyclical addition of a progestogen is not necessary if the patient has had a hysterectomy or in the case of tibolone.

Oestrogens are no longer used to *suppress lactation* because of their association with thromboembolism.

HORMONE REPLACEMENT THERAPY (HRT). Menopausal *vasomotor symptoms* and menopausal *vaginitis* are alleviated by administration of small doses of oestrogen. There is also good evidence that small doses of oestrogen given for several years starting in the perimenopausal period will diminish post-menopausal *osteoporosis* and reduce the incidence of *stroke and myocardial infarction*. There is an increased risk of *endometrial cancer* (countered by cyclical progestogen, see below) and, after some years of use, possibly a slightly increased risk of *breast cancer*.

Hormone replacement therapy (HRT) is indicated for menopausal women whose lives are inconvenienced by *vaginal atrophy* or *vasomotor instability*. Vaginal atrophy may respond to a short course of oestrogen cream given for a few weeks and repeated if necessary. Oral therapy is needed for vasomotor symptoms and should be given for at least a year; in a woman with a uterus cyclical progestogen should be added to reduce the risk of endometrial cancer (see above). Hormone replacement therapy is also indicated for women with *early natural or surgical menopause (before age 45)*, since they are at high risk of osteoporosis; in a woman with a uterus cyclical progestogen should

again be added to reduce the risk of endometrial cancer (see above); hormone replacement therapy should be given to the age of at least 50 and possibly for a further 10 years.

Long-term hormone replacement therapy in general is almost certainly favourable in risk benefit terms for menopausal women *without a uterus* because they do not require cyclical progestogen therapy; it should probably be continued for about 10 years. The picture is less clear for menopausal women *with a uterus* because the need for cyclical administration of progestogen may blunt the protective effect of low-dose oestrogen against myocardial infarction and stroke; any effect of the progestogen (favourable or otherwise) on breast cancer is not yet known. Nevertheless, risk factors for osteoporosis should be borne in mind and, if there are several, consideration given to hormone replacement therapy. Risk factors include *recent corticosteroid therapy or any disease predisposing to osteoporosis, family history, thinness, lack of exercise, alcoholism or smoking, and fracture of a hip or forearm before the age of 65; women of Afro-Caribbean origin appear to be less susceptible than those who are white or Asian.*

Choice. The choice of oestrogen for hormone replacement therapy is not straightforward and depends on an overall balance of indication, risk, and convenience. Vaginitis in a woman with a uterus can be treated for only a few weeks with an oestrogen, without addition of cyclical progestogen; this constraint includes topical cream (see section 7.2.1) since a significant amount is absorbed through the vaginal mucosa. Oestrogen therapy alone is suitable for long-term continuous therapy in a woman without a uterus. A woman with a uterus requires a regimen of oestrogen with cyclical progestogen for the last 10 to 13 days of the cycle (see below). All oral preparations of oestrogen are subject to first-pass metabolism in the intestine and liver, therefore subcutaneous or transdermal administration reflects more closely endogenous hormone activity. In the case of subcutaneous implants, problems have been encountered with the recurrence of vasomotor symptoms at supraphysiological plasma concentrations; moreover, there is evidence of prolonged endometrial stimulation after discontinuation (calling for continued cyclical progestogen).

Providing calcium intake is adequate calcium supplements do not confer additional benefit on hormone replacement therapy (see section 9.5.1).

Surgery. For hormone replacement therapy the evidence of an increased thrombotic risk is questionable, which suggests that it need not normally be stopped before major elective surgery (particularly as heparin prophylaxis is usual in this age group). For reference to supraphysiological concentrations of oestradiol implants see notes above.

OESTROGENS FOR HRT

Note. Relates only to small amounts of oestrogens given for hormone replacement therapy

Indications: see notes above and under preparations

Cautions: prolonged exposure to unopposed oestrogens may increase risk of development of endometrial cancer (see notes above); hypertension, migraine (or migraine-like headaches), cardiac or renal disease; also diabetes, melanoma, otosclerosis, multiple sclerosis, systemic lupus erythematosus; history of breast nodules or fibrocystic disease—closely monitor breast status (breast cancer, see notes above); pre-existing uterine fibroids may increase in size, symptoms of endometriosis may be exacerbated; increased risk of gall bladder disease reported; porphyria (see section 9.8.2); **interactions:** Appendix 1 (oestrogens)

Contra-indications: pregnancy; oestrogen-dependent cancer, active thrombophlebitis or thromboembolic disorders, liver disease (where liver function tests have failed to return to normal), Dubin-Johnson and Rotor syndromes, undiagnosed vaginal bleeding, breast-feeding

Side-effects: nausea and vomiting, weight changes, breast enlargement and tenderness, premenstrual-like syndrome, fluid retention, changes in liver function, cholestatic jaundice, rashes and chloasma, depression, headache, contact lenses may irritate; transdermal delivery systems may cause erythema and itching, and headache has been reported on vigorous exercise

Dose: see under preparations

COUNSELLING ON PATCHES. Patch should be removed after 3–4 days and replaced with fresh patch on slightly different site; recommended sites: clean, dry, unbroken areas of skin on trunk below waistline; not to be applied on or near breasts or under waistband. If patch falls off in bath allow skin to cool before applying new patch

---

WOMEN WITH UTERUS

The following preparations contain a **progestogen** as well as an **oestrogen** and are therefore suitable for a woman with an **intact uterus**; they are **not** suitable for use as (or with) hormonal contraceptives

---

Conjugated oestrogens with progestogen

PoM **Prempak-C®** (Wyeth)

Prempak C® 0.625 Calendar pack, all s/c, 28 maroon tablets, conjugated oestrogens 625 micrograms; 12 light brown tablets, norgestrel 150 micrograms (≡ levonorgestrel 75 micrograms). Net price 3 × 40-tab pack = £12.16

Dose: menopausal symptoms (including osteoporosis prophylaxis), if uterus intact, 1 maroon tablet daily on continuous basis, starting on 1st day of menstruation (or at any time if cycles have ceased or are infrequent), and 1 brown tablet daily on days 17–28 of each 28-day treatment cycle; subsequent courses are repeated without interval

Prempak C® 1.25 Calendar pack, all s/c, 28 yellow tablets, conjugated oestrogens 1.25 mg; 12 light brown tablets, norgestrel 150 micrograms (≡ levonorgestrel 75 micrograms). Net price 3 × 40-tab pack = £12.16

Dose: see under 0.625 Calendar pack, but taking 1 yellow tablet daily on continuous basis (instead of 1 maroon tablet) if symptoms not fully controlled with lower strength

---

Mestranol with progestogen

PoM **Syntex Menophase®** (Syntex)

Tablets, 5 pink, mestranol 12.5 micrograms; 8 orange, mestranol 25 micrograms; 2 yellow, mestranol 50 micrograms; 3 green, mestranol 25 micrograms and norethisterone 1 mg; 6 blue, mestranol 30 micrograms and norethisterone 1.5 mg; 4 lavender, mestranol 20 micrograms and norethisterone 750 micrograms. Net price per pack = £3.25

Dose: menopausal symptoms (including osteoporosis prophylaxis), if uterus intact 1 tablet daily, starting with a pink tablet on Sunday, then in sequence (without interruption)

Oestradiol with progestogen

PoM **Climagest®** (Sandoz)

Climagest® 1-mg Tablets, 16 grey-blue, oestradiol valerate 1 mg; 12 white, oestradiol valerate 1 mg and norethisterone 1 mg. Net price 28-tab pack = £4.38; 3 × 28-tab pack = £12.75

Dose: menopausal symptoms (but not osteoporosis prophylaxis), 1 grey-blue tablet daily for 16 days, starting on 1st day of menstruation (or any time if cycles have ceased or are infrequent) then 1 white tablet for 12 days; subsequent courses are repeated without interval

Climagest® 2-mg Tablets, 16 blue, oestradiol valerate 2 mg; 12 yellow, oestradiol valerate 2 mg and norethisterone 1 mg. Net price 28-tab pack = £4.38; 3 × 28-tab pack = £12.75

Dose: see Climagest® 1-mg, but starting with 1 blue tablet daily (instead of 1 grey-blue tablet) if symptoms not controlled with lower strength

PoM **Cyclo-Progynova®** (Schering Health)

Cyclo-Progynova® 1-mg Tablets, all s/c, 11 beige, oestradiol valerate 1 mg; 10 brown, oestradiol valerate 1 mg and norgestrel 500 micrograms (≡ levonorgestrel 250 micrograms). Net price per pack = £3.50

Dose: menopausal symptoms (including osteoporosis prophylaxis), if uterus intact, 1 beige tablet daily for 11 days, starting on 5th day of menstruation (or at any time if cycles have ceased or are infrequent), then 1 brown tablet daily for 10 days, followed by a 7-day interval

Cyclo-Progynova® 2-mg Tablets, all s/c, 11 white, oestradiol valerate 2 mg; 10 brown, oestradiol valerate 2 mg and norgestrel 500 micrograms (≡ levonorgestrel 250 micrograms). Net price per pack = £3.50

Dose: see Cyclo-Progynova® 1-mg, but starting with 1 white tablet daily (instead of 1 beige tablet) if symptoms not fully controlled with lower strength

---

Cautionary label wordings, see inside back cover

PoM Estracombi® (Ciba)

Combination pack of 4 self-adhesive patches of *Estraderm TTS® 50* (releasing oestradiol approx. 50 micrograms/24 hours) and 4 patches of *Estragest TTS®* (releasing oestradiol approx. 50 micrograms/24 hours and norethisterone acetate 250 micrograms/24 hours). Net price per pack = £9.95. Label: 10 patient information leaflet, counselling, administration

Dose: menopausal symptoms (including osteoporosis prophylaxis) if uterus intact, starting within 5 days of onset of menstruation (or any time if cycles have ceased or are infrequent), 1 *Estraderm TTS® 50* patch to be applied twice weekly for 2 weeks followed by 1 *Estragest TTS®* patch twice weekly for 2 weeks; subsequent courses are repeated without interval

PoM Estrapak 50® (Ciba)

Calendar pack, 8 self-adhesive patches, releasing oestradiol approx. 50 micrograms/24 hours, and 12 tablets, red, norethisterone acetate 1 mg. Net price per pack = £8.45. Label: 10 patient information leaflet, counselling, administration

Dose: menopausal symptoms (including osteoporosis prophylaxis) if uterus intact, starting within 5 days of onset of menstruation (or at any time if cycles have ceased or are infrequent), apply 1 patch twice weekly on continuous basis, and take 1 tablet daily on days 15–26 of each 28-day treatment cycle

PoM Nuvelle® (Schering Health)

Tablets, all s/c, 16 white, oestradiol valerate 2 mg; 12 pink, oestradiol valerate 2 mg and levonorgestrel 75 micrograms. Net price 3 × 28-tab pack = £13.77

Dose: menopausal symptoms (including osteoporosis prophylaxis), 1 white tablet daily for 16 days, starting on 5th day of menstruation (or any time if cycles have ceased or are infrequent) then 1 pink tablet daily for 12 days; subsequent courses are repeated without interval

Oestradiol and oestriol with progestogen

PoM Trisequens® (Novo Nordisk)

Trisequens® tablets, 12 blue, oestradiol 2 mg, oestriol 1 mg; 10 white, oestradiol 2 mg, oestriol 1 mg, norethisterone acetate 1 mg; 6 red, oestradiol 1 mg, oestriol 500 micrograms. Net price 3 × 28-tab pack = £14.97

Dose: menopausal symptoms (including osteoporosis prophylaxis), if uterus intact, 1 blue tablet daily, starting on 5th day of menstruation (or at any time if cycles have ceased or are infrequent), then 1 tablet daily in sequence (without interruption)

Trisequens Forte® tablets, 12 yellow, oestradiol 4 mg, oestriol 2 mg; 10 white, oestradiol 4 mg, oestriol 2 mg, norethisterone acetate 1 mg; 6 red, oestradiol 1 mg, oestriol 500 micrograms. Net price 3 × 28-tab pack = £14.97

Dose: menopausal symptoms (but not osteoporosis prophylaxis), see under Trisequens®, starting with 1 yellow tablet daily (instead of 1 blue tablet) if symptoms not fully controlled with lower strength

WOMEN WITHOUT UTERUS

The following preparations do **not** contain a **progestogen**; if the uterus is intact they need to be given with a progestogen in which case packs incorporating a suitable progestogen tablet are preferred (see above)

Conjugated oestrogens only

PoM Premarin® (Wyeth)

Tablets, all s/c, conjugated oestrogens 625 micrograms (maroon), net price 3 × 28-tab pack = £6.07; 1.25 mg (yellow), 3 × 28-tab pack = £9.08

Dose: menopausal symptoms including osteoporosis prophylaxis, (with progestogen for 10–12 days per cycle if uterus intact), 0.625–1.25 mg daily

*Note.*Premarin® tablets 2.5 mg (purple, net price 20 = £2.30) are available for the palliative treatment of some forms of breast cancer but are now rarely used for this purpose

Oestradiol-only

PoM Oestradiol Implants (Organon)

Implant, oestradiol 25 mg, net price each = £7.26; 50 mg, each = £14.52; 100 mg, each = £27.83

Dose: by implantation, oestrogen replacement, including osteoporosis prophylaxis (with cyclical progestogen on 10–13 days of each cycle if uterus intact, see notes above), 25–100 mg as required (usually every 4–8 months) according to oestrogen levels—check before each implant

PoM Climaval® (Sandoz)

Tablets, oestradiol valerate 1 mg (grey-blue), net price 1 × 28-tab pack = £2.34, 3 × 28-tab pack = £7.02; 2 mg (blue), 1 × 28-tab pack = £2.34, 3 × 28-tab pack = £7.02

Dose: menopausal symptoms (if patient has had a hysterectomy), 1–2 daily (for up to 24 months)

PoM Estraderm TTS® (Ciba)

Patches, self-adhesive, oestradiol, *TTS 25 patch* (releasing approx. 25 micrograms/24 hours), net price, 8-patch pack = £6.75; *TTS 50 patch* (releasing approx. 50 micrograms/24 hours), 8-patch pack = £7.45; *TTS 100 patch* (releasing approx. 100 micrograms/24 hours), 8-patch pack = £8.20. Label: 10 patient information leaflet, counselling, administration

Dose: menopausal symptoms (including osteoporosis prophylaxis in case of Estraderm TTS® 50 **only**), 1 patch to be applied twice weekly on continuous basis; give progestogen on 12 days a month (unless patient has had hysterectomy); therapy should be initiated with TTS 50 for first month, subsequently adjusted to lowest effective dose

PoM Evorel® (Cilag)

Patches, self-adhesive, oestradiol (releasing approx. 50 micrograms/24 hours). Net price 8-patch pack = £7.45. Label: 10 patient information leaflet, counselling, administration

Dose: menopausal symptoms (but not osteoporosis prophylaxis), 1 patch to be applied twice weekly on a continuous basis; increased if necessary to 2 patches twice weekly after first month; give progestogen for 12 days a month (unless patient has had hysterectomy)

PoM **Progynova®** (Schering Health)

Tablets, both s/c, oestradiol valerate 1 mg (beige), net price 21-tab pack = £1.98; 2 mg (blue), 21-tab pack = £1.98

Dose: menopausal symptoms (short-term), 1 mg daily for 21 days, interval of at least 7 days before next course; increased to 2 mg daily if required

PoM **Zumenon®** (Duphar)

Tablets, blue, f/c, oestradiol 2 mg, net price 28-tab pack = £2.55

Dose: menopausal symptoms (but not osteoporosis prophylaxis), with progestogen for 10–14 days per cycle if uterus intact, starting on the 5th day of menstruation (or any time if cycles have ceased or are infrequent) 1–2 tablets daily

Oestradiol, oestriol and oestrone only
PoM **Hormonin®** (Shire)

Tablets, pink, oestradiol 600 micrograms, oestriol 270 micrograms, oestrone 1.4 mg. Net price 100 = £7.16

Dose: menopausal symptoms (including osteoporosis prophylaxis), with progestogen for 12–13 days per cycle if uterus intact, 1–2 tablets daily

Note. Hormonin® tablets can be given continuously or cyclically (21 days out of 28)

Oestriol only
PoM **Ovestin®** (Organon)

Tablets, scored, oestriol 1 mg. Net price 30-tab pack = £4.00. Label: 25

Dose: genito-urinary symptoms associated with oestrogen-deficiency states, 0.5–3 mg daily, as single dose, for up to 1 month, then 0.5–1 mg daily until restoration of epithelial integrity (short-term use)

Piperazine oestrone sulphate only
PoM **Harmogen®** (Upjohn)

Tablets, peach, scored, piperazine oestrone sulphate 1.5 mg. Net price 100 = £11.23

Dose: menopausal symptoms (including osteoporosis prophylaxis), 1.5 mg daily on continuous basis (with progestogen for 10–13 days per 28-day cycle if uterus intact); up to 3 mg daily (in single or divided doses) for vasomotor symptoms and menopausal vaginitis

TIBOLONE

Tibolone combines oestrogenic and progestogenic activity with weak androgenic activity. It has recently been introduced for the treatment of vasomotor symptoms of the menopause. It is given continuously, without cyclical progestogen.

TIBOLONE

Indications: see under Dose

Cautions: renal impairment, epilepsy, migraine, diabetes mellitus, hypercholesterolaemia; withdraw if signs of thrombo-embolic disease, abnormal liver function tests or cholestatic jaundice; see also Note below; **interactions:** Appendix 1 (tibolone)

Contra-indications: hormone-dependent tumours, history of cardiovascular or cerebrovascular disease (e.g. thrombophlebitis, thromboembolism), uninvestigated vaginal bleeding, severe liver disease, pregnancy, breast-feeding

Side-effects: weight changes, ankle oedema, dizziness, seborrhoeic dermatitis, vaginal bleeding, headache, gastro-intestinal disturbances, increased facial hair; migraine, visual disturbances, rash and pruritus also reported

Dose: vasomotor symptoms following natural or surgical menopause, 2.5 mg daily

Note. Unsuitable for use in the premenopause and as or with an oral contraceptive; also unsuitable for use within 12 months of the last menstrual period (may cause irregular bleeding); induce withdrawal bleeding with a progestogen if transferring from another form of HRT

PoM **Livial®** (Organon)

Tablets, tibolone 2.5 mg. Net price 28-tab pack = £13.20; 3 × 28-tab pack = £39.60

ETHINYLOESTRADIOL

Ethinyloestradiol has been used as hormone replacement for menopausal symptoms in a dose of 10–20 micrograms daily. This has now been largely replaced by more appropriate forms of oestrogen.

Ethinyloestradiol is occasionally used, under **specialist supervision**, for the management of *hereditary haemorrhagic telangiectasia* in a dose of 0.5–1 mg daily (but evidence of any beneficial effect is uncertain). Dose-related side-effects include nausea, fluid retention, and thrombosis. Impotence and gynaecomastia occur in men.

For use in breast cancer, see section 8.3.1

ETHINYLOESTRADIOL

Indications: see notes above

Cautions; Contra-indications; Side-effects: cardiovascular disease (sodium retention with oedema, thromboembolism), hepatic impairment (jaundice), feminising effects in men; see also under Combined Oral Contraceptives (section 7.3.1), and under Oestrogen for HRT (above)

Dose: see notes above

PoM **Ethinyloestradiol** (Non-proprietary)

Tablets, ethinyloestradiol 10 micrograms, net price 20 = £2.06; 50 micrograms, 20 = £3.01; 1 mg, 20 = £6.17

Available from Evans

STILBOESTROL

See section 8.3.1

6.4.1.2 PROGESTOGENS

There are two main groups of progestogen, *progesterone and its analogues* (allyloestrenol, dydrogesterone, hydroxyprogesterone, and medroxyprogesterone) and *testosterone analogues* (norethisterone and norgestrel). The newer progestogens (desogestrel, norgestimate, and gestodene) are all derivatives of norgestrel; levonorgestrel is the active isomer of norgestrel and has twice its potency. Progesterone and its analogues are less androgenic than the testosterone derivatives and neither progesterone nor dydrogesterone causes virilisation. Other synthetic derivatives are variably metabolised into testosterone and oestrogen; thus side-effects vary with the preparation and the dose.

Progestogens are used in many menstrual disorders, including *severe dysmenorrhoea*, and *menorrhagia*. **Norethisterone** and **dydrogesterone** may be given alone on a cyclical basis during part of the menstrual cycle or in conjunction with an oestrogen. Where contraception is also required in younger women, however, the best choice is a combined oral contraceptive (see section 7.3.1).

Where *endometriosis* requires drug treatment, it may respond to a progestogen, e.g. norethisterone, administered on a continuous basis. Danazol, gestrinone, and gonadorelin analogues are also available (see section 6.7.2).

Progestogens have been widely advocated for the alleviation of *premenstrual symptoms* but no convincing physiological basis for such treatment has been shown.

Progestogens have been used in *habitual abortion* but there is no evidence of benefit. If they are used for this purpose they should be of the true progesterone-derivative type, e.g. **hydroxyprogesterone hexanoate** to avoid any masculinisation of a female fetus.

HORMONE REPLACEMENT THERAPY. In post-menopausal women receiving *long-term oestrogen therapy for hormone replacement*, a progestogen needs to be added cyclically to prevent cystic hyperplasia of the endometrium and possible transformation to cancer. Combined packs incorporating suitable progestogen tablets are available, see p. 287.

ORAL CONTRACEPTION. Desogestrel, ethynodiol, levonorgestrel, and norethisterone are used in *combined oral contraceptives* and in *progestogen-only contraceptives* (see sections 7.3.1 and 7.3.2).

CANCER. Progestogens also have a role in *neoplastic disease* (see section 8.3.2).

ALLYLOESTRENOL

Indications: habitual abortion, but see notes above
Cautions; Contra-indications; Side-effects: see under Medroxyprogesterone Acetate and notes above
Dose: habitual abortion, 5–10 mg daily for at least one month after the end of critical period (but see notes above)

PoM **Gestanin**® (Organon)
Tablets, scored, allyloestrenol 5 mg. Net price 20 = £1.99

DESOGESTREL

Ingredient of combined oral contraceptives (section 7.3.1)

DYDROGESTERONE

Indications: see under Dose and notes above
Cautions; Contra-indications; Side-effects: see under Medroxyprogesterone Acetate and notes

above; breakthrough bleeding may occur (increase dose)
Dose: endometriosis, 10 mg 2–3 times daily from 5th to 25th day of cycle or continuously
Infertility, irregular cycles, 10 mg twice daily from 11th to 25th day for at least 6 cycles (but not recommended)
Habitual abortion, 10 mg twice daily from day 11 to day 25 of cycle until conception, then continuously until 20th week of pregnancy and gradually reduced (but see notes above)
Dysfunctional uterine bleeding, 10 mg twice daily (together with an oestrogen) for 5–7 days to arrest bleeding; 10 mg twice daily (together with an oestrogen) from 11th to 25th day of cycle to prevent bleeding
Dysmenorrhoea, 10 mg twice daily from 5th to 25th day of cycle
Amenorrhoea, 10 mg twice daily from 11th to 25th day of cycle with oestrogen therapy from 1st to 25th day of cycle
Premenstrual syndrome, 10 mg twice daily from 12th to 26th day of cycle increased if necessary (but not recommended, see notes above)
Hormone replacement therapy, with continuous oestrogen therapy, 10 mg twice daily, for the first 12–14 days of each calendar month

PoM **Duphaston**® (Duphar)
Tablets, scored, dydrogesterone 10 mg. Net price 60-tab pack = £11.87

ETHYNODIOL DIACETATE

Ingredient of combined and progestogen-only oral contraceptives (sections 7.3.1 and 7.3.2)

GESTODENE

Ingredient of combined oral contraceptives (section 7.3.1)

GESTRONOL HEXANOATE

See section 8.3.2

HYDROXYPROGESTERONE HEXANOATE

(Hydroxyprogesterone Caproate)
Indications: habitual abortion but see notes above
Cautions; Contra-indications; Side-effects: see under Medroxyprogesterone acetate and notes above
Dose: by slow intramuscular injection, 250–500 mg weekly during first half of pregnancy

PoM **Proluton* Depot**® (Schering Health)
Injection (oily), hydroxyprogesterone hexanoate 250 mg/mL. Net price 1-mL amp = £2.35; 2-mL amp = £3.69
*formerly Primolut Depot®

LEVONORGESTREL

Ingredient of combined and progestogen-only contraceptives (sections 7.3.1 and 7.3.2)

MEDROXYPROGESTERONE ACETATE

Indications: see under Dose; contraception, see section 7.3.2.2; malignant disease, see section 8.3.2

Cautions: diabetes, hypertension, cardiac or renal disease; **interactions:** Appendix 1 (progestogens)

Contra-indications: pregnancy, undiagnosed vaginal bleeding, hepatic impairment or active liver disease, severe arterial disease, breast or genital tract carcinoma; porphyria (see section 9.8.2)

Side-effects: acne, urticaria, fluid retention, weight changes, gastro-intestinal disturbances, changes in libido, breast discomfort, premenstrual symptoms, irregular menstrual cycles; also depression, insomnia, somnolence, alopecia, hirsutism, anaphylactoid-like reaction; rarely jaundice

Dose: by mouth, 2.5–10 mg daily for 5–10 days beginning on 16th–21st day of cycle, repeated for 2 cycles in dysfunctional uterine bleeding and 3 cycles in secondary amenorrhoea

Mild to moderate endometriosis, 10 mg 3 times daily for 90 consecutive days, beginning on 1st day of cycle

By deep intramuscular injection, endometriosis, 50 mg weekly or 100 mg every 2 weeks for 6 months or longer

PoM **Depo-Provera** ® **50mg/mL** (Upjohn)

Injection (aqueous suspension), medroxyprogesterone acetate 50 mg/mL. Net price 3-mL vial = £4.55; 5-mL vial = £6.85

PoM **Provera®** (Upjohn)

Tablets, all scored, medroxyprogesterone acetate 2.5 mg (orange), net price 100-tab pack = £6.44; 5 mg (blue), 100-tab pack = £12.87; 10 mg (white), 50-tab pack = £12.87, 90-tab pack = £23.20

MEGESTROL ACETATE

See section 8.3.2

NORETHISTERONE

Indications: see under Dose; HRT, see section 6.4.1.1; contraception, see sections 7.3.1 and 7.3.2; malignant disease, see section 8.3.2

Cautions; Contra-indications; Side-effects: see under Medroxyprogesterone Acetate but more virilising and greater incidence of liver disturbances and jaundice; avoid in pregnancy; exacerbation of epilepsy and migraine

Dose: endometriosis 10 mg daily starting on 5th day of cycle (increased if spotting occurs to 20–25 mg daily, reduced once bleeding has stopped)

Menorrhagia, 5 mg 3 times daily for 10 days to arrest bleeding; to prevent bleeding 5 mg twice daily from 19th to 26th day

Dysmenorrhoea, 5 mg 3 times daily from 5th to 24th day for 3–4 cycles

Premenstrual syndrome, 5 mg 2–3 times daily from 19th to 26th day for several cycles (but not recommended, see notes above)

Postponement of menstruation, 5 mg 3 times daily starting 3 days before anticipated onset (menstruation occurs 2–3 days after stopping)

Progestogenic opposition of menopausal oestrogen HRT, see under *Micronor®. HRT,* below

Tablets of 5 mg
Note. **Not** licensed for HRT purposes
PoM **Menzol®** (Schwarz)

Tablets, scored, norethisterone 5 mg. Net price 3 × 24-tab (8-day) 'Planapak' = £7.70; 3 × 60-tab (20-day) 'Planapak' = £19.35

PoM **Primolut N®** (Schering Health)

Tablets, norethisterone 5 mg. Net price 30-tab pack = £2.16

PoM **Utovlan®** (Syntex)

Tablets, scored, norethisterone 5 mg. Net price 100 = £7.52

Tablets of 1 mg for HRT purposes
PoM **Micronor®. HRT** (Cilag)

Tablets, norethisterone 1 mg
Dose: 1 tablet daily on days 15–26 of each 28-day oestrogen HRT cycle

Combined preparations, see section 6.4.1.1

NORETHISTERONE ACETATE

Ingredient of combined oral contraceptives (section 7.3.1) and combined preparations for HRT (section 6.4.1.1)

NORGESTIMATE

Ingredient of combined oral contraceptive (section 7.3.1)

NORGESTREL

Ingredient of progestogen-only oral contraceptives (section 7.3.2) and combined preparations for HRT (section 6.4.1.1)

PROGESTERONE

Indications: see under preparations

Cautions: diabetes, breast-feeding, hypertension; hepatic, cardiac, or renal disease; **interactions:** Appendix 1 (progestogens)

Contra-indications: undiagnosed vaginal bleeding, missed or incomplete abortion, severe arterial disease, mammary carcinoma; porphyria (see section 9.8.2)

Side-effects: acne, urticaria, fluid retention, weight changes, gastro-intestinal disturbances, changes in libido, breast discomfort, premenstrual symptoms, irregular menstrual cycles; also chloasma, depression, pyrexia, insomnia, somnolence, alopecia, hirsutism; rarely jaundice. Injection may be painful

PoM **Cyclogest®** (Hoechst)
Pessaries, progesterone 200 mg, net price 15 = £5.27; 400 mg, 15 = £7.63
Dose: by vagina or rectum, premenstrual syndrome, 200 mg daily to 400 mg twice daily starting at day 12–14 and continued until onset of menstruation (but not recommended, see notes above); rectally if barrier methods of contraception are used, or if vaginal infection

PoM **Gestone®** (Paines & Byrne)
Injection, progesterone 25 mg/mL, 1-mL amp = 34p; 50 mg/mL, 1-mL amp = 44p, 2-mL amp = 58p
Dose: by deep intramuscular injection into buttock, embryo transfer, consult data sheet

6.4.2   Male sex hormones and antagonists

Androgens cause masculinisation; they may be used as replacement therapy in castrated adults and in those who are hypogonadal due to either pituitary or testicular disease. In the normal male they inhibit pituitary gonadotrophin secretion and depress spermatogenesis. Androgens also have an anabolic action which led to the development of anabolic steroids (section 6.4.3).

Androgens are useless as a treatment of impotence and impaired spermatogenesis unless there is associated hypogonadism; they should not be given until the hypogonadism has been properly investigated. Treatment should be under expert supervision.

When given to patients with hypopituitarism they can lead to normal sexual development and potency but not to fertility. If fertility is desired, the usual treatment is with gonadotrophins or pulsatile gonadotrophin-releasing hormone (section 6.5.1) which will stimulate spermatogenesis as well as androgen production.

Caution should be used when androgens or chorionic gonadotrophin are used in treating boys with delayed puberty since the fusion of epiphyses is hastened and may result in short stature.

Androgens are still quite useful in occasional women with disseminated cancer of the breast despite their masculinising effects.

Intramuscular depot preparations of **testosterone esters** are preferred for replacement therapy. Testosterone enanthate or propionate or alternatively Sustanon®, which consists of a mixture of testosterone esters and has a longer duration of action, may be used. Satisfactory replacement therapy can sometimes be obtained with 1 mL of Sustanon 250®, given by intramuscular injection once a month, although more frequent dose intervals are often necessary. Implants of testosterone have been superseded for hypogonadism but are still occasionally used. Menopausal women are also sometimes

given implants of testosterone (in a dose of 50–100 mg every 4–8 months) as an adjunct to hormone replacement therapy.

Of the orally active preparations, **testosterone undecanoate** and **mesterolone** are available. Methyltestosterone and other 17α-alkyl derivatives of testosterone are no longer on the UK market because they sometimes cause dose-related cholestatic jaundice.

TESTOSTERONE AND ESTERS
Indications: see under preparations
Cautions: cardiac, renal, or hepatic impairment (see Appendix 2), elderly, ischaemic heart disease, hypertension, epilepsy, migraine, skeletal metastases (risk of hypercalcaemia), pre-pubital boys (see notes above)
Contra-indications: breast cancer in men, prostatic cancer, hypercalcaemia, pregnancy, breast-feeding, nephrosis
Side-effects: sodium retention with oedema, hypercalcaemia, increased bone growth, priapism, precocious sexual development and premature closure of epiphyses in pre-pubertal males, virilism in women, and suppression of spermatogenesis in men

Oral
PoM **Restandol®** (Organon)
Capsules, red-brown, testosterone undecanoate 40 mg in oily solution. Net price 60 = £15.78. Label: 21, 25
Dose: androgen deficiency, 120–160 mg daily for 2–3 weeks; maintenance 40–120 mg daily

Intramuscular
PoM **Primoteston Depot®** (Schering Health)
Injection (oily), testosterone enanthate 250 mg/ mL. Net price 1-mL amp = £4.13
Dose: by slow intramuscular injection, hypogonadism, initially 250 mg every 2–3 weeks; maintenance 250 mg every 3–6 weeks
Breast cancer, 250 mg every 2–3 weeks
PoM **Sustanon 100®** (Organon)
Injection (oily), testosterone propionate 20 mg, testosterone phenylpropionate 40 mg, and testosterone isocaproate 40 mg/mL. Net price 1-mL amp = £1.11
Dose: by deep intramuscular injection, androgen deficiency, 1 mL every 2 weeks
PoM **Sustanon 250®** (Organon)
Injection (oily), testosterone propionate 30 mg, testosterone phenylpropionate 60 mg, testosterone isocaproate 60 mg, and testosterone decanoate 100 mg/mL. Net price 1-mL amp = £2.61
Dose: by deep intramuscular injection, androgen deficiency, 1 mL usually every 3 weeks
PoM **Virormone®** (Paines & Byrne)
Injection, testosterone propionate 50 mg/mL. Net price 2-mL amp = 46p
Dose: by intramuscular injection, androgen deficiency, 50 mg 2–3 times weekly
Delayed puberty, 50 mg weekly
Breast cancer, 100 mg 2–3 times weekly

Implant

PoM **Testosterone** (Organon)

Implant, testosterone 100 mg, net price = £6.17; 200 mg = £11.49

Dose: by implantation, male hypogonadism, 600 mg every 6 months

Menopausal women, see notes above

MESTEROLONE

Indications: see under Dose

Cautions; Contra-indications; Side-effects: see under Testosterone Esters; spermatogenesis unimpaired

Dose: androgen deficiency, 25 mg 3–4 times daily for several months, reduced to 50–75 mg daily in divided doses for maintenance

PoM **Pro-Viron®** (Schering Health)

Tablets, scored, mesterolone 25 mg. Net price 50 = £7.91

ANTI-ANDROGENS

Cyproterone acetate is an anti-androgen used in the treatment of severe hypersexuality and sexual deviation in the male. It inhibits spermatogenesis and produces reversible infertility (but is not a male contraceptive); abnormal sperm forms are produced. Fully informed consent is recommended and an initial spermatogram. As hepatic tumours have been produced in *animal* studies, careful consideration should be given to the risk/benefit ratio before treatment. Cyproterone acetate is also used in prostatic cancer (see section 8.3.4) and in the treatment of acne and hirsutism in women (see section 13.6.2).

Finasteride is a specific inhibitor of the enzyme 5α-reductase which metabolises testosterone into the more potent androgen, dihydrotestosterone. This inhibition of testosterone metabolism leads to reduction in prostate tissue, with improvement in urinary flow rate and obstructive symptoms.

CYPROTERONE ACETATE

Indications: see notes above; prostate cancer, see section 8.3.4

Cautions: ineffective for male hypersexuality in chronic alcoholism (relevance to prostate cancer not known); blood counts initially and throughout treatment; monitor hepatic and adrenocortical function regularly; diabetes mellitus (see also Contra-indications)

DRIVING. May impair performance of skilled tasks (e.g. driving)

Contra-indications: (do not apply in prostate cancer) hepatic disease, severe diabetes (with vascular changes); sickle-cell anaemia, malignant or wasting disease, severe depression, history of thrombo-embolic disorders; youths under 18 years (may arrest bone maturation and testicular development)

Side-effects: fatigue and lassitude, breathlessness, weight changes, reduced sebum production (may clear acne), changes in hair pattern, gynaecomas-

tia (rarely leading to galactorrhoea and benign breast nodules); rarely osteoporosis; inhibition of spermatogenesis (see notes above); liver function abnormalities reported including jaundice and hepatitis

Dose: male hypersexuality, 50 mg twice daily after food

PoM **Androcur®** (Schering Health)

Tablets, scored, cyproterone acetate 50 mg. Net price 56-tab pack = £32.23. Label: 2, 21, counselling, driving

Note. Tablets containing Cyproterone acetate 50 mg are also available from Generics, Lagap

FINASTERIDE

Indications: benign prostatic hyperplasia

Cautions: obstructive uropathy, prostate cancer; use of condoms recommended if sexual partner is pregnant or is likely to become pregnant (finasteride excreted in semen); women of child-bearing potential should avoid handling crushed or broken tablets

Side-effects: impotence, decreased libido and ejaculate volume

Dose: 5 mg daily, review treatment after 6 months (may require several months treatment before benefit is obtained)

▼ PoM **Proscar®** (MSD)

Tablets, blue, f/c, finasteride 5 mg. Net price 28-tab pack = £24.90

6.4.3 Anabolic steroids

All the anabolic steroids have some androgenic activity but they cause less virilisation than androgens in women. Their protein-building property led to the hope that they might be widely useful in medicine but this hope has not been realised. They have, for example, been given for osteoporosis in women but are no longer advocated for this purpose. Their use as body builders or tonics is quite unjustified; they are abused by some athletes.

Anabolic steroids are used in the treatment of some *aplastic anaemias* (see section 9.1.3) and to reduce the itching of *chronic biliary obstruction* (see Prescribing in Terminal Care p. 12).

NANDROLONE

Indications: osteoporosis in postmenopausal women (but not recommended, see notes above); aplastic anaemia, see section 9.1.3

Cautions: cardiac and renal impairment, hepatic impairment (see Appendix 2), hypertension, diabetes mellitus, epilepsy, migraine; monitor skeletal maturation in young patients; skeletal metastases (risk of hypercalcaemia); **interactions:** Appendix 1 (anabolic steroids)

Contra-indications: severe hepatic impairment, prostate cancer, male breast cancer, pregnancy, porphyria (see section 9.8.2)

Side-effects: acne, sodium retention with oedema, virilisation with high doses including voice changes (sometimes irreversible), amenorrhoea, inhibition of spermatogenesis, premature epiphyseal closure; abnormal liver-function tests reported with high doses; liver tumours reported occasionally on prolonged treatment with anabolic steroids

Dose: see below

Cautionary label wordings, see inside back cover

PoM **Deca-Durabolin®** (Organon)
Injection (oily), nandrolone decanoate 25 mg/mL, net price 1-mL amp = £1.75; 50 mg/mL, 1-mL amp = £3.37
Dose: by deep intramuscular injection, 50 mg every 3 weeks
PoM **Deca-Durabolin 100®** , see section 9.1.3

OXYMETHOLONE
See section 9.1.3

STANOZOLOL
Indications: see under Dose
Cautions; Contra-indications; Side-effects: see under Nandrolone. Headache, dyspepsia, euphoria, depression, cramp, and occasionally hair loss, also reported; cholestatic jaundice occasionally reported
Dose: by mouth, vascular manifestations of Behcet's disease, 10 mg daily
Hereditary angioedema, 2.5–10 mg daily to control attacks, reduced for maintenance (2.5 mg 3 times weekly may be sufficient); CHILD 1–6 years initially 2.5 mg daily, 6–12 years initially 2.5–5 mg daily, reduced for maintenance
Note. In hereditary angioedema restricted to well-established cases who have experienced serious attacks (and not for premenopausal women except in life-threatening situations)

PoM **Stromba®** (Sanofi Winthrop)
Tablets, scored, stanozolol 5 mg. Net price 56-tab pack = £26.26

6.5 Hypothalamic and pituitary hormones and anti-oestrogens

Hypothalamic and pituitary hormones are described under the following section headings:
6.5.1   Hypothalamic and anterior pituitary hormones and anti-oestrogens
6.5.2   Posterior pituitary hormones and antagonists

Use of preparations in these sections requires detailed prior investigation of the patient and *should be reserved for specialist centres.*

6.5.1 Hypothalamic and anterior pituitary hormones and anti-oestrogens

ANTI-OESTROGENS

The anti-oestrogens **clomiphene, cyclofenil,** and **tamoxifen** are used in the treatment of female infertility due to oligomenorrhoea or secondary amenorrhoea (e.g. associated with polycystic ovarian disease). They induce gonadotrophin release by occupying oestrogen receptors in the hypothalamus, thereby interfering with feedback mechanisms; chorionic gonadotrophin is sometimes used as an adjunct. Patients should be warned that there is a risk of multiple pregnancy (*rarely* more than twins).

CLOMIPHENE CITRATE
Indications: anovulatory infertility—see notes above
Cautions: see notes above; polycystic ovary syndrome (cysts may enlarge during treatment), incidence of multiple births increased
Contra-indications: hepatic disease, ovarian cysts, endometrial carcinoma, pregnancy, abnormal uterine bleeding
Side-effects: visual disturbances (withdraw), ovarian hyperstimulation (withdraw), hot flushes, abdominal discomfort, occasionally nausea, vomiting, depression, insomnia, breast tenderness, weight gain, rashes, dizziness, hair loss
Dose: 50 mg daily for 5 days, starting within about 5 days of onset of menstruation (preferably on 2nd day) or at any time (normally preceded by a progestogen-induced withdrawal bleed) if cycles have ceased; second course of 100 mg daily for 5 days may be given in absence of ovulation; most patients who are going to respond will do so to first course; 3 courses should constitute adequate therapeutic trial; long-term cyclical therapy not recommended

PoM **Clomid®** (Merrell)
Tablets, yellow, scored, clomiphene citrate 50 mg. Net price 20 = £6.56
PoM **Serophene®** (Serono)
Tablets, scored, clomiphene citrate 50 mg. Net price 20 = £6.73

TAMOXIFEN
See section 8.3.4

ANTERIOR PITUITARY HORMONES

CORTICOTROPHINS

Tetracosactrin an analogue of corticotrophin (ACTH) is used to test adrenocortical function; corticotrophin itself is no longer commercially available in the UK. Failure of the plasma cortisol concentration to rise after intramuscular administration indicates adrenocortical insufficiency.

Both corticotrophin and tetracosactrin were formerly used as alternatives to corticosteroids in conditions such as Crohn's disease or rheumatoid arthritis; their value was limited by the variable and unpredictable therapeutic response and by the waning of their effect with time.

TETRACOSACTRIN
(Tetracosactide)

Indications: see notes above

Cautions; Contra-indications; Side-effects: see section 6.3.3; important risk of anaphylaxis (medical supervision; see data sheet)

PoM Synacthen® (Ciba)

Injection, tetracosactrin 250 micrograms (as acetate)/mL. Net price 1-mL amp = 93p

> *Dose:* diagnostic, *by intramuscular or intravenous injection,* 250 micrograms as a single dose

PoM Synacthen Depot® (Ciba)

Injection (aqueous suspension), tetracosactrin 1 mg (as acetate)/mL, with zinc phosphate complex; also contains benzyl alcohol. Net price 1-mL amp = £1.73

> *Dose: by intramuscular injection,* initially 1 mg daily (or every 12 hours in acute cases); subsequently reduced to 1 mg every 2–3 days, then 1 mg weekly (or 500 micrograms every 2–3 days)

GONADOTROPHINS

Follicle-stimulating hormone (FSH) and luteinising hormone (LH) together (as in **human menopausal gonadotrophin**) or follicle-stimulating hormone alone (as in **urofollitrophin**), are used in the treatment of infertile women with proven hypopituitarism or who have not responded to clomiphene, or in superovulation treatment for assisted conception (such as *in vitro* fertilisation).

The gonadotrophins are also occasionally used in the treatment of oligospermia associated with hypopituitarism. There is no justification for their use in primary gonadal failure.

Chorionic gonadotrophin has also been used in delayed puberty in the male to stimulate endogenous testosterone production, but has little advantage over testosterone (section 6.4.2).

CHORIONIC GONADOTROPHIN
(Human Chorionic Gonadotrophin; HCG)

A preparation of a glycoprotein fraction secreted by the placenta and obtained from the urine of pregnant women having the action of the pituitary luteinising hormone

Indications: see notes above

Cautions: see notes above; cardiac or renal impairment, asthma, epilepsy, migraine

Side-effects: oedema (particularly in males—reduce dose), headache, tiredness, mood changes, gynaecomastia, local reactions; sexual precocity with high doses; may aggravate ovarian hyperstimulation

Dose: by intramuscular injection, according to patient's requirements

PoM Gonadotraphon LH® (Paines & Byrne)

Injection, powder for reconstitution, chorionic gonadotrophin. Net price 500-unit amp = 98p; 1000-unit amp = £1.25; 5000-unit amp = £3.71 (all with solvent)

PoM Pregnyl® (Organon)

Injection, powder for reconstitution, chorionic gonadotrophin. Net price 1500-unit amp = £2.07; 5000-unit amp = £3.08 (both with solvent)

PoM Profasi® (Serono)

Injection, powder for reconstitution, chorionic gonadotrophin. Net price 500-unit amp = 83p; 1000-unit amp = £1.14; 2000-unit amp = £2.10; 5000-unit amp = £3.70; 10 000-unit amp = £7.39 (all with solvent)

HUMAN MENOPAUSAL GONADOTROPHINS

Purified extract of human post-menopausal urine containing follicle-stimulating hormone (FSH) and luteinising hormone (LH); the relative *in vivo* activity is designated as a ratio; the 1:1 ratio is also known as menotrophin

Indications: see notes above

Cautions: ovarian cysts, adrenal or thyroid disorders, hyperprolactinoma or pituitary tumour

Side-effects: ovarian hyperstimulation, multiple pregnancy; local reactions

Dose: by deep intramuscular injection, according to patient's response

PoM Humegon® (Organon)

Injection, powder for reconstitution, human menopausal gonadotrophins as follicle-stimulating hormone 75 units, luteinising hormone 75 units net price per amp = £8.80; follicle-stimulating hormone 150 units, luteinising hormone 150 units, 1 amp = £16.00 (both with solvent)

PoM Normegon® (Organon)

Injection, powder for reconstitution. human menopausal gonadotrophins as follicle-stimulating hormone 75 units, luteinising hormone 25 units, net price per amp = £9.75; follicle-stimulating hormone 150 units, luteinising hormone 50 units, 1 amp = £18.00 (both with solvent)

PoM Pergonal® (Serono)

Injection, powder for reconstitution, menotrophin as follicle-stimulating hormone 75 units, luteinising hormone 75 units. Net price per amp (with solvent) = £10.18

UROFOLLITROPHIN

Extract of the urine of postmenopausal women containing follicle-stimulating hormone

Indications: see notes above

Cautions; Side-effects: see under Human Menopausal Gonadotrophins

Dose: by intramuscular injection, according to patient's response

PoM Metrodin High Purity® (Serono)

Injection, powder for reconstitution, urofollitrophin as follicle-stimulating hormone, net price 75 unit amp = £18.62; 150-unit amp = £37.24 (both with solvent)

PoM Orgafol® (Organon)

Injection, powder for reconstitution, urofollitrophin as follicle stimulating hormone, net price 75-unit amp (with solvent) = £9.75

GROWTH HORMONE

Growth hormone is used in the treatment of short stature due to growth hormone deficiency (including short stature in Turner syndrome); only the human type is effective as growth hormone is species specific. Growth hormone of human origin (HGH; somatotrophin) has been replaced by a growth hormone of human sequence, **somatropin**, produced using recombinant DNA technology.

SOMATROPIN

(Biosynthetic Human Growth Hormone)

Indications: see notes above

Cautions: only patients with open epiphyses; relative deficiencies of other pituitary hormones (notably hypothyroidism); diabetes mellitus (adjustment of antidiabetic therapy may be necessary); avoid in pregnancy (theoretical risk)

Side-effects: antibody formation; local reactions (rotate subcutaneous injection sites to prevent lipo-atrophy); in Turner syndrome temporary exacerbation of lymphoedema reported

Dose: 0.5–0.7 units/kg (Turner syndrome, 1 unit/kg) weekly divided into 6 or 7 doses for *subcutaneous injection* (alternatively divided into 2 or 3 doses for *intramuscular injection*, but more painful)

PoM **Genotropin®** (Pharmacia)

Injection, powder for reconstitution, somatropin (rbe), net price 4-unit vial (with diluent) = £30.50; 12-unit vial (with diluent) = £91.50

KabiPen injection, two-compartment cartridge containing powder for reconstitution, somatropin (rbe) and diluent. Net price 16-unit cartridge = £122.00, 36-unit cartridge = £274.50. For use with NHS KabiPen® device (available free from clinics)

KabiQuick injection, two-compartment single-dose syringe containing powder for reconstitution, somatropin (rbe) and diluent. Net price 2-unit syringe = £16.00, 3-unit syringe = £24.00, 4-unit syringe = £32.00

KabiVial injection, two-compartment cartridge containing powder for reconstitution, somatropin (rbe) and diluent. Net price 4-unit vial = £30.50, 16-unit vial = £122.00

PoM **Humatrope®** (Lilly)

Injection, powder for reconstitution, somatropin (rbe) and diluent, net price 4-unit vial = £30.50; 16-unit vial = £122.00

PoM **Norditropin®** (Novo Nordisk)

Injection, powder for reconstitution, somatropin (epr), net price 12-unit vial (with diluent) = £89.21

PenSet 12 injection, powder for reconstitution, somatropin (epr), net price 12-unit vial (with diluent in cartridge and needle) = £93.68. For use with NHS Nordiject®12 device (available free from clinics)

PenSet 24 injection, powder for reconstitution, somatropin (epr), net price 24-unit vial (with diluent in cartridge and needle) = £187.35. For use with NHS Nordiject® 24 device (available free from clinics)

PoM **Saizen®** (Serono)

Injection, powder for reconstitution, somatropin (rmc), net price 4-unit vial (with diluent) = £30.50; 10-unit vial (with diluent) = £76.25

HYPOTHALAMIC HORMONES

Gonadorelin when injected intravenously in normal subjects leads to a rapid rise in plasma concentrations of both luteinising hormone (LH) and follicle-stimulating hormone (FSH). It has not proved to be very helpful, however, in distinguishing hypothalamic from pituitary lesions. Gonadorelin is also used for treatment of infertility, particularly in the female. **Gonadorelin analogues** are indicated in endometriosis and infertility (see section 6.7.2) and in breast and prostate cancer (see section 8.3.4).

Protirelin may be of value in difficult cases of hyperthyroidism but has been superseded largely by immunoassays. Failure of plasma thyrotrophin (TSH) concentration to rise after intravenous injection indicates excess circulating thyroid hormones. Impaired or absent responses also occur in some euthyroid patients with single adenoma, multinodular goitre, or endocrine exophthalmos; patients with hypopituitarism show a reduced or delayed rise.

Sermorelin, an analogue of growth hormone releasing hormone (somatorelin, GHRH), has recently been introduced as a diagnostic test for secretion of growth hormone.

GONADORELIN

(Gonadotrophin-releasing hormone; GnRH; LH–RH)

Indications: see preparations below

Side-effects: rarely, nausea, headache, abdominal pain, increased menstrual bleeding; rarely, hypersensitivity reaction on repeated administration of large doses; irritation at injection site

Dose: see under preparations

PoM **Fertiral®** (Hoechst)

Injection, gonadorelin 500 micrograms/mL. Net price 2-mL amp = £33.44

For amenorrhoea and infertility due to abnormal release of LH–RH (endogenous gonadorelin), *by pulsatile subcutaneous infusion,* initially 10–20 micrograms over 1 minute, repeated every 90 minutes until conception occurs or for max. of 6 months; *pulsatile intravenous infusion* (in association with heparin) may be required

PoM **HRF®** (Monmouth)

Injection, powder for reconstitution, gonadorelin. Net price 100-microgram vial = £13.45; 500-microgram vial = £29.39 (both with diluent) (hosp. only)

For assessment of pituitary function (adults), *by subcutaneous or intravenous injection,* 100 micrograms

---

PoM **Relefact LH-RH**® (Hoechst)

Injection, gonadorelin 100 micrograms/mL. Net price 1-mL amp = £9.44

For assessment of pituitary function, *by intravenous injection*, 100 micrograms

PoM **Relefact LH-RH/TRH**® (Hoechst)

Injection, gonadorelin 100 micrograms, protirelin 200 micrograms/mL. Net price 1-mL amp = £10.90

For assessment of anterior pituitary reserve, by *intravenous injection*, 1 mL

PROTIRELIN

(Thyrotrophin-releasing hormone; TRH)

Indications: assessment of thyroid function and thyroid stimulating hormone reserve

Cautions: severe hypopituitarism, myocardial ischaemia, bronchial asthma and obstructive airways disease, pregnancy

Side-effects: after rapid intravenous administration desire to micturate, flushing, dizziness, nausea, strange taste; transient increase in pulse rate and blood pressure; rarely bronchospasm

Dose: by intravenous injection, 200 micrograms; CHILD 1 microgram/kg

PoM **TRH-Cambridge**® (Cambridge)

Injection, protirelin 100 micrograms/mL. Net price 2-mL amp = £4.40 (hosp. only)

SERMORELIN

Indications: see notes above

Cautions: epilepsy; discontinue growth hormone therapy 1–2 weeks before test; untreated hypothyroidism, antithyroid drugs; obesity, hyperglycaemia, elevated plasma fatty acids; avoid preparations which affect release of growth hormone (includes those affecting release of somatostatin, insulin or glucocorticoids and cyclo-oxygenase inhibitors such as aspirin and indomethacin)

Contra-indications: pregnancy and breast-feeding

Side-effects: occasional facial flushing and pain at injection site

Dose: by intravenous injection, 1 microgram/kg in the morning after an overnight fast

▼ PoM **Geref 50**® (Serono)

Injection, powder for reconstitution, sermorelin 50 micrograms (as acetate). Net price per amp (with solvent) = £55.00

6.5.2 Posterior pituitary hormones and antagonists

POSTERIOR PITUITARY HORMONES

DIABETES INSIPIDUS. **Vasopressin** (antidiuretic hormone, ADH) is used in the treatment of *pituitary* ('cranial') *diabetes insipidus* as its analogues **lypressin** or **desmopressin**. Dosage is tailored to produce a slight diuresis every 24 hours to avoid water intoxication. Treatment may be required for a limited period only in diabetes insipidus following trauma or pituitary surgery.

Desmopressin has a longer duration of action than vasopressin or lypressin; unlike vasopressin and lypressin it has no vasoconstrictor effect. It is given intranasally for maintenance therapy, and by injection in the postoperative period or in unconscious patients. Desmopressin is also used in the differential diagnosis of diabetes insipidus. Following a dose of 2 micrograms intramuscularly or 20 micrograms intranasally, restoration of the ability to concentrate urine after water deprivation confirms a diagnosis of cranial diabetes insipidus. Failure to respond occurs in nephrogenic diabetes insipidus.

In *nephrogenic* and *partial pituitary diabetes insipidus* benefit may be gained from the paradoxical antidiuretic effect of thiazides (see section 2.2.1) e.g. chlorthalidone 100 mg twice daily reduced to maintenance dose of 50 mg daily.

Chlorpropamide (section 6.1.2.1) is also useful in partial pituitary diabetes insipidus, and probably acts by sensitising the renal tubules to the action of remaining endogenous vasopressin; it is given in doses of up to 350 mg daily in adults and 200 mg daily in children, care being taken to avoid hypoglycaemia. Carbamazepine (see section 4.8.1) is also sometimes useful (in a dose of 200 mg once or twice daily) [unlicensed]; its mode of action may be similar to that of chlorpropamide.

OTHER USES. Desmopressin injection is also used to boost factor VIII concentrations in mild to moderate haemophilia.

Vasopressin infusion is used to control variceal bleeding in portal hypertension, prior to more definitive treatment and with variable results. Terlipressin, a new derivative of vasopressin, is used similarly.

Oxytocin, another posterior pituitary hormone, is indicated in obstetrics (see section 7.1.1).

VASOPRESSIN

Indications: pituitary diabetes insipidus; bleeding from oesophageal varices

Cautions: heart failure, asthma, epilepsy, migraine or other conditions which might be aggravated by water retention; renal impairment (see also contra-indications); pregnancy; avoid fluid overload

Contra-indications: vascular disease (especially disease of coronary arteries) unless extreme caution, chronic nephritis (until reasonable blood nitrogen concentrations attained)

Side-effects: pallor, nausea, belching, abdominal cramps, desire to defaecate, hypersensitivity reactions, constriction of coronary arteries (may cause anginal attacks and myocardial ischaemia)

Dose: by subcutaneous or intramuscular injection, diabetes insipidus, 5–20 units every four hours

By intravenous infusion, initial control of variceal bleeding, 20 units over 15 minutes

---

Synthetic vasopressin

PoM **Pitressin®** (P-D)

Injection, argipressin (synthetic vasopressin) 20 units/mL. Net price 1-mL amp = £10.00 (hosp. only)

DESMOPRESSIN

Indications: see under Dose

Cautions: see under Vasopressin; less pressor activity, but still need for considerable caution in renal impairment, cardiovascular disease and hypertension (not indicated for nocturnal enuresis or nocturia in these circumstances); also need for considerable caution in cystic fibrosis; avoid fluid overload—in nocturia periodic blood pressure and weight checks needed to monitor for fluid overload

Side-effects: fluid retention, and hyponatraemia (in more serious cases with convulsions) on administration without restricting fluid intake; headache, nausea, vomiting, and epistaxis also reported

Dose: by mouth

Diabetes insipidus, treatment, ADULT and CHILD, initially 300 micrograms daily (in three divided doses); maintenance, 300–600 micrograms daily; range 0.2–1.2 mg daily

Primary nocturnal enuresis (with normal urine concentrating ability), ADULT and CHILD over 5 years (preferably over 7 years), 200 micrograms at bedtime, increased to 400 micrograms if lower dose not effective (**important:** see also cautions); withdraw for at least one week for reassessment after 3 months

Postoperative polyuria/polydipsia, adjust dose according to urine osmolality

Intranasally

Diabetes insipidus, diagnosis, ADULT and CHILD, 20 micrograms

Diabetes insipidus, treatment, ADULT, 10–40 micrograms daily (in one or two divided doses); CHILD, 5–20 micrograms; infants may require lower doses

Primary nocturnal enuresis (with normal urine concentrating ability), ADULT and CHILD over 5 years (preferably over 7 years), 20–40 micrograms at bedtime (**important:** see also cautions); withdraw for at least one week for reassessment after 3 months

Nocturia associated with multiple sclerosis (when other treatments have failed), ADULT (under 65 years), 10–20 micrograms at bedtime (**important:** see also cautions)

Renal function testing (empty bladder at time of testing), ADULT, 40 micrograms; CHILD (1–15 years), 20 micrograms; CHILD (under 1 year), 10 micrograms (restrict fluid intake to 50% at next two feeds to avoid fluid overload)

By injection

Diabetes insipidus, diagnosis (*subcutaneous or intramuscular*), ADULT and CHILD, 2 micrograms

Diabetes insipidus, treatment (*subcutaneous, intramuscular or intravenous*), ADULT, 1–4 micrograms daily; CHILD 400 nanograms

Renal function testing (*subcutaneous or intramuscular*), ADULT and CHILD, 2 micrograms

Mild to moderate haemophilia and von Willebrands disease, post lumbar puncture headache, fibrinolytic response testing, consult data sheet

PoM **DDAVP®** (Ferring)

Tablets, both scored, desmopressin acetate 100 micrograms, net price 90-tab pack = £45.95; 200 micrograms, 90-tab pack = £91.90

Intranasal solution, desmopressin 100 micrograms/mL. Net price 2.5-mL dropper bottle and catheter = £9.50

Injection, desmopressin 4 micrograms/mL. Net price 1-mL amp = £1.07

PoM **Desmotabs®** (Ferring)

Tablets, scored, desmopressin acetate 200 micrograms, net price 28-tab pack = £29.00

PoM **Desmospray®** (Ferring)

Nasal spray, desmopressin 10 micrograms/metered spray. Net price 5-mL unit = £22.90

Note. Children requiring dose of less than 10 micrograms should be given DDAVP® intranasal solution

LYPRESSIN

Indications: pituitary diabetes insipidus

Cautions; Contra-indications; Side-effects: see under Vasopressin; less hypersensitivity; also nasal congestion with ulceration of mucosa

Dose: intranasally, 2.5–10 units 3–7 times daily

PoM **Syntopressin®** (Sandoz)

Nasal spray, lypressin 50 units/mL, 2.5 units/squeeze. Net price 5-mL bottle = £3.40

TERLIPRESSIN

Indications: bleeding from oesophageal varices

Cautions; Contra-indications; Side-effects: see under Vasopressin, but effects are milder

Dose: by intravenous injection, 2 mg followed by 1 or 2 mg every 4 to 6 hours until bleeding is controlled, for up to 72 hours

PoM **Glypressin®** (Ferring)

Injection, terlipressin, powder for reconstitution. Net price 1-mg vial with 5 mL diluent = £19.00 (hosp. only)

ANTIDIURETIC HORMONE ANTAGONISTS

Demeclocycline (see section 5.1.3) may be used in the treatment of hyponatraemia resulting from inappropriate secretion of antidiuretic hormone. It is thought to act by directly blocking the renal tubular effect of antidiuretic hormone. Initially 0.9 to 1.2 g is given daily in divided doses, reduced to 600–900 mg daily for maintenance.

6.6 Drugs affecting bone metabolism

6.6.1 Calcitonin
6.6.2 Bisphosphonates

See also plicamycin (section 8.1.2), calcium (section 9.5.1.1), phosphorus (section 9.5.2), vitamin D (section 9.6.4), and oestrogens in postmenopausal osteoporosis (section 6.4.1.1).

6.6.1 Calcitonin

Calcitonin is involved with parathyroid hormone in the regulation of bone turnover and hence in the maintenance of calcium balance and homoeostasis. It is used to lower the plasma-calcium concentration in some patients with hypercalcaemia (notably when associated with malignant disease). In the treatment of severe Paget's disease of bone it is used mainly for relief of pain but it is also effective in relieving some of the neurological complications, for example deafness. The prolonged use of **porcine calcitonin** can lead to the production of neutralising antibodies. **Salcatonin** (synthetic salmon calcitonin) is less immunogenic and thus more suitable for long-term therapy. When changing treatment in Paget's disease, calcitonin (pork) 80 units is equivalent to salcatonin 50 units.

CALCITONIN (PORK)

Indications: Paget's disease of bone; hypercalcaemia

Cautions: see notes above; may contain trace of thyroid; skin test if history of allergy; pregnancy and breast-feeding (avoid—inhibits lactation in *animals*)

Side-effects: nausea, vomiting, flushing, tingling of hands, unpleasant taste, inflammatory reactions at injection site

Dose: hypercalcaemia, *by subcutaneous or intramuscular injection*, initially 4 units/kg daily adjusted according to clinical and biochemical response (higher doses more conveniently given as salcatonin, see below)

Paget's disease of bone, *by subcutaneous or intramuscular injection*, dose range 80 units 3 times weekly to 160 units daily in single or divided doses; in patients with bone pain or nerve compression syndromes, 80–160 units daily for 3–6 months

PoM **Calcitare®** (Rhône-Poulenc Rorer)
Injection, powder for reconstitution, porcine calcitonin. Net price 160-unit vial (with gelatin diluent) = £11.07

SALCATONIN

Indications: see under Dose (all short term)
Cautions; Side-effects: see under Calcitonin (pork) and notes above
Dose: hypercalcaemia, *by subcutaneous or intramuscular injection*, range from 5–10 units/kg daily *to* 400 units every 6–8 hours adjusted according to clinical and biochemical response (no additional benefit with over 8 units/kg every 6 hours); *by slow intravenous infusion* (Miacalcic® only), 5–10 units/kg over at least 6 hours
Paget's disease of bone, *by subcutaneous or intramuscular injection*, dose range 50 units 3 times weekly to 100 units daily, in single or divided doses; in patients with bone pain or nerve compression syndromes, 50–100 units daily for 3–6 months
Bone pain in neoplastic disease, *by subcutaneous or intramuscular injection*, 200 units every 6 hours *or* 400 units every 12 hours for 48 hours; may be repeated at discretion of physician
Postmenopausal osteoporosis, *by subcutaneous or intramuscular injection*, 100 units daily with dietary calcium and vitamin D supplements (see sections 9.5.1.1 and 9.6.4)

PoM **Calsynar®** (Rhône-Poulenc Rorer)
Injection, salcatonin 100 units/mL in saline/acetate, net price 1 mL amp = £7.92; 200 units/mL in saline/acetate, 2 mL vial = £28.47
For subcutaneous or intramuscular injection only
PoM **Miacalcic®** (Sandoz)
Injection, salcatonin 50 units/mL, net price 1 mL amp = £3.56; 100 units/mL, 1 mL amp = £7.13; 200 units/mL, 2-mL vial = £25.62
For subcutaneous or intramuscular injection and for dilution and use as an intravenous infusion

6.6.2 Bisphosphonates

Disodium etidronate is used mainly in the treatment of *Paget's disease* of bone. It is adsorbed onto hydroxyapatite crystals, so slowing both their rate of growth and dissolution, and reduces the increased rate of bone turnover associated with the disease. Disodium etidronate is also highly effective in the treatment of *hypercalcaemia of malignancy*; more recently **disodium pamidronate** and **sodium clodronate** have been introduced for this purpose as well.
Disodium etidronate is now available with calcium carbonate for *established vertebral osteoporosis*.

DISODIUM ETIDRONATE

Indications: see under Dose
Cautions: reduce dose in mild renal impairment (avoid if moderate to severe); **interactions:** Appendix 1 (bisphosphonates)
Contra-indications: moderate to severe renal impairment; pregnancy and breast-feeding; not indicated for osteoporosis in presence of hypercalcaemia or hypercalciuria
Side-effects: nausea, diarrhoea; asymptomatic hypocalcaemia; increased bone pain in Paget's

disease, also increased risk of fractures with high doses in Paget's disease (discontinue if fractures occur); rarely skin reactions (including angio-edema); abdominal pain and constipation reported; transient taste loss also reported

Dose: Paget's disease of bone, *by mouth*, 5 mg/kg as a single daily dose for up to 6 months; doses above 10 mg/kg daily for up to 3 months may be used with caution but doses above 20 mg/kg daily are not recommended

Hypercalcaemia of malignancy, *by intravenous infusion*, 7.5 mg/kg daily for 3 days; repeat once if necessary after at least 7 days; *by mouth*, on day after last intravenous dose, 20 mg/kg as a single daily dose for 30 days; max. recommended treatment period 90 days

Established vertebral osteoporosis, see under *Didronel PMO®*

COUNSELLING. Avoid food for at least 2 hours before and after oral treatment, particularly calcium-containing products e.g. milk; also avoid iron and mineral supplements

PoM Didronel® (Procter & Gamble Pharm.)
Tablets, disodium etidronate 200 mg. Net price 60-tab pack = £43.88. Counselling, food and calcium (see above)

PoM Didronel IV® (Procter & Gamble Pharm.)
Injection, disodium etidronate 50 mg/mL. For dilution and use as an infusion. Net price 6-mL amp = £9.53

With calcium carbonate
For cautions and side-effects of calcium carbonate see section 9.5.1.1

PoM Didronel PMO® (Procter & Gamble Pharm.)
Tablets, 14 white, disodium etidronate 400 mg; 76 pink, effervescent, calcium carbonate 1.25 g (Cacit®). Net price per pack = £40.20. Label: 10 patient information leaflet, counselling, food and calcium (see above)
Dose: established vertebral osteoporosis (90-day cycles) 1 etidronate daily for 14 days, then 1 calcium daily for 76 days; recommended duration of therapy, 3 years

DISODIUM PAMIDRONATE
Disodium pamidronate was formerly called aminohydroxy-propylidenediphosphonate disodium (APD)
Indications: hypercalcaemia of malignancy
Cautions: renal impairment (divide daily dose if severe); possibility of convulsions due to electrolyte disturbances; **interactions:** Appendix 1 (bis-phosphonates)
Contra-indications: pregnancy and breast-feeding
Side-effects: nausea, diarrhoea; asymptomatic hypocalcaemia; transient rise in body temperature; occasional lymphocytopenia and hypo-magnesaemia
Dose: by slow intravenous infusion, according to plasma calcium concentration 15–60 mg in single infusion or in divided doses over 2–4 days; max. 90 mg per treatment course (see Appendix 6)

PoM Aredia® (Ciba)
Injection, powder for reconstitution, disodium pamidronate, for use as an infusion. Net price 15-mg vial = £25.97; 30-mg vial = £51.94 (both with diluent)

SODIUM CLODRONATE
Indications: see under Dose
Cautions: monitor renal and hepatic function and white cell count; renal dysfunction reported in patients receiving concomitant NSAIDs; maintain adequate fluid intake during treatment; **interactions:** Appendix 1 (bisphosphonates)
Contra-indications: moderate to severe renal impairment; pregnancy and breast-feeding
Side-effects: nausea, diarrhoea; asymptomatic hypocalcaemia; skin reactions
Dose: oestolytic lesions, hypercalcaemia and bone pain associated with skeletal metastases in patients with breast cancer or multiple myeloma, *by mouth*, 1.6 g daily in single or 2 divided doses increased if necessary to a max. of 3.2 g daily

COUNSELLING. Avoid food for 1 hour before and after treatment, particularly calcium-containing products e.g. milk; also avoid iron and mineral supplements and maintain adequate fluid intake

Hypercalcaemia of malignancy, *by slow intravenous infusion*, 300 mg daily for max. 7–10 days *or* by single-dose infusion (Bonefos® only) of 1.5 g over 4-hour period

PoM Bonefos® (Boehringer Ingelheim)
Capsules, yellow, sodium clodronate 400 mg. Net price 30-cap pack = £45.59, 112-cap pack = £170.24, 120-cap pack = £182.39. Counselling, food and calcium
Concentrate (= intravenous solution), sodium clodronate 60 mg/mL, for dilution and use as infusion. Net price 5-mL amp = £14.43

PoM Loron® (Boehringer Mannheim)
Loron® capsules, sodium clodronate 400 mg. Net price 120-cap pack = £202.65. Label: 10 patient information leaflet, counselling, food and calcium
Loron 520® tablets, f/c, scored, sodium clodronate 520 mg. Net price 60-tab pack = £182.39. Label: 10 patient information leaflet, counselling, food and calcium
Dose: 2 tablets daily in single or two divided doses; may be increased to max. 4 tablets daily
Note. Due to greater bioavailability one *Loron 520®* tablet (520 mg) is equivalent to two *Loron* capsules (2 × 400 mg)

PoM Loron® for infusion (Boehringer Mannheim)
Intravenous solution, sodium clodronate 30 mg/mL, for dilution and use as infusion. Net price 10-mL amp = £14.43

6.7   Other endocrine drugs

This section includes:

6.7.1   Bromocriptine and cabergoline
6.7.2   Danazol, gestrinone, and gonadorelin analogues
6.7.3   Metyrapone and trilostane

6.7.1   Bromocriptine and cabergoline

Bromocriptine is a stimulant of dopamine receptors in the brain; it also inhibits release of prolactin by the pituitary. Bromocriptine is used for the treatment of galactorrhoea and cyclical benign breast disease, and for the treatment of prolactinomas (when it reduces both plasma prolactin concentration and tumour size). Bromocriptine also inhibits the release of growth hormone and is sometimes used in the treatment of acromegaly, the success rate is much lower than with prolactinomas.

Cabergoline has been introduced recently; it has actions and uses similar to those of bromocriptine, but its duration of action is longer. Its profile of side-effects appears to differ from that of bromocriptine, which means that patients intolerant of bromocriptine may be able to tolerate cabergoline (and *vice versa*).

Bromocriptine and cabergoline suppress lactation, but are not recommended for routine suppression (or for the relief of symptoms of postpartum pain and engorgement) that can be adequately treated with simple analgesics and breast support.

BROMOCRIPTINE

Indications: see notes above and under Dose; parkinsonism, see section 4.9.1

Cautions: specialist evaluation—monitor for pituitary enlargement, particularly during pregnancy, annual gynaecological assessment (post-menopausal, every 6 months), monitor for peptic ulceration in acromegalic patients; contraceptive advice if appropriate (oral contraceptives may increase prolactin concentrations); caution in patients with history of serious mental disorders (especially psychotic disorders) or with cardiovascular disease or Raynaud's syndrome and monitor for retroperitoneal fibrosis; hepatic and renal impairment (see appendixes 2 and 3); porphyria (see section 9.8.2); **interactions:** Appendix 1 (bromocriptine)

HYPOTENSIVE REACTIONS. Hypotensive reactions may be disturbing in some patients during the first few days of treatment and particular care should be exercised when driving or operating machinery; tolerance may be reduced by alcohol

Contra-indications: hypersensitivity to bromocriptine or other ergot alkaloids; toxaemia of pregnancy and hypertension in postpartum women or in puerperium (see also below); advise women not to breast-feed if lactation prevention fails

POSTPARTUM OR PUERPERIUM. Should not be used postpartum or in puerperium in women with high blood pressure, coronary artery disease or symptoms (or history) of serious mental disorder; monitor blood pressure carefully (especially during first few days) in postpartum women. Very rarely hypertension, myocardial infarction, seizures or stroke (both sometimes preceded by severe headache) and mental disorders have been reported in postpartum women given bromocriptine for lactation suppression—caution with antihypertensive therapy and avoid other ergot alkaloids. Discontinue immediately if hypertension, unremitting headache or signs of CNS toxicity develop

Side-effects: nausea, vomiting, constipation, headache, dizziness, postural hypotension, drowsiness, vasospasm of fingers and toes particularly in patients with Raynaud's syndrome; *high doses,* confusion, psychomotor excitation, hallucinations, dyskinesia, dry mouth, leg cramps, pleural effusions (may necessitate withdrawal of treatment), retroperitoneal fibrosis reported (monitoring required)

Dose: prevention/suppression of lactation (but see notes above and under Contra-indications), 2.5 mg on 1st day (prevention) or daily for 2–3 days (suppression); then 2.5 mg twice daily for 14 days

Hypogonadism/galactorrhoea, infertility, initially 1–1.25 mg at bedtime, increased gradually; usual dose 7.5 mg daily in divided doses, increased if necessary to a max. of 30 mg daily. Usual dose in infertility without hyperprolactinaemia, 2.5 mg twice daily

Cyclical benign breast disease and cyclical menstrual disorders (particularly breast pain), 1–1.25 mg at bedtime, increased gradually; usual dose 2.5 mg twice daily

Acromegaly, initially 1–1.25 mg at bedtime, increase gradually to 5 mg every 6 hours

Prolactinoma, initially 1–1.25 mg at bedtime; increased gradually to 5 mg every 6 hours (occasional patients may require up to 30 mg daily)

CHILD under 15, not recommended

PoM Bromocriptine (Non-proprietary)
Tablets, bromocriptine (as mesylate), 2.5 mg, net price 30-tab pack = £5.28. Label: 21, counselling, hypotensive reactions
Available from APS, Berk, Cox, K Pharm., Norton

PoM Parlodel® (Sandoz)
Tablets, both scored, bromocriptine (as mesylate) 1 mg, net price 100-tab pack = £9.05; 2.5 mg, 30-tab pack = £5.28. Label: 21, counselling, hypotensive reactions
Capsules, bromocriptine (as mesylate) 5 mg (blue/white), net price 100-cap pack = £34.34; 10 mg (white), 100-cap pack = £63.53. Label: 21, counselling, hypotensive reactions

CABERGOLINE

Indications: see notes above and under Dose

Cautions; Contra-indications; Side-effects: see under Bromocriptine (but profile of side-effects may differ, see notes above); palpitations, epigastric and abdominal pain, epistaxis and hemianopia, syncope, asthenia, hot flushes also reported; exclude pregnancy before starting and for at least 1 month after successful treatment (ovulatory cycles persist for 6 months) then monthly pregnancy tests; advise non-hormonal contraception if pregnancy not desired; discontinue if pregnancy occurs during treatment; **interactions:** Appendix 1 (cabergoline)

HYPOTENSIVE REACTIONS. Hypotensive reactions may be disturbing in some patients during the first few days of treatment and particular care should be exercised when driving or operating machinary; tolerance may be reduced by alcohol

Dose: prevention of lactation (but see notes above), during first day postpartum, 1 mg as a single dose; suppression of established lactation (but see notes above) 250 micrograms every 12 hours for 2 days

Hyperprolactinaemic disorders, 500 micrograms weekly (as a single dose or as 2 divided doses on separate days) increased at monthly intervals in steps of 500 micrograms until optimal therapeutic response (usually 1 mg weekly, range 0.25–2 mg weekly) with monthly monitoring of serum prolactin levels; reduce initial dose and increase more gradually if patient intolerant; over 1 mg weekly give as divided doses; up to 4.5 mg weekly has been used in hyperprolactinaemic patients CHILD under 16, not recommended

▼ **PoM Dostinex®** (Farmitalia Carlo Erba)
Tablets, scored, cabergoline 500 micrograms. Net price 8-tab pack = £31.46. Label: 21, counselling, hypotensive reactions

6.7.2   Danazol, gestrinone and gonadorelin analogues

Danazol inhibits pituitary gonadotrophins; it combines androgenic activity with antioestrogenic and antiprogestogenic activity. It is used in the treatment of *endometriosis* and has also been used for *menorrhagia* and other *menstrual disorders*, *mammary dysplasia*, and *gynaecomastia* where other measures proved unsatisfactory. It may also be effective in the long-term management of *hereditary angioedema* [unlicensed indication].

Gestrinone has general actions similar to those of danazol and is indicated for the treatment of endometriosis.

DANAZOL

Indications: see notes above and under Dose

Cautions: cardiac, hepatic, or renal impairment (avoid if severe), elderly, polycythaemia, epilepsy, diabetes mellitus, hypertension, migraine, lipoprotein disorder, history of thrombosis; withdraw if virilisation (may be irreversible on continued use); non-hormonal contraceptive methods should be used, if appropriate; **interactions:** Appendix 1 (danazol)

Contra-indications: pregnancy, ensure that patients with amenorrhoea are not pregnant; breast-feeding; severe hepatic, renal or cardiac impairment; thrombo-embolic disease; uninvestigated vaginal bleeding; androgen-dependent tumours; porphyria (see section 9.8.2)

Side-effects: nausea, dizziness, rashes, backache, nervousness, headache, weight gain; menstrual disturbances, flushing and reduction in breast size; skeletal muscle spasm, hair loss; androgenic effects including acne, oily skin, oedema, hirsutism, voice changes and rarely clitoral hypertrophy (see also Cautions); insulin resistance; leucopenia and thrombocytopenia reported; benign intracranial hypertension and visual disturbances also reported; rarely cholestatic jaundice

Dose: usual range 200–800 mg daily in up to 4 divided doses; in women all doses should start during menstruation, preferably on the first day

Endometriosis, initially 400 mg daily in up to 4 divided doses, adjusted according to response, usually for 6 months

Menorrhagia, 200 mg daily, usually for 3 months

Severe cyclical mastalgia, 200–300 mg daily usually for 3–6 months

Benign breast cysts, 300 mg daily usually for 3–6 months

Gynaecomastia, 400 mg daily in divided doses for 6 months (adolescents 200 mg daily, increased to 400 mg daily if no response after 2 months)

For pre-operative thinning of endometrium, 400–800 mg daily for 3–6 weeks

PoM Danazol (Non-proprietary)
Capsules, danazol 100 mg, net price 20 = £5.53; 200 mg, 20 = £11.02

Available from APS, Cox, Generics, Hillcross, Norton

PoM Danol® (Sanofi Winthrop)
Capsules, danazol 100 mg (grey/white), net price 100-cap pack = £29.74; 200 mg (pink/white), 56-cap pack = £32.98

GESTRINONE

Indications: endometriosis

Cautions; Contra-indications; Side-effects: see under Danazol; **Interactions:** Appendix 1 (gestrinone)

Dose: 2.5 mg twice weekly starting on first day of cycle with second dose 3 days later, repeated on same two days preferably at same time each week; duration of treatment usually 6 months

MISSED DOSES. one missed dose — 2.5 mg as soon as possible and maintain original sequence; two or more missed doses — discontinue, re-start on first day of new cycle (following negative pregnancy test)

PoM Dimetriose® (Roussel)
Capsules, gestrinone 2.5 mg, net price 8-cap pack = £73.12

GONADORELIN ANALOGUES

Gonadorelin analogues, after an initial stimulation phase, down-regulate pituitary gonadotrophin secretion, leading to inhibition of ovarian steroid secretion and are thus effective in the treatment of *endometriosis*

BUSERELIN

Indications: see under Dose; prostate cancer, see section 8.3.4

Contra-indications: pregnancy (use non-hormonal method of contraception), breast-feeding; undiag-nosed vaginal bleeding

Side-effects: initially menstrual-like and subsequently breakthrough bleeding, menopause-like symptoms including hot flushes, palpitations, increased sweating, vaginal dryness and change in libido; headache or migraine, nausea, mood changes including depression, changes in breast size, breast tenderness, abdominal pain, fatigue, weight changes, nervousness, dizziness, drowsiness, acne, dry skin, back pain; muscle pain; ovarian cysts (may require withdrawal); decrease in trabecular bone density (repeat courses not recommended); urticaria, rash and pruritus, constipation, vomiting, sleep disorders, leucorrhoea, paraesthesia or sensitivity of extremities, blurred vision, and changes in body hair also reported; irritation of nasal mucosa (spray formulations only)

Dose: endometriosis, 300 micrograms (one 150-microgram spray in each nostril) 3 times daily starting on 1st or 2nd day of menstruation; max. duration of treatment 6 months (do not repeat)

Pituitary densensitisation before induction of ovulation by gonadotrophins for *in vitro* fertilisation (under specialist supervision), 150 micrograms (one spray in one nostril) 4 times daily starting in early follicular phase (day 1) *or*, after exclusion of pregnancy, in midluteal phase (day 21) and continued until down-regulation achieved (usually about 2–3 weeks) then maintained for few more days during gonadotrophin administration (stopping on administration of chorionic gonadotrophin at follicular maturity)

COUNSELLING. Avoid use of nasal decongestants before and for at least 30 minutes after treatment.

PoM Suprecur® (Hoechst)
Nasal spray, buserelin 150 micrograms (as acetate)/metered spray. Net price 2 × 100-dose pack (with metered dose pumps) = £78.98. Counselling, see above

GOSERELIN

Indications: endometriosis; prostate cancer and advanced breast cancer, see section 8.3.4

Cautions; Contra-indications; Side-effects: see under Buserelin; also bruising at injection site

Dose: by subcutaneous injection into anterior abdominal wall, 3.6 mg every 28 days; max. duration of treatment 6 months (do not repeat)

Preparations
See section 8.3.4

LEUPRORELIN ACETATE

Indications: endometriosis; prostate cancer, see section 8.3.4

Cautions; Contra-indications; Side-effects: see under Buserelin; also irritation at injection site, rotate injection site periodically

Dose: by subcutaneous or by intramuscular injection, 3.75 mg every 4 weeks, starting during the first 5 days of menstrual cycle; max. duration of treatment 6 months (do not repeat)

Preparations
See section 8.3.4

NAFARELIN

Indications: see under Dose

Cautions; Contra-indications; Side-effects: see under Buserelin

Dose: women over 18 years, endometriosis, 200 micrograms twice daily as one spray in one nostril in the morning and one spray in the other nostril in the evening starting between 2nd and 4th day of menstrual cycle, max. duration of treatment 6 months (do not repeat)

Pituitary desensitisation before induction of ovulation by gonadotrophins for *in vitro* fertilisation (under specialist supervision), 400 micrograms (one spray in each nostril) twice daily starting in early follicular phase (day 2) or, after exclusion of pregnancy, in midluteal phase (day 21) and continued until down-regulation achieved (usually within 4 weeks) then maintained for few more days during gonadotrophin administration (stopping on administration of chorionic gonadotrophin at follicular maturity); discontinue if down-regulation not achieved within 12 weeks

COUNSELLING. Avoid use of nasal decongestants before and for at least 30 minutes after treatment; repeat dose if sneezing occurs during or immediately after administration

PoM Synarel® (Syntex)
Nasal spray, nafarelin 200 micrograms (as acetate)/metered spray. Net price 30-dose unit = £30.74; 60-dose unit = £53.00. Label: 10 patient information leaflet, counselling, see above

BREAST PAIN (MASTALGIA)

Once any serious underlying cause has been ruled out, most women will respond to reassurance and reduction in dietary fat; withdrawal of an oral contraceptive or of hormone replacement therapy may help resolve the pain.

Women whose symptoms persist for longer than 6 months may require drug treatment. Danazol is the most effective but may be unacceptable owing to its unpleasant side-effects (which occur in about one-third of patients). Bromocriptine (section 6.7.1) like danazol is associated with unpleasant side-effects. Gamolenic acid (section 13.5) can be useful and, with its lack of antioestrogenic side-effects, may be preferred particularly in younger women who wish to continue taking an oral contraceptive; whereas bromocriptine and danazol act within 2 months, gamolenic acid may require 8–12 weeks to take effect.

Symptoms recur in about 50% of women within 2 years of withdrawal of therapy but may be less severe.

6.7.3   Metyrapone and trilostane

Metyrapone is a competitive inhibitor of 11β-hydroxylation in the adrenal cortex; the resulting inhibition of cortisol (and to a lesser extent aldosterone) production leads to an increase in ACTH production which, in turn, leads to increased synthesis and release of cortisol precursors. It may be used as a test of anterior pituitary function.

Although most types of *Cushing's syndrome* are treated surgically, that which occasionally accompanies carcinoma of the bronchus is not usually amenable to surgery. Metyrapone has been found helpful in controlling the symptoms of the disease; it is also used in other forms of Cushing's syndrome to prepare the patient for surgery. The dosages used are either low, and tailored to cortisol production, or high, in which case corticosteroid replacement therapy is also needed.

Trilostane reversibly inhibits 3β-hydroxysteroid dehydrogenase /delta 5-4 isomerase in the adrenal cortex; the resulting inhibition of the synthesis of mineralocorticoids and glucocorticoids may be useful in *Cushing's syndrome* and *primary hyperaldosteronism*. Trilostane appears to be less effective than metyrapone for Cushing's syndrome (where it is tailored to corticosteroid production). It also has a minor role in post-menopausal breast cancer that has relapsed following initial oestrogen antagonist therapy (corticosteroid replacement therapy is also required).

See also aminoglutethimide (section 8.3.4)

METYRAPONE

Indications: see notes above and under Dose (specialist supervision)

Cautions: gross hypopituitarism (risk of precipitating acute adrenal failure); many drugs interfere with estimation of steroids

Contra-indications: adrenocortical insufficiency (see Cautions); pregnancy, breast-feeding

Side-effects: occasional nausea, vomiting, dizziness, headache, hypotension, allergy

Dose: differential diagnosis of ACTH-dependent Cushing's syndrome, 750 mg every 4 hours for 6 doses; CHILD 15 mg/kg (minimum 250 mg) every 4 hours for 6 doses

Management of Cushing's syndrome, range 0.25–6 g daily, tailored to cortisol production; see notes above

Resistant oedema due to increased aldosterone secretion in cirrhosis, nephrosis, and congestive heart failure (with glucocorticoid replacement therapy), 2.5–4.5 g daily in divided doses

PoM Metopirone® (Ciba)
Capsules, metyrapone 250 mg. Net price 20 = £4.18.
Label: 21

TRILOSTANE

Indications: see notes above and under Dose (specialist supervision)

Cautions: breast cancer (concurrent corticosteroid replacement therapy needed, see under Dose); adrenal cortical hyperfunction (tailored to cortisol and electrolytes, concurrent corticosteroid therapy may be needed, see under Dose); hepatic and renal impairment; **interactions:** Appendix 1 (trilostane)

Contra-indications: pregnancy (use non-hormonal method of contraception) and breast-feeding; children

Side-effects: flushing, tingling and swelling of mouth, rhinorrhoea, nausea, vomiting, diarrhoea, and rashes reported; rarely granulocytopenia

Dose: adrenal cortical hyperfunction, 240 mg daily in divided doses for at least 3 days then tailored according to response with regular monitoring of plasma electrolytes and circulating corticosteroids (both mineralocorticoid and glucocorticoid replacement therapy may be needed); usual dose: 120–480 mg daily (may be increased to 960 mg)

Postmenopausal breast cancer (with glucocorticoid replacement therapy) following relapse to initial oestrogen receptor antagonist therapy, initially 240 mg daily increased every 3 days in steps of 240 mg to a maintenance dose of 960 mg daily (720 mg daily if not tolerated)

PoM Modrenal® (Wanskerne)
Capsules, trilostane 60 mg (pink/black), net price 100-cap pack = £39.60; 120 mg (pink/yellow), 100-cap pack = £79.20. Label: 21

7: Drugs used in
OBSTETRICS, GYNAECOLOGY, and URINARY-TRACT DISORDERS

In this chapter, drugs are discussed under the following headings:

7.1 Drugs used in obstetrics
7.2 Treatment of vaginal and vulval conditions
7.3 Contraceptives
7.4 Drugs for genito-urinary disorders

For hormonal therapy of gynaecological disorders see sections 6.4.1, 6.5.1 and 6.7.2.

7.1 Drugs used in obstetrics

7.1.1 Prostaglandins and oxytocics
7.1.2 Mifepristone
7.1.3 Myometrial relaxants

Note. Because of the complexity of dosage regimens in obstetrics, in all cases **detailed specialist literature** should be consulted.

7.1.1 Prostaglandins and oxytocics

Prostaglandins and oxytocics are used to induce abortion or induce or augment labour and to minimise blood loss from the placental site. They include oxytocin, ergometrine, and the prostaglandins. All induce uterine contractions with varying degrees of pain according to the strength of contractions induced.

INDUCTION OF ABORTION. **Gemeprost**, administered vaginally, and **dinoprostone**, given by the extra-amniotic route, are the preferred prostaglandins for the *medical induction of late therapeutic abortion*. Gemeprost is a prostaglandin available in the form of pessaries to ripen and soften the cervix *before surgical abortion*, particularly in primigravida. Extra-amniotic **dinoprostone** is also of value as an adjunct in 'priming' the cervix prior to *suction termination* but is rarely used nowadays.

INDUCTION AND AUGMENTATION OF LABOUR. **Oxytocin** (*Syntocinon®*) is administered by slow intravenous infusion, preferably using an infusion pump, to *induce or augment labour*, usually in conjunction with amniotomy. Uterine activity must be monitored carefully and hyperstimulation avoided. Large doses of oxytocin may result in excessive fluid retention.

Dinoprostone is available as vaginal tablets and vaginal gels for the *induction of labour*. The intravenous and oral routes are rarely used.

PREVENTION AND TREATMENT OF HAEMORRHAGE. Bleeding due to *incomplete abortion* can be controlled with **ergometrine** and **oxytocin** (*Syntometrine®*) given intramuscularly, the dose being adjusted according to the patient's condition and blood loss. This is commonly used prior to surgical evacuation of the uterus, particularly when surgery is delayed. Oxytocin and ergometrine combined are more effective in early pregnancy than either drug alone.

For the routine management of the *third stage of labour* ergometrine 500 micrograms with oxytocin 5 units (*Syntometrine®* 1 mL) is given by intramuscular injection with or after delivery of the shoulders. For the prevention of postpartum haemorrhage in *high-risk cases*, intravenous injection of *either* ergometrine 125–250 micrograms alone *or* oxytocin 5–10 units is recommended, after delivery of the shoulders (repeated if necessary); alternatively intravenous infusion of oxytocin 10–20 units/500 mL can be given after delivery of the shoulders, particularly when the uterus is *atonic*. The use of **carboprost** now has an important role for severe events.

In domiciliary obstetric practice small secondary postpartum haemorrhage may be treated with **ergometrine** by mouth in a dose of 500 micrograms three times daily for 3 days.

CARBOPROST

Indications: postpartum haemorrhage due to uterine atony in patients unresponsive to ergometrine and oxytocin

Cautions: history of glaucoma or raised intra-ocular pressure, asthma, hypertension, hypotension, anaemia, jaundice, diabetes, epilepsy; uterine scars; excessive dosage may cause uterine rupture

Contra-indications: acute pelvic inflammatory disease, cardiac, renal, pulmonary, or hepatic disease

Side-effects: nausea, vomiting and diarrhoea, hyperthermia and flushing, bronchospasm; less frequent effects include raised blood pressure, dyspnoea, and pulmonary oedema; chills, headache, diaphoresis, dizziness, and erythema and pain at injection site also reported

Dose: by deep intramuscular injection, 250 micrograms repeated if necessary at intervals of 1½ hours (in severe cases the interval may be reduced but should not be less than 15 minutes); total dose should not exceed 2 mg (8 doses)

PoM **Hemabate®** (Upjohn)

Injection, carboprost as trometamol salt (tromethamine salt) 250 micrograms/mL, net price 1-mL amp = £16.50 (hosp. only)

DINOPROSTONE

Indications: see notes above

Cautions: asthma, glaucoma and raised intra-ocular pressure; excessive dosage may cause uterine rupture; continuous administration for more than 2 days not recommended; see also notes above

Contra-indications: hypertonic uterine inertia, mechanical obstruction of delivery, placenta praevia, predisposition to uterine rupture, severe toxaemia, untreated pelvic infection, fetal distress, grand multiparas and multiple pregnancy, prior history of difficult or traumatic delivery; avoid extra-amniotic route in cervicitis or vaginitis

Side-effects: nausea, vomiting, diarrhoea, flushing, shivering, headache, dizziness, temporary pyrexia and raised white blood cell count, uterine hypertonus, unduly severe uterine contractions; all dose-related and more common after intravenous administration; also local tissue reaction and erythema after intravenous administration

Dose: see under Preparations, below

IMPORTANT. Do not confuse dose of **Prostin E2**® vaginal **gel** with that of **Prostin E2**® vaginal **tablets**—not bioequivalent. In addition, do not confuse **Prostin E2**® vaginal gel with **Prepidil**® cervical gel—different site of administration and different indication—see under Preparations, below

PoM **Prepidil**® (Upjohn)

Cervical gel, dinoprostone 200 micrograms/mL in disposable syringe. Net price 2.5-mL syringe (500 micrograms) = £14.12

Dose: by cervix, pre-induction cervical softening and dilation, inserted into cervical canal (just below level of internal cervical os), 500 micrograms [single dose gel]

PoM **Prostin E2**® (Upjohn)

Tablets, dinoprostone 500 micrograms. Net price 10-tab pack = £14.93 (hosp. only)

Dose: by mouth, induction of labour, 500 micrograms, followed by 0.5–1 mg (max. 1.5 mg) at hourly intervals

Intravenous solution, for dilution and use as an infusion, dinoprostone 1 mg/mL, net price 0.75-mL amp = £13.10; 10 mg/mL, 0.5-mL amp = £16.05 (both hosp. only; rarely used, see data sheet for dose and indications)

Extra-amniotic solution, dinoprostone 10 mg/mL. Net price 0.5-mL amp (with diluent) = £16.05 (hosp. only; less commonly used nowadays, see data sheet for dose and indications)

Vaginal gel, dinoprostone 400 micrograms/mL, net price 2.5 mL (1 mg) = £14.52; 800 micrograms/mL, 2.5 mL (2 mg) = £16.00

Dose: by vagina, induction of labour, inserted high into posterior fornix (avoid administration into cervical canal), 1 mg (unfavourable primigravida 2 mg), followed after 6 hours by 1–2 mg if required; max. [gel] 3 mg (unfavourable primigravida 4 mg)

Vaginal tablets, dinoprostone 3 mg. Net price 8-vaginal tab pack = £65.04

Dose: by vagina, induction of labour, inserted high into posterior fornix, 3 mg, followed after 6–8 hours by 3 mg if labour is not established; max. 6 mg [vaginal tablets]

Note. Prostin E2 Vaginal Gel and Vaginal Tablets are **not** bioequivalent

DINOPROST

Indications: see notes above

Cautions; Contra-indications; Side-effects: see under Dinoprostone and notes above

PoM **Prostin F2 alpha**® (Upjohn)

Intra-amniotic injection, dinoprost 5 mg (as trometamol salt)/mL. Net price 4-mL amp = £19.71 (hosp. only; rarely used, see data sheet for dose and indications)

ERGOMETRINE MALEATE

Indications: see notes above

Cautions: cardiac disease, hypertension, hepatic, and renal impairment, multiple pregnancy; porphyria (see section 9.8.2)

Contra-indications: induction of labour, 1st and 2nd stages of labour, vascular disease, severe cardiac disease, impaired pulmonary function, severe hepatic and renal impairment, sepsis, severe hypertension, eclampsia

Side-effects: nausea, vomiting, headache, dizziness, tinnitus, abdominal pain, chest pain, palpitation, dyspnoea, bradycardia, transient hypertension, vasoconstriction; stroke, myocardial infarction and pulmonary oedema also reported

Dose: see notes above

PoM **Ergometrine Tablets,** ergometrine maleate 500 micrograms. Net price 20 = £5.90

Available from Evans

PoM **Ergometrine Injection,** ergometrine maleate 500 micrograms/mL. Net price 1-mL amp = 29p

With oxytocin

PoM **Syntometrine**® (Sandoz)

Injection, ergometrine maleate 500 micrograms, oxytocin 5 units/mL. Net price 1-mL amp = 18p

Dose: by intramuscular injection, 1 mL; by intravenous injection, no longer recommended

GEMEPROST

Indications: see under Dose

Cautions: obstructive airways disease, cardiovascular insufficiency, raised intra-ocular pressure, cervicitis or vaginitis

IMPORTANT. For warnings relating to use of gemeprost in a patient undergoing termination with mifepristone, see under Mifepristone

Contra-indications: hypersensitivity to gemeprost or other prostaglandins

Side-effects: vaginal bleeding and uterine pain; nausea, vomiting, or diarrhoea; headache, muscle weakness, dizziness, flushing, chills, backache, dyspnoea, chest pain, palpitations and mild pyrexia; uterine rupture reported (most commonly in multiparas or if history of uterine surgery or if given with intravenous oxytocics)

Dose: by vagina in pessaries, softening and dilation of the cervix to facilitate transcervical operative procedures in first trimester, inserted into posterior fornix, 1 mg 3 hours before surgery

Second trimester abortion, inserted into posterior fornix, 1 mg every 3 hours for max. of 5 administrations; second course may begin 24 hours after start of treatment (if treatment fails pregnancy should be terminated by another method)

Second trimester intra-uterine death, inserted into posterior fornix, 1 mg every 3 hours for max. of 5 administrations only; monitor for coagulopathy

PoM Gemeprost (Farillon)
Pessaries, gemeprost 1 mg. Net price 5-pessary pack = £112.67

OXYTOCIN

Indications: see under Dose and notes above
Cautions: hypertension, cardiovascular disorders (special need to keep infusion volume low), abnormal presentation, multiple pregnancy, high parity, previous Caesarean section; effects enhanced by concomitant prostaglandins; pressor drugs may precipitate severe hypertension
Contra-indications: hypertonic uterine action, mechanical obstruction to delivery, failed trial labour, severe toxaemia, predisposition to amniotic fluid embolism, fetal distress, and placenta praevia
Side-effects: high doses cause violent uterine contractions leading to rupture and fetal asphyxiation, arrhythmias, maternal hypertension and subarachnoid haemorrhage, water intoxication and risk of pulmonary oedema (keep infusion volume low, see also Cautions above)
Dose: by slow intravenous infusion, induction of labour and augmentation of labour in hypotonic uterine inertia, as a solution containing 1 unit per litre, 1–3 milliunits per minute, adjusted according to response

Missed abortion, as a solution containing 10–20 units/500 mL given at a rate of 10–30 drops/minute, increased in strength by 10–20 units/500 mL every hour to a max. strength of 100 units/500 mL

PoM Syntocinon® (Sandoz)
Injection, oxytocin 1 unit/mL, net price 2-mL amp = 17p; 5 units/mL, 1-mL amp = 20p; 10 units/mL, 1-mL amp = 22p, 5-mL amp = 82p
With ergometrine, see Syntometrine®, p 306

7.1.1.1 DUCTUS ARTERIOSUS

MAINTENANCE OF PATENCY
Alprostadil (prostaglandin E$_1$) is used to maintain patency of the ductus arteriosus in neonates with congenital heart defects, prior to corrective surgery in centres where intensive care is immediately available.

ALPROSTADIL

Indications: congenital heart defects in neonates prior to corrective surgery; erectile dysfunction, see section 7.4.5
Cautions: see notes above; history of haemorrhage, avoid in hyaline membrane disease, monitor arterial pressure
Side-effects: apnoea (particularly in infants under 2 kg), flushing, bradycardia, hypotension, tachycardia, cardiac arrest, oedema, diarrhoea, fever, convulsions, disseminated intravascular coagulation, hypokalaemia; cortical

proliferation of long bones, weakening of the wall of the ductus arteriosus and pulmonary artery may follow prolonged use; gastric-outlet obstruction reported
Dose: by intravenous infusion, initially 50–100 nanograms/kg/minute, then decreased to lowest effective dose

PoM Prostin VR® (Upjohn)
Intravenous solution, alprostadil 500 micrograms/mL in alcohol. For dilution and use as an infusion. Net price 1-mL amp = £62.66 (hosp. only)

CLOSURE OF DUCTUS ARTERIOSUS
Prostaglandin E$_1$ has the role of dilating the ductus arteriosus; **indomethacin** is believed to close it by inhibiting prostaglandin synthesis.

INDOMETHACIN
(Indometacin)
Indications: patent ductus arteriosus in premature infants (under specialist supervision)
Cautions: may mask symptoms of infection; may reduce urine output by 50% or more and precipitate renal insufficiency especially in infants with heart failure, sepsis, or hepatic impairment, or who are receiving nephrotoxic drugs; if urine volume reduced, discontinue until output returns to normal; may induce hyponatraemia; monitor renal function and electrolytes
Contra-indications: untreated infection, bleeding, congenital heart disease where patency of ductus arteriosus necessary for satisfactory pulmonary or systemic blood flow; thrombocytopenia, coagulation defects, necrotising enterocolitis, renal impairment
Side-effects: include haemorrhagic, renal, gastro-intestinal, metabolic, and coagulation disorders; pulmonary hypertension, fluid retention, and exacerbation of infection
Dose: by intravenous injection, over 5–10 seconds, 3 doses at intervals of 12–24 hours, age less than 48 hours, 200 micrograms/kg then 100 micrograms/kg then 100 micrograms/kg; age 2–7 days, 200 micrograms/kg then 200 micrograms/kg then 200 micrograms/kg; age over 7 days, 200 micrograms/kg then 250 micrograms/kg then 250 micrograms/kg; solution prepared with 1–2 mL sodium chloride 0.9% or water for injections (not glucose and no preservatives)
If ductus arteriosus reopens a second course of 3 injections may be given

PoM Indocid PDA® (Morson)
Injection, powder for reconstitution, indomethacin (as sodium trihydrate). Net price 3 × 1-mg vials = £22.50 (hosp. only)

7.1.2   Mifepristone

MIFEPRISTONE
Indications: medical alternative to surgical termination of intra-uterine pregnancy of up to 63 days gestation (based on first day of last menstrual period and/or ultrasound scan)
Cautions: asthma, chronic obstructive airways disease; cardiovascular disease or risk factors; prosthetic heart valves or history of infective endocarditis (prophylaxis recommended, see section 5.1 table 2); not recommended in hepatic or renal impairment; avoid aspirin and NSAIDs for at least 8–12 days after mifepristone administration

Contra-indications: pregnancy of 64 days gestation and over, suspected ectopic pregnancy; chronic adrenal failure, long-term corticosteroid therapy, haemorrhagic disorders and anticoagulant therapy; smokers over 35 years of age (smoking and alcohol must be avoided after taking and for at least 2 days after the gemeprost pessary); porphyria (see section 9.8.2)

Side-effects: vaginal bleeding (may be severe), malaise, faintness, nausea, vomiting, rashes; uterine pain after gemeprost (may be severe and require parenteral opioids); uterine and urinary-tract infections reported

Dose: by mouth, 600 mg in a single dose in presence of doctor and observed for at least 2 hours after administration; followed 36–48 hours later (unless abortion already complete) by gemeprost 1 mg by vagina as pessaries, observed for at least 6 hours after insertion with follow-up visit 8–12 days later (if treatment fails essential that pregnancy be terminated by another method)

Note. Careful monitoring essential for 6 hours after administration of gemeprost pessary (risk of profound hypotension)

▼ PoM **Mifegyne**® (Roussel)

Tablets, yellow, mifepristone 200 mg. Net price 3-tab pack = £41.83 (supplied to NHS hospitals and premises approved under Abortion Act 1967). Label: 10 patient information leaflet

7.1.3   Myometrial relaxants

Beta$_2$-adrenoceptor stimulants (beta$_2$-sympathomimetics) relax uterine muscle and are used in selected cases in an attempt to inhibit *premature delivery.*

Their main purpose is to permit a delay in delivery of at least 48 hours; no statistically significant effect on perinatal mortality has as yet been observed. The greatest benefit is gained by using the delay to administer corticosteroid therapy or to implement other measures known to improve perinatal health. They are indicated for the inhibition of *uncomplicated* premature labour *between 24 and 33 weeks* of gestation. After successful parenteral therapy oral therapy may be used for maintenance (but **not** initially).

RITODRINE HYDROCHLORIDE

Indications: uncomplicated premature labour (see notes above)

Cautions: suspected cardiac disease (physician experienced in cardiology to assess), hypertension, hyperthyroidism, hypokalaemia (special risk with potassium-depleting diuretics), diabetes mellitus (closely monitor blood glucose during intravenous treatment); mild to moderate pre-eclampsia (avoid if severe—see Contra-indications), monitor blood pressure and pulse rate (should not exceed 135–140 beats per minute) and avoid over hydration (see Appendix 6); **important:** pulmonary oedema—closely monitor state of hydration (discontinue immediately and institute diuretic therapy if pulmonary oedema occurs); beta-blockers (effect antagonised—may be used to reverse increased tendency to uterine bleeding following Caesarean section); drugs likely to enhance sympathomimetic side-effects or

induce arrhythmias, see also **interactions**, Appendix 1 (sympathomimetics *and* sympathomimetics, beta$_2$)

Contra-indications: cardiac disease, eclampsia and severe pre-eclampsia, intra-uterine infection, intra-uterine fetal death, antepartum haemorrhage (requires immediate delivery), placenta praevia, cord compression; not for use in first or second trimesters

Side-effects: nausea, vomiting, flushing, sweating, tremor; hypokalaemia, tachycardia, palpitations, and hypotension (left lateral position throughout infusion to minimise risk), increased tendency to uterine bleeding (see Cautions); pulmonary oedema (see below and under Cautions); chest pain or tightness (with or without ECG changes) and arrhythmias reported; salivary gland enlargement also reported; on prolonged administration (several weeks) leucopenia reported

Dose: by intravenous infusion (**important:** minimum fluid volume, see below), premature labour, initially 50 micrograms/minute, gradually increased to 150–350 micrograms/minute and continued for 12–48 hours after contractions have ceased; or by intramuscular injection, 10 mg every 3–8 hours continued for 12–48 hours after contractions have ceased; then by mouth, 10 mg 30 minutes before termination of intravenous infusion, repeated every 2 hours for 24 hours, followed by 10–20 mg every 4–6 hours, max.oral dose 120 mg daily

IMPORTANT. The company has issued a reminder that although *fatal pulmonary oedema* associated with ritodrine infusion is almost certainly multifactorial in origin the balance of evidence suggests that **fluid overload** is the most important single factor. The volume of infusion fluid administered should therefore be kept to a minimum (normally using dextrose 5% as the diluent), for further guidance see appendix 6. For specific guidance on infusion rates to achieve the required dose, see data sheet

PoM **Yutopar**® (Duphar)

Tablets, scored, yellow, ritodrine hydrochloride 10 mg. Net price 90-tab pack = £19.80

Injection, ritodrine hydrochloride 10 mg/mL. Net price 5-mL amp = £2.15

SALBUTAMOL

Indications: uncomplicated premature labour (see notes above); asthma, see section 3.1.1

Cautions; Contra-indications; Side-effects: see under Ritodrine Hydrochloride

Dose: by intravenous infusion, 10 micrograms/minute gradually increased to max. of 45 micrograms/minute until contractions have ceased, then gradually reduced; or by intravenous or intramuscular injection, 100–250 micrograms repeated according to patient's response; subsequently by mouth 4 mg every 6–8 hours

Preparations, see section 3.1.1.1

TERBUTALINE SULPHATE

Indications: uncomplicated premature labour (see notes above); asthma, see section 3.1.1

Cautions; Contra-indications; Side-effects: see under Ritodrine Hydrochloride

Dose: by intravenous infusion, 5 micrograms/minute (as a 0.0005% solution) for 20 minutes, gradually increased to 10 micrograms/minute (max. of 20 micrograms/minute rarely needed) until contractions have ceased, then reduced; subsequently by subcutaneous injection, 250 micrograms every 6 hours for 3 days, and then by mouth, 5 mg every 8 hours until end of 36th week of pregnancy

Preparations, see section 3.1.1.1

7.2   Treatment of vaginal and vulval conditions

7.2.1   Preparations for vaginal atrophy
7.2.2   Anti-infective drugs

Symptoms are primarily referable to the vulva, but infections almost invariably involve the vagina which should also be treated. Applications to the vulva alone are likely to give only symptomatic relief without cure.

Aqueous medicated douches may disturb normal vaginal acidity and bacterial flora.

Topical anaesthetic agents give only symptomatic relief and may cause sensitivity reactions. They are indicated only in cases of pruritus where specific local causes have been excluded.

Systemic drugs are required in the treatment of infections such as gonorrhoea and syphilis (see section 5.1).

7.2.1   Preparations for vaginal atrophy

TOPICAL HRT

Application of cream containing an oestrogen may be used on a short-term basis to improve the quality of the vaginal epithelium in menopausal atrophic vaginitis. It is **important** to bear in mind that topical oestrogens should be used in the **minimum effective amount** and treatment discontinued as soon as possible to minimise absorption of the oestrogen. If they are used on a long-term basis, **oral progestogen** is needed for 10–14 days of each month to combat endometrial hyperplasia. For a general comment on HRT, including the role of topical oestrogens, see section 6.4.1.1.

Topical oestrogens are also used prior to vaginal surgery in postmenopausal women for prolapse when there is epithelial atrophy.

OESTROGENS, TOPICAL
Indications: see notes above.
Cautions; Contra-indications; Side-effects: see Oestrogen for HRT (section 6.4.1.1); contra-indicated in pregnancy and lactation; discontinue treatment and examine patients periodically to assess need for further treatment

PoM Ortho® Dienoestrol (Cilag)
Cream, dienoestrol 0.01%. Net price 78 g with applicator = £2.61
Condoms: damages latex condoms and diaphragms
Insert 1–2 applicatorfuls daily for 1–2 weeks, then gradually reduced to 1 applicatorful 1–3 times weekly if necessary; attempts to reduce or discontinue should be made at 3–6 month intervals with re-examination

PoM Ortho-Gynest® (Cilag)
Intravaginal cream, oestriol 0.01%. Net price 78 g with applicator = £5.40
Condoms: damages latex condoms and diaphragms
Insert 1 applicatorful daily, preferably in evening; reduced to 1 applicatorful twice a week; attempts to reduce or discontinue should be made at 3–6 month intervals with re-examination

Pessaries, oestriol 500 micrograms. Net price 15 pessaries = £5.29
Condoms: damages latex condoms and diaphragms
Insert 1 pessary daily, preferably in the evening, until improvement occurs; maintenance 1 pessary twice a week; attempts to reduce or discontinue should be made at 3–6 month intervals with re-examination

PoM Ovestin® (Organon)
Intravaginal cream, oestriol 0.1%. Net price 15 g with applicator = £4.74
Condoms: effect on latex condoms and diaphragms not yet known
Insert 1 applicator-dose daily for 2–3 weeks, then reduce to twice a week (discontinue every 2–3 months for 4 weeks to assess need for further treatment); postmenopausal surgery, 1 applicator-dose daily for 2 weeks, resuming 2 weeks after surgery

PoM Premarin® (Wyeth)
Vaginal cream, conjugated oestrogens 625 micrograms/g. Net price 42.5 g with calibrated applicator = £2.19
Condoms: effect on latex condoms and diaphragms not yet known
Insert 1–2 g daily, starting on 5th day of cycle, for 3 weeks, followed by 1-week interval; if therapy long term, oral progestogen for 10–14 days at end of each cycle essential

PoM Tampovagan® (Norgine)
Pessaries, stilboestrol 500 micrograms, lactic acid 5%. Net price 10 pessaries = £5.00
Condoms: no evidence of damage to latex condoms and diaphragms
Insert 2 pessaries at night for 2–3 weeks then reduce (short-term only, see notes above)

PoM Vagifem® (Novo Nordisk)
Vaginal tablets, f/c, m/r, oestradiol 25 micrograms in disposable applicators. Net price 15-applicator pack = £14.62
Condoms: no evidence of damage to latex condoms and diaphragms
Insert 1 tablet daily for 2 weeks then reduce to 1 tablet twice weekly; discontinue after 3 months to assess need for further treatment

NON-HORMONAL PREPARATIONS

Non-hormonal preparations include the recently developed preparations (NHS Replens®, NHS Senselle®) which have a high moisture content and remain *in situ* for up to 24 hours or longer.

See section 7.2.2 for the pH-modifying preparation Aci-jel®.

NHS Replens® (Unipath)
Vaginal gel, water 78.82% in hydrophilic (pH 2.5–3.5) basis. Net price 3-applicator pack = £2.22; 12-applicator pack = £7.91
Condoms: no evidence of damage to latex condoms and diaphragms
Insert 1 applicatorful (2.5g) three times a week

NHS Senselle® (LRC)
Vaginal lubricant. Net price 10-mL pack = £1.11, 40-mL pack = £2.83
Condoms: no evidence of damage to latex condoms and diaphragms

7.2.2   Anti-infective drugs

Effective specific treatments are available for the common vaginal infections.

FUNGAL INFECTIONS

Candidal vulvitis can be treated locally with cream but is almost invariably associated with vaginal infection which should be treated as well. *Vaginal candidiasis* is treated primarily with antifungal pessaries or cream inserted high into the vagina (including the time of menstruation).

Nystatin is a well established treatment (but stains clothing yellow). One or two pessaries are inserted for 14 to 28 nights; they may be supplemented with cream for vulvitis and to treat other superficial sites of infection.

Imidazole drugs (clotrimazole, econazole, isoconazole, and miconazole) appear to be equally effective in shorter courses of 3 to 14 days according to the preparation used; single dose preparations are also available, which is an advantage when compliance is a problem. Vaginal applications may be supplemented with cream for vulvitis and to treat other superficial sites of infection.

Recurrence is common if the full course of treatment is not completed and is also particularly likely if there are predisposing factors such as antibiotic therapy, oral contraceptive use, pregnancy, or diabetes mellitus. Possible reservoirs of infection may also lead to recontamination and should be treated. These include other skin sites such as the digits, nail beds, and umbilicus as well as the gut and the bladder. The partner may also be the source of re-infection and should be treated with cream at the same time.

Oral treatment with fluconazole or itraconazole should be reserved for resistant or recurrent infection (see section 5.2); oral ketoconazole has been associated with fatal hepatotoxicity (see section 5.2 for CSM warning).

PREPARATIONS FOR VAGINAL AND VULVAL CANDIDIASIS

Side-effects: occasional local irritation

Canesten® (Baypharm)
Cream (topical), clotrimazole 1%. Net price 20 g = £1.77; 50 g = £4.15
Condoms: effect on latex condoms and diaphragms not yet known
Apply to anogenital area 2–3 times daily
PoM[1] *Vaginal cream*, clotrimazole 2%. Net price 35 g (with 5-g applicators) = £5.09
Condoms: effect on latex condoms and diaphragms not yet known
Insert 5 g twice daily for 3 days or once nightly for 6 nights
Vaginal cream (10% VC®), clotrimazole 10%. Net price 5-g applicator pack = £3.34
Condoms: effect on latex condoms and diaphragms not yet known
Insert 5 g at night as a single dose

PoM[1] *Vaginal tablets*, clotrimazole 100 mg, net price 6 tabs with applicator = £3.29; 200 mg, 3 tabs with applicator = £3.29
Insert 200 mg for 3 nights *or* 100 mg for 6 nights
Vaginal tablets (Canesten 1®), clotrimazole 500 mg. Net price 1 with applicator = £3.29
Insert 1 at night as a single dose
PoM[1] *Duopak*, clotrimazole 100-mg vaginal tablets and cream (topical) 1%. Net price 6 tabs and 20 g cream = £4.24
Condoms: effect on latex condoms and diaphragms not yet known

Ecostatin® (Squibb)
Cream (topical), econazole nitrate 1%. Net price 15 g = £1.49; 30 g = £2.75
Condoms: damages latex condoms and diaphragms
Apply to anogenital area twice daily
PoM[1] *Pessaries*, econazole nitrate 150 mg. Net price 3 with applicator = £3.96
Condoms: damages latex condoms and diaphragms
Insert 1 pessary for 3 nights
PoM[1] *Pessary (Ecostatin 1®)*, econazole nitrate 150 mg, formulated for single-dose therapy. Net price 1 pessary with applicator = £4.40
Condoms: damages latex condoms and diaphragms
Insert 1 pessary at night as a single dose
PoM[1] *Twinpack*, econazole nitrate 150-mg pessaries and cream 1%. Net price 3 pessaries and 15 g cream = £4.98
Condoms: damages latex condoms and diaphragms

Femeron® (Janssen)
Cream, miconazole nitrate 2%. Net price 15g = £1.91
Condoms: damages latex condoms and diaphragms
Apply to anogenital area twice daily
Soft pessary, miconazole nitrate 1.2 g. Net price 1 = £3.41
Condoms: damages latex condoms and diaphragms
Insert 1 pessary at night as a single dose
PoM Flagyl Compak® see section 5.1.11
PoM [1] **Gyno-Daktarin®** (Janssen)
Intravaginal cream, miconazole nitrate 2%. Net price 78 g with applicators = £4.95
Condoms: damages latex condoms and diaphragms
Insert 5-g applicatorful twice daily for 7 days; *topical*, apply to anogenital area twice daily
Pessaries, miconazole nitrate 100 mg. Net price 14 = £4.04
Condoms: damages latex condoms and diaphragms
Insert 1 pessary twice daily for 7 days
Combipack, miconazole nitrate 100-mg pessaries and cream (topical) 2%. Net price 14 pessaries and 15 g cream = £4.35
Condoms: damages latex condoms and diaphragms
Ovule (= vaginal capsule) (Gyno-Daktarin 1®), miconazole nitrate 1.2 g in a fatty basis. Net price 1 ovule (with finger stall) = £3.95
Condoms: damages latex condoms and diaphragms
Insert 1 ovule at night as a single dose

---

1. Can be sold to the public for the treatment of *vaginal candidiasis*. Until packs labelled 'P' are available, those labelled 'PoM' can be sold providing the pharmacist *deletes* **PoM** from the pack and *substitutes* a capital **P** and provides *each purchaser* with a copy of the **patient information leaflet** supplied by the Royal Pharmaceutical Society of Great Britain.

Gyno-Pevaryl® (Cilag)

Cream, econazole nitrate 1%. Net price 15 g = £1.74; 30 g = £3.45

Condoms: no evidence of damage to latex condoms and diaphragms

Insert 5-g applicatorful intravaginally and apply to vulva at night for 14 nights; males, apply to penis and under foreskin daily for 14 days

PoM[1] *Pessaries*, econazole nitrate 150 mg. Net price 3 pessaries = £3.17

Condoms: damages latex condoms and diaphragms

Insert 1 pessary for 3 nights

PoM[1] *Pessary (Gyno-Pevaryl 1®)*, econazole nitrate 150 mg, formulated for single-dose therapy. Net price 1 pessary with applicator = £4.40

Condoms: damages latex condoms and diaphragms

Insert 1 pessary at night as a single dose

PoM[1] *Combipack*, econazole nitrate 150-mg pessaries, econazole nitrate 1% cream. Net price 3 pessaries and 15 g cream = £4.98

Condoms: damages latex condoms and diaphragms

PoM[1] *CP pack (Gyno-Pevaryl 1®)*, econazole nitrate 150-mg pessary, econazole nitrate 1% cream. Net price 1 pessary and 15 g cream = £5.84

Condoms: damages latex condoms and diaphragms

Masnoderm® (Cusi)

Cream, clotrimazole 1%. Net price 20 g = £1.54

Condoms: damages latex condoms and diaphragms

Apply to anogenital area 2–3 times daily

PoM Nizoral® (Janssen)

Cream (topical), ketoconazole 2%. Net price 30 g = £3.81

Apply to anogenital area once or twice daily

PoM Nystan® (Squibb)

Cream and *Ointment*, see section 13.10.2

Gel (topical), nystatin 100 000 units/g. Net price 30 g = £2.66

Condoms: no evidence of damage to latex condoms and diaphragms

Apply to anogenital area 2–4 times daily

Vaginal cream, nystatin 100 000 units/4-g application. Net price 60 g with applicator = £2.77

Condoms: damages latex condoms and diaphragms

Insert 1–2 applicatorfuls at night for at least 14 nights

Pessaries, yellow, nystatin 100 000 units. Net price 28-pessary pack = £1.96

Condoms: no evidence of damage to latex condoms and diaphragms

Insert 1–2 pessaries at night for at least 14 nights

Tablets, see section 5.2

Pevaryl® (Cilag)

Cream, econazole nitrate 1%. Net price 30 g = £2.65

Condoms: effect on latex condoms and diaphragms not yet known

Apply to anogenital area 2–3 times daily

Lotion and *Dusting powder*, see section 13.10.2

PoM[1] Travogyn® (Schering Health)

Vaginal tablets (=pessaries), isoconazole nitrate 300 mg. Net price 2 = £3.90

Condoms: effect on latex condoms and diaphragms not yet known

Insert 2 pessaries as a single dose preferably at night

OTHER INFECTIONS

Vaginal preparations intended to restore normal acidity (Aci-Jel®) may prevent recurrence of vaginal infections and permit the re-establishment of the normal vaginal flora.

Trichomonal infections commonly involve the lower urinary tract as well as the genital system and need systemic treatment with metronidazole or tinidazole (see section 5.4.2).

Bacterial infections with Gram-negative organisms are particularly common in association with gynaecological operations and trauma. Metronidazole is effective against certain Gram-negative organisms, especially *Bacteroides* spp. and may be used prophylactically in gynaecological surgery.

Antibacterial creams such as Sultrin® are used in the treatment of mixed bacterial infections but are of unproven value; they are ineffective against *Candida* spp. and *Trichomonas vaginalis*. A cream containing clindamycin is now also available.

Acyclovir may be used in the treatment of genital infection due to *herpes simplex virus*, the HSV type 2 being a major cause of genital ulceration. It has a beneficial effect on virus shedding and healing, generally giving relief from pain and other symptoms. See section 5.3 for systemic preparations, and section 13.10.3 for cream.

PREPARATIONS FOR OTHER VAGINAL INFECTIONS

Aci-Jel® (Cilag)

Vaginal jelly, acetic acid 0.92% in a buffered (pH 4) basis. Net price 85 g with applicator = £3.37

Condoms: no evidence of damage to latex condoms and diaphragms

Non-specific infections, insert 1 applicatorful twice daily to restore vaginal acidity

Betadine® (Seton)

Cautions: avoid in pregnancy (also if planned) and in breast-feeding; renal impairment (see Appendix 3)

Side-effects: rarely sensitivity; may interfere with thyroid function

Vaginal Cleansing Kit, solution, povidone-iodine 10%. Net price 250 mL with measuring bottle and applicator = £3.51

Condoms: no evidence of damage to latex condoms and diaphragms

To be diluted and used once daily, preferably in the morning; may be used with Betadine® pessaries or vaginal gel

Pessaries, brown, povidone-iodine 200 mg. Net price 28 pessaries with applicator = £6.34

Condoms: no evidence of damage to latex condoms and diaphragms

Vaginal gel, brown, povidone-iodine 10%. Net price 80 g with applicator = £2.92

Condoms: no evidence of damage to latex condoms and diaphragms

Vaginal infections or pre-operatively, insert 1 moistened pessary night and morning for up to 14 days *or* use morning pessary with 5-g gel at night *or* morning douche with pessary (or 5-g gel) at night

---

1. See footnote 1 on p. 310

Cautionary label wordings, see inside back cover

PoM **Dalacin®** (Upjohn)
Cream, clindamycin 2% (as phosphate). Net price
40-g pack with 7 applicators = £9.05
Condoms: damages latex condoms and diaphragms
Bacterial vaginosis, insert 5-g applicatorful intravaginally at night for 7 nights

PoM **Sultrin®** (Cilag)
Contra-indications: pregnancy
Side-effects: sensitivity
Cream, sulphathiazole 3.42%, sulphacetamide
2.86%, sulphabenzamide 3.7%. Net price 78 g
with applicator = £3.48
Condoms: damages latex condoms and diaphragms
Vaginal tablets, sulphathiazole 172.5 mg, sulphacetamide 143.75 mg, sulphabenzamide 184 mg.
Net price 20 with applicator = £2.94
Condoms: effect on latex condoms and diaphragms not yet known
Bacterial vaginosis, insert 1 pessary or applicatorful of cream twice daily for 10 days, then once daily if necessary (but see also notes above)

7.3   Contraceptives

The criteria by which contraceptive methods should
be judged are effectiveness, acceptability, and freedom from side-effects.

Hormonal contraception is the most effective
method of fertility control, short of sterilisation, but
has unwanted major and minor side-effects, especially for certain groups of women.

Intra-uterine devices have a high use-effectiveness but may produce undesirable side-effects,
especially menorrhagia, or be otherwise unsuitable
in a significant proportion of women; their use is
generally inadvisable in nulliparous women
because of the increased risk of pelvic sepsis and
infertility.

Barrier methods alone (condoms, diaphragms,
and caps) are less effective but can be very reliable
for well-motivated couples if used in conjunction
with a **spermicide**. Occasionally sensitivity reactions occur. The female condom (Femidom®) is
now also available; it is prelubricated but does not
contain a spermicide.

7.3.1   Combined oral contraceptives
Oral contraceptives containing an oestrogen and a
progestogen are the most effective preparations for
general use. Their advantages include:
reliability;
avoidance of dysmenorrhoea;
less iron-deficiency anaemia;
avoidance of pre-menstrual tension;
less benign breast disease;
protection against endometrial and ovarian cancer;
protection against pelvic inflammatory disease.
The oestrogen content ranges from 20 to 50 micrograms and generally a preparation with the lowest
oestrogen and progestogen content which gives
good cycle control and minimal side-effects in the
individual patient is chosen.

SURGERY. Oestrogen-containing oral contraceptives should be discontinued (and adequate
alternative contraceptive arrangements made) 4
weeks before major elective surgery and all surgery
to the legs; they should normally be recommenced

at the first menses occurring at least 2 weeks after
full mobilisation. When discontinuation is not possible, e.g. after trauma or if, by oversight, a patient
admitted for an elective procedure is still on an oestrogen-containing oral contraceptive, some consideration should be given to subcutaneous heparin
prophylaxis. These recommendations do not apply
to minor surgery with short duration of anaesthesia,
e.g. laparoscopic sterilisation or tooth extraction, or
to women taking oestrogen-free hormonal contraceptives (whether by mouth or by injection).

STARTING ROUTINES. Usually 1 tablet daily for 21
days followed by a 7-day interval during which withdrawal bleeding occurs; the first course is usually
started on 1st day of cycle; if starting on 4th day of
cycle or later additional precautions necessary during
first 7 days[1].

Changing from high to low dose oestrogen:
start immediately after the previous course, omitting 7-day tablet free interval.

Changing from lower or same dose oestrogen:
start after 7-day break as usual.

Changing from progestogen-only tablet: start
on 1st day of menstruation or any day if amenorrhoea present.

**Secondary   amenorrhoea   (not   due   to
pregnancy):** start any day, additional precautions
necessary during first 7 days.

After childbirth in women *not* breast-feeding:
start 3 weeks postpartum (increased risk of
thrombosis if started earlier); later than 3 weeks
postpartum additional precautions necessary for
first 7 days.

After childbirth in woman breast-feeding: not
recommended, oral progestogen-only contraceptive preferred.

After abortion or miscarriage: start same day.

MISSED PILL. It is important to bear in mind that the
critical time for loss of protection is when a pill is
omitted at the *beginning* or *end* of a cycle (which
lengthens the pill-free interval). The following
advice is now recommended by family planning
organisations:

'If you forget a pill, take it as soon as you remember, and
the next one at your normal time. If you are 12 or more
hours late with any pill (especially the first in the packet)
the pill may not work. As soon as you remember, continue normal pill taking. However, you will not be protected for the next seven days and must either not have
sex or use another method such as the sheath. If these
seven days run beyond the end of your packet, start the
next packet at once when you have finished the present
one, i.e. do not have a gap between packets. This will
mean you may not have a period until the end of two
packets but this does you no harm. Nor does it matter if
you see some bleeding on tablet-taking days. If you are
using everyday (ED) pills—miss out the seven inactive
pills. If you are not sure which these are, ask your doctor.'

---

1. Formerly 14 days but family planning organisations
now consider 7 days to be enough. For ED tablets 14 days
still advised in case course accidentally started with inactive tablets.

DIARRHOEA AND VOMITING. Vomiting and severe diarrhoea can interfere with absorption and limit effectiveness. Additional precautions should therefore be used during and for 7 days after recovery. If the vomiting and diarrhoea occurs during the last 7 tablets, the next pill-free interval should be omitted (in the case of ED tablets the inactive ones should be omitted).

INTERACTIONS. The effectiveness of both *combined* and *progestogen-only* oral contraceptives may be considerably reduced by interaction with drugs that induce hepatic enzyme activity (e.g. **carbamazepine, griseofulvin, phenytoin, phenobarbitone, primidone,** and, above all, **rifampicin**).

Family Planning Association (FPA) advice relating to a *short-term course of an enzyme-inducing drug* (important: rifampicin. see also below) is that additional contraceptive precautions should be taken whilst taking the enzyme-inducing drug and for at least 7 days after stopping it; if these 7 days run beyond the end of a packet the new packet should be started immediately without a break (in the case of ED tablets the inactive ones should be omitted). **Important:** it should be noted that **rifampicin** is such a potent enzyme-inducing drug that even if a course lasts for less than 7 days the additional contraceptive precautions should be continued for at least 4 weeks after stopping it.

FPA advice relating to a *long-term course of an enzyme-inducing drug* (important: rifampicin, see also below) in a woman unable to use an alternative method of contraception is to take an oral contraceptive containing ethinyloestradiol 50 micrograms or more; 'tricycling' with standard ('monophasic') tablets (i.e. taking 3 packets without a break followed by a short tablet-free interval of 4 days) is recommended. **Important:** it should be noted that **rifampicin** is such a potent enzyme-inducing drug that an alternative method of contraception (such as an IUD) is **always** recommended. Since the excretory function of the liver does not return to normal for several weeks after stopping an enzyme-inducing drug, FPA advice relating to *withdrawal* is that appropriate contraceptive measures are required for 4 to 8 weeks after stopping.

In the case of *combined* oral contraceptives some **broad-spectrum antibiotics** (e.g. ampicillin) may interfere with oestrogen absorption. FPA advice is that additional contraceptive precautions should be taken whilst taking a *short course of a broad-spectrum antibiotic* and for 7 days after stopping. If these 7 days run beyond the end of a packet the next packet should be started immediately without a break (in the case of ED tablets the inactive ones should be omitted). If the course *exceeds 2 weeks*, resistance to this interference develops, and additional precautions become unnecessary.

REASON TO STOP IMMEDIATELY. Combined oral contraceptives should be stopped (pending investigation and treatment), if any of the following symptoms occur:

Sudden severe pain in chest (whether or not radiating to the left arm);

Sudden breathlessness (or cough with blood stained sputum);

Severe pain in calf of one leg;

Severe pain in stomach;

Unusual severe, prolonged headache—especially if first time or getting progressively worse, or associated with: sudden partial or complete loss of vision; diplopia; dysphasia; vertigo; bad fainting attack or collapse (with or without focal epilepsy); weakness or very marked numbness suddenly affecting one side or one part of body; motor disturbances.

COMBINED ORAL CONTRACEPTIVES
('COC')

Indications: contraception; menstrual symptoms, see section 6.4.1.2

Cautions: risk factor for arterial disease (avoid if two or more risk factors present) including cigarette smoking (avoid in those over 35 years), hypertension, obesity (if 50% above ideal weight for height), diabetes mellitus (avoid if either retinopathy or nephropathy present), family history of arterial disease (ischaemic heart disease, ischaemic cerebrovascular accident) especially in a first-degree relative under 45 years; varicose veins (avoid if associated with venous thrombosis); severe depression, long-term immobilisation, sickle-cell disease, inflammatory bowel disease including Crohn's disease; **interactions:** see above and Appendix 1 (contraceptives, oral)

Contra-indications: pregnancy; severe or multiple risk factors for arterial disease (see Cautions), history of arterial or venous thrombosis, valvular heart disease associated with pulmonary hypertension or risk of mural thrombi, ischaemic heart disease, severe hypertension, varicose veins (during sclerosing treatment or where history of thrombosis); conditions where risk of intravascular thrombosis is higher such as an atherogenic lipid profile (e.g. familial hyperlipidaemia together with cholesterol above 6.5 mmol/litre), or any known prothrombotic coagulation abnormality; focal migraine, severe migraine, crescendo migraine, transient cerebral ischaemic attacks without headaches; liver disease including disorders of hepatic excretion (e.g. Dubin-Johnson or Rotor syndromes), infective hepatitis (until liver function returns to normal), porphyria (see section 9.8.2), and liver adenoma; gall-stones; after evacuation of hydatidiform mole (until return to normal of urine and plasma gonadotrophin values); history of pruritus, chorea, pemphigoid gestationis, cholestatic jaundice, or deterioration of otosclerosis; breast or genital tract carcinoma; undiagnosed vaginal bleeding; breast-feeding (until weaning or for 6 months after birth)

Side-effects. nausea, vomiting, headache, breast tenderness, changes in body weight, thrombosis (more common in blood groups A, B, and AB than O), changes in libido, depression, chloasma, hypertension, contact lenses may irritate, impairment of liver function, hepatic tumours, reduced menstrual loss, 'spotting' in early cycles, absence of withdrawal bleeding; rarely photosensitivity

Dose: STARTING ROUTINES. See notes on previous page; tablet should be taken at approximately same time each day; if delayed by longer than 12 hours contraception protection may be lost

Monophasic preparations, 1 tablet daily for 21 days usually starting on first day of cycle; subsequent courses repeated after 7-day interval (during which withdrawal bleeding occurs)

Everyday monophasic (ED) preparations, 1 tablet daily starting with an active tablet on first day of cycle (withdrawal bleeding occurs when inactive tablets are taken); subsequent courses repeated without interval

Bi- and triphasic preparations, see under individual preparations in table on p.315

Combined oral contraceptives (monophasic)

Oestrogen	Progestogen	Preparations	Comments
Ethinyloestradiol 20 micrograms	Desogestrel 150 micrograms	PoM **Mercilon** (Organon) Net price 3 × 21-tab pack = £8.31	OESTROGEN. Ethinyloestradiol 20 micrograms, low strength, particularly appropriate for obese or older women (provided combined oral contraceptive is otherwise suitable)
Ethinyloestradiol 20 micrograms	Norethisterone acetate 1 mg	PoM **Loestrin 20** (P-D) Net price 3 × 21-tab pack = £2.58	
			PROGESTOGENS. Desogestrel has been reported to give better cycle control than norethisterone
Ethinyloestradiol 30 micrograms	Desogestrel 150 micrograms	PoM **Marvelon** (Organon) Net price 3 × 21-tab pack = £4.57	OESTROGEN. Ethinyloestradiol 30 micrograms, standard strength (also applies to 35 micrograms)
Ethinyloestradiol 30 micrograms	Ethynodiol diacetate 2 mg	PoM **Conova 30** (Searle) Net price 21-tab pack = 78p	PROGESTOGENS. Desogestrel and gestodene may have less adverse effects on lipids than ethynodiol, levonorgestrel and norethisterone
Ethinyloestradiol 30 micrograms	Gestodene 75 micrograms	PoM **Femodene** (Schering Health) Net price 3 × 21-tab pack = £5.70 PoM **Femodene ED** (Schering Health) Net price 3 × 28-tab (7 are inactive) pack = £5.70 PoM **Minulet** (Wyeth) Net price 3 × 21-tab pack = £5.70	
Ethinyloestradiol 30 micrograms	Levonorgestrel 150 micrograms	PoM **Microgynon 30** (Schering Health) Net price 21-tab pack = 60p PoM **Ovranette** (Wyeth) Net price 21-tab pack = 62p	
Ethinyloestradiol 30 micrograms	Levonorgestrel 250 micrograms	PoM **Eugynon 30** (Schering Health) Net price 21-tab pack = 69p PoM **Ovran 30** (Wyeth) Net price 21-tab pack = 57p	
Ethinyloestradiol 30 micrograms	Norethisterone acetate 1.5 mg	PoM **Loestrin 30** (P-D) Net price 3 × 21-tab pack = £3.78	
Ethinyloestradiol 35 micrograms	Norethisterone 500 micrograms	PoM **Brevinor** (Syntex) Net price 3 × 21-tab pack = £1.67 PoM **Ovysmen** (Ortho) Net price 3 × 21-tab pack = £1.70	OESTROGEN. Ethinyloestradiol 35 micrograms, standard strength (also applies to 30 micrograms)
Ethinyloestradiol 35 micrograms	Norethisterone 1 mg	PoM **Neocon 1/35** (Ortho) Net price 3 × 21-tab pack = £2.27 PoM **Norimin** (Syntex) Net price 3 × 21-tab pack = £1.90	PROGESTOGENS. Norgestimate may have less adverse effects on lipids than norethisterone
Ethinyloestradiol 35 micrograms	Norgestimate 250 micrograms	PoM **Cilest** (Cilag) Net price 3 × 21-tab pack = £5.70	
Ethinyloestradiol 50 micrograms	Levonorgestrel 250 micrograms	PoM **Ovran** (Wyeth) Net price 21-tab pack = 37p	OESTROGEN. Ethinyloestradiol 50 micrograms, high strength, increased contraceptive security with increased possibility of side-effects. Used mainly in circumstances of reduced bioavailability (e.g. during long-term use of enzyme-inducing antiepileptics—see FPA advice under Interactions on p. 313)
Mestranol 50 micrograms	Norethisterone 1 mg	PoM **Norinyl-1** (Syntex) Net price 3 × 21-tab pack = £1.83 PoM **Ortho-Novin 1/50** (Ortho) Net price 3 × 21-tab pack = £2.35	OESTROGEN. Mestranol 50 micrograms, as for ethinyloestradiol 50 micrograms, above

Combined oral contraceptives (bi- and triphasic)

These are more complex to take, but provide better cycle control than equivalent 'monophasic' levonorgestrel or norethisterone formulations

Ethinyloestradiol with gestodene

PoM **Triadene**® (Schering Health)
6 *beige tablets*, ethinyloestradiol 30 micrograms, gestodene 50 micrograms;
5 *dark brown tablets*, ethinyloestradiol 40 micrograms, gestodene 70 micrograms;
10 *white tablets*, ethinyloestradiol 30 micrograms, gestodene 100 micrograms.
Net price 3 × 21-tab pack = £7.95
Dose: 1 tablet daily for 21 days, starting with beige tablet marked 'start' on 1st day of cycle; repeat after 7-day interval

PoM **Tri-Minulet**® (Wyeth)
6 *beige tablets*, ethinyloestradiol 30 micrograms, gestodene 50 micrograms;
5 *dark brown tablets*, ethinyloestradiol 40 micrograms, gestodene 70 micrograms;
10 *white tablets*, ethinyloestradiol 30 micrograms, gestodene 100 micrograms.
Net price 3 × 21-tab pack = £7.95
Dose: 1 tablet daily for 21 days, starting with beige tablet marked 1 on the 1st day of the cycle; repeat after 7-day interval

Ethinyloestradiol with levonorgestrel

PoM **Logynon**® (Schering Health)
6 *light brown tablets*, ethinyloestradiol 30 micrograms, levonorgestrel 50 micrograms;
5 *white tablets*, ethinyloestradiol 40 micrograms, levonorgestrel 75 micrograms;
10 *ochre tablets*, ethinyloestradiol 30 micrograms, levonorgestrel 125 micrograms.
Net price 21-tab pack = 95p
Dose: 1 tablet daily for 21 days, starting with light brown tablet marked 1 on 1st day of cycle; repeat after 7-day interval
PoM **Logynon ED**® (Schering Health)
As for Logynon® with additional 7 white placebo tablets.
Net price 28-tab pack = 95p
Dose: 1 tablet daily starting in red sector on 1st day of cycle; continue in sequence without interruption

PoM **Trinordiol**® (Wyeth)
6 *light brown tablets*, ethinyloestradiol 30 micrograms, levonorgestrel 50 micrograms;
5 *white tablets*, ethinyloestradiol 40 micrograms, levonorgestrel 75 micrograms;
10 *ochre tablets*, ethinyloestradiol 30 micrograms, levonorgestrel 125 micrograms.
Net price 3 × 21-tab pack = £3.28
Dose: 1 tablet daily for 21 days, starting with light brown tablet marked 1 on 1st day of cycle; repeat after 7 day interval

Ethinyloestradiol with norethisterone

PoM **BiNovum**® (Ortho)
7 *white tablets*, ethinyloestradiol 35 micrograms, norethisterone 500 micrograms;
14 *peach tablets*, ethinyloestradiol 35 micrograms, norethisterone 1 mg.
Net price 3 × 21-tab pack = £2.24
Dose: 1 tablet daily for 21 days, starting with white tablet on 1st day of cycle; repeat after 7-day interval
PoM **Synphase**® (Syntex)
7 *white tablets*, ethinyloestradiol 35 micrograms, norethisterone 500 micrograms;
9 *yellow tablets*, ethinyloestradiol 35 micrograms, norethisterone 1 mg;
5 *white tablets*, ethinyloestradiol 35 micrograms, norethisterone 500 micrograms.
Net price 21-tab pack = £1.08
Dose: 1 tablet daily for 21 days, starting with white tablet marked 1 on 5th day of cycle; repeat after 7-day interval

PoM **TriNovum**® (Ortho)
7 *white tablets*, ethinyloestradiol 35 micrograms, norethisterone 500 micrograms;
7 *light peach tablets*, ethinyloestradiol 35 micrograms, norethisterone 750 micrograms;
7 *peach tablets*, ethinyloestradiol 35 micrograms, norethisterone 1 mg.
Net price 3 × 21-tab pack = £2.83
Dose: 1 tablet daily for 21 days, starting with white tablet on 1st day of cycle; repeat after 7-day interval
PoM **TriNovum ED**® (Ortho)
As for TriNovum® with additional 7 green placebo tablets.
Net price 3 × 28-tab pack = £2.97
Dose: 1 tablet daily starting in white sector on 1st day of cycle; continue in sequence without interruption

---

EMERGENCY CONTRACEPTION

HORMONAL METHOD. The hormonal (Yuzpe) method of emergency contraception is suitable for occasional use. It involves taking two tablets, each containing ethinyloestradiol 50 micrograms and levonorgestrel 250 micrograms, followed 12 hours later by a further two tablets. The method has only been established as effective if the first dose is taken within 72 hours (3 days) of the unprotected intercourse; it is less effective than insertion of an intra-uterine device. Providing any delay does not extend beyond 72 hours, the timing of the first dose should be such that the second dose can conveniently be taken at the correct interval *exactly 12 hours later*. It is not suitable for women with a history of thrombosis or for those with focal migraine at the time of presentation. Side-effects include nausea, vomiting, headache, dizziness, breast discomfort, and menstrual irregularities. If vomiting occurs within 3 hours of taking the tablets, two replacement tablets can be given with an anti-emetic (preferably not metaclopramide which is liable to cause extrapyramidal effects in young women); alternatively insertion of an intra-uterine device (see below) may be needed.

The doctor should explain to the patient:
that her next period may be *early or late*;
that she needs to use a *barrier method of contraception* until her next period;
that she must return for a *follow-up examination* usually after 3 weeks.

Pregnancy despite treatment: see Appendix 4 (contraceptives, oral)—doctor information leaflet also available

PoM **Schering PC4®** (Schering Health)

Tablets, s/c, levonorgestrel 250 micrograms, ethinyloestradiol 50 micrograms. Net price 4-tab pack = £1.40.

For post-coital contraception as an occasional emergency measure; should not be administered if menstrual bleeding overdue or if unprotected intercourse occurred more than 72 hours previously

Dose: 2 tablets as soon as possible after coitus (up to 72 hours) then 2 further tablets 12 hours later

Note. **Ovran®** (see p.314) also contains levonorgestrel 250 micrograms and ethinyloestradiol 50 micrograms but is not licensed or packed for post-coital contraception

---

IUD. An intra-uterine contraceptive device (see section 7.3.4) can be inserted up to 120 hours (5 days) after unprotected intercourse, care being taken to exclude any sexually transmitted diseases. If exposure has occurred more than 5 days previously, the device can still be inserted up to 5 days after the earliest likely calculated ovulation (i.e. within the minimum period before implantation). Insertion of an intra-uterine device is more effective than the hormonal method.

7.3.2   Progestogen-only contraceptives

7.3.2.1 ORAL PROGESTOGEN-ONLY CONTRACEPTIVES

Oral progestogen-only preparations may offer a suitable alternative when oestrogens are contra-indicated, but have a higher failure rate than combined preparations. They are suitable for older women, for heavy smokers, and for those with hypertension, valvular heart disease, diabetes mellitus, and migraine. Menstrual irregularities (oligomenorrhoea, menorrhagia) are more common but tend to resolve on long-term treatment.

INTERACTIONS. Effectiveness of oral progestogen-only preparations is not affected by broad-spectrum antibiotics but is reduced by enzyme-inducing drugs—see p.313 and Appendix 1 (contraceptives, oral).

SURGERY. All progestogen-only contraceptives (including those given by injection) are suitable for use as an alternative to combined oral contraceptives before major elective surgery.

STARTING ROUTINE. 1 tablet daily, on a continuous basis, starting on 1st day of cycle and taken at the same time each day (if delayed by longer than 3 hours contraceptive protection may be lost). Additional contraceptive precautions are not necessary when initiating treatment.

Changing from a combined oral contraceptive: start on the day following completion of the combined oral contraceptive course without a break (or in the case of ED tablets omitting the inactive ones).

After childbirth: start any time after 3 weeks postpartum (increased risk of breakthrough bleeding if started earlier)—lactation is not affected.

MISSED PILL. The following advice is now recommended by family planning organisations:

'If you forget a pill, take it as soon as you remember and carry on with the next pill at the right time. If the pill was more than three hours overdue you are not protected. Continue normal pill-taking but you must also use another method, such as the sheath, for the next 7 days[1]'.

DIARRHOEA AND VOMITING. Vomiting and severe diarrhoea can interfere with absorption and limit effectiveness. Additional precautions should be used during and for 7 days after recovery.

ORAL PROGESTOGEN-ONLY CONTRACEPTIVES
(Progestogen-only pill, 'POP')

Indications: contraception

Cautions: heart disease, past ectopic pregnancy, malabsorption syndromes, functional ovarian cysts, active liver disease, recurrent cholestatic jaundice, history of jaundice in pregnancy; **interactions:** see p.313 and Appendix 1 (contraceptives, oral)

HYPERTENSION. Monitor blood pressure regularly in women receiving progestogen-only contraceptives—but suitable for women with history of hypertension associated with combined pill (and those with other forms of hypertension providing controlled).

Contra-indications: pregnancy, undiagnosed vaginal bleeding; severe arterial disease; liver adenoma, porphyria (see section 9.8.2); after evacuation of hydatidiform mole (until return to normal of urine and plasma gonadotrophin values); breast and genital tract carcinoma

Side-effects: menstrual irregularities (see also notes above); nausea, vomiting, headache, breast discomfort, depression, skin disorders, weight changes

Dose: 1 tablet daily at same time each day, starting on 1st day of cycle then continuously; if tablet delayed for 3 hours or more it should be regarded as a 'missed pill', see notes above

---

1. Family planning organisations formerly recommended 48 hours

PoM **Femulen®** (Searle)

Tablets, ethynodiol diacetate 500 micrograms. Net price 28-tab pack = 92p

PoM **Micronor®** (Ortho)

Tablets, norethisterone 350 micrograms. Net price 3 × 28-tab pack = £1.89

PoM **Microval®** (Wyeth)

Tablets, levonorgestrel 30 micrograms. Net price 35-tab pack = £1.00

PoM **Neogest®** (Schering Health)

Tablets, brown, s/c, norgestrel 75 micrograms (≡ levonorgestrel 37.5 micrograms). Net price 35-tab pack = 78p

PoM **Norgeston®** (Schering Health)

Tablets, s/c, levonorgestrel 30 micrograms. Net price 35-tab pack = 78p

PoM **Noriday®** (Syntex)

Tablets, norethisterone 350 micrograms. Net price 3 × 28-tab pack = £1.75

7.3.2.2 PARENTERAL PROGESTOGEN- ONLY CONTRACEPTIVES

Medroxyprogesterone acetate (Depo-Provera®) is a long-acting progestogen given by intramuscular injection; it is as effective as the combined oral preparations but should never be given without *full counselling backed by the manufacturer's approved leaflet.* It is useful for short-term interim contraception, for example, before vasectomy becomes effective. It may also be used as a long-term contraceptive for women who are unable to use any other method or for those in whom other contraceptives are contra-indicated or have caused unacceptable side-effects (or have otherwise proved unsatisfactory). Delayed return of fertility and irregular cycles may occur after discontinuation of treatment but there is no evidence of permanent infertility. Heavy bleeding has been reported in patients given medroxyprogesterone acetate in the immediate puerperium (the first dose is best delayed until 6 to 7 weeks postpartum). **Norethisterone enanthate** (Noristerat®) is a long-acting progestogen given as an oily injection which provides contraception for 8 weeks to provide short-term interim contraception e.g. before vasectomy becomes effective. The **cautions** and **contra-indications** of progestogen-only contraceptives given by injection are as for the oral preparations except that as the injection also reliably inhibits ovulation, it protects against ectopic pregnancy and functional ovarian cysts. Blood pressure should be checked before each injection.

A **levonorgestrel-releasing implant system** (Norplant®) is now also available; it has comparable efficacy to injectable medroxyprogesterone acetate but lasts for 5 years. The **cautions** and **contra-indications** are again as for oral preparations, but irregular and prolonged bleeding and amenorrhoea are common; unlike the injectable preparations the method is almost immediately reversible on removal of the implants. The risk of ectopic pregnancy is believed to be reduced overall but may be relatively higher in the later years after an insertion; since functional ovarian cysts may also be more common they need to be distinguished from

ectopic pregnancy. *Full counselling backed by the manufacturer's approved leaflet is necessary.*

INTERACTIONS. Effectiveness of parenteral progestogen-only contraceptives is not affected by broad-spectrum antibiotics but may be reduced by enzyme-inducing drugs—see p.313 and Appendix 1 (contraceptives, oral)

PARENTERAL PROGESTOGEN-ONLY CONTRACEPTIVES

Indications: contraception, see also notes above and under preparations (roles vary according to preparation)

Cautions; Contra-indications; Side-effects: see notes above and under preparations; **interactions:** see notes above, p.313, and Appendix 1 (contraceptives, oral)

COUNSELLING. Full counselling backed by *manufacturer's approved leaflet* required before administration

Dose: see under preparations

Injectable preparations

PoM **Depo-Provera®** (Upjohn)

Injection (aqueous suspension), medroxyprogesterone acetate 150 mg/mL, net price 1-mL vial = £4.55. Counselling, see patient information leaflet

Dose: by deep intramuscular injection, 150 mg in first 5 days of cycle or first 6 weeks after parturition (delay until 6 weeks after parturition if breast-feeding); for long-term contraception, repeated every 3 months

Note. The 150 mg/mL strength of Depo-Provera® is also available in a 3.3mL vial for use in cancer (see section 8.3.2), and a 50 mg/mL strength is available in 1-, 3-, and 5-mL vials for endometriosis.

PoM **Noristerat®** (Schering Health)

Injection (oily), norethisterone enanthate 200 mg/mL. Net price 1-mL amp = £3.00. Counselling, see patient information leaflet

Dose: by deep intramuscular injection into gluteal muscle, short-term contraception, 200 mg in first 5 days of cycle or immediately after parturition (duration 8 weeks); may be repeated once after 8 weeks (withhold breast-feeding for neonates with severe or persistent jaundice requiring medical treatment)

Implants

▼ PoM **Norplant®** (Roussel)

Implant capsules, containing levonorgestrel 38 mg/implant capsule. Net price 6-implant capsule pack = £179.00. Counselling, see patient information leaflet

Dose: by subdermal implantation, set of 6 implant capsules inserted within first 5 days of cycle (preferably on 1st day—after 1st day additional precautions necessary for following 7 days) *or* on 21st day after parturition (after this day additional precautions necessary for following 7 days); remove within 5 years of insertion

---

Cautionary label wordings, see inside back cover

7.3.3   Spermicidal contraceptives

Spermicidal contraceptives are useful additional safeguards but do **not** give adequate protection if used alone; they are suitable for use with barrier methods. They have two components: a spermicide and a vehicle which itself may have some inhibiting effect on sperm activity.

> **CSM Advice.** Products such as petroleum jelly (vaseline), baby oil and oil-based vaginal and rectal preparations are likely to damage condoms and contraceptive diaphragms made from latex rubber, and may render them less effective as a barrier method of contraception and as a protection from sexually transmitted diseases (including AIDS).

Condoms: no evidence of harm to latex condoms and diaphragms with the products listed below

C-Film® (FP)

Film, nonoxinol '9' 67 mg in a water-soluble basis. Net price 10 films = £1.47

Delfen® (Ortho)

Foam, nonoxinol '9' 12.5%, pressurised aerosol unit in a water-miscible basis. Net price 20 g (with applicator) = £4.65

Double Check® (FP)

Pessaries, nonoxinol '9' 6% in a water-soluble basis. Net price 10 pessaries = £1.08

Note. A pack including 10 condoms, called Two's Company®, costs £2.42 but is not prescribable on NHS

Duracreme® (LRC)

Cream, nonoxinol '9' 2% in a water-soluble basis. Net price 100-g tube = £2.60; applicator = 75p

Duragel® (LRC)

Gel, nonoxinol '9' 2% in a water-soluble basis. Net price 100-g tube = £2.60; applicator = 75p

Gynol II® (Ortho)

Jelly, nonoxinol '9' 2% in a water-soluble basis. Net price 81 g = £2.61; applicator = 75p

Ortho-Creme® (Ortho)

Cream, nonoxinol '9' 2% in a water-miscible basis. Net price 70 g = £2.44; applicator = 75p

Orthoforms® (Ortho)

Pessaries, nonoxinol '9' 5% in a water-soluble basis. Net price 15 pessaries = £2.40

Ortho-Gynol® (Ortho)

Jelly, p-di-isobutylphenoxypolyethoxyethanol 1% in a water-soluble basis. Net price 81 g = £2.99; applicator = 75p

Staycept® (Syntex)

Jelly, octoxinol 1% in a water-soluble basis. Net price 80 g = £2.08

Pessaries, nonoxinol '9' 6% in a water-soluble basis. Net price 10 pessaries = £1.51

7.3.4   Contraceptive devices

INTRA-UTERINE DEVICES

The intra-uterine device (IUD) is suitable for older parous women but should be a last-resort contraceptive for young nulliparous women because of the increased risk of pelvic inflammatory disease and infertility. Inert intra-uterine devices are no longer on the UK market but may still be worn by some women.

Smaller devices have now been introduced in order to minimise side-effects; these consist of a plastic carrier wound with copper wire or fitted with copper bands; some also have a central core of silver with the aim of preventing fragmentation of the copper. Family planning organisations now recommend that the replacement time for these devices should be 5 years (8 years for Gyne-T® 380 Slimline which also has a copper collar); any copper intrauterine device licensed currently in the UK, which is fitted in a woman over the age of 40, may remain in the uterus until menopause.

The timing and technique of fitting an intrauterine device play a critical part in its subsequent performance and call for proper training and experience. Devices should not be fitted during the heavy days of the period; they are best fitted after the end of menstruation and before the calculated time of implantation. The main excess risk of infection occurs in the first 20 days after insertion and is believed to be related to pre-existing carriage of a sexually transmitted disease, therefore pre-screening (at least for chlamydia) should ideally be performed. The woman should be advised to attend *as an emergency* if she experiences sustained pain during the next 20 days.

An intra-uterine device should not be removed in mid-cycle unless an additional contraceptive was used for the previous 7 days. If removal is essential (e.g. to treat severe pelvic infection) post-coital contraception should be considered.

If an intra-uterine device fails and the woman wishes to continue to full-term the device should be removed in the first trimester if possible.

INTRA-UTERINE CONTRACEPTIVE DEVICES

Indications: see notes above

Cautions: anaemia, heavy menses, history of pelvic inflammatory disease, diabetes, valvular heart disease (antibiotic cover needed)—avoid if prosthetic valve or past attack of infective endocarditis; epilepsy, increased risk of expulsion if inserted before uterine involution; gynaecological examination before insertion, 6 weeks after (or sooner if there is a problem), then after 6 months, then yearly; remove if pregnancy occurs; anticoagulant therapy (avoid if possible); if pregnancy occurs, increased likelihood that it may be tubal

Contra-indications: pregnancy, severe anaemia, known HIV infection, very heavy menses, history of ectopic pregnancy or tubal surgery, distorted or small uterine cavity, genital malignancy, pelvic inflammatory disease, immunosuppressive therapy, *copper devices:* copper allergy, Wilson's disease, medical diathermy

Side-effects: uterine or cervical perforation, displacement, pelvic infection may be exacerbated, heavy menses, dysmenorrhoea, allergy; *on insertion:* some pain and bleeding (helped by giving an NSAID, such as ibuprofen half-an-hour before insertion); occasionally, epileptic seizure, vasovagal attack

PoM **Multiload® Cu250** (Organon)

Intra-uterine device, copper wire, surface area approx. 250 mm² wound on vertical stem of plastic carrier, 3.6 cm length, with 2 down-curving flexible arms, monofilament thread attached to base of vertical stem; preloaded in inserter. Net price, each = £6.75
For uterine length over 7 cm; replacement every 3 years (but see notes above)

PoM **Multiload® Cu250 Short** (Organon)

Intra-uterine device, as above, with vertical stem length 2.5 cm. Net price, each = £6.75
For uterine length 5–7 cm; replacement every 3 years (but see notes above)

PoM **Multiload®Cu375** (Organon)

Intra-uterine device, as above, with copper surface area approx. 375 mm². Net price, each = £8.75
For uterine length over 7 cm; replacement every 5 years (see notes above)

PoM **Novagard®** (Pharmacia)

Intra-uterine device, copper wire with silver core, surface area approx. 200 mm² wound on vertical stem of T-shaped plastic carrier, impregnated with barium sulphate for radio-opacity, monofilament thread attached to base of vertical stem; partially preloaded in inserter. Dimensions: transverse arms, vertical stem, both 3.2 cm. Net price, each = £9.90
For uterine length over 5.5 cm; replacement every 5 years (see notes above)

PoM **Nova-T®** (Schering Health)

Intra-uterine device, copper wire with silver core, surface area approx. 200 mm² wound on vertical stem of T-shaped plastic carrier, impregnated with barium sulphate for radio-opacity, threads attached to base of vertical stem. Net price, each = £9.90
For uterine length over 6.5 cm; replacement every 5 years (see notes above)

PoM **Ortho Gyne-T®** (Ortho)

Intra-uterine device, copper wire, surface area 200 mm², wound on vertical stem of T-shaped plastic carrier, impregnated with barium sulphate for radio-opacity, 2-tail plastic thread attached to base of vertical stem. Net price each = £8.99
For uterine length over 6.5 cm; replacement every 3 years (but see notes above)

PoM **Ortho Gyne-T® 380 Slimline** (Ortho)

Intra-uterine device, as above, with copper wire surface area 320 mm² and copper collar surface 30 mm² on distal portion of each arm. Net price = £9.40
For uterine length over 6.5 cm; replacement every 8 years (see notes above)

OTHER CONTRACEPTIVE DEVICES

Contraceptive caps

Type A contraceptive pessary. Opaque rubber, sizes 1 to 5 (55–75 mm rising in steps of 5 mm), net price = £6.40
Available from Lamberts (Dumas Vault Cap®)

Type B contraceptive pessary Opaque rubber, sizes 22 to 31 mm (rising in steps of 3 mm), net price = £7.45
Available from Lamberts (Prentif Cavity Rim Cervical Cap®)

Type C contraceptive pessary Opaque rubber, sizes 1 to 3 (42, 48 and 54 mm), net price = £6.40
Available from Lamberts (Vimule Cap®)

Contraceptive diaphragms

Type A Diaphragm with flat metal spring. Transparent rubber with flat metal spring, sizes 55–95 mm (rising in steps of 5 mm), net price = £5.49
Available from Cilag (Ortho-White®), LRC (Durex Flat Spring®)

Type B Diaphragm with coiled metal rim. Opaque rubber with coiled metal rim, sizes 55–95 mm (rising in steps of 5 mm), net price = £5.53
Available from Cilag (Ortho®)

Type C Arcing Spring Diaphragm. Opaque rubber with arcing spring, sizes 55–95 mm (rising in steps of 5 mm), net price = £6.29
Available from Cilag (All-Flex®), LRC (Durex Arcing Spring®)

Fertility thermometer
Fertility (Ovulation) Thermometer (Zeal)
Mercury in glass thermometer, range 35 to 39°C (graduated in 0.1°C). Net price = £1.40
For monitoring ovulation for the fertility awareness method of contraception

7.4   Drugs for genito-urinary disorders

7.4.1	Drugs for urinary retention
7.4.2	Drugs for urinary frequency, enuresis, and incontinence
7.4.3	Drugs used in urological pain
7.4.4	Bladder instillations and urological surgery
7.4.5	Drugs for impotence

For drugs used in the treatment of urinary-tract infections see section 5.1.13.

7.4.1   Drugs for urinary retention

Acute retention is painful and is treated by catheterisation.

Chronic retention is painless and often longstanding. Catheterisation is unnecessary unless there is deterioration of renal function. After the cause has initially been established and treated, drugs may be required to increase detrusor muscle tone.

ALPHA-BLOCKERS

The selective alpha-blockers **alfuzosin, indoramin, prazosin** and **terazosin** relax smooth muscle in benign prostatic hyperplasia producing an increase in urinary flow-rate and an improvement in obstructive symptoms. Side-effects of selective alpha-blockers include *sedation, dizziness* and *hypotension (notably postural hypotension, particularly after the first dose); other side-effects* associated with this group of drugs include *drowsiness, weakness* and *lack of energy, depression, headache, dry* *mouth, nausea, urinary frequency and incontinence,* and *tachycardia and palpitations.* They should be avoided in patients with *a history of orthostatic hypotension* and special care (and reduced dosage) is needed when initiating them in the *elderly,* and in *renal* and possibly *hepatic impairment.* Since selective alpha-blockers are also antihypertensive, patients receiving *antihypertensive treatment* require reduced dosage and specialist supervision (as do those with *cardiac disorders*). **Interactions:** see Appendix 1 (alpha blockers).

DRIVING. Selective alpha-blockers may cause drowsiness and so affect ability to drive or operate machinary.

ALFUZOSIN HYDROCHLORIDE

Indications; Cautions; Contra-indications; Side-effects: see notes above
Dose: 2.5 mg 3 times daily, max.10 mg daily; ELDERLY 2.5 mg twice daily initially
FIRST DOSE EFFECT. First dose may cause collapse due to hypotensive effect (therefore should be taken on retiring to bed). Patient should be warned to lie down if symptoms such as dizziness, fatigue or sweating develop, and to remain lying down until they abate completely

▼ PoM **Xatral®** (Lorex)
Tablets, f/c, alfuzosin hydrochloride 2.5 mg. Net price 60-tab pack = £19.00; 90-tab pack = £25.00. Label: 3, counselling, see dose above

INDORAMIN

Indications; Cautions; Contra-indications; Side-effects: see notes above and section 2.5.4
Dose: 20 mg twice daily; increased if necessary by 20 mg every 2 weeks to max. 100 mg daily in divided doses; ELDERLY, 20 mg at night maybe adequate

PoM **Doralese®** (Bencard)
Tablets, yellow, f/c, indoramin 20 mg. net price 60-tab pack = £9.24. Label 2

PRAZOSIN HYDROCHLORIDE

Indications; Cautions; Contra-indications; Side-effects: see notes above and section 2.5.4
Dose: initially 500 micrograms twice daily for 3–7 days, subsequently adjusted according to response; usual maintenance (and max.) 2 mg twice daily; ELDERLY initiate with lowest possible dose
FIRST DOSE EFFECT. First dose may cause collapse due to hypotensive effect (therefore should be taken on retiring to bed). Patient should be warned to lie down if symptoms such as dizziness, fatigue or sweating develop, and to remain lying down until they abate completely

PoM **Hypovase®** Benign Prostatic Hypertrophy (Invicta)
Tablets, prazosin hydrochloride 500 micrograms, net price 56-tab pack = £2.64; 1 mg (orange, scored), 56-tab pack = £3.41; 2 mg (scored), 56-tab pack = £4.63; starter pack of 8 × 500-microgram tabs with 32 × 1-mg tabs = £3.19. Label: 3, counselling, see dose above

TERAZOSIN

Indications; Cautions; Contra-indications; Side-effects: see notes above and section 2.5.4
Dose: initially 1 mg at bedtime; dose may be doubled at weekly intervals according to response, to max. 10 mg once daily; usual maintenance 5–10 mg daily
FIRST DOSE EFFECT. First dose may cause collapse due to hypotensive effect (therefore should be taken on retiring to bed). Patient should be warned to lie down if symptoms such as dizziness, fatigue or sweating develop, and to remain lying down until they abate completely

PoM **Hytrin BPH®** (Abbott)
Tablets, terazosin (as hydrochloride) 2 mg (yellow), net price 28-tab pack = £12.55; 5 mg (tan), 28-tab pack = £18.89; 10 mg (blue), 28-tab pack = £26.59; starter pack of 7 × 1-mg tab with 7 × 2-mg tab = £6.34. Label: 3, counselling, see dose above

ANTI-ANDROGENS

FINASTERIDE

See section 6.4.2

PARASYMPATHOMIMETICS

Parasympathomimetics produce the effects of parasympathetic nerve stimulation; they possess the muscarinic rather than the nicotinic effects of acetylcholine and improve voiding efficiency by increasing detrusor muscle contraction. In the absence of obstruction to the bladder outlet they have a limited role in the relief of urinary retention. Generalised parasympathomimetic side-effects such as sweating, bradycardia, and intestinal colic may occur, particularly in the elderly.

Carbachol and **bethanechol** are choline esters that have been used in postoperative urinary retention. Bethanechol has a more selective action on the bladder than carbachol but the use of both has now been superseded by catheterisation.

Distigmine inhibits the breakdown of acetylcholine. It may help patients with an upper motor neurone neurogenic bladder.

BETHANECHOL CHLORIDE

Indications: urinary retention (but see notes above)

Contra-indications: intestinal or urinary obstruction or where increased muscular activity of urinary or gastro-intestinal tract harmful; asthma, bradycardia, hyperthyroidism, recent myocardial infarction, epilepsy, hypotension, parkinsonism, vagotonia, peptic ulceration, pregnancy; **interactions:** Appendix 1 (cholinergics)

Side-effects: parasympathomimetic effects such as nausea, vomiting, sweating, blurred vision, bradycardia, and intestinal colic

Dose: 10–25 mg 3–4 times daily half an hour before food

PoM **Myotonine®** (Glenwood)

Tablets, both scored, bethanechol chloride 10 mg, net price 20 = 90p; 25 mg, 20 = £1.15. Label: 22

CARBACHOL

Indications: urinary retention, but see notes above

Contra-indications; Side-effects: see under Bethanechol Chloride but side-effects more acute

Dose: by mouth, 2 mg 3 times daily half an hour before food

By subcutaneous injection (acute symptoms, postoperative urinary retention) 250 micrograms, repeated twice if necessary at 30-minute intervals

Note. Inadvertent intravenous administration of carbachol is **extremely hazardous** and calls for emergency treatment with atropine

PoM **Carbachol** (Non-proprietary)

Tablets, carbachol 2 mg. Net price 20 = £2.39. Label: 22

Note. Supplies may be difficult to obtain

Injection, carbachol 250 micrograms/mL

DISTIGMINE BROMIDE

Indications: urinary retention (see notes above) ; myasthenia gravis, see section 10.2.1

Cautions; asthma, bradycardia, hyperthyroidism, recent myocardial infarction, epilepsy, hypotension, parkinsonism, vagotonia, peptic ulceration, pregnancy; **interactions:** Appendix 1 (cholinergics)

Contra-indications: intestinal or urinary obstruction or where increased muscular activity of urinary or gastro-intestinal tract harmful

Side-effects: see under Bethanechol Chloride, but action slower therefore side-effects less acute; see also Neostigmine (section 10.2.1)

Dose: by mouth, 5 mg daily or on alternate days, half an hour before breakfast

By intramuscular injection, 500 micrograms 12 hours after surgery to prevent urinary retention; may be repeated every 24 hours

PoM **Ubretid®** (Rhône-Poulenc Rorer)

Tablets, scored, distigmine bromide 5 mg. Net price 30-tab pack = £19.01. Label: 22

Injection, distigmine bromide 500 micrograms/mL. Net price 1-mL amp = 80p

7.4.2 Drugs for urinary frequency, enuresis, and incontinence

URINARY INCONTINENCE

Antimuscarinic drugs such as **oxybutynin** and **flavoxate** are used to treat *urinary frequency*; they increase bladder capacity by diminishing unstable detrusor contractions. All these drugs may cause dry mouth and blurred vision and may precipitate glaucoma. Oxybutynin has a high level of side-effects which limits its use; the dosage needs to be carefully assessed, particularly in the elderly. Flavoxate has less marked side-effects but is also less effective. **Propantheline** was formerly widely used in urinary incontinence but had a low response rate with a high incidence of side-effects; it is now primarily indicated in adult enuresis. The **tricyclic antidepressants** imipramine, amitriptyline, and nortriptyline (see section 4.3.1) are sometimes effective in the management of the unstable bladder because of their antimuscarinic properties.

FLAVOXATE HYDROCHLORIDE

Indications: urinary frequency and incontinence, dysuria, urgency; bladder spasms due to catheterisation

Cautions; Contra-indications: see under Oxybutynin Hydrochloride (antimuscarinic effect considerably less marked)

Side-effects: antimuscarinic side-effects (see Atropine Sulphate, section 1.2); see also notes above

Dose: 200 mg 3 times daily

PoM **Urispas®** (Syntex)

Tablets, both s/c, flavoxate hydrochloride 100 mg, net price 20 = £1.20; 200 mg, 20 = £2.40

OXYBUTYNIN HYDROCHLORIDE

Indications: urinary frequency and incontinence, neurogenic bladder instability and nocturnal enuresis

Cautions: frail elderly; hepatic or renal impairment; hyperthyroidism; cardiac disease where increase in rate undesirable; prostatic hypertrophy; hiatus hernia with reflux oesophagitis; pregnancy and breast-feeding; porphyria (see section 9.8.2); **interactions:** Appendix 1 (antimuscarinics)

Contra-indications: intestinal obstruction or atony, severe ulcerative colitis or toxic megacolon; significant bladder outflow obstruction; glaucoma

Side-effects: include dry mouth, constipation, blurred vision, nausea, abdominal discomfort, facial flushing (more marked in children), difficulty in micturition (less commonly urinary retention); also headache, dizziness, drowsiness, dry skin, diarrhoea, arrhythmia; see also notes above

Dose: 5 mg 2–3 times daily increased if necessary to max. 5 mg 4 times daily

ELDERLY 2.5–3 mg twice daily initially, increased to 5 mg twice daily according to response and tolerance

CHILD over 5 years, neurogenic bladder instability, 2.5–3 mg twice daily increased to 5 mg twice daily (max. 5 mg 3 times daily); nocturnal enuresis (preferably over 7 years, see notes below), 2.5–3 mg twice daily increased to 5 mg 2–3 times daily (last dose before bedtime)

PoM **Cystrin®** (Pharmacia)
Tablets, oxybutynin hydrochloride 3 mg, net price 100-tab pack = £16.34; 5 mg (scored), 100-tab pack = £27.24. Label: 3
PoM **Ditropan®** (S&N Pharm.)
Tablets, both blue, scored, oxybutynin hydrochloride 2.5 mg, net price 84-tab pack = £11.74; 5 mg, 84-tab pack = £22.88. Label: 3
Elixir, oxybutynin hydrochloride 2.5 mg/5 mL. Net price 150-mL pack = £4.78. Label: 3.

PROPANTHELINE BROMIDE

Indications: adult enuresis, see notes above
Cautions; Contra-indications: see under Oxybutynin Hydrochloride
Side-effects: antimuscarinic side-effects (see Atropine Sulphate, section 1.2); see also notes above
Dose: 15–30 mg 2–3 times daily one hour before meals

Preparations
See section 1.2

NOCTURNAL ENURESIS

Nocturnal enuresis is a normal occurrence in young children but persists in as many as 5% by 10 years of age. In the absence of urinary-tract infection simple measures such as bladder training or the use of an alarm system may be successful. Drug therapy is not appropriate for children under 7 years of age and should be reserved for when alternative measures have failed. The possible side-effects and potential toxicity of these drugs if taken in overdose should be borne in mind when they are prescribed.

The most widely used treatment is with tricyclics such as **amitriptyline**, **imipramine**, and less often **nortriptyline** (see section 4.3.1). They are effective, but behaviour disturbances may occur and relapse is common after withdrawal. Treatment should not normally exceed 3 months unless a full physical examination (including ECG) is given.

Desmopressin, an analogue of vasopressin, is also used for nocturnal enuresis (see section 6.5.2).

The sympathomimetic drug **ephedrine** may also be useful.

AMITRIPTYLINE HYDROCHLORIDE

See section 4.3.1

DESMOPRESSIN

See section 6.5.2

EPHEDRINE HYDROCHLORIDE

Indications: nocturnal enuresis
Cautions; Contra-indications; Side-effects: see under Ephedrine Hydrochloride (section 3.1.1.2)
Dose: CHILD 7–8 years 30 mg, 9–12 years 45 mg, 13–15 years 60 mg at bedtime

Preparations
See section 3.1.1.2

IMIPRAMINE HYDROCHLORIDE

See section 4.3.1

NORTRIPTYLINE HYDROCHLORIDE

See section 4.3.1

7.4.3   Drugs used in urological pain

The acute pain of *ureteric colic* may be relieved with **pethidine** (section 4.7.2); **diclofenac** (section 10.1.1) is also effective and compares favourably with pethidine.

Lignocaine gel is a useful topical application in *urethral pain* or to relieve the discomfort of catheterisation (see section 15.2).

ALKALINISATION OF URINE

Alkalinisation of urine may be undertaken with **sodium bicarbonate**, or alternatively with potassium citrate. The alkalinising action may relieve the discomfort of *cystitis* caused by lower urinary tract infections. Sodium bicarbonate, in particular, is also used as a urinary alkalinising agent in some metabolic and renal disorders (see section 9.2.1.3).

POTASSIUM CITRATE

Indications: relief of discomfort in mild urinary-tract infections; alkalinisation of urine
Cautions: renal impairment, cardiac disease; elderly; **interactions:** Appendix 1 (potassium salts)
Side-effects: hyperkalaemia on prolonged high dosage, mild diuresis

Potassium Citrate Mixture (BP)
(Potassium Citrate Oral Solution)
Oral solution, potassium citrate 30%, citric acid monohydrate 5% in a suitable vehicle with a lemon flavour.
Extemporaneous preparations should be recently prepared according to the following formula; potassium citrate 3 g, citric acid monohydrate 500 mg, syrup 2.5 mL,
quillaia tincture 0.1 mL, lemon spirit 0.05 mL, double-
strength chloroform water 3 mL, water to 10 mL. Contains about 28 mmol K⁺/10 mL. Label: 27
Dose: 10 mL 3 times daily well diluted with water
Note. Concentrates for preparation of Potassium Citrate
Mixture BP are available from Evans, Hillcross
Proprietary brands of potassium citrate on sale to the public for the relief of discomfort in mild urinary-tract
infections include Cystopurin® (Fisons) and
Effercitrate® (Typharm)

SODIUM BICARBONATE
Indications: relief of discomfort in mild urinary-
tract infections; alkalinisation of urine
Cautions; Side-effects: see section 1.1.2; also caution in elderly
Dose: 3 g in water every 2 hours until urinary pH
exceeds 7; maintenance of alkaline urine 5–10 g
daily

Sodium Bicarbonate Powder. Label: 13

SODIUM CITRATE
Indications: relief of discomfort in mild urinary-
tract infections
Cautions: renal impairment, cardiac disease,
pregnancy, patients on a sodium-restricted diet;
elderly
Side-effects: mild diuresis

Note. Proprietary brands of Sodium Citrate on sale to the
public for the relief of discomfort in mild urinary-tract
infections include Cymalon® (Sterling Health),
Cystemme® (Abbott), and Cystoleve® (Cupal)

ACIDIFICATION OF URINE

Acidification of urine has been undertaken with **ascorbic
acid** but it is not always reliable.
For pH-modifying solutions for the maintenance of indwelling urinary catheters, see section 7.4.4.

ASCORBIC ACID
Indications: acidification of urine but see notes above
Dose: by mouth, 4 g daily in divided doses

Preparations
See section 9.6.3

OTHER PREPARATIONS FOR URINARY DISORDERS

A terpene mixture (Rowatinex®) is claimed to be of benefit in *urolithiasis* for the expulsion of calculi.

Rowatinex® (Monmouth)
Capsules, yellow, e/c, anethol 4 mg, borneol 10 mg, camphene 15 mg, cineole 3 mg, fenchone 4 mg, pinene 31
mg. Net price 50 = £7.35. Label: 25
Dose: 1 capsule 3–4 times daily

7.4.4   Bladder instillations and urological surgery

INFECTED BLADDERS. Various solutions are available as irrigations or washouts.

Aqueous **chlorhexidine** (see section 13.11.2) is
effective against a wide range of common urinary-
tract pathogens but not against most *Pseudomonas*
spp. Solutions containing 1 in 5000 (0.02%) are
used but they may irritate the mucosa and cause
burning and haematuria (in which case they should
be discontinued); sterile **sodium chloride solution
0.9%** (physiological saline) is usually adequate and
is therefore preferred.

Bladder irrigations of **amphotericin** 100 mic-
rograms/mL (see section 5.2) may be of value in
mycotic infections.

DISSOLUTION OF BLOOD CLOTS. Clot retention is
usually treated by irrigation with sterile **sodium
chloride solution 0.9%** but sterile **sodium citrate
solution for bladder irrigation 3%** may also be
helpful. **Streptokinase-streptodornase** (Varidase
Topical®, see section 13.11.7) is an alternative.

LOCALLY ACTING CYTOTOXIC DRUGS. **Doxorubicin**
(see section 8.1.2) is used for recurrent superficial
bladder tumours, and some papillary tumours. A
solution (50 mg in 50 mL of sterile sodium chloride
solution 0.9%) is instilled monthly. Although systemic side-effects are few, it may cause frequency,
urgency, dysuria, and occasionally reduction in
bladder capacity.

Epirubicin (see section 8.1.2) is used for papillary tumours. A solution (50 mg in 50 mL of sterile
water or sodium chloride solution 0.9%) is instilled
weekly for 8 weeks (for prophylaxis, weekly for 4
weeks then monthly for 11 months).

Mitomycin (see section 8.1.2) is used for recurrent superficial bladder tumours. A solution (10 to
40 mg in 20 to 40 mL of sterile water) is instilled
weekly or three times weekly for a total of 20
doses.

Thiotepa (see section 8.1.1) is used for recurrent
superficial bladder tumours. A solution (15 to 60
mg in 60 mL of sterile water) is instilled weekly for
4 weeks then after a break of 2 weeks, at intervals
of 1 to 2 weeks for a further 4 doses. The concentration should be reduced if there is evidence of bone-
marrow suppression.

INTERSTITIAL CYSTITIS. **Dimethyl sulphoxide** may
be used for symptomatic relief in patients with
interstitial cystitis (Hunner's ulcer). 50 mL of a
50% solution (Rimso-50®) is instilled into the
bladder, retained for 15 minutes, and voided by the
patient. Treatment is repeated at intervals of 2
weeks. Bladder spasm and hypersensitivity reactions may occur and long-term use requires
ophthalmic, renal, and hepatic assessment at intervals of 6 months.

CHLORHEXIDINE
Indications: bladder washouts, see notes above and section 13.11.2

DIMETHYL SULPHOXIDE
Indications: bladder washouts, see notes above

PoM **Rimso-50®** (Britannia)
Bladder instillation, sterile, dimethyl sulphoxide 50%, in aqueous solution. Net price 50 mL = £19.80

SODIUM CHLORIDE
Indications: bladder washouts, see notes above
Available from Baxter, Kendall

SODIUM CITRATE
Indications: bladder washouts, see notes above

Sterile Sodium Citrate Solution for Bladder Irrigation, sodium citrate 3%, dilute hydrochloric acid 0.2%, in purified water, freshly boiled and cooled, and sterilised

UROLOGICAL SURGERY

Endoscopic surgery within the urinary tract requires an isotonic irrigant as there is a high risk of fluid absorption; if this occurs in excess, hypervolaemia, haemolysis, and renal failure may result. **Glycine irrigation solution 1.5%** is the irrigant of choice for transurethral resection of the prostate gland and bladder tumours; **sterile sodium chloride solution 0.9%** (physiological saline) is used for percutaneous renal surgery.

GLYCINE
Indications: bladder irrigation during urological surgery; see notes above
Cautions; Side-effects: see notes above

Glycine Irrigation Solution (Non-proprietary)
Irrigation solution, glycine 1.5% in water for injections
Available from Baxter, Kendall

MAINTENANCE OF INDWELLING URINARY CATHETERS

The deposition which occurs in catheterised patients is usually chiefly composed of phosphate and to minimise this the catheter (if latex) should be changed at least as often as every 6 weeks. If the catheter is to be left for longer periods a silicone catheter should be used. If bladder washouts are required at frequent intervals this usually indicates that the catheter needs to be changed.

CATHETER PATENCY SOLUTIONS

Chlorhexidine 0.02%. Available from CliniFlex (Uro-Tainer Chlorhexidine® , 100-mL sachet = £2.18), Galen (Uriflex C® , 100-mL sachet = £1.93)

Mandelic acid 1% Available from CliniFlex (Uro-Tainer Mandelic Acid®, 100-mL sachet = £2.18)

Sodium chloride 0.9%. Available from Clini-Flex (Uro-Tainer Sodium Chloride®, 100-mL sachet = £2.07, Uro-Tainer M®, with integral drug additive port, 50- and 100mL sachets = £2.46), Galen (Uriflex S® , 100-mL sachet = £1.82, Uriflex SP® with integral drug additive port, 100-mL sachet = £1.96)

Solution G, citric acid 3.23%, magnesium oxide 0.38%, sodium bicarbonate 0.7%, disodium edetate 0.01%. Available from CliniFlex (Uro-Tainer Suby G® , 100-mL sachet = £2.18), Galen (Uriflex G® , 100-mL sachet = £1.93)

Solution R, citric acid 6%, gluconolactone 0.6%, magnesium carbonate 2.8%, disodium edetate 0.01%. Available from CliniFlex (Uro-Tainer Solution R® , 100-mL sachet = £2.18), Galen (Uriflex R®, 100-mL sachet = £1.93)

7.4.5   Drugs for impotence

Reasons for failure to produce a satisfactory erection include psychogenic, vascular, neurogenic, and endocrine abnormalities; many drugs are also liable to induce impotence. Intracavernosal injection of vasoactive drugs under careful medical supervision is used for both diagnostic and therapeutic purposes.

PAPAVERINE and PHENTOLAMINE

Note. Recommendations in this section involve non-licensed indications.

The most effective treatment for impotence has been shown to be direct injection of the smooth muscle relaxant **papaverine** into the corpus cavernosum. The usual dose of papaverine by intracavernosal injection is 7.5 mg initially increased according to response to a range of 30–60 mg. Patients with neurological or psychogenic impotence are more sensitive to the effect of papaverine than those with vascular abnormalities. **Phentolamine** (0.25–1.25 mg) can be added if the response is inadequate.

Persistence of the erection for longer than 4 hours is an emergency requiring aspiration of the corpora; if aspiration fails, 1 mg of metaraminol can be diluted to 5 mL with sodium chloride injection 0.9% and given by careful slow injection into the corpora.

Other side-effects include vasovagal attacks and syncope; caution is needed in patients with cardiovascular disease and ischaemic attacks.

Local side-effects include haematoma and burning pain at the site of injection and fibrotic changes in the corpora cavernosa (which may lead to Peyronie-like erectile distortion).

PAPAVERINE
Indications; Cautions; Side-effects: see notes above

Note. Papaverine is available as a 'special order' [unlicensed] product, contact Boots, Martindale, Penn or regional hospital manufacturing unit

PHENTOLAMINE
Indications; Cautions; Side-effects: see notes above; phaeochromocytoma, see section 2.5.4

Note. Phentolamine is not licensed for use in erectile dysfunction

ALPROSTADIL

Alprostadil (prostaglandin E_1) is given by intracavernosal injection for the management of erectile dysfunction; it is also used as a diagnostic test

ALPROSTADIL
Indications: erectile dysfunction; neonatal congenital heart defects, see section 7.1.1.1

Cautions: prolonged erection (priapism)—patients should be instructed to report any erection lasting 4 hours or longer; treatment of prolonged erection should not be delayed more than 6 hours—metaraminol **not** recommended (may induce severe hypertensive crisis, consult data sheet); anatomical deformations of penis (painful erection more likely)

Contra-indications: predisposition to prolonged erection (as in sickle cell anaemia, multiple myeloma or leukaemia)

Side-effects: pain during erection, prolonged erection (see under Cautions), haematoma at site of injection; also fibrosis, erythema, testicular or perineal pain, penile deviations, haemosiderin deposits in the penis; systemic effects reported (sometimes due to faulty injection technique) include blood pressure changes, postural hypotension, arrhythmias, dizziness, headache, vagal shock and collapse

Dose: by direct *intracavernous injection,* 2.5 micrograms increasing in steps of 2.5 micrograms to obtain dose suitable for producing an erection not lasting more than 1 hour; usual range 10–20 micrograms; max. 60 micrograms (max. frequency of injection not more than once in any 1 day and not more than 3 times in any 1 week)

Note. The first dose must be given by medically trained personnel; self administration may only be undertaken after proper training

▼ PoM **Caverject**® (Upjohn)

Injection, powder for reconstitution, alprostadil. Net price 20-microgram vial (with diluent) = £9.95 (hosp. only)

7.5 Appliances for urinary disorders

For details of **appliances for urinary disorders,** see Appendix 8.

8: Drugs used in the treatment of
MALIGNANT DISEASE and for IMMUNOSUPPRESSION

In this chapter, drug treatment is discussed under the following headings:

8.1 Cytotoxic drugs
8.2 Drugs affecting the immune response
8.3 Sex hormones and hormone antagonists in malignant disease

Malignant disease may be treated by surgery, radio-therapy, and/or chemotherapy. Certain tumours are highly sensitive to chemotherapy but many are not, and inappropriate drug administration in these circumstances can only increase morbidity or mortality.

8.1 Cytotoxic drugs

8.1.1 Alkylating drugs
8.1.2 Cytotoxic antibiotics
8.1.3 Antimetabolites
8.1.4 Vinca alkaloids and etoposide
8.1.5 Other antineoplastic drugs

Great care is needed when prescribing these drugs as damage to normal tissue, which may be irreversible, is an almost invariable consequence of their use. These drugs should rarely, if ever, be used empirically in a patient with cancer, and administration should always be regarded as a clinical trial with clear objectives in mind.

CRM guidelines on cytotoxic drug handling:

1. Trained personnel should reconstitute cytotoxics;
2. Reconstitution should be carried out in designated areas;
3. Protective clothing (including gloves) should be worn;
4. The eyes should be protected and means of first aid should be specified;
5. Pregnant staff should not handle cytotoxics;
6. Adequate care should be taken in the disposal of waste material, including syringes, containers, and absorbent material.

In a minority of cancers, chemotherapy may result in cure, or marked prolongation of survival. Here short-term drug-related toxicity, which may be severe, is acceptable. However, for the majority of patients, modest survival prolongation or palliation of symptoms will be the aim, and an attempt should be made to use relatively non-toxic treatments, or to consider the use of other effective modalities, e.g. radiotherapy.

Cytotoxics may be used either singly, or in combination. In the latter case, the initial letters of the drug names, or proprietary names, identify the regimen used. Drug combinations are frequently more toxic than single drugs but may have the advantage in certain tumours of enhanced response and increased survival. However for some tumours, single-agent chemotherapy remains the treatment of choice.

Most cytotoxic drugs are teratogenic, and all may cause life-threatening toxicity; administration should, where possible, be confined to those experienced in their use.

Because of the complexity of dosage regimens in the treatment of malignant disease, dose statements have been omitted from some of the drug entries in this chapter. *In all cases detailed specialist literature should be consulted.*

Prescriptions should **not** be repeated except on the instructions of a specialist.

Cytotoxic drugs fall naturally into a number of classes, each with characteristic antitumour activity, sites of action, and toxicity. A knowledge of sites of metabolism and excretion is important, as impaired drug handling as a result of disease is not uncommon and may result in enhanced toxic effects. A number of side-effects are characteristic of particular agents or groups of drugs, e.g. neurotoxicity of vinca alkaloids, and details will be provided in the appropriate sections. Most toxic effects are, however, common to many of these drugs and will be briefly outlined here.

EXTRAVASATION OF INTRAVENOUS DRUGS. A number of drugs will cause severe local tissue necrosis if leakage into the extravascular compartment occurs. Recommended modes of administration must be adhered to. Infusion of vesicant drugs should be stopped immediately if local pain is experienced. Where doubt exists as to whether significant leakage has occurred, the infusion should be discontinued and the cannula resited in another vein. There are no proven antidotes for extravasation, but general recommendations include elevation of the limb and application of ice packs three or four times daily until pain and swelling settle; if ulceration occurs plastic surgery may be required.

HYPERURICAEMIA. Hyperuricaemia, which can result in uric acid crystal formation in the urinary tract with associated renal dysfunction is a complication of the treatment of non-Hodgkin's lymphoma and leukaemia. Allopurinol (see section 10.1.4) should be started 24 hours before treating such tumours, and should be continued for 7 to 10 days (it is not required again unless further therapy is given for tumour relapse); patients should be adequately hydrated. The dose of mercaptopurine or azathioprine should be reduced if allopurinol needs to be given concomitantly (see Appendix 1).

NAUSEA AND VOMITING. Nausea and vomiting is a source of considerable distress to many patients receiving chemotherapy. It should be anticipated and, where possible, prevented with anti-emetic treatment tailored to the chemotherapy regimen and the response of the patient.

If first-line anti-emetics are ineffective treatment should be escalated as below. Hospital admission may be necessary.

Group 1: severe emesis unlikely
Drugs in this group include alkylating drugs by mouth, intravenous fluorouracil, vinca alkaloids, and methotrexate.

Phenothiazines (e.g. prochlorperazine) or domperidone, given by mouth, when necessary, will often suffice. Premedication with these drugs is often useful before intravenous chemotherapy, treatment being continued for up to 24 hours afterwards. Both prochlorperazine and domperidone are also available as suppositories which is useful for patients who develop vomiting despite oral therapy.

Group 2: moderate emesis
Drugs in this group include intravenous cyclophosphamide and doxorubicin; premedication is essential for all drugs in this group. Most patients can be treated on an out-patient basis therefore, if possible, the anti-emetics should be given by mouth.

Anti emetics in group 1 are given when necessary but it is usually preferable to give in addition dexamethasone 10 mg by mouth before and 6 hours after chemotherapy, and/or lorazepam 1 to 2 mg by mouth given similarly. Lorazepam has the advantage of causing drowsiness and amnesia, but patients cannot drive after it. Nabilone is little used and may cause dysphoria. Ondansetron may also have a valuable role.

Patients in group 1 with an unsatisfactory response can be transferred to drugs in this group.

Group 3: severe emesis
Drugs in this group include mustine, dacarbazine, and cisplatin. They commonly cause severe emesis, particularly if used in combination.

A simple well-tolerated anti-emetic regimen is dexamethasone 10 mg by mouth with lorazepam 1 to 2 mg by mouth, given before and 6 hours after chemotherapy. Out-patients should be warned not to drive. Dexamethasone and lorazepam can also be given intravenously to inpatients; the dose of lorazepam is titrated according to the patient's level of consciousness (drowsiness should be obtained with 2 to 4 mg). This regimen should be avoided in patients with chronic chest disease and care is necessary in the elderly.

The specific ($5HT_3$) serotonin antagonists (i.e. granisetron, ondansetron, tropisetron) are perhaps the most effective drugs for controlling early emesis associated with drugs in this group, but are relatively ineffective at controlling late (after 24 hours) emesis. Intravenous administration of a single dose, usually with dexamethasone, is widely used for patients in this group together with other anti-emetics (e.g. lorazepam, domperidone) as required.

Intravenous high-dose metoclopramide (see section 4.6) has now been largely replaced by the $5HT_3$ antagonists.

Patients in group 2 with an unsatisfactory response can be transferred to drugs in this group.

BONE-MARROW SUPPRESSION. All cytotoxic drugs except vincristine and bleomycin cause marrow depression. This commonly occurs 7 to 10 days after administration, but is delayed for certain drugs, such as carmustine, lomustine, and melphalan. Peripheral blood counts must be checked prior to each treatment, and doses should be reduced or therapy delayed if marrow recovery has not occurred. Fever occurring in a neutropenic patient (neutrophil count less than 0.8×10^9/litre) is an indication for immediate parenteral broad-spectrum antibiotic therapy (see section 5.1, Table 1), once appropriate bacteriological investigations have taken place.

ALOPECIA. Reversible hair loss is a common complication, although it varies in degree between drugs and individual patients. No pharmacological methods of preventing this are available.

REPRODUCTIVE FUNCTION. Most cytotoxic drugs are teratogenic and should not be administered during pregnancy, especially during the first trimester (but for transplant therapy, see below).

Contraceptive advice should be offered where appropriate before cytotoxic therapy begins (and should cover the duration of contraception required after therapy has ended). Regimens that do not contain an alkylating drug may have less effect on fertility, but those with an alkylating drug carry the risk of causing permanent male sterility (there is no effect on potency). Pre-treatment counselling and consideration of sperm storage may be appropriate. Females are less severely affected, though the span of reproductive life may be shortened by the onset of a premature menopause. No increase in fetal abnormalities or abortion-rate has been recorded in patients who remain fertile after cytotoxic chemotherapy.

Transplant therapy. Female transplanted patients immunosuppressed with azathioprine should not discontinue it on becoming pregnant; there is no evidence that azathioprine used properly is teratogenic. There is less experience of cyclosporin in pregnancy but it does not appear to be any more harmful than azathioprine. Any risk to the offspring of azathioprine-treated men is small.

8.1.1 Alkylating drugs

Extensive experience is available with these drugs, which are among the most widely used in cancer chemotherapy. They act by damaging DNA, thus interfering with cell replication. In addition to the side-effects common to many cytotoxic drugs (section 8.1), there are two problems associated with prolonged usage. Firstly, gametogenesis is often severely affected (see above). Secondly, prolonged use of these drugs, particularly when combined with extensive irradiation, is associated with a marked increase in the incidence of acute non-lymphocytic leukaemia.

Cyclophosphamide is widely used in the treatment of chronic lymphocytic leukaemia, the lymphomas, and solid tumours. It is given *by mouth* or *intravenously* and is inactive until metabolised by the liver. A urinary metabolite of cyclophosphamide, acrolein, may cause haemorrhagic cystitis; this is a rare but very serious complication; if it occurs cyclophosphamide is not normally used again. An increased fluid intake, for 24–48 hours after intravenous injection, will help avoid this complication. When high-dose therapy (e.g. more than 2 g intravenously) is used mesna (given initially intravenously then by mouth) will also help prevent this.

Ifosfamide is related to cyclophosphamide and is given *intravenously*; it is *routinely* given with mesna to reduce urothelial toxicity.

Chlorambucil is commonly used to treat chronic lymphocytic leukaemia, the indolent non-Hodgkin's lymphomas, Hodgkin's disease, and ovarian cancer. It is given *by mouth*. Side-effects, apart from marrow suppression, are uncommon, although rashes may occur.

Melphalan is used to treat myeloma and occasionally solid tumours and lymphomas. It is usually given *by mouth*, but may also be given *intravenously*. Marrow toxicity is delayed and it is usually given at intervals of 4–6 weeks.

Busulphan is used almost exclusively to treat chronic myeloid leukaemia and is given *by mouth*. Frequent blood counts are necessary as excessive myelosuppression may result in irreversible bone-marrow aplasia. Hyperpigmentation of the skin is a common side-effect and, rarely, progressive pulmonary fibrosis may occur.

Lomustine is a lipid-soluble nitrosourea and is given *by mouth*. It is mainly used to treat Hodgkin's disease and certain solid tumours. Marrow toxicity is delayed, and the drug is therefore given at intervals of 4 to 6 weeks. Permanent marrow damage may occur with prolonged use. Nausea and vomiting are common and moderately severe.

Carmustine is given *intravenously*. It has similar activity and toxicities to lomustine and is most commonly given to patients with myeloma, lymphoma, and brain tumours. Cumulative renal damage and delayed pulmonary fibrosis may occur.

Mustine is now much less commonly used. It is a very toxic drug which causes severe vomiting. The freshly prepared injection must be given into a fast-running *intravenous infusion*. Local extravasation causes severe tissue necrosis.

Estramustine is a stable combination of an oestrogen and mustine, designed to deliver mustine to the oestrogen receptor site of a tumour, for example prostate cancer. It is given *by mouth* and has both a local cytotoxic effect and (by reducing testosterone concentrations) a hormonal effect.

Treosulfan is given *by mouth* or *intravenously* and is used to treat ovarian cancer.

Thiotepa is usually used as an *intracavitary* drug for the treatment of malignant effusions or bladder cancer (see section 7.4.4). It is also occasionally used to treat breast cancer, but requires parenteral administration.

Mitobronitol is occasionally used to treat chronic myeloid leukaemia; it is available on a named-patient basis only (as *Myelobromol®*, Sinclair).

BUSULPHAN

Indications: chronic myeloid leukaemia
Cautions; Side-effects: see section 8.1 and notes above; avoid in porphyria (see section 9.8.2)
Dose: induction of remission, 60 micrograms/kg to max. 4 mg daily; maintenance, 0.5–2 mg daily

PoM **Myleran®** (Wellcome)
Tablets, busulphan 500 micrograms, net price 25 = £3.53; 2 mg, 25 = £5.32

CARMUSTINE

Indications: see notes above
Cautions; Side-effects: see section 8.1 and notes above; irritant to tissues

PoM **BiCNU®** (Bristol-Myers)
Injection, powder for reconstitution, carmustine. Net price 100-mg vial (with diluent) = £12.50

CHLORAMBUCIL

Indications: see notes above (for use as an immunosuppressant see section 8.2.1)
Cautions; Side-effects: see section 8.1 and notes above; caution in renal impairment; avoid in porphyria (see section 9.8.2)
Dose: used alone, usually 100–200 micrograms/kg daily for 4–8 weeks

PoM **Leukeran®** (Wellcome)
Tablets, both yellow, chlorambucil 2 mg, net price 25 = £8.55; 5 mg, 25 = £13.04

CYCLOPHOSPHAMIDE

Indications: see notes above
Cautions; Side-effects: see section 8.1 and notes above; reduce dose in renal impairment; avoid in porphyria (see section 9.8.2); **interactions:** Appendix 1 (cyclophosphamide)

PoM **Cyclophosphamide** (Pharmacia)
Tablets, pink, s/c, cyclophosphamide (anhydrous) 50 mg. Net price 20 = £2.12. Label: 27
Injection, powder for reconstitution, cyclophosphamide. Net price 107-mg vial = £1.06; 214-mg vial = £1.50; 535-mg vial = £2.62; 1.07-g vial = £4.58
PoM **Endoxana®** (ASTA Medica)
Tablets, s/c, cyclophosphamide 50 mg, net price 100-tab pack = £10.50 Label: 27
Injection, powder for reconstitution, cyclophosphamide. Net price 100-mg vial = 93p; 200-mg vial = £1.34; 500-mg vial = £2.34; 1-g vial = £4.09

ESTRAMUSTINE PHOSPHATE

Indications: prostate cancer
Cautions: see section 8.1
Contra-indications: peptic ulceration, severe liver or cardiac disease
Side-effects: see section 8.1; also gynaecomastia, altered liver function, cardiovascular disorders (angina and rare reports of myocardial infarction)
Dose: 0.14–1.4 g daily in divided doses (usual initial dose 560 mg daily)
COUNSELLING. Each dose should be taken not less than 1 hour before or 2 hours after meals and should not be taken with dairy products

PoM **Estracyt®** (Pharmacia)
Capsules, estramustine phosphate 140 mg (as disodium salt). Net price 100-cap pack = £149.46. Label: 23 counselling, see above

IFOSFAMIDE

Indications: see notes above
Cautions; Side-effects: see section 8.1 and notes under Cyclophosphamide; reduce dose in renal impairment; **interactions:** Appendix 1 (cyclophosphamide and ifosfamide)

PoM **Mitoxana®** (ASTA Medica)
Injection, powder for reconstitution, ifosfamide. Net price 1-g vial = £15.13; 2-g vial = £27.95 (hosp. only)

LOMUSTINE

Indications: see notes above
Cautions; Side-effects: see section 8.1 and notes above
Dose: used alone, 120–130 mg/m² body-surface every 6–8 weeks

PoM **CCNU®** (Lundbeck)
Capsules, lomustine 10 mg (blue/white), net price 20 = £9.42; 40 mg (blue), 20 = £23.69

MELPHALAN

Indications: myelomatosis; see also notes above
Cautions; Side-effects: see section 8.1 and notes above; reduce dose in renal impairment; **interactions:** Appendix 1 (melphalan)
Dose: by mouth,150–300 micrograms/kg daily for 4–6 days, repeated after 4–8 weeks

PoM **Alkeran®** (Wellcome)
Tablets, melphalan 2 mg, net price 25 = £11.73; 5 mg, 25 = £20.75
Injection, powder for reconstitution, melphalan 50 mg (as hydrochloride). Net price 50-mg vial (with solvent-diluent) = £28.26

MUSTINE HYDROCHLORIDE

(Chlormethine Hydrochloride)
Indications: Hodgkin's disease—see notes above
Cautions; Side-effects: see section 8.1 and notes above; irritant to tissues (also caution in handling—vesicant and a nasal irritant)

PoM **Mustine Hydrochloride** (Boots)
Injection, powder for reconstitution, mustine hydrochloride. Net price 10-mg vial = £15.00

THIOTEPA

Indications: see notes above and section 7.4.4
Cautions; Side-effects: see section 8.1; **interactions:** Appendix 1 (thiotepa)

PoM **Thiotepa** (Lederle)
Injection, powder for reconstitution, thiotepa, net price 15-mg vial = £4.85

TREOSULFAN

Indications: see notes above
Cautions; Side-effects: see section 8.1
Dose: by mouth, courses of 1–2 g daily in 4 divided doses to provide total dose of 21–28 g over initial 8 weeks

PoM **Treosulfan** (Medac)
Capsules, treosulfan 250 mg. Net price 20 = £23.00. Label: 25
Injection, powder for reconstitution, treosulfan. Net price 5 g in infusion bottle with transfer needle = £54.60

UROTHELIAL TOXICITY

Urothelial toxicity, commonly manifest by haemorrhagic cystitis, is a problem peculiar to the use of cyclophosphamide or ifosfamide and is caused by a metabolite (acrolein). **Mesna** reacts specifically with this metabolite in the urinary tract, preventing toxicity. Mesna is given simultaneously with cyclophosphamide or ifosfamide, and further doses are given *by mouth* or *intravenously* 4 and 8 hours after treatment.

MESNA

Indications: see notes above
Side-effects: above max. therapeutic doses, gastro-intestinal disturbances, fatigue, headache, limb pains, depression, irritability, lack of energy, rash

PoM **Uromitexan®** (ASTA Medica)
Injection, mesna 100 mg/mL. Net price 4-mL amp = £1.56; 10-mL amp = £3.39
Note. For oral administration contents of ampoule are taken in fruit juice

8.1.2 Cytotoxic antibiotics

Drugs within this group are widely used. Many cytotoxic antibiotics act as radiomimetics and simultaneous use of radiotherapy should be **avoided** as it may result in markedly enhanced normal tissue toxicity.

Doxorubicin is one of the most successful and widely used antitumour drugs, and is used to treat the acute leukaemias, lymphomas, and a variety of solid tumours. It is given by fast running *infusion,* commonly at 21-day intervals. Local extravasation will cause severe tissue necrosis. Common toxic effects include nausea and vomiting, myelosuppression, alopecia, and mucositis. This drug is largely excreted by the biliary tract, and an elevated bilirubin concentration is an indication for reducing the dose. Supraventricular tachycardia related to drug administration is an uncommon complication. Higher cumulative doses are associated with development of a cardiomyopathy. It is customary to limit total cumulative doses to 450 mg/m^2 body-surface area as symptomatic and potentially fatal heart failure is increasingly common above this level. Patients with pre-existing cardiac disease, the elderly, and those who have received myocardial irradiation should be treated cautiously. Cardiac monitoring, for example by sequential radionuclide ejection fraction measurement, may assist in safely limiting total dosage. Evidence is available to suggest that weekly low dose administration may be associated with less cardiac damage. Doxorubicin is also given by *bladder instillation* (see section 7.4.4).

Epirubicin is structurally related to doxorubicin and clinical trials suggest that it is as effective in the treatment of breast cancer. A maximum cumulative dose of 0.9–1 g/m^2 is recommended to help avoid cardiotoxicity. Like doxorubicin it is given *intravenously* and by *bladder instillation* (see section 7.4.4).

Aclarubicin and **idarubicin** are newly introduced anthracyclines with general properties similar to those of doxorubicin. They are both given *intravenously*. Idarubicin may also be given *by mouth*.

Mitozantrone is structurally related to doxorubicin and preliminary work suggests that it has equal activity in breast cancer. It is given *intravenously* and is well tolerated apart from myelosuppression and dose-related cardiotoxicity; cardiac examinations are recommended after a cumulative dose of 160 mg/m^2 if this complication is to be avoided.

Bleomycin is given *intravenously* or *intramuscularly* to treat the lymphomas, certain solid tumours and, by the *intracavitary route*, malignant effusions. It is unusual in that it causes little marrow suppression. Dermatological toxicity is common; increased pigmentation particularly affecting the flexures and subcutaneous sclerotic plaques may occur. Mucositis is also relatively common and an association with Raynaud's phenomenon is reported. Hypersensitivity reactions manifest by chills and fevers commonly occur a few hours after drug administration and may be prevented by simultaneous administration of a corticosteroid, for example hydrocortisone intravenously. The principal problem associated with the use of bleomycin is progressive pulmonary fibrosis. This is dose related, occurring more commonly at cumulative doses greater than 300 units and in the elderly. Basal lung crepitations or suspicious chest X-ray changes are an indication to stop therapy with this drug. Patients who have received extensive treatment with bleomycin (e.g. cumulative dose more than 100 units) may be at risk of developing respiratory failure if a general anaesthetic is given with

high inspired oxygen concentrations. Anaesthetists should be warned of this.

Dactinomycin is principally used to treat paediatric cancers; it is given *intravenously*. Its side-effects are similar to those of doxorubicin, except that cardiac toxicity is not a problem.

Plicamycin (mithramycin) is no longer used as a cytotoxic, but has found a useful (though diminishing) role in low dose in the emergency therapy of hypercalcaemia due to malignant disease (for general management of hypercalcaemia, see section 9.5.1.2). It is given *intravenously*.

Mitomycin is given *intravenously* to treat upper gastro-intestinal and breast cancers. It causes delayed marrow toxicity and is usually administered at 6-weekly intervals. Prolonged use may result in permanent marrow damage. It is a relatively toxic drug and may cause lung fibrosis and renal damage. It is also given by *bladder instillation* (see section 7.4.4).

ACLARUBICIN

Indications: acute non-lymphocytic leukaemia in patients who have relapsed or are resistant or refractory to first-line chemotherapy

Cautions; Side-effects: see section 8.1 and notes above; caution in hepatic and renal impairment; irritant to tissues

PoM Aclacin® (Lundbeck)
Injection, powder for reconstitution, aclarubicin 20 mg (as hydrochloride). Net price 20-mg vial = £29.20

BLEOMYCIN

Indications: squamous cell carcinoma; see also notes above

Cautions; Side-effects: see section 8.1 and notes above; reduce dose in renal impairment; also caution in handling—irritant to skin

PoM Bleomycin (Lundbeck)
Injection, powder for reconstitution, bleomycin (as sulphate). Net price 15-unit amp = £16.29
Note. Ampoules previously labelled as containing '15 mg' of bleomycin contained 15 units. The ampoules are now labelled only as units.

DACTINOMYCIN
(Actinomycin D)
Indications: see notes above
Cautions; Side-effects: see section 8.1 and notes above; irritant to tissues

PoM Cosmegen Lyovac® (MSD)
Injection, powder for reconstitution, dactinomycin, net price 500-microgram vial = £1.50

DOXORUBICIN HYDROCHLORIDE

Indications: see notes above and section 7.4.4

Cautions; Side-effects: see section 8.1 and notes above; reduce dose in hepatic impairment; also caution in handling—irritant to skin and tissues; **interactions:** see Appendix 1 (doxorubicin)

PoM **Doxorubicin Rapid Dissolution**
(Pharmacia)

Injection, powder for reconstitution, doxorubicin hydrochloride, net price 10-mg vial = £18.72; 50-mg vial = £93.60

*Note.*This preparation has replaced Adriamycin®

PoM **Doxorubicin Solution for Injection**
(Pharmacia)

Injection, doxorubicin hydrochloride 2 mg/mL, net price 5-ml vial = £20.60; 25-mL vial = £103.00

Various strengths and sizes also available from David Bull

EPIRUBICIN HYDROCHLORIDE

Indications: see notes above and section 7.4.4

Cautions; Side-effects: see section 8.1 and notes above; reduce dose in hepatic impairment; irritant to tissues

PoM **Pharmorubicin® Rapid Dissolution**
(Pharmacia)

Injection, powder for reconstitution, epirubicin hydrochloride. Net price 10-mg vial = £16.85; 20-mg vial = £33.70; 50-mg vial = £84.24

PoM **Pharmorubicin® Solution for Injection**
(Pharmacia)

Injection, epirubicin hydrochloride 2 mg/mL, net price 5-mL vial = £18.54; 25-mL vial = £92.70

IDARUBICIN HYDROCHLORIDE

Indications: advanced breast cancer after failure of frontline chemotherapy (not including anthracyclines); acute leukaemias—see notes above

Cautions; Side-effects: see section 8.1 and notes above; caution in hepatic and renal impairment; also caution in handling—irritant to skin and tissues

PoM **Zavedos®** (Pharmacia)

Capsules, idarubicin hydrochloride, 5 mg (orange), net price 1-cap pack = £28.80; 10 mg (red/white), 1-cap pack = £57.60; 25 mg (orange/white), 1-cap pack = £144.00. Label: 25

Injection, powder for reconstitution, idarubicin hydrochloride, net price 5 mg vial = £72.80; 10-mg vial = £145.60

MITOMYCIN

Indications: see notes above and section 7.4.4

Cautions; Side-effects: see section 8.1 and notes above; irritant to tissues

PoM **Mitomycin C Kyowa®** (Kyowa Hakko)

Injection, powder for reconstitution, mitomycin. Net price 2-mg vial = £6.16; 10-mg vial = £20.28; 20-mg vial = £38.68 (hosp. only)

MITOZANTRONE

(Mitoxantrone)

Indications: see notes above

Cautions; Side-effects: see section 8.1 and notes above; intrathecal administration not recommended

PoM **Novantrone®** (Lederle)

Intravenous infusion, mitozantrone 2 mg (as hydrochloride)/mL, net price 10-mL vial = £150.43; 12.5-mL vial = £188.05; 15-mL vial = £225.60

PLICAMYCIN

(Mithramycin)

Indications: refractory hypercalcaemia associated with malignancy—see notes above

Cautions; Side-effects: see section 8.1 and notes above; caution in hepatic or renal impairment (see Appendixes 2 and 3); irritant to tissues

Dose: by intravenous infusion, 25 micrograms/kg daily for 3–4 days, repeated if necessary at intervals of 7 days or longer; maintenance, 25 micrograms/kg 1–3 times each week

PoM **Mithracin®** (Pfizer)

Injection, powder for reconstitution, plicamycin, net price 2.5-mg vial = £7.51 (hosp. only)

8.1.3 Antimetabolites

Antimetabolites are incorporated into new nuclear material or combine irreversibly with vital cellular enzymes, preventing normal cellular division.

Methotrexate inhibits the enzyme dihydrofolate reductase, essential for the synthesis of purines and pyrimidines. It is given *by mouth, intravenously, intramuscularly,* or *intrathecally.* High-dose methotrexate cannot generally be recommended except in clinical trials.

Methotrexate is used as maintenance therapy for childhood acute lymphoblastic leukaemia. Other uses include choriocarcinoma, non-Hodgkin lymphomas, and a number of solid tumours. Intrathecal methotrexate is used in the CNS prophylaxis of childhood acute lymphoblastic leukaemia, and as a therapy for established meningeal cancer or lymphoma.

Methotrexate causes myelosuppression, mucositis, and rarely pneumonitis. It is **contra-indicated** if significant renal impairment is present, as the kidney is its route of excretion. It should also be **avoided** if a significant pleural effusion or ascites is present as it tends to accumulate at these sites, and its subsequent return to the circulation will be associated with myelosuppression. For similar reasons blood counts should be carefully monitored when intrathecal methotrexate is given.

Oral or parenteral folinic acid (see below) will help prevent, and speed recovery from, methotrexate mucositis or myelosuppression.

Cytarabine acts by interfering with pyrimidine synthesis. It is given *subcutaneously, intravenously,* or *intrathecally.* Its predominant use is in the induction of remission of acute myeloblastic leukaemia. It is a potent myelosuppressant and requires careful haematological monitoring.

Fluorouracil may be given *by mouth* but is usually given *intravenously*. It is used to treat a number of solid tumours, including colon and breast cancer. It may also be used topically for certain malignant skin lesions. Toxicity is unusual, but may include myelosuppression, mucositis, and rarely a cerebellar syndrome. It is also used *topically* as a cream.

Mercaptopurine is used almost exclusively as maintenance therapy for the acute leukaemias. The dose should be reduced if the patient is receiving concurrent allopurinol as this drug interferes with the metabolism of mercaptopurine.

Thioguanine is given *by mouth* to induce remission in acute myeloid leukaemia.

Azathioprine, a derivative of the antimetabolite mercaptopurine is given *by mouth*. It is commonly used as an immunosuppressant (section 8.2.1).

CYTARABINE

Indications: acute leukaemias
Cautions; Side-effects: see section 8.1 and notes above

PoM Cytarabine (Non-proprietary)
Injection, cytarabine 20 mg/mL. Net price 5-mL vial = £3.73
Injection, cytarabine 100 mg/mL. Net price 1-mL vial = £3.73; 10-mL vial = £36.73
Injection, powder for reconstitution, cytarabine. Net price 500-mg vial (with diluent) = £17.19; 1-g vial = £34.28; 1-g vial (with diluent) = £34.49
Available from David Bull
PoM Alexan® (Pfizer)
Injection, cytarabine 20 mg/mL. Net price 2-mL amp = £1.16; 5-mL amp = £2.91
PoM Alexan® 100 (Pfizer)
Injection, cytarabine 100 mg/mL. Net price 1-mL amp = £2.65; 10-mL amp = £26.46. For intravenous infusion only
PoM Cytosar® (Upjohn)
Injection, powder for reconstitution, cytarabine. Net price 100-mg vial = £3.01, 100-mg vial (with diluent) = £3.17; 500-mg vial = £14.95, 500-mg vial (with diluent) = £15.45. For intravenous injection or infusion and subcutaneous injection only

FLUOROURACIL

Indications: see notes above
Cautions; Side-effects: see section 8.1; also caution in handling—irritant; **interactions:** Appendix 1 (fluorouracil)
Dose: by mouth, maintenance 15 mg/kg weekly; max. in one day 1 g

PoM Fluorouracil (Non-proprietary)
Injection, fluorouracil 25 mg/mL (as sodium salt). Net price 10-mL vial = £2.00; 20-mL vial = £3.85; 100-mL vial = £18.67
Available from David Bull

PoM Fluoro-uracil (Roche)
Capsules, blue/orange, fluorouracil 250 mg. Net price 30-cap pack = £35.38. Label: 21
Injection, fluorouracil 25 mg/mL (as sodium salt). Net price 10-mL amp = £1.26
*Note.*The injection solution can also be given by mouth in fruit juice
PoM Efudix® (Roche)
Cream, fluorouracil 5%. Net price 20 g = £4.13

MERCAPTOPURINE

Indications: acute leukaemias
Cautions; Side-effects: see section 8.1 and notes above; reduce dose in renal impairment; avoid in porphyria (see section 9.8.2); **interactions:** Appendix 1 (mercaptopurine)
Dose: initially 2.5 mg/kg daily

PoM Puri-Nethol® (Wellcome)
Tablets, fawn, scored, mercaptopurine 50 mg. Net price 25 = £19.22

METHOTREXATE

Indications: see notes above and under Dose; rheumatoid arthritis, see section 10.1.3; psoriasis, see section 13.5.2
Cautions; Side-effects: see section 8.1 and notes above; reduce dose in renal impairment; dose-related toxicity in hepatic impairment; porphyria (see section 9.8.2); **interactions:** Appendix 1 (methotrexate)
Dose: by mouth, leukaemia in children (maintenance), 15 mg/m² weekly in combination with other drugs

PoM Methotrexate (Lederle)
Tablets, yellow, scored, methotrexate 2.5 mg, net price 20 = £2.12. Counselling, NSAIDs, see p.439
Injection, methotrexate 25 mg (as sodium salt)/mL. Net price 1-mL vial = £1.89; 2-mL vial = £2.62; 4-mL vial = £5.01; 8-mL vial = £10.02; 20-mL vial = £25.07; 40-mL vial = £44.57; 200-mL vial = £200.57
Note. Various strengths and sizes also available from David Bull
PoM Maxtrex® (Pharmacia)
Tablets, both yellow, scored, methotrexate 2.5 mg, net price 20 = £2.09; 10 mg, 20 = £9.46. Counselling, NSAIDs, see p.439

THIOGUANINE

Indications: acute leukaemias
Cautions; Side-effects: see section 8.1 and notes above; reduce dose in renal impairment
Dose: initially 2–2.5 mg/kg daily

PoM Lanvis® (Wellcome)
Tablets, yellow, scored, thioguanine 40 mg. Net price 25-tab pack = £46.48

FOLINIC ACID RESCUE

Folinic acid (leucovorin) is used to counteract the folate-antagonist action of methotrexate and thus speed recovery from methotrexate-induced mucositis or myelosuppression. It is generally given 24 hours after the methotrexate, in a dose of 15 mg by mouth every 6 hours, for 2–8 doses (depending on the dose of methotrexate). It does not counteract the antibacterial activity of folate antagonists such as trimethoprim.

Folinic acid also interacts with fluorouracil; when the two are used together in metastatic colonic cancer a favourable effect has been demonstrated on response-rate.

FOLINIC ACID

Indications: see notes above
Cautions: avoid simultaneous administration of methotrexate; as for Folic Acid (section 9.1.2) **not** indicated for pernicious anaemia or other megaloblastic anaemias where vitamin B_{12} deficient
Side-effects: rarely, pyrexia after parenteral administration
Dose: as an antidote to methotrexate (started 8–24 hours after the beginning of methotrexate infusion), in general up to 120 mg in divided doses over 12–24 hours *by intramuscular or intravenous injection or infusion*, followed by 12–15 mg *intramuscularly or* 15 mg *by mouth* every 6 hours for the next 48–72 hours
Suspected methotrexate overdosage, immediate administration of an equal or higher dose of folinic acid

PoM **Calcium Folinate** (Non-proprietary)
Tablets, scored, folinic acid (as calcium salt) 15 mg Available from David Bull (net price 10-tab pack = £36.75), Lagap (net price 10-tab pack = £49.84)
PoM **Calcium Leucovorin** (Lederle)
Tablets, scored, folinic acid 15 mg (as calcium salt). Net price 10-tab pack = £41.22
Injection, folinic acid 3 mg (as calcium salt)/mL. Net price 1-mL amp = £1.06; 350-mg vial (Lederfolin® Solution) = £90.98
Various strengths and sizes also available from David Bull
Injection, powder for reconstitution, folinic acid (as calcium salt). Net price 15-mg vial = £4.46; 30-mg vial = £8.36; 350-mg vial (Lederfolin®) = £90.98

PoM **Refolinon®** (Pharmacia)
Tablets, yellow, scored, folinic acid 15 mg (as calcium salt). Net price 30 = £94.50
Injection, folinic acid 3 mg (as calcium salt)/mL. Net price 10-mL amp = £5.70

8.1.4 Vinca alkaloids and etoposide

These interfere with microtubule assembly, causing metaphase arrest. All have similar activity but vary in the predominant site of toxicity.

The vinca alkaloids are used to treat the acute leukaemias, lymphomas, and some solid tumours (e.g. breast and lung cancer). They commonly cause peripheral and autonomic neuropathy. This side-effect is most obvious with vincristine, and is manifest by peripheral paraesthesia, loss of deep tendon reflexes, and abdominal bloating and constipation. If these symptoms are severe, doses should be reduced. Significant new motor weakness is a **contra-indication** to further use of these drugs. Recovery of the nervous system is generally slow but complete. Intrathecal administration of **all** vinca alkaloids is **contra-indicated** (usually fatal).

Vincristine causes virtually no myelosuppression. Its use may be associated with alopecia; hyponatraemia, as a result of inappropriate ADH secretion, has been described. It is given *intravenously.*

Vinblastine is a more myelosuppressive drug than vincristine, but causes less neurotoxicity. It is given *intravenously.*

Vindesine is the most recent addition to the vinca alkaloid group. It has a similar range of clinical activity, and side-effects intermediate between those of the above two drugs. It is given *intravenously.*

Etoposide may be given *by mouth* or *intravenously,* the dose when used orally being double that when given intravenously. There is evidence to suggest that administration in divided doses over 3–5 days may be beneficial; courses may not be repeated more frequently than at intervals of 21 days. It has useful activity in small cell carcinoma of the bronchus, the lymphomas, and testicular teratoma. Toxic effects include alopecia, myelosuppression, nausea, and vomiting.

ETOPOSIDE

Indications: see notes above
Cautions; Contra-indications; Side-effects: see section 8.1 and notes above; irritant to tissues

PoM **Vepesid®** (Bristol-Myers)
Capsules, etoposide 50 mg, net price 20 = £113.95; 100 mg, 10-cap pack = £99.57
Injection, etoposide 20 mg/mL. To be diluted. Net price 5-mL vial = £14.58
Caution: may dissolve certain types of filter

VINBLASTINE SULPHATE

Indications: see notes above
Cautions; Contra-indications; Side-effects: see section 8.1 and notes above; caution in handling—avoid contact with eyes; irritant to tissues
Note. IMPORTANT. Intrathecal injection **contra-indicated**

PoM **Vinblastine** (Non-proprietary)
Injection, vinblastine sulphate 1 mg/mL. Net price 10-mL vial = £12.71
Available from David Bull

PoM **Velbe**® (Lilly)

Injection, powder for reconstitution, vinblastine sulphate. Net price 10-mg amp (with diluent) = £14.15

VINCRISTINE SULPHATE

Indications: see notes above

Cautions; Contra-indications; Side-effects: see section 8.1 and notes above; caution in handling—avoid contact with eyes; irritant to tissues

Note. IMPORTANT. Intrathecal injection **contra-indicated**

PoM **Vincristine** (Non-proprietary)

Injection, vincristine sulphate 1 mg/mL. Net price 1-mL vial = £10.29; 2-mL vial = £19.95; 5-mL vial = £41.58; 1-mL syringe = £11.01; 2-mL syringe = £19.95

Available from David Bull

PoM **Oncovin**® (Lilly)

Injection, vincristine sulphate 1 mg/mL, net price 1-mL vial = £14.18; 2-mL vial = £28.05

VINDESINE SULPHATE

Indications: see notes above

Cautions; Contra-indications; Side-effects: see section 8.1 and notes above; caution in handling—avoid contact with eyes; irritant to tissues

Note. IMPORTANT. Intrathecal injection **contra-indicated**

PoM **Eldisine**® (Lilly)

Injection, powder for reconstitution, vindesine sulphate, net price 5-mg vial (with diluent) = £78.30 (hosp. only)

8.1.5   Other antineoplastic drugs

AMSACRINE

Amsacrine has an action and toxic effects similar to those of doxorubicin (section 8.1.2) and is given *intravenously*. It is used in acute myeloid leukaemia. Side-effects include myelosuppression and mucositis; electrolytes should be monitored as fatal arrhythmias have occurred in association with hypokalaemia.

AMSACRINE

Indications: see notes above

Cautions; Side-effects: see section 8.1 and notes above; reduce dose in renal or hepatic impairment; also caution in handling—irritant to skin and tissues

PoM **Amsidine**® (P-D)

Concentrate for intravenous infusion, amsacrine 5 mg (as lactate)/mL, when reconstituted by mixing two solutions. Net price 1.5-mL amp with 13.5-mL vial = £30.90. (hosp. only)

Note. Use glass apparatus for reconstitution

CARBOPLATIN

Carboplatin, a derivative of cisplatin which has probably equivalent activity in ovarian cancer, is given *intravenously*. It is also active in small cell lung cancer and is under trial in a variety of other malignancies. Carboplatin is better tolerated than cisplatin; nausea and vomiting are reduced in severity and nephrotoxicity, neurotoxicity, and ototoxicity are much less of a problem than with cisplatin. It is, however, more myelosuppressive than cisplatin.

CARBOPLATIN

Indications: see notes above

Cautions; Side-effects: see section 8.1 and notes above; reduce dose in renal impairment

PoM **Paraplatin**® (Bristol-Myers)

Injection, carboplatin 10 mg/mL. Net price 5-mL vial = £22.86; 15-mL vial = £65.83; 45-mL vial = £197.48

CISPLATIN

Cisplatin has an alkylating action and is given *intravenously*. It has useful antitumour activity in certain solid tumours including ovarian cancer and testicular teratoma. It is, however, a toxic drug. Common problems include severe nausea and vomiting, nephrotoxicity (pretreatment hydration mandatory and renal function should be closely monitored), myelotoxicity, ototoxicity (high tone hearing loss and tinnitus), peripheral neuropathy, and hypomagnesaemia. These toxic effects commonly necessitate dose reduction or drug withdrawal. It is preferable that treatment with this drug be supervised by specialists familiar with its use.

CISPLATIN

Indications: see notes above

Cautions; Side-effects: see section 8.1 and notes above; reduce dose in renal impairment; **interactions:** Appendix 1 (cisplatin)

PoM **Cisplatin** (Non-proprietary)

Injection, cisplatin 1 mg/mL. Net price 10-mL vial = £5.51; 50-mL vial = £27.29; 100-mL vial = £54.02

Available from David Bull

Injection, powder for reconstitution, cisplatin. Net price 50-mg vial = £17.00

Available from Pharmacia

CRISANTASPASE

Crisantaspase is the enzyme asparaginase produced by *Erwinia chrysanthemi*. It is given *intramuscularly* or *subcutaneously* almost exclusively in acute lymphoblastic leukaemia. Facilities for the management of anaphylaxis should be available Side-effects also include nausea, vomiting, CNS depression, and liver function and blood lipid changes; careful monitoring is therefore necessary and the urine is tested for glucose to exclude hyperglycaemia.

CRISANTASPASE

Indications; Cautions; Side-effects: see notes above

PoM **Erwinase®** (Porton)
Injection, powder for reconstitution, crisantaspase. Net price 20 × 10 000-unit vial = £858.00

DACARBAZINE

Dacarbazine is not commonly used on account of its toxicity. It has been used to treat melanoma and, in combination therapy, the soft tissue sarcomas. It is also a component of a commonly used combination for Hodgkin's disease (ABVD—doxorubicin [Adriamycin®], bleomycin, vinblastine, and dacarbazine). It is given *intravenously*. The predominant side-effects are myelosuppression and intense nausea and vomiting.

DACARBAZINE

Indications: see notes above
Cautions; Side-effects: see section 8.1; also caution in handling—irritant to skin and tissues

PoM **DTIC-Dome®** (Bayer)
Injection, powder for reconstitution, dacarbazine. Net price 100-mg vial = £4.83; 200-mg vial = £7.40

HYDROXYUREA

Hydroxyurea is an orally active drug used mainly in the treatment of chronic myeloid leukaemia. It is occasionally used for polycythaemia (the usual treatment is venesection). Myelosuppression, nausea, and skin reactions are the most common toxic effects.

HYDROXYUREA

Indications: see notes above
Cautions; Side-effects: see section 8.1 and notes above
Dose: 20–30 mg/kg daily *or* 80 mg/kg every third day

PoM **Hydrea®** (Squibb)
Capsules, pink/green, hydroxyurea 500 mg. Net price 20 = £2.39

PACLITAXEL

Paclitaxel is the first of a new group of drugs termed the taxanes. It is given by *intravenous infusion*. It is licensed only for patients with ovarian cancer in whom standard platinum-containing therapy has failed (generally taken to indicate patients

with an initially poor response or whose disease progresses within six months of treatment). Paclitaxel is relatively toxic and it is recommended that its use be confined to experienced specialists. Routine premedication with a corticosteroid, an antihistamine and a histamine H_2 receptor antagonist is recommended to prevent severe hypersensitivity reactions; despite premedication these reactions may still rarely occur, more commonly only bradycardia or asymptomatic hypotension occur.

In addition to hypersensitivity side-effects of paclitaxel include myelosuppression, peripheral neuropathy, and cardiac conduction defects with arrhythmias (which are nearly always asymptomatic). It also causes alopecia and muscle pain; nausea and vomiting is mild to moderate.

Only a minority of patients respond to paclitaxel, but the responses are sometimes prolonged.

PACLITAXEL

Indications: metastatic ovarian cancer where standard platinum-containing therapy has failed
Cautions; Contra-indications; Side-effects: see section 8.1 and notes above

▼ PoM **Taxol®** (Bristol-Myers, Squibb)
Concentrate for intravenous infusion, paclitaxel 6 mg/mL. Net price 5-mL vial = £124.79 (hosp. only)
Note. Contains polyethoxylated castor oil which has been associated with anaphylaxis

---

PENTOSTATIN

Pentostatin is highly active in hairy cell leukaemia. It is given *intravenously* on alternate weeks and is capable of inducing prolonged complete remission. It is potentially toxic, causing myelosuppression, immunosuppression and a number of other side-effects which may be severe. Its use is probably best confined to specialist centres

PENTOSTATIN

Indications: see notes above
Cautions; Contra-indications; Side-effects: see section 8.1 and notes above

▼ PoM **Nipent®** (Lederle)
Injection, powder for reconstitution, pentostatin. Net price 10-mg vial = £774.00

PROCARBAZINE

Procarbazine is most often used in Hodgkin's disease, for example in MOPP (mustine, vincristine [Oncovin®], procarbazine, and prednisolone) chemotherapy. It is given *by mouth*. Toxic effects include nausea, myelosuppression, and a hypersensitivity rash preventing further use of this drug. It is a mild monoamine-oxidase inhibitor but dietary restriction is not considered necessary. Alcohol ingestion may cause a disulfiram-like reaction.

Cautionary label wordings, see inside back cover

PROCARBAZINE

Indications: see notes above

Cautions; Side-effects: see section 8.1 and notes above; reduce dose in renal impairment; **interactions:** Appendix 1 (procarbazine)

Dose: initially 50 mg daily, increased by 50 mg daily to 250–300 mg daily in divided doses; maintenance (on remission) 50–150 mg daily to cumulative total of at least 6 g

PoM Natulan® (Cambridge)

Capsules, ivory, procarbazine 50 mg (as hydrochloride). Net price 50-cap pack = £12.00. Label: 4

RAZOXANE

Razoxane has limited activity in the leukaemias, and is little used.

RAZOXANE

Indications: see notes above

Cautions; Side-effects: see section 8.1

Dose: acute leukaemias, 150–500 mg/m^2 daily for 3–5 days

PoM Razoxin® (Zeneca)

Tablets, scored, razoxane 125 mg. Net price 30-tab pack = £26.87

8.2   Drugs affecting the immune response

8.2.1	Cytotoxic immunosuppressants
8.2.2	Corticosteroids and other immunosuppressants
8.2.3	Immunostimulants
8.2.4	Interferons
8.2.5	Aldesleukin

8.2.1   Cytotoxic immunosuppressants

These drugs are used to suppress rejection in organ transplant recipients and are also used to treat a variety of auto-immune and collagen diseases (see section 10.1.3). They are non-specific in their action and careful monitoring of peripheral blood counts is required, with dose adjustments for marrow toxicity. Patients receiving these drugs will be prone to atypical infections.

Azathioprine is widely used for transplant recipients and is also used to treat a number of auto-immune conditions, usually when corticosteroid therapy alone has provided inadequate control. This drug is metabolised to mercaptopurine, and doses should be reduced when concurrent therapy with allopurinol is given. The predominant toxic effect is myelosuppression, although hepatic toxicity is also well recognised.

Cyclophosphamide and **chlorambucil** (section 8.1.1) are less commonly prescribed as immunosuppressants.

AZATHIOPRINE

Indications: see notes above

Cautions: should not be prescribed unless adequate monitoring available throughout duration of treatment; monitoring required includes full blood counts carried out at least weekly for the first 8 weeks (more frequently with higher doses or if hepatic or renal impairment) then at least every 3 months thereafter; reduce dose in severe hepatic and renal impairment and in elderly; **interactions:** Appendix 1 (azathioprine)

BONE MARROW SUPPRESSION. Patients should be warned to report immediately any evidence of infection, unexpected bruising or bleeding, or other manifestations of bone marrow suppression

Contra-indications: hypersensitivity to azathioprine or mercaptopurine (see also under Side-effects); decision to maintain or discontinue pregnancy depends on condition being treated (see also p.327) but as general rule should not be initiated during pregnancy

Side-effects: hypersensitivity reactions–including malaise, dizziness, vomiting, fever, rigors, muscular pains, arthralgia, disturbed liver function, cholestatic jaundice, arrhythmias and hypotension (calling for immediate and permanent withdrawal); dose-related bone marrow suppression (see also Cautions); hair loss and increased susceptibility to infections in transplant recipients also receiving corticosteroids; nausea; rarely pancreatitis and pneumonitis

Dose: by mouth or *intravenously,* initially, rarely more than 3 mg/kg daily, reduced according to response; maintenance 1–3 mg/kg daily; consider withdrawal if no improvement in 3 months

Suppression of transplant rejection, loading dose, *by mouth* or *intravenously* up to 5 mg/kg; maintenance 1–4 mg/kg daily

Note. Intravenous injection is alkaline and very irritant, intravenous route should therefore be used **only** if oral route not feasible, see also Appendix 6

PoM Azathioprine (Non-proprietary)

Tablets, azathioprine 50 mg. Net price 20 = £6.43. Label: 21

Available from APS, Ashbourne (Immunoprin®), Berk (Berkaprine®), Cox, CP, Hillcross, K Pharm., Lagap, Penn (Azamune®)

PoM Imuran® (Wellcome)

Tablets, both f/c, azathioprine 25 mg (orange), net price 100-tab pack = £39.35; 50 mg (yellow), 100-tab pack = £65.61. Label: 21

Injection, powder for reconstitution, azathioprine (as sodium salt). Net price 50-mg vial = £16.54

8.2.2   Corticosteroids and other immunosuppressants

Prednisolone is widely used in oncology. It has a marked antitumour effect in acute lymphoblastic leukaemia, Hodgkin's disease, and the non-Hodgkin lymphomas. It is also active in hormone-sensitive breast cancer and may cause useful disease regression. Finally, it has a role in the palliation of

---

symptomatic end-stage malignant disease when it may produce a sense of well-being.

The corticosteroids are also powerful immunosuppressants. They are used to prevent organ transplant rejection, and in high dose to treat rejection episodes. For notes on corticosteroids see section 6.3. For warnings on live vaccines see section 14.1.

Cyclosporin is a fungal metabolite and potent immunosuppressant which is virtually non-myelotoxic but markedly nephrotoxic. It has found particular use in the field of organ and tissue transplantation, for prevention of graft rejection following bone marrow, kidney, liver, pancreas, heart, and heart-lung transplantation, and for prophylaxis of graft-versus-host disease.

CYCLOSPORIN
(Ciclosporin)

Indications: see notes above, and under Dose; atopic dermatitis and psoriasis, see section 13.5.2; rheumatoid arthritis, see section 10.1.3

Cautions: monitor kidney function—dose dependent increase in serum creatinine and urea during first few weeks may necessitate dose reduction in transplant patients (exclude rejection if kidney transplant) or discontinuation in non-transplant patients; monitor liver function (dosage adjustment based on bilirubin and liver enzymes may be needed); monitor blood pressure—discontinue if hypertension develops that cannot be controlled by antihypertensives; hyperuricaemia; monitor serum potassium especially in marked renal dysfunction (and avoid high dietary potassium); measure blood lipids before and after 1 month—if increases, restrict dietary fat and (if appropriate) reduce dose; pregnancy and breast-feeding (see Appendixes 4 and 5); porphyria (see section 9.8.2); preferably avoid other immunosuppressants except corticosteroids (over-suppression may increase susceptibility to infection and lymphoma); **interactions:** Appendix 1 (cyclosporin)

ADDITIONAL CAUTIONS IN ATOPIC DERMATITIS AND PSORIASIS, see section 13.5.2 and in RHEUMATOID ARTHRITIS, see section 10.1.3

Side-effects: commonly dose-dependent increase in serum creatinine and urea during first few weeks (see also under Cautions), and less commonly renal structural changes on long-term administration; also hypertrichosis, tremor, hypertension (especially in heart transplant patients) hepatic dysfunction, fatigue, gingival hypertrophy, gastro-intestinal disturbances, and burning sensation in hands and feet (usually during first week); *occasionally* headache, rash (possibly allergic), mild anaemia, hyperkalaemia, hyperuricaemia, hypomagnesaemia, weight increase, oedema, pancreatitis, neuropathy, confusion, paraesthesia, convulsions, dysmenorrhoea or amenorrhoea; muscle weakness, cramps, myopathy, gynaecomastia, colitis also reported; thrombocytopenia (sometimes with haemolytic uraemic syndrome) also reported; incidence of malignancies and lymphoproliferative disorders

similar to that with conventional immunosuppressive therapy

Dose: organ transplantation, used alone, 10–15 mg/kg as a single dose *by mouth* 4–12 hours before transplantation followed by 10–15 mg/kg daily for 1–2 weeks post-operatively then reduced to 2–6 mg/kg daily for maintenance (dose should be adjusted by monitoring blood concentrations and renal function; dose lower if given concomitantly with other immunosuppressant therapy (e.g. corticosteroids); if necessary one-third oral dose can be given *by intravenous infusion* over 2–6 hours

Bone-marrow transplantation, prevention and treatment of graft-versus-host disease, 3–5 mg/kg daily *by intravenous infusion* over 2–6 hours from day before transplantation to 2 weeks post-operatively (or 12.5–15 mg/kg daily *by mouth*) then 12.5 mg/kg daily *by mouth* for 3–6 months then tailed off

COUNSELLING. Total daily dose may be taken as a single dose (transplant recipients) or in 2 divided doses. To mask taste, mix with cold milk, cold chocolate drink, cola, or orange juice immediately before taking (and rinse with more to ensure total dose). Do not use plastic cup. Keep medicine measure away from other liquids (including water)

PoM Sandimmun® (Sandoz)

Capsules, cyclosporin 25 mg (pale pink), net price 30-cap pack = £20.54; 50 mg (yellow), 30-cap pack = £40.22; 100 mg (dusky pink), 30-cap pack = £76.33

Oral solution, oily, yellow, sugar-free, cyclosporin 100 mg/mL. Net price 50 mL = £114.38. Counselling, administration

Concentrate for intravenous infusion (oily), cyclosporin 50 mg/mL. To be diluted before use. Net price 1-mL amp = £1.77; 5-mL amp = £8.38

Note. Contains polyethoxylated castor oil which has been associated with anaphylaxis—observe for at least 30 minutes after starting infusion and at frequent intervals thereafter

PREDNISOLONE
See section 6.3.4

8.2.3   Immunostimulants

A suspension of inactivated *Corynebacterium parvum* organisms (Coparvax®) was formerly used by the intracavitary route to treat malignant effusions. It has now been discontinued.

8.2.4   Interferons

Interferons are naturally occurring proteins with complex effects on immunity and cell function. Recently alfa interferon (formerly called lymphoblastoid interferon) has shown some antitumour effect in certain lymphomas and solid tumours. The precise role of interferons in cancer treatment is controversial and often ill-defined. They are toxic and their use is often best confined to trials designed to evaluate their antitumour efficacy. Side-effects are dose-related, but commonly include influenza-like symptoms, lethargy, and depression. Myelosuppression may also occur, particularly affecting granulocyte counts. Cardiovascular problems (hypotension, hypertension, and arrhythmias), and hepatotoxicity have been reported. Other side-effects include thyroid abnormalities, psoriasiform rash, confusion, and coma and seizures (usually with high doses in the elderly).

INTERFERON ALFA

Indications: see under preparations
Cautions; Contra-indications; Side-effects: see notes above—but for full details (including dosage details) consult data sheets; pregnancy (Appendix 4); **interactions:** Appendix 1 (interferons)

PoM Intron A® (Schering-Plough)
Injection, interferon alfa-2b (rbe) 5-million units/mL, net price 2-mL vial = £56.52; 5-mL vial = £141.30. For subcutaneous and intramuscular injection
Injection, powder for reconstitution, interferon alfa-2b (rbe). Net price 1-million unit vial, 5 = £33.90; 3-million unit vial =£16.96; 5-million unit vial = £28.26; 10-million unit vial = £56.52; 30-million unit vial = £169.56 (all with water for injection). For subcutaneous and intramuscular injection
Both for use in AIDS-related Kaposi's sarcoma, hairy cell leukaemia, non-Hodgkins lymphoma, chronic myelogenous leukaemia, condyloma acuminata (intralesional injection), chronic active hepatitis B, and maintenance of remission in multiple myeloma

PoM Roferon-A® (Roche)
Injection, powder for reconstitution, interferon alfa-2a (rbe). Net price 3 million-unit vial = £16.96; 4.5 million-unit vial = £25.44; 9 million-unit vial = £50.88; 18 million-unit vial = £101.77 (all with syringe, needles, and water for injection). For subcutaneous and intramuscular injection
For use in AIDS-related Kaposi's sarcoma, hairy cell leukaemia, chronic myelogenous leukaemia, recurrent or metastatic renal cell carcinoma, progressive cutaneous T-cell lymphoma and chronic active hepatitis B

PoM Wellferon® (Wellcome)
Injection, interferon alfa-N1 (lns) 3 million units/mL, net price 1-mL vial = £16.96; 10 million units/mL, net price 1-mL vial = £56.52. For subcutaneous and intramuscular injection
For use in hairy cell leukaemia and chronic active hepatitis B

INTERFERON GAMMA
See section 14.5

8.2.5   Aldesleukin

Aldesleukin (recombinant interleukin-2) is licensed for use by intravenous infusion in metastatic renal cell carcinoma. This is a very toxic drug which, although responsible for tumour shrinkage in a

small proportion of patients, has not been shown to increase survival. Toxicity is universal and often severe. A common acute problem is the development of a capillary leak syndrome causing pulmonary oedema and hypotension. Bone marrow, hepatic, renal, thyroid, and CNS toxicity is also common. It is for use in **specialist units only**.
Interactions: Appendix 1 (aldesleukin)

▼ **PoM Proleukin®** (EuroCetus)
Injection, powder for reconstitution, aldesleukin. Net price 18-million unit vial = £125.00
For metastatic renal cell carcinoma, **excluding** patients in whom all three of the following prognostic factors are present; performance status of Eastern Co-operative Oncology Group of 1 or greater, more than one organ with metastatic disease sites, and a period of less than 24 months between initial diagnosis of primary tumour and date of evaluation of treatment.

8.3   Sex hormones and hormone antagonists in malignant disease

8.3.1	Oestrogens
8.3.2	Progestogens
8.3.3	Androgens
8.3.4	Hormone antagonists

Hormonal manipulation has an important role in the treatment of metastatic breast, prostate, and endometrial cancer, and a more marginal role in the treatment of hypernephroma. These treatments are not curative, but may provide excellent palliation of symptoms in selected patients, sometimes for a period of years. Tumour response, and treatment toxicity should be carefully monitored and treatment changed if progression occurs or side-effects exceed benefit.

8.3.1   Oestrogens

Stilboestrol has a decreasing role in the treatment of prostate cancer because of its side-effects. It is also occasionally used in postmenopausal women with breast cancer. Toxicity is common and dose-related side-effects include nausea, fluid retention, and venous and arterial thrombosis. Impotence and gynaecomastia always occur in men, and withdrawal bleeding may be a problem in women. Hypercalcaemia and bone pain may also occur in breast cancer.

Fosfestrol is also used for prostate cancer; it is activated by the enzyme acid phosphatase to produce stilboestrol. Side-effects are as for stilboestrol; in addition, perineal pain may complicate intravenous use.

Ethinyloestradiol is the most potent oestrogen available; unlike other oestrogens it is only slowly metabolised in the liver. It is used in breast cancer.

Polyestradiol is a long-acting oestrogen.

STILBOESTROL
(Diethylstilbestrol)

Indications: see notes above

Cautions; Side-effects: cardiovascular disease (sodium retention with oedema, thromboembolism), hepatic impairment (jaundice), feminising effects in men; see also notes above

Dose: breast cancer, 10–20 mg daily
Prostate cancer, 1–3 mg daily

PoM **Stilboestrol** (Non-proprietary)
Tablets, stilboestrol 1 mg, net price 56 = £7.57; 5 mg, 28 = £6.44
Available from APS (Apstil®)

ETHINYLOESTRADIOL

Indications: see notes above; other indications, see section 6.4.1.1

Cautions; Side-effects: see under Stilboestrol and notes above

Dose: breast cancer, 1–3 mg daily

Preparations
See section 6.4.1.1

FOSFESTROL TETRASODIUM

Indications: prostate cancer

Cautions; Contra-indications; Side-effects: see under Stilboestrol and notes above; nausea and vomiting; after intravenous injection, perineal irritation and pain in bony metastases

Dose: by slow intravenous injection, 552–1104 mg daily for at least 5 days; maintenance 276 mg 1–4 times weekly

By mouth, maintenance 100–200 mg 3 times daily, reducing to 100–300 mg daily in divided doses

PoM **Honvan®** (ASTA Medica)
Tablets, fosfestrol tetrasodium 100 mg. Net price 20 – £2.47
Injection, fosfestrol tetrasodium 55.2 mg/mL. Net price 5-mL amp = £1.19

POLYESTRADIOL PHOSPHATE

Indications: prostate cancer

Cautions; Side-effects: see under Stilboestrol and notes above

Dose: by deep intramuscular injection, 80–160 mg every 4 weeks; maintenance 40–80 mg

PoM **Estradurin®** (Pharmacia)
Injection, powder for reconstitution, polyestradiol phosphate (with mepivacaine and nicotinamide). Net price 80-mg vial (with diluent) = £3.86

8.3.2 Progestogens

Progestogens are used largely as second- or third-line therapy in breast cancer. They are also used to treat endometrial cancer and hypernephroma, but are little used for prostate cancer. **Medroxyprogesterone** or **megestrol** are usually chosen and can be

given orally; high-dose or parenteral treatment cannot be recommended. Side-effects are mild but may include nausea, fluid retention, and weight gain.

GESTRONOL HEXANOATE
(Gestonorone Caproate)

Indications: see notes above; benign prostatic hypertrophy

Cautions; Contra-indications; Side-effects: see under Medroxyprogesterone acetate (section 6.4.1.2) and notes above

Dose: endometrial cancer, *by intramuscular injection,* 200–400 mg every 5–7 days
Benign prostatic hypertrophy, *by intramuscular injection,* 200 mg every week, increased to 300–400 mg every week if necessary

PoM **Depostat®** (Schering Health)
Injection (oily), gestronol hexanoate 100 mg/mL. Net price 2-mL amp = £4.28

MEDROXYPROGESTERONE ACETATE

Indications: see notes above; other indications, see section 6.4.1.2

Cautions; Contra-indications; Side-effects: see section 6.4.1.2 and notes above; glucocorticoid effects at high dose may lead to a cushingoid syndrome

Dose: by mouth, endometrial, prostate, and renal cancer, 100–500 mg daily; breast cancer, various doses in range 0.4–1.5 g daily
By deep intramuscular injection into the gluteal muscle, various doses in range 1 g daily down to 250 mg weekly

PoM **Depo-Provera®** (Upjohn)
Injection, medroxyprogesterone acetate 150 mg/mL. Net price 3.3-mL (500-mg) vial = £12.49
PoM **Farlutal®** (Pharmacia)
Tablets, both scored, medroxyprogesterone acetate 100 mg, net price 20 = £8.12; 250 mg, 50 = £50.73
Tablets, scored, medroxyprogesterone acetate 500 mg. Net price 56 = £113.63. Label: 27
Injection, medroxyprogesterone acetate 200 mg/mL. Net price 2.5-mL vial = £13.88; 5-mL vial = £23.14
PoM **Provera®** (Upjohn)
Tablets, medroxyprogesterone acetate 100 mg (scored), net price 30-tab pack = £12.49; 200 mg (scored), 30-tab pack = £24.71; 400 mg, 30-tab pack = £48.89
Tablets, medroxyprogesterone acetate 2.5 mg, 5 mg and 10 mg, see section 6.4.1.2

MEGESTROL ACETATE

Indications: see notes above

Cautions; Contra-indications; Side-effects: see under Medroxyprogesterone acetate (section 6.4.1.2) and notes above

Dose: breast cancer, 160 mg daily in single or divided doses; endometrial cancer, 40–320 mg daily in divided doses

PoM **Megace®** (Bristol-Myers)

Tablets, both scored, megestrol acetate 40 mg, net price 20 = £5.08; 160 mg (off-white), 30-tab pack = £29.30

NORETHISTERONE

Indications: see notes above; other indications, see section 6.4.1.2

Cautions; Contra-indications; Side-effects: see section 6.4.1.2 and notes above

Dose: breast cancer, 40 mg daily, increased to 60 mg daily if required

Preparations

See section 6.4.1.2

8.3.3   Androgens

The androgens are given parenterally and are occasionally still used as second- or third-line therapy for metastatic breast cancer.

TESTOSTERONE ESTERS

Indications: see notes above; other indications, see section 6.4.2

Cautions; Contra-indications; Side-effects: see under Testosterone and Esters (section 6.4.2)

Dose: see under Preparations

PoM **Primoteston Depot®** (Schering Health)

See section 6.4.2

PoM **Virormone®** (Paines & Byrne)

See section 6.4.2

8.3.4   Hormone antagonists

8.3.4.1 BREAST CANCER

BREAST CANCER. **Tamoxifen** is an oestrogen receptor antagonist and at a dose of 20 mg daily is the hormonal treatment of choice for breast cancer in postmenopausal women with metastatic disease; it is also increasingly commonly used as a first-line treatment for premenopausal women. Overall, approximately 30% of patients with metastatic breast cancer respond to hormonal manipulation. This figure is increased to 60% in patients with oestrogen receptor positive tumours; receptor negative tumours respond in less than 10%.

Adjuvant hormonal treatment with tamoxifen 20 mg daily is also the treatment of choice in postmenopausal patients with high-risk breast cancer after treatment of the primary. Such treatment has consistently prolonged the period between diagnosis and the development of metastases and has also clearly increased survival. Tamoxifen is also increasingly commonly used as adjuvant treatment for premenopausal women with early breast cancer.

Side-effects are unusual with tamoxifen but patients with bony metastases may experience an exacerbation of pain, sometimes associated with hypercalcaemia. This reaction commonly precedes tumour response. Amenorrhoea commonly develops in premenopausal women.

Patients with non-threatening metastases unresponsive to tamoxifen may still respond to a secondary hormonal treatment. Certainly patients who initially respond to tamoxifen should receive second-line hormone treatment. No clear guidelines are available; for premenopausal patients oophorectomy or a progestogen (section 8.3.2) may be used; for postmenopausal patients a progestogen or aminoglutethimide (see below) may be used. Patients who respond can be given further hormones on relapse; refractory patients are better treated with chemotherapy or palliative therapy.

Aminoglutethimide has largely replaced adrenalectomy in postmenopausal women with breast cancer; it acts predominantly by inhibiting the conversion of androgens to oestrogens in the peripheral tissues. Corticosteroid replacement therapy is necessary (see section 6.3.1). Early toxicity is common and may include drowsiness, drug fever, and a morbilliform eruption; these side-effects generally settle spontaneously. The dose of aminoglutethimide is usually increased to 500 mg daily over 2 to 4 weeks. Hepatic enzyme induction occurs, and may require modification of the doses of other drugs (e.g. oral anticoagulants).

Trilostane (section 6.7.3) is also indicated for postmenopausal breast cancer. It is quite well tolerated but diarrhoea and abdominal discomfort may be a problem. Like aminoglutethimide, trilostane is an adrenal antagonist therefore corticosteroid replacement therapy is needed.

Formestane, an inhibitor of the enzyme aromatase (which metabolises androgens to oestrogens) is indicated for breast cancer in women with natural or artificial postmenopausal status.

Goserelin, a gonadorelin analogue is now also indicated for management of advanced breast cancer in premenopausal women.

AMINOGLUTETHIMIDE

Indications: see notes above and under Dose

Cautions: see notes above; porphyria (see section 9.8.2); **interactions:** Appendix 1 (aminoglutethimide)

Contra-indications: pregnancy and breast-feeding

Side-effects: see notes above; dizziness, somnolence, lethargy; unsteadiness at higher doses; less frequently nausea, vomiting, diarrhoea; rash (sometimes with fever) reported; allergic alveolitis and blood disorders (regular blood counts) also reported; altered thyroid function

Dose: breast or prostate cancer, 250 mg daily, increased once a week to max. 250 mg 4 times daily (lower doses may be adequate, see notes above); given with a glucocorticoid (and sometimes with a mineralocorticoid as well)

Cushing's syndrome due to malignant disease, 250 mg daily, increased gradually to 1 g daily in divided doses (occasionally 1.5–2 g daily); glucocorticoid given only if necessary

PoM **Orimeten**® (Ciba)
Tablets, scored, aminoglutethimide 250 mg. Net price 56-tab pack = £18.38

FORMESTANE
Indications: advanced breast cancer in women with natural or artificial postmenopausal status
Cautions: no studies performed in diabetes mellitus (monitor blood glucose)
DRIVING. Drowsiness may affect performance of skilled tasks (e.g. driving)
Contra-indications: not indicated for premenopausal women; pregnancy and breast-feeding
Side-effects: occasionally rash, pruritus, exanthema, hot flushes; facial hypertrichosis, alopecia, lethargy, drowsiness, emotional lability, headache, dizziness, oedema of lower leg, thrombophlebitis, vaginal bleeding, pelvic cramps, nausea, vomiting, constipation, arthralgia, muscle cramps, sore throat, and anaphylactoid reaction also reported; pain and irritation common at injection site (with occasional sterile abscess and haematoma)
Dose: by deep intramuscular injection in the gluteal muscle, 250 mg every 2 weeks (alternate sites)

▼ PoM **Lentaron**® (Ciba)
Injection, powder for reconstitution, formestane 250 mg. Net price 250-mg vial (with diluent) = £72.73. Counselling, driving

GOSERELIN
See section 8.3.4.2

TAMOXIFEN
Indications: see under Dose and notes above
Cautions: occasional cystic ovarian swellings in premenopausal women, occasional hypercalcaemia if bony metastases; porphyria (see section 9.8.2); **Interactions:** Appendix 1 (tamoxifen)
ENDOMETRIAL CHANGES. An increased incidence of endometrial changes, including hyperplasia, polyps and cancer, has been reported in association with tamoxifen. Abnormal vaginal bleeding including menstrual irregularities, vaginal discharge and symptoms such as pelvic pain or pressure in those receiving (or who have previously received) tamoxifen should be promptly investigated.
Contra-indications: pregnancy (exclude before commencing) and breast-feeding
Side-effects: hot flushes, vaginal bleeding (important: see also Cautions) or suppression of menstruation in some pre-menopausal women, vaginal discharge, pruritus vulvae, gastro-intestinal disturbances, light-headedness, tumour flare, falls in platelet counts; occasionally fluid retention, alopecia; also visual disturbances (including corneal changes, cataracts, retinopathy); liver

enzyme changes (rarely fatty liver, cholestasis, hepatitis); see also notes above
Dose: breast cancer, see notes above
Anovulatory infertility, 20 mg daily on second, third, fourth and fifth days of cycle; if necessary increased to 40 mg daily then 80 mg daily for subsequent courses; if cycles irregular, start initial course on any day, with subsequent course starting 45 days later *or* on second day of cycle if menstruation occurs

PoM **Tamoxifen** (Non-proprietary)
Tablets, tamoxifen (as citrate) 10 mg, net price 30-tab pack = £3.21; 20 mg, 30-tab pack = £4.55; 40 mg, 30-tab pack = £19.00
Various strengths available from APS, Ashbourne (Oestrifen®), Berk (Emblon®), Cox, CP, K Pharm., Lagap, Lederle (Noltam®), Pharmacia (Tamofen®)
PoM **Nolvadex**® (Zeneca)
Tablets, tamoxifen (as citrate) 10 mg, net price 30-tab pack = £6.05; 20 mg (Nolvadex-D®), 30-tab pack = £9.12; 40 mg (scored, Nolvadex-Forte®), 30-tab pack = £21.45

TRILOSTANE
See section 6.7.3

8.3.4.2 PROSTATE CANCER

PROSTATE CANCER. Metastatic cancer of the prostate is commonly responsive to hormonal treatment designed to deprive the cancer of androgen. Treatment is probably best reserved for symptomatic metastatic disease. The standard treatment is bilateral subcapsular orchidectomy, which commonly results in responses lasting 12–18 months. Alternatively, a gonadorelin analogue such as **buserelin**, **goserelin**, or **leuprorelin** may be given. These are as effective as orchidectomy or **stilboestrol** (section 8.3.1) but are expensive and require parenteral administration, at least initially. They cause initial stimulation of luteinising hormone release by the pituitary, which in turn causes testosterone secretion by the testis; this is followed by inhibition of luteinising hormone release with achievement of an anorchic state. During the first 1 to 2 weeks of treatment a number of patients develop a tumour 'flare' which may cause spinal cord compression or increased bone pain. When such problems are anticipated, alternative treatments (e.g. orchidectomy) or the additional use of an anti-androgen such as cyproterone acetate or flutamide (see below) are recommended; anti-androgen treatment should be started 3 days before the gonadorelin analogue and continued for at least 3 weeks. Other side-effects of gonadorelin analogues are similar to those of orchidectomy.

Cyproterone acetate is an anti-androgen which has been used as first-line therapy; it has a number of theoretical advantages, but is expensive. **Flutamide** is also an anti-androgen; it can be used for prostate cancer and has a role in preventing and treating the 'flare' which can occur in patients treated with gonadorelin analogues.

Alternatives after orchidectomy include cyproterone acetate or prednisolone. Such second-line treatment may palliate symptoms, but rarely results in appreciable disease regression.

AMINOGLUTETHIMIDE

See section 8.3.4.1

BUSERELIN

Indications: prostate cancer; other indications, see section 6.7.2

Cautions: during first month monitor patients at risk of ureteric obstruction or spinal cord compression, see notes above

Side-effects: initial increase in bone pain (due to transient increases in plasma testosterone); hot flushes, decreased libido, depression, headache, dizziness, nausea, vomiting, and diarrhoea, infrequent gynaecomastia, urticaria; irritation of nasal mucosa (spray formulation only)

Dose: by subcutaneous injection, 500 micrograms every 8 hours for 7 days, then *intranasally,* 1 spray into each nostril 6 times daily

COUNSELLING. Avoid use of nasal decongestants before and for at least 30 minutes after treatment.

PoM Suprefact® (Hoechst)

Injection, buserelin 1 mg (as acetate)/mL. Net price 2 × 5.5-mL vial = £29.61

Nasal spray, buserelin 100 micrograms (as acetate)/metered spray. Net price treatment pack of 4 × 10-g bottle with spray pump = £97.42. Counselling, see above

CYPROTERONE ACETATE

Indications: prostate cancer, see notes above; other indications, see section 6.4.2

Cautions: in prostate cancer, blood counts initially and throughout treatment, monitor hepatic and adrenocortical function; risk of recurrence of thromboembolic disease; diabetes mellitus, sickle-cell anaemia, severe depression (in other indications some of these are contra-indicated, see section 6.4.2)

Contra-indications: none in prostate cancer; for contra-indications relating to other indications see section 6.4.2

Side-effects: see section 6.4.2

Dose: prostate cancer, 300 mg daily in 2–3 divided doses after food

PoM Cyprostat® (Schering Health)

Tablets, scored, cyproterone acetate 50 mg net price 168-tab pack = £96.70; 100 mg, 84-tab pack = £96.70. Label: 3, 21

Note. Tablets containing Cyproterone Acetate 50 mg are also available from Generics, Lagap

FLUTAMIDE

Indications: prostate cancer, see notes above

Cautions: cardiac disease (sodium retention with oedema); monitor hepatic function (hepatotoxic); **interactions:** Appendix 1 (flutamide)

Side-effects: gynaecomastia (sometimes with galactorrhoea); nausea, vomiting, diarrhoea, increased appetite, insomnia, tiredness; other side-effects reported include decreased libido, inhibition of spermatogenesis, gastric and chest pain, headache, dizziness, oedema, blurred vision, thirst, rashes, pruritus, haemolytic anaemia, systemic lupus erythematosus-like syndrome, and lymphoedema; hepatic injury (with transaminase abnormalities, cholestatic jaundice, hepatic necrosis, encephalopathy and occasional fatality) reported

Dose: 250 mg 3 times daily (see also notes above)

PoM Drogenil® (Schering-Plough)

Tablets, yellow, scored, flutamide 250 mg, net price 84-tab pack = £110.00

GOSERELIN

Indications: prostate cancer; advanced breast cancer; endometriosis, see section 6.7.2

Cautions; Side-effects: see under Buserelin; also rashes (reversible without stopping therapy); bruising at injection site; rarely hypercalcaemia in breast cancer patients

Dose: by subcutaneous injection into anterior abdominal wall, 3.6 mg every 28 days

PoM Zoladex® (Zeneca)

Implant, goserelin 3.6 mg (as acetate) in syringe applicator. Net price each = £122.27

LEUPRORELIN ACETATE

Indications: prostate cancer; endometriosis, see section 6.7.2

Cautions; Side-effects: see under Buserelin; also, infrequently, peripheral oedema, fatigue, nausea, irritation at injection site; rotate injection site periodically

Dose: by subcutaneous or by intramuscular injection, 3.75 mg every 4 weeks (see also notes above)

PoM Prostap SR® (Lederle)

Injection (microcapsule powder for aqueous suspension), leuprorelin acetate, net price 3.75-mg vial with 2-mL vehicle-filled syringe = £125.40

8.3.4.3 GASTRO-ENTEROPANCREATIC TUMOURS

Octreotide is a long-acting analogue of the hypothalamic release-inhibiting hormone somatostatin; it is indicated for the relief of symptoms associated with gastro-enteropancreatic endocrine tumours and for the short-term treatment of acromegaly before intervention.

OCTREOTIDE

Indications: see under Dose

Cautions: occasional sudden escape from symptomatic control with rapid recurrence of severe symptoms; in insulinoma may increase depth and duration of hypoglycaemia (close observation initially and with dose changes; marked fluctuations may be reduced by increasing administration frequency); in diabetes mellitus may reduce insulin or oral antidiabetic requirements; monitor thyroid function on long-term therapy; ultrasonic examination of gall bladder before and at intervals of 6–12 months during treatment; avoid abrupt withdrawal (see side-effects below); **interactions:** Appendix 1 (octreotide)

Contra-indications: pregnancy (unless compelling reasons) and breast-feeding

Side-effects: gastro-intestinal disturbances including anorexia, nausea, vomiting, abdominal pain and bloating, flatulence, diarrhoea, and steatorrhoea; symptoms may be reduced by injecting between meals or at bedtime; impairment of postprandial glucose tolerance (rarely persistent hyperglycaemia on chronic administration); hepatic disturbance reported; gall stone formation reported after long-term treatment (abrupt withdrawal may result in biliary hypercontractility with associated biliary colic and pancreatitis); pain and irritation at injection site (rotate sites)

Dose: symptoms associated with carcinoid tumours with features of carcinoid syndrome, VIPomas, glucagonomas, *by subcutaneous injection*, initially 50 micrograms once or twice daily, gradually increased according to response to 200 micrograms 3 times daily (higher doses required exceptionally); maintenance doses variable; in carcinoid tumours discontinue after 1 week if no effect; if rapid response required, initial dose *by intravenous injection* (with ECG monitoring and after dilution to a concentration of 10–50% with sodium chloride 0.9% injection)

Acromegaly, *by subcutaneous injection*, 100–200 micrograms 3 times daily

PoM **Sandostatin**® (Sandoz)
Injection, octreotide (as acetate) 50 micrograms/mL, net price 1-mL amp = £2.90;
  100 micrograms/mL, 1-mL amp = £5.46;
  200 micrograms/mL, 5-mL vial = £54.39;
  500 micrograms/mL, 1-mL amp = £26.45

9: Drugs affecting
NUTRITION and BLOOD

In this chapter drugs and preparations are discussed under the following headings:

9.1 Anaemias and some other blood disorders
9.2 Fluids and electrolytes
9.3 Intravenous nutrition
9.4 Oral nutrition
9.5 Minerals
9.6 Vitamins
9.7 Bitters and tonics
9.8 Metabolic disorders

9.1 Anaemias and some other blood disorders

9.1.1 Iron-deficiency anaemias
9.1.2 Megaloblastic anaemias
9.1.3 Hypoplastic and haemolytic anaemias
9.1.4 Autoimmune thrombocytopenic purpura
9.1.5 G6PD deficiency
9.1.6 Drugs used in neutropenia

Before initiating treatment for anaemia it is essential to determine which type is present. Iron salts may be harmful and result in iron overload if given alone to patients with anaemias other than those due to iron deficiency.

9.1.1 Iron-deficiency anaemias

9.1.1.1 Oral iron
9.1.1.2 Parenteral iron

Treatment is only justified in the presence of a demonstrable iron-deficiency state.
Prophylaxis is justifiable in pregnancy, menorrhagia, after subtotal or total gastrectomy, and in the management of low birth-weight infants such as premature babies, twins, and in infants delivered by caesarean section.

9.1.1.1 ORAL IRON

Iron salts should be given by mouth unless there are good reasons for using another route.

Ferrous salts show only marginal differences between one another in efficiency of absorption of iron, but ferric salts are much less well absorbed. Haemoglobin regeneration rate is little affected by the type of salt used provided sufficient iron is given, and in most patients the time factor is not critical. Choice of preparation is thus usually decided by incidence of side-effects and cost.

The oral dose of elemental iron for deficiency should be 100 to 200 mg daily. It is customary to give this as dried **ferrous sulphate**, 200 mg (≡ 65 mg elemental iron) three times daily; a dose of ferrous sulphate 200 mg once or twice daily may be effective for prophylaxis or for mild iron defi-

ciency. If side-effects arise, dosage can be reduced or a change made to an alternative iron salt. It should be remembered, however, that an apparent improvement in tolerance on changing to another salt may be due to its lower content of elemental iron. The incidence of side-effects due to ferrous sulphate is no greater than with other iron salts when compared on the basis of equivalent amounts of elemental iron.

Iron content of different iron salts

Iron salt	Amount	Content of ferrous iron
Ferrous fumarate	200 mg	65 mg
Ferrous gluconate	300 mg	35 mg
Ferrous succinate	100 mg	35 mg
Ferrous sulphate	300 mg	60 mg
Ferrous sulphate, dried	200 mg	65 mg

THERAPEUTIC RESPONSE. The haemoglobin concentration should rise by about 100–200 mg per 100 mL (1–2 g per litre) per day. After the haemoglobin has risen to normal, treatment should be continued for a further three months in an attempt to replenish the iron stores. Epithelial tissue changes such as atrophic glossitis and koilonychia are usually improved although the response is often slow.

COMPOUND PREPARATIONS. Some oral preparations contain ascorbic acid to aid absorption, or the iron is in the form of a chelate, which can be shown experimentally to produce a modest increase in absorption of iron. However, the therapeutic advantage is minimal and cost may be increased.

There is neither theoretical nor clinical justification for the inclusion of other therapeutically active ingredients, such as the B group of vitamins (except folic acid for pregnant women, see Iron and Folic Acid below).

MODIFIED-RELEASE CAPSULES AND TABLETS. These are designed to release iron gradually as the capsule or tablet passes along the gut so that a smaller amount of iron is present in the lumen at any one time. It is claimed that each dose unit contains enough iron for 24 hours, thus permitting once daily dosage.

These preparations are likely to carry the iron past the first part of the duodenum into an area of the gut where conditions for iron absorption are poor. The low incidence of side-effects may well be because of the small amounts of iron available under these conditions and so the preparations have no therapeutic advantage and should not be used.

SIDE-EFFECTS. Because iron salts are astringent, gastro-intestinal irritation may occur. Nausea and epigastric pain are dose-related but the relationship

---

|

between dose and altered bowel habit (constipation or diarrhoea) is less clear. Oral iron, particularly modified-release preparations may exacerbate diarrhoea in patients with inflammatory bowel disease; care is also needed in patients with intestinal strictures and diverticulae.

Iron preparations taken orally may have a constipating effect particularly in older patients, occasionally leading to faecal impaction.

FERROUS SULPHATE

Indications: iron-deficiency anaemia
Cautions: pregnancy; **interactions:** Appendix 1 (iron)
Side-effects: see notes above
Dose: see under preparations below
COUNSELLING. Although iron preparations are best absorbed on an empty stomach they may be taken after food to reduce gastro-intestinal side-effects; they may discolour stools

Ferrous Sulphate (Non-proprietary)
Tablets, coated, dried ferrous sulphate 200 mg (65 mg iron), net price 20 = 12p
Dose: prophylactic, 1 tablet daily; therapeutic, 1 tablet 2–3 times daily
Ferrous Sulphate Oral Solution, Paediatric, BP
(Paediatric Ferrous Sulphate Mixture)
Mixture, ferrous sulphate 1.2% and a suitable antioxidant in a suitable vehicle with an orange flavour. Extemporaneous preparations should be recently prepared according to the following formula: ferrous sulphate 60 mg, ascorbic acid 10 mg, orange syrup 0.5 mL, double-strength chloroform water 2.5 mL, water to 5 mL
Dose: therapeutic, CHILD up to 1 year, 5 mL 3 times daily; 1–5 years, 10 mL 3 times daily; 6–12 years, 15 mL 3 times daily *or* 25 mL twice daily. To be taken well diluted with water

Modified-release preparations
Feospan® (Evans)
Spansule® (= capsules m/r), clear/red, enclosing green and brown pellets, dried ferrous sulphate 150 mg (47 mg iron). Net price 30-cap pack = 90p. Label: 25
Dose: 1–2 capsules daily; CHILD over 1 year 1 capsule daily; can be opened and sprinkled on food
Ferrograd® (Abbott)
Filmtabs® (= tablets f/c), m/r, red, dried ferrous sulphate 325 mg (105 mg iron). Net price 30-tab pack – 54p. Label: 25
Dose: 1 tablet daily before food
Slow-Fe® (Ciba)
Tablets, m/r, dried ferrous sulphate 160 mg (50 mg iron). Net price 28-tab pack = 25p. Label: 25
Dose: prophylactic, 1 tablet daily; therapeutic, 2 tablets daily; CHILD over 6 years, 1 tablet daily

FERROUS FUMARATE

Indications; Cautions; Side-effects: see under Ferrous Sulphate
Dose: see under preparations below

Fersaday® (Goldshield)
Tablets, orange, f/c, ferrous fumarate 322 mg (100 mg iron). Net price 28-tab pack = 70p
Dose: prophylactic, 1 tablet daily; therapeutic, 1 tablet twice daily

Fersamal® (Forley)
Tablets, brown, ferrous fumarate 200 mg (65 mg iron). Net price 20 = 29p
Dose: 1–2 tablets 3 times daily
Syrup, brown, ferrous fumarate 140 mg (45 mg iron)/5 mL. Net price 200 mL = £3.60
Dose: 10–20 mL twice daily; PREMATURE INFANT 0.6–2.4 mL/kg daily; CHILD up to 6 years 2.5–5 mL twice daily
Galfer® (Galen)
Capsules, red/green, ferrous fumarate 305 mg (100 mg iron). Net price 20 = 36p
Dose: 1 capsule 1–2 times daily before food
Syrup, brown, sugar-free ferrous fumarate 140 mg (45 mg iron)/5 mL. Net price 300 mL = £4.86
Dose: 10 mL 1–2 times daily before food; CHILD (full-term infant and young child) 2.5–5 mL 1–2 times daily

FERROUS GLUCONATE

Indications; Cautions; Side-effects: see under Ferrous Sulphate
Dose: see under preparations below

Ferrous Gluconate (Non-proprietary)
Tablets, red, coated, ferrous gluconate 300 mg (35 mg iron). Net price 20 = 13p
Dose: prophylactic, 2 tablets daily before food; therapeutic, 4–6 tablets daily in divided doses before food; CHILD 6–12 years, prophylactic and therapeutic, 1–3 tablets daily
Fergon® (Sanofi Winthrop)
Tablets, red, s/c, ferrous gluconate 300 mg (35 mg iron). Net price 20 = 43p
Dose: see above

FERROUS GLYCINE SULPHATE

Indications; Cautions; Side-effects: see under Ferrous Sulphate
Dose: see under preparations below

Plesmet® (Link)
Syrup, ferrous glycine sulphate equivalent to 25 mg iron/5 mL. Net price 100 mL = £1.00
Dose: 5–10 mL 3 times daily; CHILD 2.5–5 mL 1–3 times daily, according to age

Modified-release preparations
Ferrocontin Continus® (ASTA Medica)
Tablets, m/r, red, f/c, ferrous glycine sulphate equivalent to 100 mg iron. Net price 30-tab pack = 54p. Label: 25
Dose: 1 tablet daily

POLYSACCHARIDE-IRON COMPLEX

Indications; Cautions; Side-effects: see under Ferrous Sulphate
Dose: see under preparations below

Niferex® (Tillomed)

Elixir, brown, sugar-free, polysaccharide-iron complex equivalent to 100 mg of iron/5 mL. Net price 240-mL pack = £5.05; 30-mL dropper bottle for paediatric use = £2.16. Counselling, use of dropper

Dose: prophylactic, 2.5 mL daily; therapeutic, 5 mL daily; INFANT, 1 drop (from dropper bottle) per pound body-weight 3 times daily; CHILD 2–6 years, 2.5 mL daily, 6–12 years 5 mL daily

Niferex-150® (Tillomed)

Capsules, brown/orange, polysaccharide-iron complex equivalent to 150 mg of iron. Net price 20 = £2.28

Dose: 1–2 capsules daily

SODIUM IRONEDETATE

Indications; Cautions; Side-effects: see under Ferrous Sulphate

Dose: see under preparations below

Sytron® (Link)

Elixir, sugar-free, sodium ironedetate 190 mg equivalent, and 27.5 mg of iron/5 mL. Net price 100 mL = 99p

Dose: 5 mL increasing gradually to 10 mL 3 times daily; INFANT and PREMATURE INFANT 2.5 mL twice daily (smaller doses should be used initially); CHILD 1–5 years 2.5 mL 3 times daily, 6–12 years 5 mL 3 times daily

---

IRON AND FOLIC ACID

These preparations are used for the prevention of iron and folic acid deficiencies in pregnancy. The prophylactic dose in pregnancy is the equivalent of approximately 100 mg of iron with folic acid 200–500 micrograms daily.

It is important to note that the small doses of folic acid contained in these preparations are inadequate for the treatment of megaloblastic anaemias.

Fefol® (Evans)

Spansule® (=capsules m/r), clear/green, enclosing brown, yellow, and white pellets, dried ferrous sulphate 150 mg (47 mg iron), folic acid 500 micrograms. Net price 30-cap pack = £1.00. Label: 25

Dose: 1 capsule daily

Ferrocap-F 350® (Consolidated)

Capsules, m/r, pink, enclosing brown, white, and yellow granules, ferrous fumarate 330 mg (110 mg iron), folic acid 350 micrograms. Net price 30-cap pack = £1.25. Label: 25

Dose: 1 capsule daily

Ferrocontin Folic Continus® (ASTA Medica)

Tablets, orange, f/c, ferrous glycine sulphate equivalent to 100 mg iron for sustained release, folic acid 500 micrograms. Net price 30-tab pack = 60p. Label: 25

Dose: 1 tablet daily

Ferrograd Folic® (Abbott)

Filmtabs® (= tablets f/c), red/yellow, dried ferrous sulphate 325 mg (105 mg iron) for sustained release, folic acid 350 micrograms. Net price 30-tab pack = 60p. Label: 25

Dose: 1 tablet daily before food

Folex-350® (Rybar)

Tablets, pink, s/c, ferrous fumarate 308 mg (100 mg iron), folic acid 350 micrograms. Net price 30-tab pack = 60p

Dose: 1 tablet daily

Galfer FA® (Galen)

Capsules, red/yellow, ferrous fumarate 305 mg (100 mg iron), folic acid 350 micrograms. Net price 20 = 40p

Dose: 1 capsule daily before food

PoM **Lexpec with Iron-M®** (RP Drugs)

Syrup, brown, sugar-free, ferric ammonium citrate equivalent to 80 mg iron, folic acid 500 micrograms/5 mL. Net price 125 mL = £6.40

Dose: 5–10 mL daily before food

Note. Lexpec with Iron-M® contains five times less folic acid than Lexpec with Iron®

Meterfolic® (Sinclair)

Tablets, grey, f/c, ferrous fumarate equivalent to 100 mg iron, folic acid 400 micrograms. Net price 30-tab pack = £1.03

Dose: 1 tablet 1–2 times daily

Pregaday® (Evans)

Tablets, brown, f/c, ferrous fumarate equivalent to 100 mg iron, folic acid 350 micrograms. Net price 28-tab pack = 51p

Dose: 1 tablet daily

Pregnavite Forte F, see compound iron preparations

PoM **Slow-Fe Folic®** (Ciba)

Tablets, m/r, ivory, f/c, dried ferrous sulphate 160 mg (50 mg iron), folic acid 400 micrograms. Net price 28-tab pack = 28p. Label: 25

Dose: 1–2 tablets daily

Higher folic acid content

Appropriate in context of prevention of *recurrence of neural tube defects*, see recommendations on p.348. *Caution:* has the theoretical disadvantage of masking anaemia due to vitamin-B$_{12}$ deficiency (which could allow vitamin-B$_{12}$ neuropathy to develop).

PoM **Ferfolic SV®** (Sinclair)

Tablets, pink, ferrous gluconate 250 mg (30 mg iron), folic acid 4 mg, ascorbic acid 10 mg. Net price 20 = 85p

Dose: anaemia, 1–3 tablets daily after food

Prophylaxis of neural tube defects in women known to be at risk, 1 tablet daily started before conception and continued for at least first trimester; see also recommendations on p.348

PoM **Folicin®**, see under Compound Iron Preparations

PoM **Lexpec with Iron®** (RP Drugs)

Syrup, brown, sugar-free, ferric ammonium citrate equivalent to 80 mg iron, folic acid 2.5 mg/5 mL. Net price 125 mL = £6.60

Dose: 5–10 mL daily before food

Note. Lexpec with Iron® contains five times as much folic acid as Lexpec with Iron-M®

COMPOUND IRON PREPARATIONS

There is no justification for prescribing compound iron preparations, except for preparations of iron and folic acid for prophylactic use in pregnancy (see above).

Ferrous Sulphate Tablets, Compound, green, s/c, dried ferrous sulphate equivalent to 170 mg of FeSO$_4$, copper sulphate 2.5 mg, manganese sulphate 2.5 mg. Net price 20 tabs = 30p

Dose: 1–2 tablets daily

NHS **Fefol-Vit**® (Evans)

Spansule® (= capsules m/r), clear/white, enclosing brown, orange, yellow, and white pellets, dried ferrous sulphate 150 mg (47 mg iron) with vitamins B group (including folic acid 500 micrograms) and C. Net price 30-cap pack = £1.82. Label: 25

Dose: 1 capsule daily during pregnancy

Fefol Z® (Evans)

Spansule® (= capsules m/r), blue/clear, enclosing brown, yellow, and white pellets, dried ferrous sulphate 150 mg (47 mg iron), folic acid 500 micrograms, zinc sulphate monohydrate 61.8 mg (22.5 mg zinc). Net price 30-cap pack = £1.79. Label: 25

Dose: 1 capsule daily during pregnancy

NHS **Ferrograd C**® (Abbott)

Filmtabs® (= tablets f/c), red, dried ferrous sulphate 325 mg (105 mg iron) for sustained release, ascorbic acid 500 mg (as sodium salt). Net price 30-tab pack = £1.56. Label: 25

Dose: 1 tablet daily before food

NHS **Fesovit Z**® (Evans)

Spansule® (= capsules m/r), orange/clear, enclosing brown, orange, and white pellets, dried ferrous sulphate 150 mg (47 mg iron), zinc sulphate monohydrate 61.8 mg (22.5 mg zinc) with vitamins B group and C. Net price 30-cap pack = £2.80. Label: 25

Dose: 1–2 capsules daily; CHILD over 1 year 1 capsule daily

PoM **Folicin**® (Link)

Tablets, s/c, dried ferrous sulphate 200 mg (60 mg iron), folic acid 2.5 mg with minerals. Net price 20 = 30p

Dose: 1–2 tablets daily during pregnancy

NHS **Givitol**® (Galen)

Capsules, red/maroon, ferrous fumarate 305 mg (100 mg iron) with vitamins B group and C. Net price 20 = 82p

Dose: 1 capsule daily before food

NHS ***Pregnavite Forte F**® (Goldshield)

Tablets, lilac, s/c, dried ferrous sulphate 84 mg (25.2 mg iron), folic acid 120 micrograms, vitamin A 1333 units, thiamine hydrochloride 500 micrograms, riboflavine 500 micrograms, nicotinamide 5 mg, pyridoxine hydrochloride 330 micrograms, ascorbic acid 13.3 mg, vitamin D 133 units, calcium phosphate 160 mg. Net price 84-tab pack = £2.95

Dose: 1 tablet 3 times daily during or after food

* except to reduce the risk of spina bifida or anencephaly in babies born to women who have previously given birth to one of more babies (or aborted a fetus) with a neural tube defect and endorsed 'SLS' ('S2B' in Scotland); **important** but see Department of Health recommendations on p. 348

9.1.1.2 PARENTERAL IRON

The only valid reason for administering iron **parenterally** is failure of oral therapy due to lack of patient cooperation, severe gastro-intestinal side-effects, continuing severe blood loss or malabsorption. Provided that the oral iron preparation is taken reliably and is absorbed, then the haemoglobin response is not significantly faster with the parenteral route. The need for a more rapid cure of the anaemia is therefore not met by parenteral administration of iron.

A suitable parenteral preparation contains a complex of iron, sorbitol and citric acid as **iron sorbitol injection** (Jectofer®). It is **not** suitable for intravenous injection and, although the low mean molecular weight allows rapid absorption from the injection site, excretion in the saliva and substantial urinary losses also occur.

It is usual to give a course of *deep intramuscular* injections. The manufacturer's dosage schedules should be consulted; these usually include a supplement for reconstitution of iron stores.

To prevent leakage along the needle track with subsequent staining of the skin, intramuscular injections should be deep with suitable technique.

IRON SORBITOL INJECTION

Contains 5% (50 mg /mL) of iron

Indications: iron-deficiency anaemia

Cautions: oral iron should be stopped at least 24 hours before; other injectable iron preparations should be stopped a week before; urine may darken on standing

Contra-indications: liver disease, kidney disease (particularly pyelonephritis), untreated urinary-tract infections; preferably avoid in patients with pre-existing cardiac abnormalities (e.g. angina or arrhythmias)

Side-effects: occasionally severe arrhythmias

Dose: *by deep intramuscular injection,* see notes above and manufacturer's literature

PoM **Jectofer**® (Astra)

Injection, iron sorbitol injection. Net price 2-mL amp = 47p

9.1.2 Drugs used in megaloblastic anaemias

Most megaloblastic anaemias are due to lack of either vitamin B_{12} or folate and it is essential to establish in every case which deficiency is present and the underlying cause. In emergencies, where delay might be dangerous, it is sometimes necessary to administer both substances after the bone marrow test while plasma assay results are awaited. Normally, however, appropriate treatment should be instituted only when the results of tests are available.

The most common cause of megaloblastic anaemia in the UK is *pernicious anaemia* in which lack of gastric intrinsic factor due to an auto-immune gastritis causes malabsorption of vitamin B_{12}.

Vitamin B_{12} is also needed in the treatment of megaloblastosis due to *prolonged nitrous oxide anaesthesia,* which inactivates the vitamin, and in the rare syndrome of *congenital transcobalamin II deficiency.*

Vitamin B_{12} should be given prophylactically after *total gastrectomy* or *total ileal resection* (or after *partial gastrectomy* if a vitamin B_{12} absorption test shows vitamin B_{12} malabsorption).

Apart from dietary deficiency, all other causes of vitamin-B_{12} deficiency are attributable to *malabsorption* so there is little place for the use of vitamin B_{12} orally and none for vitamin B_{12} intrinsic factor complexes given by mouth.

Hydroxocobalamin has completely replaced cyanocobalamin as the form of vitamin B_{12} of choice for therapy; it is retained in the body longer than cyanocobalamin and thus for maintenance therapy need only be given at intervals of 3 months.

Although a haematological response in vitamin-B_{12} deficiency may be obtained by small doses, it is customary to start treatment with 1 mg by intramuscular injection repeated 5 times at intervals of 2 to 3 days to replenish the depleted body stores. Thereafter, maintenance treatment, which is usually for life, can be instituted. There is no evidence that larger doses provide any additional benefit in vitamin-B_{12} neuropathy.

Folic acid has few indications for long-term therapy since most causes of folate deficiency are self-limiting or will yield to a short course of treatment. It should not be used in undiagnosed megaloblastic anaemia unless vitamin B_{12} is administered concurrently otherwise neuropathy may be precipitated (see above).

In *folate-deficient megaloblastic anaemia* (e.g. due to poor nutrition, pregnancy, or antiepileptics), standard treatment to bring about a haematological remission and replenish body stores, is oral administration of folic acid 5 mg daily for 4 months; up to 15 mg daily may be necessary in malabsorption states.

For *prophylaxis in chronic haemolytic states or in renal dialysis*, it is sufficient to give folic acid 5 mg daily or even weekly, depending on the diet and the rate of haemolysis.

For *prophylaxis in pregnancy* the dose of folic acid is 200–500 micrograms daily (see Iron and Folic Acid, section 9.1.1.1). See also below.

PREVENTION OF NEURAL TUBE DEFECTS. Recommendations of an expert advisory group of the Department of Health include the advice that:

To prevent *recurrence of neural tube defect* women who wish to become pregnant (or who are at risk of becoming pregnant) should be advised to take folic acid supplements at a dose of 5 mg daily (reduced to 4 mg daily if a suitable preparation becomes available); supplementation should continue until the twelfth week of pregnancy. Women receiving antiepileptic therapy need individual counselling by their doctor before starting folic acid.

To prevent *first occurrence of neural tube defect* women who are planning a pregnancy should be advised to take folic acid as a medicinal or food supplement at a dose of 400 micrograms daily before conception and during the first 12 weeks of pregnancy. Women who have not been supplementing and who suspect they are pregnant should start at once and continue until the twelfth week of pregnancy.

There is **no** justification for prescribing multiple-ingredient vitamin preparations containing vitamin B_{12} or folic acid.

HYDROXOCOBALAMIN

Indications: Pernicious anaemia, other causes of vitamin-B_{12} deficiency, subacute combined degeneration of the spinal cord

Cautions: should not be given before diagnosis fully established but see also notes above

Dose: by intramuscular injection, initially 1 mg repeated 5 times at intervals of 2–3 days; maintenance dose 1 mg every 3 months; CHILD, dosage as for adult

PoM **Hydroxocobalamin Injection,** hydroxocobalamin 1 mg/mL. Net price 1-mL amp = £1.36

Note. The BP directs that when vitamin B_{12} injection is prescribed or demanded hydroxocobalamin injection shall be dispensed or supplied

The brand names NHS Cobalin-H® (Link) and NHS Neo-Cytamen® (Evans) are used for hydroxocobalamin injection

CYANOCOBALAMIN

Indications: see notes above

Dose: by mouth, vitamin-B_{12} deficiency of dietary origin, 50–150 micrograms or more daily taken between meals; CHILD 35–50 micrograms twice daily

By intramuscular injection, initially 1 mg repeated 10 times at intervals of 2–3 days, maintenance 1 mg every month, but see notes above

Cyanocobalamin (Non-proprietary)

NHS *Tablets,* cyanocobalamin 50 micrograms. Net price 50-tab pack = £2.14

* except to treat or prevent vitamin-B_{12} deficiency in a patient who is a vegan or who has a proven vitamin-B_{12} deficiency of dietary origin and endorsed 'SLS' ('S2B' in Scotland)

Note. The brand name NHS Cytacon® (Goldshield) is used for cyanocobalamin tablets

NHS *Liquid,* cyanocobalamin 35 micrograms/5 mL. Net price 200 mL = £2.14

Note. The brand name NHS Cytacon® (Goldshield) is used for cyanocobalamin liquid

PoM *Injection,* cyanocobalamin 1 mg/mL. Net price 1-mL amp = £1.00

Note. The BP directs that when vitamin B_{12} injection is prescribed or demanded hydroxocobalamin injection shall be dispensed or supplied

The brand name NHS Cytamen® (Evans) is used for cyanocobalamin injection

FOLIC ACID

Indications: see notes above

Cautions: should never be given alone in the treatment of Addisonian pernicious anaemia and other vitamin B_{12}-deficiency states because it may precipitate the onset of subacute combined degeneration of the spinal cord. Do not use in malignant disease unless megaloblastic anaemia due to folate deficiency is an important complication (some malignant tumours are folate-dependent); **interactions:** Appendix 1 (vitamins)

Dose: initially, 5 mg daily for 4 months (see notes above); maintenance, 5 mg every 1–7 days depending on underlying disease; CHILD up to 1 year, 500 micrograms/kg daily; over 1 year, as adult dose

Prevention of neural tube defects, see notes above

PoM ¹**Folic Acid Tablets,** folic acid 5 mg, net price 20 = 7p

1. Can be sold to the public provided daily doses do not exceed 500 micrograms

Note. Preparations containing folic acid 400 micrograms are also on sale to the public (as food supplements)

PoM **Lexpec®** (RP Drugs)

Syrup, sugar-free, folic acid 2.5 mg/5 mL. Net price 125 mL = £5.85

FOLINIC ACID
See section 8.1.3

9.1.3   Drugs used in hypoplastic, haemolytic, and renal anaemias

Anabolic steroids, pyridoxine, antilymphocyte immunoglobulin, and various corticosteroids are used in hypoplastic and haemolytic anaemias.

The place of **anabolic steroids** in the therapy of *aplastic anaemia* remains somewhat controversial and their effectiveness is unclear. There is a wide variation in the reported successful responses. Occasional patients, however, do seem to derive benefit. Since nandrolone decanoate requires intramuscular injection it is unsuitable in aplastic anaemia or cytotoxic aplasia because of the low platelet count; it is customary to prescribe oxymetholone in doses of the order of 2–3 mg/kg daily, and to continue therapy for at least 3 to 6 months. At these dose levels, virilising side-effects may be expected in female patients and in children. Controlled trials have shown that antilymphocyte globulin produces a response in 50% of acquired cases; higher response rates have been reported when cyclosporin is given as well.

It is unlikely that dietary deprivation of **pyridoxine** (section 9.6.2) produces haematological effects in man. However, certain forms of *sideroblastic anaemia* respond to pharmacological doses, possibly reflecting its role as a co-enzyme during haemoglobin synthesis. Pyridoxine is indicated in both *idiopathic acquired* and *hereditary sideroblastic anaemias*. Although complete cures have not been reported, some increase in haemoglobin may occur; the dose required is usually high, up to 400 mg daily. *Reversible sideroblastic anaemias* respond to treatment of the underlying cause but in pregnancy, haemolytic anaemias, and alcohol dependence, or during isoniazid treatment, pyridoxine is also indicated.

Corticosteroids (see section 6.3) have an important place in the management of a wide variety of haematological disorders. They include conditions with an immune basis such as *auto-immune haemolytic anaemia*, *immune thrombocytopenias* and *neutropenias*, and *major transfusion reactions*. They are also used in chemotherapy schedules for many types of lymphoma, *lymphoid leukaemias*, and *paraproteinaemias*, including *myelomatosis*. Corticosteroids are used in *aplastic anaemias*, where their value is more debatable.

NANDROLONE
Indications: aplastic anaemia but see notes above; postmenopausal osteoporosis, see section 6.4.3
Cautions; Contra-indications; Side-effects: see section 6.4.3
Dose: by deep intramuscular injection, aplastic anaemia (but not recommended, see notes above), nandrolone decanoate 50–100 mg weekly
PoM **Deca-Durabolin 100®** (Organon)
Injection (oily), nandrolone decanoate 100 mg/mL. Net price 1-mL amp = £6.68

OXYMETHOLONE
Indications: aplastic anaemia; see notes above
Cautions: monitor liver function (if altered, reduce dose or discontinue); renal impairment (see also Contra-indications), cardiac impairment; long-term treatment especially in the young (risk of hepatic tumours); elderly men (risk of prostate hypertrophy or carcinoma); monitor serum iron and iron binding capacity; monitor serum cholesterol (particularly if history of myocardial infarction and coronary artery disease); diabetes mellitus; **interactions:** Appendix 1 (anabolic steroids)
Contra-indications: breast or prostate cancer in men; breast cancer with hypercalcaemia in women; pregnancy; breast-feeding; nephrosis or nephrotic phase of nephritis; hepatic impairment (see Appendix 2); infants; porphyria (see section 9.8.2)
Side-effects: nausea, vomiting, diarrhoea; excitation, sleeplessness; chills, muscle cramps; acne; liver toxicity including jaundice and pruritus, hepatocellular carcinoma, and hepatic coma; oedema, congestive heart failure; premature closure of epiphyses; virilisation in women and prepubertal children; amenorrhoea, impairment of fertility; hypercalcaemia; blood lipid changes
Dose: aplastic anaemia, 2–3 mg/kg daily in divided doses; CHILD 2–3 mg/kg daily (less in Fanconi's anaemia)
See also notes above

PoM **Anapolon 50®** (Syntex)
Tablets, scored, oxymetholone 50 mg. Net price 20 = £14.46

ERYTHROPOIETIN

Epoetin (recombinant human erythropoietin) is used for the anaemia associated with erythropoietin deficiency in chronic renal failure. The clinical efficacy of epoetin alfa and epoetin beta is similar and they can be used interchangeably.

Other factors which contribute to the anaemia of chronic renal failure such as iron or folate deficiency should be corrected; aluminium toxicity, concurrent infection or other inflammatory disease may also impair the response to epoetin.

EPOETIN ALFA and BETA
(Recombinant human erythropoietins)
Indications: see under preparations, below
Cautions: inadequately treated or poorly controlled blood pressure (monitor closely blood pressure, haemoglobin, and electrolytes), interrupt treatment if blood pressure uncontrolled; exclude other causes of anaemia (e.g. folic acid or vitamin B_{12} deficiency) and give iron supplements if necessary; ischaemic vascular disease; thrombocytosis (monitor platelet count for first 8 weeks); history of convulsions; malignant disease;

chronic liver failure; sudden stabbing migraine-like pain is warning of hypertensive crisis; increase in heparin dose may be needed; pregnancy and breast-feeding

Contra-indications: uncontrolled hypertension

Side-effects: dose-dependent increase in blood pressure or aggravation of hypertension; in isolated patients with normal or low blood pressure, hypertensive crisis with encephalopathy-like symptoms and generalised tonic-clonic seizures requiring immediate medical attention; dose-dependent increase in platelet count (but thrombocytosis rare) regressing during treatment; influenza-like symptoms (may be reduced if intravenous injection given over 5 minutes); shunt thrombosis especially if tendency to hypotension or arteriovenous shunt complications; isolated reports of hyperkalaemia, increase in plasma creatinine, urea and phosphate, convulsions, skin reactions, palpebral oedema, myocardial infarction, anaphylaxis

Dose: aimed at increasing haemoglobin concentration at rate not exceeding $2 g/100 mL/month$ to stable level of $10–12 g/100 mL$ ($9.5–11 g/100 mL$ in children); see under preparations, below

Note. Although epoetin alfa and beta are clinically indistinguishable the prescriber must specify which is required

Epoetin alfa
PoM Eprex® (Cilag)
Injection, epoetin alfa 2000 units/mL, net price 0.5-mL (1000-unit) vial = £8.78, 0.5-mL (1000-unit) pre-filled syringe = £9.23, 1-mL (2000-unit) vial = £17.55; 4000 units/mL, 0.5-mL (2000-unit) pre-filled syringe = £18.00, 1-mL (4000-unit) vial = £35.10; 10 000 units/mL, 0.3-mL (3000-unit) pre-filled syringe = £26.78, 0.4-mL (4000-unit) pre-filled syringe = £35.55, 1-mL (10 000-unit) vial = £87.75, 1-mL (10 000-unit) pre-filled syringe = £88.20

Dose: anaemia associated with chronic renal failure in patients on haemodialysis, *by subcutaneous injection* (max. 1 mL per injection site) or *by intravenous injection* over 2 minutes, initially 50 units/kg 3 times weekly increased according to response in steps of 25 units/kg at intervals of 4 weeks; omit one of the weekly doses if haemoglobin rise exceeds 2 g/100 mL per month with the initial dose; max. 600 units/kg weekly in 3 divided doses; maintenance dose (when haemoglobin concentration of 10–12 g/100 mL achieved), usually 100–300 units/kg weekly in 2–3 divided doses; CHILD (intravenous route only) initially as for adults; maintenance dose (when haemoglobin concentration of 9.5–11 g/100 mL achieved), under 10 kg usually 75–150 units/kg 3 times weekly, 10–30 kg usually 60–150 units/kg 3 times weekly, over 30 kg usually 30–100 units/kg 3 times weekly

Anaemia associated with chronic renal failure in adults on peritoneal dialysis, *by subcutaneous injection* (max. 1 mL per injection site) or *by intravenous injection* over 2 minutes, initially 50 units/kg twice weekly increased according to response in steps of 25 units/kg at intervals of 4 weeks; maintenance dose (when haemoglobin concentration of 10–12 g/100 mL achieved), 50–100 units/kg weekly in 2 equally divided doses

Severe symptomatic anaemia of renal origin in adults with renal insufficiency not yet on dialysis, preferably *by subcutaneous injection* (max. 1 mL per injection site), initially 50 units/kg 3 times weekly increased according to response in steps of 25 units/kg at intervals of 4 weeks; max. 600 units/kg weekly in 3 divided doses; maintenance dose (when haemoglobin concentration of 10–12 g/100 mL achieved), 50–100 units/kg weekly in 3 divided doses

Note. Subcutaneous dose generally about 20–30% lower than intravenous; when changing route give same dose then adjust according to weekly haemoglobin measurements

Epoetin beta
PoM Recormon® (Boehringer Mannheim)
Injection, powder for reconstitution, epoetin beta. Net price 1000-unit vial = £8.78; 2000-unit vial = £17.55; 5000-unit vial = £43.88 (all with water for injections)

Note. Avoid contact of reconstituted injection with glass; use only plastic materials

Recormon® S injection (for subcutaneous use), powder for reconstitution, epoetin beta. Net price 1000-unit vial = £8.78; 2000-unit vial = £17.55 (both with syringe and water for injections)

Dose: anaemia associated with chronic renal failure in dialysis patients, severe symptomatic anaemia of renal origin in patients not yet on dialysis, ADULT and CHILD over 2 years,

By subcutaneous injection, initially 20 units/kg 3 times weekly for 4 weeks, increased according to response at monthly intervals in steps of 20 units/kg; maintenance dose (when haemoglobin concentration of 10–12 g/100 mL achieved), initially reduce dose by half then adjust according to response at intervals of 1–2 weeks

By intravenous injection over 2 minutes, initially 40 units/kg 3 times weekly for 4 weeks, increased if initial haemoglobin rise less than 1 g/100 mL per month to 80 units/kg 3 times weekly with further increases if needed at monthly intervals in steps of 20 units/kg; maintenance dose (when haemoglobin concentration of 10–12 g/100 mL achieved), initially reduce dose by half then adjust according to response at intervals of 1–2 weeks

Max. by either route 720 units/kg weekly

IRON OVERLOAD

Severe tissue iron overload may occur in aplastic and other refractory anaemias, mainly as the result of repeated blood transfusions. It is a particular problem in refractory anaemias with hyperplastic bone marrow, especially *thalassaemia major*, where excessive iron absorption from the gut and inappropriate iron therapy may add to the tissue siderosis.

Venesection therapy is contra-indicated, but the long-term administration of the iron chelating compound **desferrioxamine mesylate** is useful. Subcutaneous infusions of desferrioxamine (20–40 mg/kg over 12 hours) are given on 5 to 7 nights each week. Desferrioxamine (up to 2 g per unit of blood) may also be given through the infusion line at the time of blood transfusion.

Iron excretion induced by desferrioxamine is enhanced by administration of vitamin C (section 9.6.3) in a dose of 200 mg daily (100 mg in infants); it should be given separately from food since it also enhances iron absorption. In patients with cardiac abnormalities vitamin C should be avoided for 1–2 weeks after starting desferrioxamine treatment.

Infusion of desferrioxamine may be used to treat *aluminium overload* in dialysis patients; theoretically 100 mg of desferrioxamine binds with 4.1 mg of aluminium.

Orally active iron chelators are under clinical study but are not available for general use.

DESFERRIOXAMINE MESYLATE

Indications: see notes above; iron poisoning, see Emergency Treatment of Poisoning

Cautions: renal impairment, eye and ear examinations; aluminium-related encephalopathy (may exacerbate neurological dysfunction), pregnancy, breast-feeding; **interactions:** Appendix 1 (desferrioxamine)

Side-effects: gastro-intestinal disturbances; arrhythmias, hypotension (especially when given too rapidly by intravenous injection); anaphylaxis; dizziness, convulsions; Yersinia infection more frequent; disturbances of hearing and vision (including lens opacity and retinopathy); skin reactions; pain on intramuscular injection

Dose: see notes above; iron poisoning, see Emergency Treatment of Poisoning

Note. For full details and warnings relating to administration, consult data sheet

Preparations

See under Emergency Treatment of Poisoning

9.1.4   Drugs used in autoimmune thrombocytopenic purpura

It is usual to commence the treatment of autoimmune (idiopathic) thrombocytopenic purpura with corticosteroids, e.g. prednisolone of the order of 1 mg/kg daily, gradually reducing the dosage over the subsequent weeks. In patients who fail to achieve a satisfactory platelet count or relapse when corticosteroid dosage is reduced or withdrawn, splenectomy is considered.

Other therapy that has been tried in refractory cases includes azathioprine (see section 8.2.1), cyclophosphamide (see section 8.1.1), vincristine or vinblastine (see section 8.1.4) (or vinblastine-loaded platelets), cyclosporin (see section 8.2.2), and danazol (section 6.7.3). Intravenous immunoglobulins (see section 14.5), have also been used in refractory cases or where a temporary rapid rise in platelets is needed, as in pregnancy or pre-operatively. For patients with chronic severe thrombocytopenia refractory to other therapy, tranexamic acid (see section 2.11) may be given to reduce the severity of haemorrhage.

9.1.5   G6PD deficiency

Glucose 6-phosphate dehydrogenase (G6PD) deficiency is highly prevalent in populations originating from most parts of Africa, from most parts of Asia, from Oceania, and from Southern Europe; it can also be encountered, rarely, in any other population.

When prescribing drugs for patients who are G6PD deficient, the following three points should be kept in mind:

1. G6PD deficiency is genetically heterogeneous; different genetic variants entail different susceptibility to the haemolytic risk from drugs; thus, a drug found to be safe in some G6PD-deficient subjects may not be equally safe in others;
2. no test specifically designed to identify potential risk in G6PD-deficient subjects is currently carried out by manufacturers;
3. the risk and severity of haemolysis is almost always dose-related.

The table below should be read with these points in mind. Whenever possible, a test for G6PD deficiency should be done before prescribing a drug in the list, especially if the patient belongs to a population group in which G6PD deficiency is common.

A very small group of G6PD-deficient individuals, with chronic non-spherocytic haemolytic anaemia, have haemolysis even in the absence of an exogenous trigger. These patients must be regarded as being at high risk of severe exacerbation of haemolysis following administration of any of the drugs listed below.

Drugs with definite risk of haemolysis in most G6PD-deficient subjects

Dapsone and other sulphones (higher doses for dermatitis herpetiformis more likely to cause problems)
Methylene blue
Niridazole [not on UK market]
Nitrofurantoin
Pamaquin [not on UK market]
Primaquine (30 mg weekly for 8 weeks has been found to be without undue harmful effects in Afro and Asian people, see section 5.4.1)
4-Quinolones (including ciprofloxacin and nalidixic acid)
Sulphonamides (including co-trimoxazole; some sulphonamides, e.g. sulphadiazine, have been tested and found not to be haemolytic in many G6PD-deficient subjects)

Drugs with possible risk of haemolysis in some G6PD-deficient subjects

Aspirin (acceptable in a dose of at least 1 g daily in most G6PD-deficient subjects)
Chloroquine (acceptable in acute malaria)
Menadione, water-soluble derivatives (e.g. menadiol sodium phosphate)
Probenecid
Quinidine (acceptable in acute malaria)
Quinine (acceptable in acute malaria)

Note. Mothballs may contain naphthalene which also causes haemolysis in subjects with G6PD-deficiency.

9.1.6   Drugs used in neutropenia

Filgrastim (recombinant human granulocyte-colony stimulating factor) may reduce the duration of neutropenia associated with the use of cancer chemotherapy and thereby reduce the incidence of associated sepsis. Filgrastim has, however, no routine indication at present and is expensive; it should only be administered by those experienced in its use.

Lenograstim (recombinant human granulocyte-colony stimulating factor) and **molgramostim** (recombinant human granulocyte macrophage-colony stimulating factor) have now also been introduced.

FILGRASTIM

(Recombinant human granulocyte-colony stimulating factor, G-CSF)

Indications: (specialist use only) reduction of neutropenia and incidence of febrile neutropenia in cytotoxic chemotherapy of non-myeloid malignancy; reduction in duration of neutropenia (and associated sequelae) in myeloablative therapy followed by bone-marrow transplantation; severe congenital neutropenia, cyclic neutropenia, or idiopathic neutropenia and history of severe or recurrent infections (distinguish carefully from other haematological disorders)

Cautions: tumours with myeloid characteristics (risk of tumour growth), pre-malignant myeloid conditions; reduced myeloid precursors; monitor leucocyte count (discontinue treatment if leucocytosis, see data sheet); monitor platelet count and haemoglobin; osteoporotic bone disease (monitor bone density if given for more than 6 months); does not prevent other toxic effects of high-dose chemotherapy; pregnancy, breast-feeding

Contra-indications: severe congenital neutropenia (Kostman's syndrome) with abnormal cytogenetics

Side-effects: musculoskeletal pain, transient hypotension, disturbances in liver enzymes and serum uric acid; urinary abnormalities including dysuria; allergic reactions (more common after intravenous infusion), proteinuria and haematuria reported; on long-term use cutaneous vasculitis also reported, also splenic enlargement, headache, diarrhoea, anaemia and epistaxis

Dose: cytotoxic-induced neutropenia, *by subcutaneous injection or by intravenous infusion* (over 30 minutes), 500 000 units/kg daily started not less than 24 hours after cytotoxic chemotherapy, continued until neutrophil count in normal range, usually for up to 14 days

Myeloablative therapy followed by bone-marrow transplantation, *by intravenous infusion* over 30 minutes or over 24 hours *or by subcutaneous infusion* over 24 hours, 1 million units/kg daily, started not less than 24 hours following cytotoxic chemotherapy (and within 24 hours of bone-marrow infusion), then adjusted according to absolute neutrophil count (see data sheet)

Severe chronic neutropenia, by *subcutaneous injection*, ADULT and CHILD, in severe congenital neutropenia, initially 1.2 million units/kg daily in single or divided doses (initially 500 000 units/kg daily in idiopathic or cyclic neutropenia), adjusted according to response (see data sheet)

▼ PoM **Neupogen**® (Amgen, Roche)
Injection, filgrastim 30 million units (300 micrograms)/mL; net price 1-mL vial = £77.03, 1.6-mL (48 million-unit) vial = £122.85

LENOGRASTIM

(Recombinant human granulocyte-colony stimulating factor, rHuG-CSF)

Indications: (specialist use only) reduction in the duration of neutropenia and associated complications

following bone-marrow transplantation for non-myeloid malignancy or following treatment with cytotoxic chemotherapy associated with a significant incidence of febrile neutropenia

Cautions; Side-effects: see under Filgrastim

Dose: following bone-marrow transplantation, *by intravenous infusion*, ADULT and CHILD over 2 years 19.2 million units/m^2 daily started the day after transplantation, continued until neutrophil count stable in acceptable range (max. 28 days)

Cytotoxic-induced neutropenia, *by subcutaneous injection*, ADULT and CHILD over 2 years 19.2 million units/m^2 daily started the day after completion of chemotherapy, continued until neutrophil count stable in acceptable range (max. 28 days)

▼ PoM **Granocyte**® (Chugai)
Injection, powder for reconstitution, lenograstim, net price 33.6 million-unit (263-microgram) vial (with 1-mL amp water for injections) = £77.03

MOLGRAMOSTIM

(Recombinant human granulocyte macrophage-colony stimulating factor, GM-CSF)

Indications: (specialist use only) reduction of severity of neutropenia (and risk of infection) in cytotoxic chemotherapy; acceleration of myeloid recovery following bone-marrow transplantation; neutropenia in patients treated with ganciclovir in AIDS-related cytomegalovirus retinitis

Cautions: monitor serum albumin concentration and full blood count including differential white cell, platelet and haemoglobin; monitor closely patients with pulmonary disease; history of or predisposition to autoimmune disease; pregnancy and breast-feeding; not yet recommended for patients under 18 years

Contra-indications: myeloid malignancies

Side-effects: nausea, diarrhoea, vomiting, anorexia; dyspnoea; asthenia, fatigue; rash, fever, rigors, musculoskeletal pain; local reaction following subcutaneous injection; also reported, non-specific chest pain, stomatitis, headache, increased sweating, abdominal pain, pruritus, peripheral oedema, paraesthesia, and myalgia; serious reactions reported include anaphylaxis, cardiac failure, capillary leak syndrome, cerebrovascular disorders, confusion, convulsions, hypotension, cardiac rhythm abnormalities, intracranial hypertension, pericardial effusion, pericarditis, pleural effusion, pulmonary oedema, syncope

Dose: cytotoxic chemotherapy, *by subcutaneous injection*, 60 000–110 000 units/kg daily, starting 24 hours after last dose of chemotherapy, continued for 7–10 days

Bone-marrow transplantation, *by intravenous infusion*, 110 000 units/kg daily, starting day after transplantation, continued until absolute neutrophil count in desirable range (see data sheet); max. duration of treatment 30 days

Adjunct in ganciclovir treatment, *by subcutaneous injection*, 60 000 units/kg daily for 5 days then adjusted to maintain desirable absolute neutrophil count and white blood cell count

▼ PoM **Leucomax**® (Sandoz, Schering-Plough)
Injection, powder for reconstitution, molgramostim, net price 1.67 million-unit (150-microgram) vial = £38.51; 3.33 million-unit (300-microgram) vial = £77.02; 7.77 million-unit (700-microgram) vial = £179.89

9.2 Fluids and electrolytes

9.2.1 Oral administration
9.2.2 Intravenous administration
9.2.3 Plasma and plasma substitutes

The following tables give a selection of useful electrolyte values:

Electrolyte concentrations—intravenous fluids

Intravenous infusion	Millimoles per litre				
	Na^+	K^+	HCO_3^-	Cl^-	Ca^{2+}
Normal Plasma Values	142	4.5	26	103	2.5
Sodium Chloride 0.9%	150	—	—	150	—
Compound Sodium Lactate (Hartmann's)	131	5	29	111	2
Sodium Chloride 0.18% and Glucose 4%	30	—	—	30	—
Potassium Chloride 0.3% and Glucose 5%	—	40	—	40	—
Potassium Chloride 0.3% and Sodium Chloride 0.9%	150	40	—	190	—
To correct metabolic acidosis					
Sodium Bicarbonate 1.26%	150	—	150	—	—
Sodium Bicarbonate 8.4% for cardiac arrest	1000	—	1000	—	—
Sodium Lactate (M/6)	167	—	167	—	—

Millimoles of each ion in 1 gram of salt

Electrolyte		mmol/g approx.
Ammonium chloride		18.7
Calcium chloride ($CaCl_2,2H_2O$)	Ca	6.8
	Cl	13.6
Potassium bicarbonate		10
Potassium chloride		13.4
Sodium bicarbonate		11.9
Sodium chloride		17.1
Sodium lactate		8.9

Electrolyte content—gastro-intestinal secretions

Type of fluid	Millimoles per litre				
	H^+	Na^+	K^+	HCO_3^-	Cl^-
Gastric	40–60	20–80	5–20	—	100–150
Biliary	—	120–140	5–15	30–50	80–120
Pancreatic	—	120–140	5–15	70–110	40–80
Small bowel	—	120–140	5–15	20–40	90–130

Faeces, vomit, or aspiration should be saved and analysed where possible if abnormal losses are suspected; where this is impracticable the approximations above may be helpful in planning replacement therapy

9.2.1 Oral administration

9.2.1.1 Oral potassium
9.2.1.2 Oral sodium and water
9.2.1.3 Oral bicarbonate

Sodium and potassium salts, which may be given by mouth to prevent deficiencies or to treat established deficiencies of mild or moderate degree, are discussed in this section. Oral preparations for removing excess potassium and preparations for oral rehydration therapy are also included here. Oral bicarbonate, for metabolic acidosis, is also described in this section.

For reference to calcium, magnesium, and phosphate, see section 9.5.

9.2.1.1 ORAL POTASSIUM

Compensation for potassium loss is especially necessary:

1. in those taking digoxin or anti-arrhythmic drugs, where potassium depletion may induce arrhythmias;
2. in patients in whom secondary hyperaldosteronism occurs, e.g. renal artery stenosis, cirrhosis of the liver, the nephrotic syndrome, and severe heart failure;
3. in patients with excessive losses of potassium in the faeces, e.g. chronic diarrhoea associated with intestinal malabsorption or laxative abuse.

Measures to compensate for potassium loss may also be required in the elderly since they frequently take inadequate amounts of potassium in the diet (but see below for warning on renal insufficiency). Measures may also be required during long-term administration of drugs known to induce potassium loss (e.g. corticosteroids). Potassium supplements are seldom required with the small doses of diuretics given to treat hypertension; potassium-sparing diuretics (rather than potassium supplements) are recommended for prevention of hypokalaemia due to diuretics such as frusemide or the thiazides when these are given to eliminate oedema.

DOSAGE. If potassium salts are used for the *prevention of hypokalaemia*, then doses of potassium chloride 2 to 4 g (approx. 25 to 50 mmol) daily by mouth are suitable in patients taking a normal diet. Smaller doses must be used if there is renal insufficiency (common in the elderly) otherwise there is danger of hyperkalaemia. Potassium salts cause nausea and vomiting therefore poor compliance is a major limitation to their effectiveness; where appropriate, potassium-sparing diuretics are preferable.

When there is *established potassium depletion* or when the plasma-potassium concentration is less than 3.5 mmol/litre, larger doses of 10 to 15 g (approx. 135 to 200 mmol) daily of potassium chloride may be required over periods of days or weeks. Potassium depletion is frequently associated with chloride depletion and with metabolic alkalosis, and these disorders require correction.

ADMINISTRATION. Potassium salts are preferably given as a liquid (or effervescent) preparation, rather than modified-release tablets; they should be given as the chloride (the use of effervescent potassium tablets BPC 1968 should be restricted to *hyperchloraemic states*, section 9.2.1.3).

Salt substitutes. A number of salt substitutes which contain significant amounts of potassium chloride are readily available as health food products (e.g. Losalt and Ruthmol). These should not be used by patients with renal failure as potassium intoxication may result.

POTASSIUM BICARBONATE
Section 9.2.1.3

POTASSIUM CHLORIDE
Indications: potassium depletion (see notes above)
Cautions: intestinal stricture, history of peptic ulcer, hiatus hernia (for sustained-release preparations); **interactions:** Appendix 1 (potassium salts)
Contra-indications: renal failure, plasma potassium concentrations above 5 mmol/litre
Side-effects: nausea and vomiting (severe symptoms may indicate obstruction), oesophageal or small bowel ulceration
Dose: see notes above

Note. Do not confuse Effervescent Potassium Tablets BPC 1968 (section 9.2.1.3) with effervescent potassium chloride tablets. Effervescent Potassium Tablets BPC 1968 do not contain chloride ions and their use should be restricted to hyperchloraemic states (section 9.2.1.3). Effervescent Potassium Chloride Tablets BP are usually available in two strengths, one containing 6.7 mmol each of K⁺ and Cl⁻ (corresponding to Kloref®), the other containing 12 mmol K⁺ and 8 mmol Cl⁻ (corresponding to Sando-K®). Generic prescriptions must specify the strength required.

Kay-Cee-L® (Geistlich)
Syrup, red, sugar-free, potassium chloride 7.5% (1 mmol/mL each of K⁺ and Cl⁻). Net price 500 mL = £3.00. Label: 21
Kloref® (Cox)
Tablets, effervescent, betaine hydrochloride, potassium benzoate, bicarbonate, and chloride, equivalent to potassium chloride 500 mg (6.7 mmol each of K⁺ and Cl⁻). Net price 50 = £1.66. Label: 13, 21
Kloref-S® (Cox)
Granules, effervescent, sugar-free, betaine hydrochloride, potassium bicarbonate and chloride equivalent to potassium chloride 1.5 g (20 mmol each of K⁺ and Cl⁻)/sachet. Net price 30 sachets = £3.30. Label: 13, 21
Sando-K® (Sandoz)
Tablets, effervescent, potassium bicarbonate and chloride equivalent to potassium 470 mg (12 mmol of K⁺) and chloride 285 mg (8 mmol of Cl⁻). Net price 20 = 34p. Label: 13, 21

Modified-release preparations
Avoid unless effervescent tablets or liquid preparations inappropriate
Slow-K® (Ciba)
Tablets, m/r, orange, s/c, potassium chloride 600 mg (8 mmol each of K⁺ and Cl⁻). Net price 20 = 10p. Label: 25, 27, counselling, swallow whole with fluid during meals while sitting or standing

POTASSIUM CITRATE
See section 7.4.3

POTASSIUM REMOVAL

Ion-exchange resins may be used to remove excess potassium in *mild hyperkalaemia* or in *moderate hyperkalaemia* when there are not ECG changes; intravenous therapy is required in emergencies (section 9.2.2).

POLYSTYRENE SULPHONATE RESINS
Indications: hyperkalaemia associated with anuria or severe oliguria, and in dialysis patients
Cautions: children (impaction of resin with excessive dosage or inadequate dilution)
Contra-indications: avoid calcium-containing resin in hyperparathyroidism, multiple myeloma, sarcoidosis, or metastatic carcinoma; avoid sodium-containing resin in congestive heart failure and severe renal impairment
Side-effects: rectal ulceration following rectal administration
Dose: by mouth, 15 g 3–4 times daily in water (not fruit juice which has a high K⁺ content)
By rectum, as an enema, 30 g in methylcellulose solution, retained for 9 hours
CHILD, either route, 0.5–1 g/kg daily
Calcium Resonium® (Sanofi Winthrop)
Powder, buff, calcium polystyrene sulphonate. Net price 300 g = £43.23. Label: 13
Resonium A® (Sanofi Winthrop)
Powder, buff, sodium polystyrene sulphonate. Net price 454 g = £58.53. Label: 13

9.2.1.2 ORAL SODIUM AND WATER

Sodium chloride is indicated in states of sodium depletion and usually needs to be given intravenously (section 9.2.2). In chronic conditions associated with mild or moderate degrees of sodium depletion, e.g. in salt-losing bowel or renal disease, oral supplements of sodium chloride or bicarbonate (section 9.2.1.3), according to the acid-base status of the patient, may be sufficient.

SODIUM BICARBONATE
Section 9.2.1.3

SODIUM CHLORIDE
Indications: sodium depletion; see also section 9.2.2.

Slow Sodium® (Ciba)
Tablets, m/r, sodium chloride 600 mg (approx. 10 mmol each of Na⁺ and Cl⁻). Net price 20 = 11p. Label: 25

ORAL REHYDRATION THERAPY (ORT)

As a worldwide problem *diarrhoea* is by far the most important indication for fluid and electrolyte replacement. Intestinal absorption of sodium and water is enhanced by glucose (and other carbohydrates). Replacement of fluid and electrolytes lost through diarrhoea can therefore be achieved by giving solutions containing sodium, potassium, and glucose.

Oral rehydration solutions should:

enhance the absorption of water and electrolytes;
replace the electrolyte deficit adequately and safely;
contain an alkalising agent to counter acidosis;
be slightly hypo-osmolar (about 250 mmol/litre);
be simple to use in hospital and at home;
be palatable and acceptable, especially to children;
be readily available.

It is the policy of the World Health Organization (WHO) to promote a single oral rehydration solution but use it flexibly (e.g. by giving extra water between drinks of oral rehydration solution to moderately dehydrated infants).

Oral rehydration solutions used in the UK are lower in sodium (35–60 mmol/litre) and higher in glucose (up to 200 mmol/litre) than the WHO formulation. They are of benefit for *mild to moderate diarrhoea*, when the body's homoeostatic mechanisms are still working and will not be harmful, but they may be suboptimal in correction of fluid loss and electrolyte imbalance. In the *more severe diarrhoeas* the WHO formulation is marginally more effective in correcting dehydration; it carries no danger of hypernatraemia if used correctly. In acute diarrhoea normal feeding can continue as soon as the fluid deficit has been corrected; breast-feeding in particular should be offered between oral rehydration drinks.

For intravenous rehydration see section 9.2.2

ORAL REHYDRATION SALTS (ORS)

Indications: fluid and electrolyte loss in diarrhoea, see notes above

Dose: according to fluid loss, usually 200–400 mL solution after every loose motion; INFANT 1–1½ times usual feed volume; CHILD 200 mL after every loose motion

UK formulations

Note. After reconstitution any unused solution should be discarded no later than 1 hour after preparation unless stored in a refrigerator when it may be kept for up to 24 hours.

Diocalm Junior® (SmithKline Beecham Healthcare)

Oral powder, sodium chloride 350 mg, potassium chloride 300 mg, sodium citrate 590 mg, anhydrous glucose 4 g/sachet. Net price 5-sachet pack (orange-flavoured) = £1.22

Reconstitute one sachet with 200 mL of water (freshly boiled and cooled for infants)

Note. Five sachets reconstituted with 1 litre of water provide Na$^+$ 60 mmol, K$^+$ 20 mmol, Cl$^-$ 50 mmol, citrate 10 mmol, and glucose 111 mmol

Dioralyte® (Rhône-Poulenc Rorer)

Effervescent tablets, sodium chloride 117 mg, sodium bicarbonate 336 mg, potassium chloride 186 mg, citric acid anhydrous 384 mg, anhydrous glucose 1.62 g. Net price 10-tab pack (blackcurrant- or citrus-flavoured) = £1.17

Reconstitute 2 tablets with 200 mL of water (only for adults and for children over 1 year)

Note. Ten tablets when reconstituted with 1 litre of water provide Na$^+$ 60 mmol, K$^+$ 25 mmol, Cl$^-$ 45 mmol, citrate 20 mmol, and glucose 90 mmol

Oral powder, sodium chloride 470 mg, potassium chloride 300 mg, disodium hydrogen citrate 530 mg, glucose 3.56 g/sachet. Net price 20 sachet-pack (blackcurrant- or citrus-flavoured or plain) = £4.07

Reconstitute one sachet with 200 mL of water (freshly boiled and cooled for infants).

Note. Five sachets reconstituted with 1 litre of water provide Na$^+$ 60 mmol, K$^+$ 20 mmol, Cl$^-$ 60 mmol, citrate 10 mmol, and glucose 90 mmol

Electrolade® (Roche)

Oral powder, sodium chloride 236 mg, potassium chloride 300 mg, sodium bicarbonate 500 mg, anhydrous glucose 4 g/sachet (banana- or melon-flavoured). Net price 20-sachet pack = £3.99

Reconstitute one sachet with 200 mL of water (freshly boiled and cooled for infants)

Note. Five sachets when reconstituted with 1 litre of water provide Na$^+$ 50 mmol, K$^+$ 20 mmol, Cl$^-$ 40 mmol, HCO$_3^-$ 30 mmol, and glucose 111 mmol

Gluco-lyte® (Cupal)

Oral powder, sodium chloride 200 mg, potassium chloride 300 mg, sodium bicarbonate 300 mg, glucose 8 g/sachet. Net price 6 sachets = £1.34

Reconstitute one sachet with 200 mL of water (freshly boiled and cooled for infants)

Note. Five sachets when reconstituted with 1 litre of water provide Na$^+$ 35 mmol, K$^+$ 20 mmol, Cl$^-$ 37 mmol, HCO$_3^-$ 18 mmol, and glucose 200 mmol (corresponds to Oral Rehydration Salts—Formula A, BP)

Rapolyte® (Janssen)

Oral powder, sodium chloride 350 mg, potassium chloride 300 mg, sodium citrate 580 mg, anhydrous glucose 4 g/sachet. Net price 5-sachet pack (raspberry-flavoured) = £1.23

Reconstitute one sachet with 200 mL of water (freshly boiled and cooled for infants)

Note. Five sachets reconstituted with 1 litre of water provide Na$^+$ 60 mmol, K$^+$ 20 mmol, Cl$^-$ 50 mmol, citrate 10 mmol, and glucose 111 mmol

Rehidrat® (Searle)

Oral powder, sodium chloride 440 mg, potassium chloride 380 mg, sodium bicarbonate 420 mg, citric acid 440 mg, glucose 4.09 g, sucrose 8.07 g, fructose 70 mg/sachet. Net price 24-sachet pack (orange, blackcurrant or lemon and lime flavour) = £6.44; 16-sachet pack (mixed flavours) = £4.29

Note. Lemon and lime version stains vomit green; blackcurrant version contains greater amounts of glucose (4.13 g) and sucrose (8.17 g), and less fructose (10 mg)

Reconstitute one sachet with 250 mL of water (freshly boiled and cooled for infants)

Note. Four sachets when reconstituted with 1 litre of water provide Na$^+$ 50 mmol, K$^+$ 20 mmol, Cl$^-$ 50 mmol, HCO$_3^-$ 20 mmol, citrate 9 mmol, glucose approx. 91 mmol, sucrose approx. 94 mmol, and fructose approx. 1–2 mmol

WHO formulations
WHO Oral Rehydration Salts

Oral powder, sodium chloride 3.5 g, potassium chloride 1.5 g, sodium citrate 2.9 g, anhydrous glucose 20 g. To be dissolved in sufficient water to produce 1 litre (providing Na^+ 90 mol, K^+ 20 mol, Cl^- 80 mmol, citrate 10 mmol, glucose 111 mmol/litre)

Note. Recommended by the WHO and the United Nations Childrens Fund but not commonly used in the UK. Corresponds to Oral Rehydration Salts—Citrate (Formula C) BP; the alternative WHO formulation corresponds to Oral Rehydration Salts—Bicarbonate (Formula B) BP and is less stable

9.2.1.3 ORAL BICARBONATE

Sodium bicarbonate is given by mouth for *chronic acidotic states* such as uraemic acidosis or renal tubular acidosis. The dose for correction of metabolic acidosis is not predictable and the response must be assessed; 4.8 g daily (57 mmol each of Na^+ and HCO_3^-) or more may be required. For severe metabolic acidosis, sodium bicarbonate can be given intravenously (section 9.2.2).

Sodium bicarbonate may also be used to make the pH of the urine alkaline (see section 7.4.3); for use in dyspepsia see section 1.1.2.

Sodium supplements may increase blood pressure or cause fluid retention and pulmonary oedema in those at risk; hypokalaemia may be exacerbated.

Where *hyperchloraemic acidosis* is associated with potassium deficiency, as in some renal tubular and gastro-intestinal disorders it may be appropriate to give oral **potassium bicarbonate**, although acute or severe deficiency should be managed by intravenous therapy.

SODIUM BICARBONATE

Indications: see notes above

Cautions: see notes above; avoid in respiratory acidosis; **interactions:** Appendix 1 (antacids and adsorbents)

Dose: see notes above

Sodium Bicarbonate (Non-proprietary)

Capsules, sodium bicarbonate 500 mg (approx. 6 mmol each of Na^+ and HCO_3^-). Net price 20 = 44p

Available from Norton

Tablets, sodium bicarbonate 300 mg, net price 20 tabs = 37p

POTASSIUM BICARBONATE

Indications: see notes above

Cautions: cardiac disease, renal impairment; **interactions:** Appendix 1 (potassium salts)

Contra-indications: hypochloraemia; plasma potassium concentration above 5 mmol/litre

Side-effects: nausea and vomiting

Dose: see notes above

Potassium Tablets, Effervescent, potassium bicarbonate 500 mg, potassium acid tartrate 300 mg, each tablet providing 6.5 mmol of K^+. To be dissolved in water before administration. Net price 100 = £3.11. Label: 13, 21

Note. These tablets do not contain chloride; for effervescent tablets containing potassium and chloride, see under Potassium Chloride, section 9.2.1.1

WATER

The term water used without qualification means either potable water freshly drawn direct from the public supply and suitable for drinking or freshly boiled and cooled purified water. The latter should be used if the public supply is from a local storage tank or if the potable water is unsuitable for a particular preparation. (Water for injections, section 9.2.2.)

9.2.2   Intravenous administration

Solutions of electrolytes are given intravenously, to meet normal fluid and electrolyte requirements or to replenish substantial deficits or continuing losses, when the patient is nauseated or vomiting and is unable to take adequate amounts by mouth.

In an individual patient the nature and severity of the electrolyte imbalance must be assessed from the history and clinical and biochemical examination. Sodium, potassium, chloride, magnesium, phosphate, and water depletion can occur singly and in combination with or without disturbances of acid-base balance; for reference to the use of magnesium and phosphates, see section 9.5.

Isotonic solutions may be infused safely into a peripheral vein. Solutions more concentrated than plasma, for example 20% glucose are best given through an indwelling catheter positioned in a large vein.

INTRAVENOUS SODIUM

Sodium chloride in isotonic solution provides the most important extracellular ions in near physiological concentration and is indicated in *sodium depletion* which may arise from such conditions as gastro-enteritis, diabetic ketoacidosis, ileus, and ascites. In a severe deficit of from 4 to 8 litres, 2 to 3 litres of isotonic sodium chloride may be given over 2 to 3 hours; thereafter infusion can usually be at a slower rate.

Excessive administration should be avoided; the jugular venous pressure should be assessed, the bases of the lungs should be examined for crepitations, and in elderly or seriously ill patients it is often helpful to monitor the right atrial (central) venous pressure.

Compound sodium lactate (Hartmann's solution) can be used instead of isotonic sodium chloride solution during surgery or in the initial management of the injured or wounded.

Sodium chloride and glucose solutions are indicated when there is combined *water and sodium depletion*. A 1:1 mixture of isotonic sodium chloride and 5% glucose allows some of the water (free of sodium) to enter body cells which suffer most from dehydration while the sodium salt with a volume of water determined by the normal plasma Na^+ remains extracellular. An example of combined sodium chloride and water depletion occurs in persistent vomiting.

SODIUM CHLORIDE

Indications: electrolyte imbalance, also section 9.2.1.2

Cautions: restrict intake in impaired renal function, cardiac failure, hypertension, peripheral and pulmonary oedema, toxaemia of pregnancy

Side-effects: administration of large doses may give rise to sodium accumulation and oedema

Dose: see notes above

PoM **Sodium Chloride Intravenous Infusion,** usual strength sodium chloride 0.9% (9 g, 150 mmol each of Na^+ and Cl^-/litre), this strength being supplied when normal saline for injection is requested. Net price 2-mL amp = 30p; 5-mL amp = 32p; 10-mL amp = 35p; 20-mL amp = 67p; 50-mL amp = £1.52

In hospitals, 500- and 1000-mL packs, and sometimes other sizes, are available

Note. The term 'normal saline' should **not** be used to describe sodium chloride intravenous infusion 0.9%; the term 'physiological saline' is acceptable but it is preferable to give the composition (i.e. sodium chloride intravenous infusion 0.9%).

With other ingredients

PoM **Sodium Chloride and Glucose Intravenous Infusion,** usual strength sodium chloride 0.18% (1.8 g, 30 mmol each of Na^+ and Cl^-/litre) and 4% of anhydrous glucose

In hospitals, 500- and 1000-mL packs, and sometimes other sizes are available

PoM **Ringer's Solution for Injection,** calcium chloride (dihydrate) 322 micrograms, potassium chloride 300 micrograms, sodium chloride 8.6 mg/mL, providing the following ions (in mmol/litre), Ca^{2+} 2.2, K^+ 4, Na^+ 147, Cl^- 156

In hospitals, 500- and 1000-mL packs, and sometimes other sizes, are available

PoM **Sodium Lactate Intravenous Infusion, Compound** (Hartmann's Solution for Injection; Ringer-Lactate Solution for Injection), sodium chloride 0.6%, sodium lactate 0.25%, potassium chloride 0.04%, calcium chloride 0.027% (containing Na^+ 131 mmol, K^+ 5 mmol, Ca^{2+} 2 mmol, HCO_3^- (as lactate) 29 mmol, Cl^- 111 mmol/litre)

In hospitals, 500- and 1000-mL packs, and sometimes other sizes, are available

INTRAVENOUS GLUCOSE

Glucose solutions (5%) are mainly used to replace water deficits and should be given alone when there is no significant loss of electrolytes. Average water requirements in a healthy adult are 1.5 to 2.5 litres daily and this is needed to balance unavoidable losses of water through the skin and lungs and to provide sufficient for urinary excretion. Water depletion (dehydration) tends to occur when these losses are not matched by a comparable intake, as for example may occur in coma or dysphagia or in the aged or apathetic who may not drink water in sufficient amount on their own initiative.

Excessive loss of water without loss of electrolytes is uncommon, occurring in fevers, hyperthyroidism, and in uncommon water-losing renal states such as diabetes insipidus or hypercalcaemia. The volume of glucose solution needed to replenish deficits varies with the severity of the disorder, but usually lies within the range of 2 to 10 litres.

Glucose solutions are also given in regimens with calcium, bicarbonate, and insulin for the emergency management of *hyperkalaemia*. They are also given, after correction of hyperglycaemia, during treatment of diabetic ketoacidosis, when they must be accompanied by continuing insulin infusion.

GLUCOSE
(Dextrose Monohydrate)

Note. Glucose BP is the monohydrate but Glucose Intravenous Infusion BP is a sterile solution of anhydrous glucose or glucose monohydrate, potency being expressed in terms of anhydrous glucose

Indications: fluid replacement (see notes above), provision of energy (section 9.3)

Side-effects: glucose injections especially if hypertonic may have a low pH and may cause venous irritation and thrombophlebitis

Dose: water replacement, see notes above; energy source, 1–3 litres daily of 20–50% solution

PoM **Glucose Intravenous Infusion,** glucose or anhydrous glucose (potency expressed in terms of anhydrous glucose), usual strength 5% (50 mg/mL). 25% solution, net price 25-mL amp = £2.21; 50% solution, 25-mL amp = £3.11, 50-mL amp = £2.45

In hospitals, 500- and 1000-mL packs, and sometimes other sizes, are available; also available from IMS (Min-I-Jet® Glucose, 50% in 50-ml disposable syringe).

INTRAVENOUS POTASSIUM

Potassium chloride and sodium chloride intravenous infusion and **potassium chloride and glucose** intravenous infusion are used to correct severe *hypokalaemia* and depletion and when sufficient potassium cannot be taken by mouth. Potassium chloride, as ampoules containing 1.5 g (20 mmol K^+) in 10 mL[1], may be added to 500 mL of sodium chloride or glucose intravenous infusion; the solution then contains 40 mmol/ litre and may be given slowly over 2 to 3 hours with ECG monitoring in difficult cases[2]. Repeated measurements of plasma potassium are necessary to determine whether further infusions are required and to avoid the development of hyperkalaemia; this is especially liable to occur in renal failure.

1. **Important**: mix infusion solution **thoroughly** after adding potassium chloride; use ready-prepared solutions when possible
2. Higher concentrations may be given in severe cases but require infusion pump control

POTASSIUM CHLORIDE

Indications: electrolyte imbalance; see also oral potassium supplements, section 9.2.1.1

Cautions: for intravenous infusion the concentration of solution should not usually exceed 3.2 g (43 mmol)/litre

Side-effects: rapid infusion toxic to heart

Dose: by slow intravenous infusion, depending on the deficit or the daily maintenance requirements, see also notes above

PoM **Potassium Chloride and Glucose Intravenous Infusion,** usual strength potassium chloride 0.3% (3 g, 40 mmol each of K^+ and Cl^-/litre) with 5% of anhydrous glucose

In hospitals, 500- and 1000-mL packs, and sometimes other sizes, are available

PoM **Potassium Chloride and Sodium Chloride Intravenous Infusion,** usual strength potassium chloride 0.3% (3 g/litre) and sodium chloride 0.9% (9 g/litre), containing 40 mmol of K^+, 150 mmol of Na^+, and 190 mmol of Cl^-/litre

In hospitals, 500- and 1000-mL packs, and sometimes other sizes, are available

PoM **Potassium Chloride, Sodium Chloride, and Glucose Intravenous Infusion,** sodium chloride 0.18% (1.8 g, 30 mmol of Na^+/litre) with 4% of anhydrous glucose and usually sufficient potassium chloride to provide 10–40 mmol of K^+/litre (to be specified by the prescriber)

In hospitals, 500- and 1000-mL packs, and sometimes other sizes, are available

PoM **Potassium Chloride Solution, Strong,** (sterile), potassium chloride 15% (150 mg, approximately 2 mmol each of K^+ and Cl^-/mL). Net price 10-mL amp = 81p

IMPORTANT. Must be diluted with **not less** than 50 times its volume of sodium chloride intravenous infusion 0.9% or other suitable diluent and **mixed well**

Solutions containing 10 and 20% of potassium chloride are also available in both 5- and 10-mL ampoules.

BICARBONATE AND LACTATE

Sodium bicarbonate is used to control severe *metabolic acidosis* (as in renal failure). Since this condition is usually attended by sodium depletion, it is reasonable to correct this first by the administration of isotonic sodium chloride intravenous infusion, provided the kidneys are not primarily affected and the degree of acidosis is not so severe as to impair renal function. In these circumstances, isotonic sodium chloride alone is usually effective as it restores the ability of the kidneys to generate bicarbonate. In renal acidosis or in severe metabolic acidosis of any origin (for example blood pH < 7.1) sodium bicarbonate (1.26%) may be infused with isotonic sodium chloride when the acidosis remains unresponsive to correction of anoxia or fluid depletion; a total volume of up to 6 litres (4 litres of sodium chloride and 2 litres of sodium bicarbonate) may be necessary in the adult. In severe shock due for example to cardiac arrest (see section 2.7), metabolic acidosis may develop without sodium depletion; in these circumstances sodium bicarbonate is best given in a small volume of hypertonic

solution, such as 50 mL of 8.4% solution intravenously; plasma pH should be monitored.

Sodium bicarbonate infusion is also used in the emergency management of *hyperkalaemia* (see also under Glucose).

Sodium lactate intravenous infusion is obsolete in metabolic acidosis, and carries the risk of producing lactic acidosis, particularly in seriously ill patients with poor tissue perfusion or impaired hepatic function.

SODIUM BICARBONATE

Indications: metabolic acidosis

Dose: by slow intravenous injection, a strong solution (up to 8.4%), or *by continuous intravenous infusion,* a weaker solution (usually 1.26%), an amount appropriate to the body base deficit (see notes above)

PoM **Sodium Bicarbonate Intravenous Infusion,** usual strength sodium bicarbonate 1.26% (12.6 g, 150 mmol each of Na^+ and HCO_3^-/litre); various other strengths available

In hospitals, 500- and 1000-mL packs, and sometimes other sizes, are available

PoM **Min-I-Jet® Sodium Bicarbonate** (IMS)

Intravenous injection, sodium bicarbonate in disposable syringe, net price 4.2%, 10 mL = £4.81; 8.4%, 10 mL = £5.19, 50 mL = £7.75

SODIUM LACTATE

Indications: diabetic coma, diminished alkali reserve (but see notes above)

PoM **Sodium Lactate Intravenous Infusion,** sodium lactate M/6, contains the following ions (in mmol/litre), Na^+ 167, HCO_3^- (as lactate) 167

WATER

PoM **Water for Injections.** Net price 1-mL amp = 12p; 2-mL amp = 14p; 5-mL amp = 20p; 20-mL amp = 51p; 50-mL amp = £1.03

9.2.3   Plasma and plasma substitutes

Plasma and albumin solutions, prepared from whole blood, contain soluble proteins and electrolytes but no clotting factors, blood group antibodies, or pseudocholinesterases; they may be given without regard to the recipient's blood group.

Plasma and albumin solutions are used for the treatment of hypoproteinaemia and the low plasma volume associated with conditions such as burns; concentrated albumin solutions may also be used to obtain a diuresis in hypoalbuminaemic patients (e.g. in hepatic cirrhosis). Plasma substitutes are more appropriate for acute blood loss (e.g. haematemesis).

ALBUMIN SOLUTION

(Human Albumin Solution)

A solution containing protein derived from plasma, serum, or normal placentas; at least 95% of the protein is albumin. The solution may be isotonic (containing 4–5% protein) or concentrated (containing 15–25% protein).

Indications: see under preparations, below

Cautions: history of cardiac or circulatory disease (administer slowly to avoid rapid rise in blood pressure and cardiac failure, and monitor cardiovascular and respiratory function); correct dehydration when administering concentrated solution

Contra-indications: cardiac failure; severe anaemia

Side-effects: allergic reactions with nausea, vomiting, increased salivation, fever, and chills reported

Isotonic solutions

Indications: acute or sub-acute loss of plasma volume e.g. in burns, pancreatitis, trauma, and complications of surgery; plasma exchange

Available as: *Human Albumin Solution 4.5%* (50-, 100-, 250-, and 400-mL bottles—Immuno); *Albuminar-5®* (500-mL vials—Armour); *Albutein®* 5% (250- and 500-mL vials—Alpha); *Buminate®* 5.0% (250- and 500-mL bottles—Baxter); *Zenalb®* 4.5 (50-, 100-, 250-, and 500-mL bottles—BPL)

Concentrated solutions (20–25%)

Indications: severe hypoalbuminaemia associated with low plasma volume and generalised oedema where salt and water restriction with plasma volume expansion are required; adjunct in the treatment of hyperbilirubinaemia by exchange transfusion in the newborn

Available as: *Albumin Solution 20%* (100-mL vials—SNBTS); *Human Albumin Solution 20%* (10-, 50-, and 100-mL vials—Immuno); *Albutein®* 20% (50 and 100-mL vials—Alpha); *Albutein®* 25% (20-, 50-, and 100-mL vials—Alpha); *Buminate®* 20% (50- and 100-mL vials—Baxter); *Zenalb®* 20 (5-, 50-, and 100-mL bottles—BPL)

PLASMA PROTEIN SOLUTION

(Plasma Protein Fraction, PPF)

An isotonic solution containing 4–5% protein derived from plasma or serum; at least 85% of the protein is albumin.

Indications: see notes above

Cautions; Contra-indications; Side-effects: see under Albumin Solution

Preparations

Available as: *Plasma Protein Solution 4.5%* (100- and 500-mL bottles—SNBTS); *Plasmatein®* 5% (250- and 500-mL vials—Alpha)

PLASMA SUBSTITUTES

Dextrans, **gelatin**, and the etherified starches, **hetastarch** and **pentastarch** are macromolecular substances which are slowly metabolised; they may be used at the outset to expand and maintain blood volume in shock arising from conditions such as burns or septicaemia. They are rarely needed when shock is due to sodium and water depletion as, in these circumstances, the shock responds to water and electrolyte repletion. They should not be used to maintain plasma volume in conditions such as burns or peritonitis where there is loss of plasma protein, water and electrolytes over periods of several days or weeks. In these situations, plasma or plasma protein fractions containing large amounts of albumin should be given. Plasma substitutes may be used as an immediate short-term measure until blood is available.

Dextrans may interfere with blood group cross-matching or biochemical measurements and these should be carried out before infusion is begun. Dextran 70 by intravenous infusion is used predominantly for volume expansion. Dextran 40 intravenous infusion is used in an attempt to improve peripheral blood flow in ischaemic disease of the limbs and peripheral thrombo-embolism.

> **Dosage.** Because of the complex requirements relating to blood volume expansion and the primary significance of blood, plasma protein, and electrolyte replacement, detailed dose statements have been omitted. *In all cases specialist literature should be consulted.*

DEXTRAN 40 INTRAVENOUS INFUSION

Dextrans of weight average molecular weight about '40 000' 10% in glucose intravenous infusion 5% or in sodium chloride intravenous infusion 0.9%

Indications: conditions associated with peripheral local slowing of the blood flow, prophylaxis of post-surgical thrombo-embolic disease

Cautions; Contra-indications; Side-effects: see under Dextran 70 Intravenous Infusion; correct dehydration before infusion and give adequate fluids during therapy; very special care in those at risk of vascular overloading

Dose: by intravenous infusion, initially 500–1000 mL; further doses are given according to the patient's condition (see notes above)

PoM **Gentran 40®** (Baxter)

Intravenous infusion, dextran 40 intravenous infusion in glucose intravenous infusion 5% or in sodium chloride intravenous infusion 0.9%. Net price 500-mL bottle (both) = £4.90

PoM **Rheomacrodex®** (Pharmacia)

Intravenous infusion, dextran 40 intravenous infusion in glucose intravenous infusion 5% or in sodium chloride intravenous infusion 0.9%. Net price 500-mL bottle (both) = £6.35

DEXTRAN 70 INTRAVENOUS INFUSION

Dextrans of weight average molecular weight about '70 000' 6% in glucose intravenous infusion 5% or in sodium chloride intravenous infusion 0.9%

Indications: short-term blood volume expansion; prophylaxis of post-surgical thrombo-embolic disease

Cautions: congestive heart failure, renal impairment; blood samples for cross-matching should ideally be taken before infusion

Contra-indications: severe congestive heart failure; renal failure; bleeding disorders such as thrombocytopenia and hypofibrinogenaemia

Side-effects: rarely anaphylactoid reactions

Dose: by intravenous infusion, after moderate to severe haemorrhage, 500–1000 mL rapidly initially followed by 500 mL later if necessary; severe burns, up to 3000 mL in the first few days with electrolytes (see also notes above)

PoM Gentran 70® (Baxter)

Intravenous infusion, dextran 70 intravenous infusion in glucose intravenous infusion 5% or in sodium chloride intravenous infusion 0.9%. Net price 500-mL bottle (both) = £4.90

PoM Macrodex® (Pharmacia)

Intravenous infusion, dextran 70 intravenous infusion in glucose intravenous infusion 5% or in sodium chloride intravenous infusion 0.9%. Net price 500-mL bottle (both) = £4.01

GELATIN

Note. The gelatin is partially degraded

Indications: low blood volume

Cautions; Contra-indications; Side-effects: see under Dextran 70 Intravenous Infusion

Dose: by intravenous infusion, initially 500–1000 mL of a 3.5–4% solution (see notes above)

PoM Gelofusine® (Braun)

Intravenous infusion, succinylated gelatin (modified fluid gelatin, average molecular weight 30 000) 4%, sodium chloride 0.9%. Net price 500-mL bottle = £4.06

PoM Haemaccel® (Hoechst)

Intravenous infusion, polygeline (degraded and modified gelatin, average molecular weight 35 000) 35 g, Na^+145 mmol, K^+ 5.1 mmol, Ca^{2+} 6.25 mmol, Cl^- 145 mmol/litre. Net price 500-mL bottle = £3.71

ETHERIFIED STARCH

A starch composed of more than 90% of amylopectin that has been etherified with hydroxyethyl groups; hetastarch has a higher degree of etherification than pentastarch

Indications: low blood volume

Cautions; Contra-indications; Side-effects: see under Dextran 70 Intravenous Infusion; pruritus reported

Dose: see under preparations below

Hetastarch

PoM Elohes® 6% (Oxford Nutrition)

Intravenous infusion, hetastarch (weight average molecular weight 200 000) 6% in sodium chloride intravenous infusion 0.9%. Net price 500-mL Monoflac® bag = £9.75

Dose: by intravenous infusion, 500–1000 mL; usual daily max. 1500 mL (see notes above)

PoM HAES-steril® (Fresenius)

Intravenous infusion, hetastarch (weight average molecular weight 200 000), net price (both in sodium chloride intravenous infusion 0.9%) 6%, 500 mL = £10.50; 10%, 500 mL = £16.50

Dose: by intravenous infusion, usual range 500–1000 mL (see notes above)

PoM Hespan® (Du Pont)

Intravenous infusion, hetastarch (weight average molecular weight 450 000) 6% in sodium chloride intravenous infusion 0.9%. Net price 500-mL Steriflex® bag = £16.30

Dose: by intravenous infusion, 500–1000 mL; usual daily max. 1500 mL (see notes above)

Pentastarch

PoM Pentaspan® (Du Pont)

Intravenous infusion, pentastarch (weight average molecular weight 250 000) 10% in sodium chloride intravenous infusion 0.9%. Net price 500-mL Intraflex bag = £11.25

Dose: by intravenous infusion, 500–2000 mL; usual daily max. 2000 mL (see notes above)

9.3   Intravenous nutrition

When adequate feeding via the alimentary tract is not possible, nutrients may be given by intravenous infusion. This may be in addition to ordinary oral or tube feeding—**supplemental parenteral nutrition**, or may be the sole source of nutrition—**total parenteral nutrition** (TPN). Indications for this method include preparation of undernourished patients for surgery, chemotherapy, or radiation therapy; severe or prolonged disorders of the gastro-intestinal tract; major surgery, trauma, or burns; prolonged coma or refusal to eat; and some patients with renal or hepatic failure. The composition of proprietary preparations available is in the table below.

Protein is given as mixtures of essential and non-essential synthetic L-amino acids. Ideally, all essential amino acids should be included with a wide variety of non-essential ones to provide sufficient nitrogen together with electrolytes (see also section 9.2.2). Available solutions vary in their composition of amino acids; they often contain an energy source (usually glucose) and electrolytes.

Energy is provided in a ratio of 0.6 to 1.1 megajoules (150–250 kcals) per gram of protein nitrogen. Energy requirements must be met if amino acids are to be utilised for tissue maintenance. Although it has long been held that carbohydrate has a greater nitrogen-sparing effect than fat, recent studies have shown that a mixture of both energy sources, usually 30 to 50% as fat, gives better utilisation of amino acid solutions than glucose alone.

Proprietary Infusion Fluids for Parenteral Feeding

Preparation	Nitrogen g/litre	[1]Energy kJ/litre	Electrolytes mmol/litre					Other components/litre
			K+	Mg2+	Na+	Acet-	Cl-	
Aminoplasmal L5 (Braun) Net price 500 mL = £7.50	8.03		25	2.5	48	59	31	acid phosphate 9 mmol, malate 7.5 mmol
Aminoplasmal L10 (Braun) Net price 500 mL = £14.20	16.06		25	2.5	48	59	62	acid phosphate 9 mmol, malate 7.5 mmol
Aminoplasmal Ped (Braun) Net price 100 mL = £5.25; 250 mL = £6.50	7.4		25	2.5	50	27	15	
Aminoplex 5 (Geistlich) Net price 1000 mL = £11.95	5.0	3600	28	4	35	28	43	ethanol 5%, sorbitol 125 g, malic acid 1.85 g
Aminoplex 12 (Geistlich) Net price 500 mL = £11.31; 1000 mL = £19.07	12.44		30	2.5	35	5	67	malic acid 4.6 g
Aminoplex 14 (Geistlich) Net price 500 mL = £10.36	13.4		30		35		79	vitamins, malic acid 5.36 g
Aminoplex 24 (Geistlich) Net price 250 mL = £9.79; 500 mL = £17.28	24.9		30	2.5	35	5	67	malic acid 4.5 g
FreAmine III 8.5% (Fresenius) Net price 500 mL = £11.99; 1000 mL = £21.06	13.0				10	72	<3	phosphate 10 mmol
FreAmine III 10% (Fresenius) Net price 500 mL = £13.60; 1000 mL = £23.50	15.3				10	88	<2	phosphate 20 mmol
FreAmine HBC 6.9% (Fresenius) Net price 750 mL = £14.43	9.73				10	57	<3	
Glucoplex 1000 (Geistlich) Net price 500 mL = £3.30; 1000 mL = £4.71		4200	30	2.5	50		67	acid phosphate 18 mmol, Zn2+ 0.046 mmol, anhydrous glucose 240 g
Glucoplex 1600 (Geistlich) Net price 500 mL = £3.64; 1000 mL = £4.88		6700	30	2.5	50		67	acid phosphate 18 mmol, Zn2+ 0.046 mmol, anhydrous glucose 400 g
Hepanutrin (Geistlich) Net price 500 mL = £15.74	15.6							
HeplexAmine 8% (Fresenius) Net price 500 mL = £16.28	12				10	61	<3	phosphate 10 mmol
Hyperamine 30 (Braun) Net price 500 mL = £21.60	30				5			
Intrafusin 22 (Pharmacia) Net price 500 mL = £14.24	22.8							
Intralipid 10% (Pharmacia) Net price 100 mL = £3.90; 500 mL = £8.58		4600						fractionated soya oil 100 g, glycerol 22.5 g, phosphate 15 mmol
Intralipid 20% (Pharmacia) Net price 100 mL = £5.85; 250 mL = £9.65; 500 mL = £12.87		8400						fractionated soya oil 200 g, glycerol 22.5 g, phosphate 15 mmol
Intralipid 30% (Pharmacia) Net price 333 mL = £14.40		12600						fractionated soya oil 300 g, glycerol 16.7 g, phosphate 15 mmol
Ivelip 10% (Clintec) Net price 100 mL = £4.78; 500 mL = £9.51		4600						soya oil 100 g, glycerol 25 g
Ivelip 20% (Clintec) Net price 100 mL = £6.58; 500 mL = £14.53; 1000 mL = £25.84		8400						soya oil 200 g, glycerol 25 g
[2]Lipofundin MCT/LCT 10% (Braun) Net price 100 mL = £6.40; 500 mL = £10.50		4430						soya oil 50 g, medium chain triglycerides 50 g
[2]Lipofundin MCT/LCT 20% (Braun) Net price 100 mL = £7.30; 250 mL = £9.80; 500 mL = £16.00		8000						soya oil 100 g, medium chain triglycerides 100 g
Lipofundin S 10% (Braun) Net price 100 mL = £6.00; 500 mL = £9.80		4470						soya oil 100 g
Lipofundin S 20% (Braun) Net price 100 mL = £7.00; 500 mL = £15.30		8520						soya oil 200 g
Nephramine 5.4% (Fresenius) Net price 250 mL = £14.72	6.4				5	44	<3	essential amino acids only
Nutracel 400 (Clintec) Net price 500 mL = £2.54		3400	18		0.16		66	Ca2+ 15 mmol, Mn2+ 0.08 mmol, Zn2+ 0.08 mmol, anhydrous glucose 200 g
Nutracel 800 (Clintec) Net price 1000 mL = £4.39		3400	9		0.08		33	Ca2+ 7.5 mmol, Mn2+ 0.04 mmol, Zn2+ 0.04 mmol, anhydrous glucose 200 g

1. Excludes protein- or amino acid-derived energy
2. Treatment with Lipofundin MCT/LCT should be limited to up to 10 days
Note: 1000 kcal = 4.1868 MJ; 1 MJ (1000 kJ) = 238.8 kcal. All entries are **PoM**

Proprietary Infusion Fluids for Parenteral Feeding (*continued*)

Preparation	Nitrogen g/litre	[1]Energy kJ/litre	Electrolytes mmol/litre					Other components/litre
			K+	Mg2+	Na+	Acet-	Cl-	
Plasma-Lyte 148 (water) (Baxter) Net price 1000 mL = £1.63			5	1.5	140	27	98	gluconate 23 mmol
Plasma-Lyte 148 (dextrose 5%) (Baxter) Net price 1000 mL = £1.63		840	5	1.5	140	27	98	gluconate 23 mmol, anhydrous glucose 50 g
Plasma-Lyte M (dextrose 5%) (Baxter) Net price 1000 mL = £1.36		840	16	1.5	40	12	40	Ca2+ 2.5 mmol, lactate 12 mmol, anhydrous glucose 50 g
[2]Primene 10% (Clintec) Net price 100 mL = £6.05; 250 mL = £8.29	15						15.6	
Soyacal 10% (Alpha) Net price 50 mL = £2.75; 100 mL = £4.25; 250 mL = £7.25; 500 mL = £9.50		4600						purified soya oil 100 g, glycerol 22.1 g
Soyacal 20% (Alpha) Net price 50 mL = £4.25; 100 mL = £6.50; 250 mL = £10.75; 500 mL = £14.00		8400						purified soya oil 200 g, glycerol 22.1 g
Synthamin 9 (Clintec) Net price 500 mL = £6.97; 1000 mL = £12.92	9.1		60	5	70	100	70	acid phosphate 30 mmol
Synthamin 14 (Clintec) Net price 500 mL = £10.09; 1000 mL = £17.94; 3000 mL = £51.29	14.0		60	5	70	140	70	acid phosphate 30 mmol
Synthamin 14 without electrolytes (Clintec) Net price 500 mL = £10.34; 1000 mL = £18.33	14.0					68	34	
Synthamin 17 (Clintec) Net price 500 mL = £13.26; 1000 mL = £24.08	16.5		60	5	70	150	70	acid phosphate 30 mmol
Synthamin 17 without electrolytes (Clintec) Net price 500 mL = £13.26	16.5					82	40	
Synthamix 9/800X (Clintec) Net price 2000 mL = £34.13	4.55	1680	30	7	35	50	51.5	acid phosphate 15 mmol, Zn2+ 0.02 mmol, Ca2+ 3.75 mmol, Mn2+ 0.02 mmol, anhydrous glucose 100 g
Synthamix 9/1800X (Clintec) Net price 2500 mL = £35.59	3.64	3024	24	5.6	28	40	41.2	acid phosphate 12 mmol, Zn2+ 0.016 mmol, Ca2+ 3 mmol, Mn2+ 0.016 mmol, anhydrous glucose 180 g
Synthamix 14/1200X (Clintec) Net price 2000 mL = £37.54	7	2520	30	7	35	70	51.5	acid phosphate 15 mmol, Zn2+ 0.02 mmol, Ca2+ 3.75 mmol, Mn2+ 0.02 mmol, anhydrous glucose 150 g
Synthamix 14/2200X (Clintec) Net price 2500 mL = £39.00	5.6	3696	24	5.6	28	56	41.2	acid phosphate 12 mmol, Zn2+ 0.016 mmol, Ca2+ 3 mmol, Mn2+ 0.016 mmol, anhydrous glucose 220 g
Vamin 9 (Pharmacia) Net price 500 mL = £5.85; 1000 mL = £10.04	9.4		20	1.5	50		50	Ca2+ 2.5 mmol
Vamin 9 glucose (Pharmacia) Net price 100 mL = £3.02; 500 mL = £6.14; 1000 mL = £11.02	9.4	1700	20	1.5	50		50	Ca2+ 2.5 mmol, anhydrous glucose 100 g
Vamin 14 (Pharmacia) Net price 500 mL = £8.63; 1000 mL = £14.67	13.5		50	8	100	135	100	Ca2+ 5 mmol, SO4 2- 8 mmol
Vamin 14 (electrolyte-free) (Pharmacia) Net price 500 mL = £8.29; 1000 mL = £14.67	13.5							
Vamin 18 (electrolyte-free) (Pharmacia) Net price 500 mL = £10.97; 1000 mL = £19.74	18							
Vaminolact (Pharmacia) Net price 100 mL = £3.36; 500 mL = £7.75	9.3							
Vitrimix KV (Pharmacia) Net price (combined pack of Intralipid 20% 250 mL and Vamin 9 glucose 750 mL) = £19.40	7.0	3340	15	1.1	38		38	Ca2+ 1.9 mmol, anhydrous glucose 75 g

1. Excludes protein- or amino acid-derived energy
2. For use in neonates and children only
   Note. 1000 kcal = 4.1868 MJ; 1 MJ (1000 kJ) = 238.8 kcal. All entries are PoM

Glucose is the preferred source of carbohydrate, but if more than 180 g is given per day frequent monitoring of blood glucose is required, and insulin may be necessary. Glucose in various strengths from 10 to 50% must be infused through a central venous catheter to avoid thrombosis. Preparations are available with useful added ions and trace elements, e.g. Glucoplex®.

Fructose and sorbitol have been used in an attempt to avoid the problem of hyperosmolar hyperglycaemic non-ketotic acidosis but other metabolic problems may occur, as with xylitol and ethanol which are now rarely used.

Fat emulsions have the advantages of a high energy to fluid volume ratio, neutral pH, and iso-osmolarity with plasma, and provide essential fatty acids. Available preparations are soya bean oil emulsions. Several days of adaptation may be required to attain maximal utilisation. Reactions include occasional febrile episodes (usually only with 20% emulsions) and rare anaphylactic responses. Interference with biochemical measurements such as those for blood gases and calcium may occur if samples are taken before fat has been cleared. Daily checks are necessary to ensure complete clearance from the plasma in conditions where fat metabolism may be disturbed. **Additives may only be mixed with fat emulsions where compatibility is known.**

Total parenteral nutrition (TPN) requires the use of a solution containing amino acids, glucose, fat, electrolytes, trace elements, and vitamins. This is now provided by the pharmacy in the form of the 3-litre bag. The solution is infused through a central venous catheter inserted under full surgical precautions. Only nutritional fluids should be given by this line. Loading doses of vitamin B₁₂ and folic acid are advised and other vitamins are given parenterally twice weekly.

Before starting, the patient should be well oxygenated with a near normal circulating blood volume, renal function, and acid-base status. Appropriate biochemical tests should have been carried out beforehand and serious deficits corrected. Nutritional and electrolyte status must be monitored throughout treatment

SUPPLEMENTARY PREPARATIONS

Administraion. Because of the complex requirements relating to parenteral nutrition full details relating to administration have been omitted. In all cases *data sheets and specialist literature should be consulted.*

PoM Addiphos® (Pharmacia)
Solution, sterile, phosphate 40 mmol, K⁺ 30 mmol, Na⁺ 30 mmol/20 mL. For addition to Vamin® solutions and glucose intravenous infusions. Net price 20-mL vial = £1.15

PoM Additrace® (Pharmacia)
Solution, trace elements for addition to Vamin® solutions, traces of Fe³⁺, Zn²⁺, Mn²⁺, Cu²⁺, Cr³⁺, Se⁴⁺, Mo⁶⁺, F⁻, I⁻. For adult use. Net price 10-mL amp = £1.75

PoM Multibionta® (Merck)
Solution, ascorbic acid 500 mg, dexpanthenol 25 mg, nicotinamide 100 mg, pyridoxine hydrochloride 15 mg, riboflavine sodium phosphate 10 mg, thiamine hydrochloride 50 mg, tocopheryl acetate 5 mg, vitamin A 10 000 units. For addition to infusion solutions. Net price 10-mL amp = £1.61
Contra-indications: not for use in neonates owing to presence of benzyl alcohol as additive

PoM Ped-El® (Pharmacia)
Solution, sterile, Ca²⁺, Cu²⁺, Fe³⁺, Mg²⁺, Mn²⁺, Zn²⁺, Cl⁻, F⁻, I⁻, P. For addition to Vamin® solutions. For paediatric use. Net price 20-mL vial = £1.55
Cautions: long-term use (risk of manganese toxicity); long-term use acceptable provided baseline blood (or serum) manganese concentration normal or low—monitor manganese concentration regularly and discontinue if raised or if cholestasis develops; **contra-indicated** if biochemical or clinical evidence of liver impairment (especially cholestasis); in neonates serum aluminium monitoring also recommended

PoM Solivito N® (Pharmacia)
Solution, powder for reconstitution, biotin 60 micrograms, cyanocobalamin 5 micrograms, folic acid 400 micrograms, glycine 300 mg, nicotinamide 40 mg, pyridoxine hydrochloride 4.9 mg, riboflavine sodium phosphate 4.9 mg, sodium ascorbate 113 mg, sodium pantothenate 16.5 mg, thiamine mononitrate 3.1 mg. Dissolve in water for injections or glucose intravenous infusion for adding to glucose intravenous infusion or Intralipid®; dissolve in Vitlipid N® or Intralipid® for adding to Intralipid® only. Net price per vial = £1.75

PoM Vitlipid N® (Pharmacia)
Emulsion, adult, vitamin A 330 units, ergocalciferol 20 units, dl-alpha tocopherol 1 unit, phytomenadione 15 micrograms/mL. For addition to Intralipid®. Net price 10 mL amp = £1.71
Emulsion, infant, vitamin A 230 units, ergocalciferol 40 units, dl-alpha tocopherol 0.7 unit, phytomenadione 20 micrograms/mL. For addition to Intralipid®. Net price 10-mL amp = £1.71

9.4   Oral nutrition

9.4.1   Foods for special diets
9.4.2   Enteral nutrition

9.4.1   Foods for special diets

These are preparations that have been modified to eliminate a particular constituent from a food or are nutrient mixtures formulated as substitutes for the food. They are for patients who either cannot tolerate or cannot metabolise certain common constituents of food.

PHENYLKETONURIA. Phenylketonuria (phenylalaninaemia), which results from the inability to metabolise phenylalanine, is managed by restricting its dietary intake to a small amount sufficient for tissue building and repair. Aspartame (as a sweetener in some foods and medicines) contributes to the phenylalanine intake and may affect control of phenylketonuria. Where the presence of aspartame is specified on a data sheet this is indicated in the BNF against the preparation.

COELIAC DISEASE. Coeliac disease, which results from an intolerance to gluten, is managed by completely eliminating gluten from the diet.

> **ACBS.** In certain clinical conditions some foods may have the characteristics of drugs and the Advisory Committee on Borderline Substances advises as to the circumstances in which such foods may be regarded as drugs and so can be prescribed in the NHS. Prescriptions for these foods issued in accordance with the advice of this committee and endorsed 'ACBS' will normally not be investigated. See Appendix 7 for details of these foods and a listing by clinical condition (consult Drug Tariff for late amendments).

Preparations
See Appendix 7

9.4.2   Enteral nutrition

The body's reserves of protein rapidly become exhausted in severely ill patients, especially during chronic illness or in those with severe burns, extensive trauma, pancreatitis, or intestinal fistula. Much can be achieved by frequent meals and by persuading the patient to take supplementary snacks of ordinary food between the meals.

However, extra calories, protein, other nutrients, and vitamins are often best given by supplementing ordinary meals with sip or tube feeds of one of the nutritionally complete foods.

When patients cannot feed normally at all, for example patients with severe facial injury, oesophageal obstruction, or coma, a diet composed solely of nutritionally complete foods must be given. This is planned by a dietitian who will take into account the protein and total energy requirement of the patient and decide on the form and relative contribution of carbohydrate and fat to the energy requirements.

There are a number of nutritionally complete foods available and their use reduces an otherwise heavy workload in hospital or in the home. Most contain protein derived from milk or soya. Some contain protein hydrolysates or free amino acids and are only appropriate for patients who have diminished ability to break down protein, as may be the case in inflammatory bowel disease or pancreatic insufficiency.

Even when nutritionally complete feeds are being given it may be important to monitor water and electrolyte balance. Extra minerals (e.g. magnesium and zinc) may be needed in patients where gastrointestinal secretions are being lost. Additional vitamins may also be needed. Regular haematological and biochemical tests may be needed particularly in the unstable patient.

Some feeds are supplemented with vitamin K; for drug interactions of vitamin K see Appendix 1 (vitamins).

CHILDREN. Infants and young children have special requirements and in most situations liquid feeds prepared for adults are totally unsuitable and should not be given. Expert advice should be sought.

Preparations
See Appendix 7

9.5   Minerals

9.5.1   Calcium and magnesium
9.5.2   Phosphorus
9.5.3   Fluoride
9.5.4   Zinc

See section 9.1.1 for iron salts.

9.5.1   Calcium and magnesium

9.5.1.1 Calcium supplements
9.5.1.2 Hypercalcaemia
9.5.1.3 Magnesium

9.5.1.1 CALCIUM SUPPLEMENTS

Calcium supplements are usually only required where dietary calcium intake is deficient. This dietary requirement varies with age and is relatively greater in childhood, pregnancy, and lactation, due to an increased demand, and in old age, due to impaired absorption. In osteoporosis a daily supplement of 800 mg (20 mmol) calcium (as a suitable salt) may reduce the rate of bone loss, but larger doses have not been shown to be more effective. Patients with hypoparathyroidism rarely require calcium supplements after the early stages of stabilisation on vitamin D (section 9.6.4).

In hypocalcaemic tetany an initial intravenous injection of 10 mL (2.25 mmol) of calcium gluconate injection 10% may be followed by the continuous infusion of about 40 mL (9 mmol) daily, but plasma calcium should be monitored. This regimen can also be used, immediately but temporarily, to reduce the toxic effects of hyperkalaemia.

Calcium may also be used in cardiac resuscitation (see section 2.7).

CALCIUM SALTS
Indications: see notes above; calcium deficiency
Cautions: renal impairment; sarcoidosis; **interactions:** Appendix 1 (calcium salts)
Contra-indications: conditions associated with hypercalcaemia and hypercalciuria (eg. some forms of malignant disease)

Side-effects: mild gastro-intestinal disturbances; bradycardia, arrhythmias, and irritation after intravenous injection

Dose: by mouth, daily in divided doses, see notes above

By *deep intramuscular injection or by slow intravenous injection*, acute hypocalcaemia, calcium gluconate 1–2 g (2.25–4.5 mmol of Ca^{2+})

CHILD obtain paediatric advice; intramuscular route not recommended

Oral preparations

Calcium Gluconate (Non-proprietary)

Tablets, calcium gluconate 600 mg (53.4 mg calcium or 1.35 mmol Ca^{2+}). Net price 20 = 55p. Label: 24

Effervescent tablets, calcium gluconate 1 g (89 mg calcium or 2.25 mmol Ca^{2+}). Net price 100 = £6.16. Label: 13

Note. Each tablet usually contains 4.46 mmol Na^+

Calcium Lactate (Non-proprietary)

Tablets, calcium lactate 300 mg (39 mg calcium or 1 mmol Ca^{2+}). Net price 20 = 29p

Cacit® (Procter & Gamble Pharm.)

Tablets, effervescent, pink, calcium carbonate 1.25 g, providing calcium citrate when dispersed in water (500 mg calcium or 12.6 mmol Ca^{2+}). Net price 76-tab pack = £16.72. Label: 13

Calcichew® (Shire)

Tablets (both chewable), calcium carbonate 1.25 g (500 mg calcium or 12.6 mmol Ca^{2+}), net price 100-tab pack = £10.97; 2.5 g (*Calcichew Forte®*, 1 g calcium or 25 mmol Ca^{2+}), 100-tab pack = £21.94. Label: 24

Additives: include aspartame

Calcidrink® (Shire)

Granules, effervescent, calcium carbonate 2.52 g (1 g calcium or 25 mmol Ca^{2+}). Net price 30-sachet pack = £8.48. Label: 13

Calcium-500 (Renacare)

Tablets, pink, f/c, calcium carbonate 1.25 g (500 mg calcium or 12.5 mmol Ca^{2+}). Net price 100-tab pack = £8.26. Label: 25

Calcium-Sandoz® (Sandoz)

Syrup, calcium glubionate 1.09 g, calcium lactobionate 723 mg (108.3 mg calcium or 2.7 mmol Ca^{2+})/5 mL. Net price 100 mL = 49p

Citrical® (Shire)

Granules, calcium carbonate 1.26 g (500 mg calcium or 12.6 mmolCa^{2+})/sachet. Net price 90-sachet pack = £23.40. Label: 13

Ossopan® (Sanofi Winthrop)

Tablets, buff, f/c, hydroxyapatite 830 mg (calcium 178 mg or 4.4 mmol Ca^{2+}). Net price 50 = £10.09

Granules, brown, hydroxyapatite 3.32 g (calcium 712 mg or 17.8 mmol Ca^{2+})/sachet. Net price 28-sachet pack = £18.04

Sandocal® (Sandoz)

Sandocal-400 tablets, effervescent, calcium lactate gluconate 930 mg, calcium carbonate 700 mg, anhydrous citric acid 1.189 g, providing calcium 400 mg (10 mmol Ca^{2+}). Net price 5 × 20-tab pack = £7.20. Label: 13

Sandocal-1000 tablets, effervescent, calcium lactate gluconate 2.327 g, calcium carbonate 1.75 g, anhydrous citric acid 2.973 g providing 1 g calcium (25 mmol Ca^{2+}). Net price 3 × 10-tab pack = £6.45. Label: 13

Titralac®, section 9.5.2.2

Parenteral preparations

PoM **Calcium Gluconate** (Non-proprietary)

Injection, calcium gluconate 10% (8.9 mg calcium or 220 micromol Ca^{2+}/mL. Net price 10-mL amp = 46p

PoM **Calcium-Sandoz®** (Sandoz)

Injection, calcium glubionate equivalent to 10% of calcium gluconate (9.3 mg calcium or 225 micromol Ca^{2+}/mL). Net price 10-mL amp = 27p

PoM **Min-I-Jet® Calcium Chloride 10%** (IMS)

Injection, calcium chloride 100 mg/mL (27.3 mg calcium or 680 micromol Ca^{2+}/mL). Net price 10-mL disposable syringe = £4.02

9.5.1.2 HYPERCALCAEMIA

Severe hypercalcaemia calls for urgent treatment before detailed investigation of the cause. After rehydration (if necessary with intravenous infusion of **sodium chloride 0.9%**) a **loop diuretic** may be given to increase urinary calcium excretion. Drugs (such as thiazides and vitamin D compounds) which promote hypercalcaemia, should be discontinued and dietary calcium should be restricted.

If *severe hypercalcaemia persists* drugs which inhibit mobilisation of calcium from the skeleton may be required. The **bisphosphonates** are useful and disodium pamidronate (see section 6.6.2) is probably the most effective; it is probably as effective as plicamycin, yet is less toxic and has a much longer effect. **Plicamycin** (see section 8.1.2) is probably the most rapidly effective drug but cannot be given continuously for more than a few days because of marrow toxicity; the duration of its hypocalcaemic effect is unpredictable but can last several days.

Corticosteroids (see section 6.3) are widely given, but may only be useful where hypercalcaemia is due to sarcoidosis or vitamin D intoxication; they often take several days to achieve the desired effect.

Calcitonin (see section 6.6.1) is relatively non-toxic but is expensive and its effect can wear off after a few days despite continued use; it is rarely effective where bisphosphonates have failed to reduce serum calcium adequately.

Intravenous chelating drugs such as **trisodium edetate** are rarely used; they usually cause pain in the limb receiving the infusion and may cause renal damage.

After treatment of severe hypercalcaemia the underlying cause must be established. *Further treatment* is governed by the same principles as for initial therapy. Salt and water depletion and drugs promoting hypercalcaemia should be avoided; oral administration of a bisphosphonate may be useful. **Sodium cellulose phosphate**, which binds calcium in the gut, is rarely helpful, and any associated increase in serum phosphate may be harmful. Similarly, oral and intravenous phosphate may only achieve a reduction in serum calcium by precipitating calcium phosphate in the tissues, resulting in nephrocalcinosis and impairment of renal function. Parathyroidectomy may be indicated for hyperparathyroidism.

BISPHOSPHONATES
See section 6.6.2

CALCITONIN
See section 6.6.1

CORTICOSTEROIDS
See section 6.3.4

PLICAMYCIN
See section 8.1.2

SODIUM CELLULOSE PHOSPHATE
Indications: reduction of calcium absorption from food in conditions such as hypercalciuria and hypercalcaemia (but see also notes above)

Cautions: renal impairment (avoid if severe); pregnancy and breast-feeding; growing children

Contra-indications: congestive heart failure and other conditions in which low sodium intake essential, severe renal impairment

Side-effects: occasional diarrhoea; magnesium deficiency reported

Dose: 5 g 3 times daily with meals; CHILD 10 g daily in 3 divided doses with meals

Calcisorb® (3M)
Sachets, sodium cellulose phosphate 5 g. Net price 90-sachet pack = £18.72. Label: 13, 21, counselling, may be sprinkled on food

TRISODIUM EDETATE
Indications: hypercalcaemia (but see notes above); lime burns in the eye (see under Preparations)

Cautions: plasma-calcium determinations required; caution in tuberculosis

Contra-indications: impaired renal function

Side-effects: nausea, diarrhoea, cramp; in overdosage renal damage

Dose: hypercalcaemia, *by slow intravenous infusion,* up to 70 mg/kg daily over 2–3 hours

PoM Limclair® (Sinclair)
Injection, trisodium edetate 200 mg/mL. Net price 5-mL amp = £4.76

For topical use in the eye, dilute 1 mL to 50 mL with sterile purified water

9.5.1.3 MAGNESIUM

Magnesium is an essential constituent of a vast number of enzyme systems, in particular those involved in energy generation. Most of it is found in the skeleton in the calcium apatite crystal lattice.

Magnesium salts are not well absorbed from the gastro-intestinal tract which explains the use of magnesium sulphate (section 1.6.4) as an osmotic laxative.

Magnesium is mainly excreted by the kidneys and is therefore retained in renal failure.

The effects of hypermagnesaemia and of hypomagnesaemia are similar to those of hyperkalaemia and hypokalaemia; hypocalcaemia is usually associated with hypomagnesaemia.

Oral magnesium salts are occasionally required on a long-term basis in patients with malabsorption.

Parenteral magnesium chloride or sulphate is occasionally needed to correct magnesium deficiency in alcoholism or that has arisen from prolonged diarrhoea or vomiting which has been treated with parenteral fluid and nutrition without magnesium supplements; magnesium of the order of 35–75 mmol is given by slow intravenous infusion (in glucose 5%) on the first day followed by 25 mmol on subsequent days (a cumulative total of up to 160 mmol may be required). Repeated measurements of plasma magnesium are advisable to determine the rate and duration of the infusion. The dose should be reduced in renal failure. For maintenance (e.g. for intravenous nutrition) parenteral doses of magnesium are of the order of 10–20 mmol daily (often about 12 mmol daily).

Magnesium sulphate has also been recommended for the emergency treatment of *serious arrhythmias,* especially in the presence of hypokalaemia (when hypomagnesaemia may also be present) and when salvos of rapid ventricular tachycardia show the characteristic twisting wave front known as *torsades de pointes.* The usual dose of magnesium sulphate is intravenous injection of 8 mmol over 10–15 minutes (repeated once if necessary). Recent (unconfirmed) studies have also demonstrated a sustained reduction in mortality in patients with *suspected myocardial infarction* given an initial intravenous injection of magnesium sulphate 8 mmol over 20 minutes followed by an intravenous infusion of 65–72 mmol over the following 24 hours. Provided the initial intravenous injection is given slowly to reduce the incidence of flushing, intravenous magnesium sulphate has few side-effects.

PoM Magnesium Sulphate (Non-proprietary)
Injection, magnesium sulphate 50% (49.3 mg magnesium or 2.03 mmol Mg^{2+}/mL). Net price 2-mL amp = £4.18

9.5.2 Phosphorus

9.5.2.1 Phosphate supplements
9.5.2.2 Phosphate-binding agents

9.5.2.1 PHOSPHATE SUPPLEMENTS

Oral phosphate supplements may be required in addition to vitamin D in a small minority of patients with hypophosphataemic vitamin D-resistant rickets. Diarrhoea is a common side-effect and should prompt a reduction in dosage.

Phosphate infusion is occasionally needed in alcohol dependence or in phosphate deficiency arising from use of parenteral nutrition deficient in phosphate supplements; phosphate depletion also occurs in severe diabetic ketoacidosis. For *established hypophosphataemia*, monobasic potassium hydrogen phosphate may be infused at a maximum rate of 9 mmol every 12 hours. Excessive doses of phosphates may cause hypocalcaemia and metastatic calcification; it is **essential** to monitor closely plasma concentrations of calcium, phosphate, potassium, and other electrolytes.

Phosphate-Sandoz® (Sandoz)
Tablets, effervescent, anhydrous sodium acid phosphate 1.936 g, sodium bicarbonate 350 mg, potassium bicarbonate 315 mg, equivalent to phosphorus 500 mg (16.1 mmol phosphate), sodium 468.8 mg (20.4 mmol Na$^+$), potassium 123 mg (3.1 mmol K$^+$). Net price 20 = 73p. Label: 13

9.5.2.2 PHOSPHATE-BINDING AGENTS

Aluminium-containing and calcium-containing antacids are used as phosphate-binding agents in the management of hyperphosphataemia complicating renal failure. Calcium-containing phosphate-binding agents are contra-indicated in hypercalcaemia or hypercalciuria. Phosphate-binding agents which contain aluminium may increase plasma aluminium in dialysis patients.

ALUMINIUM HYDROXIDE
Indications: hyperphosphataemia
Cautions: hyperaluminaemia; see also notes above; **interactions:** Appendix 1 (antacids and adsorbents)

Aluminium Hydroxide (Non-proprietary)
Mixture (gel), about 4% w/w Al$_2$O$_3$ in water. Net price 200 mL = 41p
Dose: hyperphosphataemia, 20–100 mL according to requirements of patient; antacid, see section 1.1.1
Note. The brand name NHS Aludrox® (Charwell) is used for aluminium hydroxide mixture, net price 200 mL = 80p. For NHS Aludrox® tablets see preparations with magnesium, section 1.1.1

Alu-Cap® (3M)
Capsules, green/red, dried aluminium hydroxide 475 mg (low Na$^+$). Net price 120-cap pack = £4.22
Dose: phosphate-binding agent in renal failure, 4–20 capsules daily in divided doses with meals; antacid, see section 1.1.1

CALCIUM CARBONATE
Indications: hyperphosphataemia
Cautions: see notes above; **interactions:** Appendix 1 (calcium salts)
Side-effects: hypercalcaemia

Calcichew®, section 9.5.1.1
Calcium-500, section 9.5.1.1
Titralac® (3M)
Tablets, calcium carbonate 420 mg (168 mg calcium or 4.2 mmol Ca^{2+}), glycine 180 mg. Net price 180-tab pack = £2.94
Dose: calcium supplement, or phosphate-binding agent (with meals) in renal failure, according to the requirements of the patient

9.5.3 Fluoride

Availability of adequate fluoride confers significant resistance to dental caries. It is now considered that the topical action of fluoride on enamel and plaque is more important than the systemic effect.

Where the natural fluoride content of the drinking water is significantly less than 1 mg per litre (one part per million) artificial fluoridation is the most economical method of supplementing fluoride intake.

Daily administration of tablets or drops is a suitable alternative, but systemic fluoride supplements should not be prescribed without prior reference to the fluoride content of the local water supply; they are not advisable when the water contains more than 700 micrograms per litre (0.7 parts per million). In addition, the British Association for the Study of Community Dentistry now recommends that infants need not receive fluoride supplements until the age of 6 months.

Use of dentifrices which incorporate sodium fluoride and/or monofluorophosphate is also a convenient source of fluoride.

Individuals who are either particularly caries prone or medically compromised may be given additional protection by use of fluoride rinses or by application of fluoride gels. Rinses may be used daily or weekly; daily use of a less concentrated rinse is more effective than weekly use of a more concentrated one. Gels must be applied on a regular basis under professional supervision; extreme caution is necessary to prevent the child from swallowing any excess. Less concentrated gels have recently become available for home use. Varnishes are also available and are particularly valuable for young or handicapped children since they adhere to the teeth and set in the presence of moisture.

SODIUM FLUORIDE

Note. Sodium fluoride 2.2 mg provides approx. 1 mg fluoride ion

Indications: prophylaxis of dental caries—see notes above

Contra-indications: not for areas where drinking water is fluoridated

Side-effects: occasional white flecks on teeth with recommended doses; rarely yellowish-brown discoloration if recommended doses are exceeded

Dose: expressed as fluoride ion (F⁻):

Water content less than 300 micrograms F⁻/litre (0.3 parts per million), CHILD up to 6 months none; 6 months–2 years 250 micrograms F⁻ daily, 2–4 years 500 micrograms F⁻ daily, over 4 years 1 mg F⁻ daily

Water content between 300 and 700 micrograms F⁻/litre (0.3–0.7 parts per million), CHILD up to 2 years none, 2–4 years 250 micrograms F⁻ daily, over 4 years 500 micrograms F⁻ daily

Water content above 700 micrograms F⁻/litre (0.7 parts per million), supplements not advised (see notes above)

Tablets

COUNSELLING. Tablets should be sucked or dissolved in the mouth and taken preferably in the evening

There are arrangements for health authorities to supply fluoride tablets in the course of pre-school dental schemes, and they may also be supplied in school dental schemes.

En-De-Kay® (Stafford-Miller)

Fluotabs 2–4 years, natural orange-flavoured, scored, sodium fluoride 1.1 mg (500 micrograms F⁻). Net price 200-tab pack = £1.83

Fluotabs 4+ years, natural orange-flavoured, scored, sodium fluoride 2.2 mg (1 mg F⁻). Net price 200-tab pack = £1.83

Fluor-a-day® (Dental Health)

Tablets, buff, sodium fluoride 1.1 mg (500 micrograms F⁻), net price 200-tab pack = £1.61; 2.2 mg (1 mg F⁻), 200-tab pack = £1.61

FluoriGard® (Colgate-Palmolive)

Tablets 0.5, purple, grape-flavoured, scored, sodium fluoride 1.1 mg (500 micrograms F⁻). Net price 200-tab pack = £1.79

Tablets 1.0, orange, orange-flavoured, scored, sodium fluoride 2.2 mg (1 mg F⁻). Net price 200-tab pack = £1.79

Oral-B Fluoride® (Oral-B Labs)

Tablets, sodium fluoride 1.1 mg (500 micrograms F⁻), net price 200-tab pack = £1.95; 2.2 mg (1 mg F⁻) (pink), 200-tab pack = £1.95

Oral drops

Note. Fluoride supplements not considered necessary below 6 months of age (see notes above)

En-De-Kay® (Stafford-Miller)

Fluodrops® (= paediatric drops), sugar-free, sodium fluoride 550 micrograms (250 micrograms F⁻)/0.15 mL. Net price 60 mL = £1.36

Note. Corresponds to Sodium Fluoride Drops DPF 0.37% equivalent to sodium fluoride 80 micrograms (F⁻ 36 micrograms)/drop

FluoriGard® (Colgate-Palmolive)

Drops, sugar-free, sodium fluoride 275 micrograms (125 micrograms F⁻)/drop. Net price 30 mL = £1.41

Note. Corresponds to Sodium Fluoride Drops DPF 0.84% equivalent to sodium fluoride 275 micrograms (F⁻ 125 micrograms)/drop

Mouthwashes

Rinse mouth for 1 minute and spit out

COUNSELLING. Avoid eating, drinking, or rinsing mouth for 15 minutes after use

PoM En-De-Kay® (Stafford-Miller)

Daily fluoride mouthrinse (= mouthwash), blue, sodium fluoride 0.05%. Net price 250 mL = £1.31

CHILD 6 years and over, for *daily* use, rinse with 10 mL

Fluorinse (= mouthwash), red, sodium fluoride 2%. Net price 100 mL = £2.73. Counselling, see above

CHILD 8 years and over, for *daily* use, dilute 5 drops to 10 mL of water; for *weekly* use, dilute 20 drops to 10 mL

PoM FluoriGard® (Colgate-Palmolive)

Daily dental rinse (= mouthwash), blue, sodium fluoride 0.05%. Net price 500 mL = £2.45. Counselling, see above

CHILD 6 years and over, for *daily* use, rinse with 10 mL

Weekly dental rinse (= mouthwash), blue, sodium fluoride 0.2%. Net price 150 mL = £1.83. Counselling, see above

CHILD 6 years and over, for *weekly* use, rinse with 10 mL

9.5.4   Zinc

Oral zinc therapy should only be given when there is good evidence of deficiency (hypoproteinaemia spuriously lowers plasma-zinc concentrations). Zinc deficiency can occur in individuals on inadequate diets, in malabsorption, with increased body loss due to trauma, burns and protein-losing conditions, and during intravenous feeding. Therapy should continue until clinical improvement occurs and be replaced by dietary measures unless there is severe malabsorption, metabolic disease, or continuing zinc loss. Side-effects of zinc salts are abdominal pain and dyspepsia.

ZINC SALTS

Indications; Cautions; Side-effects: see notes above; **interactions:** Appendix 1 (zinc)

Solvazinc® (Thames)

Effervescent tablets, yellow-white, zinc sulphate 200 mg (45 mg zinc). Net price 30 = £3.60. Label: 13, 21

Dose: 1 tablet in water 1–3 times daily after food

Zincomed® (Medo)

Capsules, blue/white, zinc sulphate 220 mg. Net price 30-cap pack = 99p. Label: 21

Dose: 1 capsule 3 times daily after food

Z Span® (Goldshield)

Spansule® (= capsules m/r), blue/clear, enclosing white and grey pellets, zinc sulphate monohydrate 61.8 mg (22.5 mg zinc). Net price 30-cap pack = £2.20. Label: 25

Dose: adults and children over 1 year, 1–3 capsules daily as required; can be opened and pellets sprinkled on cool food; not to be chewed

9.6 Vitamins

9.6.1	Vitamin A
9.6.2	Vitamin B group
9.6.3	Vitamin C
9.6.4	Vitamin D
9.6.5	Vitamin E
9.6.6	Vitamin K
9.6.7	Multivitamin preparations

Vitamins are used for the prevention and treatment of specific deficiency states or where the diet is known to be inadequate; they may be prescribed in the NHS to prevent or treat deficiency but not as dietary supplements.

Their use as general 'pick-me-ups' is of unproven value and, in the case of preparations containing vitamin A or D, may actually be harmful if patients take more than the prescribed dose. The 'fad' for mega-vitamin therapy with water-soluble vitamins, such as ascorbic acid and pyridoxine, is unscientific and can be harmful.

Dietary reference values for vitamins are available in the Department of Health publication:

Dietary Reference Values for Food Energy and Nutrients for the United Kingdom: Report of the Panel on Dietary Reference Values of the Committee on Medical Aspects of Food Policy. *Report on Health and Social Subjects 41*. London: HMSO, 1991

9.6.1 Vitamin A

Deficiency of vitamin A (retinol) is rare in Britain even in disorders of fat absorption.

Massive overdose can cause rough skin, dry hair, an enlarged liver, and a raised erythrocyte sedimentation rate and raised serum calcium and serum alkaline phosphatase concentrations.

In view of evidence suggesting that high levels of vitamin A may cause birth defects, women who are (or may become) pregnant are advised not to take vitamin A supplements (including tablets and fish-liver oil drops), except on the advice of a doctor or an antenatal clinic; nor should they eat liver or products such as liver paté or liver sausage.

VITAMIN A

(Retinol)

Indications; Cautions; Side-effects: see notes above

Dose: see notes above and under preparations

Vitamins A and D

Halibut-liver Oil (Non-proprietary)

Capsules, vitamin A 4000 units [also contains vitamin D]. Net price 20 = 12p

Available from Thornton & Ross

Vitamins A and D (Non-proprietary)

Capsules, vitamin A 4000 units, vitamin D 400 units. Net price 20 = 50p

Available from CP

NHS **Halycitrol®** (LAB)

Emulsion, vitamin A 4600 units, vitamin D 380 units/5 mL. Net price 114 mL = £1.20

Dose: 5 mL daily but see notes above

Vitamins A, D, and C for children

Children's Vitamin Drops (Hough)

Oral drops, ascorbic acid (as sodium ascorbate) 20 mg, vitamin A 700 units, vitamin D 300 units/5 drops.

Recommended by Department of Health for routine supplementation in young children. Available direct to public under the Welfare Food Scheme from maternity and child health clinics and welfare food distribution centres; not available on prescription

Dose: CHILD 1 month–5 years, 5 drops daily

Note. The Department of Health recommends these drops for children aged 6 months to 2 years (preferably 5 years particularly in winter and early spring); some infants from 1 month of age may also benefit (for details see *Present Day Practice in Infant Feeding* 3rd Report)

Minadex® (Seven Seas)

Oral drops, ascorbic acid 15 mg, vitamin A 750 units, vitamin D 200 units/0.14 mL. Net price 25-mL pack with pipette = £1.05, 50-mL pack with pipette = £1.97

Dose: INFANT and CHILD under 5 years, 0.28 mL (upper level on graduated pipette) daily; INFANT fed on vitamin D-fortified milk, CHILD over 5 years and ADULT, 0.14 mL (lower level on graduated pipette) daily

Vitamin A injection

PoM **Ro-A-Vit®** (Cambridge)

Injection, vitamin A (retinol) 50 000 units (as palmitate)/mL. Net price 2-mL amp = £1.69

Dose: by deep intramuscular injection, deficiency, 100 000 units monthly, increased to weekly in acute deficiency states; courses no longer than 6 weeks interval

Liver disease, 100 000 units every 2–4 months

INFANT under 1 year and CHILD 50 000 units monthly

Note. Contains polyethoxylated castor oil which has been associated with anaphylaxis; do **not** mix or dilute

Cautions: children, liver disease (specialist use), see also notes above

9.6.2 Vitamin B group

Deficiency of the B vitamins, other than deficiency of vitamin B_{12} (section 9.1.2) is rare in Britain and is usually treated by preparations containing thiamine (B_1), riboflavine (B_2), and nicotinamide, which is used in preference to nicotinic acid, as it does not cause vasodilatation. Other members (or substances traditionally classified as members) of the vitamin B complex such as aminobenzoic acid, biotin, choline, inositol, and pantothenic acid or panthenol may be included in vitamin B preparations but there is no evidence of their value.

The severe deficiency states Wernicke's encephalopathy and Korsakoff's psychosis, especially as seen in chronic alcoholism, are best treated by the parenteral administration of B vitamins (Pabrinex®); anaphylaxis has been reported with these preparations (see CSM advice, below).

As with other vitamins of the B group, pyridoxine (B_6) deficiency is rare, but it may occur during isoniazid therapy and is characterised by peripheral neuritis. High doses of pyridoxine are given in some metabolic disorders, such as hyperoxaluria, and it is also used in sideroblastic anaemia (section 9.1.3). Pyridoxine has been tried in a wide variety of other disorders, including the premenstrual syndrome, but there is little sound evidence to support the claims, and overdosage induces toxic effects.

RIBOFLAVINE
(Vitamin B_2)
Indications: see notes above

Preparations
Injections of vitamins B and C, see under Thiamine

Oral vitamin B complex preparations, see below

THIAMINE
(Vitamin B_1)
Indications: see notes above
Cautions: anaphylactic shock may occasionally follow injection (see CSM advice below)
Dose: mild chronic deficiency, 10–25 mg daily; severe deficiency, 200–300 mg daily

CSM advice
Since potentially serious allergic adverse reactions may occur during, or shortly after, administration, the CSM has recommended that:

1. Use be restricted to patients in whom parenteral treatment is essential;

2. Intravenous injections should be administered slowly (over 10 minutes);

3. Facilities for treating anaphylaxis should be available when administered.

Thiamine (Non-proprietary)
Tablets, thiamine hydrochloride 25 mg, net price 20 = 17p; 50 mg, 20 = 28p; 100 mg, 20 = 47p; 300 mg, 20 = 74p
Available from Roche (NHS Benerva®)

PoM Pabrinex® (Link)
Parenteral vitamins B and C for rapid correction of severe depletion or malabsorption (e.g in alcoholism, after acute infections, postoperatively, or in psychiatric states), maintenance of vitamins B and C in chronic intermittent haemodialysis

Dose: see CSM advice above
Coma or delirium from alcohol, from opioids, or from barbiturates, collapse following narcosis, by intravenous injection or infusion of *I/V High potency,* 2-3 pairs every 8 hours
Psychosis following narcosis or electroconvulsive therapy, toxicity from acute infections, by intravenous injection or infusion of *I/V High potency* or by deep intramuscular injection into the gluteal muscle of *I/M High potency,* 1 pair twice daily for up to 7 days
Haemodialysis, by intravenous infusion of *I/V High potency* (in sodium chloride intravenous infusion 0.9%) 1 pair every 2 weeks

I/M High potency injection, for intramuscular use only, ascorbic acid 500 mg, nicotinamide 160 mg, pyridoxine hydrochloride 50 mg, riboflavine 4 mg, thiamine hydrochloride 250 mg/7 mL. Net price 7 mL (in 2 amps) = £1.94

I/V High potency injection, for intravenous use only, ascorbic acid 500 mg, anhydrous glucose 1 g, nicotinamide 160 mg, pyridoxine hydrochloride 50 mg, riboflavine 4 mg, thiamine hydrochloride 250 mg/10 mL. Net price 10 mL (in 2 amps) = £1.74

Oral vitamin B complex preparations, see below

PYRIDOXINE HYDROCHLORIDE
(Vitamin B_6)
Indications: see under Dose
Cautions: **interactions:** Appendix 1 (vitamins)
Dose: deficiency states, 20–50 mg up to 3 times daily
Isoniazid neuropathy, prophylaxis 10 mg daily; therapeutic, 50 mg three times daily
Idiopathic sideroblastic anaemia, 100–400 mg daily in divided doses
Premenstrual syndrome, 50–100 mg daily (but see notes above)

Pyridoxine (Non-proprietary)
Tablets, pyridoxine hydrochloride 10 mg, net price 20 = 33p; 20 mg, 20 = 33p; 50 mg, 20 = 31p
Available from Hillcross, Roche Consumer Health (NHS Benadon®)

NHS Complement Continus® (Napp)
Tablets, m/r, yellow, pyridoxine hydrochloride 100 mg. Net price 28-tab pack = £1.92. Label: 25

Injections of vitamins B and C, see under Thiamine

NICOTINAMIDE
Indications: see notes above

Nicotinamide (Non-proprietary)
Tablets, nicotinamide 50 mg. Net price 20 = 27p

Injections of vitamins B and C, see under Thiamine

NICOTINIC ACID
See section 2.12

FOLIC ACID

See section 9.1.2

FOLINIC ACID

See section 8.1.3

VITAMIN B$_{12}$

See section 9.1.2

ORAL VITAMIN B COMPLEX PREPARATIONS

Note. Other multivitamin preparations are in section 9.6.7.

Vitamin B Tablets, Compound, nicotinamide   15 mg, riboflavine 1 mg, thiamine hydrochloride 1 mg. Net price 20 = 7p
Dose: prophylactic, 1–2 tablets daily

Vitamin B Tablets, Compound, Strong, brown, f/c or s/c, nicotinamide 20 mg, pyridoxine hydrochloride 2 mg, riboflavine 2 mg, thiamine hydrochloride 5 mg. Net price 20 = 10p
Dose: treatment of vitamin B deficiency, 1 2 tablets 3 times daily

NHS Becosym® (Roche Consumer Health)
Tablets, brown, f/c, vitamin B tablets, compound, strong. Net price 20 = 29p
Forte tablets, brown, f/c, thiamine hydrochloride 15 mg, riboflavine 15 mg, nicotinamide 50 mg, pyridoxine hydrochloride 10 mg. Net price 20 = 64p

NHS Benerva Compound® (Roche Consumer Health)
Tablets, yellow, vitamin B tablets, compound. Net price 20 = 12p

NHS Vigranon B® (Wallace Mfg)
Syrup, thiamine hydrochloride 5 mg, riboflavine 2 mg, nicotinamide 20 mg, pyridoxine hydrochloride 2 mg, panthenol 3 mg/5 mL. Net price 150 mL = £1.38

OTHER COMPOUNDS

Potassium aminobenzoate has been used in the treatment of various disorders associated with excessive fibrosis such as scleroderma but its therapeutic value is **doubtful.**

Potaba® (Glenwood)
Capsules, red/white, potassium aminobenzoate 500 mg. Net price 20 = £1.06. Label: 21
Tablets, potassium aminobenzoate 500 mg. Net price 20 = 83p. Label: 21
Envules® (= powder in sachets), potassium aminobenzoate 3 g. Net price 40 sachets = £12.70. Label: 13, 21
Dose: Peyronie's disease, scleroderma, 12 g daily in divided doses after food

---

9.6.3   Vitamin C

(Ascorbic acid)

Vitamin C therapy is essential in scurvy, but less florid manifestations of vitamin C deficiency are commonly found, especially in the elderly. It is rarely necessary to prescribe more than 100 mg daily except early in the treatment of scurvy.

Claims that vitamin C ameliorates colds or promotes wound healing have not been proved.

ASCORBIC ACID

Indications: prevention and treatment of scurvy
Dose: prophylactic, 25–75 mg daily; therapeutic, not less than 250 mg daily in divided doses

Ascorbic Acid (Non-proprietary)
Tablets, ascorbic acid 25 mg, net price 20 = 10p; 50 mg, 20 = 8p; 100 mg, 20 = 29p; 200 mg, 20 = 40p; 500 mg (label: 24), 20 = 76p
Available from APS, Roche Consumer Health (NHS Redoxon®)
Tablets, effervescent, ascorbic acid 1 g. Net price 10-tab pack = 92p. Label: 13
Available from Roche Consumer Health (NHS Redoxon®)
Injection, ascorbic acid 100 mg/mL. Net price 5-mL amp = £2.28

For children's welfare vitamin drops containing vitamin C with A and D, see vitamin A

9.6.4   Vitamin D

Note. The term Vitamin D is used for a range of compounds which possess the property of preventing or curing rickets. They include ergocalciferol (calciferol, vitamin D$_2$), cholecalciferol (vitamin D$_3$), dihydrotachysterol, alfacalcidol (1α-hydroxycholecalciferol), and calcitriol (1,25-dihydroxycholecalciferol).

Simple vitamin D *deficiency,* which is not uncommon in Asians consuming unleavened bread and in the elderly living alone, can be prevented by taking an oral supplement of only 10 micrograms (400 units) of **ergocalciferol** (calciferol, vitamin D$_2$) daily. Since there is no plain tablet of this strength available **calcium and ergocalciferol tablets** can be given (although the calcium is unnecessary).

Vitamin D deficiency caused by *intestinal malabsorption* or *chronic liver disease* usually requires vitamin D in pharmacological doses, such as **calciferol tablets** up to 1 mg (40 000 units) daily; the hypocalcaemia of *hypoparathyroidism* often requires doses of up to 2.5 mg (100 000 units) daily in order to achieve normocalcaemia. The newer vitamin D derivatives, **alfacalcidol** and **calcitriol,** have a shorter duration of action, and therefore have the advantage that problems associated with hypercalcaemia due to excessive dosage are shorter lasting and easier to treat.

Vitamin D requires hydroxylation by the kidney to its active form therefore the hydroxylated derivatives **alfacalcidol** or **calcitriol** should be prescribed if patients with *severe renal impairment* require vitamin D therapy.

Important. All patients receiving pharmacological doses of vitamin D should have the plasma calcium concentration checked at intervals (initially weekly) and whenever nausea or vomiting are present. Breast milk from women taking pharmacological doses of vitamin D may cause hypercalcaemia if given to an infant.

ERGOCALCIFEROL
(Calciferol, Vitamin D$_2$)

Indications: see notes above

Cautions: take care to ensure correct dose in infants; monitor plasma calcium in patients receiving high doses and in renal impairment

Contra-indications: hypercalcaemia; metastatic calcification

Side-effects: symptoms of overdosage include anorexia, lassitude, nausea and vomiting, diarrhoea, weight loss, polyuria, sweating, headache, thirst, vertigo, and raised concentrations of calcium and phosphate in plasma and urine

Dose: see notes above

Daily supplements

Note. There is no plain vitamin D tablet available for treating simple deficiency (see notes above). Alternatives include vitamins capsules (see 9.6.7), preparations of vitamins A and D (see 9.6.1), and calcium and ergocalciferol tablets (see below).

Calcium and Ergocalciferol (Non-proprietary) (Calcium and Vitamin D)

Tablets[1], calcium lactate 300 mg, calcium phosphate 150 mg (97 mg calcium or 2.4 mmol Ca^{2+}), ergocalciferol 10 micrograms (400 units). Net price 20 = 17p. Counselling, crush before administration or may be chewed

1. Calcium with Vitamin D Tablets (BPC) which contained ergocalciferol 12.5 micrograms (500 units) have been replaced by Calcium and Ergocalciferol Tablets

Calcichew D3® (Shire)

Tablets (chewable), calcium carbonate 1.26 g (500 mg calcium or 12.6 mmol Ca^{2+}), cholecalciferol 5 micrograms (200 units). Net price 100-tab pack = £13.65. Label: 24

Additives: include aspartame

Pharmacological strengths (see notes above)

Calciferol (Non-proprietary)

Tablets, cholecalciferol or ergocalciferol 250 micrograms (10 000 units), net price 20 = £2.60; 1.25 mg (50 000 units) may also be available

Available from Evans

Note. The BP directs that when high-strength calciferol tablets are prescribed or demanded, tablets containing 250 micrograms shall be dispensed or supplied, and when strong calciferol tablets are prescribed or demanded it should be **confirmed** that tablets containing 1.25 mg are intended. To avoid **errors** arising from the use of these titles prescribers should **abandon** them and **specify strength required**

PoM *Injection,* cholecalciferol or ergocalciferol, 7.5 mg (300 000 units)/mL in oil. Net price 1-mL amp = £5.92, 2-mL amp = £7.07

ALFACALCIDOL
(1α-Hydroxycholecalciferol)

Indications: see notes above

Cautions; Contra-indications; Side-effects: see under Ergocalciferol

Dose: by mouth or by intravenous injection over 30 seconds, ADULT and CHILD over 20 kg, initially 1 microgram daily (elderly 500 nanograms), adjusted to avoid hypercalcaemia; maintenance, usually 0.25–1 microgram daily; NEONATE and PREMATURE INFANT initially 50–100 nanograms/kg daily, CHILD under 20 kg initially 50 nanograms/kg daily

PoM **AlfaD**® (Du Pont)

Capsules, alfacalcidol 250 nanograms (pink), net price 100-cap pack = £12.08; 1 microgram (orange), 30-cap pack = £10.80

PoM **One-Alpha**® (Leo)

Capsules, alfacalcidol 250 nanograms, net price 20 = £2.36; 1 microgram (brown), 20 = £7.02

Solution, sugar-free, alfacalcidol 200 nanograms/mL. Net price 60 mL = £15.19 (with oral syringe)

Injection, alfacalcidol 2 micrograms/mL, net price 0.5-mL amp = £2.43, 1-mL amp = £4.63

Note. Contains propylene glycol and should be used with caution in small premature infants

CALCITRIOL
(1,25-Dihydroxycholecalciferol)

Indications: see notes above

Cautions; Contra-indications; Side-effects: see under Ergocalciferol

Dose: see under preparations below

PoM **Calcijex**® (Abbott)

Injection, calcitriol 1 microgram/mL, net price 1-mL amp = £5.71; 2 micrograms/mL, 1-mL amp = £11.42

Dose: hypocalcaemia in dialysis patients with chronic renal failure, by intravenous injection (or injection through catheter) after haemodialysis, initially 500 nanograms (approx. 10 nanograms/kg) 3 times a week, increased if necessary in steps of 250–500 nanograms at intervals of 2–4 weeks; usual dose 0.5–3 micrograms 3 times a week; CHILD not established

PoM **Rocaltrol**® (Roche)

Capsules, calcitriol 250 nanograms (red/white), net price 20 = £4.31; 500 nanograms (red), 20 = £7.71

Dose: ADULT, initially 250 nanograms daily or on alternate days, increased if necessary in steps of 250 nanograms at intervals of 2–4 weeks; usual dose 0.5–1 micrograms daily; CHILD not established

CHOLECALCIFEROL
(Vitamin D$_3$)

Indications; Cautions; Contra-indications; Side-effects: see under Ergocalciferol—alternative to ergocalciferol in calciferol tablets and injection

DIHYDROTACHYSTEROL
Cautions; Contra-indications; Side-effects: see under Ergocalciferol

AT 10® (Sanofi Winthrop)
Oral solution, dihydrotachysterol 250 micrograms/mL. Net price 15-mL dropper bottle = £21.27
Dose: acute, chronic, and latent forms of hypocalcaemic tetany due to hypoparathyroidism, consult data sheet

9.6.5 Vitamin E
(Tocopherols)

The daily requirement of vitamin E has not been well defined but is probably about 3 to 15 mg daily. There is little evidence that oral supplements of vitamin E are essential in adults, even where there is fat malabsorption secondary to cholestasis. In young children with congenital cholestasis, abnormally low vitamin E concentrations may be found in association with neuromuscular abnormalities, which usually respond only to the parenteral administration of vitamin E.

Vitamin E has been tried for various other conditions but there is no scientific evidence of its value. High doses have been associated with adverse effects.

ALPHA TOCOPHERYL ACETATE
Indications: see notes above
Cautions: predisposition to thrombosis; increased risk of necrotising enterocolitis in premature infants weighing less than 1.5 kg
Side-effects: diarrhoea and abdominal pain with doses more than 1 g daily

Vitamin E Suspension (Cambridge)
Suspension, alpha tocopheryl acetate 500 mg/5 mL. Net price 100 mL = £7.93
Dose: malabsorption in cystic fibrosis, 100–200 mg daily; CHILD under 1 year 50 mg daily; 1 year and over, 100 mg daily
Malabsorption in abetalipoproteinaemia, ADULT and CHILD 50 100 mg/kg daily
Malabsorption in chronic cholestasis, INFANT 150–200 mg/kg daily

9.6.6 Vitamin K

Vitamin K is necessary for the production of blood clotting factors and proteins necessary for the normal calcification of bone.

Because vitamin K is fat soluble, patients with *fat malabsorption*, especially in biliary obstruction or hepatic disease, may become deficient. For oral administration to prevent vitamin-K deficiency in malabsorption syndromes, a water-soluble preparation, **menadiol sodium phosphate** must be used; the usual dose is about 10 mg daily.

For *prophylaxis against vitamin K deficiency bleeding in infants* the Department of Health has advised that paediatricians and midwives and other health care professionals with responsibilities in this area of practice should establish locally agreed policies for each maternity service.

A report of an Expert Committee advising on the administration of vitamin K to infants has been published by the British Paediatric Association and is available from:
British Paediatric Association,
5 St Andrew's Place,
London NW1 4LB.

Oral coumarin *anticoagulants* act by interfering with vitamin K metabolism in the hepatic cells and their effects can be antagonised by giving vitamin K; for British Society for Haematology Guidelines, see section 2.8.2.

MENADIOL SODIUM PHOSPHATE
Indications; Dose: see notes above
Cautions: G6PD deficiency (see section 9.1.5) and vitamin E deficiency (risk of haemolysis); **interactions:** Appendix 1 (vitamins)
Contra-indications: neonates and infants, late pregnancy

Synkavit® (Cambridge)
Tablets, scored, menadiol sodium phosphate equivalent to 10 mg of menadiol phosphate. Net price 20 = 93p

PHYTOMENADIONE
(Vitamin K$_1$)
Indications; Dose: see notes above
Cautions: intravenous injections (see section 2.8.2) should be given very slowly; **interactions:** Appendix 1 (vitamins)

Konakion® (Roche)
Tablets, s/c, phytomenadione 10 mg. Net price 25-tab pack = £4.62. To be chewed or allowed to dissolve slowly in the mouth (Label: 24)
PoM *Injection*, phytomenadione 2 mg/mL, net price 0.5-mL amp = 24p; 10 mg/mL, 1-mL amp = 45p
Note. Contains polyethoxylated castor oil which has been associated with anaphylaxis

9.6.7 Multivitamin preparations

Vitamins Capsules, ascorbic acid 15 mg, nicotinamide 7.5 mg, riboflavine 500 micrograms, thiamine hydrochloride 1 mg, vitamin A 2500 units, vitamin D 300 units. Net price 20 = 15p
Abidec® (W L)
Drops, vitamins A, B group, C, and D. Net price 25 mL (with dropper) = £1.64
NHS **BC 500®** (Whitehall)
Tablets, orange, f/c, vitamins B group and C. Net price 30 = £1.96
NHS **Calcimax®** (Wallace Mfg)
Syrup, brown, vitamins B group, C, and D. Net price 150 mL = £1.68
NHS **Concavit®** (Wallace Mfg)
Capsules, vitamins A, B group, C, D, and E. Net price 20 = £1.11
Drops and *syrup*, vitamins A, B group, C, and D. Net price drops 15 mL = £1.60; syrup 150 mL = £1.88

Dalivit® (Eastern)

Oral drops, vitamins A, B group, C, and D. Net price 2 × 15 mL = £1.40

ℕℍ⅁ Octovit® (Goldshield)

Tablets, maroon, f/c, dried ferrous sulphate (10 mg iron) with vitamins A, B group, C, D, E, and minerals. Net price 14-tab pack = £2.55

ℕℍ⅁ Orovite® (SmithKline Beecham Healthcare)

Tablets, maroon, s/c, vitamins B group and C. Net price 25-tab pack = £1.85

ℕℍ⅁ Orovite 7® (SmithKline Beecham Healthcare)

Granules, orange, vitamins A, B group, C, and D. Net price 10-sachet pack = £1.49, 30-sachet pack = £4.22. Label: 13

VITAMIN AND MINERAL SUPPLEMENTS AND ADJUNCTS TO SYNTHETIC DIETS

Forceval® (Unigreg)

Capsules, brown/red, vitamins (ascorbic acid 60 mg, biotin 100 micrograms, cyanocobalamin 3 micrograms, folic acid 300 micrograms, nicotinamide 18 mg, pantothenic acid 4 mg, pyridoxine 2 mg, riboflavine 1.6 mg, thiamine 1.2 mg, vitamin A 2500 units, vitamin D_2 400 units, vitamin E 10 mg, vitamin K_1 70 micrograms), minerals and trace elements (calcium 100 mg, chromium 200 micrograms, copper 2 mg, iodine 140 micrograms, iron 12 mg, magnesium 30 mg, manganese 3 mg, molybdenum 250 micrograms, phosphorus 77 mg, potassium 4 mg, selenium 50 micrograms, zinc 15 mg). Net price 30-cap pack = £5.39, 45-cap pack = £7.70; 90-cap pack = £14.70

Dose: vitamin and mineral deficiency and as adjunct in synthetic diets, 1 capsule daily

Junior capsules, brown, vitamins (ascorbic acid 25 mg, biotin 50 micrograms, cyanocobalamin 2 micrograms, folic acid 100 micrograms, nicotinamide 7.5 mg, pantothenic acid 2 mg, pyridoxine 1 mg, riboflavine 1 mg, thiamine 1.5 mg, vitamin A 1250 units, vitamin D_2 200 units, vitamin E 5 mg, vitamin K_1 25 micrograms), minerals and trace elements (chromium 50 micrograms, copper 1 mg, iodine 75 micrograms, iron 5 mg, magnesium 1 mg, manganese 1.25 mg, molybdenum 50 micrograms, selenium 25 micrograms, zinc 5 mg). Net price 30-cap pack = £4.05, 60-cap pack = £7.70

Dose: vitamin and mineral deficiency and as adjunct in synthetic diets, CHILD over 5 years, 2 capsules daily

Ketovite® (Paines & Byrne)

PoM *Tablets*, yellow, ascorbic acid 16.6 mg, riboflavine 1 mg, thiamine hydrochloride 1 mg, pyridoxine hydrochloride 330 micrograms, nicotinamide 3.3 mg, calcium pantothenate 1.16 mg, alpha tocopheryl acetate 5 mg, inositol 50 mg, biotin 170 micrograms, folic acid 250 micrograms, acetomenaphthone 500 micrograms. Net price 100-tab pack = £4.17

Dose: prevention of deficiency in disorders of carbohydrate or amino acid metabolism, 1 tablet 3 times daily; with Ketovite® Liquid as vitamin supplement with synthetic diets

Liquid, pink, sugar-free, vitamin A 2500 units, ergocalciferol 400 units, choline chloride 150 mg, cyanocobalamin 12.5 micrograms/5 mL. Net price 150-mL pack = £2.70

Dose: prevention of deficiency in disorders of carbohydrate or amino acid metabolism, 5 mL daily; with Ketovite® Tablets as vitamin supplement with synthetic diets

9.7   Bitters and tonics

Mixtures containing simple and aromatic bitters, such as alkaline gentian mixture, are traditional remedies for loss of appetite. All depend on suggestion.

Gentian Mixture, Acid, BP

Mixture, concentrated compound gentian infusion 10%, dilute hydrochloric acid 5% in a suitable vehicle. Extemporaneous preparations should be recently prepared according to the following formula: concentrated compound gentian infusion 1 mL, dilute hydrochloric acid 0.5 mL, doublestrength chloroform water 5 mL, water to 10 mL

Dose: 10 mL 3 times daily in water before meals

Gentian Mixture, Alkaline, BP

(Alkaline Gentian Oral Solution)

Mixture, concentrated compound gentian infusion 10%, sodium bicarbonate 5% in a suitable vehicle. Extemporaneous preparations should be recently prepared according to the following formula: concentrated compound gentian infusion 1 mL, sodium bicarbonate 500 mg, doublestrength chloroform water 5 mL, water to 10 mL

Dose: 10 mL 3 times daily in water before meals

ℕℍ⅁ Effico® (Pharmax)

Tonic, green, thiamine hydrochloride 180 micrograms, nicotinamide 2.1 mg, caffeine 20.2 mg, compound gentian infusion 0.31 mL/5 mL. Net price 300-mL pack = £1.71, 500-mL pack = £2.31

ℕℍ⅁ Labiton® (LAB)

Tonic, brown, thiamine hydrochloride 375 micrograms, caffeine 3.5 mg, kola nut dried extract 3.025 mg, alcohol 1.4 mL/5 mL. Net price 200 mL = £1.63

ℕℍ⅁ Metatone® (W-L)

Tonic, thiamine hydrochloride 500 micrograms, calcium glycerophosphate 45.6 mg, manganese glycerophosphate 5.7 mg, potassium glycerophosphate 45.6 mg, sodium glycerophosphate 22.8 mg/5 mL. Net price 300 mL = £1.71

9.8   Metabolic disorders

9.8.1   Wilson's disease and carnitine deficiency

9.8.2   Acute porphyrias

This section covers drugs used in metabolic disorders and not readily classified elsewhere.

9.8.1   Wilson's disease and carnitine deficiency

WILSON'S DISEASE

Penicillamine (see also section 10.1.3) is used in Wilson's disease (hepatolenticular degeneration) to aid the elimination of copper ions. See below for other indications.

Trientine is used for the treatment of Wilson's disease only, in patients intolerant of penicillamine; it is **not** an alternative to penicillamine for rheumatoid arthritis or cystinuria.

PENICILLAMINE

Indications: see under Dose below
Cautions; Contra-indications; Side-effects: see section 10.1.3
Dose: Wilson's disease, 1.5–2 g daily in divided doses before food; max. 2 g daily for 1 year; maintenance 0.75–1 g daily; ELDERLY, 20 mg/kg daily in divided doses; CHILD, up to 20 mg/kg daily in divided doses, minimum 500 mg daily
Chronic active hepatitis (after disease controlled with corticosteroids), initially 500 mg daily in divided doses slowly increased over 3 months; usual maintenance dose 1.25 g daily; ELDERLY not recommended
Cystinuria, therapeutic, 1–3 g daily in divided doses before food, adjusted to maintain urinary cystine below 200 mg/litre. Prophylactic (maintain urinary cystine below 300 mg/litre) 0.5–1 g at bedtime; maintain adequate fluid intake (at least 3 litres daily); CHILD and ELDERLY minimum dose to maintain urinary cystine below 200 mg/litre
Severe active rheumatoid arthritis, see section 10.1.3
Copper and lead poisioning, see Emergency Treatment of Poisoning

Preparations
See section 10.1.3

TRIENTINE DIHYDROCHLORIDE

Indications: Wilson's disease in patients intolerant of penicillamine
Cautions: see notes above; pregnancy; **Interactions:** Appendix 1 (trientine)
Side-effects: nausea; penicillamine-induced systemic lupus erythematosus may not resolve on transfer to trientine
Dose: 1.2–2.4 g daily in 2–4 divided doses before food

▼ PoM **Trientine Dihydrochloride Capsules,**
trientine dihydrochloride 300 mg. Label: 6, 22
Available from K & K-Greeff
Note. The CSM has requested that in addition to the usual CSM reporting request special records should also be kept by the pharmacist

Carnitine is available for the management of primary or secondary carnitine deficiency.

CARNITINE

Indications: primary and secondary carnitine deficiency
Cautions: renal impairment; pregnancy (but appropriate to use) and breast-feeding
Side-effects: nausea, vomiting, abdominal pain, diarrhoea, body odour; side-effects may be dose-related—monitor tolerance during first week and after any dose increase
Dose: by mouth, 1–3 g daily in divided doses (usual max. 3 g daily—higher doses occasionally required); CHILD (under 12 years, as Paediatric solution) 100 mg/kg daily (usual max. 3 g daily—higher doses occasionally required)
By intravenous injection over 2–3 minutes, ADULT and CHILD, according to requirement, 100 mg/kg daily (usual max. 3 g daily—higher doses occasionally required)

▼ PoM **Carnitor** (Co-Pharma)
Tablets, L-carnitine 330 mg. Net price 90-tab pack = £105.00
Chewable tablets, L-carnitine 1 g. Net price 10-tab pack = £35.00
Oral liquid, L-carnitine 1 g/10-mL single-dose bottle. Net price 10 × 10-mL single-dose bottle = £35.00
Paediatric solution, L-carnitine 30%. Net price 20 mL = £21.00
Injection, L-carnitine 200 mg/mL. Net price 5-mL amp = £19.92

9.8.2 Acute porphyrias

The acute porphyrias (acute intermittent porphyria, variegate porphyria, hereditary coproporphyria and plumboporphyria) are hereditary disorders of haem biosynthesis; they have a prevalence of about 1 in 10 000 of the population.

Great care must be taken when prescribing for patients with acute porphyria since many drugs can induce acute porphyric crises. Since acute porphyrias are hereditary, relatives of affected individuals should be screened and advised about the potential danger of certain drugs.

The following list contains drugs on the UK market that have been classified as 'unsafe' in porphyria because they have been shown to be porphyrinogenic in animals or *in vitro*, or have been associated with acute attacks in patients.

Further information may be obtained from:
Porphyria Research Unit
Western Infirmary
Glasgow G11 6NT

Drugs unsafe for use in acute porphyrias

Note. Quite modest changes in chemical structure can lead to changes in porphyrinogenicity but where possible general statements have been made about groups of drugs; these should be checked first

Drug groups (please check **first**)

Amphetamines	Barbiturates[3]	Diuretics[6]	Menopausal Steroids[5]
Anabolic Steroids	Benzodiazepines[4]	Ergot Derivatives[7]	Mercury Compounds
Antidepressants[1]	Cephalosporins	Gold Salts	Progestogens
Antihistamines[2]	Contraceptives, steroid[5]	Hormone Replacement Therapy[5]	Sulphonamides[8]
			Sulphonylureas

Individual Drugs (please check groups above **first**)

Alcohol	Danazol	Isoniazid	Oxyphenbutazone
Alcuronium	Dapsone	Ketoconazole	Oxytetracycline
Aluminium-containing Antacids[9]	Dexfenfluramine	Lignocaine	Pentazocine[11]
	Dextropropoxyphene[11]	Lisinopril	Phenoxybenzamine
Aminoglutethimide	Diclofenac	Loxapine	Phenylbutazone
Amiodarone	Diethylpropion	Mebeverine	Phenytoin
Azapropazone	Diltiazem	Mefenamic Acid	Piroxicam
Baclofen	Doxycycline	Meprobamate	Pivampicillin[12]
Bromocriptine	Econazole	Mercaptopurine	Prilocaine
Busulphan	Enalapril	Methotrexate	Probenecid
Captopril	Enflurane	Methyldopa	Pyrazinamide
Carbamazepine	Erythromycin	Metoclopramide	Rifampicin
Carisoprodol	Ethamsylate	Metyrapone	Simvastatin
Chlorambucil	Ethionamide	Miconazole	Sulphinpyrazone
Chloramphenicol	Ethosuximide	Mifepristone	Sulpiride
Chlormezanone	Etomidate	Minoxidil	Tamoxifen
Chloroform[10]	Fenfluramine	Nalidixic Acid	Theophylline[13]
Clonidine	Flucloxacillin	Nifedipine	Thioridazine
Cocaine	Flupenthixol	Nitrofurantoin	Tinidazole
Colistin	Griseofulvin	Orphenadrine	Trimethoprim
Cyclophosphamide	Halothane	Oxybutynin	Valproate[4]
Cycloserine	Hydralazine	Oxycodone	Verapamil
Cyclosporin	Hyoscine	Oxymetazoline	Zuclopenthixol
	Isometheptene Mucate		

1. Includes tricyclic (and related) and MAOIs.
2. Most antihistamines should be avoided but chlorpheniramine and cyclizine thought to be safe.
3. Includes methohexitone, primidone, and thiopentone.
4. Status epilepticus has been treated successfully with intravenous diazepam; where essential, seizure prophylaxis has been undertaken with clonazepam or valproate.
5. Includes both progestogen-only and combined (progestogen content probably more hazardous than oestrogen).
6. Acetazolamide, amiloride, bumetanide, and triamterene have been used.
7. Includes ergometrine (oxytocin probably safe), lysuride and pergolide.
8. Includes co-trimoxazole and sulphasalazine.
9. Absorption limited but magnesium-containing antacids preferable.
10. Small amounts in medicines probably safe.
11. Morphine, diamorphine, codeine, dihydrocodeine, and pethidine are thought to be safe.
12. Ampicillin and amoxycillin probably safe.
13. Includes aminophylline.

10: Drugs used in the treatment of
MUSCULOSKELETAL and JOINT DISEASES

In this chapter, drug treatment is discussed under the following headings:

10.1 Drugs used in rheumatic diseases and gout
10.2 Drugs used in neuromuscular disorders
10.3 Drugs for the relief of soft-tissue inflammation

For treatment of septic arthritis see section 5.1, table 1.

10.1 Drugs used in rheumatic diseases and gout

10.1.1 Non-steroidal anti-inflammatory drugs
10.1.2 Corticosteroids
10.1.3 Drugs which suppress the rheumatic disease process
10.1.4 Drugs for the treatment of gout

Most rheumatic diseases require symptomatic treatment with non-steroidal anti-inflammatory drugs (NSAIDs) to relieve pain and stiffness.

In certain circumstances corticosteroids may be used to suppress inflammation.

Drugs are also available which may affect the disease process itself and favourably influence the outcome. For *rheumatoid arthritis* these include penicillamine, gold salts, antimalarials (chloroquine and hydroxychloroquine), immunosuppressants (azathioprine, chlorambucil, cyclophosphamide, and methotrexate), and sulphasalazine; they are sometimes known as second-line or disease-modifying antirheumatic drugs. For *psoriatic arthritis* they include gold salts, azathioprine, and methotrexate, and for *gout* they include uricosuric drugs and allopurinol.

10.1.1 Non-steroidal anti-inflammatory drugs (NSAIDs)

In *single doses* NSAIDs have analgesic activity comparable to that of paracetamol (see section 4.7.1) and can therefore be taken on demand for mild or intermittent pain or as a supplement to regular treatment. In regular *full dosage* they have both a lasting analgesic and an anti-inflammatory effect. This combination makes them particularly useful for the treatment of continuous or regular pain associated with inflammation. Therefore, although paracetamol often gives adequate pain control in osteoarthritis, NSAIDs are more appropriate than paracetamol or the opioid analgesics in the *inflammatory arthritides* (e.g. rheumatoid arthritis) and in some cases of advanced osteoarthritis. They may also be of benefit in the less well defined conditions of *back pain* and *soft-tissue disorders*.

Differences in anti-inflammatory activity between different NSAIDs are small, but there is considerable variation in individual patient response. About 60% of patients will respond to any NSAID. Among the rest, those who do not respond to one may well respond to another. Therefore it is often necessary to try several drugs before finding one to suit a particular patient. Most NSAIDs should produce an effect within a few days. If used for analgesia alone they should be changed if no response is obtained after a week; if an anti-inflammatory action is also required they should be changed if no response is obtained after three weeks.

The main differences between NSAIDs are in the incidence and type of side-effects. Before treatment is started the prescriber should weigh efficacy against possible side-effects.

ASPIRIN AND THE SALICYLATES

Aspirin[1] was the traditional first choice anti-inflammatory analgesic but most physicians now prefer to start treatment with another NSAID which may be better tolerated and more convenient for the patient.

In regular high dosage aspirin has about the same anti-inflammatory effect as other NSAIDs. The required dose for active inflammatory joint disease is 3.6 g or more daily. There is little anti-inflammatory effect with less than 3 g daily. Gastro-intestinal side-effects such as nausea, dyspepsia, and gastro-intestinal bleeding may occur with any dosage of aspirin but anti-inflammatory doses are associated with a much higher incidence of side-effects. Gastro-intestinal side-effects may be minimised by taking the dose after food. Numerous formulations are available which improve gastric tolerance and minimise occult bleeding, including dispersible and enteric-coated preparations.

Anti-inflammatory doses of aspirin may also cause mild chronic salicylate intoxication (salicylism) characterised by dizziness, tinnitus, and deafness; these symptoms may be controlled by reducing the dosage.

Benorylate, an aspirin-paracetamol ester, is broken down after absorption from the gastro-intestinal tract. It need only be given twice daily and gastric tolerance is slightly better than with aspirin.

---

1. Owing to an association with Reye's syndrome the CSM has recommended that aspirin-containing preparations should no longer be given to children under the age of 12 years, unless specifically indicated, e.g. for juvenile arthritis (Still's disease). It is **important** to advise families that aspirin is not a suitable medicine for children with minor illnesses.

Prices are **net**, see p. 1

ASPIRIN
(Acetylsalicylic Acid)

Indications: pain and inflammation in rheumatic disease and other musculoskeletal disorders (including juvenile arthritis); see also section 4.7.1; antiplatelet, see section 2.9

Cautions: asthma, allergic disease, uncontrolled hypertension, hepatic or renal impairment (avoid if severe), dehydration, pregnancy (particularly at term) (see also Appendix 4), elderly; G6PD-deficiency (see section 9.1.5); **interactions:** Appendix 1 (aspirin)

REYE'S SYNDROME. Owing to an association with Reye's syndrome the CSM has recommended that aspirin-containing preparations should no longer be given to children under the age of 12 years, unless specifically indicated, e.g. for juvenile arthritis (Still's disease). It is **important** to advise families that aspirin is not a suitable medicine for children with minor illnesses.

Contra-indications: gastro-intestinal ulceration; children under 12 years (except for juvenile arthritis) and breast-feeding (association with Reye's syndrome, see above); haemophilia and other bleeding disorders; not for treatment of gout

HYPERSENSITIVITY. Aspirin and other NSAIDs are **contra-indicated** in patients with a history of hypersensitivity to aspirin or any other NSAID—*which includes those* in whom attacks of *asthma, angioedema, urticaria or rhinitis* have been precipitated by aspirin or any other NSAID

Side-effects: common with anti-inflammatory doses; gastro-intestinal discomfort or nausea, ulceration with occult bleeding (but occasionally major haemorrhage); also other haemorrhage (e.g. subconjunctival); hearing disturbances such as tinnitus (leading rarely to deafness), vertigo, mental confusion, hypersensitivity reactions (angioedema, bronchospasm and rashes); increased bleeding time; rarely oedema, myocarditis, blood disorders, particularly thrombocytopenia; overdosage: see Emergency Treatment of Poisoning, p.20

Dose: 0.3–1 g every 4 hours; max. in acute conditions 8 g daily; CHILD, juvenile arthritis, up to 80 mg/kg daily in 5–6 divided doses, increased in acute exacerbations to 130 mg/kg. Doses should be taken after food

Preparations
See section 4.7.1

BENORYLATE
(Benorilate)

(Aspirin-paracetamol ester; 2 g benorylate is equivalent to approximately 1.15 g aspirin and 970 mg paracetamol)

Indications: pain and inflammation in rheumatic disease and other musculoskeletal disorders; mild to moderate pain; pyrexia

Cautions; Contra-indications; Side-effects: see under Aspirin (above) and Paracetamol (section 4.7.1)

Dose: rheumatic disease, 4–8 g daily divided into 2–3 doses; max. 6 g daily for elderly.
Mild to moderate pain, 2 g twice daily preferably after food

Benoral® (Sanofi Winthrop)
Tablets, benorylate 750 mg. Net price 100-tab pack = £8.36. Label: 21, 31
Granules, benorylate 2 g/sachet. Net price 60 sachet-pack = £13.77. Label: 13, 21, 31
Suspension, sugar-free, benorylate 2 g/5 mL. Net price 300 mL = £11.86. Label: 21, 31
Note. Generic versions of benorylate tablets and suspension are available from various manufacturers

---

OTHER NSAIDs

Ibuprofen is a propionic acid derivative with anti-inflammatory, analgesic, and antipyretic properties. It has fewer side-effects than other NSAIDs but its anti-inflammatory properties are weaker. Doses of 1.6 to 2.4 g daily are needed for rheumatoid arthritis and it is unsuitable for conditions where inflammation is prominent such as acute gout.

Other propionic acid derivatives:

Naproxen has emerged as one of the first choices as it combines good efficacy with a low incidence of side-effects (but more than ibuprofen, see CSM comment on next page) and administration is only twice daily.

Fenbufen is claimed to be associated with less gastro-intestinal bleeding, but there is a high risk of rashes (see p.382).

Fenoprofen is as effective as naproxen, and **flurbiprofen** may be slightly more effective. Both are associated with slightly more gastro-intestinal side-effects than ibuprofen.

Ketoprofen has anti-inflammatory properties similar to ibuprofen and has more side-effects (see also CSM comment on next page).

Tiaprofenic acid is as effective as naproxen; it has more side-effects than ibuprofen (**important:** reports of severe cystitis, see CSM advice on p.385).

Drugs with properties similar to those of propionic acid derivatives:

Azapropazone is similar in effect to naproxen; it has a tendency to cause rashes and is associated with an increased risk of severe gastro-intestinal toxicity (**important:** see CSM restrictions on p.380).

Diclofenac has an action similar to that of naproxen; its side-effects are also similar.

Diflunisal is an aspirin derivative but its clinical effect more closely resembles that of the propionic acid derivatives than that of its parent compound. Its long duration of action allows twice-daily administration.

Etodolac is comparable in effect to naproxen; side-effects appear to be comparable to those of ibuprofen but long-term data are awaited.

Indomethacin has an action equal to or superior to that of naproxen, but with a high incidence of side-effects including headaches, dizziness, and gastro-intestinal disturbances (see also CSM comment opposite).

Mefenamic acid is a related analgesic but its anti-inflammatory properties are minor and side-effects differ in that diarrhoea and occasionally

---

haemolytic anaemia may occur which necessitate discontinuation of treatment.

Nabumetone is comparable in effect to naproxen; side-effects appear to be comparable to those of ibuprofen but long-term data are awaited.

Phenylbutazone is a potent anti-inflammatory drug but because of occasional serious side-effects its use is limited to the hospital treatment of ankylosing spondylitis. In addition to its gastric side-effects it has two rare but dangerous side-effects. It causes fluid retention and, in predisposed patients, may precipitate cardiac failure. It also causes agranulocytosis (which may occur within the first few days of treatment) and aplastic anaemia. In ankylosing spondylitis prolonged administration may be necessary but it should not be used unless other drugs have failed.

Piroxicam is as effective as naproxen and has a prolonged duration of action which permits once-daily administration. It has more gastro-intestinal side-effects than ibuprofen, especially in the elderly (see also CSM comment opposite).

Sulindac is similar in tolerance to naproxen.

Tenoxicam is similar in activity and tolerance to naproxen. Its long half-life allows once-daily administration.

Tolmetin is comparable in effect to ibuprofen.

CAUTIONS. NSAIDs should be used with caution in the *elderly*, in *allergic disorders* (they are **contra-indicated** in patients with a history of hypersensitivity to aspirin or any other NSAID—*which includes those* in whom attacks of *asthma, angioedema, urticaria or rhinitis* have been precipitated by aspirin or any other NSAID), and during *pregnancy.*

In patients with *renal, cardiac, or hepatic impairment* caution is required since the use of NSAIDs may result in deterioration of renal function (see also under Side-effects, below); the dose should be kept as **low as possible** and renal function should be **monitored**.

NSAIDs should not be given to patients with *active peptic ulceration*, see also **CSM advice** below. While it is preferable to avoid them in patients with current or previous gastro-intestinal ulceration, and to withdraw them if gastro-intestinal lesions develop, nevertheless patients with serious rheumatic diseases (e.g. rheumatoid arthritis) are usually dependent on NSAIDs for effective relief of pain and stiffness. Administration of histamine H_2-receptor blocking drugs (see section 1.3.1) or misoprostol (see section 1.3.4) may permit recommencement of a NSAID without further gastro-intestinal problems.

SIDE-EFFECTS. Side-effects are variable in severity and frequency. Gastro-intestinal discomfort, nausea, diarrhoea, and occasionally bleeding and ulceration occur; dyspepsia may be minimised by taking these drugs with food or milk. Other side-effects include hypersensitivity reactions (particularly angioedema, bronchospasm, and rashes), headache, dizziness, vertigo, hearing disturbances such as tinnitus, and haematuria. Blood disorders have also occurred. Fluid retention may occur

(rarely precipitating congestive heart failure in elderly patients). Reversible acute renal failure may be provoked by NSAIDs especially in patients with pre-existing renal impairment (**important**, see also under Cautions above). Rarely, papillary necrosis or interstitial fibrosis associated with NSAIDs may lead to renal failure. Aseptic meningitis has been reported rarely with NSAIDs; patients with connective tissue disorders such as systemic lupus erythematosus may be especially susceptible. Hepatic damage is another rare side-effect.

Overdosage: see Emergency Treatment of Poisoning, p. 20.

CSM advice (g.i. side-effects).

Recent evidence on the relative safety of 7 oral NSAIDs has indicated differences in the risks of serious upper gastro-intestinal side-effects. **Azapropazone** is associated with the *highest risk* (**important**: see also restrictions on p. 380) and **ibuprofen** with the *lowest*; **piroxicam, ketoprofen, indomethacin, naproxen** and **diclofenac** are associated with *intermediate risks* (possibly higher in the case of piroxicam). There are insufficient data to reach clear conclusions on other available oral NSAIDs.

Recommendations are that NSAIDs associated with low risk should *generally be preferred*, to start at the *lowest recommended dose, not to use more than one* oral NSAID at a time, and to remember that all NSAIDs are *contra-indicated* in patients with peptic ulceration.

Previous recommendations of the CSM have included the advice that in patients with a history of peptic ulcer disease and in the elderly, NSAIDs should be given only after other forms of treatment have been carefully considered.

CSM warning (asthma).

Any degree of worsening of asthma may be related to the ingestion of NSAIDs, either prescribed or (in the case of ibuprofen and others) purchased over the counter.

IBUPROFEN

Indications: pain and inflammation in rheumatic disease (including juvenile arthritis) and other musculoskeletal disorders; mild to moderate pain including dysmenorrhoea; postoperative analgesia; fever and pain in children see section 4.7.1

Cautions; Side-effects: see notes above; **interactions:** Appendix 1 (NSAIDs)

HYPERSENSITIVITY. NSAIDs are **contra-indicated** in patients with a history of hypersensitivity to aspirin or any other NSAID—*which includes those* in whom attacks of *asthma, angioedema, urticaria or rhinitis* have been precipitated by aspirin or any other NSAID

Dose: initially 1.2–1.8 g daily in 3–4 divided doses preferably after food; increased if necessary to max. of 2.4 g daily; maintenance dose of 0.6–1.2 g daily may be adequate; CHILD 20 mg/kg daily in divided doses (juvenile arthritis, up to 40 mg/kg daily), not recommended for children under 7 kg

---

PoM Ibuprofen (Non-proprietary)

Tablets, coated, ibuprofen 200 mg, net price 20 = 16p; 400 mg, 20 = 33p; 600 mg, 20 = 75p. Label: 21

Various strengths available from APS (Apsifen®), Ashbourne (Arthrofen®), Berk (Lidifen®), Cox, DDSA (Ebufac®), Isis (Isisfen®), K Pharm., Lagap (Ibular®), Medipharma (Ibumed®), Norton, Rima (Rimafen®), Upjohn (Motrin®, including an 800-mg strength)

Note. Proprietary brands of ibuprofen preparations are on sale to the public; brand names include Anadin Ibuprofen®, Cuprofen®, Ibrufhalal®, Inoven®, Junifen®, Librofem®, Migrafen®, Novaprin®, Nurofen®, Pacifene®, PhorPain®, Proflex®, Relcofen®

PoM Brufen® (Boots)

Tablets, all magenta, ibuprofen 200 mg (s/c), net price 20 = 58p; 400 mg (s/c), 20 = £1.17; 600 mg (f/c), 20 = £1.85. Label: 21

Syrup, orange, ibuprofen 100 mg/5 mL. Net price 500 mL = £7.34. Label: 21

Dose: 20 mg/kg daily in divided doses *or* 1–2 years 2.5 mL 3–4 times daily, 3–7 years 5 mL 3–4 times daily, 8–12 years 10 mL 3–4 times daily; not recommended for children weighing less than 7 kg; juvenile rheumatoid arthritis up to 40 mg/kg daily in divided doses

Granules, effervescent, ibuprofen 600 mg/sachet. Net price 20-sachet pack = £5.15. Label: 13, 21

Note. Contains sodium approx. 9 mmol/sachet

PoM Junifen Sugar-Free® : see section 4.7.1

Modified release
PoM Brufen Retard® (Boots)

Tablets, m/r, f/c, ibuprofen 800 mg, net price 56-tab pack = £11.76. Label: 25, 27

Dose: 2 tablets daily, preferably in the early evening, increased in severe cases to 3 tablets daily in 2 divided doses

PoM Fenbid® (Goldshield)

Spansule® (= capsule m/r), maroon/pink, enclosing off-white pellets, ibuprofen 300 mg. Net price 120-cap pack = £9.64. Label: 25

Dose: 1–3 capsules every 12 hours

With codeine
For an adverse comment on compound analgesic preparations, see p. 180. For details of the **side-effects, cautions,** and **contra-indications** of opioid analgesics, see p. 185 (**important:** the elderly are particularly susceptible to opioid side-effects).

PoM Codafen Continus® (Napp)

Tablets, white/pink, ibuprofen 300 mg (m/r), codeine phosphate 20 mg. Net price 112-tab pack = £12.57. Label: 2, 21, 25

Dose: 1–2 tablets every 12 hours; max. 3 tablets every 12 hours

Topical preparations: section 10.3.2

ACEMETACIN

(Glycolic acid ester of indomethacin)

Indications: pain and inflammation in rheumatic disease and other musculoskeletal disorders; post-operative analgesia

Cautions; Side-effects: see under Indomethacin

Dose: 120 mg daily in divided doses with food, increased if necessary to 180 mg daily

PoM Emflex® (Merck)

Capsules, yellow/orange, acemetacin 60 mg, net price 90-cap pack = £22.48. Label: 21, counselling, driving

AZAPROPAZONE

Indications: see under CSM restrictions, below

CSM RESTRICTIONS. CSM *has restricted* azapropazone to use in rheumatoid arthritis, ankylosing spondylitis and acute gout only when other NSAIDs have been tried and failed, *has* **contra-indicated** it in patients with a history of peptic ulceration, and *has reduced* the maximum daily dose to 600 mg for rheumatoid arthritis and ankylosing spondylitis in patients over 60

Cautions; Side-effects: see notes above; also contra-indicated if history of peptic ulceration, inflammatory bowel disease or blood disorder; for specific restrictions and contra-indications relating to renal impairment see under Dose; photosensitivity may occur. Avoid in porphyria (see section 9.8.2); **important:** reports of serious enhancement of effect of warfarin; other **interactions:** Appendix 1 (NSAIDs)

PHOTOSENSITIVITY. CSM has reminded of need to advise patients taking azapropazone to avoid direct exposure to sunlight (or to use sunblock preparations)

Dose:
Rheumatoid arthritis and ankylosing spondylitis only, 1.2 g daily in 2 or 4 divided doses; in renal impairment or in elderly 300 mg twice daily, avoid altogether in severe renal impairment
Acute gout (always ensure increased fluid intake), 1.8 g daily in divided doses until acute symptoms subside (usually by 4th day) *then* 1.2 g daily in divided doses until symptoms resolve—consider appropriate alternative therapy if they persist; in mild renal impairment or in elderly, 1.8 g daily for first 24 hours then 1.2 g daily in divided doses reducing to max. 600 mg daily in divided doses as soon as possible (preferably by 4th day) *then* continuing only until acute symptoms resolve—consider appropriate alternative therapy if they persist, and *avoid altogether for gout* in moderate to severe renal impairment and *avoid for gout in elderly* even in mild renal impairment

PoM Rheumox® (Wyeth)

Capsules, orange, azapropazone 300 mg. Net price 20 = £2.86. Label: 11 (also photosensitivity counselling, see above), 21

Tablets, orange, f/c, scored, azapropazone 600 mg. Net price 20 = £4.98. Label: 11 (also photosensitivity counselling, see above), 21

DICLOFENAC SODIUM

Indications: pain and inflammation in rheumatic disease (including juvenile arthritis) and other musculoskeletal disorders; acute gout

Cautions; Side-effects: see notes above; porphyria (see section 9.8.2); pain may occur at injection site (occasionally tissue damage); suppositories may cause irritation; **interactions:** Appendix 1 (NSAIDs)

Dose: by mouth, 75–150 mg daily in 2–3 divided doses, preferably after food

By deep intramuscular injection into the gluteal muscle, acute exacerbations and post-operative, 75 mg once daily (twice daily in severe cases) for max. of 2 days

Ureteric colic, 75 mg then a further 75 mg after 30 minutes if necessary

By rectum in suppositories, 100 mg, usually at night

Max. total daily dose by any route 150 mg

CHILD 1 year or over, juvenile arthritis, *by mouth or by rectum,* 1–3 mg/kg daily in divided doses (25 mg e/c tablets or 12.5 mg suppositories only)

PoM Diclofenac Sodium (Non-proprietary)
Tablets, both e/c, diclofenac sodium 25 mg, net price 20 = £1.88; 50 mg, 20 = £3.65. Label: 5, 25
Available from APS, Ashbourne (Diclozip®), Berk, Cox, Eastern (Volraman®), Isis (Isclofen®, 50 mg), K Pharm., Lagap (Rhumalgan®), Norton, Shire (Valenac®), Sterwin

PoM Voltarol® (Geigy)
Tablets, both e/c, diclofenac sodium 25 mg (yellow), net price 84-tab pack = £7.88; 50 mg (brown), 84-tab pack = £15.32. Label: 5, 25
Dispersible tablets, pink, diclofenac, equivalent to diclofenac sodium 50 mg, net price 21-tab pack = £4.68. Label: 13, 21
Note. Voltarol Dispersible tablets are more suitable for **short-term** use in acute conditions for which treatment required for no more than 3 months (no information on use beyond 3 months)
Injection, diclofenac sodium 25 mg/mL. Net price 3-mL amp = 79p
Suppositories, diclofenac sodium 100 mg. Net price 10 = £3.11
Paediatric suppositories, diclofenac sodium 12.5 mg. Net price 10 = 59p
Emulgel® gel, section 10.3.2

Modified release
PoM Diclomax Retard® (P-D)
Capsules, m/r, diclofenac sodium 100 mg. Net price 28-tab pack = £9.36. Label: 21, 25
Dose: 1 capsule daily preferably with food
PoM Motifene® 75 mg (Panpharma)
Capsules, e/c, m/r, diclofenac sodium 75 mg (enclosing e/c pellets containing diclofenac sodium 25 mg and m/r pellets containing diclofenac sodium 50 mg). Net price 56-cap pack = £14.99. Label: 25
Dose: 1 capsule 1-2 times daily
PoM Voltarol® 75 mg SR and Retard (Geigy)
Tablets, both m/r, diclofenac sodium 75 mg (*Voltarol® 75 mg SR,* pink), net price 28-tab pack = £9.37, 56-tab pack = £18.74; 100 mg (*Voltarol Retard®,* red), net price 28-tab pack = £12.49. Label: 21, 25
Note. Modified-release tablets containing diclofenac sodium 100 mg available from Berk (*Flamrase® SR*), net

price 28-tab pack = £12.18; Lagap (*Rhumalgan SR®*), net price 30-tab pack = £13.38

With misoprostol
For cautions, contra-indications, and side-effects of misoprostol, see section 1.3.4

PoM Arthrotec® (Searle)
Tablets, e/c, diclofenac sodium 50 mg, misoprostol 200 micrograms. Net price 60-tab pack = £14.98; 140-tab pack = £34.95 (hosp. only). Label: 21, 25
Dose: patients requiring diclofenac for rheumatoid arthritis or osteoarthrosis, with prophylaxis against NSAID-induced gastroduodenal ulceration, 1 tablet 2–3 times daily with food

DIFLUNISAL

Indications: pain and inflammation in rheumatic disease and other musculoskeletal disorders; mild to moderate pain including dysmenorrhoea
Cautions; Side-effects: see notes above; breast-feeding; **interactions:** Appendix 1 (NSAIDs)
Dose: mild to moderate pain, initially 1 g, then 500 mg every 12 hours (increased to max. 500 mg every 8 hours if necessary)
Osteoarthrosis, rheumatoid arthritis, 0.5–1 g daily as a single daily dose *or* in 2 divided doses
Dysmenorrhoea, initially 1 g, then 500 mg every 12 hours

PoM Diflunisal (Non-proprietary)
Tablets, coated, diflunisal 250 mg, net price 20 = £1.80; 500 mg, 20 = £3.61. Label: 21, 25, counselling, avoid aluminium hydroxide
Available from APS
PoM Dolobid® (Morson)
Tablets, both f/c, diflunisal 250 mg (peach), net price 20 = £1.80; 500 mg (orange), 20 = £3.61. Label: 21, 25, counselling, avoid aluminium hydroxide

ETODOLAC

Indications: pain and inflammation in rheumatoid arthritis and osteoarthrosis
Cautions; Side-effects: see notes above; **interactions:** Appendix 1 (NSAIDs)
Dose: 200 mg or 300 mg twice daily *or* 400 mg or 600 mg once daily; max. 600 mg daily

PoM Lodine® (Wyeth)
Capsules, etodolac 200 mg (light- and dark-grey), net price 60-cap pack = £12.24; 300 mg (light-grey), 60-cap pack = £16.89. Label: 21
Tablets, brown, f/c, etodolac 200 mg. Net price 60-tab pack = £12.24. Label: 21

Modified release
PoM Lodine SR® (Wyeth)
Tablets, m/r, light-grey, etodolac 600 mg. Net price 30-tab pack = £17.70. Label : 25
Dose: 1 tablet daily

FENBUFEN

Indications: pain and inflammation in rheumatic disease and other musculoskeletal disorders

Cautions; Side-effects: see notes above, but high risk of rashes (discontinue immediately); erythema multiforme and Stevens-Johnson syndrome reported; also allergic interstitial lung disorders (may follow rashes); **interactions:** Appendix 1 (NSAIDs)

Dose: 300 mg in the morning and 600 mg at bedtime *or* 450 mg twice daily

PoM **Lederfen®** (Lederle)

Capsules, dark blue, fenbufen 300 mg. Net price 84-cap pack = £19.12. Label: 21

Note. Fenbufen capsules also available from APS, Ashbourne (Fenbuzip®), Cox, Norton

Tablets, both light blue, f/c, fenbufen 300 mg, net price 84-tab pack = £19.12; 450 mg, 56-tab pack = £19.12. Label: 21

Note. Fenbufen tablets also available from APS, Ashbourne (Fenbuzip®), Cox (450 mg), Norton

Effervescent tablets, fenbufen 450 mg (*Lederfen F®*). Net price 56-tab pack = £24.24. Label: 13, 21

FENOPROFEN

Indications: pain and inflammation in rheumatic disease and other musculoskeletal disorders; mild to moderate pain

Cautions; Side-effects: see notes above; upper respiratory infection and nasopharyngitis reported; **interactions:** Appendix 1 (NSAIDs)

Dose: 200–600 mg 3–4 times daily with food; max. 3 g daily

PoM **Fenopron®** (Dista)

Tablets, both orange, fenoprofen (as calcium salt) 300 mg (*Fenopron®* 300), net price 100 = £8.61; 600 mg (*Fenopron®* 600, scored), 100 = £16.67. Label: 21

PoM **Progesic®** (Lilly)

Tablets, yellow, fenoprofen 200 mg (as calcium salt). Net price 100 = £15.16. Label: 21

FLURBIPROFEN

Indications: pain and inflammation in rheumatic disease and other musculoskeletal disorders; mild to moderate pain including dysmenorrhoea; postoperative analgesia

Cautions; Side-effects: see notes above; local irritation on rectal administration; **interactions:** Appendix 1 (NSAIDs)

Dose: by mouth or by rectum in suppositories, 150–200 mg, daily in divided doses, increased in acute conditions to 300 mg daily

Dysmenorrhoea, initially 100 mg, then 50–100 mg every 4–6 hours; max. 300 mg daily

PoM **Froben®** (Boots)

Tablets, both yellow, s/c, flurbiprofen 50 mg, net price 20 = £1.51; 100 mg, 20 = £3.13. Label: 21

Note. Flurbiprofen tablets also available from APS, Cox, Du Pont, Lagap, Norton

Suppositories, flurbiprofen 100 mg. Net price 12 = £2.90

Modified release

PoM **Froben SR®** (Boots)

Capsules, m/r, yellow, enclosing off-white beads, flurbiprofen 200 mg. Net price 30-cap pack = £10.88. Label: 21, 25

Dose: rheumatic disease, 1 capsule daily, preferably in the evening

INDOMETHACIN

(Indometacin)

Indications: pain and moderate to severe inflammation in rheumatic disease and other acute musculoskeletal disorders; acute gout; dysmenorrhoea; closure of ductus arteriosus (section 7.1.1.1)

Cautions: see notes above; breast-feeding, epilepsy, parkinsonism, psychiatric disturbances; during prolonged therapy ophthalmic and blood examinations are particularly advisable; avoid rectal administration in proctitis and haemorrhoids; **interactions:** Appendix 1 (NSAIDs)

DRIVING. Dizziness may affect performance of skilled tasks (e.g. driving)

Side-effects: see notes above; frequently gastrointestinal disturbances (including diarrhoea), headache, dizziness, and light-headedness; gastrointestinal ulceration and bleeding; rarely, drowsiness, confusion, insomnia, convulsions, psychiatric disturbances, depression, syncope, blood disorders (particularly thrombocytopenia), hypertension, hyperglycaemia, blurred vision, corneal deposits, peripheral neuropathy. On rectal administration pruritus, discomfort, bleeding

Dose: by mouth, rheumatic disease, 50–200 mg daily in divided doses, with food

Acute gout, 150–200 mg daily in divided doses

Dysmenorrhoea, up to 75 mg daily

By rectum in suppositories, 100 mg at night and in the morning if required

Combined oral and rectal treatment, max. total daily dose 150–200 mg

PoM **Indomethacin** (Non-proprietary)

Capsules, indomethacin 25 mg, net price 20 = 21p; 50 mg, 20 = 57p. Label: 21, counselling, driving, see above

Available from APS, Ashbourne (Indomax®), Berk (Imbrilon®), Cox, CP, DDSA (Artracin®), Galen (Mobilan®), K Pharm., Morson (Indocid®), Rima (Rimacid®)

Suspension, sugar-free, indomethacin 25 mg/5 mL. Net price 200 mL = £3.12. Label: 21, counselling, driving, see above

Available from Morson (Indocid®)

Suppositories, indomethacin 100 mg. Net price 10 = £1.11. Counselling, driving, see above

Available from Berk (Imbrilon®), Cox, Morson (Indocid®), Norton

---

Modified release
PoM Indomethacin m/r preparations
Capsules, m/r, indomethacin 75 mg. Net price 20 =
£3.34. Label: 21, 25, counselling, driving, see
above
Dose: 1 capsule 1–2 times daily
Available from Ashbourne (Indomax 75 SR®, 28-cap
pack), CP (Rheumacin LA®), Generics (Slo-Indo®),
Pharmacia (Indomod®, 30-cap pack; also 25- mg
strength), Lagap (Indolar SR®), Morson (Indocid-R®)
Tablets, m/r, indomethacin 25 mg (*Flexin-25
Continus*®, green), net price 56-tab pack = £7.15;
50 mg (*Flexin-LS Continus*®, red), 28-tab pack =
£7.15; 75 mg (*Flexin Continus*®, yellow), 28-tab
pack = £10.21. Label: 21, 25, counselling, driving, see above
Dose: initially 75 mg daily, adjusted in steps of 25–
50 mg; range 25–200 mg daily in 1–2 divided doses;
dysmenorrhoea, up to 75 mg daily
Available from Napp

KETOPROFEN

Indications: pain and mild inflammation in rheumatic disease and other musculoskeletal disorders, and after orthopaedic surgery; acute gout;
dysmenorrhoea
Cautions; Side-effects: see notes above; pain may
occur at injection site (occasionally tissue damage); suppositories may cause rectal irritation;
interactions: Appendix 1 (NSAIDs)
Dose: by mouth, rheumatic disease, 100–200 mg
daily in 2–4 divided doses with food
Pain and dysmenorrhoea, 50 mg up to 3 times
daily
By rectum in suppositories, rheumatic disease,
100 mg at bedtime
Combined oral and rectal treatment, max. total
daily dose 200 mg
By deep intramuscular injection into the gluteal
muscle, 50–100 mg every 4 hours (max. 200 mg
in 24 hours) for up to 3 days

PoM Alrheumat® (Bayer)
Capsules, off white, ketoprofen 50 mg. Net price
20 = £1.22. Label: 21
PoM Orudis® (Rhône-Poulenc Rorer)
Capsules, ketoprofen 50 mg (green/purple), net
price 112-cap pack = £7.86; 100 mg (pink), 56-
cap pack = £7.89. Label: 21
Suppositories, ketoprofen 100 mg. Net price 10 =
£3.45
PoM Oruvail® (Rhône-Poulenc Rorer)
Injection, ketoprofen 50 mg /mL. Net price 2-mL
amp = 73p
Gel, section 10.3.2

Modified release
PoM Oruvail® (Rhône-Poulenc Rorer)
Capsules, both m/r, enclosing white pellets, ketoprofen 100 mg (pink/purple), net price 56-cap
pack = £15.73; 150 mg (pink), 28-cap pack =
£9.81; 100-cap pack = £33.25; 200 mg (pink/
white), 28-cap pack = £15.99. Label: 21, 25
Note. Modified-release capsules containing ketoprofen
100 mg and 200 mg also available from APS (Keto-
vail®), Du Pont (Ketoprofen CR®), Lagap (Larafen
CR®-200 mg)

KETOROLAC TROMETAMOL
See section 15.1.4.2

MEFENAMIC ACID
Indications: mild to moderate pain in rheumatoid
arthritis (including juvenile arthritis), osteoarthrosis, and related conditions; dysmenorrhoea
Cautions: see notes above; also contra-indicated
in inflammatory bowel disease; blood tests
required during long-term treatment; porphyria
(see section 9.8.2); **interactions:** Appendix 1
(NSAIDs)
Side-effects: see notes above; drowsiness; diarrhoea or rashes (withdraw treatment); thrombocytopenia, haemolytic anaemia; convulsions in
overdosage
Dose: 500 mg 3 times daily preferably after food;
CHILD over 6 months, 25 mg/kg daily in divided
doses for not longer than 7 days, except in juvenile arthritis

PoM Mefenamic Acid (Non-proprietary)
Capsules, mefenamic acid 250 mg. Net price 20 =
71p. Label: 21
Available from APS, Ashbourne (Dysman 250®), Berk
(Contraflam®), Cox, K Pharm., Lagap, Norton, P-D
(Ponstan®), Sterwin
Tablets, mefenamic acid 500 mg, net price 20 =
£2.07. Label: 21
Available from APS, Ashbourne (Dysman® 500), Berk,
Cox, K.Pharm, Norton, P-D (Ponstan Forte®).
Paediatric oral suspension, mefenamic acid
50 mg/5 mL. Net price 125 mL = £3.37. Label: 21
Available from P-D (Ponstan®)

NABUMETONE
Indications: pain and inflammation in osteoarthrosis and rheumatoid arthritis
Cautions; Side-effects: see notes above; **interactions:** Appendix 1 (NSAIDs)
Dose: 1 g at night, in severe conditions 0.5–1 g in
morning as well; elderly 0.5 1 g daily

PoM Relifex® (Bencard)
Tablets, red, f /c, nabumetone 500 mg. Net price
56-tab pack = £16.46. Label: 21, 25
Suspension, sugar-free, nabumetone 500 mg /5 mL.
Net price 300-mL pack = £22.93. Label: 21

NAPROXEN
Indications: pain and inflammation in rheumatic
disease (including juvenile arthritis) and other
musculoskeletal disorders; acute gout
Cautions; Side-effects: see notes above; suppositories may cause rectal irritation and occasional
bleeding; **interactions:** Appendix 1 (NSAIDs)

Dose: by mouth, 0.5–1 g daily in 2 divided doses *or* 1 g once daily; CHILD (over 5 years), juvenile arthritis, 10 mg/kg daily in 2 divided doses

Acute musculoskeletal disorders, 500 mg initially, then 250 mg every 6–8 hours as required; max. dose after first day 1.25 g daily

Acute gout, 750 mg initially, then 250 mg every 8 hours until attack has passed

By rectum in suppositories, 500 mg at bedtime; if necessary 500 mg in morning as well

PoM **Naproxen** (Non-proprietary)

Tablets, naproxen 250 mg, net price 20 = 95p; 500 mg, 20 = £1.44. Label: 21

Available from APS, Ashbourne (Arthrosin®), Berk (Timpron®), BHR (Prosaid®), Cox, CP (Arthroxen®), K Pharm., Lagap (Laraflex®), Norton, Shire (Valrox®), Sterwin

PoM **Naprosyn®** (Syntex)

Tablets, all scored, naproxen 250 mg (buff), net price 20 = £2.43; 375 mg (pink), 60-tab pack = £10.97; 500 mg (buff), 60-tab pack = £14.61. Label: 21

Tablets, all e/c, (*Naprosyn EC®*), naproxen 250 mg, net price 56-tab pack = £6.83; 375 mg, 56-tab pack = £10.24; 500 mg, 56-tab pack = £13.65. Label: 5, 25

Suspension, orange, naproxen 125 mg/5 mL. Contains about 1.7 mmol Na+/5 mL. Net price 100 mL = £2.12. Label: 21

Granules, naproxen 500 mg/sachet. Net price 60 sachets = £18.98. Label: 13, 21

Suppositories, naproxen 500 mg. Net price 10 = £3.18

PoM **Nycopren®** (Nycomed)

Tablets, both e/c, naproxen 250 mg (scored), net price 20 = £2.07; 500 mg, 60-tab pack = £12.41. Label: 5, 25

PoM **Synflex®** (Syntex)

Tablets, orange, naproxen sodium 275 mg. Net price 20 = £2.83. Label: 21

Note. 275 mg naproxen sodium ≡ 250 mg naproxen

Dose: musculoskeletal disorders, postoperative analgesia, 550 mg twice daily when necessary, preferably after food; max. 1.1 g daily

Dysmenorrhoea, initially 550 mg then 275 mg every 6–8 hours as required; max. of 1.375 g on 1st day and 1.1 g daily thereafter

Modified release

PoM **Naprosyn® S/R** (Syntex)

Tablets, m/r, f/c, scored, naproxen 500 mg (as sodium salt), net price 56-tab pack = £15.29. Label: 25

Dose: rheumatic and musculoskeletal disorders, 1–2 tablets once daily

With misoprostol

For cautions, contra-indications, and side-effects of misoprostol, see section 1.3.4

PoM **Napratec®** (Searle)

Combination pack, 56 yellow scored tablets, naproxen 500 mg; 56 white scored tablets, misoprostol 200 micrograms. Net price = £19.80. Label: 21

Dose: patients requiring naproxen for rheumatoid arthritis, osteoarthritis, or ankylosing spondylitis, with prophylaxis against NSAID-induced gastroduodenal ulceration, 1 naproxen 500-mg tablet and 1 misoprostol 200-microgram tablet taken together twice daily with food

PHENYLBUTAZONE

Indications: ankylosing spondylitis when other therapy is unsuitable

Cautions: blood counts before and during treatment if for more than 7 days; elderly (reduce dose); breast-feeding; withdraw treatment if acute pulmonary syndrome including fever and dyspnoea occurs; may aggravate systemic lupus erythematosus; see also notes above; **interactions:** Appendix 1 (NSAIDs)

Contra-indications: cardiovascular disease, renal and hepatic impairment; pregnancy; history of peptic ulceration, gastro-intestinal haemorrhage, or blood disorders; porphyria (see section 9.8.2); Sjögren's syndrome; thyroid disease; children under 14

Side-effects: see notes above; parotitis, stomatitis, goitre, pancreatitis, hepatitis, nephritis, visual disturbances; rarely leucopenia, thrombocytopenia, agranulocytosis, aplastic anaemia, erythema multiforme (Stevens-Johnson syndrome), toxic epidermal necrolysis (Lyell's syndrome)

Dose: initially 200 mg 2–3 times daily for 2 days, with or after food, then reduced to minimum effective, usually 100 mg 2–3 times daily

Not for children under 14 years

PoM **Butacote®** (Geigy)

Tablets, pale blue, e/c, s/c, phenylbutazone 100 mg, net price 20 = 40p (hosp. only). Label: 5, 21, 25

PIROXICAM

Indications: pain and inflammation in rheumatic disease (including juvenile arthritis) and other musculoskeletal disorders; acute gout

Cautions: see notes above; porphyria (see section 9.8.2); **interactions:** Appendix 1 (NSAIDs)

Side-effects: see notes above; pain may occur at injection site (occasionally tissue damage); pancreatitis reported

Dose: by mouth or by rectum, rheumatic disease, initially 20 mg daily, maintenance 10–30 mg daily, in single or divided doses

CHILD (over 6 years) *by mouth*, juvenile arthritis, less than 15 kg, 5 mg daily; 16–25 kg, 10 mg; 26–45 kg; over 46 kg, 20 mg

Acute musculoskeletal disorders, 40 mg daily in single or divided doses for 2 days, then 20 mg daily for 7–14 days

Acute gout, 40 mg initially, then 40 mg daily in single or divided doses for 4–6 days

By deep intramuscular injection into gluteal muscle, for initial treatment of acute conditions, as dose by mouth (on short-term basis)

PoM Piroxicam (Non-proprietary)

Capsules, piroxicam 10 mg, net price 20 = £1.56; 20 mg, 20 = £3.13. Label: 21

Available from APS, Ashbourne (Pirozip®), Berk (Flamatrol®), Cox, CP, K Pharm., Lagap (Larapam®), Norton

PoM Feldene® (Pfizer)

Capsules, piroxicam 10 mg (maroon/blue), net price 56-cap pack = £6.00; 20 mg (maroon), 28-cap pack = £6.00. Label: 21

Tablets, (Feldene Melt®), piroxicam 20 mg, net price 28-tab pack = £9.83. Label: 10 patient information leaflet, 21

Note. Feldene Melt® tablets can be taken by placing on tongue or by swallowing; contain aspartame equivalent to phenylalanine 140 micrograms/tablet (see section 9.4.1)

Dispersible tablets, piroxicam 10 mg (scored), net price 56-tab pack = £9.75; 20 mg, 28-tab pack = £9.75. Label: 13, 21

Injection, piroxicam 20 mg/mL. Net price 1-mL amp = 70p

Suppositories, piroxicam 20 mg. Net price 10 = £5.20

Gel, section 10.3.2

SULINDAC

Indications: pain and inflammation in rheumatic disease and other musculoskeletal disorders; acute gout

Cautions; Side-effects: see notes above; caution if history of renal stones; ensure adequate hydration; **interactions:** Appendix 1 (NSAIDs)

Dose: 200 mg twice daily with food (may be reduced according to response); max. 400 mg daily; acute gout should respond within 7 days; limit treatment of peri-articular disorders to 7–10 days

PoM Clinoril® (MSD)

Tablets, both yellow, scored, sulindac 100 mg, net price 20 = £2.24; 200 mg, 20 = £4.32. Label: 21

Note. Sulindac tablets also available from APS, Generics

TENOXICAM

Indications: pain and inflammation in rheumatic disease and other musculoskeletal disorders

Cautions; Side-effects: see notes above; **interactions:** Appendix 1 (NSAIDs)

Dose: by mouth, rheumatic disease, 20 mg daily Acute musculoskeletal disorders, 20 mg daily for 7 days; max. 14 days

By intravenous or intramuscular injection, for initial treatment for 1–2 days, as dose by mouth

PoM Mobiflex® (Roche)

Tablets, red-brown, f/c, tenoxicam 20 mg. Net price 28-tab pack = £14.10. Label: 21

Effervescent tablets, tenoxicam 20 mg. Net price 10-tab pack = £5.90. Label: 13, 21

Milk Granules (= granules), tenoxicam 20 mg/sachet. Net price 10-sachet pack = £5.90. Label: 13, 21

Injection, powder for reconstitution, tenoxicam 20 mg. Net price per amp (with solvent) = 93p

TIAPROFENIC ACID

Indications: pain and inflammation in rheumatic disease and other musculoskeletal disorders

Cautions; Side-effects: see notes above; bladder irritation reported, see below; **interactions:** Appendix 1 (NSAIDs)

CSM ADVICE. Following reports of **severe cystitis** associated with tiaprofenic acid the CSM has recommended that tiaprofenic acid *should not be given* to patients with pre-existing urinary tract disorders and *should be stopped* if urinary symptoms develop. Patients *should be advised* to stop taking tiaprofenic acid and to report to their doctor promptly if they develop urinary tract symptoms (such as increased frequency, nocturia, urgency, pain on urinating, or blood in urine)

Dose: 600 mg daily in 2–3 divided doses

PoM Surgam® (Roussel)

Tablets, tiaprofenic acid 200 mg, net price 84-tab pack = £15.89; 300 mg, 56-tab pack = £15.89. Label: 21

Note. Tiaprofenic acid tablets also available from Cox

Modified release

PoM Surgam SA® (Roussel)

Capsules, m/r, maroon/pink enclosing white pellets, tiaprofenic acid 300 mg. Net price 56-cap pack = £15.89. Label: 25

Dose: 2 capsules once daily

TOLMETIN

Indications: pain and inflammation in rheumatic disease (including juvenile arthritis) and other musculoskeletal disorders

Cautions; Side-effects: see notes above; **interactions:** Appendix 1 (NSAIDs)

Dose: 0.6–1.8 g daily in 2–4 divided doses; max. 30 mg/kg daily up to 1.8 g

CHILD, juvenile arthritis, 20–25 mg/kg daily in 3–4 divided doses; max. 30 mg/kg daily up to 1.8 g

PoM Tolectin® (Cilag)

Capsules, tolmetin (as sodium salt) 200 mg (ivory/orange), net price 90-cap pack = £15.97; 400 mg (orange), 90 cap = £23.97. Label: 21

10.1.2   Corticosteroids

10.1.2.1 SYSTEMIC CORTICOSTEROIDS

The general actions and uses of the corticosteroids are described in section 6.3. Treatment with corticosteroids in rheumatic diseases should be reserved for specific indications, e.g. when other anti-inflammatory drugs are unsuccessful.

In severe, possibly life-threatening, situations a high initial dose of corticosteroid is given to induce remission and the dose then gradually reduced to the lowest maintenance dose that will control the disease or, if possible, discontinued altogether. A major problem is that relapse may occur as dosage reduction is made, particularly if this is carried out too rapidly. The tendency is therefore to increase and maintain dosage and consequently the patient becomes dependent on corticosteroids. For this reason pulse doses of corticosteroids (e.g. methyl-prednisolone (as sodium succinate) up to 1 g intravenously on three consecutive days) is in current use to suppress highly active inflammatory disease while longer term and slower acting medication is being commenced.

Prednisolone is used for most purposes; it has the advantage over the more potent corticosteroids (see section 6.3.2) of permitting finer dosage adjustments. To minimise side-effects the maintenance dose of prednisolone should be kept as low as possible, usually 7.5 mg daily and seldom exceeding 10 mg daily.

Polymyalgia rheumatica and *temporal (giant cell) arteritis* are always treated with corticosteroids. The usual initial dose of prednisolone in polymyalgia rheumatica is 10 to 15 mg daily and in temporal arteritis 40 to 60 mg daily (the higher dose being used if visual symptoms occur). Treatment should be continued until remission occurs and doses then gradually reduced to a maintenance level of about 7.5 mg–10 mg daily. Relapse is common if therapy is stopped within 3 years but most patients can discontinue treatment after approximately 3 to 6 years after which recurrences become rare.

Polyarteritis nodosa and *polymyositis* are usually treated with corticosteroids. An initial dose of 60 mg of prednisolone daily is often used and reduced to a maintenance dose of 10 to 15 mg daily.

Systemic lupus erythematosus is treated with corticosteroids when necessary using a similar dosage regimen to that for polyarteritis nodosa and polymyositis (above). Patients with pleurisy, pericarditis, or other systemic manifestations will respond to corticosteroids. It may then be possible to reduce the dosage; alternate-day treatment is sometimes adequate, and the drug may be gradually withdrawn. In some mild cases corticosteroid treatment may be stopped after a few months. Many mild cases of systemic lupus erythematosus do not require corticosteroid treatment. Alternative treatment with anti-inflammatory analgesics, and possibly chloroquine, should be considered.

Since effective doses of systemic corticosteroids may cause Cushing's syndrome these drugs should **not** be used to suppress symptoms of *rheumatoid arthritis* unless alternative anti-inflammatory drugs and drugs which may affect the disease process (section 10.1.3) have proved unsuccessful, with increasing disability due to the inflammatory process. The smallest effective dose should be used and increased if necessary, but should not exceed the equivalent of prednisolone 7.5 or 10 mg daily. Attempts should always be made gradually to reduce the dose. Corticosteroids in low dosage may be useful in the elderly patient, and similar nocturnal doses may relieve morning stiffness.

Ankylosing spondylitis should not be treated with long-term corticosteroids; rarely, pulse doses may be needed and may be useful in extremely active disease that does not respond to conventional treatment.

10.1.2.2 LOCAL CORTICOSTEROID INJECTIONS

Corticosteroids are injected locally for an anti-inflammatory effect. In inflammatory conditions of the joints, particularly in rheumatoid arthritis, they are given by *intra-articular injection* to relieve pain, increase mobility, and reduce deformity in one or a few joints. Full aseptic precautions are essential; infected areas should be avoided. Occasionally an acute inflammatory reaction develops after an intra-articular or soft-tissue injection of a corticosteroid. This may be a reaction to the microcrystalline suspension of the corticosteroid used, but must be distinguished from sepsis introduced into the injection site. An almost insoluble compound such as triamcinolone hexacetonide has a long-acting (depot) effect and is preferred for intra-articular injection.

Smaller amounts of corticosteroids may also be injected directly into soft tissues for the relief of inflammation in conditions such as *tennis* or *golfer's elbow* or *compression neuropathies*. In *tendinitis*, injections should be made into the tendon sheath and not directly into the tendon (due to the absence of a true tendon sheath, the Achilles tendon should not be injected). A soluble preparation (e.g. containing betamethasone or dexamethasone sodium phosphate) is preferred for injection into the carpal tunnel.

Cortisone acetate is **not** effective for local injection and hydrocortisone acetate or one of the synthetic analogues such as triamcinolone hexacetonide is generally used. The risk of necrosis and muscle wasting may be slightly increased with triamcinolone; flushing has been reported with intra-articular corticosteroid injections. Charcot-like arthropathies have also been reported (particularly following repeated intra-articular injections).

Corticosteroid injections are also injected into soft tissues for the treatment of skin lesions (see section 13.4).

LOCAL CORTICOSTEROID INJECTIONS

Indications: local inflammation of joints and soft tissues (for details, see individual data sheets)

Cautions; Contra-indications; Side-effects: see notes above (for details see also individual data sheets)

Dose: see under preparations

Dose calculated as dexamethasone sodium phosphate

PoM Dexamethasone (Organon)

Injection, dexamethasone sodium phosphate 5 mg/mL (≡ dexamethasone 4 mg/mL ≡ dexamethasone phosphate 4.8 mg/mL). Net price 1-mL amp = 83p; 2-mL vial = £1.27

Dose: by intra-articular or soft-tissue injection (for details see data sheet), 0.4–4 mg (calculated as dexamethasone sodium phosphate) according to size; where appropriate may be repeated at intervals of 3–21 days acccording to response

Dose calculated as dexamethasone phosphate

PoM Decadron® (MSD)

Injection, dexamethasone phosphate 4 mg/mL (≡ dexamethasone 3.33 mg/mL ≡ dexamethasone sodium phosphate 4.17 mg/mL). Net price 2-mL vial = £1.76

Dose: by intra-articular or soft-tissue injection (for details see data sheet), 0.4–4 mg (calculated as dexamethasone phosphate) according to size (*soft-tissue infiltration* 2–6 mg); where appropriate may be repeated at intervals of 3–21 days

Note. Injection containing Dexamethasone phosphate 4 mg/mL (as sodium phosphate) is also available from David Bull

Hydrocortisone acetate

PoM Hydrocortistab® (Boots)

Injection, (aqueous suspension), hydrocortisone acetate 25 mg/mL. Net price 1-mL amp = £1.05

Dose: by intra-articular or soft-tissue injection (for details see data sheet), 5–50 mg according to size; where appropriate may be repeated at intervals of 21 days; not more than 3 joints should be treated on any one day; CHILD 5–30 mg (divided)

Methylprednisolone acetate

PoM Depo-Medrone® (Upjohn)

Injection (aqueous suspension), methylprednisolone acetate 40 mg/mL. Net price 1-mL vial = £2.73; 2-mL vial = £4.90; 3-mL vial = £7.11

Dose: by intra-articular or soft-tissue injection (for details see data sheet), 4–80 mg, according to size; where appropriate may be repeated at intervals of 7–35 days

PoM Depo-Medrone® with Lidocaine (Upjohn)

Injection (aqueous suspension), methylprednisolone acetate 40 mg, lignocaine hydrochloride 10 mg/mL. Net price 1-mL vial = £2.70; 2-mL vial = £4.90

Dose: as for Depo-Medrone®

Prednisolone acetate

PoM Deltastab® (Boots)

Injection (aqueous suspension), prednisolone acetate 25 mg/mL. Net price 1-mL amp = £1.05

Dose: by intra-articular or soft-tissue injection (for details see data sheet), 5–25 mg according to size; not more than 3 joints should be treated on any one day; where appropriate may be repeated when relapse occurs

Triamcinolone acetonide

PoM Adcortyl® Intra-articular / Intradermal (Squibb)

Injection (aqueous suspension), triamcinolone acetonide 10 mg/mL. Net price 1-mL amp = £1.02; 5-mL vial = £4.14

Dose: by intra-articular injection or soft-tissue injection (for details see data sheet), 2.5–15 mg according to size (for larger doses use *Kenalog®* instead); where appropriate may be repeated when relapse occurs

By intradermal injection, (for details see data sheet): 2–3 mg; max. 5 mg at any one site (total max. 30 mg); where appropriate may be repeated at intervals of 1–2 weeks

CHILD under 6 years not recommended

PoM Kenalog® Intra-articular / Intramuscular (Squibb)

Injection (aqueous suspension), triamcinolone acetonide 40 mg/mL. Net price 1-mL vial = £1.70

Dose: by intra-articular or soft-tissue injection , (for details see data sheet), 5–40 mg according to size; total max. 80 mg (for doses below 5 mg use *Adcortyl® Intra-articular/Intradermal* instead); where appropriate may be repeated when relapse occurs; CHILD under 6 years not recommended

Triamcinolone hexacetonide

PoM Lederspan® (Lederle)

Injection (aqueous suspension), triamcinolone hexacetonide 5 mg/mL. Net price 5-mL vial = £2.85

Dose: by intradermal injection (for details see data sheet), up to 500 micrograms/square inch of affected skin

Injection (aqueous suspension), triamcinolone hexacetonide 20 mg/mL. Net price 1-mL vial = £2.48; 5 mL vial = £9.65

Dose: by intra-articular or soft-tissue injection (for details see data sheet), 2–30 mg according to size; where appropriate may be repeated at intervals of 21–28 days; for *intradermal injection*, see above

10.1.3   Drugs which suppress the rheumatic disease process

Certain drugs such as gold, penicillamine, hydroxychloroquine, chloroquine, immunosuppressants, and sulphasalazine may suppress the disease process in *rheumatoid arthritis*, as may gold and immunosuppressants in *psoriatic arthritis*. Unlike NSAIDs they do not produce an immediate therapeutic effect but require 4 to 6 months of treatment for a full response. If one of these drugs does not lead to objective benefit within 6 months, it should be discontinued.

These drugs may improve not only the symptoms and signs of inflammatory joint disease but also extra-articular manifestations such as vasculitis. They reduce the erythrocyte sedimentation rate and sometimes the titre of rheumatoid factor. Some (e.g. the immunosuppressants) may retard erosive damage as judged radiologically.

These drugs are used in rheumatoid arthritis where treatment with NSAIDs has been unsuccessful, so that there is evidence of disease progression including continuing active joint inflammation and worsening radiological changes. Since, in the first few months, the course of rheumatoid arthritis is unpredictable, it is usual to delay treatment for about 6 months depending on the progress of the disease, but treatment should be initiated before joint damage becomes irreversible.

Penicillamine and immunosuppressants are also sometimes used in rheumatoid arthritis where there are troublesome extra-articular features such as vasculitis, and in patients who are taking excessive doses of corticosteroids. Where the response is satisfactory there is often a striking reduction in requirements of both corticosteroids and other drugs. Gold, penicillamine, and related drugs may also be used to treat *juvenile arthritis* (Still's disease) when indications are similar.

Gold and penicillamine are effective in *palindromic rheumatism* and chloroquine is sometimes used to treat *systemic* and *discoid lupus erythematosus*.

GOLD

Gold may be given by intramuscular injection as sodium aurothiomalate or by mouth as auranofin.

Sodium aurothiomalate must be given by deep intramuscular injection and the area gently massaged. A test dose of 10 mg must be given followed by doses of 50 mg at weekly intervals until there is definite evidence of remission. Benefit is not to be expected until about 300 to 500 mg has been given; if there is no remission after 1 g has been given it should be discontinued. In patients who do respond, the interval between injections is then gradually increased to 4 weeks and treatment is continued for up to 5 years after complete remission. If relapse occurs dosage may be immediately increased to 50 mg weekly and only once control has been obtained again should the dosage be reduced. It is important to avoid complete relapse since second courses of gold are not usually effective. Children may be given 1 mg/kg weekly to a maximum of 50 mg weekly, the intervals being gradually increased to 4 weeks according to response; an initial test dose is given corresponding to one-tenth to one-fifth of the calculated dose.

Auranofin is given by mouth. If there is no response after 9 months treatment should be discontinued.

Gold therapy should be discontinued in the presence of blood disorders or proteinuria (associated with immune complex nephritis) which is repeatedly above 300 mg/litre without other cause (such as urinary-tract infection). Urine tests and full blood counts (including total and differential white cell and platelet counts) must therefore be performed before each intramuscular injection; in the case of oral treatment the urine and blood tests should be carried out monthly. Rashes with pruritus often occur after 2 to 6 months of intramuscular treatment and may necessitate discontinuation of treatment; the most common side-effect of oral therapy, diarrhoea with or without nausea or abdominal pain, may respond to bulking agents (such as bran) or temporary reduction in dosage.

SODIUM AUROTHIOMALATE

Indications: active progressive rheumatoid arthritis, juvenile arthritis

Cautions: see notes above; patients should report pruritus, metallic taste, fever, sore throat or tongue, buccal ulceration, purpura, epistaxis, bleeding gums, bruising, menorrhagia, diarrhoea; renal and hepatic impairment, elderly, history of urticaria, eczema, colitis, drugs which cause blood disorders; annual chest X-ray; **interactions:** Appendix 1 (gold)

Contra-indications: severe renal and hepatic disease (see notes above); history of blood disorders or bone marrow aplasia, exfoliative dermatitis,

systemic lupus erythematosus, necrotising enterocolitis, pulmonary fibrosis; pregnancy and breast-feeding (see Appendixes 4 and 5); porphyria (see section 9.8.2)

Side-effects: severe reactions (occasionally fatal) in up to 5% of patients; mouth ulcers, skin reactions, proteinuria, blood disorders (sometimes sudden and fatal); rarely colitis, peripheral neuritis, pulmonary fibrosis, hepatotoxicity with cholestatic jaundice, alopecia

Dose: by deep intramuscular injection, administered on expert advice, see notes above

PoM Myocrisin® (Rhône-Poulenc Rorer)
Injection, sodium aurothiomalate 20 mg/mL, net price 0.5-mL (10-mg) amp = £1.31; 40 mg/mL, 0.5-mL (20-mg) amp = £1.91; 100 mg/mL, 0.5-mL (50-mg) amp = £3.87

AURANOFIN

Indications: active progressive rheumatoid arthritis when NSAIDs inadequate alone

Cautions; Contra-indications: see under Sodium Aurothiomalate; also caution in inflammatory bowel disease

BLOOD COUNTS. Withdraw if platelets fall below 100 000/mm³ or if signs and symptoms suggestive of thrombocytopenia occur, see also notes above

Side-effects: diarrhoea most common (reduced by bulking agents such as bran); see also under Sodium Aurothiomalate

Dose: administered on expert advice, 6 mg daily (initially in 2 divided doses then if tolerated as single dose), if response inadequate after 6 months, increase to 9 mg daily (in 3 divided doses), discontinue if no response after a further 3 months

COUNSELLING. Warn patient to tell doctor immediately if sore throat, mouth ulcers, bruising, fever. malaise, rash, diarrhoea or non-specific illness develops

PoM Ridaura® (Bencard)
Tablets, pale yellow, f/c, auranofin 3 mg. Net price 60-tab pack = £28.00. Label: 21, counselling, blood disorder symptoms (see above)

PENICILLAMINE

Penicillamine has a similar action to gold, and more patients are able to continue treatment than with gold but side-effects occur frequently. An initial dose of 125 to 250 mg daily before food is given for 1 month, increased by this amount every 4 to12 weeks until remission occurs. Penicillamine should be discontinued if there is no improvement within 1 year. The usual maintenance dose is 500 to 750 mg daily, but up to 1.5 g may rarely be required.

Patients should be warned not to expect improvement for at least 6 to 12 weeks after treatment is initiated. If remission has been sustained for 6 months, reduction of dosage by 125 to 250 mg every 12 weeks may be attempted.

Blood counts, including platelets, and urine examinations should be carried out every 1 or 2 weeks for the first 2 months then every 4 weeks to detect blood disorders and proteinuria. A reduction in platelet count indicates that treatment with penicillamine should be stopped, subsequently re-introduced at a lower dosage level and then, if possible, gradually increased. Proteinuria, associated with immune complex nephritis, occurs in up to 30% of patients, but may resolve despite continuation of treatment; treatment may be continued provided that renal function tests remain normal, oedema is absent, and the 24-hour urinary excretion of protein does not exceed 2 g.

Nausea may occur but is not usually a problem provided that penicillamine is taken before food or on retiring and that low initial doses are used and only gradually increased. Loss of taste may occur about 6 weeks after treatment is started but usually returns 6 weeks later irrespective of whether or not treatment is discontinued; mineral supplements are not recommended. Rashes are a common side-effect. Those which occur in the first few months of treatment disappear when the drug is stopped and treatment may then be re-introduced at a lower dose level and gradually increased. Late rashes are more resistant and often necessitate discontinuation of treatment.

There is some evidence that patients who are hypersensitive to penicillin may have a higher risk of penicillamine reactions.

PENICILLAMINE

Indications: see notes above and under Dose

Cautions: see notes above; renal impairment (see Appendix 3), pregnancy (see Appendix 4); avoid concurrent gold, chloroquine, hydroxychloroquine, or immunosuppressive treatment; avoid oral iron within 2 hours of a dose; **interactions:** Appendix 1 (penicillamine)

BLOOD COUNTS and URINE TESTS. See notes above. Longer intervals may be adequate in cystinuria and Wilson's disease. Consider withdrawal if platelets fall below 120000 or white blood cells below 2500/mm³ or if 3 successive falls within normal range (can restart at reduced dose when counts return to normal but permanent withdrawal necessary if recurrence of neutropenia or thrombocytopenia)

COUNSELLING. Warn patient to tell doctor immediately if sore throat, mouth ulcers, bruising, fever, malaise, rash, or non-specific illness develops.

Contra-indications: hypersensitivity (except in life-threatening situation when desensitisation may be attempted—see data sheet); lupus erythematosus

Side-effects: (see also notes above) initially nausea, anorexia, fever, and skin reactions; taste loss (mineral supplements not recommended); blood disorders including thrombocytopenia, neutropenia, agranulocytosis and aplastic anaemia; proteinuria, rarely haematuria (withdraw immediately); haemolytic anaemia, nephrotic syndrome, lupus erythematosus-like syndrome, myasthenia gravis-like syndrome, pemphigus, Goodpasture's syndrome, and Stevens-Johnson syndrome also reported; in non-rheumatoid con-

ditions rheumatoid arthritis-like syndrome also reported; late rashes (reduce dose or withdraw treatment)

Dose: severe active rheumatoid arthritis, administered on expert advice, ADULT initially 125–250 mg daily before food for 1 month increased by similar amounts at intervals of not less than 4 weeks to usual maintenance of 500–750 mg daily; max. 1.5 g daily; ELDERLY initially 50–125 mg daily before food for 1 month increased by similar amounts at intervals of not less than 4 weeks; max. 1 g daily; CHILD initially 50 mg daily before food for 1 month increased at intervals of not less than 4 weeks to maintenance of 15–20 mg/kg daily

Wilson's disease, chronic active hepatitis, and cystinuria, see section 9.8

Copper and lead poisoning, see Emergency Treatment of Poisoning, p.24

PoM Penicillamine (Non-proprietary)
Tablets, penicillamine 125 mg, net price 20 = £2.02; 250 mg, 20 = £3.49. Label: 6, 22, counselling, blood disorder symptoms (see above)
Available from APS, Cox, Evans, K Pharm.

PoM Distamine® (Dista)
Tablets, all f/c, penicillamine 50 mg (scored), net price 20 = £1.09; 125 mg, 20 = £2.17; 250 mg, 20 = £3.74. Label: 6, 22, counselling, blood disorder symptoms (see above)

PoM Pendramine® (ASTA Medica)
Tablets, both scored, f/c, penicillamine 125 mg, net price 20 = £1.80; 250 mg, 20 = £3.27. Label: 6, 22, counselling, blood disorder symptoms (see above)

ANTIMALARIALS

Chloroquine and **hydroxychloroquine** have a similar action to, and are better tolerated than, gold or penicillamine; retinopathy is rare provided the doses given below are not exceeded.

These drugs should not be used for psoriatic arthritis. It should also be noted that it is difficult to distinguish ageing changes from drug-induced retinopathy in the elderly.

Mepacrine (see section 5.4.4) is sometimes used in discoid lupus erythematosus.

CHLOROQUINE

Indications: active rheumatoid arthritis (including juvenile arthritis), systemic and discoid lupus erythematosus; malaria, see section 5.4.1

Cautions: hepatic and renal impairment, pregnancy (but for malaria benefit outweighs risk, see Appendix 4, Antimalarials), porphyria, may exacerbate psoriasis, neurological disorders (especially history of epilepsy), may aggravate myasthenia gravis, severe gastro-intestinal disorders, G6PD deficiency (see section 9.1.5); elderly (see notes above); avoid concurrent hepatotoxic drugs—other **interactions:** Appendix 1 (chloroquine)

Advice of College of Ophthalmologists on long-term therapy.

1. Eye examination before long-term chloroquine or hydroxychloroquine to establish baseline;
2. Patient to stop taking and seek immediate advice from prescribing medical practitioner or general practitioner or ophthalmologist if any disturbance of vision noted;
3. Prescribing medical practitioner to be responsible for monitoring if considered necessary;
4. If monitoring considered necessary, *once monthly Amsler testing by patient* may detect premaculopathy (visual disturbance in absence of ophthalmoscopically visible macular changes—which is frequently reversible).

Ocular toxicity very unlikely with chloroquine phosphate not exceeding 4 mg/kg daily (= chloroquine base approx. 2.5 mg/kg daily) or hydroxychloroquine sulphate not exceeding 6.5 mg/kg daily.

To avoid excessive dosage in obese patients special care needed to *calculate on basis of lean body-weight.*

Side-effects: gastro-intestinal disturbances, headache; also visual disturbances, irreversible retinal damage, corneal opacities, depigmentation or loss of hair, skin reactions, ECG changes; rarely blood disorders (thrombocytopenia, agranulocytosis and aplastic anaemia), psychosis reported; *important:* very toxic in overdosage—immediate advice from poisons centres essential (see also p.22)

Dose: administered on expert advice, chloroquine (base) 150 mg daily; max. 2.5 mg/kg daily, see recommendations above; CHILD, up to 3 mg/kg daily

Note. Chloroquine base 150 mg ≡ chloroquine sulphate 200 mg ≡ chloroquine phosphate 250 mg (approx.).

Preparations: see section 5.4.1

HYDROXYCHLOROQUINE SULPHATE

Indications: active rheumatoid arthritis (including juvenile arthritis), systemic and discoid lupus erythematosus

Cautions; Side-effects: see under Chloroquine and notes (above)

Dose: administered on expert advice, initially 400 mg daily in divided doses; maintenance 200–400 mg daily; max. 6.5 mg/kg daily, see recommendations above; CHILD, up to 6.5 mg/kg daily

PoM Plaquenil® (Sanofi Winthrop)
Tablets, orange, s/c, hydroxychloroquine sulphate 200 mg. Net price 56-tab pack = £18.88. Label: 5

IMMUNOSUPPRESSANTS

When used in *rheumatoid arthritis* **immunosuppressants** have a similar action to gold and are useful alternatives in cases that have failed to respond to gold, penicillamine, chloroquine, or hydroxychloroquine.

Azathioprine (see section 8.2.1) is usually chosen and is usually given in a dose of 1.5 to 2.5 mg/kg daily in divided doses. Blood counts are needed

to detect possible neutropenia and/or thrombocytopenia which is usually resolved by reducing the dose. Nausea, vomiting, and diarrhoea may occur, usually starting early during the course of treatment, and may necessitate withdrawal of the drug; herpes zoster infection may also occur.

Methotrexate has also been shown to be effective. It is usually given in an initial dose of 2.5 mg by mouth once a week, increased slowly to a maximum of 15 mg once a week (occasionally 20 mg), subject to regular full blood counts (including differential white cell count and platelet count) and liver-function tests.

Cyclosporin has also been shown to be effective and is now also licensed for severe active rheumatoid arthritis when conventional therapy is inappropriate or ineffective.

Chlorambucil (see section 8.1.1) is another immunosuppressant which is used in rheumatoid arthritis [unlicensed indication]; a dose of 100 to 200 micrograms/kg daily is usually given initially; most patients require between 2.5 and 7.5 mg daily. Regular blood counts including platelets should be carried out. **Cyclophosphamide** (see section 8.1.1) is more toxic but may be used at a dose of 1 to 1.5 mg/kg daily for rheumatoid arthritis with severe systemic manifestations [unlicensed indication].

Immunosuppressants are also used in the management of severe cases of *systemic lupus erythematosus* and other connective tissue disorders. They are often given in conjunction with corticosteroids for patients with severe or progressive renal disease though the evidence for their benefit is doubtful. They may be used in cases of *polymyositis* which are resistant to corticosteroids. They are used for their corticosteroid-sparing effect in patients whose corticosteroid requirements are excessive. **Azathioprine** is usually used but **chlorambucil** is an alternative.

Azathioprine and methotrexate are used in the treatment of *psoriatic arthropathy* for severe or progressive cases which are not controlled with anti-inflammatory drugs. There is an impression that **azathioprine** is the more effective for psoriatic arthritis and that **methotrexate** is the more effective for skin manifestations.

AZATHIOPRINE

Indications: see notes above; transplantation rejection, see section 8.2.1

Cautions; Contra-indications; Side-effects: see under Azathioprine, section 8.2.1

Dose: by mouth, initially, rarely more than 3 mg/kg daily, reduced according to response; maintenance 1–3 mg/kg daily; consider withdrawal if no improvement within 3 months

Preparations : see section 8.2.1

CYCLOSPORIN
(Ciclosporin)

Indications: severe active rheumatoid arthritis when conventional therapy inappropriate or ineffective; graft-versus host disease, see section 8.2.2; atopic dermatitis and psoriasis, see section 13.5.2.

Cautions; Side-effects: see section 8.2.2

ADDITIONAL CAUTIONS IN RHEUMATOID ARTHRITIS. *Contra-indicated* in abnormal renal function, hypertension not under control (see also below), infections not under control, and malignancy. Measure serum creatinine at least twice before treatment and monitor every 2 weeks for first 3 months, then every 4 weeks (or more frequently if dose increased or concomitant NSAIDs introduced or increased (see also *interactions:* Appendix 1 (cyclosporin)), reducing dose if serum creatinine increases more than 30% above baseline in more than 1 measurement; if above 50%, reducing dose by 50% (even if within normal range) and discontinuing if reduction not successful within 1 month; monitor blood pressure (discontinue if hypertension develops that cannot be controlled by antihypertensive therapy); monitor hepatic function if concomitant NSAIDs given.

Dose: ADULT over 18 years *by mouth,* administered in accordance with expert advice initially, 2.5 mg/kg daily in 2 divided doses, if necessary increased gradually after 6 weeks to max. 4 mg/kg daily (discontinuing if response still insufficient after 3 months); dose adjusted according to response for maintenance and treatment reviewed after 6 months (continue only if benefits outweigh risks); CHILD and under 18 years, not recommended

COUNSELLING. Total daily dose to be taken in 2 divided doses. To mask taste, mix with cold milk, cold chocolate drink, cola, or orange juice immediately before taking (and rinse with more to ensure total dose). Do not use plastic cup. Keep medicine measure away from other liquids (including water)

Preparations:
See section 8.2.2

METHOTREXATE

Indications: severe active rheumatoid arthritis unresponsive to conventional therapy; malignant disease, see section 8.1.3; psoriasis, see section 13.5.2

Cautions; Contra-indications; Side-effects: p 439
PULMONARY TOXICITY. Pulmonary toxicity may be a special problem in rheumatoid arthritis (patient to contact doctor if dyspnoea or cough). For other special warnings, including counselling advice relating to interaction with aspirin and NSAIDs, see p.439.

Dose: by mouth, 7.5 mg once weekly (as a single dose *or* divided into 3 doses of 2.5 mg given at intervals of 12 hours), adjusted according to response; max. total weekly dose 20 mg

Preparations
See section 8.1.3

SULPHASALAZINE

Sulphasalazine was initially introduced for the treatment of rheumatoid arthritis. Recent re-evaluation has confirmed that it has a beneficial effect in suppressing the inflammatory activity of rheumatoid arthritis. Side-effects include rashes, gastrointestinal intolerance and, especially in patients with rheumatoid arthritis, occasional leucopenia, neutropenia, and thrombocytopenia. These haematological abnormalities occur usually in the first 3 to 6 months of treatment and are reversible on cessation of treatment. Close monitoring of full blood counts (including differential white cell count and platelet count) is necessary initially, and at monthly intervals during the first 3 months (liver function tests also being performed at monthly intervals for the first 3 months).

SULPHASALAZINE
(Sulfasalazine)

Indications: active rheumatoid arthritis; ulcerative colitis, see section 1.5 and notes above

Cautions; Contra-indications; Side-effects: see section 1.5 and notes above
BLOOD DISORDERS. CSM has reminded of need to warn patient to report immediately if sore throat, fever, malaise or non-specific illness develops. Treatment should be stopped immediately if suspicion or laboratory evidence of blood disorder

Dose: by mouth, administered on expert advice, as enteric-coated tablets, initially 500 mg daily, increased by 500 mg at intervals of 1 week to a max. of 2–3 g daily in divided doses

PoM Salazopyrin EN-Tabs® (Pharmacia)
Tablets, e/c, yellow, f/c, sulphasalazine 500 mg. Net price 125-tab pack = £12.75. Label: 5, 14, 25, counselling, blood disorder symptoms (see above), contact lenses may be stained

10.1.4   Drugs for treatment of gout

It is important to distinguish drugs used for the treatment of acute attacks of gout from those used in the long-term control of the disease. The latter exacerbate and prolong the acute manifestations if started during an attack.

ACUTE ATTACKS

Acute attacks of gout are usually treated with high doses of **NSAIDs** such as azapropazone (**important:** see CSM restrictions on p.380), diclofenac, indomethacin, ketoprofen, naproxen, piroxicam, or sulindac (section 10.1.1). Colchicine is an alternative. Aspirin is *not* indicated in gout. Allopurinol and uricosurics are not effective in treating an acute attack and may prolong it indefinitely if started during the acute episode.

Colchicine is probably as effective as NSAIDs. Its use is limited by the development of toxicity at higher doses, but it is of value in patients with heart failure since, unlike NSAIDs, it does not induce fluid retention; moreover it can be given to patients receiving anticoagulants.

COLCHICINE

Indications: acute gout, short-term prophylaxis during initial therapy with allopurinol and uricosuric drugs

Cautions: gastro-intestinal disease, renal impairment, pregnancy and breast-feeding; **interactions:** Appendix 1 (colchicine)

Side-effects: most common are nausea, vomiting, and abdominal pain; excessive doses may also cause profuse diarrhoea, gastro-intestinal haemorrhage, rashes, and renal damage. Rarely peripheral neuritis, alopecia, and with prolonged treatment blood disorders

Dose: 1 mg initially, followed by 500 micrograms every 2–3 hours until relief of pain is obtained or vomiting or diarrhoea occurs, or until a total dose of 10 mg has been reached. The course should not be repeated within 3 days

Prevention of attacks during initial treatment with allopurinol or uricosuric drugs, 500 micrograms 2–3 times daily

PoM **Colchicine** (Non-proprietary)

Tablets, colchicine 500 micrograms, net price 20 = £2.87

Available from CP, Evans

INTERVAL TREATMENT

For long-term ('interval') control of gout the formation of uric acid from purines may be reduced with the **xanthine-oxidase inhibitor** allopurinol, or the **uricosuric drugs** probenecid or sulphinpyrazone may be used to increase the excretion of uric acid in the urine. Treatment should be continued indefinitely once the decision has been made to prevent further attacks of gout by correcting the hyperuricaemia. These drugs should never be started during an acute attack. The initiation of treatment may precipitate an acute attack therefore colchicine or an anti-inflammatory analgesic should be used as a prophylactic and continued for at least one month after the hyperuricaemia has been corrected (usually about 3 months of prophylaxis).

Allopurinol is a convenient well tolerated drug which is now widely used. It is especially useful in patients with renal impairment or urate stones where uricosuric drugs cannot be used. It is usually given once daily, as the active metabolite of allopurinol has a long half-life, but doses over 300 mg daily should be divided. Allopurinol treatment should not be started until an acute attack of gout has completely subsided, as further attacks may be precipitated. It is well tolerated in most patients but may occasionally cause rashes. Allopurinol is *not* indicated for the treatment of asymptomatic hyperuricaemia.

The uricosuric drugs include **probenecid** and **sulphinpyrazone**. They can be used instead of allopurinol, or in conjunction with it in cases that are resistant to treatment.

If an acute attack develops in a patient taking allopurinol or a uricosuric the treatment should continue at the same dosage while the acute attack is treated in its own right.

Aspirin and salicylates antagonise the uricosuric drugs; they do not antagonise allopurinol but are nevertheless *not* indicated in gout.

Crystallisation of urate in the urine may occur with the uricosuric drugs and it is important to ensure that there is an adequate urine output especially in the first few weeks of treatment. As an additional precaution the urine may be rendered alkaline.

The **NSAIDs** are described in section 10.1.1.

ALLOPURINOL

Indications: prophylaxis of gout and of uric acid and calcium oxalate renal stones

Cautions: administer prophylactic colchicine or NSAID (*not* aspirin or salicylates) until at least 1 month after hyperuricaemia corrected; ensure adequate fluid intake (2 litres/day); hepatic and renal impairment (see Appendix 3). In neoplastic conditions treatment with allopurinol (if required) should be commenced before cytotoxic drugs are given; **interactions:** Appendix 1 (allopurinol)

Contra-indications: not a treatment for acute gout but continue if attack develops when already receiving allopurinol, and treat attack separately (see notes above)

Side-effects: rashes (**withdraw** therapy; if rash mild re-introduce cautiously but **discontinue** immediately if recurrence—skin reactions associated with exfoliation, fever, lymphadenopathy, arthralgia, and eosinophilia, resembling Stevens-Johnson or Lyell's syndrome, occur rarely); gastro-intestinal disorders. Rarely malaise, headache, vertigo, drowsiness, taste disturbances, hypertension, symptomless xanthine deposits in muscle, alopecia, hepatotoxicity, paraesthesia and neuropathy

Dose: initially 100 mg daily as a single dose, after food, gradually increased over 1–3 weeks according to the plasma or urinary uric acid concentration, to about 300 mg daily; usual maintenance dose 200–600 mg daily, rarely 900 mg daily, divided into doses of not more than 300 mg; CHILD (in neoplastic conditions, enzyme disorders) 10–20 mg/kg daily

PoM **Allopurinol** (Non-proprietary)

Tablets, allopurinol 100 mg, net price 20 = 26p; 300 mg, 20 = 52p. Label: 8, 21, 27

Available from APS, Ashbourne (Xanthomax®), Berk (Caplenal®), Cox, CP, DDSA (Cosuric®), K Pharm., Norton, Rima (Rimapurinol®), Roche (Hamarin®)

PoM **Zyloric®** (Wellcome)

Tablets, allopurinol 100 mg, net price 100-tab pack = £10.96; 300 mg, 28-tab pack = £7.86. Label: 8, 21, 27

PROBENECID

Indications: gout prophylaxis (to correct hyperuricaemia); reduction of tubular excretion of penicillins and certain cephalosporins, see section 5.1

Cautions, during initial gout therapy administer prophylactic colchicine or NSAID (*not* aspirin or salicylates), ensure adequate fluid intake (about 2 litres daily), render urine alkaline if uric acid overload is high; peptic ulceration, renal impairment (avoid if severe); transient false-positive Benedict's test; G6PD-deficiency (see section 9.1.5); **interactions:** Appendix 1 (probenecid)

Contra-indications: history of blood disorders, nephrolithiasis, porphyria (see section 9.8.2), acute gout attack; avoid aspirin and salicylates

Side-effects: infrequent; occasionally nausea and vomiting, urinary frequency, headache, flushing, dizziness, rashes; rarely hypersensitivity, nephrotic syndrome, hepatic necrosis, aplastic anaemia

Dose: uricosuric therapy, initially 250 mg twice daily after food, increased after a week to 500 mg twice daily then up to 2 g daily in 2–4 divided doses according to plasma-uric acid concentration and reduced for maintenance

PoM Benemid® (MSD)
Tablets, scored, probenecid 500 mg. Net price 20 = 66p. Label: 12, 21, 27

SULPHINPYRAZONE
(Sulfinpyrazone)

Indications: gout prophylaxis, hyperuricaemia

Cautions; Contra-indications: see under Probenecid; regular blood counts advisable; avoid in hypersensitivity to NSAIDs; cardiac disease (may cause salt and water retention); **interactions:** Appendix 1 (sulphinpyrazone)

Side-effects: gastro-intestinal disturbances, occasionally allergic skin reactions, salt and water retention; rarely blood disorders, gastro-intestinal ulceration and bleeding, acute renal failure, raised liver enzymes, jaundice and hepatitis

Dose: initially 100–200 mg daily with food (or milk) increasing over 2–3 weeks to 600 mg daily (rarely 800 mg daily), continued until serum uric acid concentration normal then reduced for maintenance (maintenance dose may be as low as 200 mg daily)

PoM Anturan® (Geigy)
Tablets, both yellow, s/c, sulphinpyrazone 100 mg, net price 20 = 94p; 200 mg, 84-tab pack = £7.82. Label: 12, 21

10.2 Drugs used in neuromuscular disorders

10.2.1 Drugs which enhance neuromuscular transmission

Anticholinesterases are used as first-line treatment in *myasthenia gravis*.

Corticosteroids are only given concomitantly if anticholinesterase treatment is failing.

Plasmapheresis may produce temporary remission in otherwise unresponsive patients.

ANTICHOLINESTERASES

Anticholinesterase drugs are used to enhance neuromuscular transmission in voluntary and involuntary muscle in myasthenia gravis. They prolong the action of acetylcholine by inhibiting the action of the enzyme acetylcholinesterase. Excessive dosage of these drugs may impair neuromuscular transmission and precipitate 'cholinergic crises' by causing a depolarising block. This may be difficult to distinguish from a worsening myasthenic state.

Side-effects of anticholinesterases are due to their parasympathomimetic action. Muscarinic effects include increased sweating, salivary, and gastric secretion, also increased gastro-intestinal and uterine motility, and bradycardia. These effects are antagonised by atropine.

Edrophonium has a very brief action and is therefore used mainly for the diagnosis of myasthenia gravis. A single test-dose usually causes substantial improvement in muscle power (lasting about 5 minutes) in patients with the disease (if respiration already impaired, *only* in conjunction with someone skilled at intubation).

It can also be used to determine whether a patient with myasthenia is receiving inadequate or excessive treatment with cholinergic drugs. If treatment is excessive an injection of edrophonium will either have no effect or will intensify symptoms (if respiration already impaired, *only* in conjunction with someone skilled at intubation). Conversely, transient improvement may be seen if the patient is being inadequately treated. The test is best performed just before the next dose of anticholinesterase.

Neostigmine produces a therapeutic effect for up to 4 hours. Its pronounced muscarinic action is a disadvantage, and administration of an antimuscarinic drug such as atropine or propantheline may be required to prevent colic, excessive salivation, or diarrhoea. In severe disease neostigmine may be given every 2 hours. The maximum that most patients can tolerate is 180 mg daily.

Pyridostigmine is less powerful and slower in action than neostigmine but it has a longer duration of action. It is preferable to neostigmine because of its smoother action and the need for less frequent dosage. It is particularly preferred in patients whose muscles are weak on wakening. It has a comparatively mild gastro-intestinal effect but an antimuscarinic drug may still be required. It is inadvisable to exceed a daily dose of 720 mg.

Distigmine has the most protracted action but the danger of a 'cholinergic crisis' caused by accumulation of the drug is greater than with shorter-acting drugs.

Neostigmine and edrophonium are also used to reverse the actions of the non-depolarising muscle relaxants (see section 15.1.6).

NEOSTIGMINE

Indications: myasthenia gravis; other indications, see section 15.1.6

Cautions: asthma (*extreme* caution), bradycardia, recent myocardial infarction, epilepsy, hypotension, parkinsonism, vagotonia, peptic ulceration, renal impairment, pregnancy and breast-feeding. Atropine or other antidote to muscarinic effects may be necessary (particularly when neostigmine is given by injection), but it should not be given routinely as it may mask signs of overdosage; **interactions:** Appendix 1 (cholinergics)

Contra-indications: intestinal or urinary obstruction

Side-effects: nausea, vomiting, increased salivation, diarrhoea, abdominal cramps (more marked with higher doses). Signs of overdosage are increased gastro-intestinal discomfort, bronchial secretions, and sweating, involuntary defaecation and micturition, miosis, nystagmus, bradycardia, hypotension, agitation, excessive dreaming, and weakness eventually leading to fasciculation and paralysis

Dose: by mouth, neostigmine bromide 15–30 mg at suitable intervals throughout day, total daily dose 75–300 mg (but see also notes above); NEONATE 1–5 mg every 4 hours, half an hour before feeds; CHILD up to 6 years initially 7.5 mg, 6–12 years initially 15 mg, usual total daily dose 15–90 mg

By subcutaneous or intramuscular injection, neostigmine methylsulphate 1–2.5 mg at suitable intervals throughout day (usual total daily dose 5–20 mg); NEONATE 50–250 micrograms every 4 hours half an hour before feeds; CHILD 200–500 micrograms as required

PoM **Prostigmin**® (Roche)

Tablets, scored, neostigmine bromide 15 mg. Net price 20 = 53p

Injection, neostigmine methylsulphate 500 micrograms/mL, net price 1-mL amp = 16p; 2.5 mg/mL, 1-mL amp = 16p

DISTIGMINE BROMIDE

Indications: myasthenia gravis; urinary retention and other indications, see section 7.4.1

Cautions; Contra-indications; Side-effects: see under Neostigmine

Dose: initially 5 mg daily half an hour before breakfast, increased at intervals of 3–4 days if necessary to a max. of 20 mg daily; CHILD up to 10 mg daily according to age

Preparations

See section 7.4.1

EDROPHONIUM CHLORIDE

Indications: see under Dose and notes above; surgery, see section 15.1.6

Cautions; Contra-indications; Side-effects: see under Neostigmine; have resuscitation facilities; *extreme* caution in respiratory distress (see notes above) and in asthma

Note. Severe cholinergic reactions can be counteracted by injection of atropine sulphate (which should always be available)

Dose: diagnosis of myasthenia gravis, *by intravenous injection,* 2 mg followed after 30 seconds (if no adverse reaction has occurred) by 8 mg; in adults without suitable veins, *by intramuscular injection,* 10 mg

Detection of overdosage or underdosage of cholinergic drugs, *by intravenous injection,* 2 mg (best before next dose of anticholinesterase, see notes above)

CHILD *by intravenous injection* 20 micrograms / kg followed after 30 seconds (if no adverse reaction has occurred) by 80 micrograms/kg

PoM **Camsilon**¹® (Cambridge)

Injection, edrophonium chloride 10 mg/mL. Net price 1-mL amp = 90p

1. Formerly Tensilon®

PYRIDOSTIGMINE BROMIDE

Indications: myasthenia gravis

Cautions; Contra-indications; Side-effects: see under Neostigmine; weaker muscarinic action

Dose: by mouth, 30–120 mg at suitable intervals throughout day, total daily dose 0.3–1.2 g (but see also notes above); NEONATE 5–10 mg every 4 hours, ½–1 hour before feeds; CHILD up to 6 years initially 30 mg, 6–12 years initially 60 mg, usual total daily dose 30–360 mg

PoM **Mestinon**® (Roche)

Tablets, scored, pyridostigmine bromide 60 mg. Net price 20 = £1.11

IMMUNOSUPPRESSANT THERAPY

Corticosteroids (see section 6.3) are established as treatment for myasthenia gravis where *thymectomy* is inadvisable or to reduce the risk of surgery beforehand. The initial dose may be high (up to 100 mg **prednisolone** daily) but most advise starting with a smaller dose (20 mg prednisolone daily) and gradually increasing it. There is grave risk of exacerbation of the myasthenia during the initial stages of therapy, particularly in the first 2-3 weeks, therefore inpatient supervision is essential. Improvement usually begins after about 2 weeks on the high-dose regimen. In some patients a prolonged remission may be induced, but often patients need a maintenance dose of 10–40 mg of prednisolone daily; alternate-day therapy is popular. Patients who need a corticosteroid may benefit from the addition of **azathioprine** (see section 8.2.1) in a dose of 2 mg/kg daily which may allow a reduction in corticosteroid dosage.

10.2.2   Skeletal muscle relaxants

Drugs described below are used for the relief of chronic muscle spasm or spasticity; they are not indicated for spasm associated with minor injuries. They act principally on the central nervous system with the exception of dantrolene which has a peripheral site of action. They differ in action from the muscle relaxants used in anaesthesia (see section 15.1.5) which block transmission at the neuromuscular junction.

The underlying cause of spasticity should be treated and any aggravating factors (e.g. pressure sores, infection) remedied. Skeletal muscle relaxants are effective in most forms of spasticity except the rare alpha variety. The major disadvantage of treatment with these drugs is that reduction in muscle tone can cause a loss of splinting action of the spastic leg and trunk muscles and sometimes lead to an increase in disability.

Dantrolene acts directly on skeletal muscle and produces fewer central adverse effects making it a drug of choice. The dose should be increased slowly.

Baclofen inhibits transmission at spinal level and also depresses the central nervous system. The dose should be increased slowly to avoid the major side-effects of sedation and hypotonia (other adverse events are uncommon).

Diazepam may also be used. Sedation and, occasionally, extensor hypotonus are disadvantages. Other benzodiazepines also have muscle-relaxant properties. Muscle-relaxant doses of benzodiazepines are similar to anxiolytic doses (see section 4.1.2).

Quinine salts (see section 5.4.1) 200 to 300 mg at bedtime are effective in relieving nocturnal leg cramps. **Important:** they are very toxic in overdosage and accidental fatalities have occurred in children—immediate expert advice is essential (see also p.22).

BACLOFEN

Indications: chronic severe spasticity of voluntary muscle

Cautions: psychiatric illness, cerebrovascular disease, elderly; respiratory, hepatic, or renal impairment, epilepsy; hypertonic bladder sphincter; pregnancy; avoid abrupt withdrawal; porphyria (see section 9.8.2); **interactions:** Appendix 1 (muscle relaxants)

DRIVING. Drowsiness may affect performance of skilled tasks (e.g. driving); effects of alcohol enhanced

Contra-indications: peptic ulceration

Side-effects: frequently sedation, drowsiness, nausea; occasionally lightheadedness, lassitude, confusion, dizziness, ataxia, hallucinations, headache, euphoria, insomnia, depression, tremor, nystagmus, paraesthesias, convulsions, muscular pain and weakness, respiratory or cardiovascular depression, hypotension, gastro-intestinal and urinary disturbances; rarely visual disorders, taste alterations, increased sweating, rash, altered liver function, and paradoxical increase in spasticity

Dose: 5 mg 3 times daily, preferably after food, gradually increased; max. 100 mg daily; CHILD 0.75–2 mg/kg daily (over 10 years, max. 2.5 mg/kg daily) *or* 2.5 mg 4 times daily increased gradually according to age to maintenance: 1–2 years 10–20 mg daily, 2–6 years 20–30 mg daily, 6–10 years 30–60 mg daily

PoM **Baclofen** (Non-proprietary)
Tablets, baclofen 10 mg. Net price 20 = £1.35. Label: 2, 8
Available from APS, Ashbourne (Baclospas®), Berk, Cox, CP, Evans, K Pharm., Lagap, Norton

PoM **Lioresal®** (Geigy)
Tablets, scored, baclofen 10 mg. Net price 20 = £1.96. Label: 2, 8
Additives: include gluten
Liquid, sugar-free, baclofen 5 mg/5 mL. Net price 300 mL = £6.16. Label: 2, 8

DANTROLENE SODIUM

Indications: chronic severe spasticity of voluntary muscle

Cautions: impaired cardiac and pulmonary function; test liver function before and at intervals during therapy; therapeutic effect may take a few weeks to develop but if treatment is ineffective it should be discontinued after 4–6 weeks. Avoid when spasticity is useful, for example, locomotion; **interactions:** Appendix 1 (muscle relaxants).

DRIVING. Drowsiness may affect performance of skilled tasks (e.g. driving); effects of alcohol enhanced

Contra-indications: hepatic impairment (may cause severe liver damage); acute muscle spasm

Side-effects: transient drowsiness, dizziness, weakness, malaise, fatigue, diarrhoea (withdraw if severe, discontinue treatment if recurs on re-introduction), anorexia, nausea, headache, rash; less frequently constipation, dysphagia, speech and visual disturbances, confusion, nervousness, insomnia, depression, seizures, chills, fever, increased urinary frequency; rarely, tachycardia, erratic blood pressure, dyspnoea, haematuria, possible crystalluria, urinary incontinence or retention, pleural effusion, pericarditis, dose-related hepatotoxicity (occasionally fatal) may be more common in women over 30 especially those taking oestrogens

Dose: initially 25 mg daily, may be increased at weekly intervals to max. of 100 mg 4 times daily; usual dose 75 mg 3 times daily; CHILD not recommended

PoM **Dantrium®** (Procter & Gamble Pharm.)
Capsules, both orange/brown, dantrolene sodium 25 mg, net price 20 = £3.42; 100 mg, 20 = £11.97. Label: 2
Injection—see section 15.1.8

DIAZEPAM

Indications: muscle spasm of varied aetiology, including tetanus; other indications, see sections 4.1.2, 4.8, 15.1.4.1

Cautions; Contra-indications; Side-effects: see section 4.1.2; also hypotonia; special precautions for intravenous injection (see section 4.8.2)

Dose: by mouth, 2–15 mg daily in divided doses, increased if necessary in spastic conditions to 60 mg daily according to response

Cerebral spasticity in selected cases, CHILD 2–40 mg daily in divided doses

By intramuscular or by slow intravenous injection (into a large vein at a rate of not more than 5 mg/minute), in acute muscle spasm, 10 mg repeated if necessary after 4 hours

Tetanus, ADULT and CHILD, *by intravenous injection,* 100–300 micrograms/kg repeated every 1–4 hours; *by intravenous infusion* (*or by nasoduodenal tube*), 3–10 mg/kg over 24 hours, adjusted according to response

Preparations

See section 4.1.2

OTHER MUSCLE RELAXANTS

The clinical efficacy of carisoprodol, chlormezanone and meprobamate (see section 4.1.2), methocarbamol, and orphenadrine as muscle relaxants is **not** well established although they have been included in compound analgesic preparations.

CARISOPRODOL

Indications: short-term symptomatic relief of muscle spasm (but see notes above)

Cautions; Contra-indications; Side-effects: see under Meprobamate, section 4.1.2. Drowsiness is common; avoid in porphyria (see section 9.8.2)

Dose: 350 mg 3 times daily; ELDERLY half adult dose or less

PoM **Carisoma®** (Pharmax)
Tablets, carisoprodol 125 mg, net price 20 = £1.49; 350 mg, 20 = £1.64. Label: 2

METHOCARBAMOL

Indications: short-term symptomatic relief of muscle spasm (but see notes above)

Cautions: hepatic and renal impairment (avoid injection in renal impairment)

DRIVING. Drowsiness may affect performance of skilled tasks (e.g. driving); effects of alcohol enhanced

Contra-indications: coma or pre-coma, brain damage, epilepsy, myasthenia gravis

Side-effects: lassitude, light-headedness, dizziness, restlessness, anxiety, confusion, drowsiness, nausea, allergic rash or angioedema, convulsions

Dose: by mouth, 1.5 g 4 times daily (elderly 750 mg or less); may be reduced to 750 mg 3 times daily

By slow intravenous injection or by infusion, 1–3 g (max. rate 300 mg/min.); max. dose 3 g (elderly, 1.5 g) daily for 3 days

PoM **Robaxin®** (Shire)
750 Tablets, scored, methocarbamol 750 mg. Net price 20 = £2.30. Label: 2
Injection, methocarbamol 100 mg/mL in aqueous macrogol '300'. Net price 10-mL amp = £1.36
PoM **Robaxisal Forte®** : see section 4.7.1

ORPHENADRINE CITRATE

Indications: short-term symptomatic relief of muscle spasm (but see notes above)

Cautions: see under Benzhexol Hydrochloride, section 4.9.2. Avoid in children; porphyria (see section 9.8.2); reduce dose in elderly

Side-effects: dry mouth and other antimuscarinic side-effects; see also Orphenadrine Hydrochloride, section 4.9.2

Dose: by intramuscular or by slow intravenous injection (over 5 minutes), 60 mg repeated after 12 hours if necessary

PoM **Norflex®** (3M)
Injection, orphenadrine citrate 30 mg/mL. Net price 2-mL amp = 60p

10.3   Drugs for the relief of soft-tissue inflammation

10.3.1   Enzymes
10.3.2   Rubefacients and other topical antirheumatics

10.3.1   Enzymes

Hyaluronidase is used to render the tissues more easily permeable to injected fluids, e.g. for introduction of fluids by subcutaneous infusion (termed hypodermoclysis).

HYALURONIDASE

Indications: enhance permeation of subcutaneous or intramuscular injections, local anaesthetics and subcutaneous infusions; promote resorption of excess fluids and blood

Cautions: infants or elderly (control speed and total volume and avoid overhydration especially in renal impairment)

Contra-indications: do not apply direct to cornea; avoid sites where infection or malignancy; not for anaesthesia in unexplained premature labour; not to be used to reduce swelling of bites or stings; not for intravenous administration

Side-effects: occasional severe allergy

Dose: With subcutaneous or intramuscular injection, 1500 units mixed with the injection fluid (ensure compatibility)

With local anaesthetics, 1500 units mixed with local anaesthetic solution (ophthalmology, 15 units/mL)

Hypodermoclysis, 1500 units administered before 500-1000 mL infusion fluid

Extravasation or haematoma, 1500 units infiltrated into affected area (as soon as possible after extravasation)

PoM **Hyalase®** (CP)
Injection, powder for reconstitution, hyaluronidase (ovine). Net price 1500-unit amp = £4.43

10.3.2 Rubefacients and other topical antirheumatics

Rubefacients act by counter-irritation. Pain, whether superficial or deep-seated, is relieved by any method which itself produces irritation of the skin. Counter-irritation is comforting in painful lesions of the muscles, tendons, and joints, and in non-articular rheumatism. Rubefacients probably all act through the same essential mechanism and differ mainly in intensity and duration of action.

Topical **NSAIDs** (e.g. benzydamine, felbinac, ibuprofen, salicylamide) may provide some slight relief of pain in musculoskeletal conditions.

TOPICAL NSAIDs AND COUNTER-IRRITANTS

CAUTIONS. Apply with gentle massage only. Avoid contact with eyes, mucous membranes, and inflamed or broken skin; discontinue if rash develops. Hands should be washed immediately after use. Not for use with occlusive dressings. Topical application of large amounts may result in systemic effects including hypersensitivity and asthma (renal disease has also been reported). Not generally suitable for children. Patient packs carry a warning to avoid during pregnancy or breast-feeding.
HYPERSENSITIVITY. For NSAID hypersensitivity and asthma warning, see p.379
PHOTOSENSITIVITY. Patients should be advised against excessive exposure to sunlight of area treated in order to avoid possibility of photosensitivity

Algesal® (Duphar)
Cream, diethylamine salicylate 10%. Net price 50 g = 75p. Apply three times daily
Algipan® (Whitehall)
Spray application, methyl nicotinate 1.5%, glycol salicylate 10%. Net price 135-mL aerosol spray = £1.59. Label: 15
Aspellin® (Fisons)
Liniment, ammonium salicylate 1%, camphor 0.6%, menthol 1.4%, ethyl and methyl salicylate 0.54%. Net price 125 mL = 87p; 500 mL = £2.98
Balmosa® (Pharmax)
Cream, camphor 4%, capsicum oleoresin 0.035%, menthol 2%, methyl salicylate 4%. Net price 40 g = 68p
Difflam® (3M)
Cream, benzydamine hydrochloride 3%. Net price 15 g = £1.05 (hosp. only); 100 g = £7.00. Apply 3–6 times daily for up to 10 days
PoM **Feldene®** (Pfizer)
Gel, piroxicam 0.5%. Net price 60 g = £5.00; 112 g = £7.84 (also 7.5 g starter pack, hosp. only)
Apply 3–4 times daily; therapy should be reviewed after 4 weeks
Ibugel® (Dermal)
Gel, ibuprofen 5%. Net price 100 g = £6.53
Apply up to 3 times daily

Intralgin® (3M)
Gel, benzocaine 2%, salicylamide 5% in an alcoholic vehicle. net price 50 g = 49p
Movelat® (Panpharma)
Cream, heparinoid 0.2%, salicylic acid 2%. Net price 100 g = £4.14. Apply up to 4 times daily
Gel, ingredients as for cream but in a colourless gel basis. Net price 100 g = £4.14. Apply up to 4 times daily
PoM **Oruvail®** (Rhône-Poulenc Rorer)
Gel, ketoprofen 2.5%. Net price 100 g = £6.78
Apply 2–4 times daily for up to 7 days (usual recommended dose 15 g daily)
Proflex® (Zyma)
Cream, ibuprofen 5%. Net price 100 g = £6.50
Apply 3–4 times daily
Transvasin® (Seton)
Cream, ethyl nicotinate 2%, hexyl nicotinate 2%, tetrahydrofurfuryl salicylate 14%. Net price 40 g = 77p; 80 g = £1.38
Apply at least twice daily
Spray application, hydroxyethyl salicylate 5%, diethylamine salicylate 5%, methyl nicotinate 1%. Net price 125 mL = £1.28
PoM **Traxam®** (Lederle)
Foam, felbinac 3.17%. Net price 100 g = £7.00. Label:15
Gel, felbinac 3%. Net price 50 g = £7.00
Apply 2–4 times daily; max. 25 g daily; therapy should be reviewed after 14 days
Note. Felbinac is an active metabolite of the NSAID fenbufen
PoM **Voltarol Emulgel®** (Geigy)
Gel, diclofenac diethylammonium salt 1.16% (equivalent to diclofenac sodium 1%). Net price 20 g (hosp. only) = £1.55; 100 g = £7.00. Apply 3–4 times daily; therapy should be reviewed after 14 days (or after 28 days for osteoarthritis)

COUNTER-IRRITANT FOR POST-HERPETIC NEURALGIA

Axsain® (Euroderma)
Cream, capsaicin 0.075%. Net price 45 g = £15.04. For post-herpetic neuralgia (**important: after** lesions have healed), apply up to 3–4 times daily

POULTICES

Kaolin Poultice, heavy kaolin 52.7%, thymol 0.05%, boric acid 4.5%, peppermint oil 0.05%, methyl salicylate 0.2%, glycerol 42.5%. Net price 200 g = £1.57
Warm and apply directly or between layers of muslin; avoid application of overheated poultice
Kaolin Poultice K/L Pack® (K/L)
Kaolin poultice. Net price 4 × 100-g pouches = £5.50

For list of topical NSAIDs and counter-irritants on sale to public see next page

Topical NSAIDs and counter-irritants on sale to the public (unless otherwise specified, not prescribable on NHS) together with their significant ingredients include:

Algesal® (diethylamine salicylate; prescribable on NHS), **Algipan Rub®** (capsicin, glycol salicylate, methyl nicotinate), **Algipan Spray®** (glycol salicylate, methyl nicotinate; prescribable on NHS), **Aspellin®** (ammonium salicylate, camphor, ethyl salicylate, methyl salicylate, menthol; prescribable on NHS)

Balmosa® (camphor, capsicum oleoresin, menthol, methyl salicylate; prescribable on NHS), **Bengués Balsam®** (menthol, methyl salicylate), **BN Liniment®** (turpentine oil, strong ammonia solution, ammonium chloride), **Boots Pain Relief Balm®** (ethyl nicotinate, glycol monosalicylate, nonylic acid vanillylamide), **Boots Pain Relief Embrocation®** (camphor, turpentine oil)

Cremalgin® (capsicin, glycol salicylate, methyl nicotinate)

Deep Freeze Cold Gel® (menthol), **Deep Freeze Pain Relief Spray®** (dichlorodifluoromethane, trichlorofluoromethane), **Deep Heat Extra Strength®**, **Deep Heat Massage Liniment®**, **Deep Heat Maximum®**, **Deep Heat Pre-Sport Rub®** (menthol, methyl salicylate), **Deep Heat Rub®** (eucalyptus oil, menthol, methyl salicylate, turpentine oil), **Deep Heat Spray Relief®** (glycol salicylate, ethyl salicylate, methyl salicylate, methyl nicotinate), **Difflam® Cream** (benzydamine; prescribable on NHS), **Dubam Cream®** (methyl salicylate, menthol, cineole), **Dubam Spray®** (ethyl salicylate, methyl salicylate, glycol salicylate, methyl nicotinate)

Elliman's Universal Embrocation® (acetic acid, turpentine oil)

Fiery Jack Cream® (capsicum oleoresin, diethylamine salicylate, glycol salicylate, methyl nicotinate), **Fiery Jack Ointment®** (capsicum oleoresin)

Goddard's White Oil Embrocation® (dilute acetic acid, dilute ammonia solution, turpentine oil)

Ibuleve, **Ibuleve Sports Gel®** (ibuprofen), **Intralgin®** (benzocaine, salicylamide; prescribable on NHS)

Lloyds Cream® (diethyl salicylate)

Movelat® (heparinoid, salicylic acid; prescribable on NHS)

Nasciodine® (camphor, iodine, menthol, methyl salicylate, turpentine oil), **Nella Red Oil®** (clove oil, mustard oil, methyl nicotinate)

Oruvail® Gel (ketoprofen 30-g tube; 100-g tube prescribable on NHS (PoM)

PR Freeze Spray® (dichlorodifluoromethane, trichlorofluoromethane), **PR Heat Spray®** (ethyl nicotinate, methyl salicylate, camphor); **Proflex®** (ibuprofen; prescribable on NHS), **Proflex Pain Relief®** (ibuprofen)

Radian-B Muscle Lotion®, **Radian-B Heat Spray®** (ammonium salicylate, camphor, menthol, salicylic acid), **Radian-B Muscle Rub®** (camphor, capsicin, menthol, methyl salicylate), **Ralgex Cream®** (capsicin, glycol monosalicylate, methyl nicotinate), **Ralgex Freeze Spray®** (methoxymethane, glycol monosalicylate, isopentane), **Ralgex Low Odour Spray®** (glycol monosalicylate, methyl nicotinate), **Ralgex Spray®** (ethyl salicylate, methyl salicylate, glycol monosalicylate, methyl nicotinate), **Ralgex Stick®** (capsicin, ethyl salicylate, methyl salicylate, glycol salicylate, menthol)

Salonair® (benzyl nicotinate, camphor, glycol salicylate, menthol, methyl salicylate, squalane), **Salonpas Plasters®** (glycol salicylate, methyl salicylate)

Tiger Balm Red Extra Strength® (camphor, clove oil, cajuput oil, cinnamon oil, menthol, peppermint oil), **Tiger Balm®** (cajuput oil, camphor, clove oil, menthol, peppermint oil), **Transvasin Cream®** (ethyl nicotinate, hexyl nicotinate, thurfyl salicylate; prescribable on NHS), **Transvasin Spray®** (diethylamine salicylate, hydroxyethyl salicylate, methyl nicotinate; prescribable on NHS)

Zam-Buk® (camphor, eucalyptus oil, thyme oil, colophony)

11:Drugs acting on the
EYE

In this chapter, drug treatment is discussed under the following headings:

The entries in this chapter generally relate only to local eye treatment. Systemic indications and side-effects of many of the drugs are given elsewhere (see index).

OTHER PREPARATIONS. Subconjunctival injection may be used to administer anti-infective drugs, mydriatics, or corticosteroids for conditions not responding to topical therapy. The drug diffuses through the sclera to the anterior and posterior chambers and vitreous humour in higher concentration than can be achieved by absorption from eye-drops. However, because the dose-volume is limited (usually not more than 1 mL), this route is suitable only for drugs which are readily soluble.

Drugs such as antibiotics and corticosteroids may be administered systemically to treat an eye condition.

Suitable plastic devices which gradually release a specified amount of drug over a period of, say, 1 week are also used (e.g. Ocuserts®).

11.1   Administration of drugs to the eye

EYE-DROPS AND EYE OINTMENTS. When administered in the form of eye-drops, drugs penetrate the globe, probably through the cornea. However, systemic effects, which are usually undesirable, may well arise from absorption of drugs into the general circulation via conjunctival vessels or from the nasal mucosa after the excess of the preparation has drained down through the tear ducts. For example, timolol (a beta-blocker), administered as eye-drops may induce bronchospasm or bradycardia in susceptible individuals.

Eye ointments are often applied to lid margins for blepharitis. They may also be used in the conjunctival sac for other conditions especially where a prolonged action is required.

When two different preparations in the form of eye-drops are required at the same time of day, for example pilocarpine and timolol in glaucoma, dilution and overflow may occur when one immediately follows the other. The patient should therefore leave an interval of a few minutes. At night, an eye ointment for the second drug will reduce the problem.

Generally it is inadvisable for patients to continue to wear contact lenses, particularly hydrophilic (soft) contact lenses when receiving eye-drops. For warnings relating to eye-drops and contact lenses, see section 11.9.

EYE LOTIONS. These are solutions for the irrigation of the conjuctival sac. They act mechanically to flush out irritants or foreign bodies as a first-aid treatment. Sterile sodium chloride 0.9% solution (section 11.8.2) is usually used. In emergency, tap water drawn freshly from the main (not stored water) will suffice.

11.2   Control of microbial contamination

Preparations for the eye should be sterile when issued. Eye-drops in multiple-application containers are suitably preserved but care should be taken to avoid contamination of the contents during use.

Eye-drops in multiple-application containers for *domiciliary use* should not be used for more than 4 weeks after first opening (unless otherwise stated).

Eye-drops for use in *hospital wards* should be discarded 1 week after opening. Individual containers should be provided for each patient and when both eyes are being treated, a separate container should be used for each eye. Containers used before an operation should be discarded at the time of the operation and fresh containers supplied. A fresh supply should also be provided upon discharge from hospital.

Eye-drops used in *out-patient departments* should be discarded at the end of each day. In clinics for eye diseases and in accident and emergency departments, where the dangers of infection are high, single-application packs should be used; if a multiple-application pack is used, it should be discarded after single use.

Diagnostic dyes (e.g. fluorescein) should be used only from single-application packs.

In *eye surgery* it is wise to use single-application containers. Preparations used during intra-ocular procedures and others that may penetrate into the anterior chamber must be isotonic and without preservatives and buffered if necessary to a neutral pH. Large volume intravenous infusion preparations are not suitable for this purpose. For all surgical procedures, a previously unopened container is used for each patient.

11.3   Anti-infective eye preparations

11.3.1   Antibacterials
11.3.2   Antifungals
11.3.3   Antivirals

EYE INFECTIONS. Most acute superficial eye infections can be treated topically. Blepharitis and conjunctivitis are often caused by staphylococci; keratitis and endophthalmitis may be bacterial, viral, or fungal.

Bacterial *blepharitis* is treated by application of an antibacterial eye ointment to the conjunctival sac or to the lid margins but systemic treatment may occasionally be required.

Acute *infective conjunctivitis* is treated with antibacterial eye-drops and eye ointment. A poor response might indicate viral or allergic conjunctivitis. *Gonococcal conjunctivitis* is treated with systemic and topical antibiotics.

Corneal ulcer and *keratitis* require specialist treatment and may call for subconjunctival or systemic administration of antibiotics.

Endophthalmitis is a medical emergency which also calls for specialist management and often requires parenteral, subconjunctival, or intraocular administration of antibiotics.

11.3.1   Antibacterials

Bacterial infections are generally treated topically with eye-drops and eye ointments.

Chloramphenicol has a broad spectrum of activity and is the drug of choice for *superficial eye infections*. Other antibiotics with a broad spectrum of activity include **framycetin**, **gentamicin**, and **neomycin**, and also **ciprofloxacin**, **norfloxacin** and **ofloxacin**. Gentamicin and tobramycin (and possibly ciprofloxacin, norfloxacin, and ofloxacin) are effective for infections caused by *Pseudomonas aeruginosa*.

Ciprofloxacin eye-drops have recently been licensed for *corneal ulcers*; intensive application (especially in the first 2 days) is required throughout the day and night.

Chlortetracycline and **tetracycline** are used in the treatment of *chlamydial infections* including *trachoma*.

Fusidic acid is useful for staphylococcal infections.

Propamidine isethionate is of little value in bacterial infections but is specific for the rare but devastating condition of *acanthamoeba keratitis* (neomycin may be used as an adjunct).

WITH CORTICOSTEROIDS. Many antibiotic preparations also incorporate a corticosteroid but such mixtures should **not** be used unless a patient is under close specialist supervision. In particular they should not be prescribed for undiagnosed 'red eye' which is sometimes caused by the herpes simplex virus and may be difficult to diagnose (section 11.4).

ADMINISTRATION
Eye-drops. Apply at least every 2 hours then reduce frequency as infection is controlled and continue for 48 hours after healing.
Eye ointment. Apply *either* at night (if eye-drops used during the day) *or* 3–4 times daily (if eye ointment used alone).

CHLORAMPHENICOL

Indications; Administration: see notes above
Side-effects: transient stinging; rare reports of aplastic anaemia

PoM Chloramphenicol (Non-proprietary)
Eye-drops, chloramphenicol 0.5%. Net price 10 mL = 56p
Eye ointment, chloramphenicol 1%. Net price 4 g = 71p

PoM Chloromycetin® (P-D)
Ophthalmic ointment (= eye ointment), chloramphenicol 1%. Net price 4 g = 67p
Redidrops (= eye-drops), chloramphenicol 0.5%. Net price 5 mL = £1.10; 10 mL = £1.18
Additives: include phenylmercuric acetate

PoM Sno Phenicol® (S&N Pharm.)
Eye-drops, chloramphenicol 0.5%, in a viscous vehicle. Net price 10 mL = £1.08
Additives: include chlorhexidine acetate

Single use
PoM Minims® Chloramphenicol (S&N Pharm.)
Eye-drops, chloramphenicol 0.5%. Net price 20 × 0.5 mL = £5.90

CHLORTETRACYCLINE

Indications: local treatment of infections, including trachoma (see notes above and under Tetracycline)
Administration: see notes above

PoM Aureomycin® (Lederle)
Ophthalmic ointment (= eye ointment), chlortetracycline hydrochloride 1%. Net price 3.5 g = 92p

CIPROFLOXACIN

Indications: superficial bacterial infections, see notes above; corneal ulcers
Side-effects: local burning and itching; lid margin crusting
Administration: superficial bacterial infection, see notes above
Corneal ulcer, apply throughout day and night, first day 2 drops every 15 minutes for 6 hours then every 30 minutes for the rest of the day, second day apply 2 drops every hour, third to fourteenth days apply 2 drops every 4 hours; if longer treatment required physician to decide frequency (max. duration of treatment 21 days)

▼ PoM **Ciloxan**® (Alcon)
Ophthalmic solution (= eye-drops), ciprofloxacin (as hydrochloride) 0.3%. Net price 5 mL = £4.94
Additives: include benzalkonium chloride

FRAMYCETIN SULPHATE
Indications; Administration: see notes above

PoM **Soframycin**® (Roussel)
Eye-drops, framycetin sulphate 0.5%. Net price 8 mL = £2.15
Additives: include phenylmercuric nitrate
Eye ointment, framycetin sulphate 0.5%. Net price 5 g = 88p

FUSIDIC ACID
Indications: see notes above

PoM **Fucithalmic**® (Leo)
Eye-drops, m/r, fusidic acid 1% in gel basis (liquifies on contact with eye). Net price 5 g = £2.19
Additives: include benzalkonium chloride
Apply twice daily

GENTAMICIN
Indications; Administration: see notes above

PoM **Cidomycin**® (Roussel)
Drops (for ear or eye), gentamicin 0.3% (as sulphate). Net price 8 mL = £1.31
Additives: include benzalkonium chloride, disodium edetate
Eye ointment, gentamicin 0.3% (as sulphate), net price 5 g = £1.97
PoM **Garamycin**® (Schering-Plough)
Drops (for ear or eye), gentamicin 0.3% (as sulphate). Net price 10 mL = £1.79
Additives: include benzalkonium chloride
PoM **Genticin**® (Roche)
Drops (for ear or eye), gentamicin 0.3% (as sulphate). Net price 10 mL = £2.00
Additives: include benzalkonium chloride

Single use
PoM **Minims**® **Gentamicin** (S&N Pharm.)
Eye-drops, gentamicin 0.3% (as sulphate). Net price 20 × 0.5 mL = £5.75

NEOMYCIN SULPHATE
Indications; Administration: see notes above

PoM **Neomycin** (Non-proprietary)
Eye-drops, neomycin sulphate 0.5% (3500 units/mL). Net price 10 mL = £2.00
Eye ointment, neomycin sulphate 0.5% (3500 units/g). Net price 3 g = 89p
PoM **Neosporin**® (Cusi)
Eye-drops, gramicidin 25 units, neomycin sulphate 1700 units, polymyxin B sulphate 5000 units/mL. Net price 5 mL = £5.36
Additives: include thiomersal
Apply 2–4 times daily or more frequently if required

Single use
PoM **Minims**® **Neomycin Sulphate** (S&N Pharm.)
Eye-drops, neomycin sulphate 0.5%. Net price 20 × 0.5 mL = £5.75

NORFLOXACIN
Indications; Administration: see notes above
Side-effects: local burning and smarting; rarely conjunctival hyperaemia, chemosis (conjunctival oedema) and photophobia, bitter taste

PoM **Noroxin**® (MSD)
Ophthalmic solution (= eye-drops), norfloxacin 0.3%. Net price 5 mL = £1.97
Additives: include benzalkonium chloride

OFLOXACIN
Indications; Administration: see notes above
Side-effects: local irritation including photophobia; dizziness, numbness, nausea and headache reported

▼ PoM **Exocin**® (Allergan)
Ophthalmic solution (= eye-drops), ofloxacin 0.3%. Net price 5 mL = £2.27
Additives: include benzalkonium chloride

POLYMYXIN B SULPHATE
Indications; Administration: see notes above

PoM **Polyfax**® (Cusi)
Eye ointment, polymyxin B sulphate 10 000 units, bacitracin zinc 500 units/g. Net price 4 g = £3.41
PoM **Polytrim**® (Cusi)
Eye-drops, trimethoprim 0.1%, polymyxin B sulphate 10 000 units/mL. Net price 5 mL = £3.19
Additives: include thiomersal
Eye ointment, trimethoprim 0.5%, polymyxin B sulphate 10 000 units/g. Net price 4 g = £3.19

PROPAMIDINE ISETHIONATE
Indications: local treatment of infections (but see notes above)

Brolene® (Rhône-Poulenc Rorer)
Eye-drops, propamidine isethionate 0.1%. Net price 10 mL = £1.78
Apply 4 times daily
Note. Eye-drops containing propamidine isethionate 0.1% also available from Typharm (Golden Eye Drops)
Eye ointment, dibromopropamidine isethionate 0.15%. Net price 5 g = £1.90
Apply 1–2 times daily
Note. Eye ointment containing dibromopropamidine isethionate 0.15% also available from Typharm (Golden Eye Ointment)

Cautionary label wordings, see inside back cover

Prices are **net**, see p.1

TETRACYCLINE HYDROCHLORIDE

Indications; Administration: see notes above

TRACHOMA. For mass antitrachoma treatment, the World Health Organization recommends **tetracycline hydrochloride** eye ointment applied to both eyes twice daily for 5 days in each month for 6 months. Chlortetracycline eye ointment may also be used but chloramphenicol is not as effective.

For active trachoma in the individual, one or both of the following are effective. (i) For adults, orally administered sulphonamides for 2 weeks or the long-acting sulphadimethoxine (no longer on UK market) 1 g initially followed by 500 mg daily for 10 days (see section 5.1.8). For children, erythromycin should be used (see section 5.1.5). (ii) Tetracycline eye ointment three times daily for 6 weeks.

PoM Achromycin® (Lederle)

Ointment (for ear or eye), tetracycline hydrochloride 1%. Net price 3.5 g = 68p

TOBRAMYCIN

Indications; Administration: see notes above

PoM Tobralex® (Alcon)

Eye-drops, tobramycin 0.3%. Net price 5 mL = £1.39

Additives: include benzalkonium chloride

11.3.2   Antifungals

Fungal infections of the cornea are rare but tend to occur after agricultural injuries, especially in hot and humid climates. Orbital mycosis is rare, and when it occurs is usually due to direct spread of infection from the paranasal sinuses. Increasing age, debility, or immunosuppression by drugs, for example, following renal transplantation, may encourage fungal proliferation in many parts of the body. The spread of infection via the bloodstream occasionally produces a metastatic endophthalmitis.

A wide range of fungi are capable of producing ocular mycosis and may be identified by appropriate laboratory procedures.

Antifungal preparations for the eye are not generally available. Treatment will normally be carried out at specialist centres, but requests for information about supplies of preparations not available commercially should be addressed to the District Pharmaceutical Officer (or equivalent in Scotland or Northern Ireland) or to Moorfields Eye Hospital, City Road, London EC1V 2PD (071-253 3411).

11.3.3   Antivirals

Herpes simplex infections producing, for example, dendritic corneal ulcer can be treated with **acyclovir**; alternatively **idoxuridine** may be used.

ACYCLOVIR

Indications: local treatment of herpes simplex infections

Administration: apply 5 times daily (continue for at least 3 days after complete healing)

PoM Zovirax® (Wellcome)

Eye ointment, acyclovir 3%. Net price 4.5 g = £10.67

Tablets and *injection,* see section 5.3

Cream, see section 13.10.3

IDOXURIDINE

Indications: local treatment of herpes simplex infections

Contra-indications: pregnancy (toxicity in *animal* studies)

Administration: apply eye ointment every 4 hours

PoM Idoxene® (Spodefell)

Eye ointment, idoxuridine 0.5%. Net price 3 g = £2.45

11.4   Corticosteroids and other anti-inflammatory preparations

11.4.1   Corticosteroids

11.4.2   Other anti-inflammatory preparations

11.4.1   Corticosteroids

Corticosteroids administered topically, by subconjunctival injection, and systemically have an important place in treating uveitis and scleritis; they are also used to reduce post-operative inflammation following eye operations.

Topical corticosteroids should normally only be used under expert supervision; they should not be prescribed for undiagnosed 'red eye'. There are two main dangers from topical corticosteroids. First the 'red eye' may be caused by herpes simplex virus which produces a dendritic ulcer; corticosteroids aggravate the condition which may lead to loss of vision or even loss of the eye. Second, again arising from the use of eye-drop formulations, a 'steroid glaucoma' may be produced, after a few weeks treatment, in patients predisposed to chronic simple glaucoma. Use of a combination product containing a corticosteroid with an anti-infective is rarely justified.

Systemic corticosteroids can usefully be given on an alternate-day basis to minimise side-effects. The risk of producing glaucoma is not great, but 'steroid cataract' is a very high risk (75%) if more than 15 mg of prednisolone or equivalent is given daily for several years. The longer the duration, the greater is the risk. A dose of less then 10 mg per day is usually safe.

BETAMETHASONE

Indications: local treatment of inflammation (short-term)

Cautions; Side-effects: see notes above

Administration: apply eye-drops every 1–2 hours until controlled then reduce frequency, eye ointment 2–4 times daily or at night when used with eye-drops

PoM Betnesol® (Evans)

Drops (for ear, eye, or nose), betamethasone sodium phosphate 0.1%. Net price 10 mL = £1.31
Additives: include benzalkonium chloride
Eye ointment, betamethasone sodium phosphate 0.1%. Net price 3 g = 56p

PoM Betnesol-N® (Evans)

Drops (for ear, eye, or nose), see section 12.1.1
Eye ointment, betamethasone sodium phosphate 0.1%, neomycin sulphate 0.5%. Net price 3 g = 64p

PoM Vista-Methasone® (Daniels)

Drops (for ear, eye, or nose), betamethasone sodium phosphate 0.1%. Net price 5 mL = £1.05; 10 mL = £1.28
Additives: include benzalkonium chloride

PoM Vista-Methasone N® (Daniels)

Drops (for ear, eye, or nose), see section 12.1.1

CLOBETASONE BUTYRATE

Indications: local treatment of inflammation (short-term)

Cautions; Side-effects: see notes above; reduced tendency to raise intra-ocular pressure

Administration: apply eye-drops 4 times daily; severe conditions every 1–2 hours until controlled then reduce frequency

PoM Eumovate® (Cusi)

Eye-drops, clobetasone butyrate 0.1%. Net price 10 mL = £3.61
Additives: include benzalkonium chloride

PoM Eumovate-N® (Cusi)

Eye-drops, clobetasone butyrate 0.1%, neomycin sulphate 0.5%. Net price 10 mL = £3.75
Additives: include benzalkonium chloride

DEXAMETHASONE

Indications: local treatment of inflammation (short-term)

Cautions; Side-effects: see notes above

Administration: apply eye-drops 4–6 times daily; severe conditions every hour until controlled then reduce frequency

PoM Maxidex® (Alcon)

Eye-drops, dexamethasone 0.1%, hypromellose 0.5%. Net price 5 mL = £1.49; 10 mL = £2.95
Additives: include benzalkonium chloride

PoM Maxitrol® (Alcon)

Eye-drops, dexamethasone 0.1%, hypromellose 0.5%, neomycin 0.35% (as sulphate), polymyxin B sulphate 6000 units/mL. Net price 5 mL = £1.77
Additives: include benzalkonium chloride
Eye ointment, dexamethasone 0.1%, neomycin 0.35% (as sulphate), polymyxin B sulphate 6000 units/g. Net price 3.5 g = £1.52
Additives: include hydroxybenzoates

PoM Sofradex® (Roussel)

Drops and ointment (for ear or eye), see section 12.1.1

FLUOROMETHOLONE

Indications: local treatment of inflammation (short-term)

Cautions; Side-effects: see notes above; reduced tendency to raise intra-ocular pressure

Administration: apply eye-drops 2–4 times daily (initially every hour for 24–48 hours then reduce frequency)

PoM FML® (Allergan)

Ophthalmic suspension (= eye-drops), fluorometholone 0.1%, polyvinyl alcohol (Liquifilm®) 1.4%. Net price 5 mL = £1.79; 10 mL = £3.09
Additives: include benzalkonium chloride, disodium edetate, polysorbate 80

PoM FML-Neo® (Allergan)

Eye-drops, fluorometholone 0.1%, neomycin sulphate 0.5%, polyvinyl alcohol (Liquifilm®) 1.4%. Net price 5 mL = £2.08
Additives: include benzalkonium chloride, disodium edetate, polysorbate 80

HYDROCORTISONE ACETATE

Indications: local treatment of inflammation (short-term)

Cautions; Side-effects: see notes above

PoM Hydrocortisone (Non-proprietary)

Eye-drops, hydrocortisone acetate 1%. Net price 10 mL = £2.15
Eye ointment, hydrocortisone acetate 0.5%, net price 3 g = £1.11; 1%, 3 g = £1.10; 2.5%, 3 g = £1.35

PoM Chloromycetin Hydrocortisone® (P-D)

Eye ointment, chloramphenicol 1%, hydrocortisone acetate 0.5%. Net price 4 g = 70p

PoM Neo-Cortef® (Cusi)

Drops and *ointment* (for ear or eye), see section 12.1.1
Note. Eye-drops containing hydrocortisone acetate 1.5% and neomycin sulphate 0.5% also available from Daniels

---

PREDNISOLONE

Indications: local treatment of inflammation (short-term)

Cautions; Side-effects: see notes above

Administration: apply eye-drops every 1–2 hours until controlled then reduce frequency

PoM Pred Forte® (Allergan)

Eye-drops, prednisolone acetate 1%. Net price 5 mL = £1.59; 10 mL = £3.19
Additives: include benzalkonium chloride, disodium edetate, polysorbate 80
Apply 2–4 times daily

PoM Predsol® (Evans)

Drops (for ear or eye), prednisolone sodium phosphate 0.5%. Net price 10 mL = £1.31
Additives: include benzalkonium chloride

PoM Predsol-N® (Evans)

Drops (for ear or eye), see section 12.1.1

Single use
PoM Minims® Prednisolone (S&N Pharm.)

Eye-drops, prednisolone sodium phosphate 0.5%. Net price 20 × 0.5 mL = £5.75

11.4.2   Other anti-inflammatory preparations

Other preparations used for the topical treatment of inflammation and allergic conjunctivitis include antihistamines, lodoxamide, and sodium cromoglycate.

Topical preparations of **antihistamines** such as eye-drops containing antazoline sulphate (with xylometazoline hydrochloride as Otrivine-Antistin®) may be used for short-term treatment of allergic conjunctivitis.

Sodium cromoglycate eye-drops may be useful for vernal catarrh and other allergic forms of conjunctivitis.

Lodoxamide eye-drops have been introduced for allergic conjunctival conditions including seasonal allergic conjunctivitis and vernal catarrh.

ANTAZOLINE
Indications: allergic conjunctivitis

Otrivine-Antistin® (CIBA Vision)
Eye-drops, antazoline sulphate 0.5%, xylometazoline hydrochloride 0.05%. Net price 10 mL = £1.83
Additives: include benzalkonium chloride, disodium edetate
Apply 2–3 times daily

PoM **Vasocon A®** (CIBA Vision)
Eye-drops, antazoline phosphate 0.5%, naphazoline hydrochloride 0.05%. Net price 10 mL = £2.41
Additives: include benzalkonium chloride, disodium edetate
Apply every 3–4 hours

LODOXAMIDE
Indications: allergic conjunctivitis
Side-effects: mild transient burning, stinging, itching, and lachrymation
Administration: ADULT and CHILD over 4 years, apply eye drops 4 times daily

▼ PoM **Alomide®** (Galen)
Ophthalmic solution (= eye-drops), lodoxamide 0.1% (as trometamol). Net price 10 mL = £5.48
Additives: include benzalkonium chloride, disodium edetate

SODIUM CROMOGLYCATE
Indications: allergic conjunctivitis
Administration: apply eye-drops 4 times daily, eye ointment 2–3 times daily

PoM ¹**Sodium Cromoglycate** (Non-proprietary)
Eye-drops, sodium cromoglycate 2%. Net price 13.5 mL = £5.15
Available from Baker Norton (Hay-Crom®), Fisons (Opticrom® Aqueous), Novex (Vividrin®)
Eye ointment, sodium cromoglycate 4%. Net price 5 g = £7.25
Available from Fisons (Opticrom®)
1. Sodium cromoglycate 2% eye-drops and 4% eye ointment can be sold to the public (in max. pack sizes of 10 mL for eye-drops and 5 g for eye ointment) for treatment of acute seasonal (allergic) conjunctivitis; proprietary brands of eye-drops on sale to the public include *Broleze®, Clariteyes®, Opticrom® Allergy,* and *Optrex® Hayfever Allergy*

11.5   Mydriatics and cycloplegics

Antimuscarinics dilate the pupil and paralyse the ciliary muscle; they vary in potency and duration of action. The relative potencies and durations of action of the principal drugs, in ascending order, are:

tropicamide (3 hours)
cyclopentolate, hyoscine, homatropine (all up to 24 hours)
atropine (7 days or longer)

Short-acting, relatively weak mydriatics, such as **tropicamide 0.5%,** facilitate the examination of the fundus of the eye. **Cyclopentolate** 1% or **atropine** are preferable for producing cycloplegia for refraction in young children. Atropine 1% (in ointment form) is sometimes preferred for children under 5 years of age. Atropine is also used for the treatment of Iridocyclitis mainly to prevent posterior synechiae, often with phenylephrine 10% eye-drops (2.5% in children, elderly, and those with cardiac disease).

CAUTIONS AND SIDE-EFFECTS. Contact dermatitis is not uncommon with the antimuscarinic mydriatic drugs, especially atropine. In addition, toxic systemic reactions to atropine (and hyoscine) and cyclopentolate may occur in the very young and the very old.

Darkly pigmented iris is more resistant to pupillary dilatation and caution should be exercised to avoid overdosage.

Mydriasis may precipitate acute closed-angle ('congestive') glaucoma in a few patients, usually aged over 60 years, who are predisposed to the condition because of a shallow anterior chamber.

Interactions. Phenylephrine may interact with systemically administered monoamine-oxidase inhibitors; see also Appendix 1 (sympathomimetics).

DRIVING. Patients should be warned not to drive for 1 to 2 hours after mydriasis.

ANTIMUSCARINICS

ATROPINE SULPHATE
Indications: refraction procedures in young children; see also notes above
Cautions: action persistent, may precipitate glaucoma; see also notes above

PoM **Atropine** (Non-proprietary)
Eye-drops, atropine sulphate 1%. Net price 10 mL = 78p
Eye ointment, atropine sulphate 1%. Net price 3 g = £1.28
PoM **Isopto Atropine®** (Alcon)
Eye-drops, atropine sulphate 1%, hypromellose 0.5%. Net price 5 mL = 99p
Additives: include benzalkonium chloride

Single use
PoM **Minims® Atropine Sulphate** (S&N Pharm.)
Eye-drops, atropine sulphate 1%. Net price 20 ×
0.5 mL = £4.92

CYCLOPENTOLATE HYDROCHLORIDE
Indications: see notes above
Cautions: patients with raised intra-ocular pressure; see notes above

PoM **Mydrilate®** (Boehringer Ingelheim)
Eye-drops, cyclopentolate hydrochloride 0.5%, net
price 5 mL = 73p; 1%, 5 mL = 98p
Additives: include benzalkonium chloride

Single use
PoM **Minims® Cyclopentolate** (S&N Pharm.)
Eye-drops, cyclopentolate hydrochloride 0.5 and
1%. Net price 20 × 0.5 mL (both) = £4.92

HOMATROPINE HYDROBROMIDE
Indications; Cautions: see notes above

PoM **Homatropine** (Non-proprietary)
Eye-drops, homatropine hydrobromide 1%, net
price 10 mL = £1.82; 2%, 10 mL = £2.04

Single use
PoM **Minims® Homatropine Hydrobromide**
(S&N Pharm.)
Eye-drops, homatropine hydrobromide 2%. Net
price 20 × 0.5 mL = £5.75

HYOSCINE HYDROBROMIDE
Indications; Cautions: see notes above

PoM **Hyoscine** (Non-proprietary)
Eye-drops, hyoscine hydrobromide 0.25%. Net
price 10 mL = 85p

TROPICAMIDE
Indications; Cautions: see notes above

PoM **Mydriacyl®** (Alcon)
Eye-drops, tropicamide 0.5%, net price 5 mL =
£1.36; 1%, 5 mL = £1.68
Additives: include benzalkonium chloride

Single use
PoM **Minims® Tropicamide** (S&N Pharm.)
Eye-drops, tropicamide 0.5 and 1%. Net price 20 ×
0.5 mL (both) = £5.75
PoM **NODS® Tropicamide** (S&N Pharm.)
Ophthalmic applicator strips, tropicamide
125 micrograms. Net price 25 individually
wrapped strips = £4.31
Administration: 1 strip placed in lower conjunctival sac
Note. In terms of mydriatic and cycloplegic effect, one
125-microgram strip is equivalent to 1 drop of tropicamide 1% eye-drops

SYMPATHOMIMETICS

ADRENALINE
Section 11.6

PHENYLEPHRINE HYDROCHLORIDE
Indications; Cautions: see notes above

Phenylephrine (Non-proprietary)
Eye-drops, phenylephrine hydrochloride 10%. Net
price 10 mL = £2.30
Available from Daniels
See also under Hypromellose (section 11.8.1)

Single use
Minims® Phenylephrine Hydrochloride
(S&N Pharm.)
Eye-drops, phenylephrine hydrochloride 2.5%,
net price 20 × 0.5 mL = £5.75; 10%, 20 × 0.5 mL
= £5.75

11.6   Treatment of glaucoma

An abnormally high intra-ocular pressure, glaucoma, may result in blindness. In virtually all cases, rise in pressure is due to reduced outflow of aqueous humour, the inflow remaining constant.

Glaucoma is treated by the application of eye-drops containing beta-blockers, miotics, or adrenaline (and guanethidine). Acetazolamide and dichlorphenamide are given by mouth and, in emergency or before surgery, mannitol may be given by intravenous infusion.

Probably the commonest condition is *chronic simple glaucoma* where the obstruction is in the trabecular meshwork. It is commonly first treated with a topical beta-blocker and other drugs added as necessary to control the intra-ocular pressure e.g. adrenaline or pilocarpine.

If supplementary topical treatment is required after *iridectomy* or a drainage operation in either open-angle or closed-angle glaucoma, a beta-blocker is preferred to pilocarpine. This is because of the risk that posterior synechiae will be formed as a result of the miotic effect of pilocarpine, especially in closed-angle glaucoma. It is then also advantageous to utilise the mydriatic side-effect of adrenaline.

MIOTICS

The small pupil is an unfortunate side-effect of these drugs (except when pilocarpine is used temporarily prior to operation for *closed-angle glaucoma*). The key factor is the opening up of the inefficient drainage channels in the trabecular meshwork resulting from contraction or spasm of the ciliary muscle. This also produces accommodation spasm that may result in blurring of vision and browache (a particular disadvantage in patients under 40 years of age).

Pilocarpine has a duration of action of 3 to 4 hours. **Physostigmine** is more potent; it is still used with pilocarpine but is not usually used alone. **Carbachol** is sometimes used to lower intra-ocular pressure, usually in conjunction with other miotics such as physostigmine.

Demecarium bromide (as *Tosmilen®*, Sinclair) and **ecothiopate iodide** (as *Phospholine Iodide®*, Cusi) are no longer on the UK market but are still available on a named-patient basis for use under expert supervision.

Generalised parasympathomimetic side effects such as sweating, bradycardia and intestinal colic may follow systemic absorption of these eye-drops; other effects may include hypersalivation and bronchospasm.

CARBACHOL

Indications: see notes above
Administration: apply eye-drops up to 4 times daily

PoM Isopto Carbachol® (Alcon)
Eye-drops, carbachol 3%, hypromellose 1%. Net price 10 mL = £1.76
Additives: include benzalkonium chloride

PHYSOSTIGMINE SULPHATE
(Eserine)
Indications; Side-effects: see notes above
Administration: apply eye-drops 2–6 times daily

PoM Physostigmine (Non-proprietary)
Eye-drops, physostigmine sulphate 0.25%, net price 10 mL = £2.50; 0.5%, 10 mL = £2.74
May no longer be available

PILOCARPINE

Indications; Side-effects: see notes above
Administration: apply eye-drops 3–6 times daily

PoM Pilocarpine (Non-proprietary)
Eye-drops, pilocarpine hydrochloride 0.5%, net price 10 mL = £1.24; 1%, 10 mL = £1.00; 2%, 10 mL = £1.07; 3%, 10 mL = £1.24; 4%, 10 mL = £1.37
PoM Isopto Carpine® (Alcon)
Eye-drops, all with hypromellose 0.5%; pilocarpine hydrochloride 0.5%, net price 10 mL = 73p; 1%, 10 mL = 81p; 2%, 10 mL = 90p; 3%, 10 mL = 97p; 4%, 10 mL = £1.04
Additives: include benzalkonium chloride
PoM Sno Pilo® (S&N Pharm.)
Eye-drops, in a viscous vehicle, pilocarpine hydrochloride 1%, net price 10 mL = £1.04; 2%, 10 mL = £1.14; 4%, 10 mL = £1.36
Additives: include benzalkonium chloride

Single use
PoM Minims® Pilocarpine Nitrate (S&N Pharm.)
Eye-drops, pilocarpine nitrate 1, 2, and 4%. Net price 20 × 0.5 mL (all) = £4.92

Modified release
PoM Ocusert® (Cusi)
Pilo-20 ocular insert, m/r, pilocarpine 20 micrograms released per hour for 1 week. Net price pack of 8 inserts = £35.08. Counselling, method of use
Pilo-40 ocular insert, m/r, pilocarpine 40 micrograms released per hour for 1 week. Net price pack of 8 inserts = £40.90. Counselling, method of use

ADRENALINE/GUANETHIDINE

Adrenaline probably acts both by reducing the rate of production of aqueous humour and by increasing the outflow through the trabecular meshwork. It is contra-indicated in closed-angle glaucoma because it is a mydriatic, unless an iridectomy has been carried out. Side-effects include severe smarting and redness of the eye; adrenaline should be used with caution in patients with hypertension and heart disease.

Dipivefrine is a prodrug of adrenaline. It is stated to pass more rapidly through the cornea and is then converted to the active form.

Guanethidine enhances and prolongs the effects of adrenaline. Prolonged use, particularly of the higher strengths may result in conjunctival fibrosis with secondary corneal changes; the conjunctiva and cornea should be examined at least every six months.

ADRENALINE

Indications; Contra-indications: see notes above
Administration: apply eye-drops 1–2 times daily

PoM Eppy® (S&N Pharm.)
Eye-drops, adrenaline 1%. Net price 7.5 mL = £4.06
Additives: include benzalkonium chloride, also acetylcysteine as antioxidant
PoM Simplene® (S&N Pharm.)
Eye-drops, adrenaline, in a viscous vehicle, 0.5%, net price 7.5 mL = £3.45; 1%, 7.5 mL = £3.79
Additives: include benzalkonium chloride, also acetylcysteine as antioxidant

DIPIVEFRINE HYDROCHLORIDE

Indications; Contra-indications: as for Adrenaline, see notes above
Administration: apply 1 drop twice daily

PoM Propine® (Allergan)
Eye-drops, dipivefrine hydrochloride 0.1%. Net price 5 mL = £3.99, 10 mL = £4.99
Additives: include benzalkonium chloride, disodium edetate

GUANETHIDINE MONOSULPHATE

Indications; Cautions: see notes above
Administration: apply eye-drops 1–2 times daily

PoM **Ganda®** (S&N Pharm.)

Eye-drops '1 + 0.2', guanethidine monosulphate 1%, adrenaline 0.2% in a viscous vehicle. Net price 7.5 mL = £4.49

Additives: include benzalkonium chloride

Eye-drops '3 + 0.5', guanethidine monosulphate 3%, adrenaline 0.5% in a viscous vehicle. Net price 7.5 mL = £5.86

Additives: include benzalkonium chloride

BETA-BLOCKERS

Topical application of a beta-blocker to the eye reduces intra-ocular pressure effectively in *chronic simple glaucoma*, probably by reducing the rate of production of aqueous humour. Administration by mouth also reduces intra-ocular pressure but this route is not used (see comment under Systemic Drugs).

Beta-blockers used as eye-drops include **timolol** and, more recently, **betaxolol, carteolol, levobunolol**, and **metipranolol**.

CAUTIONS, CONTRA-INDICATIONS AND SIDE-EFFECTS. Systemic absorption may follow topical application therefore eye-drops containing a beta-blocker are contra-indicated in patients with bradycardia, heart block, or heart failure. **Important:** for a warning to avoid in asthma see CSM advice below. Consider also other cautions, contra-indications and side-effects of beta-blockers (p.72). Local side-effects of eye-drops include transitory dry eyes and allergic blepharoconjunctivitis.

CSM advice. The CSM has advised that beta-blockers, even those with apparent cardioselectivity, should not be used in patients with asthma or a history of obstructive airways disease, unless no alternative treatment is available. In such cases the risk of inducing bronchospasm should be appreciated and appropriate precautions taken.

INTERACTIONS. Since systemic absorption may follow topical application the possibility of interactions, in particular, with drugs such as verapamil should be borne in mind. See also section 2.3.2 and Appendix 1 (beta-blockers).

BETAXOLOL HYDROCHLORIDE

Indications; Cautions; Contra-indications; Side-effects: see notes above

Administration: apply eye-drops twice daily

PoM **Betoptic®** (Alcon)

Eye-drops, betaxolol 0.5% (as hydrochloride). Net price 5 mL = £5.17

Additives: include benzalkonium chloride

CARTEOLOL HYDROCHLORIDE

Indications; Cautions; Contra-indications; Side-effects: see notes above

Administration: apply eye-drops twice daily

PoM **Teoptic®** (CIBA Vision)

Eye-drops, carteolol hydrochloride 1%, net price 5 mL = £4.83; 2%, 5 mL = £5.67

Additives: include benzalkonium chloride

LEVOBUNOLOL HYDROCHLORIDE

Indications; Cautions; Contra-indications; Side-effects: see notes above

Administration: apply eye-drops once or twice daily

PoM **Betagan®** (Allergan)

Eye-drops, levobunolol hydrochloride 0.5%, polyvinyl alcohol (Liquifilm®) 1.4%. Net price 5-mL bottle with C Cap® = £4.88

Additives: include benzalkonium chloride, disodium edetate

Unit dose eye-drops, levobunolol hydrochloride 0.5%, polyvinyl alcohol (Liquifilm®) 1.4%. Net price 30 × 0.4 mL = £10.45

Additives: include disodium edetate

METIPRANOLOL

Indications; Cautions; Contra-indications; Side-effects: see notes above but in chronic open angle glaucoma **restricted** to patients allergic to preservatives or to those wearing soft contact lenses (in whom benzalkonium chloride should be avoided); granulomatous anterior uveitis reported (discontinue treatment)

Administration: apply eye-drops twice daily

PoM **Minims® Metipranolol** (S&N Pharm.)

Eye-drops, metipranolol 0.1%, net price 20 × 0.5 mL = £10.19; 0.3%, 20 × 0.5 mL = £11.09

TIMOLOL MALEATE

Indications; Cautions; Contra-indications; Side-effects: see notes above

Administration: apply eye-drops twice daily

PoM **Timoptol®** (MSD)

Eye-drops, in Ocumeter® metered-dose unit, timolol (as maleate) 0.25%, net price 5 mL = £5.18; 0.5%, 5 mL = £5.82

Additives: include benzalkonium chloride

Unit dose eye-drops, timolol (as maleate) 0.25%, net price 30 × 0.25 mL = £9.60; 0.5%, 30 × 0.25 mL = £10.97

PoM **Glaucol®** (Baker Norton)

Unit dose eye-drops, timolol (as maleate) 0.25%, net price 30 unit-dose vials = £5.18; 0.5%, 30 unit-dose vials = £5.82

SYSTEMIC DRUGS

The side-effects of beta-blockers are probably sufficient to prevent their being prescribed by the ophthalmologist for administration by mouth. Hence **acetazolamide** will retain a significant place in treatment. It inhibits carbonic anhydrase, thus reducing the bicarbonate in aqueous humour and the water secreted with it, resulting in a fall in the intra-ocular pressure. **Dichlorphenamide** has a similar but more prolonged action. Both these drugs have a diuretic action and a moderate incidence of side-effects, giving rise, especially in the elderly, to paraesthesia, hypokalaemia, lack of appetite, drowsiness and depression; rashes and blood disorders occur rarely. Intravenous hypertonic **mannitol**, or **glycerol** by mouth, are useful short-term ocular hypotensive drugs. Acetazolamide by intramuscular or preferably intravenous injection is also useful in the pre-operative treatment of closed-angle glaucoma.

ACETAZOLAMIDE

Indications; Side-effects: see notes above

Cautions: avoid in severe renal impairment; pregnancy; not generally recommended for prolonged administration but if given blood counts needed; **interactions:** Appendix 1 (acetazolamide)

Dose: by mouth or by intravenous injection, 0.25–1 g daily in divided doses

By intramuscular injection, as for intravenous injection but preferably avoided because of alkaline pH

PoM **Diamox®** (Storz)

Tablets, acetazolamide 250 mg. Net price 20 = £1.91. Label: 3

Sodium Parenteral (= injection), powder for reconstitution, acetazolamide (as sodium salt). Net price 500-mg vial = £14.76

PoM **Diamox® SR** (Storz)

Capsules, m/r, two-tone orange, enclosing orange f/c pellets, acetazolamide 250 mg. Net price 28-cap pack = £10.50. Label: 3, 25

Dose: 1–2 capsules daily

DICHLORPHENAMIDE

Indications; Cautions; Side-effects: see under Acetazolamide and notes above

Dose: initially 100–200 mg, then 100 mg every 12 hours, adjusted according to the patient's response

PoM **Daranide®** (MSD)

Tablets, yellow, scored, dichlorphenamide 50 mg. Net price 20 = 95p

11.7   Local anaesthetics

Oxybuprocaine and amethocaine are probably the most widely used topical local anaesthetics. Proxymetacaine causes less initial stinging and is useful for children. Cocaine was formerly used in surgery; its toxicity to corneal epithelium was its main drawback. Oxybuprocaine or a combined preparation of lignocaine and fluorescein is used for tonometry. Lignocaine, with or without adrenaline, is injected into the eyelids for minor surgery, while retrobulbar or peribulbar injections are used for surgery of the globe itself.

AMETHOCAINE HYDROCHLORIDE

Indications: local anaesthetic

PoM **Amethocaine Eye-drops,** amethocaine hydrochloride 0.5%, net price 10 mL = £2.50; 1%, 10 mL = £2.80

Single use

PoM **Minims® Amethocaine Hydrochloride** (S&N Pharm.)

Eye-drops, amethocaine hydrochloride 0.5 and 1%. Net price 20 × 0.5 mL (both) = £5.75

LIGNOCAINE HYDROCHLORIDE

Indications: local anaesthetic

PoM **Minims® Lignocaine and Fluorescein** (S&N Pharm.)

Eye-drops, lignocaine hydrochloride 4%, fluorescein sodium 0.25%. Net price 20 × 0.5 mL = £6.93

OXYBUPROCAINE HYDROCHLORIDE

Indications: local anaesthetic

PoM **Minims® Benoxinate (Oxybuprocaine) Hydrochloride** (S&N Pharm.)

Eye-drops, oxybuprocaine hydrochloride 0.4%. Net price 20 × 0.5 mL = £4.92

PROXYMETACAINE HYDROCHLORIDE

Indications: local anaesthetic

PoM **Ophthaine®** (Squibb)

Eye-drops, proxymetacaine hydrochloride 0.5%. Net price 15 mL = £4.49

Additives: include benzalkonium chloride, chlorbutol

11.8   Miscellaneous ophthalmic preparations

11.8.1   Preparations for tear deficiency

Chronically sore eyes associated with reduced tear secretion, usually in cases of rheumatoid arthritis (Sjögren's syndrome), often respond to hypromellose eye-drops and mucolytic agents.

ACETYLCYSTEINE

Indications: tear deficiency, impaired mucus production

Administration: apply eye-drops 3–4 times daily

PoM **Ilube®** (Cusi)

Eye-drops, acetylcysteine 5%, hypromellose 0.35%. Net price 10 mL = £4.63

Additives: include benzalkonium chloride, disodium edetate

CARBOMER

A synthetic high molecular weight polymer of acrylic acid cross-linked with either allylsucrose or allyl ethers of pentaerythritol

Indications: dry eyes including keratoconjunctivitis sicca, unstable tear film

Administration: apply 3–4 times daily or as required

Viscotears® (CIBA Vision)
Liquid gel (= eye-drops), carbomer 940 (polyacrylic acid) 0.2%. Net price 10 g = £2.95
Additives: include cetrimide, disodium edetate

HYDROXYETHYLCELLULOSE
Indications: tear deficiency

Minims® Artificial Tears (S&N Pharm.)
Eye-drops, hydroxyethylcellulose 0.44%. Net price 20 × 0.5 mL = £5.75

HYPROMELLOSE
Indications: tear deficiency

Hypromellose (Non-proprietary)
Eye-drops, hypromellose '4000' (or '4500' or '5000') 0.3%. Net price 10 mL = 56p
Isopto Alkaline® (Alcon)
Eye-drops, hypromellose 1%. Net price 10 mL = 99p
Additives: include benzalkonium chloride
Isopto Plain® (Alcon)
Eye-drops, hypromellose 0.5%. Net price 10 mL = 85p
Additives: include benzalkonium chloride
Tears Naturale® (Alcon)
Eye-drops, dextran '70' 0.1%, hypromellose 0.3%. Net price 15 mL = £1.68
Additives: include benzalkonium chloride, disodium edetate

With phenylephrine
Isopto Frin® (Alcon)
Eye-drops, phenylephrine hydrochloride 0.12%, hypromellose 0.5%. Net price 10 mL = £1.14
Additives: include benzethonium chloride

LIQUID PARAFFIN
Indications: tear deficiency

Lacri-Lube® (Allergan)
Eye ointment, white soft paraffin, liquid paraffin. Net price 3.5 g = £1.99, 5 g = £2.59
Additives: include wool fat derivatives

POLYVINYL ALCOHOL
Indications: tear deficiency

Hypotears® (CIBA Vision)
Eye-drops, macrogol '8000' 2%, polyvinyl alcohol 1%. Net price 10 mL = £1.85
Additives: include benzalkonium chloride, disodium edetate

Liquifilm Tears® (Allergan)
Ophthalmic solution (= eye-drops), polyvinyl alcohol 1.4%. Net price 15 mL = £1.69
Additives: include benzalkonium chloride, disodium edetate
Preservative-free ophthalmic solution (= eye-drops), polyvinyl alcohol 1.4%, povidone 0.6%. Net price 30 × 0.4 mL = £5.60
Sno Tears® (S&N Pharm.)
Eye-drops, polyvinyl alcohol 1.4%. Net price 10 mL = £1.10
Additives: include benzalkonium chloride, disodium edetate

11.8.2 Other preparations

Zinc sulphate is a traditional astringent which has been used in eye-drops for treatment of excessive lachrymation.

Simple eye ointment is a bland sterile preparation which may be used to soften crusts in blepharitis or as a bland lubricant at night.

Fluorescein sodium and **rose bengal** are used in diagnostic procedures and for locating damaged areas of the cornea due to injury or disease. Rose bengal is much more efficient for the diagnosis of conjunctival epithelial damage.

Certain eye-drops, e.g. benzylpenicillin, colistin, desferrioxamine, and trisodium edetate (see also section 9.5.1.2), may be prepared aseptically from material supplied for injection.

ACETYLCHOLINE CHLORIDE
Indications: cataract surgery, penetrating keratoplasty, iridectomy, and other anterior segment surgery requiring rapid miosis

PoM Miochol® (CIBA Vision)
Solution for intra-ocular irrigation, acetylcholine chloride 1%, mannitol 3% when reconstituted. Net price 2 mL -vial = £8.32

APRACLONIDINE
Note. Apraclonidine is a derivative of clonidine
Indications: control or prevention of postoperative elevation of intraocular pressure after anterior segment laser surgery
Cautions: severe cardiovascular disease (including hypertension); history of vasovagal attack; pregnancy and breast-feeding; exaggerated reduction in intra-ocular pressure should be closely monitored; **interactions:** Appendix 1 (apraclonidine)
DRIVING. Drowsiness may affect performance of skilled tasks (e.g. driving)
Side-effects: hyperaemia, lid retraction, conjunctival blanching, mydriasis; since systemic absorption may follow topical application, potential for cardiovascular effects (see Cautions)
Administration: apply 1 drop 1 hour before laser procedure then 1 drop immediately after completion of procedure; CHILD not recommended

▼ PoM **Iopidine**® (Alcon)
Ophthalmic solution (= eye-drops), apraclonidine 1% (as hydrochloride). Net price 12 × 2 single use 0.25-mL units = £81.90

CHYMOTRYPSIN

Indications: zonulolysis in intracapsular cataract extraction

PoM **Zonulysin**® (Henleys)
Injection, powder for reconstitution, alphachymotrypsin 300 USP units (≡ 1.5 microkatals). Net price per vial (with diluent) = £9.50

DICLOFENAC SODIUM

Indications: inhibition of intraoperative miosis during cataract surgery (but does not possess intrinsic mydriatic properties); postoperative inflammation in cataract surgery

▼ PoM **Voltarol**® **Ophtha** (CIBA Vision)
Eye-drops, diclofenac sodium 0.1%. Net price pack of 4 single-dose units = £3.99, pack of 40 single-dose units = £39.90

FLURBIPROFEN SODIUM

Indications: inhibition of intraoperative miosis (but does not possess intrinsic mydriatic properties)

▼ PoM **Ocufen**® (Allergan)
Ophthalmic solution (= eye-drops), flurbiprofen sodium 0.03%, polyvinyl alcohol (Liquifilm®) 1.4%. Net price 10 × 0.4 mL = £38.90

PARAFFIN, YELLOW, SOFT

Indications: see notes above

Lubrifilm® (Cusi)
Eye ointment, yellow soft paraffin 80%, liquid paraffin 10%, wool fat 10%. Net price 4 g = £1.68
Simple Eye Ointment, liquid paraffin 10%, wool fat 10%, in yellow soft paraffin. Net price 4 g = £1.30

SODIUM CHLORIDE

Indications: irrigation, including first-aid removal of harmful substances

Sodium Chloride 0.9% Solutions
See section 13.11.1
Balanced Salt Solution
Solution (sterile), sodium chloride 0.64%, sodium acetate 0.39%, sodium citrate 0.17%, calcium chloride 0.048%, magnesium chloride 0.03%, potassium chloride 0.075%.
Available from Alcon (15 mL and 30 mL) and from CIBA Vision (15 mL)

Single use
Minims® **Sodium Chloride** (S&N Pharm.)
Eye-drops, sodium chloride 0.9%. Net price 20 × 0.5 mL = £4.92

SODIUM HYALURONATE

A visco-elastic polymer normally present in the aqueous and vitreous humour
Indications: used during surgical procedures on the eye
Side-effects: occasional hypersensitivity (avian origin); occasional transient rise in intra-ocular pressure

PoM **Healonid**® (Pharmacia)
Injection, sodium hyaluronate 10 mg/mL in disposable syringes, net price 0.5 mL = £44.87, 0.75 mL = £67.24

ZINC SULPHATE

Indications; Cautions: see notes above

Zinc Sulphate (Non-proprietary)
Eye-drops, zinc sulphate 0.25%. Net price 10 mL = £2.00
Note. Eye-drops containing zinc sulphate 0.25% also available from Rhône-Poulenc Rorer (Sootheye® with Autodrop®)

DIAGNOSTIC PREPARATIONS

FLUORESCEIN SODIUM

Indications: detection of lesions and foreign bodies

Minims® **Fluorescein Sodium** (S&N Pharm.)
Eye-drops, fluorescein sodium 1 or 2%. Net price 20 × 0.5 mL (both) = £4.92

ROSE BENGAL

Indications: detection of lesions and foreign bodies

Minims® **Rose Bengal** (S&N Pharm.)
Eye-drops, rose bengal 1%. Net price 20 × 0.5 mL = £5.75

11.9   Contact lenses

Many patients wear these lenses and special care is required in prescribing eye preparations for them. Unless medically indicated the lenses should not be worn during treatment. If the patient is wearing hard lenses the use of eye-drops containing anti-inflammatory drugs over long periods of time is to be deprecated. Some drugs can spoil hydrophilic soft lenses. Therefore unless eye-drops are specifically indicated as safe to use with hydrophilic contact lenses, the lenses should be removed before instillation and not worn during the period of treatment.

12:Drugs used in the treatment of diseases of the
EAR, NOSE, and OROPHARYNX

In this chapter, drug treatment is discussed under the following headings:

12.1 Drugs acting on the ear
12.2 Drugs acting on the nose
12.3 Drugs acting on the oropharynx

12.1 Drugs acting on the ear

12.1.1 Otitis externa
12.1.2 Otitis media
12.1.3 Removal of ear wax

12.1.1 Otitis externa

Otitis externa is an inflammatory reaction of the meatal skin. It is important to exclude an underlying chronic otitis media before treatment is commenced. Many cases recover after thorough cleansing of the external ear canal by suction, dry mopping, or gentle syringing. A frequent problem in resistant cases is the difficulty in applying lotions and ointments satisfactorily to the relatively inaccessible affected skin. The most effective method is to introduce a ribbon gauze dressing soaked with **corticosteroid** ear drops or with an astringent such as **aluminium acetate** solution. When this is not practical, the ear should be gently cleaned with a probe covered in cotton wool and the patient encouraged to lie with the affected ear uppermost for ten minutes after the canal has been filled with a liberal quantity of the appropriate solution.

If infection is present, a topical anti-infective which is not used systemically (such as **neomycin** or **clioquinol**) may be used, but for only about a week as excessive use may result in fungal infections; these may be difficult to treat and require expert advice. Sensitivity to the anti-infective or solvent may occur and resistance to antibacterials is a possibility with prolonged use. **Chloramphenicol** may also be used but the ear drops contain propylene glycol and cause sensitivity in about 10% of patients (the eye ointment can be used instead [unlicensed indication]). Solutions containing an anti-infective and a corticosteroid (such as Locorten-Vioform®) are used for treating cases where infection is present with inflammation and eczema. The CSM has warned that when otitis externa is treated topically with preparations containing chlorhexidine, aminoglycosides (e.g. neomycin, framycetin), or polymyxins in patients who have a perforation of the tympanic membrane (ear drum), there is an increased risk of drug-induced deafness. It is therefore important to ensure that there is no perforation in such patients before prescription of these preparations. In the presence of a perforation many specialists, however, do use these drops cautiously in patients with *otitis media*, see section 12.1.2.

An acute infection may cause severe pain and a systemic antibiotic is required with a simple analgesic such as paracetamol. When a resistant staphylococcal infection (a boil) is present in the external auditory meatus, **flucloxacillin** is the drug of choice (see section 5.1, Table 1).

The skin of the pinna adjacent to the ear canal is often affected by eczema. Topical corticosteroid creams and ointments (see section 13.4) are then required, but prolonged use should be avoided.

ASTRINGENT PREPARATIONS

ALUMINIUM ACETATE
Indications: inflammation in otitis externa (see notes above)

Aluminium Acetate Ear drops (13%) consists of aluminium acetate solution, BP.
Insert into the meatus or apply on a gauze wick which should be kept saturated with the ear drops
Available from manufacturers of 'special order' products
Aluminium Acetate Ear drops (8%)
Prepared by diluting 8 parts of aluminium acetate solution, BP, with 5 parts of purified water, freshly boiled and cooled; it must be freshly prepared. Directions as above

ANTI-INFLAMMATORY PREPARATIONS

BETAMETHASONE SODIUM PHOSPHATE
Indications: eczematous inflammation in otitis externa (see notes above)
Cautions: avoid prolonged use
Contra-indications: untreated infection

PoM Betnesol® (Evans)
Drops (for ear, eye, or nose), betamethasone sodium phosphate 0.1%. Net price 10 mL = £1.31
Additives: include benzalkonium chloride
Ear, apply 2–3 drops every 2–3 hours; reduce frequency when relief obtained; *eye*, see section 11.4.1; *nose*, see section 12.2.1
PoM Vista-Methasone® (Daniels)
Drops (for ear, eye, or nose), betamethasone sodium phosphate 0.1%. Net price 5 mL = £1.05; 10 mL = £1.28
Additives: include benzalkonium chloride
Ear, apply 2–3 drops every 3–4 hours; reduce frequency when relief obtained; *eye*, see section 11.4.1; *nose*, see section 12.2.1

PREDNISOLONE SODIUM PHOSPHATE
Indications: eczematous inflammation in otitis externa (see notes above)
Cautions: avoid prolonged use
Contra-indications: untreated infection

PoM Predsol® (Evans)

Drops (for ear or eye), prednisolone sodium phosphate 0.5%. Net price 10 mL = £1.31

Additives: include benzalkonium chloride

Ear, apply 2–3 drops every 2–3 hours; reduce frequency when relief obtained; *eye*, see section 11.4.1

ANTI-INFECTIVE PREPARATIONS

CHLORAMPHENICOL

Indications: bacterial infection in otitis externa (but see notes above)

Cautions: avoid prolonged use (see notes above)

Side-effects: high incidence of sensitivity reactions to vehicle

PoM Chloramphenicol (Non-proprietary)

Ear drops, chloramphenicol 5% in propylene glycol. Net price 10 mL = £1.10

Apply 2–3 drops into the ear 2–3 times daily

CLIOQUINOL

Indications: mild bacterial or fungal infections in otitis externa (see notes above)

Cautions: avoid prolonged use (see notes above)

Side-effects: local sensitivity; stains skin and clothing

With corticosteroid

PoM Locorten-Vioform® (Zyma)

Ear drops, clioquinol 1%, flumethasone pivalate 0.02%. Net price 7.5 mL = £1.02

Apply 2–3 drops into the ear twice daily for up to 7–10 days

CLOTRIMAZOLE

Indications: fungal infection in otitis externa (see notes above)

Side-effects: occasional skin irritation or sensitivity

Canesten® (Baypharm)

Solution, clotrimazole 1% in polyethylene glycol (macrogol 400). Net price 20 mL = £2.32

Ear, apply 2–3 times daily continuing for at least 14 days after disappearance of infection; *skin*, see section 13.10.2

FRAMYCETIN SULPHATE

Indications; Cautions; Side-effects: see under Gentamicin

Preparations

Ingredient of compound anti-infective ear preparations (see next page)

GENTAMICIN

Indications: bacterial infection in otitis externa (see notes above)

Cautions: avoid prolonged use; slight risk of ototoxicity increased if perforated eardrum (see notes above); pregnancy and breast-feeding

Side-effects: local sensitivity

PoM Cidomycin® (Roussel)

Drops (for ear or eye), gentamicin 0.3% (as sulphate). Net price 8 mL = £1.31

Additives: include benzalkonium chloride, disodium edetate

Ear, apply 2–4 drops 3–4 times daily and at night; *eye*, see section 11.3.1

PoM Garamycin® (Schering-Plough)

Drops (for ear or eye), gentamicin 0.3% (as sulphate). Net price 10 mL = £1.79

Additives: include benzalkonium chloride

Ear, apply 3–4 drops 3–4 times daily; reduce frequency when relief obtained; *eye*, see section 11.3.1

PoM Genticin® (Roche)

Drops (for ear or eye), gentamicin 0.3% (as sulphate). Net price 10 mL = £2.00

Additives: include benzalkonium chloride

Ear, apply 2–3 drops 3–4 times daily and at night; *eye*, see section 11.3.1

With corticosteroid

PoM Gentisone HC® (Roche)

Ear drops, gentamicin 0.3% (as sulphate), hydrocortisone acetate 1%. Net price 10 mL = £4.00

Additives: include benzalkonium chloride

Apply 2–4 drops into the ear 3–4 times daily and at night

NEOMYCIN SULPHATE

Indications: bacterial infection in otitis externa (see notes above)

Cautions: avoid prolonged use (see notes above); slight risk of ototoxicity increased if perforated eardrum (see notes above)

Side-effects: local sensitivity

With corticosteroid

PoM Audicort® (Lederle)

Ear drops, neomycin (as neomycin undecenoate) 0.35%, triamcinolone acetonide 0.1%. Net price 10 mL = £7.31

Apply 2–5 drops into the ear 3–4 times daily; CHILD not recommended

PoM Betnesol-N® (Evans)

Drops (for ear, eye, or nose), betamethasone sodium phosphate 0.1%, neomycin sulphate 0.5%. Net price 10 mL = £1.35

Additives: include benzalkonium chloride

Ear, apply 2–3 drops 3–4 times daily; *eye*, see section 11.4.1; *nose*, section 12.2.3

PoM Neo-Cortef® (Cusi)

Drops (for ear or eye), hydrocortisone acetate 1.5%, neomycin sulphate 0.5%. Net price 5 mL = £4.24

Additives: include miripirium chloride (myristyl-gamma-picolinium chloride)

Ear, apply 2–3 drops 3–4 times daily; *eye*, see section 11.4.1

Ointment (for ear or eye), hydrocortisone acetate 1.5%, neomycin sulphate 0.5%. Net price 3.9 g = £3.33

Ear, apply 1–2 times daily; *eye*, see section 11.4.1

PoM Otomize® (Stafford-Miller)

Ear spray, dexamethasone 0.1%, neomycin sulphate 3250 units/mL, glacial acetic acid 2%. Net price 5-mL pump-action aerosol unit = £3.85

Apply 1 metered spray into the ear 3 times daily

PoM Predsol-N® (Evans)

Drops (for ear or eye), neomycin sulphate 0.5%, prednisolone sodium phosphate 0.5%. Net price 10 mL = £1.20

Additives: include thiomersal

Ear, apply 2–3 drops 3–4 times daily; *eye*, see section 11.4.1

PoM Vista-Methasone N® (Daniels)

Drops (for ear, eye, or nose), betamethasone sodium phosphate 0.1%, neomycin sulphate 0.5%. Net price 5 mL = £1.12; 10 mL = £1.33

Additives: include thiomersal

Ear, apply 2–3 drops every 3–4 hours; reduce frequency when relief obtained; *eye*, see section 11.4.1; *nose*, section 12.2.3

TETRACYCLINE HYDROCHLORIDE

Indications: susceptible bacterial infection in otitis externa (see notes above)

Cautions: avoid prolonged use

Side-effects: local sensitivity; stains skin and clothing

PoM Achromycin® (Lederle)

Ointment (for ear or eye), tetracycline hydrochloride 1%. Net price 3.5 g = 68p

Ear, apply 1–2 times daily; *eye*, see section 11.3.1

OTHER COMPOUND ANTI-INFECTIVE PREPARATIONS

PoM Otosporin® (Wellcome)

Ear drops, hydrocortisone 1%, neomycin sulphate 0.439%, polymyxin B sulphate 0.119%. Net price 5 mL = £2.15; 10 mL = £4.30

Apply 3 drops into the ear 3–4 times daily

PoM Sofradex® (Roussel)

Drops (for ear or eye), dexamethasone (as sodium metasulphobenzoate) 0.05%, framycetin sulphate 0.5%, gramicidin 0.005%. Net price 10 mL = £3.90

Ear, apply 2–3 drops 3–4 times daily; *eye*, see section 11.4.1

Ointment (for ear or eye), dexamethasone 0.05%, framycetin sulphate 0.5%, gramicidin 0.005%. Net price 3 g = £1.95

Ear, apply 1–2 times daily; *eye*, see section 11.4.1

PoM Terra-Cortril® (Pfizer)

Ear suspension (= ear drops), hydrocortisone acetate 15 mg, oxytetracycline 5 mg (as hydrochloride), polymyxin B sulphate 10 000 units/mL. Net price 5 mL = £2.06

Apply 2–4 drops into the ear 3 times daily

PoM Tri-Adcortyl Otic® (Squibb)

Ear ointment, gramicidin 0.025%, neomycin 0.25% (as sulphate), nystatin 3.33%, triamcinolone acetonide 0.1% in Plastibase®. Net price 10 g = £1.58

Apply into the ear 2–4 times daily

OTHER AURAL PREPARATIONS

Choline salicylate is a mild analgesic but it is of doubtful value when applied topically. There is no place for the use of local anaesthetics in ear drops.

Audax® (Napp)

Ear drops, choline salicylate 20%, glycerol 12.6%. Net price 8 mL = £1.67

12.1.2   Otitis media

Acute otitis media is the commonest cause of severe pain in small children and recurrent attacks, especially in infants, are particularly distressing. *Otitis media with effusion* ('glue ear') is present in about 10% of the child population and in 90% of children with cleft palates; this condition should be referred to hospital because of the risk of permanent damage to middle ear function and impaired language development. Chronic otitis media is thought to be a legacy from untreated or resistant cases of otitis media with effusion.

Local treatment of *acute otitis media* is ineffective and there is no place for drops containing a local anaesthetic. Many attacks are viral in origin and need only treatment with a **simple analgesic** such as paracetamol for pain. Severe attacks of bacterial origin should be treated with **systemic antibiotics**; bacterial examination of any discharge is helpful in selecting the appropriate treatment (see section 5.1, Table 1). Again, simple analgesics such as paracetamol are used to relieve pain. In *recurrent acute otitis media* a daily dose of a prophylactic antibiotic (trimethoprim or erythromycin) during the winter months can be tried.

The organisms recovered from patients with *chronic otitis media* are often opportunists living in the debris, keratin, and necrotic bone present in the middle ear and mastoid. Thorough cleansing with an aural suction tube may completely control infection of many years duration. Acute exacerbations of chronic infection may require systemic antibiotics (see section 5.1, Table 1). A swab should be taken to determine the organism present and its antibiotic sensitivity. Unfortunately the culture often produces *Pseudomonas aeruginosa* and *Proteus* spp, sensitive only to parenteral antibiotics. Local debridement of the meatal and middle ear contents may then be followed by topical treatment with ribbon gauze dressings as for otitis externa (section 12.1.1). This is particularly true with infections in mastoid cavities when dusting powders can also be tried.

In the presence of a perforation, however, many specialists use ear drops containing **aminoglycosides** (e.g. neomycin) or **polymyxins**, if the otitis media has failed to settle with systemic antibiotics; it is considered that the pus in the middle ear associated with otitis media carries a higher risk of ototoxicity than the drops themselves.

12.1.3   Removal of ear wax

Wax is a normal bodily secretion which provides a protective film on the meatal skin and need only be removed if it causes deafness or interferes with a proper view of the ear drum. As a general rule syringing is best avoided in patients with a history of recurring otitis externa, a perforated ear drum, or previous ear surgery. A person who has hearing only in one ear should not have that ear syringed because even a very slight risk of damage is unacceptable in this situation.

Wax may be removed by syringing with warm water. If necessary, wax can be softened with sim-

---

ple remedies such as **olive oil** or **almond oil** before syringing. The patient should lie with the affected ear uppermost for 5 to 10 minutes after a generous amount of the solution has been introduced into the ear. Some proprietary preparations containing organic solvents can cause irritation of the meatal skin, and in most cases the simple remedies which are indicated above are just as effective and less likely to cause irritation. **Docusate sodium** is an ingredient in a number of proprietary preparations.

Almond Oil
Allow to warm to room temperature before use.
Olive Oil
Allow to warm to room temperature before use.
Sodium Bicarbonate Ear Drops, BP
Ear drops, sodium bicarbonate 5%
> Extemporaneous preparations should be recently prepared according to the following formula: sodium bicarbonate 500 mg, glycerol 3 mL, freshly boiled and cooled purified water to 10 mL

Cerumol® (LAB)
Ear drops, chlorbutol 5%, paradichlorobenzene 2%, arachis oil 57%. Net price 11 mL = £1.07

Dioctyl® (Schwarz)
Ear drops, docusate sodium 5% in macrogol. Net price 10 mL = £1.40

Exterol® (Dermal)
Ear drops, urea-hydrogen peroxide complex 5% in glycerol. Net price 8 mL = £1.89

Molcer® (Wallace Mfg)
Ear drops, docusate sodium 5%. Net price 15 mL = £1.08

Otex® (DDD)
Ear drops, urea hydrogen peroxide 5%. Net price 8 mL = £1.83

Waxsol® (Norgine)
Ear drops, docusate sodium 0.5%. Net price 10 mL = 98p

12.2   Drugs acting on the nose

12.2.1 Drugs used in nasal allergy
12.2.2 Topical nasal decongestants
12.2.3 Anti-infective nasal preparations

Rhinitis is often self-limiting and sinusitis is best treated with antibiotics (see section 5.1, Table 1). There are few indications for the use of sprays and drops except in allergic rhinitis where topical preparations of corticosteroids or sodium cromoglycate have much to offer. Most other preparations contain sympathomimetic drugs which may damage the nasal cilia and their prolonged use causes mucosal oedema and severe nasal obstruction (rhinitis medicamentosa). Symptomatic relief in chronic nasal obstruction may be obtained with **systemic nasal decongestants** (see section 3.10). Douching the nose with salt and water is **not** recommended.

12.2.1   Drugs used in nasal allergy

Mild cases are controlled by **oral antihistamines** and **systemic nasal decongestants** (see sections 3.4.1 and 3.10). Many patients with severe symptoms can now expect relief from topical preparations of **corticosteroids** or **sodium cromoglycate**.

Although sodium cromoglycate is less effective than a topical corticosteroid, it is often the first choice in children. Treatment should begin 2 to 3 weeks before the hay fever season commences and may have to be continued for months or even years in some patients. No significant side-effects have been reported. Very disabling symptoms occasionally justify the use of **systemic corticosteroids** for short periods (see section 6.3), for example in students taking important examinations. They may also be used at the beginning of a course of treatment with a corticosteroid spray to relieve severe mucosal oedema and allow the spray to penetrate the nasal cavity.

Azelastine is an antihistamine available as a nasal spray for allergic rhinitis. It is less effective than a topical corticosteroid but probably more effective than cromoglycate.

AZELASTINE HYDROCHLORIDE
Indications: allergic rhinitis
Side-effects: irritation of nasal mucosa; taste disturbance

PoM Rhinolast® (ASTA Medica)
Aqueous nasal spray, azelastine hydrochloride 140 micrograms (0.14 mL)/metered spray. Net price 20 mL (with metered pump) = £12.48
> Apply 140 micrograms (1 spray) into each nostril twice daily; CHILD not recommended

---

BECLOMETHASONE DIPROPIONATE
(Beclometasone Dipropionate)
Indications: allergic and vasomotor rhinitis
Cautions: untreated nasal infection, prolonged use in children, previous treatment with corticosteroids by mouth
Side-effects: sneezing after administration; rarely dryness and irritation of nose and throat, epistaxis

PoM [1]Beconase® (A&H)
Beconase® nasal spray (aerosol), beclomethasone dipropionate 50 micrograms/metered spray. Net price 200-spray unit with applicator = £5.01
Additives: include CFC propellants
> ADULT and CHILD over 6 years, apply 100 micrograms (2 sprays) into each nostril twice daily *or* 50 micrograms (1 spray) into each nostril 3–4 times daily; max. total 400 micrograms (8 sprays) daily

Beconase® aqueous nasal spray (aqueous suspension), beclomethasone dipropionate 50 micrograms/metered spray. Net price 200-spray unit with applicator = £5.01
> ADULT and CHILD over 6 years, apply 100 micrograms (2 sprays) into each nostril twice daily *or* 50 micrograms (1 spray) into each nostril 3–4 times daily; max. total 400 micrograms (8 sprays) daily
> 1. Can be sold to the public for nasal administration (other than by aerosol) if supplied for the treatment of seasonal allergic rhinitis in adults and children over 12 years subject to max. single dose of 100 micrograms per nostril, max. daily dose of 200 micrograms per nostril, and a pack size limit of 200 doses; a proprietary brand (Beconase® Hayfever) is on sale to the public

---

BETAMETHASONE SODIUM PHOSPHATE

Indications; Cautions; Side-effects: see under Beclomethasone Dipropionate

PoM **Betnesol®** (Evans)

Drops (for ear, eye, or nose), betamethasone sodium phosphate 0.1%. Net price 10 mL = £1.31

Additives: include benzalkonium chloride

Nose, apply 2–3 drops into each nostril 2–3 times daily; *ear*, section 12.1.1; *eye*, see section 11.4.1

PoM **Vista-Methasone®** (Daniels)

Drops (for ear, eye, or nose), betamethasone sodium phosphate 0.1%. Net price 5 mL = £1.05, 10 mL = £1.28

Additives: include benzalkonium chloride

Nose, apply 2–3 drops into each nostril twice daily; *ear*, section 12.1.1; *eye*, see section 11.4.1

BUDESONIDE

Indications: allergic and vasomotor rhinitis

Cautions: see under Beclomethasone Dipropionate; also patients with pulmonary tuberculosis

Side-effects: see under Beclomethasone Dipropionate

PoM **Rhinocort®** (Astra)

Rhinocort® nasal aerosol, budesonide 50 micrograms/metered spray, 200-spray unit with nasal adaptor. Net price complete unit = £5.66

Additives: include CFC propellants

ADULT and CHILD over 6 years, apply 200 micrograms (4 sprays) into each nostril once daily in the morning *or* 100 micrograms (2 sprays) into each nostril twice daily, reduced for maintenance

Rhinocort Aqua® nasal spray, budesonide 100 micrograms/metered spray. Net price 100-spray unit = £6.00

ADULT and CHILD over 12 years, apply 200 micrograms (2 sprays) into each nostril once daily in the morning *or* 100 micrograms (1 spray) into each nostril twice daily, reduced for maintenance

FLUNISOLIDE

Indications; Cautions; Side-effects: see under Beclomethasone Dipropionate

PoM **Syntaris®** (Syntex)

Aqueous nasal spray, flunisolide 25 micrograms/0.1 mL metered spray. Net price 240-spray unit with pump and applicator = £5.50

Apply 50 micrograms (2 sprays) into each nostril 2–3 times daily; CHILD over 5 years 25 micrograms (1 spray) into each nostril 3 times daily, reduced for maintenance

FLUTICASONE PROPIONATE

Indications: allergic rhinitis

Cautions; Side-effects: see under Beclomethasone Dipropionate

PoM **Flixonase®** (A&H)

Aqueous nasal spray, fluticasone propionate 50 micrograms/metered spray. Net price 120-spray unit with applicator = £11.43

ADULT and CHILD over 12 years, apply 100 micrograms (2 sprays) into each nostril once daily, preferably in the morning, increased to twice daily if required; max. total 8 sprays daily; CHILD 4–11 years, 50 micrograms (1 spray) into each nostril once daily, increased to twice daily if required; max. total 4 sprays daily

SODIUM CROMOGLYCATE

(Sodium Cromoglicate)

Indications: prophylaxis of allergic rhinitis (see notes above)

Side-effects: local irritation; rarely transient bronchospasm

Rynacrom® (Fisons)

Nasal drops, sodium cromoglycate 2%. Net price 15 mL = £5.08

ADULT and CHILD, instil 2 drops into each nostril 6 times daily

4% aqueous nasal spray, sodium cromoglycate 4% (5.2 mg/squeeze). Net price 22 mL with pump = £8.46

ADULT and CHILD, apply 1 squeeze into each nostril 2–4 times daily

Rynacrom Compound® (Fisons)

Nasal spray, sodium cromoglycate 2% (2.6 mg/metered spray) and xylometazoline hydrochloride 0.025% (32.5 micrograms/metered spray). Net price 26 mL with pump = £6.66

Apply 1 spray into each nostril 4 times daily

Note. A proprietary brand of sodium cromoglycate 2% and xylometazoline hydrochloride 0.025% (Resiston One®) is on sale to the public

Vividrin® (Novex)

Nasal spray, sodium cromoglycate 2%. Net price 15 mL = £5.45

Additives: include benzalkonium chloride

ADULT and CHILD, apply 1 spray into each nostril 4–6 times daily

12.2.2 Topical nasal decongestants

The nasal mucosa is sensitive to changes in the atmospheric temperature and humidity and these alone may cause slight nasal congestion. The nose and nasal sinuses produce a litre of mucus in 24 hours and much of this finds its way silently into the stomach via the nasopharynx. Slight changes in the nasal airway, accompanied by an awareness of mucus passing along the nasopharynx causes some patients to be inaccurately diagnosed as suffering from chronic sinusitis. These symptoms are particularly noticeable in the later stages of the common cold for which there is no effective treatment at the moment; the temptation to use nasal drops should be resisted. **Sodium chloride** 0.9% given as nasal drops may relieve nasal congestion by helping to liquefy mucous secretions.

Symptomatic relief from the nasal congestion associated with vasomotor rhinitis, nasal polypi, and the common cold can be obtained by the short-term use (usually not longer than 7 days) of decongestant nasal drops and sprays. These all contain sympathomimetic drugs which exert their effect by vasoconstriction of the mucosal blood vessels which in turn reduces the thickness of the nasal mucosa. They are of limited value as they can give rise to a rebound phenomenon as their effects wear off, due to a secondary vasodilatation with a subsequent temporary increase in nasal congestion. This in turn tempts the further use of the decongestant, leading to a vicious circle of events. **Ephedrine nasal drops** is the safest sympathomimetic preparation and can give relief for several hours. The more potent sympathomimetic drugs oxymetazoline, phenylephrine, and xylometazoline are more likely to cause a rebound effect. **All** of these preparations may cause a hypertensive crisis if used during treatment with a monoamine-oxidase inhibitor.

Non-allergic watery rhinorrhoea often responds well to treatment with **ipratropium bromide**.

Inhalations of **warm moist air** are useful in the treatment of symptoms of acute infective conditions, and the use of compounds containing volatile substances such as menthol and eucalyptus may encourage their use (see section 3.8). There is no evidence that nasal preparations containing antihistamines and anti-infective agents have any therapeutic effect.

Systemic nasal decongestants—see section 3.10.

SYMPATHOMIMETICS

EPHEDRINE HYDROCHLORIDE

Indications: nasal congestion

Cautions: avoid excessive or prolonged use; caution in infants under 3 months (no good evidence of value—if irritation occurs might narrow nasal passage); **interactions:** Appendix 1 (sympathomimetics)

Side-effects: local irritation; after excessive use tolerance with diminished effect, rebound congestion

Administration: see below

Ephedrine Nasal Drops, BP

Nasal drops, ephedrine hydrochloride in a suitable aqueous vehicle

Note. The BP directs that if no strength is specified 0.5% drops should be supplied; net price 10 mL = 95p

Instil 1–2 drops into each nostril up to 3 or 4 times daily when required

---

XYLOMETAZOLINE HYDROCHLORIDE

Indications: nasal congestion

Cautions; Side-effects: see under Ephedrine Hydrochloride

Xylometazoline Nasal Drops, xylometazoline hydrochloride 0.1%, net price 10 mL = £1.19

Instil 2–3 drops into each nostril 2–3 times daily when required; max. duration 7 days; not recommended for children under 12 years

Xylometazoline Nasal Drops, Paediatric, xylometazoline hydrochloride 0.05%, net price 10 mL = £1.19

CHILD over 3 months instil 1–2 drops into each nostril 1–2 times daily when required (not recommended for infants under 3 months of age, doctor's advice only under 2 years); max. duration 7 days

Note. The brand name NHSOtrivine® (Zyma) is used for xylometazoline adult nasal drops 0.1%, children's nasal drops 0.05%, and adult nasal spray 0.1%

Sympathomimetic nasal preparations on sale to the public (not prescribable on the NHS) include: **Afrazine®** (oxymetazoline), **Dristan®** (oxymetazoline), **Fenox®** (phenylephrine), **Otrivine®** (xylometazoline—prescribable in non-proprietary form as nasal drops, see above), **Sudafed®** nasal spray (oxymetazoline)

ANTIMUSCARINIC

IPRATROPIUM BROMIDE

Indications: watery rhinorrhoea associated with perennial rhinitis

Cautions; Side-effects: see section 3.1.2; avoid spraying near eyes

Administration: apply 20–40 micrograms (1–2 puffs) into affected nostril up to 4 times daily; not recommended for children under 12 years

PoM **Rinatec®** (Boehringer Ingelheim)

Nasal spray, ipratropium bromide 20 micrograms/metered spray. Net price 200-dose unit = £4.59

12.2.3   Anti-infective nasal preparations

There is **no** evidence that topical anti-infective nasal preparations have any therapeutic value; for elimination of nasal staphylococci, see below.

Systemic treatment of sinusitis—see section 5.1, Table 1.

PoM **Betnesol-N®** (Evans)

Drops (for ear, eye, or nose), betamethasone sodium phosphate 0.1%, neomycin sulphate 0.5%. Net price 10 mL = £1.35

Additives: include benzalkonium chloride

Nose, apply 2–3 drops into each nostril 2–3 times daily; *eye,* see section 11.4.1; *ear,* see section 12.1.1

PoM **Dexa-Rhinaspray®** (Boehringer Ingelheim)

Nasal inhalation, dexamethasone 21-isonicotinate 20 micrograms, neomycin sulphate 100 micrograms, tramazoline hydrochloride 120 micrograms/metered inhalation. Net price 125-dose unit = £1.95

PoM **Locabiotal®** (Servier)

Aerosol spray, fusafungine 125 micrograms/metered inhalation. Net price 200-dose unit with nasal and oral adaptors = £1.55

PoM **Vista-Methasone N®** (Daniels)

Drops (for ear, eye, or nose), betamethasone sodium phosphate 0.1%, neomycin sulphate 0.5%. Net price 5 mL = £1.12, 10 mL = £1.33

Additives: include thiomersal

Nose, apply 2–3 drops into each nostril twice daily; *eye,* see section 11.4.1; *ear,* see section 12.1.1

NASAL STAPHYLOCOCCI

Elimination of organisms such as staphylococci from the nasal vestibule can be achieved by the use of a cream containing **chlorhexidine and neomycin** (Naseptin®), but re-colonisation frequently occurs. Coagulase-positive staphylococci can be obtained from the noses of 40% of the population.

A nasal ointment containing **mupirocin** is also available; it should probably be kept in reserve for resistant cases. To avoid the development of resistance its use in hospital should, if possible, be avoided and it should not be used for longer than 10 days.

PoM Bactroban Nasal® (Beecham)
Nasal ointment, mupirocin 2% in white soft paraffin basis. Net price 3 g = £5.15
For eradication of nasal carriage of staphylococci, including methicillin-resistant *Staphylococcus aureus* (MRSA), apply 2–3 times daily to the inner surface of each nostril

PoM Naseptin® (Zeneca)
Cream, chlorhexidine hydrochloride 0.1%, neomycin sulphate 0.5%. Do not dilute. Net price 15 g = 99p
For eradication of nasal carriage of staphylococci, apply to nostrils 4 times daily for 10 days; for preventing nasal carriage of staphylococci apply to nostrils twice daily

12.3 Drugs acting on the oropharynx

12.3.1 Drugs for oral ulceration and inflammation
12.3.2 Oropharyngeal anti-infective drugs
12.3.3 Lozenges, sprays, and gels
12.3.4 Mouthwashes, gargles, and dentifrices

12.3.1 Drugs for oral ulceration and inflammation

Ulceration of the oral mucosa may be caused by trauma (physical or chemical), recurrent aphthae, infections, carcinoma, dermatological disorders, nutritional deficiencies, gastro-intestinal disease, haematopoietic disorders, and drug therapy. It is important to establish the diagnosis in each case as the majority of these lesions require specific management in addition to local treatment. Patients with an unexplained mouth ulcer of more than 3 weeks' duration require urgent referral to hospital to exclude oral cancer. Local treatment aims at protecting the ulcerated area, or at relieving pain or reducing inflammation.

SIMPLE MOUTHWASHES. A **saline** or **compound thymol glycerin** mouthwash may relieve the pain of traumatic ulceration. The mouthwash is made up with warm water and used at frequent intervals until the discomfort and swelling subsides.

ANTISEPTIC MOUTHWASHES. Secondary bacterial infection may be a feature of any mucosal ulceration; it can increase discomfort and delay healing. Use of a **chlorhexidine** or **povidone-iodine** mouthwash is often beneficial and may accelerate healing of recurrent aphthae.

MECHANICAL PROTECTION. **Carmellose gelatin paste** may relieve some discomfort arising from ulceration by protecting the ulcer site. The paste adheres to the mucosa, but is difficult to apply effectively to some parts of the mouth.

CORTICOSTEROIDS. Topical corticosteroid therapy may be used for different forms of oral ulceration. In the case of aphthous ulcers it is most effective if applied in the 'prodromal' phase.

Thrush or other types of candidiasis are recognised complications of corticosteroid treatment.

Hydrocortisone lozenges are allowed to dissolve next to an ulcer and are useful in recurrent aphthae, erosive lichen planus, discoid lupus erythematosus, and benign mucous membrane pemphigoid.

Triamcinolone dental paste is designed to keep the corticosteroid in contact with the mucosa for long enough to permit penetration of the lesion, but is difficult for patients to apply properly.

Systemic corticosteroid therapy is reserved for severe conditions such as pemphigus vulgaris (see section 6.3.4).

LOCAL ANALGESICS. Local analgesics have a limited role in the management of oral ulceration. When applied topically their action is of a relatively short duration so that analgesia cannot be maintained continuously throughout the day. The main indication for a topical local analgesic is to relieve the pain of otherwise intractable oral ulceration particularly when it is due to major aphthae. For this purpose lignocaine 5% ointment or lozenges containing a local anaesthetic are applied to the ulcer. When local anaesthetics are used in the mouth care must be taken not to produce anaesthesia of the pharynx before meals as this might lead to choking.

Benzydamine mouthwash or spray may be useful in palliating the discomfort associated with a variety of ulcerative conditions. It has also been found to be effective in reducing the discomfort of post-irradiation mucositis. Some patients find the full-strength mouthwash causes some stinging and, for them, it should be diluted with an equal volume of water.

Choline salicylate dental gel has some analgesic action and may provide relief for recurrent aphthae, but excessive application or confinement under a denture irritates the mucosa and can itself cause ulceration. Benefit in teething may merely be due to pressure of application (comparable with biting a teething ring); excessive use can lead to salicylate poisoning.

OTHER PREPARATIONS. **Carbenoxolone** gel or mouthwash may be of some value. **Tetracycline** rinsed in the mouth may also be of value.

BENZYDAMINE HYDROCHLORIDE

Indications: painful inflammatory conditions of oropharynx

Side-effects: occasional numbness or stinging

Difflam® (3M)

Oral rinse, green, benzydamine hydrochloride 0.15%. Net price 300 mL = £4.10

Rinse or gargle, using 15 mL (diluted if stinging occurs) every 1½–3 hours as required, usually for not more than 7 days; not suitable for children under 12 years

Spray, benzydamine hydrochloride 0.15%. Net price 30-mL unit = £3.57

ADULT, 4–8 puffs onto affected area every 1½–3 hours; CHILD under 6 years 1 puff per 4 kg to max. 4 puffs every 1½–3 hours; 6–12 years 4 puffs every 1½–3 hours

CARBENOXOLONE SODIUM

Indications: mild oral and perioral lesions

Bioral Gel® (Sterling Health)

Gel, carbenoxolone sodium 2% in adhesive basis. Net price 5 g = £2.00

Apply after meals and at bedtime

PoM Bioplex® (Thames)

Mouthwash granules, carbenoxolone sodium 1% (20 mg/sachet). Net price 24 × 2-g sachets = £9.60

For mouth ulcers, rinse with 1 sachet in 30–50 mL of warm water 3 times daily and at bedtime

CARMELLOSE SODIUM

Indications: mechanical protection of oral and perioral lesions

Orabase® (ConvaTec)

Oral paste, carmellose sodium 16.58%, pectin 16.58%, gelatin 16.58%, in Plastibase®. Net price 30 g = £1.64; 100 g = £3.63

Apply a thin layer when necessary after meals

Orahesive® (ConvaTec)

Powder, carmellose sodium, pectin, gelatin, equal parts. Net price 25 g = £1.88

Sprinkle on the affected area

CORTICOSTEROIDS

Indications: oral and perioral lesions

Contra-indications: untreated oral infection

Side-effects: occasional exacerbation of local infection

PoM Adcortyl in Orabase® (Squibb)

Oral paste, triamcinolone acetonide 0.1% in adhesive basis. Net price 10 g = £1.27

ADULT and CHILD, apply a thin layer 2–4 times daily; do not rub in; use limited to 5 days for children and short-term use also advised for elderly

Corlan® (Evans)

Pellets (= lozenges), hydrocortisone 2.5 mg (as sodium succinate). Net price 20 = £1.40

ADULT and CHILD, 1 lozenge 4 times daily, allowed to dissolve slowly in the mouth in contact with the ulcer; if ulcers recur rapidly treatment may be continued for a period at reduced dosage

LOCAL ANAESTHETICS

Indications: relief of pain in oral lesions

Cautions: avoid prolonged use; hypersensitivity

Lozenges containing local anaesthetics are available with antiseptics, see section 12.3.3

SALICYLATES

Indications: mild oral and perioral lesions

Cautions: frequent application, especially in children, may give rise to salicylate poisoning

Note. CSM warning on aspirin and Reye's syndrome does not apply to non-aspirin salicylates or to topical preparations such as teething gels

Choline salicylate

Choline Salicylate Dental Gel, BP

Oral gel, choline salicylate 8.7% in a flavoured gel basis

Available as Bonjela® (R&C), net price 15 g (sugar-free) = £1.23; Teejel® (Seton), 10 g = 83p

Apply ½-inch of gel with gentle massage not more often than every 3 hours; CHILD over 4 months ¼-inch of gel not more often than every 3 hours; max. 6 applications daily

Salicylic acid

Pyralvex® (Norgine)

Oral paint, brown, anthraquinone glycosides 5%, salicylic acid 1%. Net price 10 mL with brush = £1.41

Apply 3–4 times daily

TETRACYCLINE

Indications: severe recurrent aphthous ulceration; oral herpes (section 12.3.2)

Side-effects: fungal superinfection

For side-effects, cautions and contra-indications relating to systemic administration of tetracyclines see section 5.1.3

Local application

For preparation of a mouthwash, the contents of a 250-mg tetracycline capsule (see section 5.1.3) can be stirred into a small amount of water, then held in the mouth for 2–3 minutes 3 times daily for not longer than 3 days followed by a break of at least 3 days before treatment is recommenced (to avoid oral thrush); it should preferably not be swallowed

Note. Tetracycline stains teeth; avoid in children under 12 years of age

12.3.2   Oropharyngeal anti-infective drugs

The most common cause of a sore throat is a viral infection which does not benefit from anti-infective treatment. Streptococcal sore throats require systemic **penicillin** therapy (see section 5.1.1). Acute ulcerative gingivitis (Vincent's infection) responds to systemic **metronidazole** 200 mg 3 times daily for 3 days (see section 5.1.11).

Preparations administered in the dental surgery for the local treatment of periodontal disease include gels of metronidazole (*Elyzol*®, Dumex) and of minocycline (*Dentomycin*®, Lederle).

FUNGAL INFECTIONS

Candida albicans may cause thrush and other forms of stomatitis which are sometimes a sequel to the use of broad-spectrum antibiotics or cytotoxics; withdrawing the causative drug may lead to rapid resolution. Otherwise, **nystatin, amphotericin,** or **miconazole** may be effective.

AMPHOTERICIN

Indications: oral and perioral fungal infections

PoM Fungilin® (Squibb)
Lozenges, yellow, amphotericin 10 mg. Net price 6 × 10 lozenge-pack = £3.95. Label: 9, 24, counselling, after food
Dissolve 1 lozenge slowly in the mouth 4 times daily, may require 10–15 days' treatment (continued for 48 hours after lesions have resolved); increase to 8 daily if infection severe
Suspension, yellow, sugar-free, amphotericin 100 mg/mL. Net price 12 mL with pipette = £2.31. Label: 9, counselling, use of pipette, hold in mouth, after food
Place 1 mL in the mouth after food and retain near lesions 4 times daily for 14 days (continued for 48 hours after lesions have resolved)

MICONAZOLE

Indications: oral fungal infections
Cautions: pregnancy; avoid in porphyria (see section 9.8.2); **interactions:** Appendix 1 (miconazole)

PoM ¹Daktarin® (Janssen)
Oral gel, sugar-free, miconazole 25 mg/mL. Net price 80 g = £5.00. Label: 9, counselling, hold in mouth, after food
Place 5 10 mL in the mouth after food 4 times daily; retain near lesions; CHILD under 2 years 2.5 mL twice daily, 2–6 years 5 mL twice daily, over 6 years 5 mL 4 times daily
Localised lesions, smear affected area with clean finger; a 15 g tube (net price £1.95) also available
1. 15-g tube can be sold to the public
Tablets—see section 5.2

NYSTATIN

Indications: oral and perioral fungal infections
Dose: (as pastilles or as suspension) 100 000 units 4 times daily after food, usually for 7 days (continued for 48 hours after lesions have resolved)
Note. Immunosuppressed patients may require higher doses (e.g. 500 000 units 4 times daily)

PoM Nystan® (Squibb)
Pastilles, yellow/brown, nystatin 100 000 units. Net price 28 pastille-pack = £3.24. Label: 9, 24, counselling, after food
Suspension, yellow, nystatin 100 000 units/mL. Net price 30 mL with pipette = £2.05. Label: 9, counselling, use of pipette, hold in mouth, after food

Suspension, gluten-, lactose-, and sugar-free, nystatin 100 000 units/mL when reconstituted with water. Measure with pipette. Net price 24 mL with pipette = £1.67. Label: 9, counselling, use of pipette, hold in mouth, after food

PoM Nystatin-Dome® (Lagap)
Suspension, yellow, nystatin 100 000 units/mL. Net price 30 mL with 1-mL spoon = £2.50. Label: 9, counselling, use of 1-mL spoon, hold in mouth, after food

VIRAL INFECTIONS

The management of herpes infections of the mouth is a soft diet, adequate fluid intake, analgesics as required, and the use of **chlorhexidine** mouthwash (Corsodyl®, section 12.3.4) to control plaque accumulation if toothbrushing is painful. In the case of severe herpetic stomatitis, systemic **acyclovir** is required (see section 5.3).

Herpes infections of the mouth may also respond to **tetracycline** (section 12.3.1) rinsed in the mouth.

Idoxuridine 0.1% paint has been superseded by more effective preparations.

ACYCLOVIR
See section 5.3

TETRACYCLINE
Section 12.3.1

12.3.3 Lozenges, sprays, and gels

There is no convincing evidence that antiseptic lozenges and sprays have a beneficial action and they sometimes irritate and cause sore tongue and sore lips. Some of these preparations also contain local anaesthetics which relieve pain but may cause sensitisation.

In particular preparations containing clioquinol are not recommended.

Bradosol® (Zyma)
Lozenges, sugar-free, green, benzalkonium chloride 500 micrograms. Net price 20 lozenges = £1.02
Dequadin® (Crookes)
Lozenges, orange, dequalinium chloride 250 micrograms. Net price 20 lozenges = 66p
Labosept® (LAB)
Pastilles, red, dequalinium chloride 250 micrograms. Net price 20 pastilles = 68p
PoM Locabiotal® (Servier)
Aerosol spray, section 12.2.3
Merocets® (Merrell)
Lozenges, yellow, cetylpyridinium chloride 0.066%. Net price 24 lozenges = 94p

Clioquinol
Oralcer® (Vitabiotics)
Lozenges, ivory, ascorbic acid 6 mg, clioquinol 35 mg. Net price 20 lozenges = £1.15

Cautionary label wordings, see inside back cover

With local anaesthetic

Bradosol Plus® (Zyma)

Lozenges, green, lignocaine hydrochloride 5 mg, domiphen bromide 500 micrograms. Net price 24 lozenges = £1.18

Adults and children over 12 years, 1 lozenge sucked every 2–3 hours; max. 8 lozenges daily

Dequacaine® (Crookes)

Lozenges, amber, benzocaine 10 mg, dequalinium chloride 250 micrograms. Net price 24 lozenges = £1.16

Adults and children over 12 years, 1 lozenge sucked every 2 hours or as required; max. 8 lozenges daily

Eludril® (Chefaro)

Aerosol spray, amethocaine hydrochloride 0.015%, chlorhexidine gluconate 0.05%. Net price 55 mL = £2.29

Adults and children over 12 years, 1 spray 3–4 times daily; not immediately before food

Medilave® (Martindale)

Gel, benzocaine 1%, cetylpyridinium chloride 0.01%. Net price 10 g = 61p

Adults, apply thin layer 3–4 times daily; no longer recommended for children under 12 years

Merocaine® (Merrell)

Lozenges, green, benzocaine 10 mg, cetylpyridinium chloride 1.4 mg. Net price 24 lozenges = £1.05

Adults and children over 12 years, 1 lozenge sucked every 2 hours or as required; max. 8 lozenges daily

Tyrozets® (MSD)

Lozenges, pink, benzocaine 5 mg, tyrothricin 1 mg. Net price 24 lozenges = 66p

1 lozenge sucked every 3 hours (max. 8 lozenges daily); reduce dose in children (not for children under 3 years)

Vicks Ultra Chloraseptic® (Procter & Gamble)

Throat spray, benzocaine 1 mg/metered spray. Net price 15 mL = £2.53

Adults and children over 13 years, 3 sprays every 2–3 hours (max. 24 sprays daily); child 6–12 years, 1 spray every 2–3 hours (max. 8 sprays daily)

For teething

Calgel® (Wellcome)

Teething gel, lignocaine hydrochloride 0.33%, cetylpyridinium chloride 0.1%. Net price 10 g = 93p

Apply small quantity to gum up to 6 times daily (no longer recommended for infants under 3 months)

12.3.4   Mouthwashes, gargles, and dentifrices

Mouthwashes have a mechanical cleansing action and freshen the mouth. Warm **compound sodium chloride mouthwash** or **compound thymol glycerin** is as useful as any.

Mouthwashes containing an oxidising agent, such as hydrogen peroxide, may be useful in the treatment of acute ulcerative gingivitis (Vincent's infection) as the organisms involved are anaerobes. It also has a mechanical cleansing effect due to frothing when in contact with oral debris. **Sodium perborate** is similar in effect to hydrogen peroxide.

There is evidence that **chlorhexidine** has a specific effect in inhibiting the formation of plaque on teeth. A chlorhexidine mouthwash may be useful as an adjunct to other oral hygiene measures in cases of oral infection or when toothbrushing is not possible.

There is no convincing evidence that gargles are effective.

CETYLPYRIDINIUM CHLORIDE
Indications: oral hygiene

Merocet® (Merrell)

Solution (= mouthwash or gargle), yellow, cetylpyridinium chloride 0.05%. Net price 200 mL = £1.49

To be used undiluted or diluted with an equal volume of warm water

CHLORHEXIDINE GLUCONATE
Indications: oral hygiene; plaque inhibition

Side-effects: idiosyncratic mucosal irritation; reversible brown staining of teeth

Corsodyl® (SmithKline Beecham)

Dental gel, chlorhexidine gluconate 1%. Net price 50 g = 91p

Brush on the teeth once or twice daily

Mouthwash, chlorhexidine gluconate 0.2% (aniseed or mint-flavoured). Net price 300 mL = £1.38

Rinse the mouth with 10 mL for about 1 minute twice daily

Oral spray, chlorhexidine gluconate 0.2% (mint-flavoured). Net price 60 mL = £3.08

Apply as required to tooth and gingival surfaces using up to max. 12 actuations (approx. 0.14 mL/actutation) twice daily

Eludril® (Chefaro)

Mouthwash, chlorhexidine gluconate 0.1%, chlorbutol 0.5%. Net price 90 mL = £1.16; 250 mL = £2.35; 500 mL = £4.14

Use 10–15 mL in a third of a tumblerful of warm water 2–3 times daily

HEXETIDINE
Indications: oral hygiene

Oraldene® (W-L)

Mouthwash or *gargle*, red, hexetidine 0.1%. Net price 100 mL = 93p; 200 mL = £1.51

Use 15 mL undiluted 2–3 times daily

OXIDISING AGENTS
Indications: oral hygiene, see notes above

Hydrogen Peroxide Mouthwash, DPF, consists of Hydrogen Peroxide Solution 6% (≡ approx. 20 volume) BP

Rinse the mouth for 2–3 minutes with 15 mL in half a tumblerful of warm water 2–3 times daily

Bocasan® (Oral-B Labs)

Mouthwash, sodium perborate 68.6% (buffered). Net price 20 × 1.7-g sachet-pack = £1.68

Use 1 sachet in 30 mL of water 3 times daily after meals

Cautions: Do not use for longer than 7 days because of possible absorption of borate; not recommended in renal impairment or for children under 5 years

---

PHENOL

Indications: oral hygiene

Chloraseptic® (Procter & Gamble)

Mouthwash/gargle, green, phenol 1.4%. Net price 150 mL = £2.18

Use every 2 hours if necessary, undiluted or diluted with an equal volume of water as a mouthwash or gargle (CHILD 6–12 years on doctor's advice only; under 6 years not recommended)

Vicks Ultra Chloraseptic, see section 12.3.3

POVIDONE-IODINE

Indications: oral hygiene

Cautions: pregnancy; breast-feeding

Contra-indications: avoid regular use in patients with thyroid disorders or those receiving lithium therapy

Side-effects: idiosyncratic mucosal irritation and hypersensitivity reactions; may interfere with thyroid-function tests and with tests for occult blood

Betadine® (Seton)

Mouthwash or *gargle,* amber, povidone-iodine 1%. Net price 250 mL = £1.17

Adults and children over 6 years, up to 10 mL undiluted or diluted with an equal quantity of warm water for up to 30 seconds up to 4 times daily for up to 14 days

SODIUM CHLORIDE

Indications: oral hygiene, see notes above

Sodium Chloride Mouthwash, Compound, BP

Mouthwash, sodium bicarbonate 1%, sodium chloride 1.5% in a suitable vehicle with a peppermint flavour.

Extemporaneous preparations should be prepared according to the following formula: sodium chloride 1.5 g, sodium bicarbonate 1 g, concentrated peppermint emulsion 2.5 mL, double strength chloroform water 50 mL, water to 100 mL.

To be diluted with an equal volume of warm water

THYMOL

Indications: oral hygiene, see notes above

Compound Thymol Glycerin, BP 1988, glycerol 10%, thymol 0.05% with colouring and flavouring

To be used undiluted or diluted with 3 volumes of warm water

Mouthwash Solution-tablets, consist of tablets which may contain antimicrobial, colouring, and flavouring agents in a suitable soluble effervescent basis to make a mouthwash suitable for dental purposes.

Dissolve 1 tablet in a tumblerful of warm water

OTHER PREPARATIONS FOR OROPHARYNGEAL USE

Artificial saliva may be indicated for dry mouth. Of the proprietary preparations available, Luborant® is licensed for any condition giving rise to a dry mouth; Saliva Orthana®, Salivace®, and Glandosane® have ACBS approval for dry mouth associated only with radiotherapy or sicca syndrome. Salivix® pastilles are also available and have similar ACBS approval.

Glandosane® (Fresenius)

Aerosol spray, carmellose sodium 500 mg, sorbitol 1.5 g, potassium chloride 60 mg, sodium chloride 42.2 mg, magnesium chloride 2.6 mg, calcium chloride 7.3 mg, and dipotassium hydrogen phosphate 17.1 mg/50 g. Net price 50-mL unit (neutral, lemon or peppermint flavoured) = £3.95

ACBS: patients suffering from dry mouth as a result of having (or having undergone) radiotherapy, or sicca syndrome, spray onto oral and pharyngeal mucosa as required

Luborant® (Antigen)

Oral spray, pink, sorbitol 1.8 g, carmellose sodium (sodium carboxymethylcellulose) 390 mg, dibasic potassium phosphate 48.23 mg, potassium chloride 37.5 mg, monobasic potassium phosphate 21.97 mg, calcium chloride 9.972 mg, magnesium chloride 3.528 mg, sodium fluoride 258 micrograms/60 mL, with preservatives and colouring agents. Net price 60-mL unit = £3.96

Saliva deficiency, 2–3 sprays onto oral mucosa up to 4 times daily, or as directed

Saliva Orthana® (Nycomed)

Aerosol spray, gastric mucin (porcine) 3.5%, with preservatives and flavouring agents. Net price 450 mL bottle (with empty 50-mL spray bottle) = £25.10, 450 mL refill = £24.68; also 50 mL spray bottle (hosp. only)

Lozenges, mucin 63 mg, xylitol 39 mg, in a sorbitol basis. Net price 10 × 45-lozenge pack = £25.07

ACBS: patients suffering from dry mouth as a result of having (or having undergone) radiotherapy, or sicca syndrome, spray 2–3 times onto oral and pharyngeal mucosa, when required

Note. Saliva Orthana® aerosol spray is available with fluoride (sodium fluoride 4.2 mg /litre) and without fluoride; the lozenges do not contain fluoride

Salivace® (Penn)

Oral spray, carmellose sodium (sodium carboxymethylcellulose), xylitol, calcium chloride, dibasic potassium phosphate, sodium chloride, potassium chloride, and methyl hydroxybenzoate. Net price 100 mL = £4.95

ACBS: patients suffering from dry mouth as a result of having (or having undergone) radiotherapy, or sicca syndrome, 1–2 sprays onto oral mucosa as required

Salivix® (Thames)

Pastilles, sugar-free, reddish-amber, acacia, malic acid and other ingredients. Net price 50-pastille pack = £2.30

ACBS: patients suffering from dry mouth as a result of having (or having undergone) radiotherapy, or sicca syndrome, suck 1 pastille when required

13: Drugs acting on the
SKIN

In this chapter, drug treatment is discussed under the following headings:

13.1 Vehicles
13.2 Emollient and barrier preparations
13.3 Local anaesthetics and antipruritics
13.4 Topical corticosteroids
13.5 Preparations for eczema and psoriasis
13.6 Preparations for acne
13.7 Preparations for warts and calluses
13.8 Sunscreens and camouflagers
13.9 Shampoos and some other scalp preparations
13.10 Anti-infective skin preparations
13.11 Disinfectants and cleansers
13.12 Antiperspirants
13.13 Wound management products
13.14 Topical circulatory preparations

Suitable quantities of dermatological preparations to be prescribed for specific areas of the body are:

	Creams and Ointments	Lotions
Face	5 to 15 g	100 mL
Both hands	25 to 50 g	200 mL
Scalp	50 to 100 g	200 mL
Both arms or both legs	100 to 200 g	200 mL
Body	200 g	500 mL
Groins and genitalia	15 to 25 g	100 mL

These amounts are usually suitable for 2 to 4 weeks. The recommendations do not apply to corticosteroid preparations which should be applied thinly. Corticosteroid creams and ointments are available in various pack sizes, commonly 15 g or 30 g, while corticosteroid lotions are usually packed in 20- or 100-mL sizes.

ADDITIVES. The following additives in topical preparations may be associated with sensitisation, particularly of eczematous skin. Details of whether they are contained in preparations listed in the BNF are given after the preparation entry.

Most commonly	Less commonly	Rarely[2]
Wool fat and related substances[1]	Benzyl alcohol	Beeswax
Chlorocresol	Butylated hydroxyanisole	Edetic acid (EDTA)
Ethylenediamine	Butylated hydroxytoluene	Isopropyl palmitate
Fragrances	Hydroxybenzoates (parabens)	
	Polysorbates	
	Propylene glycol	
	Sorbic acid	

1. Purified versions of wool fat have reduced the problem, but it remains significant
2. Non-dermatologists can reasonably disregard the substances in this category

13.1 Vehicles

Both vehicle and active ingredients are important in the treatment of skin conditions; it is being increasingly recognised that the vehicle alone may have more than a mere placebo effect. The vehicle affects the degree of hydration of the skin, has a mild anti-inflammatory effect, and aids the penetration of active drug in the preparation.

The vehicle may take the form of an *application, collodion, cream, dusting powder, lotion, ointment,* or *paste*:

Applications are usually viscous solutions, emulsions, or suspensions for application to the skin.

Collodions are painted on the skin and allowed to dry to leave a flexible film over the site of application.

Creams are essentially miscible with the skin secretion. They may contain an antimicrobial preservative unless the active ingredient or basis has sufficient intrinsic bactericidal or fungicidal activity. Generally, creams are cosmetically more acceptable than ointments as they are less greasy and easier to apply.

Dusting powders are finely divided powders that contain one or more active ingredients with or without auxiliary substances. They are intended to be applied to skin for therapeutic, prophylactic or lubricant purposes. Dusting powder intended for large open wounds or severely injured skin should be sterile.

Lotions may be preferred to ointments or creams when it is intended to apply a thin layer of the preparation over a large or hairy area. *Shake lotions* (such as calamine lotion) containing insoluble powders have a cooling effect and leave a deposit of inert powder on the skin surface.

Ointments are greasy preparations which are normally anhydrous and insoluble in water, and are more occlusive than creams. They are particularly suitable for chronic, dry lesions. The most commonly used ointment bases consist of soft paraffin or a combination of soft, liquid and hard paraffin. Some modern ointment bases have both *hydrophilic and lipophilic* properties; they may have occlusive properties on the skin surface, encourage hydration, and also be miscible with water; they often have a mild anti-inflammatory effect. *Water-soluble ointments* contain macrogols which are freely soluble in water and are therefore readily washed off; they have a limited but useful application in circumstances where ready removal is desirable.

Pastes are stiff preparations containing a high proportion of finely powdered solids such as zinc oxide and starch. They are used for circumscribed lesions such as those which occur in lichen simplex, chronic eczema, or psoriasis. They are less occlusive than ointments and can be used to protect subacute, lichenified, or excoriated skin.

DILUTION. The BP directs that creams and ointments should **not** normally be diluted but that should dilution be necessary care should be taken, in particular, to prevent microbial contamination. The appropriate diluent should be used and heating should be avoided during mixing; excessive dilution may affect the stability of some creams. Diluted creams should normally be used within 2 weeks of their preparation.

13.2 Emollient and barrier preparations

13.2.1 Emollients
13.2.2 Barrier preparations
13.2.3 Dusting powders

BORDERLINE SUBSTANCES. The preparations marked 'ACBS' are regarded as drugs when prescribed in accordance with the advice of the Advisory Committee on Borderline Substances for the clinical conditions listed. Prescriptions issued in accordance with this advice and endorsed 'ACBS' will normally not be investigated. See Appendix 7 for listing by clinical condition.

13.2.1 Emollients

Emollients soothe, smooth and hydrate the skin and are indicated for all dry scaling disorders (such as ichthyosis). Their effects are short-lived and they should be applied frequently even after improvement occurs. They are useful in dry eczematous disorders, and to a lesser extent in psoriasis (section 13.5.2). Simple preparations such as **aqueous cream** are often as effective as the more complex proprietary formulations; in general, the choice depends on patient preference. Some ingredients may cause sensitisation, notably hydrous wool fat (lanolin) or antibacterials and this should be suspected if an eczematous reaction occurs.

Camphor, menthol, and phenol have a mild antipruritic effect when used in emollient preparations. Calamine and zinc oxide may also be included as they slightly enhance therapeutic efficacy; they are particularly useful in dry eczema. Zinc and titanium preparations have mild astringent properties. Thickening agents such as talc and kaolin may also be included. Preparations containing an antibacterial should be avoided unless infection is present (section 13.10).

Urea is employed as a hydrating agent. It is used in scaling conditions and may be useful in elderly patients and infantile eczemas. It is often used with other topical agents such as corticosteroids to enhance penetration.

Aqueous Cream, BP, emulsifying ointment 30%, phenoxyethanol 1% in freshly boiled and cooled purified water. Net price 100 g = 30p

Emulsifying Ointment, BP, emulsifying wax 30%, white soft paraffin 50%, liquid paraffin 20%. Net price 100 g = 31p

Hydrous Ointment, BP (oily cream), dried magnesium sulphate 0.5%, phenoxyethanol 1%, wool alcohols ointment 50%, in freshly boiled and cooled purified water. Net price 100 g = 34p

Paraffin, White Soft, BP (white petroleum jelly). Net price 100 g = 35p

Paraffin, Yellow Soft, BP (yellow petroleum jelly). Net price 100 g = 35p

Zinc Cream, BP, zinc oxide 32%, arachis oil 32%, calcium hydroxide 0.045%, oleic acid 0.5%, wool fat 8%, in freshly boiled and cooled purified water. Net price 50 g = 19p
For napkin and urinary rash and eczematous conditions

Zinc Ointment, BP, zinc oxide 15%, in simple ointment. Net price 25 g = 12p
For napkin and urinary rash and eczematous conditions

Zinc and Castor Oil Ointment, BP, zinc oxide 7.5%, castor oil 50%, arachis oil 30.5%, white beeswax 10%, cetostearyl alcohol 2%. Net price 25 g = 13p
For napkin and urinary rash

Alcoderm® (Novex)
Cream, containing liquid paraffin, cetyl alcohol, stearyl alcohol, sodium lauryl sulphate, carbomer, triethanolamine, sorbitan monostearate, sorbitol, spermaceti, silicone fluid. Net price 60 g = £2.40
Additives: include hydroxybenzoates (parabens), isopropyl palmitate
Lotion, water-miscible, ingredients as above. Net price 120 mL = £2.86

Aveeno® (Bioglan)
Cream, colloidal oatmeal, white oat fraction in emollient basis. Net price 100 mL = £3.10
ACBS: For endogenous and exogenous eczema, xeroderma, ichthyosis, and senile pruritus associated with dry skin
Additives: include benzyl alcohol

Diprobase® (Schering-Plough)
Cream, cetomacrogol 2.25%, cetostearyl alcohol 7.2%, liquid paraffin 6%, white soft paraffin 15%, water-miscible basis used for Diprosone® cream. Net price 50 g = £1.61; 500-g dispenser = £6.92
For dry skin conditions
Additives: include chlorocresol
Ointment, liquid paraffin 5%, white soft paraffin 95%, basis used for Diprosone® ointment. Net price 50 g = £1.61
Additives: none as listed in section 13.1

Dermalex® —section 13.10.5

Drapolene® —section 13.2.2

E45® (Crookes)
Cream, light liquid paraffin 12.6%, white soft paraffin 14.5%, wool fat 1% in self-emulsifying monostearin. Net price 50 g – £1.09; 125 g – £2.20; 500 g – £5.17.
For dry skin conditions
Additives: include hydroxybenzoates (parabens)
Wash E45, soap substitute, zinc oxide 5% in an emollient basis. Net price 150 mL = £2.29.
ACBS: for endogenous and exogenous eczema, xeroderma, ichthyosis and senile pruritus associated with dry skin
Additives: include butylated hydroxytoluene

Hewletts Cream® (Bioglan)
Cream, hydrous wool fat 4%, zinc oxide 8%. Net price 35 g = £1.13; 400 g = £4.53
For nursing hygiene and care of skin
Additives: include fragrance

Humiderm® (BritCair)
Cream, pyrrolidone carboxylic acid 5% (as sodium salt). Net price 60 g = £3.71.
For dry skin conditions
Additives: include hydroxybenzoates (parabens), propylene glycol

Hydromol® (Quinoderm Ltd)
Cream, arachis oil 10%, isopropyl myristate 5%, liquid paraffin 10%, sodium pyrrolidone carboxylate 2.5%, sodium lactate 1%. Net price 50 g = £2.04; 100 g = £3.40; 500 g = £10.94.
For dry skin conditions
Additives: include hydroxybenzoates (parabens)

Kamillosan® (Norgine)
Ointment, chamomile extracts 10.5%. Net price 5 g = 57p (hosp. only); 24 g = £1.64.
For napkin rash, sore nipples and chapped hands
Additives: include beeswax, hydroxybenzoates (parabens), wool fat

Keri® (Bristol-Myers)
Lotion, mineral oil 16%, with lanolin oil. Net price 190-mL pump pack = £3.56; 380-mL pump pack = £5.81.
For dry skin conditions and napkin rash
Additives: include hydroxybenzoates (parabens), propylene glycol, fragrance

Lacticare® (Stiefel)
Lotion, lactic acid 5%, sodium pyrrolidone carboxylate 2.5%. Net price 150 mL = £3.19.
For dry skin conditions
Additives: include isopropyl palmitate, fragrance

Lipobase® (Yamanouchi)
Cream, fatty cream basis used for Locoid Lipocream®. Net price 50 g = £2.05
Additives: include hydroxybenzoates (parabens)

Massé Breast Cream® (Cilag)
Cream (water-miscible), containing arachis oil, cetyl alcohol, glycerol, glyceryl monostearate, wool fat, polysorbate 60, potassium hydroxide, sorbitan monostearate, stearic acid. Net price 28 g = £1.40.
For pre- and post-natal nipple care
Additives: include hydroxybenzoates (parabens)

Morhulin® (Seton)
Ointment, cod-liver oil 11.4%, zinc oxide 38%, in a basis containing wool fat and paraffin. Net price 50 g = £1.02; 350 g = £4.90.
For minor wounds, varicose ulcers, and pressure sores
Additives: include wool fat derivative

Neutrogena® Dermatological Cream (Neutrogena)
Cream, glycerol 40% in an emollient basis. Net price 100 g = £3.34.
For dry skin conditions
Additives: include hydroxybenzoates (parabens)

Oilatum® (Stiefel)
Cream, arachis oil 21%. Net price 40 g = £1.79; 80 g = £2.78
Additives: include fragrance
Shower emollient (gel), light liquid paraffin 70%. Net price 125 g = £4.84
Additives: include fragrance

Sudocrem® (Tosara)
Cream, benzyl alcohol 0.39%, benzyl benzoate 1.01%, benzyl cinnamate 0.15%, wool fat 4%, zinc oxide 15.25%. Net price 30 g = 69p; 60 g = 74p; 125 g = £1.25; 250 g = £2.23; 400 g = £3.27.
For napkin rash and pressure sores
Additives: include beeswax (synthetic), polysorbates, propylene glycol, fragrance

Ultrabase® (Schering Health)
Cream, water-miscible, containing liquid paraffin and white soft paraffin. Net price 50 g = £1.05; 500-g dispenser = £6.89.
For dry skin conditions
Additives: include hydroxybenzoates (parabens), disodium edetate, fragrance

Unguentum Merck® (Merck)
Cream (hydrophilic and lipophilic), cetostearyl alcohol 9%, glyceryl monostearate 3%, saturated neutral oil 2%, liquid paraffin 3%, white soft paraffin 32%, propylene glycol 5%, polysorbate '40' 8%, silicic acid 0.1%, sorbic acid 0.2%. Net price 50 g = £1.59; 100 g = £3.13; 200 mL = £6.19; 500 g = £9.55.
For dry skin conditions and napkin rash

Vaseline Dermacare® (Elida Gibbs)
Cream, dimethicone 1%, white soft paraffin 15%. Net price 100 mL = £1.47
ACBS: for endogenous and exogenous eczema, xeroderma, ichthyosis and senile pruritus associated with dry skin
Additives: include hydroxybenzoates (parabens)
Lotion, dimethicone 1%, liquid paraffin 4%, white soft paraffin 5% in an emollient basis. Net price 75 mL = £1.18; 200 mL = £2.29
ACBS: as for Vaseline Dermacare® Cream
Additives: include disodium edetate, hydroxybenzoates (parabens), wool fat

Preparations containing urea
Aquadrate® (Procter & Gamble Pharm.)
Cream, urea 10%. Net price 30 g = £1.59; 100 g = £4.79
Additives: none as listed in section 13.1
For dry scaling and itching skin, apply thinly and rub into area when required

Calmurid® (Novex)
Cream, urea 10%, lactic acid 5%. Diluent aqueous cream, life of diluted cream 14 days. Net price 100 g = £4.36; 400-g dispenser = £15.63
Additives: none as listed in section 13.1
Apply a thick layer for 3–5 minutes, massage into area, and remove excess, usually twice daily. Use half-strength cream for 1 week if stinging occurs

Nutraplus® (Novex)
Cream, urea 10%. Net price 60 g = £2.62
Additives: include hydroxybenzoates, propylene glycol
For dry scaling and itching skin, apply 2–3 times daily

13.2.1.1 EMOLLIENT BATH ADDITIVES

Alpha Keri Bath® (Bristol-Myers)
Bath oil, liquid paraffin 91.7%, oil-soluble fraction of wool fat 3%. Net price 240 mL = £3.45; 480 mL = £6.43
Additives: include fragrance
Add 10–20 mL/bath (infants 5 mL)

Aveeno® (Bioglan)
Aveeno® Bath oil, colloidal oatmeal, white oat fraction in emollient basis. Net price 250 mL = £3.20
ACBS: for endogenous and exogenous eczema, xeroderma, ichthyosis, and senile pruritus associated with dry skin
Additives: include beeswax, fragrance
Add 20–30 mL/bath
Aveeno Oilated® Bath additive, oatmeal, white oat fraction in emollient basis. Net price 10 × 50-g sachets = £5.67
ACBS: as for Aveeno® Bath oil
Additives: none as listed in section 13.1
Add 1 sachet/bath (infants half sachet)
Aveeno Regular® Bath additive, oat meal, white oat fraction in emollient basis. Net price 10 × 50-g sachets = £5.67
ACBS: as for Aveeno® Bath oil
Additives: none as listed in section 13.1
Add 1 sachet/bath (infants half sachet)

Balmandol® (S&N Pharm.)
Bath oil, almond oil 30%, light liquid paraffin 69.6%. Net price 225 mL = £3.59; 500 mL = £7.18
Additives: include butylated hydroxyanisole, fragrance
Add 15–30 mL/bath

Balneum® (Merck)

Balneum® *bath oil*, soya oil 84.75%. Net price
200 mL = £2.79; 500 mL = £6.06; 1 litre = £11.70
For dry skin conditions including those associated with
dermatitis and eczema; add 20 mL/bath
Additives: include butylated hydroxytoluene, propylene glycol,
fragrance

Balneum Plus® *bath oil*, soya oil 82.95%, mixed lau-
romacrogols 15%. Net price 500 mL = £8.33
For dry skin conditions including those associated with
dermatitis and eczema where pruritus also experienced;
add 20 mL/bath
Additives: include butylated hydroxytoluene, propylene glycol,
fragrance

Balneum with Tar®—section 13.5.1

Bath E45® (Crookes)

Bath oil, cetyl dimethicone 5%. Net price 150 mL =
£2.29
ACBS: for endogenous and exogenous eczema, xeroderma, ichthyosis, and senile pruritus associated with
dry skin
Additives: include butylated hydroxyanisole
Add 15 mL/bath

Diprobath® (Schering-Plough)

Bath additive, isopropyl myristate 39%, light liquid
paraffin 46%. Net price 500 mL = £8.34.
Additives: none as listed in section 13.1
Add 25 mL/bath (infants 10 mL)

Emmolate® (Bio-Medical)

Bath oil, acetylated wool alcohols 5%, liquid paraffin
65%. Net price 200 mL = £2.25 (hosp. only)
Additives: none as listed in section 13.1
Add 15–20 mL/bath

Emulsiderm® (Dermal)

Liquid emulsion, liquid paraffin 25%, isopropyl myristate 25%, benzalkonium chloride 0.5%. Net price
250 mL (with 10-mL measure) = £4.33; 1 litre (with
30-mL measure) = £11.57
Additives: include polysorbate 60
Add 30 mL/bath (infants 15 mL)

Hydromol Emollient® (Quinoderm Ltd)

Bath additive, isopropyl myristate 13%, light liquid
paraffin 37.8%. Net price 150 mL = £1.64; 350 mL =
£3.06; 1 litre = £7.09
Additives: none as listed in section 13.1
Add 1–3 capfuls/bath (infants ½–2 capfuls)

Oilatum® (Stiefel)

Oilatum Emollient® *bath additive* (emulsion),
acetylated wool alcohols 5%, liquid paraffin 63.4%.
Net price 250 mL = £2.75; 500 mL = £4.57
For dry skin conditions including dermatitis; add 5–
15 mL/bath
Additives: include isopropyl palmitate, fragrance

Oilatum Plus®bath additive, benzalkonium chloride
6%, triclosan 2%, light liquid paraffin 52.5%. Net
price 500 mL = £7.86
For topical treatment of eczema including eczema at risk
from infection; add 1–2 capfuls/bath (infants over 6
months 1 capful)
Additives: include wool fat, isopropyl palmitate

Savlon® Bath Oil (Zyma)

Savlon® Bath oil, acetylated wool alcohols 5%, liquid
paraffin 65%. Net price 150 mL = £2.28
Add 15–20 mL/bath

13.2.2   Barrier preparations

Barrier preparations often contain water-repellent
substances such as **dimethicone** or other silicones.
They are used for areas around stomata (see also
Appendix 8), sore areas in the elderly, bedsores, etc.
They are no substitute for adequate nursing care,
and it is doubtful if they are any more effective than
the traditional compound **zinc ointments**.

NAPKIN RASH. Barrier creams and ointments are
used to give protection against napkin rash which is
usually a local dermatitis. The first line of treatment
is to ensure that napkins are changed frequently,
and that tightly fitting rubber pants are avoided.
The rash may clear when left exposed to the air and
a napkin rash preparation (see preparations below)
may be helpful. If the rash is associated with a
fungal infection, an antifungal cream such as clotrimazole cream (see section 13.10.2) is useful. A
mild corticosteroid such as hydrocortisone may be
useful but treatment should be limited to a week or
less and it should be remembered that napkins and
plastic pants may act as an occlusive dressing and
increase absorption (for cautions see hydrocortisone p.427).

Conotrane® (Yamanouchi)

Cream, benzalkonium chloride 0.1%, dimethicone
'350' 22%. Net price 50 g = 61p; 100 g = 99p; 500 g
= £3.74.
For napkin and urinary rash and pressure sores
Additives: include fragrance

Drapolene® (Wellcome)

Cream, benzalkonium chloride 0.02%, cetrimide
0.2% in a water-miscible basis. Net price 55 g =
85p; 100 g = £1.34; 125 g = £1.41; 500 g = £6.12.
For napkin rash
Additives: include chlorocresol, wool fat

Metanium® (Bengué)

Ointment, titanium dioxide 20%, titanium peroxide
5%, titanium salicylate 3%, titanium tannate 0.1%, in
a silicone basis. Net price 25 g = 76p.
For napkin rash and related disorders
Additives: none as listed in section 13.1

Savlon® Nappy Rash Cream (Zyma)

Savlon® Nappy Rash cream, dimethicone '1000'
10%, cetrimide 0.3%. Net price 50 g = 83p; 100 g =
£1.40.
For napkin rash
Additives: include butylated hydroxytoluene, hydroxybenzoates
(parabens)

Siopel® (Zeneca)

Barrier cream, dimethicone '1000' 10%, cetrimide
0.3%. Net price 50 g = 62p.
For dermatoses, colostomy and ileostomy care, urinary
rash, and related conditions
Additives: include butylated hydroxytoluene, hydroxybenzoates
(parabens)

Sprilon® (Perstorp)

Spray application, dimethicone 1.04%, zinc oxide
12.5%, in a basis containing wool fat, wool alcohols,
cetostearyl alcohol, dextran, white soft paraffin, liquid paraffin, propellants. Net price 115-g pressurised
aerosol unit = £3.71.
For urinary rash, pressure sores, and ileostomy
Caution: flammable

Vasogen® (Pharmax)

Barrier cream, dimethicone 20%, calamine 1.5%,
zinc oxide 7.5%. Net price 50 g= 70p; 100 g = £1.20.
For napkin and urinary rash, pressure sores, and pruritus
ani
Additives: include hydroxybenzoates (parabens), wool fat

13.2.3   Dusting powders

Dusting powders are used in folds where friction may
occur between opposing skin surfaces. They should not
be applied in areas that are very moist as they tend to
cake and abrade the skin. **Talc** acts as a lubricant powder but does not absorb moisture whereas **starch** is less
lubricant but absorbs water. Other inert powders such

as kaolin or zinc oxide may also be used in the formulation of dusting powders. See also section 13.11 for antiseptic dusting powders.

Talc Dusting Powder, BP, starch 10% in sterilised purified talc. Net price 100 g = 39p
Zinc, Starch and Talc Dusting-powder, BPC, zinc oxide 25%, starch 25%, sterilised purified talc 50%. Net price 50 g = 16p
ZeaSORB® (Stiefel)
Dusting powder, aldioxa 0.2%, chloroxylenol 0.5%, pulverised maize core 45%. Net price 50 g = £2.15
Additives: include fragrance

13.3   Local anaesthetics and antipruritics

Pruritus may be caused by systemic disease (such as drug hypersensitivity, obstructive jaundice, endocrine disease, and certain malignant diseases) as well as by skin disease (e.g. psoriasis, eczema, urticaria, and scabies). Where possible the underlying causes should be treated. There is no really effective topical antipruritic. **Calamine** preparations are widely prescribed for pruritus, and **emollient** preparations (section 13.2.1) may also be of value. **Crotamiton** does not appear to be any more effective than calamine.

Insect stings are also best treated with calamine preparations or emollients. Topical antihistamines and local anaesthetics may cause sensitisation and are only marginally effective.

For preparations used in *pruritus ani*, see section 1.7.1.

CALAMINE
Indications: pruritus

Calamine Cream, Aqueous, BP, calamine   4%, zinc oxide3%, liquid paraffin 20%, self-emulsifying glyceryl monostearate 5%, cetomacrogol emulsifying wax 5%, phenoxyethanol 0.5%, freshly boiled and cooled purified water 62.5%. Net price 100mL = 48p
Calamine Lotion, BP, calamine 15%, zinc oxide 5%, glycerol 5%, bentonite 3%, sodium citrate 0.5%, liquefied phenol 0.5%, in freshly boiled and cooled purified water. Net price 200 mL = 52p
Calamine Lotion, Oily, BP1980, calamine 5%, arachis oil 50%, oleic acid 0.5%, wool fat 1%, in calcium hydroxide solution. Net price 200 mL = 80p

CROTAMITON
Indications: pruritus (including pruritus after scabies), but see notes above
Cautions: avoid use near eyes and broken skin
Contra-indications: acute exudative dermatoses

Eurax® (Zyma)
Cream, crotamiton 10%. Net price 30 g = £1.77; 100 g = £2.99
Additives: include beeswax, hydroxybenzoates (parabens), fragrance
Lotion, crotamiton 10%. Net price 100 mL = £2.29
Additives: include propylene glycol, sorbic acid, fragrance

LOCAL ANAESTHETICS
Indications: relief of local pain, see notes above. See section 15.2 for use in surface anaesthesia
Cautions: may cause hypersensitivity
Note. Topical local anaesthetic preparations may be absorbed, especially through mucosal surfaces, therefore excessive application should be avoided, particularly in infants and children

Anethaine® (Torbet)
Cream, amethocaine hydrochloride 1%. Net price 25 g = £1.34
Additives: include fragrance
Solarcaine® (Schering-Plough)
Cream, benzocaine 1%, triclosan 0.2%. Net price 25 mL = £1.55
Additives: include benzyl alcohol, disodium edetate
Lotion, benzocaine 0.5%, triclosan 0.2%. Net price 75 mL = £2.04
Additives: include disodium edetate, hydroxybenzoates (parabens)
Spray (= application), benzocaine 2.86%, triclosan 0.057%, pressurised aerosol unit. Net price 95 g = £2.60
Additives: include propylene glycol
Xylocaine® (Astra)
Ointment, see section 15.2

TOPICAL ANTIHISTAMINES
Indications: see notes above
Cautions: may cause hypersensitivity; avoid in eczema; photosensitivity (diphenhydramine); use for longer than 3 days not recommended

The following is a list of topical antihistamine preparations on sale to the public, together with their significant ingredients:
Anthisan® (mepyramine), **Caladryl®** cream and lotion (calamine, camphor, diphenhydramine), **Cupal Insect Bite Ointment®** (antazoline), **Histergan® Cream** (diphenhydramine), **R.B.C®** (antazoline, calamine, camphor, cetrimide, menthol), **Wasp-Eze®** (benzocaine, mepyramine)

13.4   Topical corticosteroids

Topical corticosteroids are used for the treatment of inflammatory conditions of the skin other than those due to an infection, in particular the *eczematous disorders.* Corticosteroids suppress various components of the inflammatory reaction while in use; they are in no sense curative, and when treatment is discontinued a rebound exacerbation of the condition may occur. They are indicated for the relief of symptoms and for the suppression of signs of the disorder when potentially less harmful measures are ineffective.

Corticosteroids are of no value in the treatment of *urticaria* and are **contra-indicated** in *rosacea* and in *ulcerative conditions* as they worsen the condition. They should not be used indiscriminately in *pruritus.*

Systemic or potent topical corticosteroids should be avoided or given only under specialist supervision *in psoriasis* because, although they may suppress the psoriasis in the short term, relapse or vigorous rebound occurs on withdrawal (sometimes precipitating severe pustular psoriasis). Topical use of potent corticosteroids on widespread psoriasis also inevitably leads to systemic as well as to local side-effects. It is reasonable, however, to prescribe a weaker corticosteroid (such as hydrocortisone) for short periods (perhaps up to 8 weeks) for *flexural , scalp* and *facial psoriasis* (**important:** not more potent than hydrocortisone 1% on the face).

In general, the most potent topical corticosteroids should be reserved for recalcitrant dermatoses such as *chronic discoid lupus erythematosus, lichen simplex chronicus, hypertrophic lichen planus*, and *palmar plantar pustulosis*. With rare exceptions, potent corticosteroids should not be used on the face as they may precipitate a rosacea-like disorder and aggravate pre-existing rosacea.

Intradermal corticosteroid injections (see section 10.1.2.2) are more effective than the very potent topical corticosteroid preparations and they should be reserved for severe cases where there are localised lesions (such as *keloid scars* or *hypertrophic lichen planus*) and topical treatment has failed. Their effects may last for several weeks or even months. Particular care is needed with the injection technique in order to avoid severe skin atrophy.

SIDE-EFFECTS. Unlike the *potent* and *very potent* groups, the *moderate* and *mild* groups are rarely associated with side-effects. The more potent the preparation the more care is required, as absorption through the skin can cause severe pituitary-adrenal-axis suppression and hypercorticism (see section 6.3.3), both of which depend on the area of the body treated and the duration of the treatment. It must also be remembered that absorption is greatest from areas of thin skin, raw surfaces, and intertriginous areas, and is increased by occlusion.

Local side-effects include:

(a) spread and worsening of untreated infection;
(b) thinning of the skin which may be restored over a period of time although the original structure may never return;
(c) irreversible striae atrophicae;
(d) increased hair growth;
(e) perioral dermatitis, an inflammatory papular disorder on the face of young women;
(f) acne at the site of application in some patients;
(g) mild depigmentation and vellus hair.

CHOICE OF FORMULATION. *Water miscible* creams are suitable for moist or weeping lesions whereas *ointments* are generally chosen for dry, lichenified or scaly lesions or where a more occlusive effect is required. *Lotions* may be useful when minimal application to a large area is required. *Occlusive polythene dressings* have been used to increase the effect, but they also increase the risk of side-effects. The *inclusion of urea* increases the penetration of the corticosteroid.

USE IN CHILDREN. Children, especially babies, are particularly susceptible to side-effects. The more potent corticosteroids are **contra-indicated** in infants under 1 year, and in general should be **avoided** in paediatric treatment or if necessary used with great care for short periods; a mild cortico-

steroid such as hydrocortisone is useful for treating napkin rash (see section 13.2.2) and for infantile eczemas (but see caution below)

COMPOUND PREPARATIONS. The advantages of including other substances with corticosteroids in topical preparations are debatable. The commonest ones are the **antibacterials**.

Topical corticosteroid potencies

Potency	Examples
Mild	Hydrocortisone 1%
Moderately potent	Clobetasone butyrate 0.05%
Potent	Betamethasone 0.1% (as valerate) Hydrocortisone butyrate
Very potent	Clobetasol propionate 0.05%

The preparation containing the **least potent** drug at the **lowest strength** which is effective is the one of choice; dilution should be avoided whenever possible.

HYDROCORTISONE

Indications: mild inflammatory skin disorders such as eczema (but for over-the-counter preparations, see next page); napkin rash, see notes above and section 13.2.2

Cautions: see notes above; also avoid prolonged use in infants and children (extreme caution in dermatoses of infancy including napkin rash—where possible treatment should be limited to 5–7 days), avoid prolonged use on the face (and keep away from eyes); more potent corticosteroids **contra-indicated** in infants under 1 year (see also notes above)

PSORIASIS. Risks of more potent corticosteroids in psoriasis include possibility of rebound relapse, development of generalised pustular psoriasis, and local and systemic toxicity, see also section 13.5.2; they are specifically **contra-indicated** in widespread plaque psoriasis

Contra-indications: untreated bacterial, fungal, or viral skin lesions; acne, rosacea, perioral dermatitis; not recommended for acne vulgaris (more potent corticosteroids specifically **contra-indicated**)

Side-effects: see notes above

Administration: apply thinly 2–3 times daily, reducing frequency as condition responds

PoM Hydrocortisone (Non-proprietary)
Cream, hydrocortisone 0.5%, net price, 15 g = 33p; 30 g = 60p; 1%, 15 g = 38p. Label: 28. Potency: mild
Ointment, hydrocortisone 0.5%, net price 15 g = 35p; 30 g = 60p; 1%, 15 g = 38p. Label: 28. Potency: mild
When hydrocortisone cream or ointment is prescribed and no strength is stated, the 1% strength should be supplied

The following is a list of skin creams and ointments that contain hydrocortisone alone or with other ingredients: **Dermacort®** (hydrocortisone 0.1%, cream), **Eurax Hc®** (hydrocortisone 0.25%; crotamiton 10%, cream), **Hc45®** (hydrocortisone acetate 1%, cream), **Lanacort®** (hydrocortisone acetate 1%, cream and ointment). They can be sold to the public for treatment of allergic contact dermatitis, irritant dermatitis, and insect bite reactions.

Cautions: not for children under 10 years or in pregnancy, without medical advice

Contra-indications: eyes/face, anogenital region, broken or infected skin (including cold sores, acne, and athlete's foot)

Administration: apply sparingly over small area 1–2 times daily for max. of 1 week

Labelling must state. If the condition is not improved, consult your doctor.

Proprietary hydrocortisone preparations

Note. The preparations listed below are PoM; those on sale to the public (with restrictions) are specified above.

PoM **Cobadex®** (Cox)

Cream, hydrocortisone 1%, dimethicone '350' 20%. Net price 20 g = £2.10. Label: 28. Potency: mild

Additives: include hydroxybenzoates (parabens), polysorbate 80, propylene glycol

PoM **Dioderm®** (Dermal)

Cream, hydrocortisone 0.1%. Net price 30 g = £2.59. Label: 28. Potency: mild

Additives: include propylene glycol

Note. Although this contains only 0.1% hydrocortisone, the formulation is designed to provide a clinical activity comparable to that of Hydrocortisone Cream 1% BP

PoM **Efcortelan®** (Glaxo)

Cream, hydrocortisone 0.5%, net price, 30 g = 60p; 1%, 30 g = 74p; 2.5%, 30 g = £1.66. Label: 28. Potency: mild

Additives: include chlorocresol

Ointment, hydrocortisone 0.5%, net price, 30 g = 60p; 1%, 30 g = 74p; 2.5%, 30 g = £1.66. Label: 28. Potency: mild

Additives: none as listed in section 13.1

PoM **Hydrocortistab®** (Boots)

Cream, hydrocortisone acetate 1%. Net price 15 g = 35p. Label: 28. Potency: mild

Additives: include chlorocresol

Ointment, hydrocortisone 1%. Net price 15 g = 35p. Label: 28. Potency: mild

Additives: none as listed in section 13.1

PoM **Hydrocortisyl®** (Roussel)

Cream, hydrocortisone 1%. Net price 15 g = 27p. Label: 28. Potency: mild

Additives: include chlorocresol

Ointment, hydrocortisone 1%. Net price 15 g = 27p. Label: 28. Potency: mild

Additives: include wool fat

PoM **Mildison®** (Yamanouchi)

Lipocream, hydrocortisone 1%. Net price 30 g = £2.19. Label: 28. Potency: mild

Additives: include hydroxybenzoates (parabens)

Compound preparations

Note. Compound preparations with coal tar, section 13.5.1

PoM **Alphaderm®** (Procter & Gamble Pharm.)

Cream, hydrocortisone 1%, urea 10%. Net price 30 g = £2.36; 100 g = £7.32. Label: 28. Potency: moderate

Additives: none as listed in section 13.1

PoM **Calmurid HC®** (Novex)

Cream, hydrocortisone 1%, urea 10%, lactic acid 5%. Net price 30 g = £2.33; 100 g = £6.75. Label: 28. Potency: moderate

Additives: none as listed in section 13.1

Note. Manufacturer advises dilute to half-strength with aqueous cream for 1 week if stinging occurs then transfer to undiluted preparation (but see section 13.1 for advice to avoid dilution where possible)

PoM **Epifoam®** (Stafford-Miller)

Foam (= application), hydrocortisone acetate 1%, pramoxine hydrochloride 1%, in a muco-adherent basis (pressurised aerosol pack). Net price 12-g unit (approx. 20 applications of 5 mL) = £2.74. Label: 28. Potency: mild

Additives: include hydroxybenzoates, propylene glycol

For perineal trauma including post-episiotomy pain and discomfort, apply on a pad 3–4 times daily

PoM **Eurax-Hydrocortisone®** (Zyma)

Cream, hydrocortisone 0.25%, crotamiton 10%. Net price 30 g = 91p. Label: 28. Potency: mild

Additives: include hydroxybenzoates (parabens), propylene glycol, fragrance

Note. A 15-g tube is on sale to the public for treatment of contact dermatitis and insect bites (Eurax Hc®)

PoM **Hydrocal®** (Bioglan)

Cream, hydrocortisone acetate 1%, in a basis containing calamine. Net price 25 g = £3.99. Label: 28. Potency: mild

Additives: include hydroxybenzoates (parabens), polysorbates

With antimicrobials

See notes above for comment on compound preparations

PoM **Canesten HC®** (Baypharm)

Cream, hydrocortisone 1%, clotrimazole 1%. Net price 30 g = £3.10. Label: 28. Potency: mild

Additives: include benzyl alcohol

PoM **Daktacort®** (Janssen)

Cream, hydrocortisone 1%, miconazole nitrate 2%. Net price 30 g = £2.24. Label: 28. Potency: mild

Additives: include butylated hydroxyanisole, disodium edetate

Ointment, hydrocortisone 1%, miconazole nitrate 2%. Net price 30 g = £3.10. Label: 28. Potency: mild

Additives: none as listed in section 13.1

PoM **Econacort®** (Squibb)

Cream, hydrocortisone 1%, econazole nitrate 1%. Net price 30 g = £2.25. Label: 28. Potency: mild

Additives: include butylated hydroxyanisole

PoM **Fucidin H®** (Leo)

Cream, hydrocortisone acetate 1%, fusidic acid 2%. Net price 15 g = £3.22; 30 g = £5.55. Label: 28. Potency: mild

Additives: include butylated hydroxyanisole, potassium sorbate

Gel, hydrocortisone acetate 1%, fusidic acid 2%. Net price 15 g = £2.84; 30 g = £4.93. Label: 28. Potency: mild

Additives: include hydroxybenzoates (parabens), polysorbate 80

Ointment, hydrocortisone acetate 1%, sodium fusidate 2%. Net price 15 g = £2.63; 30 g = £4.56. Label: 28. Potency: mild

Additives: include wool fat

PoM Gregoderm® (Unigreg)

Ointment, hydrocortisone 1%, neomycin sulphate 0.4%, nystatin 100 000 units/g, polymyxin B sulphate 7250 units/g. Net price 15 g = £2.51. Label: 28. Potency: mild

Additives: none as listed in section 13.1

PoM Nystaform-HC® (Bayer)

Cream, hydrocortisone 0.5%, nystatin 100 000 units/g, chlorhexidine hydrochloride 1%. Net price 30 g = £2.66. Label: 28. Potency: mild

Additives: include benzyl alcohol, polysorbate 60

Ointment, hydrocortisone 1%, nystatin 100 000 units/g, chlorhexidine acetate 1%. Net price 30 g = £2.66. Label: 28. Potency: mild

Additives: none as listed in section 13.1

PoM Quinocort® (Quinoderm Ltd)

Cream, hydrocortisone 1%, potassium hydroxyquinoline sulphate 0.5%. Net price 30 g = £1.56. Label: 28. Potency: mild

Additives: include edetic acid (EDTA), chlorocresol

PoM Terra-Cortril® (Pfizer)

Topical ointment, hydrocortisone 1%, oxytetracycline 3% (as hydrochloride). Net price 15 g = £1.01; 30 g = £1.82. Label: 28. Potency: mild

Additives: none as listed in section 13.1

Spray application, hydrocortisone 50 mg, oxytetracycline 150 mg (as hydrochloride) in a pressurised aerosol unit, net price 30-mL = £1.44; double these amounts in 60-mL unit, net price = £2.50. Label: 28. Potency: mild

Additives: none as listed in section 13.1

PoM Terra-Cortril Nystatin® (Pfizer)

Cream, hydrocortisone 1%, nystatin 100 000 units/g, oxytetracycline 3% (as calcium salt). Net price 30 g = £2.01. Label: 28. Potency: mild

Additives: include hydroxybenzoates (parabens), polysorbate, propylene glycol, fragrance

PoM Timodine® (R&C)

Cream, hydrocortisone 0.5%, nystatin 100 000 units/g, benzalkonium chloride solution 0.2%, dimethicone '350' 10%. Net price 30 g = £2.38. Label: 28. Potency: mild

Additives: include butylated hydroxyanisole, hydroxybenzoates (parabens), sorbic acid

PoM Tri-Cicatrin® (Wellcome)

Ointment, hydrocortisone 1%, bacitracin zinc 250 units/g, neomycin sulphate 3400 units/g, nystatin 100 000 units/g. Net price 15 g = £2.24; 30 g = £4.47. Label: 28. Potency: mild

Additives: none as listed in section 13.1

PoM Vioform-Hydrocortisone® (Zyma)

Cream, hydrocortisone 1%, clioquinol 3%. Net price 30 g = £1.53. Label: 28. Potency: mild

Additives: none as listed in section 13.1

Ointment, hydrocortisone 1%, clioquinol 3%. Net price 30 g = £1.53. Label: 28. Potency: mild

Additives: none as listed in section 13.1

Caution: stains clothing

HYDROCORTISONE BUTYRATE

Indications: severe inflammatory skin disorders such as eczema unresponsive to less potent corticosteroids; psoriasis, see notes above

Cautions; Contra-indications; Side-effects: see under Hydrocortisone and notes above

Administration: apply thinly 2–4 times daily (1–2 times daily for scalp lotion), reducing frequency as condition responds

PoM Locoid® (Yamanouchi)

Cream, hydrocortisone butyrate 0.1%. Net price 30 g = £2.27; 100 g = £6.95. Label: 28. Potency: potent

Additives: include hydroxybenzoates (parabens)

Lipocream, hydrocortisone butyrate 0.1%. Net price 30 g = £2.38; 100 g = £7.29. Label: 28. Potency: potent

Additives: include hydroxybenzoates (parabens)

Note. For bland cream basis see Lipobase®, section 13.2.1

Ointment, hydrocortisone butyrate 0.1%. Net price 30 g = £2.27; 100 g = £6.95. Label: 28. Potency: potent

Additives: none as listed in section 13.1

Scalp lotion, hydrocortisone butyrate 0.1%, in an aqueous isopropyl alcohol basis. Net price 30 mL = £3.20; 100 mL = £9.81. Label: 15, 28. Potency: potent

Additives: none as listed in section 13.1

With antimicrobials

See notes above for comment on compound preparations

PoM Locoid C® (Yamanouchi)

Cream, hydrocortisone butyrate 0.1%, chlorquinaldol 3%. Net price 30 g = £2.97. Label: 28. Potency: potent

Additives: none as listed in section 13.1

Ointment, ingredients as for cream, in a greasy basis. Net price 30 g = £2.97. Label: 28. Potency: potent

Additives: none as listed in section 13.1

ALCLOMETASONE DIPROPIONATE

Indications: inflammatory skin disorders such as eczema

Cautions; Contra-indications; Side-effects: see under Hydrocortisone and notes above

Administration: apply thinly 2–3 times daily, reducing frequency as condition responds

PoM Modrasone® (Schering-Plough)

Cream, alclometasone dipropionate 0.05%. Net price 15 g = £1.66; 50 g = £4.68. Label: 28. Potency: moderate

Additives: include chlorocresol, propylene glycol

Ointment, alclometasone dipropionate 0.05%. Net price 15 g = £1.66; 50 g = £4.68. Label: 28. Potency: moderate

Additives: include beeswax, propylene glycol

BECLOMETHASONE DIPROPIONATE

Indications: severe inflammatory skin disorders such as eczema unresponsive to less potent corticosteroids; psoriasis, see notes above

Cautions; Contra-indications; Side-effects: see under Hydrocortisone and notes above

Administration: apply thinly twice daily, reducing frequency as condition responds

PoM **Propaderm®** (Glaxo)
Cream, beclomethasone dipropionate 0.025%.
Net price 30 g = £1.58. Label: 28. Potency: potent
Additives: include chlorocresol
Ointment, beclomethasone dipropionate 0.025%.
Net price 30 g = £1.58. Label: 28. Potency: potent
Additives: include propylene glycol

BETAMETHASONE ESTERS

Indications: severe inflammatory skin disorders
such as eczema unresponsive to less potent corticosteroids; psoriasis, see notes above
Cautions; Contra-indications; Side-effects: see
under Hydrocortisone and notes above. Application of more than 100 g per week of 0.1% preparation is likely to cause adrenal suppression
Administration: apply thinly 2–3 times daily (1–2
times daily for scalp lotion), reducing frequency
as condition responds

PoM **Betamethasone Valerate** (Non-proprietary)
Cream, betamethasone 0.1% (as valerate). Net
price 30 g = £1.40. Label: 28. Potency: potent
Ointment, betamethasone 0.1% (as valerate). Net
price 30 g = £1.40. Label: 28. Potency: potent
PoM **Betnovate®** (Glaxo)
Cream, betamethasone 0.1% (as valerate), in a
water-miscible basis. Net price 30 g = £1.40;
100 g = £3.95; 100 g pump-dispenser = £4.45.
Label: 28. Potency: potent
Additives: include chlorocresol
Ointment, betamethasone 0.1% (as valerate), in an
anhydrous paraffin basis. Net price 30 g = £1.40;
100 g = £3.95; 100 g pump-dispenser = £4.45.
Label: 28. Potency: potent
Additives: none as listed in section 13.1
Lotion, betamethasone 0.1% (as valerate). Net
price 100 mL = £4.75. Label: 28. Potency: potent
Additives: include hydroxybenzoates (parabens)
Scalp application, betamethasone 0.1% (as valer-
ate). Net price 100 mL = £5.18. Label: 15, 28.
Potency: potent
Additives: none as listed in section 13.1
PoM **Betnovate-RD®** (Glaxo)
Cream, betamethasone 0.025% (as valerate) in a
water-miscible basis (1 in 4 dilution of
Betnovate® cream). Net price 100 g = £3.26.
Label: 28. Potency: moderate
Additives: include chlorocresol
Ointment, betamethasone 0.025% (as valerate) in
an anhydrous paraffin basis (1 in 4 dilution of
Betnovate® ointment). Net price 100 g = £3.26.
Label: 28. Potency: moderate
Additives: none as listed in section 13.1
PoM **Diprosone®** (Schering-Plough)
Cream, betamethasone 0.05% (as dipropionate).
Net price 30 g = £2.51; 100 g = £7.12. Label: 28.
Potency: potent
Additives: include chlorocresol
Ointment, betamethasone 0.05% (as dipropionate).
Net price 30 g = £2.51; 100 g = £7.12. Label: 28.
Potency: potent
Additives: none as listed in section 13.1
Lotion, betamethasone 0.05% (as dipropionate).
Net price 30 mL = £3.17; 100 mL = £9.07. Label:
28. Potency: potent
Additives: none as listed in section 13.1

With salicylic acid
See notes above for comment on compound preparations
PoM **Diprosalic®** (Schering-Plough)
Ointment, betamethasone 0.05% (as dipropionate),
salicylic acid 3%. Net price 30 g = £3.30; 100 g =
£9.50. Label: 28. Potency:potent
Additives: none as listed in section 13.1
Apply thinly 1–2 times daily; max. 60 g per week
Scalp application, betamethasone 0.05% (as
dipropionate), salicylic acid 2%, in an alcoholic
basis. Net price 100 mL = £10.50. Label: 28.
Potency: potent
Additives: include disodium edetate
Apply a few drops 1–2 times daily

With antimicrobials
See notes above for comment on compound preparations
PoM **Betnovate-C®** (Glaxo)
Cream, betamethasone 0.1% (as valerate), clio-
quinol 3%. Net price 30 g = £1.72. Label: 28.
Potency: potent
Additives: include chlorocresol
Ointment, betamethasone 0.1% (as valerate), clio-
quinol 3%. Net price 30 g = £1.72. Label: 28.
Potency: potent
Additives: none as listed in section 13.1
Caution: stains clothing
PoM **Betnovate-N®** (Glaxo)
Cream, betamethasone 0.1% (as valerate), neo-
mycin sulphate 0.5%. Net price 30 g = £1.72;
100 g = £4.77. Label: 28. Potency: potent
Additives: include chlorocresol
Ointment, betamethasone 0.1% (as valerate), neo-
mycin sulphate 0.5%. Net price 30 g = £1.72;
100 g = £4.77. Label: 28. Potency: potent
Additives: none as listed in section 13.1
PoM **Fucibet®** (Leo)
Cream, betamethasone 0.1% (as valerate), fusidic
acid 2%. Net price 15 g = £3.74; 30 g = £6.32.
Label: 28. Potency: potent
Additives: include chlorocresol
PoM **Lotriderm®** (Schering-Plough)
Cream, betamethasone 0.05% (as dipropionate),
clotrimazole 1%. Net price 15 g = £3.40. Label:
28. Potency: potent
Additives: include benzyl alcohol, propylene glycol

BUDESONIDE

Indications: severe inflammatory skin disorders
such as eczema; psoriasis, see notes above
Cautions; Contra-indications; Side-effects: see
under Hydrocortisone and notes above
Administration: apply thinly 2–3 times daily

PoM **Preferid®** (Yamanouchi)
Cream, budesonide 0.025%. Net price 30 g =
£2.96; 100 g = £9.06. Label: 28. Potency: potent
Additives: include sorbic acid
Ointment, budesonide 0.025%. Net price 30 g =
£2.96; 100 g = £9.06. Label: 28. Potency: potent
Additives: include white beeswax, propylene glycol

CLOBETASOL PROPIONATE

Indications: short-term treatment only of severe resistant inflammatory skin disorders such as recalcitrant eczema unresponsive to less potent corticosteroids; psoriasis, see notes above

Cautions; Contra-indications; Side-effects: see under Hydrocortisone and notes above. Not more than 50 g of 0.05% preparation should be applied per week

Administration: apply thinly 1–2 times daily for up to 4 weeks, reducing frequency as condition responds

PoM Dermovate® (Glaxo)
Cream, clobetasol propionate 0.05%. Net price 30 g = £2.56; 100 g = £7.52. Label: 28. Potency: very potent
Additives: include beeswax (or beeswax substitute), chlorocresol, propylene glycol
Ointment, clobetasol propionate 0.05%. Net price 30 g = £2.56; 100 g = £7.52. Label: 28. Potency: very potent
Additives: include propylene glycol
Scalp application, clobetasol propionate 0.05%, in a thickened alcoholic basis. Net price 30 mL = £2.93; 100 mL = £9.91. Label: 15, 28. Potency: very potent
Additives: none as listed insection 13.1

With antimicrobials
See notes above for comment on compound preparations
PoM Dermovate-NN® (Glaxo)
Cream, clobetasol propionate 0.05%, neomycin sulphate 0.5%, nystatin 100 000 units/g. Net price 30 g = £3.50. Label: 28. Potency: very potent
Additives: include beeswax substitute
Ointment, ingredients as for cream, in a paraffin basis. Net price 30 g = £3.50. Label: 28. Potency: very potent
Additives: none as listed in section 13.1

CLOBETASONE BUTYRATE

Indications: eczema and dermatitis of all types; maintenance between courses of more potent corticosteroids
Cautions; Contra-indications; Side-effects: see under Hydrocortisone and notes above
Administration: apply thinly up to 4 times daily, reducing frequency as condition responds

PoM Eumovate® (Glaxo)
Cream, clobetasone butyrate 0.05%. Net price 30 g = £1.76; 100 g = £5.16. Label: 28. Potency: moderate
Additives: include beeswax substitute, chlorocresol
Ointment, clobetasone butyrate 0.05%. Net price 30 g = £1.76; 100 g = £5.16. Label: 28. Potency: moderate
Additives: none as listed in section 13.1

With antimicrobials
See notes above for comment on compound preparations
PoM Trimovate® (Glaxo)
Cream, clobetasone butyrate 0.05%, oxytetracycline 3% (as calcium salt), nystatin 100 000 units/g. Net price 30 g = £3.13. Label: 28. Potency: moderate
Additives: include chlorocresol

DESOXYMETHASONE
(Desoximetasone)

Indications: severe acute inflammatory, allergic, and chronic skin disorders; psoriasis, see notes above
Cautions; Contra-indications; Side-effects: see under Hydrocortisone and notes above
Administration: apply thinly 2–3 times daily reducing frequency as condition responds

PoM Stiedex® (Stiefel)
Oily cream, desoxymethasone 0.25%. Net price 30 g = £3.43. Label: 28. Potency: potent
Additives: include wool fat
LP Oily cream, desoxymethasone 0.05%. Net price 30 g = £2.86; 100 g = £8.58. Label:28. Potency: moderate
Additives: include edetic acid (EDTA), wool fat
Lotion, desoxymethasone 0.25%, salicylic acid 1%. Net price 50 mL = £8.05. Label: 28. Potency: potent
Additives: include disodium edetate, propylene glycol

DIFLUCORTOLONE VALERATE

Indications: severe inflammatory skin disorders such as eczema unresponsive to less potent corticosteroids; high strength (0.3%), short-term treatment of severe exacerbations; psoriasis, see notes above
Cautions; Contra-indications; Side-effects: see under Hydrocortisone and notes above; not more than 60 g of 0.3% applied per week
Administration: apply thinly 2–3 times daily for up to 4 weeks (0.1% preparations) or 2 weeks (0.3% preparations), reducing strength and frequency as condition responds

PoM Nerisone® (Schering Health)
Cream, diflucortolone valerate 0.1%. Net price 30 g = £2.56. Label: 28. Potency: potent
Additives: include disodium edetate, hydroxybenzoates (parabens)
Oily cream, diflucortolone valerate 0.1%. Net price 30 g = £2.56. Label: 28. Potency: potent
Additives: none as listed in section 13.1
Ointment, diflucortolone valerate 0.1%. Net price 30 g = £2.56. Label: 28. Potency: potent
Additives: none as listed in section 13.1
PoM Nerisone Forte® (Schering Health)
Oily cream, diflucortolone valerate 0.3%. Net price 15 g = £2.09. Label: 28. Potency: very potent
Additives: none as listed in section 13.1
Ointment, diflucortolone valerate 0.3%. Net price 15 g = £2.09. Label: 28. Potency: very potent
Additives: none as listed in section 13.1

FLUCLOROLONE ACETONIDE

Indications: severe inflammatory skin disorders such as eczema unresponsive to less potent corticosteroids; psoriasis, see notes above
Cautions; Contra-indications; Side-effects: see under Hydrocortisone and notes above
Administration: apply thinly twice daily, reducing frequency as condition responds

PoM Topilar® (Bioglan)

Cream, fluclorolone acetonide 0.025%. Net price 30 g = £2.97; 100 g = £8.39. Label: 28. Potency: potent

Additives: include propylene glycol

Ointment, fluclorolone acetonide 0.025%. Net price 30 g = £2.97; 100 g = £8.39. Label: 28. Potency: potent

Additives: include propylene glycol, wool fat

FLUOCINOLONE ACETONIDE

Indications: inflammatory skin disorders such as eczema, 0.0025–0.01% in milder conditions, 0.025% in severe conditions; psoriasis, see notes above

Cautions; Contra-indications; Side-effects: see under Hydrocortisone and notes above

Administration: apply thinly 2–3 times daily, reducing strength and frequency as condition responds

PoM Synalar® (Zeneca)

Cream, fluocinolone acetonide 0.025%. Net price 15 g = 76p; 30 g = £1.37; 50 g = £2.05. Label: 28. Potency: potent

Additives: include benzyl alcohol, polysorbates, propylene glycol

Gel, fluocinolone acetonide 0.025%. Net price 30 g = £1.45. For use on scalp and other hairy areas. Label: 28. Potency: potent

Additives: include hydroxybenzoates (parabens), propylene glycol

Ointment, fluocinolone acetonide 0.025%. Net price 15 g = 76p; 30 g = £1.37; 50 g = £2.05. Label: 28. Potency: potent

Additives: include propylene glycol, wool fat

PoM Synalar 1 in 4 Dilution® (Zeneca)

Cream, fluocinolone acetonide 0.00625%. Net price 50 g = £1.56. Label: 28. Potency: moderate

Additives: include benzyl alcohol, polysorbates, propylene glycol

Ointment, fluocinolone acetonide 0.00625%. Net price 50 g = £1.83. Label: 28. Potency: moderate

Additives: include propylene glycol, wool fat

PoM Synalar 1 in 10 Dilution® (Zeneca)

Cream, fluocinolone acetonide 0.0025%. Net price 50 g = £1.48. Label: 28. Potency: mild

Additives: include benzyl alcohol, polysorbates, propylene glycol

With antibacterials
See notes above for comment on compound preparations

PoM Synalar C® (Zeneca)

Cream, fluocinolone acetonide 0.025%, clioquinol 3%. Net price 15 g = 94p. Label: 28. Potency: potent

Additives: include disodium edetate, hydroxybenzoates (parabens), polysorbates, propylene glycol

Ointment, ingredients as for cream. Net price 15 g = 94p. Label: 28. Potency: potent.

Caution: stains clothing

Additives: include propylene glycol, wool fat

PoM Synalar N® (Zeneca)

Cream, fluocinolone acetonide 0.025%, neomycin sulphate 0.5%. Net price 15 g = 81p; 30 g = £1.41. Label: 28. Potency: potent

Additives: include hydroxybenzoates (parabens), polysorbates, propylene glycol

Ointment, ingredients as for cream, in a greasy basis. Net price 15 g = 81p; 30 g = £1.41. Label: 28. Potency: potent

Additives: include propylene glycol, wool fat

FLUOCINONIDE

Indications: severe inflammatory skin disorders such as eczema unresponsive to less potent corticosteroids; psoriasis, see notes above

Cautions; Contra-indications; Side-effects: see under Hydrocortisone and notes above

Administration: apply thinly 3–4 times daily (1–2 times daily for scalp lotion), reducing frequency as condition responds

PoM Metosyn® (Zeneca)

FAPG cream, fluocinonide 0.05%. Net price 25 g = £1.22; 100 g = £4.59. Label: 28. Potency: potent

Additives: include propylene glycol

Ointment, fluocinonide 0.05%. Net price 25 g = £1.22; 100 g = £4.59. Label: 28. Potency: potent

Additives: include propylene glycol, wool fat

Scalp lotion, fluocinonide 0.05% in a propylene glycol-alcohol basis. Net price 30 mL (with applicator) = £1.56. Label: 15, 28. Potency: potent

Additives: include propylene glycol

FLUOCORTOLONE

Indications: 0.25%—severe inflammatory skin disorders such as eczema unresponsive to less potent corticosteroids; 0.1%—milder inflammatory skin disorders; psoriasis, see notes above

Cautions; Contra-indications; Side-effects: see under Hydrocortisone and notes above

Administration: apply thinly 2–3 times daily, reducing strength and frequency as condition responds

PoM Ultradil Plain® (Schering Health)

Cream, fluocortolone hexanoate 0.1%, fluocortolone pivalate 0.1%. Net price 50 g = £2.86. Label: 28. Potency: moderate

Additives: include disodium edetate, hydroxybenzoates (parabens), fragrance

Ointment, fluocortolone hexanoate 0.1%, fluocortolone pivalate 0.1%. Net price 50 g = £2.86. Label: 28. Potency: moderate

Additives: include wool fat, fragrance

PoM Ultralanum Plain® (Schering Health)

Cream, fluocortolone hexanoate 0.25%, fluocortolone pivalate 0.25%. Net price 50 g = £4.65. Label: 28. Potency: moderate

Additives: include disodium edetate, hydroxybenzoates (parabens), fragrance

Ointment, fluocortolone 0.25%, fluocortolone hexanoate 0.25%. Net price 50 g = £4.65. Label: 28. Potency: moderate

Additives: include wool fat, fragrance

FLURANDRENOLONE

(Fludroxycortide)

Indications: inflammatory skin disorders such as eczema

Cautions; Contra-indications; Side-effects: see under Hydrocortisone and notes above

Administration: apply thinly 2–3 times daily, reducing strength and frequency as condition responds

PoM **Haelan®** (Dista)

Cream, flurandrenolone 0.0125%. Net price 60 g = £2.97. Label: 28. Potency: moderate

Additives: include propylene glycol

Ointment, flurandrenolone 0.0125%. Net price 60 g = £2.97. Label: 28. Potency: moderate

Additives: include beeswax, polysorbate

NHS *Tape,* polythene adhesive film impregnated with flurandrenolone 4 micrograms/cm². Net price 7.5 cm × 50 cm = £2.70; 7.5 cm × 200 cm = £9.08

For chronic localised recalcitrant dermatoses (but not acute or weeping), cut tape to fit lesion, apply to clean, dry skin shorn of hair, usually for 12 of each 24 hours

With antibacterials

See notes above for comment on compound preparations

PoM **Haelan-C®** (Dista)

Cream, flurandrenolone 0.0125%, clioquinol 3%. Net price 30 g = £2.02. Label: 28. Potency: moderate

Additives: include hydroxybenzoates (parabens), disodium edetate

Ointment, flurandrenolone 0.0125%, clioquinol 3%. Net price 30 g = £2.02. Label: 28. Potency: moderate

Additives: none as listed in section 13.1

Caution: clioquinol stains clothing

FLUTICASONE PROPIONATE

Indications: inflammatory skin disorders such as dermatitis and eczema unresponsive to less potent corticosteroids

Cautions; Contra-indications; Side-effects: see under Hydrocortisone and notes above

Administration: apply thinly once daily

▼ PoM **Cutivate®** (Glaxo)

Cream, fluticasone propionate 0.05%. Net price 15 g = £2.35; 50 g = £6.95. Label: 28. Potency: potent

Additives: include propylene glycol

HALCINONIDE

Indications: short-term treatment only of severe resistant inflammatory skin disorders such as recalcitrant eczemas unresponsive to less potent corticosteroids; psoriasis, see notes above

Cautions; Contra-indications; Side-effects: see under Hydrocortisone and notes above

Administration: apply thinly 2–3 times daily, reducing frequency as condition responds

PoM **Halciderm Topical®** (Squibb)

Cream, halcinonide 0.1%. Net price 30 g = £3.40. Label: 28. Potency: very potent

Additives: include propylene glycol

METHYLPREDNISOLONE ACETATE

Indications: inflammatory skin disorders such as eczema

Cautions; Contra-indications; Side-effects: see under Hydrocortisone

With antimicrobial

See notes above for comment on compound preparations

PoM **Neo-Medrone®** (Upjohn)

Cream, methylprednisolone acetate 0.25%, neomycin sulphate 0.5%. Net price 15 g = £1.44. Label: 28. Potency: mild

Additives: include butylated hydroxyanisole, butylated hydroxytoluene, hydroxybenzoates (parabens), fragrance

Apply thinly 1–3 times daily

MOMETASONE FUROATE

Indications: severe inflammatory skin disorders such as eczema unresponsive to less potent corticosteroids; psoriasis, see notes above

Cautions; Contra-indications; Side-effects: see under Hydrocortisone and notes above

Administration: apply thinly once daily (to scalp in case of lotion)

▼ PoM **Elocon®** (Schering-Plough)

Cream, mometasone furoate 0.1%. Net price 30 g = £4.88. Label: 28. Potency: potent

Additives: none as listed in section 13.1

Ointment, mometasone furoate 0.1%. Net price 30 g = £4.88. Label: 28. Potency: potent

Additives: none as listed in section 13.1

Lotion, mometasone furoate 0.1% in an aqueous isopropyl alcohol basis. Net price 30 mL = £4.88. Label: 28. Potency: potent

Additives: include propylene glycol

TRIAMCINOLONE ACETONIDE

Indications: severe inflammatory skin disorders such as eczema unresponsive to less potent corticosteroids; psoriasis, see notes above

Cautions; Contra-indications; Side-effects: see under Hydrocortisone and notes above

Administration: apply thinly 2–4 times daily, reducing frequency as condition responds

PoM **Adcortyl®** (Squibb)

Cream, triamcinolone acetonide 0.1%. Net price 30 g = £1.59. Label: 28. Potency: potent

Additives: include benzyl alcohol, propylene glycol

Ointment, triamcinolone acetonide 0.1%. Net price 30 g = £1.59. Label: 28. Potency: potent

Additives: none as listed in section 13.1

PoM **Ledercort®** (Lederle)

Cream, triamcinolone acetonide 0.1%. Net price 15 g = £1.68. Label: 28. Potency: potent

Additives: include benzyl alcohol

With antimicrobials
See notes above for comment on compound preparations

PoM Adcortyl with Graneodin® (Squibb)
Cream, triamcinolone acetonide 0.1%, gramicidin 0.025%, neomycin 0.25% (as sulphate). Net price 25 g = £3.00. Label: 28. Potency: potent
Additives: include benzyl alcohol, propylene glycol

PoM Aureocort® (Lederle)
Cream, triamcinolone acetonide 0.1%, chlortetracycline hydrochloride 3% (as chlortetracycline), in a water-miscible basis. Net price 15 g = £2.70. Label: 28. Potency: potent
Additives: include chlorocresol
Ointment, triamcinolone acetonide 0.1%, chlortetracycline hydrochloride 3%, in an anhydrous greasy basis containing wool fat and white soft paraffin. Net price 15 g = £2.70. Label: 28. Potency: potent
Additives: include hydroxybenzoates (parabens), wool fat
Caution: stains clothing

PoM Nystadermal® (Squibb)
Cream, triamcinolone acetonide 0.1%, nystatin 100 000 units/g. Net price 15 g = £2.27. Label: 28. Potency: potent
Additives: include benzyl alcohol, propylene glycol, fragrance

PoM Pevaryl TC® (Cilag)
Cream, triamcinolone 0.1%, econazole nitrate 1%. Net price 15 g = £4.00. Label: 28. Potency: potent
Additives: include butylated hydroxyanisole, disodium edetate, benzoic acid

PoM Tri-Adcortyl® (Squibb)
Cream, triamcinolone acetonide 0.1%, gramicidin 0.025%, neomycin 0.25% (as sulphate), nystatin 100 000 units/g. Net price 30 g = £3.15. Label: 28. Potency: potent
Additives: include benzyl alcohol, ethylenediamine, propylene glycol, fragrance
Ointment, ingredients as for cream, in an ointment basis. Net price 30 g = £3.15. Label: 28. Potency: potent
Additives: none as listed in section 13.1

13.5   Preparations for eczema and psoriasis

13.5.1   Preparations for eczema
13.5.2   Preparations for psoriasis

13.5.1   Preparations for eczema

Eczema ('dermatitis') is due to a particular type of epidermal inflammation and is caused by a wide variety of factors; where possible the causative factors should be established and removed. In many cases no underlying factor can be identified (atopic eczema).

Dry, fissured, scaly lesions are treated with bland **emollients** (section 13.2.1) which are often all that is necessary to allay irritation and permit healing. Preparations containing zinc oxide and calamine are sometimes useful; zinc may have a weak anti-eczematous action. Preparations such as **emulsifying ointment** are used as soap substitutes and in the bath. **Keratolytics** such as salicylic acid, followed by coal tar are used in chronic eczematous conditions where there is marked thickening of the skin and pronounced scaling.

Weeping eczemas may be treated with corticosteroids (section 13.4) ; they are, however, commonly secondarily infected. Wet dressings of **potassium permanganate** (0.01%) (section 13.11.6) are applied; if a large area is involved, potassium permanganate baths are taken. When necessary **topical antibacterials** are used (section 13.10.1) but those which are not given systemically should be chosen.

Coal tar is more active than salicylic acid and has anti-inflammatory, antipruritic and keratolytic properties. It is used in psoriasis and eczema. Coal tar has superseded wood tar as it is more active. The formulation and strength chosen depends on patient acceptability and severity of the condition; the 'thicker' the patch of eczema or psoriasis the stronger the concentration of coal tar required. **Coal tar paste** or **zinc and coal tar paste** are generally suitable for most cases but are limited by their unpleasant appearance and smell and they may not be used on the face. Some of the newer preparations are less unsightly and may be preferred. Preparations such as Carbo-Dome® are suitable for treating the face. **Zinc paste and coal tar bandage** (section 13.13.1) is useful for treating the limbs. **Tar shampoos** are described in section 13.9. When lesions are extensive coal tar baths are useful. Combinations of coal tar with zinc or salicylic acid have no advantage over the simpler preparations. Preparations containing hydrocortisone and coal tar are useful in eczemas.

Ichthammol has a milder action than coal tar and has been used in the less acute forms of eczema. It can be applied conveniently to flexures of the limbs as **zinc paste and ichthammol bandage** (section 13.13.1).

Cyclosporin (section 13.5.2) is now available for *severe resistant atopic dermatitis*; its use calls for specialist care in a hospital context.

For comment on the role of **corticosteroids** see section 13.4. For comment on **gamolenic acid** see p.435

COAL TAR

Indications: chronic eczema and psoriasis
Cautions: avoid eyes and broken or inflamed skin
Side-effects: skin irritation and acne-like eruptions, photosensitivity; stains skin, hair, and fabric
Administration: apply 1–3 times daily starting with low-strength preparations
Note. For shampoo preparations see section 13.9; impregnated dressings see section 13.13.1

Ointments and similar preparations
Calamine and Coal Tar Ointment, BP, calamine 12.5 g, strong coal tar solution 2.5 g, zinc oxide 12.5 g, hydrous wool fat 25 g, white soft paraffin 47.5 g
Apply 1–2 times daily

Coal Tar and Salicylic Acid Ointment, BP, coal tar 2 g, salicylic acid 2 g, emulsifying wax 11.4 g, white soft paraffin 19 g, coconut oil 54 g, polysorbate '80' 4 g, liquid paraffin 7.6 g
Apply 1–2 times daily

Coal Tar Paste, BP, strong coal tar solution 7.5%, in compound zinc paste
Apply 1–2 times daily

Zinc and Coal Tar Paste, BP, zinc oxide 6%, coal tar 6%, emulsifying wax 5%, starch 38%, yellow soft paraffin 45%
Apply 1–2 times daily

Alphosyl® (Stafford-Miller)
Cream, coal tar extract 5%, allantoin 2%, in a vanishing-cream basis. Net price 100 g = £2.44
Additives: include beeswax, hydroxybenzoates (parabens), isopropyl palmitate, propylene glycol
Apply 2–4 times daily
Lotion, coal tar extract 5%, allantoin 2%. Net price 250 mL = £2.21
Additives: include isopropyl palmitate, propylene glycol
For application to skin or scalp, 2–4 times daily

Carbo-Dome® (Lagap)
Cream, coal tar solution 10%, in a water-miscible basis. Net price 30 g = £1.97; 100 g = £5.95
Additives: include beeswax, hydroxybenzoates (parabens)
Apply 2–3 times daily

Clinitar® (Shire)
Cream, coal tar extract 1%. Net price 100 g = £5.37
Additives: include isopropyl palmitate, propylene glycol
Apply 1–2 times daily

Cocois® (Bioglan)
Scalp ointment, coal tar solution 12%, salicylic acid 2%, precipitated sulphur 4%, in a coconut oil emollient basis. Net price 40 g (with applicator nozzle) = £4.25; 100 g = £7.98
Additives: none as listed in section 13.1
Use once weekly as necessary (if severe use daily for first 3–7 days), shampoo off after 1 hour; CHILD 6–12 years, medical supervision required (not recommended under 6 years)

Gelcosal® (Quinoderm Ltd)
Gel, strong coal tar solution 5%, pine tar 5%, salicylic acid 2%. Net price 50 g = £3.12
Additives: none as listed in section 13.1
Apply twice daily

Gelcotar® (Quinoderm Ltd)
Gel, strong coal tar solution 5%, pine tar 5%. Net price 50 g = £2.83; 500 g = £14.74
Additives: none as listed in section 13.1
Apply twice daily
Liquid, see section 13.9

Pragmatar® (Bioglan)
Cream, cetyl alcohol-coal tar distillate 4%, salicylic acid 3%, sulphur (precipitated) 3%. Net price 25 g = £2.17; 100 g = £6.99
Additives: include fragrance
Apply thinly daily; for scalp apply weekly to clean hair or in severe cases daily. Dilute with a few drops of water before application to infants

Psoriderm® (Dermal)
Cream, coal tar 6%, lecithin 0.4%. Net price 225 mL = £3.24
Additives: include hydroxybenzoates (parabens), isopropyl palmitate, propylene glycol
Apply 1–2 times daily
Scalp lotion—section 13.9

PsoriGel® (Novex)
Gel, coal tar solution USP 7.5% in an alcoholic emollient basis. Net price 90 g = £3.81
Additives: include propylene glycol
Apply 1–2 times daily

Bath preparations
Coal Tar Solution, BP, coal tar 20%, polysorbate '80' 5%, in alcohol (96%). Net price 100 mL = 58p
Use 100 mL in a bath
Note. Strong Coal Tar Solution BP contains coal tar 40%

Balneum with Tar® (Merck)
Bath oil, coal tar distillate 30%, soya oil 55%. Net price 200 mL = £3.23.
For psoriasis and eczema
Additives: none as listed in section 13.1
Use 1 measure (20 mL) in bath (infants 10 mL)

Polytar Emollient® (Stiefel)
Bath additive, coal tar solution 2.5%, arachis oil extract of coal tar 7.5%, tar 7.5%, cade oil 7.5%, liquid paraffin 35%. Net price 350 mL = £4.87.
For psoriasis, eczema, atopic and pruritic dermatoses
Additives: include isopropyl palmitate
Use 2–4 capfuls in bath and soak for 20 minutes

Psoriderm® (Dermal)
Bath emulsion, coal tar 40%. Net price 200 mL = £2.88.
For psoriasis
Additives: include polysorbate 20
Use 30 mL in a bath and soak for 5 minutes

Coal tar and corticosteroid preparations
PoM **Alphosyl HC®** (Stafford-Miller)
Cream, coal tar extract 5%, hydrocortisone 0.5%, allantoin 2%. Net price 30 g = £1.66; 100 g = £4.73.
Label: 28. Potency: mild
Additives: include beeswax, hydroxybenzoates (parabens), isopropyl palmitate, wool fat
Apply thinly twice daily; CHILD under 5 years not recommended

PoM **Carbo-Cort®** (Lagap)
Cream, coal tar solution 3%, hydrocortisone 0.25%. Net price 30 g = £3.61. Label: 28. Potency: mild
Additives: include beeswax, hydroxybenzoates (parabens)
Apply thinly 2–3 times daily

PoM **Tarcortin®** (Stafford-Miller)
Cream, coal tar extract 5%, hydrocortisone 0.5%. Net price 100 g = £3.08. Label: 28. Potency: mild
Additives: include hydroxybenzoates (parabens), isopropyl palmitate, propylene glycol, polysorbates, fragrance
Apply thinly 2–4 times daily

ICHTHAMMOL
Indications: chronic eczema
Side-effects: skin irritation and sensitisation
Administration: apply 1–3 times daily

Ichthammol Ointment, BP 1980, ichthammol 10%, yellow soft paraffin 45%, wool fat 45%. Net price 25 g = 19p

Zinc and Ichthammol Cream, BP, ichthammol 5%, cetostearyl alcohol 3%, wool fat 10%, in zinc cream. Net price 100 g = 63p

Zinc Paste and Ichthammol Bandage, BP (Ichthopaste®, Icthaband®), see section 13.13.1

SALICYLIC ACID
See section 13.5.2

GAMOLENIC ACID

Gamolenic acid has been claimed to improve patients with eczema and in particular atopic dermatitis. However, the evidence in favour of a useful therapeutic effect is poor.

GAMOLENIC ACID
Indications: see under preparations
Cautions: history of epilepsy, concomitant treatment with epileptogenic drugs e.g. phenothiazines; pregnancy
Side-effects: occasional nausea, indigestion, headache
Dose: see below

PoM **Epogam®** (Searle)
Capsules, gamolenic acid 40 mg in evening primrose oil. Net price 240-cap pack = £24.41. Counselling, see below
Additives: include vitamin E 10 mg as *in vivo* antoxidant
Dose: symptomatic relief of atopic eczema 4–6 capsules twice daily; CHILD 1–12 years 2–4 capsules twice daily
Paediatric capsules, gamolenic acid 80 mg in evening primrose oil. Net price 60-cap pack = £15.41. Counselling, see below
Additives: include vitamin E 20 mg as *in vivo* antoxidant
Dose: symptomatic relief of atopic eczema CHILD over 1 year, 1–2 capsules twice daily
COUNSELLING. Capsules may be cut open and contents swallowed or taken on bread; paediatric capsules have 'snip-off' neck for convenience of administration

Mastalgia
(for advice see p. 303).
PoM **Efamast®** (Searle)
Capsules, gamolenic acid 40 mg in evening primrose oil. Net price 224-cap pack = £23.72
Additives: include vitamin E 10 mg as *in vivo* antoxidant
Dose: symptomatic relief of cyclical and non-cyclical mastalgia, 3–4 capsules twice daily, usually for 8-12 weeks then stopped or continued at lower maintenance dose

13.5.2   Preparations for psoriasis

Psoriasis is characterised by epidermal thickening and scaling. It has less tendency to heal spontaneously than eczema. For mild conditions, treatment, other than reassurance and an **emollient**, may be unnecessary.

In more troublesome cases of psoriasis, local application of **salicylic acid** (see below), **coal tar** (see section 13.5.1), or **dithranol** (see below) may have a beneficial effect. **Calcipotriol** (see below) is now also widely used.

Salicylic acid may be used in all hyperkeratotic and scaling conditions to enhance the rate of loss of surface scale. Preparations containing salicylic acid 2% are used initially and then gradually increased to concentrations of 3 to 6%. Side-effects are few but include irritant contact sensitivity, or, when large areas are treated, salicylism (see section 10.1.1).

Dithranol is used in psoriasis and is the most potent topical preparation available for this condition. The preparation is applied carefully to the lesion, covered with a dressing, and left for one hour. Applications are preferably left on the skin overnight but short contact applications of 30 minutes to an hour are also effective and are more convenient; usual concentrations are 0.1–2%. Dithranol must be used with caution as it can cause quite severe skin irritation. For this reason it must be applied only to the lesions and it is customary to start with low concentrations and gradually build up to the maximum concentration which produces a therapeutic effect without irritation. Hands should be washed thoroughly after use. Some patients are intolerant to dithranol even in low concentrations; it is important to recognise them early in treatment. Fair skin is more sensitive than dark skin. Proprietary preparations such as Dithrocream® are most commonly used as they may cause less staining and irritation than dithranol paste. Dithranol and urea combinations (Psoradrate®) may improve skin texture by rehydration. **Dithranol triacetate** has no advantage over traditional preparations. *Ingram's method* of applying dithranol is sometimes used in hospital. The patient soaks in a warm bath containing coal tar solution 1 in 800 and after drying is exposed to ultraviolet radiation B (UVB) to produce a slight erythema. **Dithranol paste** is applied to the lesions and the normal skin protected by applying talc and stockinette dressings. The procedure is repeated daily.

UVB phototherapy is also effective by itself in mild to moderate psoriasis.

Calcipotriol is a vitamin D derivative that is now widely used for topical application for mild to moderate psoriasis affecting up to 40% of skin area; a scalp solution is now also available.

PUVA, photochemotherapy using psoralens with long-wave ultraviolet irradiation (UVA), is an effective method of treating some patients with psoriasis. Special lamps are required, and a psoralen, generally methoxsalen [unlicensed] is given by mouth about 2 hours beforehand, to sensitise the skin to the effects of irradiation. A course of PUVA may last 4 to 6 weeks and requires a variable number of treatments. Treatment is only available in specialist centres; it has to be carefully regulated, owing to the short-term hazard of severe burning and the long-term hazards of cataract formation, accelerated ageing, and the development of skin cancer.

Acitretin is a retinoid given by mouth for the treatment of *severe resistant or complicated psoriasis* and some of the *congenital disorders of keratinisation* including Darier's disease (keratosis follicularis). It is a metabolite of **etretinate** (which it has replaced). It should be prescribed **only** by, or under the supervision of, a consultant dermatologist and is available to hospitals (or specified retail pharmacies) **only**. It is a retinoid (a vitamin A derivative) with marked effects on keratinising epithelia. A therapeutic effect occurs after 2 to 4 weeks with maximum benefit after 4 to 6 weeks. Acitretin treats only manifestations not the ultimate causes of these diseases, but treatment should be limited to a period of 6 to 9 months with a 3- to 4-month rest period before repeating treatment. Most patients suffer from dryness and cracking of the lips. Other side-effects include a mild transient increase in the rate of hair fall (reversible on withdrawal), occasional generalised pruritus, paronychia, and nose bleeds. There is a tendency for the plasma lipids to rise in some patients. Acitretin is **teratogenic** and must be **avoided** in pregnancy. Contraceptive meas-

---

·

ures must be taken at least **1 month before** and during treatment by women who may become pregnant and for at least **two years after** a course of the drug.

An antimetabolite, usually **methotrexate**, may also be used for *severe resistant psoriasis*, but this must again always be done under hospital supervision, the dose being adjusted according to severity of the condition and in accordance with haematological and biochemical measurements; the usual dose is 10 to 25 mg of methotrexate weekly, by mouth.

Cyclosporin is now also available for *severe resistant psoriasis* and once again its use calls for specialist care in a hospital context.

For comment on the limited role of **corticosteroids** in psoriasis, see section 13.4.

TOPICAL PREPARATIONS FOR PSORIASIS

CALCIPOTRIOL

Indications: see under Administration
Cautions: pregnancy; avoid use on face and inadvertent transfer to other body areas; wash hands thoroughly after application; risk of hypercalcaemia if more than 100 g weekly used (reported with less in generalised pustular or erythrodermic exfoliative psoriasis)
Contra-indications: disorders of calcium metabolism
Side-effects: local irritation; also dermatitis, pruritus, erythema, aggravation of psoriasis, photosensitivity; rarely facial or perioral dermatitis; hypercalcaemia (see Cautions)
Administration: cream or *ointment,* mild to moderate plaque psoriasis affecting up to 40% of skin area, apply twice daily; max. 100 g weekly (less with *scalp solution,* see below); CHILD not recommended

PoM **Dovonex**® (Leo)
Cream, calcipotriol 50 micrograms/g. Net price 30 g = £7.75; 100 g = £22.28
Additives: include disodium edetate
Ointment, calcipotriol 50 micrograms/g. Net price 30 g = £7.75; 100 g = £22.28
Additives: include disodium edetate, propylene glycol
Scalp solution, calcipotriol 50 micrograms/mL. Net price 60 mL = £22.28
Additives: include propylene glycol
Scalp solution, apply to scalp twice daily; max. 60 mL weekly (may be less with cream or ointment, see below); CHILD not recommended
MAX. WHEN PREPARATIONS USED TOGETHER. Max. total calcipotriol 5 mg in any one week (e.g. *scalp solution* 60 mL with *cream* or *ointment* 30 g or *cream* or *ointment* 60 g with *scalp solution* 30 mL)

COAL TAR
See section 13.5.1

DITHRANOL
Indications: subacute and chronic psoriasis, see notes above
Cautions: avoid use near eyes; see also notes above
Contra-indications: hypersensitivity; acute and pustular psoriasis
Side-effects: local burning sensation and irritation; stains skin, hair, and fabrics
Administration: see notes above

PoM * **Dithranol Ointment, BP** dithranol, in yellow soft paraffin; usual strengths 0.1–2%. Part of basis may be replaced by hard paraffin if a stiffer preparation is required. Label: 28
* PoM if dithranol content more than 1%, otherwise P
Dithranol Paste, BP, dithranol in zinc and salicylic acid (Lassar's) paste. Usual strengths 0.1–1% of dithranol. Label: 28
Alphodith® (Stafford-Miller)
Ointment, dithranol 0.4%, net price 50 g = £3.41; 1%, 50 g = £4.14; PoM2%, 50 g = £5.85; PoM3%, 50 g = £8.29. Label: 10 patient information leaflet, 28. For application to skin or scalp
Additives: none as listed in section 13.1
Anthranol® (Stiefel)
Ointment, dithranol 0.4%, net price 50 g = £3.50; 1%, 50 g = £4.25; PoM2%, 50 g = £6.00. Label: 28. For application to skin or scalp
Additives: include salicylic acid 0.5% as an antioxidant
Dithrocream® (Dermal)
Cream, dithranol 0.1%, net price 50 g = £3.86; 0.25%, 50 g = £4.14; 0.5%, 50 g = £4.77; 1%, 50 g = £5.55; PoM 2%, 50 g = £6.95. Label: 28. For application to skin or scalp
Additives: include chlorocresol
Dithrolan® (Dermal)
Ointment, dithranol 0.5%, salicylic acid 0.5%. Net price 90 g = £5.35. Label: 28
Additives: none as listed in section 13.1
Psoradrate® (Procter & Gamble Pharm.)
Cream, dithranol in a powder-in-cream basis containing urea. 0.1%, net price 30 g = £2.48, 100 g = £7.40; 0.2%, 30 g = £2.74, 100 g = £8.50. Label: 28
Additives: include polysorbate 40
Psorin® (Thames)
Ointment, dithranol 0.11%, crude coal tar 1%, salicylic acid 1.6%. Net price 50 g = £5.30, 100 g = £10.50. Label: 28
Additives: include beeswax, wool fat

SALICYLIC ACID
Indications: hyperkeratoses
Cautions: see notes above; avoid broken or inflamed skin
Side-effects: sensitivity, excessive drying, irritation, systemic effects after prolonged use (see section 10.1.1)

Salicylic Acid Collodion, BP —section 13.7

Salicylic Acid Ointment, BP, salicylic acid 2%, in wool alcohols ointment. Net price 25 g = 16p
Apply twice daily

Cautionary label wordings, see inside back cover

Zinc and Salicylic Acid Paste, BP (Lassar's Paste), zinc oxide 24%, salicylic acid 2%, starch 24%, white soft paraffin 50%. Net price 25 g = 16p

Apply twice daily

ORAL RETINOIDS FOR PSORIASIS

ACITRETIN

Note. Acitretin is a metabolite of etretinate

Indications: severe extensive psoriasis resistant to other forms of therapy; palmo-plantar pustular psoriasis; severe congenital ichthyosis; severe Darier's disease (keratosis follicularis)

Cautions: exclude pregnancy before starting—patients should avoid pregnancy at least 1 month before, during, and for at least 2 years after treatment, should avoid tetracycline, high doses of vitamin A (more than 4000–5000 units daily) and use of keratolytics, and should not donate blood during or for 1 year after stopping therapy (teratogenic risk); monitor hepatic function and plasma lipids (especially in hypertriglyceridaemia) at start, 1 month after initiating treatment, and then at intervals of 3 months; diabetes (can alter glucose tolerance—initial frequent blood glucose checks); radiographic assessment on long-term treatment; investigate atypical musculoskeletal symptoms; not recommended for children except under exceptional circumstances (premature epiphyseal closure reported); patients should avoid excessive exposure to sunlight and unsupervised use of sunlamps; **interactions:** Appendix 1 (acitretin)

Contra-indications: hepatic and renal impairment; pregnancy (**important teratogenic risk:** see Cautions and Appendix 4); breast-feeding

Side-effects: (mainly dose-related) dryness of mucous membranes (sometimes erosion), of skin (sometimes scaling, thinning, erythema especially of face, and pruritus), and of conjunctiva (sometimes conjunctivitis and decreased tolerance of contact lenses); other side-effects reported include palmar and plantar exfoliation, epistaxis, epidermal fragility, paronychia, granulomatous lesions, reversible hair thinning and alopecia, myalgia and arthralgia, occasional nausea, headache, malaise, drowsiness and sweating; benign intracranial hypertension (**avoid** concomitant tetracyclines); photosensitivity, mood changes and blood disorders (including thrombocytopenia and anaemia) reported for etretinate, raised liver enzymes, rarely jaundice and hepatitis (**avoid** concomitant methotrexate); raised triglycerides; decreased night vision reported; skeletal hyperostosis and extraosseous calcification reported following long-term administration of etretinate (and premature epiphyseal closure in children, see Cautions)

Dose: administered in accordance with expert advice, initially 25–30 mg daily (Darier's disease 10 mg daily) for 2–4 weeks, then adjusted according to response, usually within range 25–50 mg daily (in some cases up to max. 75 mg daily) for further 6–8 weeks (in Darier's disease and ichthyosis not more than 50 mg daily for up to 6 months); CHILD (**important:** exceptional circumstances only, see Cautions), 500 micrograms/kg daily (occasionally up to 1 mg/kg daily to max. 35 mg daily for limited periods) with careful monitoring of musculoskeletal development

▼ PoM **Neotigason®** (Roche)

Capsules, acitretin 10 mg (brown/white), net price 56-cap pack = £26.53; 25 mg (brown/yellow), 56-cap pack = £61.57 (**hosp. or specified retail pharmacy only**—see data sheet for details, specialist dermatological supervision). Label: 10 patient information leaflet, 21

ETRETINATE

Note. Etretinate is a derivative of tretinoin which is a form of Vitamin A

Indications; Cautions; Contra-indications; Side-effects: see under Acitretin

TERATOGENIC RISK. It is **important** to bear in mind that pregnancy must continue to be **avoided** for **2 years** after stopping treatment (nor should blood be donated for 2 years after stopping)

PoM **Tigason®** (Roche)
Product discontinued

ORAL IMMUNOSUPPRESSANTS FOR PSORIASIS

CYCLOSPORIN

(Ciclosporin)

Indications: see under Dose; transplantation and graft-versus-host disease, see section 8.2.2

Cautions; Side-effects: see section 8.2.2

ADDITIONAL CAUTIONS IN ATOPIC DERMATITIS AND PSORIASIS. **Contra-indicated** in abnormal renal function, hypertension not under control (see also below), infections not under control, and malignancy (see also below). Dermatological and physical examination, including blood pressure and renal function measurements required at least twice before starting; discontinue if hypertension develops that cannot be controlled by dose reduction or antihypertensive therapy; avoid excessive exposure to sunlight and use of UVB or PUVA; *in atopic dermatitis,* also allow herpes simplex infections to clear before starting (if they occur during treatment withdraw if severe); *Staphylococcus aureus* skin infections not absolute contra-indication providing controlled (but avoid erythromycin unless no other alternative—see also **interactions:** Appendix 1 (cyclosporin); monitor serum creatinine every 2 weeks throughout; *in psoriasis,* also exclude malignancies (including those of skin and cervix) before starting (biopsy any lesions not typical of psoriasis) and treat patients with malignant or pre-malignant conditions of skin only after appropriate treatment (and if no other option); monitor serum creatinine every 2 weeks for first 3 months then every 2 months (monthly if dose more than 2.5 mg/kg daily), reducing dose by 25–50% if increases more than 30% above baseline (even if within normal range) and discontinuing if reduction not successful within 1 month; also discontinue if lymphoproliferative disorder develops

---

Dose: ADULT over 16 years *by mouth*, administered in accordance with expert advice

Short-term treatment (max. 8 weeks) of severe atopic dermatitis where conventional therapy ineffective or inappropriate, initially 2.5 mg/kg daily in 2 divided doses, if good initial response not achieved within 2 weeks, increase rapidly to max. 5 mg/kg daily; initial dose of 5 mg/kg daily if very severe; CHILD under 16 years not recommended

Severe psoriasis where conventional therapy ineffective or inappropriate, initially 2.5 mg/kg daily in 2 divided doses, increased gradually to max. 5 mg/kg daily if no improvement within 1 month (discontinue if response still insufficient after 6 weeks); initial dose of 5 mg/kg daily justified if condition requires rapid improvement; CHILD and under 16 years not recommended

COUNSELLING. Total daily dose to be taken in 2 divided doses. To mask taste, mix with cold milk, cold chocolate drink, cola or orange juice immediately before taking (and rinse with more to ensure total dose). Do not use plastic cup. Keep medicine measure away from other liquids (including water)

Preparations

See section 8.2.2

METHOTREXATE

Indications: severe uncontrolled psoriasis unresponsive to conventional therapy; malignant disease, see section 8.1.3; rheumatoid arthritis, see section 10.1.3

Cautions; Side-effects: methotrexate is an antimetabolite with severe haematological, pulmonary, gastro-intestinal, and other toxicity for use only by specialists (see also notes above, section 8.1.3, and data sheet); investigations required before starting include complete haematological analysis, renal function tests (contra-indicated if significant impairment, see section 8.1.3 and Appendix 3), liver function tests (contra-indicated if abnormalities, see below and Appendix 2) followed by constant monitoring during treatment; also **contra-indicated** in pregnancy (avoid conception, for at least 6 months after stopping) and breast-feeding (see Cytotoxic drugs, Appendixes 4 and 5) and immunodeficiency syndromes; extreme caution in peptic ulceration, ulcerative colitis, diarrhoea and ulcerative stomatitis (withdraw if stomatitis develops—may be first sign of gastro-intestinal toxicity); photosensitivity—lesions of psoriasis aggravated by UV radiation (skin ulceration reported); **interactions:** see below and Appendix 1 (methotrexate)

BLOOD COUNT. Haematopoietic suppression may occur abruptly (with apparently safe dosage); any profound drop in white cell or platelet count calls for immediate withdrawal of methotrexate and introduction of supportive treatment

LIVER TOXICITY. Particular attention should be paid to the possible development of liver toxicity by carrying out liver function tests before starting methotrexate and every 2–4 months during therapy. Treatment should not be started or should be discontinued if any abnormality of liver function tests or liver biopsy is present or develops during therapy. Abnormalities may return to normal

within 2 weeks after which treatment may be recommenced if judged appropriate

PULMONARY TOXICITY. May be special problem in rheumatoid arthritis (patient to contact doctor immediately if dyspnoea or cough)

ASPIRIN and other NSAIDS. Concurrent administration of aspirin or other NSAIDs may reduce excretion of methotrexate and increase its toxicity. If aspirin or other NSAIDs are given concurrently the dose of methotrexate should be carefully monitored. Patients should be advised to avoid self-medication with over-the-counter aspirin or ibuprofen

Dose: by mouth, 10–25 mg once weekly, adjusted according to response; ELDERLY consider dose reduction (extreme caution); CHILD not recommended

Preparations

See section 8.1.3

13.6   Preparations for acne

13.6.1   Topical preparations for acne

Most topical preparations are intended for removing follicular plugs and reducing skin flora.

In mild acne it may be enough to cleanse the skin regularly and use a keratolytic such as retinoic acid or salicylic acid.

Failing that, topical application of an antibacterial such as benzoyl peroxide or an antibiotic such as erythromycin or clindamycin may be adequate.

CLEANSERS AND ABRASIVES FOR ACNE

The skin is cleansed regularly with detergent solutions (section 13.11.3). Abrasives may also be used but their effectiveness is uncertain.

In mild acne the exfoliating action of regular cleansing of the affected skin may be adequate. Abrasives are of very limited value, they represent an extreme form of cleansing and their peeling action may have a marginal effect in reducing comedones.

ABRASIVE AGENTS

Indications: cleansing in acne vulgaris

Cautions: avoid contact with eyes; discontinue use temporarily if skin becomes irritated

Contra-indications: superficial venules, telangiectasia

Brasivol® (Stiefel)

Paste No. 1, aluminium oxide 38.09% in fine particles, in a soap-detergent basis; *Paste No. 2,* aluminium oxide 52.2% in medium particles, net price 75 g (both) = £2.49

Additives: include fragrance

Use instead of soap 1–3 times daily, starting with fine grade

Ionax Scrub® (Novex)

Gel, polyethylene granules 21.9%, benzalkonium chloride 0.25% in a foaming aqueous alcoholic basis. Net price 60 g = £3.13

Additives: include propylene glycol

Use instead of soap 1–2 times daily

For control and hygiene of acne and cleansing of the skin prior to acne treatment

KERATOLYTICS FOR ACNE

Cleansing is followed by application of **anti-bacterials** and **keratolytics**; thick greasy preparations should not be used. Preparations usually contain benzoyl peroxide, hydroxyquinoline, salicylic acid, or a topical retinoid. Many of these irritate the skin but it is doubtful if a therapeutic effect can be obtained without some degree of irritation (subsides with continued treatment).

Azelaic acid is effective in mild to moderate acne; it owes its action both to antibacterial and to keratolytic activity and can be tried if benzoyl peroxide does not work.

Preparations containing sulphur are obsolete and should be avoided.

AZELAIC ACID

Indications: acne vulgaris

Cautions: pregnancy, breast-feeding; avoid contact with eyes

Side-effects: local irritation (reduce frequency or discontinue use temporarily); rarely photosensitisation

▼ PoM **Skinoren®** (Schering Health)

Cream, azelaic acid 20%, net price 30 g = £5.00
Additives: include propylene glycol
Apply to clean skin twice daily (sensitive skin, once daily for first week); period of treatment should not exceed 6 months

BENZOYL PEROXIDE

Indications: acne vulgaris

Cautions: avoid contact with eyes, mouth, and mucous membranes; may bleach fabrics

Side-effects: skin irritation

Administration: apply 1–2 times daily to clean skin, starting treatment with lower-strength preparations

Acetoxyl® (Stiefel)

Gel, benzoyl peroxide in an aqueous-acetone-gel basis, 2.5% ('*2.5' Gel*), net price 40 g = £1.59; 5% ('*5' Gel*), 40 g = £1.76
Additives: include propylene glycol

Acnecide® (Novex)

Gel, benzoyl peroxide, in an aqueous gel basis, 5% ('*5' Gel*), net price 60 g = £3.75; 10% ('*10' Gel*), 60 g = £4.12
Additives: include propylene glycol

Acnegel® (Stiefel)

Gel, benzoyl peroxide in an aqueous alcoholic basis, 5% net price 50 g = £2.17; 10% ('*Forte' Gel*), 50 g = £2.38
Additives: none as listed in section 13.1

Benoxyl® (Stiefel)

Cream, benzoyl peroxide, in a non-greasy basis, 5% ('*5' Cream*), net price 40 g = £1.29
Additives: include isopropyl palmitate, propylene glycol

Lotion, benzoyl peroxide, in a non-greasy basis, 5% ('*5' Lotion*), net price 30 mL = £1.03; 10% ('*10' Lotion*), 30 mL = £1.09
Additives: include isopropyl palmitate, propylene glycol

Benzagel® (Bioglan)

Gel, benzoyl peroxide 5% ('*5' Gel*), net price 40 g = £2.67; 10% ('*10' Gel*), 40 g = £3.05
Additives: include fragrance

Nericur® (Schering Health)

Gel, benzoyl peroxide, in an aqueous gel basis, 5% ('*5' Gel*), net price 30 g = £1.45; 10% ('*10' Gel*), 30 g = £1.60
Additives: include propylene glycol

Panoxyl® (Stiefel)

Aquagel (= aqueous gel), benzoyl peroxide 2.5% ('*2.5' Aquagel*), net price 40 g = £1.72; 5% ('*5' Aquagel*), 40 g = £1.92; 10% ('*10' Aquagel*), 40 g = £2.12.
Additives: include propylene glycol

Gel, benzoyl peroxide, in an aqueous alcoholic basis, 5% ('*5' Gel*), net price 40 g = £1.44; 10% ('*10' Gel*), 40 g = £1.63
Additives: include fragrance

Wash, benzoyl peroxide, in a detergent basis, 10% ('*10' Wash*), net price 150 mL = £3.50
Additives: none as listed in section 13.1

With antimicrobials

Acnidazil® (Cilag)

Cream, benzoyl peroxide 5%, miconazole nitrate 2%. Net price 15 g = £2.10; 30 g = £3.40
Additives: include polysorbate 20, propylene glycol

PoM **Benzamycin®** (Bioglan)

Gel, pack for reconstitution, providing erythromycin 3% and benzoyl peroxide 5%. Net price per pack to provide 23.3 g = £7.99
Additives: none as listed in section 13.1
Apply to clean skin twice daily (very fair skin, initially once daily at night)

Quinoderm® (Quinoderm Ltd)

Cream, benzoyl peroxide 10%, potassium hydroxyquinoline sulphate 0.5%, in an astringent vanishing-cream basis. Net price 25 g = £1.24; 50 g = £1.86
Additives: include edetic acid (EDTA)

Cream 5, benzoyl peroxide 5%, potassium hydroxyquinoline sulphate 0.5%, in an astringent vanishing-cream basis. Net price 50 g = £1.69
Additives: include edetic acid (EDTA)

Lotio-gel 5%, benzoyl peroxide 5%, potassium hydroxyquinoline sulphate 0.5%, in an astringent creamy basis. Net price 30 mL = £1.47
Additives: include edetic acid (EDTA)

SALICYLIC ACID

Indications: acne vulgaris

Cautions: avoid contact with mouth, eyes, mucous membranes; systemic effects after excessive use (see section 10.1.1)

Side-effects: local irritation

Acnisal® (Euroderma)

Topical solution, salicylic acid 2% in a detergent basis. Net price 177 mL = £4.50. Use up to 3 times daily
Additives: include benzyl alcohol, hydroxybenzoates (parabens)

SULPHUR

Cautions: avoid contact with eyes, mouth, and mucous membranes; causes skin irritation

With resorcinol
Prolonged application of resorcinol may interfere with thyroid function therefore not recommended
Eskamel® (Goldshield)
Cream, resorcinol 2%, sulphur 8%, in a non-greasy flesh-coloured basis. Net price 25 g = £1.90
Additives: include propylene glycol, fragrance

With salicylic acid
See above for cautions relating to salicylic acid
Salicylic Acid and Sulphur Cream, BP 1980, salicylic acid 2%, precipitated sulphur 2%, in aqueous cream
Salicylic Acid and Sulphur Ointment, BPC, salicylic acid 3%, precipitated sulphur 3%, in hydrous ointment (oily cream)

TOPICAL ANTIBIOTICS FOR ACNE

Topical antibiotics are also used for mild to moderately severe acne. Topical preparations of erythromycin, tetracycline, and clindamycin seem to be quite useful for many patients with the milder forms of acne; they can produce mild irritation of the skin but rarely sensitise.

Cross resistance, especially between erythromycin and clindamycin is an increasing problem. To avoid this:

when possible use non-antibiotic antimicrobials (such as benzoyl peroxide);

avoid concomitant treatment with different oral and topical antibiotics;

if a particular antibiotic is effective, use it for repeat courses.

Topical chloramphenicol and neomycin are not suitable owing to sensitisation.

ANTIBIOTICS

Indications: acne vulgaris
Cautions: alcoholic preparations are not suitable for use with benzoyl peroxide
DURATION OF TREATMENT. Usual max. duration of treatment 10–12 weeks to minimise problems with antibiotic resistance (but course may be repeated after interval of few weeks)

Benzamycin® see under Benzoyl peroxide above
PoM Dalacin T® (Upjohn)
Topical solution, clindamycin (as phosphate) 1%, in an aqueous alcoholic basis. Net price 30 mL (with applicator) = £4.54
Additives: include propylene glycol
Apply to clean skin twice daily
Lotion, clindamycin (as phosphate) 1% in an aqueous basis. Net price 30 mL = £5.32
Additives: include hydroxybenzoates (parabens)
Apply to clean skin twice daily
PoM Stiemycin® (Stiefel)
Solution, erythromycin 2% in an alcoholic basis. Net price 50 mL = £9.00
Additives: include propylene glycol
Apply to clean skin twice daily

PoM Topicycline® (Monmouth)
Solution, powder for reconstitution, tetracycline hydrochloride, 4-epitetracycline hydrochloride, providing tetracycline hydrochloride 2.2 mg/mL when reconstituted with solvent containing *n*-decyl methyl sulphoxide and citric acid in 40% alcohol. Net price per pack of powder and solvent to provide 70 mL = £7.70
Additives: none as listed in section 13.1
Apply to clean skin twice daily
PoM Zineryt® (Yamanouchi)
Topical solution, powder for reconstitution, erythromycin 40 mg, zinc acetate 12 mg/mL when reconstituted with solvent containing ethanol. Net price per pack of powder and solvent to provide 30 mL = £8.04; 90 mL = £22.91
Additives: none as listed in section 13.1.
Apply to clean skin twice daily

TOPICAL RETINOIDS FOR ACNE

Topical application of **tretinoin** (which is the acid form of vitamin A) or of its isomer **isotretinoin** modifies keratinisation so as to reduce pilosebaceous duct occlusion. This is useful in treating acne, but patients should be warned that some redness and skin peeling may occur after application for several days. Isotretinoin is also given by mouth, see section 13.6.2 for **additional warnings**.

ISOTRETINOIN

Note. Isotretinoin is an isomer of tretinoin
Indications; Cautions; Contra-indications; Side-effects (after topical application only): see under Tretinoin and notes above
IMPORTANT. For **indications**, **cautions**, **contra-indications** and **side-effects** of isotretinoin **when given by mouth**, see next page
Administration: apply thinly to clean skin 1–2 times daily

PoM Isotrex® (Stiefel)
Gel, isotretinoin 0.05%. Net price 30 g = £6.96.
Label: 10 patient information leaflet
Additives: include butylated hydroxytoluene

TRETINOIN

Note. Tretinoin is the acid form of vitamin A
Indications: acne vulgaris
Cautions: avoid contact with eyes, mouth, and mucous membranes; do not use simultaneously with other peeling agents (can be alternated every 12 hours with benzoyl peroxide); do not use with ultra-violet lamps (and minimise exposure to sunlight)
Contra-indications: pregnancy, eczema, broken or sunburned skin; personal or family history of cutaneous epithelioma
Side-effects: irritation, erythema, peeling; changes in pigmentation, photosensitivity
Administration: apply thinly to clean skin 1–2 times daily

PoM **Retin-A**® (Cilag)

Cream, tretinoin 0.025%, net price 60 g = £6.03; 0.05%, 60 g = £6.03. For dry or fair skin
Additives: include butylated hydroxytoluene, sorbic acid
Gel, tretinoin 0.01%, net price 60 g = £6.03; 0.025%, 60 g = £6.03. For severe acne, initial treatment, or dark and oily skins
Additives: include butylated hydroxytoluene
Lotion, tretinoin 0.025%. Net price 100 mL = £6.94. For application to large areas such as the back
Additives: include butylated hydroxytoluene

TOPICAL CORTICOSTEROIDS FOR ACNE

Topical **corticosteroids** should **not** be used in acne.

CORTICOSTEROIDS

Indications: not recommended (see notes above)
Cautions; Contra-indications; Side-effects: section 13.4 and notes above

PoM **Actinac**® (Roussel)

Lotion (powder for reconstitution), chloramphenicol 1.25%, hydrocortisone acetate 1.25%, allantoin 0.75%, butoxyethyl nicotinate 0.75%, precipitated sulphur 10%, when reconstituted with solvent. Discard after 21 days. Net price 2 × 6.25 g bottles powder with 2 × 20-mL bottles solvent = £9.30. Label: 28. Potency: mild
Additives: include fragrance

13.6.2   Oral preparations for acne

ORAL ANTIBIOTICS FOR ACNE

Systemic antibacterial treatment is useful. **Tetracycline** (see section 5.1.3), **erythromycin** (see section 5.1.5), and occasionally other antibacterials are used. The usual dosage regimen for tetracycline and erythromycin, taken before meals, is 500 mg twice daily for 3 months reduced to 250 mg twice daily for a further 3 months. Maximum improvement usually occurs after four to six months but in resistant cases treatment may need to be continued for two or more years. As there have been some reports of pseudomembranous colitis with tetracycline, caution is necessary in long-term administration; administration of erythromycin for longer than 14 days is occasionally associated with cholestatic jaundice.

As an alternative to tetracycline itself, **minocycline** (section 5.1.3) offers less likelihood of bacterial resistance; it is given in a dosage of 100 mg daily. **Doxycycline** may also be used in a dosage of 50 mg daily. Although **trimethoprim** is not licensed for acne it too is used, in a dosage of 100 mg twice daily.

Concomitant use of different topical and systemic antibiotics is undesirable owing to the increased likelihood of the development of bacterial resistance.

TETRACYCLINES
See section 5.1.3

ERYTHROMYCIN
See section 5.1.5

HORMONE TREATMENT FOR ACNE

Cyproterone acetate with **ethinyloestradiol** (Dianette®) contains an anti-androgen. It is no more effective than an oral broad spectrum antibiotic but is useful in women who also wish to receive oral contraception.

Improvement of acne probably occurs because of decreased sebum secretion which is under androgen control. Some women with mild to moderate idiopathic hirsutism may also benefit as hair growth is also androgen-dependent (see also section 6.4.2). It is contra-indicated in pregnancy and in a predisposition to thrombosis.

CYPROTERONE ACETATE

Indications: see notes above
Cautions; Contra-indications; Side-effects: see under Combined Oral Contraceptives (7.3.1)

With ethinyloestradiol

PoM **Dianette**® (Schering Health)

Tablets, beige, s/c, cyproterone acetate 2 mg, ethinyloestradiol 35 micrograms. Net price 21-tab pack = £4.80

Dose: 1 tablet daily for 21 days starting on 1st day of menstrual cycle and repeated after a 7-day interval, usually for several months; withdraw when acne or hirsutism completely resolved (repeat courses may be given if recurrence)

ORAL RETINOID FOR ACNE

Isotretinoin (Roaccutane®) is a retinoid used for the systemic treatment of cystic and conglobate acne and severe acne which has failed to respond to an adequate course of a systemic antimicrobial agent. It is also useful in women with acne developing in the third or fourth decades of life, since this late onset acne is frequently resistant to antibiotics.

It acts by greatly reducing sebum secretion. It should be prescribed **only** by, or under the supervision of, a consultant dermatologist, and is available to hospitals **only**. It is given in doses of 500 micrograms/kg/day for at least 16 weeks but doses may be adjusted if necessary after 4 weeks. Repeat courses are occasionally required. An exacerbation is common some 2–4 weeks after starting treatment but usually subsides after a few weeks.

Side-effects of isotretinoin include dry lips, sore eyes, nose bleeds, mild transient hair loss, and joint pains. Plasma lipids and liver function should be checked by investigation monthly as there is a tendency for the plasma lipids to rise in some patients. The drug is **teratogenic** and must **not** be given to women who are pregnant or those who may become pregnant unless there is concomitant effective contraception and then only after detailed explanation by the physician. The contraceptive measures must continue for at least **one month** after ceasing treatment with the drug.

ISOTRETINOIN

Note. Isotretinoin is an isomer of tretinoin

Indications: see notes above

Cautions: exclude pregnancy before starting—pregnancy must be avoided at least 1 month before, during, and for at least 1 month after treatment; avoid donating blood during and for at least 1 month after treatment; monitor hepatic function and plasma lipids at start, 1 month after initiating treatment, then at intervals of 3 months; avoid tetracyclines, high doses of vitamin A (more than 4000–5000 units daily) and use of keratolytics during treatment; monitor blood glucose in diabetic patients

Contra-indications: pregnancy (**important teratogenic risk:** see Cautions and Appendix 4); breast-feeding; renal or hepatic impairment; hypervitaminosis A, hyperlipidaemia

Side-effects: (mainly dose-related) dryness of skin (with scaling, thinning, erythema, pruritus), epidermal fragility (trauma may cause blistering); dryness of nasal mucosa (with mild epistaxis), of pharyngeal mucosa (with hoarseness), of conjunctiva (sometimes conjunctivitis), decreased tolerance to contact lenses; visual disturbances (papilloedema, optic neuritis, corneal opacities, cataracts, decreased night vision, photophobia, blurred vision)—expert referral and consider withdrawal; hair thinning (reversible on withdrawal); nausea, headache, malaise, drowsiness, sweating; benign intracranial hypertension (avoid concomitant tetracyclines); myalgia and arthralgia; raised liver enzymes (rarely jaundice and hepatitis); raised plasma triglycerides and cholesterol; allergic vasculitis and granulomatous lesions reported, other side-effects reported include hearing deficiency, mood changes, convulsions, menstrual irregularities, hyperuricaemia, inflammatory bowel disease, paronychia and Gram-positive infections, bone changes (including early epiphyseal closure and skeletal hyperostosis following long-term administration), thrombocytopenia, thrombocytosis, neutropenia and anaemia, and allergic vasculitis

Dose: initially 500 micrograms/kg daily in 1–2 divided doses with food for 4 weeks; if good response continue for further 8–12 weeks; if little response, up to 1 mg/kg daily for 8–12 weeks; if intolerant, reduce dose to 100–200 micrograms/kg daily

PoM **Roaccutane**® (Roche)

Capsules, isotretinoin 5 mg (red-violet/white), net price 56-cap pack = £19.08; 20 mg (red-violet/white), 56-cap pack = £54.98 (**hosp. or specified retail pharmacy only**—see data sheet for details, specialist dermatological supervision). Label: 10, patient information card, 21

13.7   Preparations for warts and calluses

The least destructive method possible should be chosen to treat these lesions as they are self-limiting and all viral warts including those on the soles of the feet (verrucas) eventually disappear spontaneously. The preparations used are keratolytics which slowly remove the hyperkeratotic layers and destroy the underlying epidermis.

Salicylic acid preparations are useful but can cause considerable irritation of the treated area. They are suitable for the removal of *warts and calluses.* An ointment containing podophyllum resin with salicylic acid (*Posalfilin*®) is available for treating *plantar warts* (for podophyllum preparations suitable for treating genital warts see next page).

Preparations containing **formaldehyde** and **glutaraldehyde** are also available but their effects are unpredictable. Formaldehyde and glutaraldehyde preparations may both irritate and sensitise the skin.

SALICYLIC ACID

Indications: see under preparations

Cautions: protect surrounding skin and avoid broken skin; not suitable for application to face, anogenital region, or large areas

Contra-indications: diabetes or if peripheral blood circulation impaired

Side-effects: skin irritation, see notes above

ADMINISTRATION. Instructions in proprietary packs generally incorporate advice to remove dead skin by gentle rubbing with a pumice stone and to cover with plaster after application (unless in collodion basis)

Salicylic Acid Collodion, BP, salicylic acid 12%, in flexible collodion. Label: 15. For warts and calluses, apply daily or on alternate days

Cuplex® (S&N Pharm.)

Gel, salicylic acid 11%, lactic acid 4%, copper acetate (= Cu^{2+} 0.0011%), in a collodion basis. Net price 5 g = £2.33. Label: 15. For plantar and mosaic warts, corns, and calluses, apply twice daily

Duofilm® (Stiefel)

Paint, salicylic acid 16.7%, lactic acid 16.7%, in flexible collodion. Net price 15 mL (with applicator) = £1.95. Label: 15. For plantar and mosaic warts, apply daily

Occlusal® (Euroderma)

Application, salicylic acid 26% in polyacrylic solution. Net price 10 mL (with applicator) = £2.41. Label: 15. For common and plantar warts, apply daily

Salactol® (Dermal)

Paint, salicylic acid 16.7%, lactic acid 16.7%, in flexible collodion. Net price 10 mL (with applicator) = £1.93. Label: 15. For warts, particularly plantar warts, verrucas, corns, and calluses, apply daily

Salatac® (Dermal)

Gel, salicylic acid 12%, lactic acid 4% in a collodion basis. Net price 8 g (with applicator) = £3.36. Label: 15. For warts, verrucas, corns, and calluses, apply daily

Verrugon® (Pickles)

Ointment, salicylic acid 50% in a paraffin basis. Net price 6 g = £1.47. For plantar warts apply daily

---

Cautionary label wordings, see inside back cover

With podophyllum
Posalfilin® (Norgine)
Ointment, podophyllum resin 20%, salicylic acid
25%. Net price 10 g = £3.12. For plantar warts
apply daily
Note. Owing to the salicylic acid content, not suitable
for anogenital warts; owing to the podophyllum content
also contra-indicated in pregnancy

FORMALDEHYDE

Indications: see under preparations
Cautions; Contra-indications; Side-effects: see
under Salicylic Acid

Formaldehyde Lotion, formaldehyde solution,
BP, 3 mL, water to 100 mL. For plantar warts,
applied at night as a soak
Veracur® (Typharm)
Gel, formaldehyde 0.75% in a water-miscible gel
basis. Net price 15 g = £1.25. For warts, particularly plantar warts, apply twice daily

GLUTARALDEHYDE

Indications: see under preparations
Cautions; Contra-indications; Side-effects: see
under Salicylic Acid, stains skin brown

Glutarol® (Dermal)
Solution (= application), glutaraldehyde 10%. Net
price 10 mL (with applicator) = £2.19. For warts,
particularly plantar warts, apply twice daily
Verucasep® (Galen)
Gel, glutaraldehyde 10%. Net price 15 g = £1.95.
For warts, particularly plantar warts, apply twice
daily

GENITAL WARTS

Podophyllum preparations may be useful for *genital warts* but can cause considerable irritation of the
treated area and can cause **severe toxicity** on excessive application (see Cautions below). They are
contra-indicated in pregnancy. Preparations containing the major active constituent **podophyllotoxin** (*Condyline®*, *Warticon®* and *Warticon Fem®*)
are now also available for genital warts.
Condyline® and *Warticon®* are suitable for self-
treatment in men; *Warticon Fem®* is suitable for
self-treatment in women.

PODOPHYLLUM

Indications: see under preparations
Cautions: avoid normal skin and open wounds;
keep away from face; very irritant to eyes;
important: see also warnings below
Contra-indications: pregnancy and breast-feeding; children
Side-effects: see notes above

PoM **Podophyllin Paint, Compound, BP,** (podophyllum resin 15% in compound benzoin tincture),
podophyllum resin 1.5 g, compound benzoin tincture
to 10 mL; 5 mL to be dispensed unless otherwise
directed. Label: 15
External genital warts, applied weekly in genitourinary
clinic (or at a general practitioner's surgery by trained
nurses after screening for other sexually transmitted diseases)
IMPORTANT. Should be allowed to stay on the treated
area for not longer than 6 hours and then washed off.
Care should be taken to avoid splashing the surrounding
skin during application (which must be covered with
soft paraffin as a protection). Where there are a large
number of warts only a few should be treated at any one
time as **severe toxicity** caused by absorption of podophyllin has been reported

Podophyllotoxin
PoM **Condyline®** (Yamanouchi)
Solution, podophyllotoxin 0.5% in alcoholic basis.
Net price 3.5 mL (with applicators) = £16.00.
Label: 15
Condylomata acuminata affecting the penis or the
female external genitalia, apply twice daily for 3 consec-
utive days; treatment may be repeated at weekly inter-
vals if necessary for a total of five 3-day treatment
courses; direct medical supervision for lesions in the
female and for lesions greater than 4 cm² in the male;
max. 50 single applications ("loops") per session (see
leaflet)
PoM **Warticon®** (Perstorp)
Solution, podophyllotoxin 0.5% in alcoholic basis.
Net price 3 mL (with applicators— *Warticon®*[for
men]; with applicators and mirror—*Warticon
Fem®* [for women]) = £14.50. Label: 15
Condylomata acuminata affecting the penis or the
female external genitalia, apply twice daily for 3 consecutive days; treatment may be repeated at weekly intervals if necessary for a total of four 3-day treatment
courses; direct medical supervision for lesions greater
than 4 cm²; max. 50 single applications ("loops") per
session (see leaflet)

13.8   Sunscreens and camouflagers

13.8.1   Sunscreening preparations
13.8.2   Camouflaging preparations

13.8.1   Sunscreening preparations

Solar ultraviolet irradiation is harmful to the skin. It
is responsible for disorders such as *polymorphic
light eruption, Hutchinson's summer prurigo,* and
the various *cutaneous porphyrias.* It also provokes
(or at least aggravates) disorders such as *rosacea*
and *lupus erythematosus.* It may also contribute to
serious skin disorders in patients *sensitised by
drugs* such as demeclocycline, phenothiazines, or
amiodarone. All these conditions (as well as *sunburn*) may occur after relatively short periods of
exposure to the sun. Exposure over longer periods
may cause more serious problems. Both *melanoma*
and *non-melanoma skin cancer* are now thought to
be caused in many instances by solar ultraviolet
irradiation. It is now also believed that exposure to
the sun causes the skin to wrinkle and develop other

---

signs *associated with ageing*. Solar ultraviolet irradiation also provokes attacks of *recurrent herpes labialis* (although it is not known whether the effect of sunlight exposure is local or systemic).

Solar ultraviolet radiation is approximately 200–400 nm in wavelength. The medium wavelengths (280–310 nm, known as UVB) cause sunburn and contribute to the long-term changes responsible for skin cancer and ageing. The long wavelengths (310–400 nm, known as UVA) do not cause sunburn but are responsible for many *photosensitivity reactions* and *photodermatoses*; they also seem to contribute to long-term damage and to be involved in the pathogenesis of *skin cancer* and *photodamage*.

Sunscreen preparations that contain substances such as aminobenzoic acid protect the skin against UVB and hence against sunburn. The sun protection factor (SPF, usually indicated in the preparation title) provides guidance on the degree of protection offered against UVB; it indicates the multiples of protection provided against burning, compared with unprotected skin; for example, an SPF of 8 should enable a person to remain 8 times longer in the sun without burning. Such preparations, however, do not prevent long-term damage associated with UVA, which might not become apparent for 10 to 20 years. Preparations that also contain reflective substances, such as titanium dioxide, provide the most effective protection against UVA. Some products now indicate the degree of protection offered against UVA with a star rating system. This system does not refer to an absolute measure but indicates the protection against UVA relative to protection against UVB for the same product. Four stars indicate that the product offers a balanced amount of UVA and UVB protection; products with three, two, or one star rating indicate that the protection offered is greater against UVB than UVA. However the usefulness of the star rating system remains controversial.

Some sunscreens, particularly aminobenzoates, may rarely cause photosensitivity reactions. Bergamot oil (which contains 5-methoxypsoralen) occasionally causes photosensitisation with subsequent pigmentation; it is suspected of increasing the incidence of skin cancers, but this has not been established.

BORDERLINE SUBSTANCES. The preparations marked 'ACBS' are regarded as drugs when prescribed for skin protection against ultraviolet radiation in abnormal cutaneous photosensitivity resulting from genetic disorders or photodermatoses, including those resulting from radiotherapy; chronic or recurrent herpes simplex labialis. Preparations with SPF less than 15 are no longer prescribable. See also Appendix 7.

Coppertone® (Scholl)

Ultrashade 23 lotion, (UVA and UVB protection; UVB-SPF23) ethylhexyl *p*-methoxycinnamate 7.5%, oxybenzone 3%, padimate-O 2.5%. Net price 150 mL = £4.46. ACBS
Additives: include hydroxybenzoates (parabens), wool fat, fragrance

Piz Buin® (Zyma)

Sunblock lotion, (UVA and UVB protection; UVB-SPF 20), ethylhexyl *p*-methoxycinnamate 7.5%, avobenzone 1.5%, titanium dioxide 3%. Net price 200 mL = £5.84. ACBS
Additives: include hydroxybenzoates (parabens), propylene glycol, fragrance

RoC® (RoC)

Total sunblock cream, (UVA and UVB protection; UVB-SPF 25), colourless or tinted, containing avobenzone, ethylhexyl *p*-methoxycinnamate. Net price 50 mL = £4.06. ACBS
Additives: include beeswax, hydroxybenzoates (parabens)

Spectraban® (Stiefel)

Lotion, (UVB protection; UVB-SPF 25) aminobenzoic acid 5%, padimate-O 3.2%, in an alcoholic basis. Net price 150 mL = £2.49. ACBS
Additives: include fragrance
Caution: flammable; stains clothing
Ultra lotion, (UVA and UVB protection; UVB-SPF 28), water resistant, avobenzone 2%, oxybenzone 3%, padimate-O 8%, titanium dioxide 2%. Net price 150 mL = £4.32. ACBS
Additives: include benzyl alcohol, disodium edetate, sorbic acid, fragrance

Sun E45® (Crookes)

Sunblock cream, (UVA and UVB protection; UVB-SPF 25), water resistant, titanium dioxide 18%. Net price 75 mL = £4.63. ACBS
Additives: include butylated hydroxytoluene, isopropyl palmitate
Ultra protection lotion, (UVA and UVB protection; UVB-SPF 15), water resistant, titanium dioxide 13.4%. Net price 150 mL = £5.71. ACBS
Additives: include butylated hydroxytoluene, isopropyl palmitate

Uvistat® (Windsor)

Lipscreen, (UVA and UVB protection; UVB-SPF 15), ethylhexyl *p*-methoxycinnamate 3%, avobenzone 4%. Net price 5-g stick = £1.53. ACBS
Additives: include butylated hydroxyanisole, fragrance
Babysun cream (UVA and UVB protection; UVB-SPF 22), water-resistant, ethylhexyl *p*-methoxy cinnamate 7%, avobenzone 4%, titanium dioxide 4.5%. Net price 50 g = £3.63, 100 g = £5.10. ACBS
Additives: include disodium edetate, hydroxybenzoates (parabens), fragrance
Cream (UVA and UVB protection; UVB-SPF 20), water-resistant, ethylhexyl *p*-methoxycinnamate 7%, avobenzone 4%, titanium dioxide 4.5%. Net price 50 g = £3.40, 100 g = £5.10. ACBS
Additives: include disodium edetate, hydroxybenzoates (parabens), fragrance
Ultrablock cream, (UVA and UVB protection; UVB-SPF 30), ethylhexyl *p*-methoxycinnamate 7.5%, avobenzone 4%, titanium dioxide 6.5%. Net price 50 g = £4.08. ACBS
Additives: include disodium edetate, hydroxybenzoates (parabens), fragrance

13.8.2 Camouflagers

Disfigurement of the skin can be very distressing to patients and have a marked psychological effect. In skilled hands, or with experience, these preparations can be very effective in concealing scars and birthmarks. The depigmented patches in vitiligo are also very disfiguring and camouflage creams are of great cosmetic value.

BORDERLINE SUBSTANCES. The preparations marked 'ACBS' are regarded as drugs when prescribed for postoperative scars and other deformities and as an adjunctive therapy in the relief of emotional disturbances due to disfiguring skin disease, such as vitiligo. See also Appendix 7.

Boots Covering Cream® (Boots)
Cream (2 shades). Net price 50 g = £1.64. ACBS
Additives:include hydroxybenzoates (parabens)
Covermark® (Cupharma)
Additives: include beeswax, hydroxybenzoates (parabens), fragrance
Classic foundation (masking cream, 10 shades). Net price 30 g = £11.23. ACBS
Finishing powder. Net price 75 g = £9.50. ACBS
Dermablend® (Baker Norton)
Cover creme. Net price 10.7 g (10 shades) = £6.25; 28.4 g (11 shades)= £10.55. ACBS
Additives: include beeswax, hydroxybenzoates (parabens)
Leg cover, (7 shades). Net price 64 g = £9.35. ACBS
Additives: include beeswax, hydroxybenzoates (parabens)
Setting powder. Net price 28 g = £9.00. ACBS
Additives: include hydroxybenzoates (parabens)
Dermacolor® (Fox)
Camouflage creme, (30 shades). Net price 30 g = £6.09. ACBS
Additives: include beeswax, wool fat, fragrance
Fixing powder, (5 shades). Net price 60 g = £4.76. ACBS
Additives: include fragrance
Keromask® (Network Management)
Masking cream, (2 shades). Net price 15 mL = £3.68. ACBS
Additives:include butylated hydroxyanisole, hydroxybenzoates (parabens), wool fat
Finishing powder. Net price 25 g = £3.68. ACBS
Additives: none as listed in section 13.1
Veil® (Blake)
Cover cream, (19 shades). Net price 19 g = £3.97; 44 g = £5.96; 70 g = £8.23. ACBS
Additives: include hydroxybenzoates (parabens), wool fat derivative
Finishing powder, translucent. Net price 35 g = £3.97. ACBS
Additives: include butylated hydroxyanisole, hydroxybenzoates (parabens)

13.9   Shampoos and some other scalp preparations

Dandruff (pityriasis capitis) is believed to be caused by follicular overgrowth with pityrosporum yeasts; it often increases at puberty. The treatment of choice is the frequent use of a mild detergent shampoo generally once or twice weekly; this rids the scalp of scale but does not have a therapeutic effect in itself. Shampoos containing antimicrobial agents such as **pyrithione zinc** have beneficial effects and are on sale to the general public. Shampoos containing **tar** extracts may be useful and they are also used in *psoriasis*, both as adjunctive treatment and for the removal of pastes etc. Shampoos containing **selenium sulphide** are of no more value than the other shampoos and should not

be used within 48 hours of applying hair colouring or permanent waving preparations. **Ketoconazole** is also useful as a shampoo (see section 13.10.2).

For more severe conditions, weak **corticosteroid** gels and lotions (section 13.4), applied to the scalp may be helpful.

Cradle cap in infants may be treated with **olive oil** or **arachis oil** applications before shampooing.

See also sections 13.5 (psoriasis and eczema), 13.10.4 (lice), and 13.10.2 (ringworm).

ADMINISTRATION. Shampoos should generally be used once to three times weekly
Alphosyl 2 in 1® (Stafford-Miller)
Shampoo, alcoholic coal tar extract 5%. Net price 125 mL = £1.81; 250 mL = £3.43.
Baltar® (Merck)
Shampoo, coal tar distillate 1.5% in soap-free basis. Net price 225 mL = £2.56; 500 mL = £4.48
Betadine® (Seton)
Shampoo solution, povidone-iodine 4%, in a surfactant solution. Net price 250 mL = £2.43.
Capasal® (Dermal)
Shampoo, coal tar 1%, coconut oil 1%, salicylic acid 0.5%. Net price 250 mL = £4.83
Capitol® (Dermal)
Gel, benzalkonium chloride 0.5%. Net price 120 g = £3.00.
Ceanel Concentrate® (Quinoderm Ltd)
Shampoo, cetrimide 10%, undecenoic acid 1%, phenylethyl alcohol 7.5%. Net price 50 mL = £1.07; 150 mL = £2.83; 500 mL = £8.33
Clinitar® (Shire)
Shampoo solution, coal tar extract 2%. Net price 100 g = £2.50
Gelcotar® (Quinoderm Ltd)
Liquid, strong coal tar solution 1.25%, cade oil 0.5%, in a shampoo basis. Net price 150 mL = £1.41; 350 mL = £2.83
Gel, see section 13.5.1
Genisol® (Roche Consumer Health)
Liquid, prepared coal tar 2% (as purified coal tar fractions), sodium sulphosuccinated undecylenic monoalkylolamide 1%. Net price 58 mL = £1.28; 250 mL = £4.10; 600 mL = £8.54
Ionil T® (Novex)
Shampoo application, benzalkonium chloride 0.2%, coal tar solution 4.25%, salicylic acid 2% in an alcoholic basis. Net price 200 mL = £2.56
Lenium® (Cilag)
Cream, selenium sulphide 2.5%. Net price 42 g = 88p; 100 g = £1.50
Meted® (Euroderma)
Shampoo, salicylic acid 3%, sulphur 5%. Net price 120 mL = £3.90
PoM **Nizoral®** shampoo—section 13.10.2
Pentrax® (Euroderma)
Shampoo, coal tar 4.3%. Net price 120 mL = £3.90
Polytar® (Stiefel)
Liquid, arachis oil extract of crude coal tar 0.3%, cade oil 0.3%, coal tar solution 0.1%, oleyl alcohol 1%, tar 0.3%. Net price 250 mL = £2.23

Polytar AF® (Stiefel)

Shampoo, arachis oil extract of coal tar 0.3%, cade oil 0.3%, coal tar solution 0.1%, pine tar 0.3%, pyrithione zinc 1%. Net price 150 mL = £4.40.

Polytar Plus® (Stiefel)

Liquid, ingredients as Polytar® liquid with hydrolysed animal protein 3%. Net price 350 mL = £3.29

Pragmatar® —section 13.5.1

Psoriderm® (Dermal)

Scalp lotion (= shampoo), coal tar 2.5%, lecithin 0.3%. Net price 250 mL = £4.85

Selsun® (Abbott)

Shampoo application, selenium sulphide 2.5%. Net price 50 mL = £1.08; 100 mL = £1.63; 150 mL = £2.21 (for adults and children over 5 years)

T/Gel® (Neutrogena)

Shampoo, coal tar extract 2%. Net price 125 mL = £2.68; 250 mL = £4.18

LITHIUM SUCCINATE

Topical application of lithium succinate in the form of an ointment has been shown to be effective in seborrhoeic dermatitis

PoM Efalith® (Searle)

Ointment, lithium succinate 8%, zinc sulphate 0.05%. Net price 20 g = £12.19

Additives: include wool fat derivative

Seborrhoeic dermatitis (adults only), apply thinly twice daily initially, then reduce

Cautions: may exacerbate psoriasis

MALE-PATTERN BALDNESS

Topical application of minoxidil may stimulate limited hair growth in a small proportion of patients but only for as long as it is used.

MINOXIDIL

Indications: male-pattern baldness (men and women)

Cautions; Contra-indications; Side-effects: see section 2.5.1 (only about 1.4% absorbed); monitor hypertensive patients closely; avoid contact with eyes, mouth and mucous membranes, broken, infected, or inflamed skin; avoid inhalation of spray mist and use with topically applied drugs known to enhance absorption; local side-effects: irritant dermatitis, allergic contact dermatitis

Administration: ADULT aged 18–65 years, apply 1 mL twice daily to dry hair and scalp (discontinue if no improvement after 1 year)

NHS PoM Regaine® (Upjohn)

Topical solution, minoxidil 2% in an aqueous alcoholic basis. Net price 60-mL bottle with applicators = £20.00

Additives: include propylene glycol

Cautions: flammable; wash hands after application

Note. The Royal Pharmaceutical Society's Law Department has reminded pharmacists that neither the safety nor the stability of mixtures of Minoxidil lotion with other products has been established, and that this fact should be drawn to the prescriber's attention before any such mixture is dispensed.

13.10 Anti-infective skin preparations

13.10.1 Antibacterial preparations

13.10.2 Antifungal preparations

13.10.3 Antiviral preparations

13.10.4 Parasiticidal preparations

13.10.5 Preparations for minor cuts and abrasions

13.10.1 Antibacterial preparations

13.10.1.1 Antibacterial preparations only used topically

13.10.1.2 Antibacterial preparations also used systemically

For many skin infections such as *erysipelas* and *cellulitis* systemic antibacterial treatment is the method of choice because the infection is too deeply sited for adequate penetration of topical preparations. For details of suitable treatment see section 5.1, table 1.

Impetigo may be treated by topical application of **fusidic acid** or **mupirocin** or, if widespread, with oral administration of **flucloxacillin** or **erythromycin** (see section 5.1, table 1). Mild antiseptics such as **povidone-iodine** (section 13.11.4) are used to remove crusts and exudate.

Although there are a great many antibacterial drugs presented in topical preparations they are potentially hazardous and frequently their use is not necessary if adequate hygienic measures can be taken. Moreover not all skin conditions that are oozing, crusted, or characterised by pustules are actually infected.

To minimise the development of resistant organisms it is advisable to limit the choice of drugs applied topically to those not used systemically. Unfortunately some of these, for example neomycin, may cause sensitisation, and there is cross-sensitivity with other aminoglycoside antibiotics, such as gentamicin. If large areas of skin are being treated, ototoxicity may also be a hazard with aminoglycosides (and also with polymyxins), particularly in children, in the elderly, and in those with renal impairment. Resistant organisms are more common in hospitals, and whenever possible swabs for examination should be taken before beginning treatment.

Mupirocin is not related to any other antibiotic in use. Although *Staphylococcus aureus* strains with low level resistance to mupirocin are emerging, it is generally useful when there is resistant infection. To avoid the development of resistance it should not be used for longer than 10 days and its use in hospital should if possible be avoided.

Silver sulphadiazine is used in the treatment of infected burns.

13.10.1.1 ANTIBACTERIAL PREPARATIONS ONLY USED TOPICALLY

FRAMYCETIN SULPHATE

Indications; Cautions; Side-effects: see under Neomycin Sulphate

LARGE OPEN WOUNDS. If large areas of skin are being treated ototoxicity may be a hazard, particularly in children, in the elderly, and in those with renal impairment

PoM **Soframycin**® (Roussel)
Ointment, framycetin sulphate 1.5%, gramicidin 0.005%, in a wool fat and paraffin basis. Net price 15 g = £1.68
Additives: include wool fat
Superficial bacterial infection, apply up to 3 times daily (short-term use)
Sofra-Tulle® *see* Framycetin Gauze Dressing, section 13.13.6

MUPIROCIN

Indications: bacterial skin infections
Cautions: see below
Administration: apply up to 3 times daily for up to 10 days

PoM **Bactroban**® (Beecham)
Ointment, mupirocin 2%. Net price 15 g = £4.08
Additives: none as listed in section 13.1
Note. Contains macrogol therefore caution in renal impairment; may sting
Nasal ointment, see section 12.2.3

NEOMYCIN SULPHATE

Indications: skin infections
Cautions; Side-effects: see notes above

LARGE OPEN WOUNDS. If large areas of skin are being treated ototoxicity may be a hazard, particularly in children, in the elderly, and in those with renal impairment

PoM **Neomycin Cream BPC**
Cream, neomycin sulphate 0.5%, cetomacrogol emulsifying ointment 30%, chlorocresol 0.1%, disodium edetate 0.01%, in freshly boiled and cooled purified water. Net price 15 g = 88p
Apply up to 3 times daily (short-term use)
PoM **Cicatrin**® (Wellcome)
Cream, neomycin sulphate 3300 units, bacitracin zinc 250 units, cysteine 2 mg, glycine 10 mg, threonine 1 mg/g. Net price 15 g = £4.52; 30 g = £8.22
Additives: include wool fat derivative
Superficial bacterial infection of skin, apply up to 3 times daily; max. 60 g daily for 3 weeks; do not repeat for at least 3 months
Dusting powder, neomycin sulphate 3300 units, bacitracin zinc 250 units, cysteine 2 mg, glycine 10 mg, threonine 1 mg/g. Net price 15 g = £4.87; 50 g = £12.31
Additives: none as listed in section 13.1
Superficial bacterial infection of skin, apply up to 3 times daily, max. 50 g daily for 4 weeks; do not repeat for at least 3 months

Aerosol, neomycin sulphate 16 500 units, bacitracin zinc 1250 units, cysteine 12 mg, glycine 60 mg/g; pressurised aerosol can. Net price 1 can = £11.74
Additives: none as listed in section 13.1
Superficial bacterial infection of skin, apply as required, max. 1 can daily for 12 weeks; do not repeat for at least 3 months
PoM **Graneodin**® (Squibb)
Ointment, neomycin sulphate 0.25%, gramicidin 0.025%. Net price 25 g = £1.47
Additives: none as listed in section 13.1
Superficial bacterial infection of skin and prophylaxis against infection following minor surgery, apply 2–4 times daily (short-term use)
PoM **Tribiotic**® (3M)
Spray application, neomycin sulphate 500 000 units, bacitracin zinc 10 000 units, polymyxin B sulphate 150 000 units/pressurised aerosol can. Net price per can (110 g) = £5.72
Additives: none as listed in section 13.1
Prevention and control of bacterial infection in surgery apply sparingly as required, max. 1 can daily for 7 days

POLYMYXINS

(Includes colistin sulphate and polymyxin B sulphate)
Indications: skin infections
Cautions; Side-effects: see notes above

LARGE OPEN WOUNDS. If large areas of skin are being treated ototoxicity may be a hazard, particularly in children, in the elderly, and in those with renal impairment

PoM **Polyfax**® (Cusi)
Ointment, polymyxin B sulphate 10 000 units, bacitracin zinc 500 units/g. Net price 20 g = £8.73
Apply 3 times daily
PoM **Colomycin**® (Pharmax)
Powder, sterile, for making topical preparations (usually 1%), colistin sulphate. Net price 1 g vial = £19.24

Other preparations
Ingredient of Tribiotic®

SILVER SULPHADIAZINE

Indications: skin infection, particularly Gram-negative infections such as pseudomonal infections in second- and third-degree burns, infected leg ulcers, and pressure sores
Cautions: hepatic and renal impairment
Contra-indications: sensitivity to sulphonamides
Side-effects: rarely allergic reactions including rashes; argyria reported following prolonged use

PoM **Flamazine**® (S&N Pharm.)
Cream, silver sulphadiazine 1%. Net price 50 g = £4.30; 250 g = £11.52; 500 g = £20.40
Additives: include polysorbates, propylene glycol
Note. Silver sulphadiazine 1% cream is also available from Norton, net price 50 g = £4.19; 250 g = £11.23; 500 g = £19.87
In burns apply daily with sterile applicator; in leg ulcers apply at least 3 times a week

13.10.1.2 ANTIBACTERIAL PREPARATIONS ALSO USED SYSTEMICALLY

CHLORTETRACYCLINE HYDROCHLORIDE

Indications: susceptible skin infections
Cautions: see notes above; overgrowth with non-susceptible organisms; stains clothing
Side-effects: rarely local hypersensitivity reactions
Administration: apply 1 to 3 times daily

PoM Aureomycin® (Lederle)
Cream, chlortetracycline hydrochloride 3% (as chlortetracycline). Net price 30 g = £1.77
Additives: include chlorocresol
Ointment, chlortetracycline hydrochloride 3%. Net price 30 g = £1.77
Additives: include hydroxybenzoates (parabens), wool fat

FUSIDIC ACID

Indications: staphylococcal skin infections
Cautions: see notes above; avoid contact with eyes
Side-effects: rarely local hypersensitivity reactions
Administration: apply 3–4 times daily

PoM Fucidin® (Leo)
Cream, fusidic acid 2%. Net price 15 g = £2.87; 30 g = £4.84
Additives: include butylated hydroxyanisole
Gel, fusidic acid 2%. Net price 15 g = £2.48; 30 g = £4.29
Additives: include hydroxybenzoates (parabens), polysorbate 80
Ointment, sodium fusidate 2%. Net price 15 g = £2.34; 30 g = £3.97
Additives: include wool fat

PoM Fucidin Intertulle® see section 13.13.6

GENTAMICIN

Indications: skin infections
Cautions; Side-effects: see notes above
LARGE OPEN WOUNDS. If large areas of skin are being treated ototoxicity may be a hazard, particularly in children, in the elderly, and in those with renal impairment
Administration: apply 3–4 times daily

PoM Cidomycin Topical® (Roussel)
Cream, gentamicin 0.3% (as sulphate). Net price 15 g = £1.71; 30 g = £3.31
Additives: include hydroxybenzoates (parabens), propylene glycol
Ointment, gentamicin 0.3% (as sulphate). Net price 15 g = £1.71; 30 g = £3.31
Additives: none as listed in section 13.1

METRONIDAZOLE

Indications: see under preparations

PoM Metrogel® (Sandoz)
Gel, metronidazole 0.75%. Net price 40 g = £17.36. Label: 10 patient information leaflet
Additives: include propylene glycol
Administration: acute inflammatory exacerbations of acne rosacea, apply thinly twice daily for 8–9 weeks; avoid contact with eyes

PoM Metrotop® (Pharmacia)
Gel, metronidazole 0.8%. Net price 15 g = £4.95; 30 g = £8.75
Additives: none as listed in section 13.1
Administration: de-odourisation of fungating malodorous tumours, apply to clean wound 1 to 2 times daily and cover (flat wounds, apply liberally; cavities, smear on paraffin gauze and pack loosely); use tube once only

TETRACYCLINE HYDROCHLORIDE

Indications; Cautions; Side-effects: see under Chlortetracycline Hydrochloride

PoM Achromycin Topical® (Lederle)
Ointment, tetracycline hydrochloride 3%. Net price 30 g = £1.44
Additives: include hydroxybenzoates (parabens), wool fat
Apply 1–3 times daily

13.10.2   Antifungal preparations

Ideally skin scrapings should be examined to confirm diagnosis before treatment is begun. Widespread or intractable fungal infections are treated systemically (see section 5.2). Most localised infections are treated with the topical preparations described below.

Nail ringworm (tinea unguium) and scalp ringworm (*T. capitis*) are best treated systemically (see section 5.2). Most other ringworm infections, including tinea pedis, may be adequately treated with topical preparations. The imidazoles **clotrimazole, econazole,** and **miconazole** are all effective and commonly used. **Sulconazole** is a recently introduced imidazole with similar properties. Combinations of imidazoles and weak corticosteroids may be of use in the treatment of some eczematous disorders and, in the first few days only, of a severely inflamed patch of ringworm. **Compound benzoic acid ointment** (Whitfield's ointment) is also quite effective but cosmetically less acceptable than the proprietary preparations. It is generally used to treat patches of ringworm (tinea) on the trunk, limbs, palms, or soles. The **undecenoates** are less effective in treating ringworm infections.

Candidal skin infections may also be treated by topical application with the broad-spectrum antifungals, clotrimazole, econazole, and miconazole. Oral preparations of some antifungals are now also available (see section 5.2), but should preferably be reserved for those who are resistant to (or intolerant of) topical preparations. **Nystatin** preparations are also equally as effective in candidiasis although they are ineffective against infections due to dermatophyte fungi (tinea).

Lotions are generally chosen for application to large and hairy areas. Ointments are best avoided on moist surfaces because of their occlusive properties. Dusting-powders have no place in the treatment of fungal infections, except for toiletry or cosmetic purposes, as they are therapeutically ineffective and may cause skin irritation.

Amorolfine is a newly introduced antifungal that differs chemically from other antifungals. It is available as a cream for fungal skin infections and a lacquer for fungal nail infections. **Terbinafine** has also been recently introduced in the form of a cream; it is also available for systemic administration (see section 5.2).

AMOROLFINE

Indications: see under preparations
Cautions: pregnancy, breast-feeding; avoid eyes, ears, and mucous membranes
Side-effects: occasional transient burning sensation, erythema, pruritus

▼ PoM **Loceryl®** (Roche)
Cream, amorolfine (as hydrochloride) 0.25%. Net price 20 g = £4.83. Label: 10 patient information leaflet
Additives: include disodium edetate
Administration: fungal skin infections, apply once daily after cleansing in the evening for at least 2–3 weeks (up to 6 weeks for foot mycosis)
Nail lacquer, amorolfine (as hydrochloride) 5%. Net price 5-mL pack (with nail files, spatulas and cleansing swabs) = £34.38. Label: 10 patient information leaflet
Administration: fungal nail infections, apply to infected nails 1–2 times weekly after filing and cleansing; allow to dry (approx. 3 minutes); treat finger nails for 6 months, toe nails for 9–12 months (review at intervals of 3 months)

BENZOIC ACID

Indications: ringworm (tinea)

Benzoic Acid Ointment, Compound, BP
(Whitfield's ointment), benzoic acid 6%, salicylic acid 3%, in emulsifying ointment
Apply twice daily

BENZOYL PEROXIDE

Indications: fungal skin infections, particularly tinea pedis

Quinoped® (Quinoderm Ltd)
Cream, benzoyl peroxide 5%, potassium hydroxyquinoline sulphate 0.5%, in an astringent basis. Net price 25 g = 96p
Additives: include edetic acid (EDTA)
Apply twice daily

CLOTRIMAZOLE

Indications: fungal skin infections
Side-effects: occasional skin irritation or sensitivity
Administration: apply 2–3 times daily continuing for 14 days after lesions have healed

Canesten® (Baypharm)
Cream, clotrimazole 1%. Net price 20 g = £1.77; 50 g = £4.15
Additives: include benzyl alcohol, polysorbate 60
Note. A generic version of clotrimazole 1% cream is available from APS, Cox
Solution, clotrimazole 1% in macrogol 400 (polyethylene glycol 400). Net price 20 mL = £2.32. For hairy areas
Additives: none as listed in section 13.1
Spray, clotrimazole 1%, in 30% isopropyl alcohol. Net price 40-mL atomiser = £4.99. Label: 15. For large or hairy areas
Additives: include propylene glycol
Dusting powder, clotrimazole 1%. Net price 30 g = £1.52
Additives: none as listed in section 13.1

Masnoderm® (Cusi)
Cream, clotrimazole 1%. Net price 20 g = £1.54
Additives: include benzyl alcohol, polysorbates

ECONAZOLE NITRATE

Indications; Side-effects: see under Clotrimazole
Administration: apply 2–3 times daily continuing for 14 days after lesions have healed; nail infections, apply daily under occlusive dressing

Ecostatin® (Squibb)
Cream, econazole nitrate 1%. Net price 15 g = £1.49; 30 g = £2.75
Additives: include butylated hydroxyanisole, fragrance
Pevaryl® (Cilag)
Cream, econazole nitrate 1%. Net price 30 g = £2.65
Additives: include butylated hydroxyanisole, fragrance
Lotion, econazole nitrate 1%. Net price 30 mL = £3.33
Additives: include butylated hydroxyanisole, fragrance
Dusting powder, econazole nitrate 1%. Net price 30 g = £2.60
Additives: none as listed in section 13.1

KETOCONAZOLE

Indications; Side-effects: see under Clotrimazole

PoM **Nizoral®** (Janssen)
Cream, ketoconazole 2%. Net price 30 g = £3.81
Additives: include polysorbates, propylene glycol
Apply 1–2 times daily, continuing for a few days after lesions have healed
Shampoo, ketoconazole 2%. Net price 120 mL = £8.75
Additives: none as listed in section 13.1
For seborrhoeic dermatitis and dandruff apply twice weekly for 2–4 weeks, for pityriasis versicolor once daily for max. 5 days; avoid for 2 weeks following topical corticosteroid treatment

MICONAZOLE NITRATE

Indications; Side-effects: see under Clotrimazole
Administration: apply twice daily continuing for 10 days after lesions have healed; nail infections, apply daily under occlusive dressing

Daktarin® (Janssen)

Cream, miconazole nitrate 2%. Net price 30 g = £2.07

Additives: include butylated hydroxyanisole

Note. A generic version of miconazole nitrate 2% cream is available from APS, Hillcross

Dusting powder, miconazole nitrate 2%. Net price 20 g = £1.72

Additives: none as listed in section 13.1

Spray powder, miconazole nitrate 0.16%, in an aerosol basis. Net price 100 g = £1.72

Additives: none as listed in section 13.1

Twin pack, 1 × 30 g pack of cream miconazole nitrate 2%, with 1 × 30 g dusting-powder miconazole nitrate 2%. Net price = £3.80

NYSTATIN

Indications: skin infections due to *Candida* spp.

Administration: apply 2–4 times daily, continuing for 7 days after lesions have healed

PoM **Nystaform®** (Bayer)

Cream, nystatin 100 000 units/g, chlorhexidine hydrochloride 1%. Net price 30 g = £2.62

Additives: include benzyl alcohol, polysorbate 60

PoM **Nystan®** (Squibb)

Cream, nystatin 100 000 units/g. Net price 30 g = £2.18

Additives: include benzyl alcohol, propylene glycol, fragrance

Gel, nystatin 100 000 units/g. Net price 30 g = £2.18

Additives: include chlorocresol, fragrance

Ointment, nystatin 100 000 units/g, in Plastibase®. Net price 30 g = £1.75

Additives: none as listed in section 13.1

PoM **Tinaderm-M®** (Schering-Plough)

Cream, nystatin 100 000 units/g, tolnaftate 1%. Net price 20 g = £1.83. For *Candida* infections and tinea

Additives: include butylated hydroxytoluene, hydroxybenzoates (parabens), fragrance

SALICYLIC ACID

Indications: fungal skin infections, particularly tinea

Side-effects: hypersensitivity reactions

Phytex® (Pharmax)

Paint, salicylic acid 1.46% (total combined), tannic acid 4.89% and boric acid 3.12% (as borotannic complex), in a vehicle containing alcohol and ethyl acetate. Net price 25 mL (with brush) = £1.29. For fungal nail infections (onychomycosis)

Additives: none as listed in section 13.1

Apply twice daily

Caution: flammable; avoid in pregnancy and children under 5 years

SULCONAZOLE NITRATE

Indications; Side-effects: see under Clotrimazole

Cautions: avoid contact with eyes (lens changes in *animals* after high oral doses)

PoM **Exelderm®** (Zeneca)

Cream, sulconazole nitrate 1%. Net price 30 g = £3.80

Apply 1–2 times daily continuing for 2–3 weeks after lesions have healed

Additives: include polysorbates, propylene glycol

TERBINAFINE

Indications: fungal skin infections

Cautions: pregnancy, breast-feeding; avoid contact with eyes

Side-effects: redness, itching, or stinging; rarely allergic reactions (discontinue)

▼ PoM **Lamisil®** (Sandoz)

Cream, terbinafine hydrochloride 1%. Net price 15 g = £4.86; 30 g = £8.76

Apply thinly 1–2 times daily for up to 1 week in tinea pedis, 1–2 weeks in tinea corporis and tinea cruris, 2 weeks in cutaneous candidiasis and pityriasis versicolor; review after 2 weeks; CHILD not recommended

Additives: include benzyl alcohol, polysorbate 60

Tablets, see section 5.2

TIOCONAZOLE

Indications: see under preparations

Side-effects: local irritation, usually during first week of treatment; discontinue if sensitivity reaction develops

Trosyl® (Pfizer)

PoM *Nail solution*, tioconazole 28%. Net price 12 mL (with applicator brush) = £27.38

Additives: none as listed in section 13.1

Administration: fungal nail infections, apply to nails and surrounding skin twice daily for up to 6 months (may be extended to 12 months)

Cream, tioconazole 1%. Net price 15 g = £1.51; 30 g = £2.78

Additives: include benzyl alcohol, polysorbate 60

Administration: fungal skin infections, apply once or twice daily for 2–4 weeks (up to 6 weeks for foot mycosis)

UNDECENOATES

Indications: skin infections, particularly tinea pedis

Monphytol® (LAB)

Paint, methyl undecenoate 5%, propyl undecenoate 0.7%, salicylic acid 3%, methyl salicylate 25%, propyl salicylate 5%, chlorbutol 3%. Net price 18 mL (with brush) = £1.17. For fungal (particularly nail) infections

Additives: none as listed in section 13.1

Apply twice daily

Mycota® (Seton)

Cream, zinc undecenoate 20%, undecenoic acid 5%. Net price 25 g = 88p

Additives: include fragrance

Dusting powder, zinc undecenoate 20%, undecenoic acid 2%. Net price 70 g = £1.36

Additives: include fragrance

Spray application, undecenoic acid 2.5%, dichlorophen 0.25% (pressurised aerosol pack). Net price 113 g = £1.39

Additives: include fragrance

Apply 1–2 times daily

13.10.3   Antiviral preparations

Acyclovir cream is indicated for the treatment of initial and recurrent labial and genital herpes simplex infections; treatment should begin as early as possible. Systemic treatment is necessary for buccal or vaginal infections; herpes zoster (shingles) also requires systemic treatment (for details of systemic use see section 5.3).

Idoxuridine solution (5% in dimethyl sulphoxide) is of little value

---

ACYCLOVIR
(Aciclovir)

Indications: see notes above

Side-effects: transient stinging or burning; occasionally erythema or drying of the skin

Cautions: avoid contact with eyes and mucous membranes

PoM Zovirax® (Wellcome)

Cream, acyclovir 5%. Net price 2 g = £8.37; 10 g = £25.22

Administration: apply to lesions every 4 hours (5 times daily) for 5 days, started at first sign of attack

Additives: include propylene glycol

Note. A 2-g tube is on sale to the public for the treatment of cold sores (Zovirax® Cold Sore Cream)

Eye ointment, see section 11.3.3

Tablets, see section 5.3

IDOXURIDINE IN DIMETHYL SULPHOXIDE

Indications: see notes above

Cautions: avoid contact with the eyes, mucous membranes, and textiles; breast-feeding (may taste unpleasant)

Contra-indications: pregnancy (toxicity in *animal* studies); not to be used in mouth

Side-effects: stinging on application, changes in taste; overuse may cause maceration

PoM Herpid® (Yamanouchi)

Application, idoxuridine 5% in dimethyl sulphoxide. Net price 5 mL (with applicator) = £6.86

Administration: Herpes simplex or herpes zoster, apply to lesions 4 times daily for 4 days, starting at first sign of attack; CHILD under 12 years, not recommended

PoM Iduridin® (Ferring)

Application, idoxuridine 5% in dimethyl sulphoxide. Net price 5 mL (with applicator) = £4.90

Administration: Herpes simplex or herpes zoster, apply to lesions 4 times daily for 4 days, starting at first sign of attack; CHILD under 12 years, not recommended

Application, idoxuridine 40% in dimethyl sulphoxide. Net price 5 mL (with applicator) = £19.00; 20 mL with dropper = £39.00

Administration: Severe herpes zoster only, apply on plain lint and retain over affected area (dermatome), changing once every 24 hours for 4 days (**not** for herpes simplex); CHILD under 12 years, not recommended

PoM Virudox® (Bioglan)

Application, idoxuridine 5% in dimethyl sulphoxide. Net price 5 mL (with applicator) = £6.19

Administration: Herpes simplex or herpes zoster, apply to lesions 4 times daily for 4 days, starting at first sign of attack; CHILD under 12 years, not recommended

13.10.4   Parasiticidal preparations

SCABIES

Lindane, **malathion** and **permethrin** are indicated for *scabies (Sarcoptes scabiei)*, but lindane should be avoided during pregnancy or breast-feeding, in young children, and in patients with low body-weight or a history of epilepsy.

Aqueous preparations are preferable to alcoholic lotions, which are not recommended owing to irritation of excoriated skin and the genitalia.

Older preparations include benzyl benzoate, which is an irritant and should be avoided in children; monosulfiram, which was liable to induce disulfiram-like reactions with alcohol has been discontinued.

APPLICATION. Although acaricides have traditionally been applied after a hot bath, this is not necessary and there is even evidence that a hot bath may increase absorption into the bloodstream, removing them from their site of action on the skin.

All members of the affected household should be treated. Treatment should be applied to the whole body paying particular attention to the webs of the fingers and toes and brushing lotion under the ends of the nails. In the case of infants and young children (up to the age of about 2 years) application should be extended to the scalp, neck, face, and ears (if the product packaging does not contra-indicate this). Providing the application is done properly lindane, malathion and permethrin need only be applied once; in the case of benzyl benzoate up to three applications on consecutive days may be needed.

ITCHING. The *itch of scabies* persists for some days after the infestation has been eliminated and antipruritic treatment may be required. Application of **crotamiton** can be used to control itching after treatment with more effective acaricides, but caution is necessary if the skin is excoriated — **calamine** is probably more suitable. Oral administration of a **sedative antihistamine** (see section 3.4.1) at night may also be useful.

HEAD LICE

Malathion and **carbaryl** are recommended for *head lice (Pediculus humanus capitis)*. Both should generally be used as lotions in preference to shampoos, which are not in contact with the hair long enough and are normally diluted too much in use to be effective; aqueous formulations are preferred for asthmatic patients and small children, to avoid alcoholic fumes. A contact time of 12 hours or overnight treatment is recommended. A 2-hour treatment is no longer regarded as sufficient to ensure death of eggs.

Permethrin and **phenothrin** are two recently introduced pyrethroids, both of which are very effective and are also recommended.

Lindane is no longer recommended because of resistant strains.

In general, treatment for head lice should preferably be repeated after 7 days to kill lice emerging from any eggs that might have survived the first application.

Most health districts operate a **rotating policy** for head lice treatment. Details of the drugs which are currently recommended for use in the different health districts can be obtained from District Pharmaceutical Officers.

A **head lice repellant** containing piperonal 2% (Rappell®) is on sale to the public.

CRAB LICE

Malathion, lindane and **carbaryl** are effective for *crab lice* (*Pthirus pubis*). Aqueous lotions should be applied to all hairy parts of the body for 12 hours or overnight; a second treatment is preferable after 7 days to kill lice emerging from surviving eggs. Alcoholic lotions are not recommended (owing to irritation of excoriated skin and the genitalia).

Aqueous **malathion** lotion is effective for *crab lice of the eye lashes* (but does not have a product licence for this indication).

BENZYL BENZOATE

Benzyl benzoate is effective for *scabies* but is not a first-choice for *scabies* (see notes above)

BENZYL BENZOATE
Indications: see notes above and under preparations
Cautions: children (see notes above), avoid contact with eyes and mucous membranes; do not use on broken or secondarily infected skin; pregnancy and breast-feeding
Side-effects: skin irritation, burning sensation especially on genitalia and excoriations, occasionally rashes

Benzyl Benzoate Application, BP, benzyl benzoate 25% in an emulsion basis. Net price 500 mL = £2.20
Administration: scabies—apply 25% application over the whole body, omitting the head and neck; repeat without bathing on the following day and wash off 24 hours later; a third application may be required in some cases
Note. Not recommended for children—dilution to reduce irritant effect also reduces efficacy (see notes above)
Available from CP, K Pharm., Rhône-Poulenc Rorer (Ascabiol®)

CARBARYL

Carbaryl is recommended for *head lice* and *crab lice* (see notes above)

CARBARYL
Indications: see notes above and under preparations
Cautions: avoid contact with eyes; do not use on broken or infected skin; alcoholic lotions **not** recommended for pediculosis in asthmatics or small children, or for crab lice (see notes above); do not use lotion more than once a week for 3 weeks at a time; children under 6 months, medical supervision required
Side-effects: skin irritation
Administration: lotion—apply to dry hair and rub into the hair and scalp or affected areas, allow to dry naturally, comb, and remove by washing 12 hours later (see also notes above); shampoo—shampoo in, leave on hair for 5 minutes, rinse, repeat, rinse, allow to dry, comb, repeat twice at intervals of 3 days

Carylderm® (Napp)
Lotion, carbaryl 0.5%, in an alcoholic basis. Net price 55 mL = £1.77; 160 mL = £3.13. Label: 15. For crab lice and head lice (alcoholic, see notes above)
Shampoo, carbaryl 1%. Net price 100 mL = £2.56. For crab lice and head lice

Clinicide® (De Witt)
Lotion, carbaryl 0.5% in an aqueous basis containing 10% alcohol. Net price 50 mL = £1.13. For crab lice and head lice

Derbac® C (Napp)
Liquid (= lotion), carbaryl 1% in an aqueous basis. Net price 50 mL = £1.77; 200 mL = £3.76. For head lice
Shampoo solution, carbaryl 0.5% in an aqueous basis. Net price 75 mL = £1.83. For head lice

Suleo-C® (Napp)
Lotion, carbaryl 0.5%, in an alcoholic basis. Net price 50 mL = £1.77; 200 mL = £3.76. Label: 15. For head lice (alcoholic, see notes above)
Shampoo, carbaryl 0.5%. Net price 75 mL = £1.83. For head lice

LINDANE

Lindane is recommended for *scabies* and *crab lice* (see notes above). It is no longer recommended for *head lice* (see notes above)

LINDANE
Indications: see notes above and under preparations
Cautions: avoid contact with eyes and mucous membranes; do not use on broken or infected skin; do not use more than once one course of treatment; pregnancy (see Appendix 4) and breast-feeding; children under 6 months, medical supervision required; see also above (under Scabies)
Side-effects: skin irritation
Administration: see preparations

Quellada® (Stafford-Miller)
Lotion, lindane 1%, in a lotion basis. Net price 100 mL = 61p; 500 mL = £2.03. For scabies
Administration: scabies, apply thinly over whole body, omitting head and neck, wash off using cool water after 24 hours; repeat if necessary after 7 days

---

Application PC, lindane 1%, in a shampoo basis. Net price 100 mL = 69p. For crab lice (but see notes above)

Administration: crab lice and head lice (but see notes above), apply to dry hair, leave for 4 minutes, add water to produce lather, rinse, towel dry, comb

MALATHION

Malathion is recommended for *scabies*, *head lice* and *crab lice* (for details see notes above)

MALATHION

Indications: see notes above and under preparations

Cautions: avoid contact with eyes; do not use on broken or infected skin; alcoholic lotions **not** recommended for pediculosis in asthmatics or small children, or for scabies or crab lice (see notes above); do not use lotion more than once a week for 3 weeks at a time; children under 6 months, medical supervision required

Side-effects: skin irritation

Administration: pediculosis—rub 0.5% lotion into dry hair, scalp, and affected area, comb, allow to dry naturally, remove by washing after 12 hours (see also notes above); apply 1% shampoo to hair for 5 minutes, rinse, repeat, rinse again, comb, repeat twice at intervals of 3 days

Scabies—apply 0.5% preparation over whole body, omitting the head and neck, and wash off after 24 hours, see also notes above

Derbac-M® (Napp)

Liquid, malathion 0.5% in an aqueous basis. Net price 50 mL = £1.77; 200 mL = £3.76. For crab lice, head lice and scabies

Prioderm® (Napp)

Lotion, malathion 0.5%, in an alcoholic basis. Net price 55 mL = £1.77; 160 mL = £3.13. Label: 15. For crab lice, head lice and scabies (alcoholic, see notes above)

Cream shampoo, malathion 1%. Net price 40 g = £1.83. For crab lice and head lice

Suleo-M® (Napp)

Lotion, malathion 0.5%, in an alcoholic basis. Net price 50 mL = £1.77; 200 mL = £3.76. Label: 15. For head lice (alcoholic, see notes above)

PERMETHRIN

Permethrin is effective for *scabies* and *head lice* (for details see notes above)

PERMETHRIN

Indications: see notes above and under preparations

Cautions: avoid contact with eyes; do not use on broken or infected skin; pregnancy and breast-feeding; children under 6 months, medical supervision required for cream rinse (head lice); children aged 2 months—2 years, medical supervision required for dermal cream (scabies)

Side-effects: pruritus, erythema, and stinging; rarely rashes and oedema

Lyclear® (Wellcome)

Cream rinse, permethrin 1% in basis containing isopropyl alcohol 20%. Net price 59 mL = £2.01

Administration: head lice, apply to clean damp hair, leave on for 10 minutes, rinse and dry; not affected by chlorine in swimming pools

Dermal cream, permethrin 5%. Net price 30 g = £5.50. Label: 10 patient information leaflet

Administration: scabies, apply over whole body (excluding head in adults), and wash off after 8–24 hours; CHILD apply over whole body including face, neck, scalp and ears. If hands are washed with soap and water within 8 hours of application, cream should be reapplied

PHENOTHRIN

Phenothrin is recommended for *head lice* and *crab lice* (for details see notes above)

PHENOTHRIN

Indications: see notes above and under preparations

Cautions: avoid contact with eyes; do not use on broken or infected skin; children under 6 months, medical supervision required; may cause wheezing in asthmatics

Side-effects: skin irritation

Full Marks® (Napp)

Lotion, phenothrin 0.2% in basis containing isopropyl alcohol 69.3%. Net price 55 mL = £1.77; 160 mL = £3.13. Label: 15

Administration: crab lice and head lice (alcoholic, see above), apply to dry hair, allow to dry naturally; shampoo after 2 hours, comb while still wet

13.10.5   Preparations for minor cuts and abrasions

Some of the preparations listed are used in minor burns, and abrasions. They are applied as necessary. Preparations containing camphor, hydrargaphen, and sulphonamides should be **avoided**. Preparations such as magnesium sulphate paste are also listed but are now rarely used to treat carbuncles and boils as these are best treated with antibiotics (see section 5.1.1.2).

Cetrimide Cream, BP, cetrimide 0.5% in a suitable water-miscible basis such as cetostearyl alcohol 5%, liquid paraffin 50% in freshly boiled and cooled purified water. Net price 50 g = 21p

Chlorhexidine Cream, BP 1988, chlorhexidine gluconate solution usually 5% (≡ chlorhexidine gluconate 1%), cetomacrogol emulsifying wax 25%, liquid paraffin 10%, in purified water, freshly boiled and cooled

Proflavine Cream, BPC, proflavine hemisulphate 0.1%, yellow beeswax 2.5%, chlorocresol 0.1%, liquid paraffin 67.3%, freshly boiled and cooled purified water 25%, wool fat 5%. Net price 100 mL = 40p

Caution: stains clothing

Anaflex® (Geistlich)

Cream, polynoxylin 10%, in a water-miscible basis. Net price 50 g = £2.71

Betadine® (Seton)

Ointment, povidone-iodine 10%, in a water-miscible basis. Net price 20 g = £1.45; 80 g = £2.92. Avoid in children under 2 years

Additives: none as listed in section 13.1

Brulidine® (Rhône-Poulenc Rorer)

Cream, dibromopropamidine isethionate 0.15%, in a water-miscible basis. Net price 25 g = 77p

Additives: include hydroxybenzoates (parabens), fragrance

Cetavlex® (Zeneca)

Cream, cetrimide 0.5%, in a water-miscible basis. Net price 50 g = 54p

Additives: include hydroxybenzoates (parabens)

Dermalex® (Sanofi Winthrop)

Skin lotion, allantoin 0.2%, hexachlorophane 0.5%, squalane 3% in an emulsion basis. Net price 100 mL = £2.00; 250 mL = £5.22.

For prevention of pressure sores and prevention and treatment of urinary rash. Avoid in children under 2 years, except under medical supervision

Additives: include butylated hydroxyanisole, edetic acid, hydroxybenzoates (parabens), wool fat, fragrance

Vesagex® (Rybar)

Cream, cetrimide 1%. Net price 500 g = £4.99

Additives: include chlorocresol, fragrance

Preparations for boils

Magnesium Sulphate Paste, BP, dried magnesium sulphate 45 g, glycerol 55 g, phenol 500 mg. Net price 25 g = 49p; 50 g = 57p. Should be stirred before use

Apply under dressing

Secaderm® —section 13.14

COLLODION

Flexible collodion may be used to seal minor cuts and wounds that have partially healed.

Collodion, Flexible, BP, castor oil 2.5%, colophony 2.5% in a collodion basis, prepared by dissolving pyroxylin (10%) in a mixture of 3 volumes of ether and 1 volume of alcohol (90%). Net price 10 mL = 16p. Label: 15 (**important:** very highly inflammable)

SURGICAL TISSUE ADHESIVE

Enbucrilate is used as a tissue adhesive for closure of minor skin wounds and sealing sutured skin wounds. Within 20 seconds of contact with tissue moisture it polymerises with an exothermic reaction into a firm adhesive bond. It must therefore be applied very thinly (to avoid heat damage) and with proper technique (poor alignment cannot be corrected). Contact with eyes, internal organs, blood vessels, and nervous tissue should be **avoided**.

Histoacryl® (Davis & Geck)

Tissue adhesive, sterile, enbucrilate with blue dye. Net price (single use) 500-mg vial = £9.60 (hosp. use only)

13.11 Disinfectants and cleansers

13.11.1 Alcohols and saline

13.11.2 Chlorhexidine salts

13.11.3 Cationic surfactants and soaps

13.11.4 Chlorine and iodine

13.11.5 Phenolics

13.11.6 Astringents, oxidisers, and dyes

13.11.7 Desloughing agents

The choice of *cleanser* is an important factor in treating skin conditions. For example, scaling disorders are best treated with **emulsifying ointment** (section 13.2.1) or other cleansers that do not irritate the skin.

Sodium chloride solution 0.9% is suitable for general cleansing of skin and wounds.

Useful *disinfectants* for skin cleansing include **cetrimide** (which has useful detergent properties), **chlorhexidine** and **potassium permanganate solution** 1 in 8000. **Povidone-iodine** is preferred to chlorinated solutions (such as dilute sodium hypochlorite solution) which are too irritant and are no longer recommended. Topical preparations of **hexachlorophane** should be used with caution in neonates and should **not** be used on large raw surfaces.

Astringent preparations, such as **potassium permanganate** solution are useful for treating eczematous reactions (section 13.5.1). Silver nitrate lotion is now rarely used as it stains the skin black and may cause toxic effects if used for prolonged periods.

13.11.1 Alcohols and saline

ALCOHOL

Indications: skin preparation before injection

Cautions: flammable; avoid broken skin; patients have suffered severe burns when diathermy has been preceded by application of alcoholic skin disinfectants.

Industrial Methylated Spirit, BP

Mixture of 19 volumes of ethanol (absolute alcohol) of an appropriate strength with 1 volume of approved wood naphtha and is Industrial Methylated Spirit of the quality known either as '66 OP' or as '74 OP'

Net price 100 mL = 18p. Label: 15

Surgical Spirit, BP, methyl salicylate 0.5 mL, diethyl phthalate 2%, castor oil 2.5%, in industrial methylated spirit. Net price 100 mL = 18p. Label: 15

SODIUM CHLORIDE

Indications: see notes above

Irriclens® (ConvaTec)

Solution in aerosol can, (sterile), sodium chloride 0.9%. Net price 240-mL can = £2.98

Normasol® (Seton)

Solution (sterile), sodium chloride 0.9%. Net price
25 × 25-mL sachet = £5.85; 6 × 100-mL sachet =
£4.29

See also section 11.8.2

Sterac® Sodium Chloride (Galen)

Solution (sterile), sodium chloride 0.9%. Net price
150 mL = 83p; 1000 mL = £1.10

Steripod® Sodium Chloride (Seton)

Steripod® sodium chloride 0.9% solution (sterile),
sodium chloride 0.9%. Net price 25 × 20-mL
sachet = £6.83

13.11.2   Chlorhexidine salts

CHLORHEXIDINE

Indications: see under preparations; bladder irrigation and catheter patency solutions (see section
7.4.4)

Cautions: avoid contact with eyes, brain, meninges and middle ear; not for use in body cavities;
alcoholic solutions not suitable before diathermy

Side-effects: occasional sensitivity

Chlorasept® (Baxter)

2000 Solution (sterile), pink, chlorhexidine acetate
0.05%. Net price 1000 mL = 79p

For cleansing and disinfecting wounds and burns

CX Antiseptic Dusting Powder® (Bio-Medical)

Dusting powder, sterile, chlorhexidine acetate 1%.
Net price 15 g = £2.25

For skin disinfection and antisepsis

Note. Chlorhexidine Dusting Powder BP 1988 contains
chlorhexidine hydrochloride 0.5% but no preparation is
available commercially

Hibiscrub® (Zeneca)

Cleansing solution, red, chlorhexidine gluconate
solution 20% (≡ 4% chlorhexidine gluconate),
perfumed, in a surfactant solution. Net price
250 mL = £1.10; 500 mL = £1.61

Use instead of soap for pre-operative hand and skin
preparation and for general hand and skin antisepsis

Hibisol® (Zeneca)

Solution, chlorhexidine gluconate solution 2.5%
(≡ 0.5% chlorhexidine gluconate), in isopropyl
alcohol 70% with emollients. Net price 500 mL =
£1.68

To be used undiluted for hand and skin disinfection

Hibitane Obstetric® (Zeneca)

Cream, chlorhexidine gluconate solution 5%
(≡ 1% chlorhexidine gluconate), in a pourable
water-miscible basis. Net price 250 mL = 98p.

For use in obstetrics and gynaecology as an antiseptic
and lubricant (for application to skin around vulva and
perineum and to hands of midwife or doctor)

Phiso-med® (Sanofi Winthrop)

Solution, chlorhexidine gluconate 4% in an emulsion basis. Net price 150 mL = £4.64.

For use as a soap substitute in acne and seborrhoeic conditions; for bathing babies in maternity units (as 1 in 10
dilution) to prevent cross-infection and for pre-operative
hand and skin preparation

Sterexidine® (Galen)

Solution (sterile), chlorhexidine gluconate 0.02%.
Net price 150 mL = 83p; 1000 mL = £1.10

For disinfection and wound cleansing

Steripod® Chlorhexidine (Seton)

Steripod® Chlorhexidine solution, chlorhexidine
gluconate solution 0.25% (≡ chlorhexidine
gluconate 0.05%). Net price 25 × 20-mL vials =
£6.83

For swabbing wounds and burns

Unisept® (Seton)

Solution (sterile), pink, chlorhexidine gluconate
0.05%. Net price 25 × 25-mL sachet = £5.85; 6 ×
100-mL sachet = £4.29

For cleansing and disinfecting wounds and burns and
swabbing in obstetrics

With cetrimide

Steripod® Chlorhexidine/Cetrimide (Seton)

Steripod® Chlorhexidine/Cetrimide solution,
chlorhexidine gluconate solution 0.075%
(≡chlorhexidine gluconate 0.015%), cetrimide
0.15%. Net price 25 × 20-mL vials = £6.83

For cleansing and disinfecting wounds and burns

Tisept® (Seton)

Solution (sterile), yellow, chlorhexidine gluconate
0.015%, cetrimide 0.15%. Net price 25 × 25-mL
sachet = £6.00; 6 × 100-mL sachet = £5.85

To be used undiluted for general skin disinfection and
wound cleansing

Travasept 100® (Baxter)

Solution (sterile), yellow, chlorhexidine acetate
0.015%, cetrimide 0.15%. Net price 500 mL =
74p; 1000 mL = 79p

To be used undiluted in skin disinfection such as wound
cleansing and obstetrics

CONCENTRATES

Hibitane 5% Concentrate® (Zeneca)

Solution, red, chlorhexidine gluconate solution
25% (≡ 5% chlorhexidine gluconate), in a perfumed aqueous solution. Net price 5 litres =
£11.46

To be used diluted 1 in 10 (0.5%) with alcohol 70% for
pre-operative skin preparation, or 1 in 100 (0.05%) with
water for general skin disinfection

Note. Alcoholic solutions not suitable before diathermy
(see Alcohol, above)

With cetrimide

Hibicet Hospital Concentrate® (Zeneca)

Solution, orange, chlorhexidine gluconate solution
7.5% (≡ chlorhexidine gluconate 1.5%), cetrimide 15%. Net price 5 litres = £8.54

To be used diluted 1 in 100 (1%) to 1 in 30 with water
for skin disinfection and wound cleansing, and diluted 1
in 30 in alcohol 70% for pre-operative skin preparation

Note. Alcoholic solutions not suitable before diathermy
(see Alcohol, above)

13.11.3   Cationic surfactants and soaps

BENZALKONIUM CHLORIDE

Indications: skin disinfection such as pre-operative skin preparation

Cautions: avoid contact with eyes

Roccal® (Sanofi Winthrop)

Solution, blue, benzalkonium chloride 1%. Net price 2.25 litres = £13.35

To be used diluted 1 in 10 to 1 in 200

Additives: include fragrance

Roccal Concentrate 10X® (Sanofi Winthrop)

Concentrate, blue, benzalkonium chloride 10%. Net price 2.25 litres = £49.49

For preparation of Roccal Solution with freshly boiled and cooled purified water

Additives: include fragrance

CETRIMIDE

Indications: skin disinfection

Cautions: avoid contact with eyes; avoid use in body cavities

Side-effects: skin irritation and occasionally sensitisation

Preparations

Ingredient of Hibicet Hospital Concentrate®, Steripod®, Tisept®, and Travasept®100, see above

SOFT SOAP

Indications: removal of adherent crusts

Soap Spirit, BP, soft soap 65% in alcohol (90%). Net price 100 mL = 37p

SUBSTITUTE SOAPS

See section 13.2.1 (emulsifying ointment); section 13.2.1.1 (emollient bath additives)

13.11.4 Chlorine and Iodine

CHLORINATED SOLUTIONS

Cautions: bleaches fabric; irritant (protect surrounding tissues with soft paraffin)

Chlorinated Lime and Boric Acid Solution, BP,

(Eusol), chlorinated lime 1.25%, boric acid 1.25%, in purified water, freshly boiled and cooled. Contains not less than 0.25% available chlorine. It must be freshly prepared. Has been used undiluted for skin disinfection, particularly in wound and ulcer cleansing but no longer recommended (too irritant)

Chlorinated Soda Solution, Surgical, BPC,

(Dakin's Solution), boric acid, chlorinated lime, sodium carbonate, sufficient of each to provide a solution containing 0.5% of available chlorine in purified water, freshly boiled and cooled. Net price 500 mL = 74p. Has been used undiluted for cleansing wounds and ulcers but no longer recommended (too irritant)

Chlorasol® (Seton)

Solution (sterile), sodium hypochlorite, containing 0.3–0.4% available chlorine. Net price 25 × 25-mL sachets = £8.99

Irritant therefore no longer recommended

IODINE COMPOUNDS

Indications: skin disinfection

Cautions: pregnancy, breast-feeding; broken skin (see below); renal impairment (see Appendix 3)

LARGE OPEN WOUNDS. The application of povidone-iodine to large wounds or severe burns may produce systemic adverse effects such as metabolic acidosis, hypernatraemia and impairment of renal function.

Contra-indications: avoid regular use in patients with thyroid disorders or those receiving lithium therapy

Side-effects: rarely sensitivity; may interfere with thyroid function tests

Betadine® (Seton)

Antiseptic paint, povidone-iodine 10% in an alcoholic solution. Net price 8 mL (with applicator brush) = £1.06

Apply undiluted to minor wounds and infections, twice daily

Alcoholic solution, povidone-iodine 10%. Net price 500 mL = £2.00

To be applied undiluted in pre- and post-operative skin disinfection; CHILD not recommended for regular use in neonates (and contra-indicated in very low birthweight infants)

Note. Flammable—caution in procedures involving hot wire cautery and diathermy

Antiseptic solution, povidone-iodine 10% in aqueous solution. Net price 500 mL = £1.83

To be applied undiluted in pre- and post-operative skin disinfection; CHILD not recommended for regular use in neonates (and contra-indicated in very low birthweight infants)

Note. Not for body cavity irrigation

Dry powder spray, povidone-iodine 2.5% in a pressurised aerosol unit. Net price 150-g unit = £2.92

For skin disinfection, particularly minor wounds and infections; CHILD under 2 years not recommended

Note. Not for use in serous cavities

Scalp and skin cleanser solution, povidone-iodine 7.5%, in a surfactant basis. Net price 250 mL = £2.43

Use for seborrhoeic conditions of scalp and acne vulgaris of face and neck 1–2 times daily; CHILD under 2 years not recommended

Skin cleanser solution, povidone-iodine 4%, in a surfactant basis. Net price 250 mL = £2.24

For infective conditions of the skin. Retain on skin for 3–5 minutes before rinsing; repeat twice daily; CHILD under 2 years not recommended

Surgical scrub, povidone-iodine 7.5%, in a nonionic surfactant basis. Net price 500 mL = £1.65

To be used as a pre-operative scrub for hands and skin; CHILD not recommended for regular use in neonates (and contra-indicated in very low birthweight infants)

Savlon® Dry Powder (Zyma)

Savlon® Dry powder spray, povidone-iodine 1.14% in a pressurised aerosol unit. Net price 50-mL unit = £1.72

For minor wounds

Videne® (DePuy)

Dusting powder, povidone-iodine 5%. Net price 15 g = £2.60

For minor wounds

13.11.5   Phenolics
HEXACHLOROPHANE
(Hexachlorophene)

Indications: see under preparations (below)
Contra-indications: avoid use on badly burned or excoriated skin; pregnancy; children under 2 years except on medical advice
Side-effects: sensitivity; rarely photosensitivity

PoM **Ster-Zac DC Skin Cleanser®** (Hough)
Cream, hexachlorophane 3%. Net price 150 mL = £3.55
Use 3–5 mL instead of soap as pre-operative scrub for hands
Additives: information not disclosed for BNF

Ster-Zac Powder® (Hough)
Dusting-powder, hexachlorophane 0.33%, zinc oxide 3%, talc 88.67%, starch 8% (sterile). Net price 30 g = 69p
Additives: information not disclosed for BNF
Prevention of neonatal staphylococcal sepsis, after ligature of cord sprinkle on perineum, groin, front of abdomen, and axillas; after cutting cord and spraying with plastic dressing, powder stump and adjacent skin; after every napkin change powder stump, adjacent skin, perineum, groin, axillas, buttocks, and front of abdomen; continue until stump drops away and wound healed
Adjunct for treatment of recurrent furunculosis, powder daily area of skin normally subject to furunculosis

TRICLOSAN
Indications: skin disinfection
Cautions: avoid contact with eyes

Manusept® (Hough)
Antibacterial hand rub, blue, triclosan 0.5%, isopropyl alcohol 70%. Net price 250 mL = £1.07; 500 mL = £1.56
For disinfection and pre-operative hand preparation
Additives: information not disclosed for BNF

Ster-Zac Bath Concentrate® (Hough)
Solution, triclosan 2%. Net price 28.5 mL = 40p; 500 mL = £4.46
For staphylococcal skin infections; prevention of cross-infection use 1 sachet/bath
Additives: information not disclosed for BNF

13.11.6   Astringents, oxidisers, and dyes

ALUMINIUM ACETATE
Indications: exudative eczematous reactions and wounds

Aluminium Acetate Lotion, aluminium acetate solution 5 mL, purified water, freshly boiled and cooled, to 100 mL. It should be freshly prepared. To be used undiluted as a wet dressing
Note. Aluminium acetate solution (13%) for the preparation of aluminium acetate lotion (0.65%) is available from Martindale, Penn, etc. (special order)

CRYSTAL VIOLET
(Gentian violet; Methylrosanilium Chloride)
Indications: see below
Cautions: stains clothes and skin
Side-effects: mucosal ulcerations

Crystal Violet Paint, BP1980, crystal   violet 0.5%, in purified water, freshly boiled and cooled. To be used undiluted
Note. Licensed for topical application on unbroken skin only; no longer recommended for application to mucous membranes or open wounds; restrictions do not apply to use for skin marking prior to surgery

HYDROGEN PEROXIDE
Indications: skin disinfection, particularly cleansing and deodorising wounds and ulcers
Cautions: large or deep wounds; avoid normal skin; bleaches fabric

Hydrogen Peroxide Solution, BP
Solution 6% (20 vols). Net price 100 mL = 20p
Solution 3% (10 vols). Net price 100 mL = 20p
Note. The BP directs that when hydrogen peroxide is prescribed, hydrogen peroxide solution 6% (20 vols) should be dispensed.
IMPORTANT. Strong solutions of hydrogen peroxide which contain 27% (90 vols) and 30% (100 vols) are only for the preparation of weaker solutions

Hioxyl® see Desloughing Agents (below)

POTASSIUM PERMANGANATE
Indications: cleansing and deodorising suppurating eczematous reactions and wounds
Cautions: irritant to mucous membranes; stains skin and clothing
Administration: wet dressings or baths, approx. 0.01% solution

Potassium Permanganate Solution, potassium permanganate 0.1% (1 in 1000) in water
To be diluted 1 in 10 to provide a 0.01% (1 in 10 000) solution

Permitabs® (Bioglan)
Solution tablets, for preparation of topical solution, potassium permanganate 400 mg. Net price 30-tab pack = £2.59
1 tablet dissolved in 4 litres of water provides a 0.01% (1 in 10 000) solution

13.11.7   Desloughing agents

Desloughing agents for ulcers are second-line treatment and the underlying causes should be treated. The main beneficial effect is removal of slough and clot and the ablation of local infection. Preparations which absorb or help promote the removal of exudate may also help (section 13.13.3). It should be noted that substances applied to an open area are easily absorbed and perilesional skin is easily sensitised. Gravitational dermatitis may be due to neomycin or lanolin sensitivity. Enzyme preparations such as streptokinase-streptodornase or alternatively dextranomer (section 13.13.8) are designed for sloughing ulcers and may help.

Aserbine® (Forley)

Cream, benzoic acid 0.025%, malic acid 0.375%, propylene glycol 1.75%, salicylic acid 0.006%. Net price 100 g = £1.17

Apply liberally to wound surface (best results with twice daily wound dressing but more frequent changes may be needed)

Additives: include hydroxybenzoates (parabens)

Solution, benzoic acid 0.15%, malic acid 2.25%, propylene glycol 40%, salicylic acid 0.0375%. Net price 500 mL = £1.76

Use as wash before each application of cream (or use as wet dressing)

Additives: include fragrance

Hioxyl® (Quinoderm Ltd)

Cream, hydrogen peroxide (stabilised) 1.5%. Net price 25 g = £1.81; 100 g = £5.66

For leg ulcers and pressure sores

Additives: none as listed in section 13.1

Apply when necessary and if necessary cover with a dressing

PoM Varidase Topical® (Lederle)

Powder, streptokinase 100 000 units, streptodornase 25 000 units. For preparing solutions for topical use. Net price per vial = £7.80; with physiological saline 20 mL (combi-pack) = £8.20

Additives: none as listed in section 13.1

Apply as wet dressing usually 1–2 times daily. Also used to dissolve clots in the bladder or urinary catheters; **contra-indicated** in active haemorrhage

13.12   Antiperspirants

Aluminium chloride is a potent antiperspirant used in the treatment of severe hyperhidrosis.

ALUMINIUM CHLORIDE

Indications: hyperhidrosis

Cautions: avoid contact with eyes; do not shave axilla or use depilatories within 12 hours of use

Side-effects: skin irritation

Administration: apply at night to dry skin, wash off on following morning, initially daily then reduce frequency as condition improves—do not bathe immediately before use

Anhydrol Forte® (Dermal)

Solution (= application), aluminium chloride hexahydrate 20% in an alcoholic basis. Net price 60-mL bottle with roll-on applicator = £2.82. Label: 15

PoM Driclor® (Stiefel)

Application, aluminium chloride hexahydrate 20% in an alcoholic basis. Net price 60-mL bottle with roll-on applicator = £2.82. Label: 15

13.13   Wound management products

13.13.1 Bandages
13.13.2 Surgical adhesive tapes
13.13.3 Adhesive dressings
13.13.4 Surgical absorbents
13.13.5 Wound dressing pads
13.13.6 Tulle dressings
13.13.7 Vapour-permeable films and membranes
13.13.8 Gel and colloid dressings
13.13.9 Foam dressings
13.13.10 Elastic hosiery

13.13.1   Bandages

RETENTION BANDAGES

Non-stretch fabric retention bandages

Open-wove Bandage, BP 1988 (types 1, 2 and 3). Cotton cloth, plain weave, warp of cotton, weft of cotton, viscose, or combination, one continuous length. Type 1, 5 m (all): 2.5 cm, net price = 26p; 5 cm = 44p; 7.5 cm = 64p; 10 cm = 82p (most suppliers) 5 m × 5 cm supplied when size not stated

Uses: protection and retention of absorbent dressings; support for minor strains, sprains; securing splints

*Note.*Type 1 bandage formerly described as Open-Wove Bandage BPC 1973; Type 2 formerly described as 'medium quality'; Type 3 formerly described as 'hospital quality'

Triangular Calico Bandage, BP 1980. Unbleached calico rt. angle triangle. 90 cm × 90 cm × 1.27 m, net price = £1.00 (most suppliers)

Uses: sling

NHS Domette Bandage, BP 1988. Fabric, plain weave, cotton warp and wool weft (hospital quality also available, all cotton). 5 m (all): 5 cm, net price = 54p; 7.5 cm = 81p; 10 cm = £1.08; 15 cm = £1.61 (Robert Bailey, Vernon-Carus)

Uses: protection and support where warmth required

Multiple Pack Dressing No. 1 (Drug Tariff). Contains absorbent cotton, absorbent cotton gauze type 13 light (sterile), open-wove bandages (banded). Net price per pack = £2.88

Multiple Pack Dressing No. 2 (Drug Tariff). As for No. 1 (above) but with larger quantities of cotton and cotton gauze and two sizes of bandages. Net price per pack = £4.84

Stretch fabric retention bandages

Cotton Conforming Bandage, BP 1988. Cotton fabric, plain weave, treated to impart some elasticity to warp and weft. 3.5 m (all):

type A, 5 cm, net price = 54p, 7.5 cm = 68p, 10 cm = 82p, 15 cm = £1.13 (S&N—*Crinx*®)

type B, 5 cm = 55p, 7.5 cm = 71p, 10 cm = 87p, 15 cm = £1.13 (J&J—*Kling*®)

Uses: retention of dressings in difficult positions (e.g. over joints)

Knitted Polyamide and Cellulose Contour Bandage, BP 1988. Fabric, knitted warp of polyamide filament, weft of cotton or viscose, fast edges, one continuous length. 4 m stretched (all): 5 cm = 16p, 7 cm = 20p, 10 cm = 23p, 15 cm = 39p (Parema—*K-Band*®)

Polyamide and Cellulose Contour Bandage, BP 1988 (formerly Nylon and Viscose Stretch Bandage). Fabric, plain weave, warp of polyamide filament, weft of cotton or viscose, fast edges, one continuous length. 4 m stretched (all)—Robinsons—*Stayform*®(5 cm = 30p, 7.5 cm = 38p, 10 cm = 43p, 15 cm = 73p); Seton—*Slinky*® (net price 5 cm = 36p, 7.5 cm = 50p, 10 cm =61p, 15 cm = 86p); S&N—*Easifix* ® (5 cm = 29p, 7.5 cm = 36p, 10 cm =42p, 15 cm = 71p)
Uses: retention of dressings

N̶H̶S̶ **Tubular Gauze Bandage, Seamless.**
Unbleached cotton yarn, positioned with applicators. 20 m roll (all): 00, net price = £1.70; 01 = £1.74; 12 = £2.33; 34 = £3.42; 56 = £4.73; 78 = £5.54; T1 = £7.98; T2 = £10.29 (Seton—*Tubegauz*®)
Uses: retention of dressings on limbs, abdomen, trunk

Elasticated Tubular Bandage, BP (formerly Elasticated Surgical Tubular Stockinette). Knitted fabric, elasticated threads of rubber-cored polyamide or polyester with cotton or cotton and viscose yarn, tubular. Lengths 50 cm and 1 m, various widths 6.25 cm–12 cm, net price 39p–£1.69 (Brevet—*Texagrip*®; JLB Textiles—*Textube*® (formerly called *Lastogrip*®); Salt—*Rediform*®; S&N—*Tensogrip*®; Seton—*Tubigrip*®; Sigma—*Sigma ETB*®). Where no brand stated by prescriber, net price of stockinette supplied not to exceed: length 50 cm, 6.25 cm = 56p, 6.75 cm = 60p, 7.5 cm = 61p, 8.75 cm = 68p, 10 cm = 69p, 12 cm = 70p; length 1 m, 6.25 cm= £1.01, 6.75 cm = £1.08, 7.5 cm = £1.10, 8.75 cm = £1.15, 10 cm = £1.15, 12 cm = £1.33
Uses: retention of dressings on limbs, abdomen, trunk

Elasticated Surgical Tubular Stockinette, Foam padded (Drug Tariff specification 25). Fabric as for Elasticated Tubular Bandage with polyurethane foam lining. Heel, elbow, knee, small, net price = £2.13, medium = £2.30, large = £2.46; sacral, small, medium, and large (all) = £10.95 (Seton—*Tubipad*®)
Uses: relief of pressure and elimination of friction in relevant area; porosity of foam lining allows normal water loss from skin surface

Elasticated Viscose Stockinette (Drug Tariff specification 46). Lightweight plain-knitted elasticated tubular bandage. Length 1 m (all): net price 5 cm (medium limb) = 70p; 7.5 cm (large limb) = 92p; 10.75 cm (OS limb, head, child trunk) = £1.49; 17.5 cm (adult trunk) = £1.87 (Seton—*Tubifast*®)
Uses: retention of dressings

Elastic Net Surgical Tubular Stockinette (Drug Tariff Specification 26). Lightweight elastic open-work net tubular fabric.
type A : arm/leg, 40 cm × 1.8 cm (size C), net price = 32p; thigh/head, 60 cm × 2.5 cm (size E) = 58p; trunk (adult), 60 cm × 4.5 cm (Size F) = 85p; trunk (OS adult) 60 cm × 5.4 cm (size G) = £1.14 (Brevet—*Netelast*®)
type B: *Setonet*® withdrawn
type C: *Macrofix*® withdrawn

Cotton Stockinette, Bleached, BP1988 (formerly Cotton Surgical Tubular Stockinette). Knitted fabric, cotton yarn, tubular. 1 m × 2.5 cm, net price = 24p; 5 cm = 36p; 7.5 cm = 44p; 6 m × 10 cm = £3.00 (J&J, Seton)
Uses: 1 m lengths, basis (with wadding) for Plaster of Paris bandages etc. ; 6 m length, compression bandage

Ribbed Cotton and Viscose Surgical Tubular Stockinette, BP 1988. Knitted fabric of 1:1 ribbed structure, singles yarn spun from blend of two-thirds cotton and one-third viscose fibres, tubular. Length 5 m (all):
type A (lightweight): arm/leg (child), arm (adult) 5 cm, net price = £1.86; arm (OS adult), leg (adult) 7.5 cm = £2.41; leg (OS adult) 10 cm = £3.21; trunk (child) 15 cm

= £4.62; trunk (adult) 20 cm = £5.32; trunk (OS adult) 25 cm = £6.39 (Seton)
type B (heavyweight): sizes as for type A, net price £1.82–£6.26 (Sallis—*Eesiban*®)
Drug Tariff specifies various combinations of sizes to provide sufficient material for part or full body coverage
Uses: protective dressings with tar-based and other nonsteroid ointments

SUPPORT AND COMPRESSION BANDAGES

Non-adhesive woven extensible bandages

Crepe Bandage, BP 1988. Fabric, plain weave, warp of wool threads and crepe-twisted cotton threads, weft of cotton threads; stretch bandage. 4.5 m stretched (all): 5 cm, net price = 77p; 7.5 cm = £1.08; 10 cm = £1.43; 15 cm = £2.04 (most suppliers)
Uses: light support system for strains, sprains, compression over paste bandages for varicose veins

Cotton Crepe Bandage, BP 1988. Fabric, plain weave, warp of crepe-twisted cotton threads, weft of cotton and/or viscose threads; stretch bandage. 4.5 m stretched (both): 7.5 cm, net price = £2.42; 10 cm = £3.13; other sizesN̶H̶S̶ (most suppliers)
Uses: light support system for strains, sprains, compression over paste bandages for varicose ulcers

N̶H̶S̶ **Cotton Stretch Bandage, BP 1988.** Fabric, plain weave, warp of crepe-twisted cotton threads, weft of cotton threads; stretch bandage, lighter than cotton crepe. 4.5 m stretched (all): 5 cm, net price = 30p; 7.5 cm = 41p; 10 cm = 54p; 15 cm = 76p (most suppliers)
Uses: light support system for strains, sprains, compression over paste bandages for varicose veins

Cotton Suspensory Bandage (Drug Tariff). Type 1: cotton net bag with draw tapes and webbing waistband; net price small, medium, and large (all) = £1.30, extra large = £1.36. Type 2: cotton net bag with elastic edge and webbing waistband; small = £1.41, medium = £1.46, large = £1.52, extra large = £1.58. Type 3: cotton net bag with elastic edge and webbing waistband with elastic insertion; small, medium, and large (all) = £1.53; extra large = £1.59
Type supplied to be endorsed
Uses: support of scrotum

N̶H̶S̶ **Cotton and Rubber Elastic Bandage, BP.** Fabric, plain weave, warp of combined cotton and rubber threads, weft of cotton threads (S&N)
Uses: provision of high compression and medium support

Heavy Cotton and Rubber Elastic Bandage, BP.
Heavy version of above with one end folded as foot loop; fastener also supplied. 1.8 m unstretched × 7.5 cm, net price = £10.38 (Marlow, Seton, S&N—*Elastoweb*®).
Uses: provision of high even compression over large surface

Elastic Web Bandage, BP (also termed Blue Line Webbing). Characteristic fabric woven ribbon fashion, warp threads of cotton and rubber with mid-line threads coloured blue, weft threads of cotton or combined cotton and viscose; may be dyed skin colour; with or without foot loop. Per m (both) 7.5 cm, net price = 70p; 10 cm = £1.00; with foot loop (Drug Tariff specification 2a) 7.5 cm each = £3.87 (Marlow, Seton)
Uses: provision of support and high compression over large surface

Elastic Web Bandage without Foot Loop (also termed Red Line Webbing)(Drug Tariff specification 2b) (Scott-Curwen). Characteristic fabric woven ribbon fashion, warp threads of cotton and rubber with mid-line threads coloured red, weft threads of cotton or combined cotton and viscose. 7.5 cm × 2.75 m (2.5 m unstretched), net price = £3.03; 7.5 cm × 3.75 m (3.5 m unstretched) = £3.66

Uses: provision of support and high compression over large surfaces

High compression extensible bandages
(Drug Tariff specification 52)

PEC High Compression Bandage (Drug Tariff). Polymide, elastane, and cotton compression (high) extensible bandage, 3.5 m unstretched (both): 7.5 cm, net price = £2.20; 10 cm = £2.85 (Seton—*Setopress*®)

Uses: high compression for varicose ulcers

VEC High Compression Bandage (Drug Tariff). Viscose, elastane, and cotton compression (high) extensible bandage, 3 m unstretched (both); 7.5 cm, net price = £2.17; 10 cm = £2.81 (S&N—*Tensopress*®)

Uses: high compression for varicose ulcers

Adhesive woven extensible bandages

Titanium dioxide elastic adhesive bandage, BP
(formerly Porous Flexible Adhesive Bandage). Woven fabric, elastic in warp (crepe-twisted cotton threads), weft of cotton and/or viscose threads, spread with adhesive mass containing titanium dioxide but free from rubber and zinc oxide. 4.5 m stretched × 7.5 cm, net price = £3.33 (Credenhill—*Credaplast*® formerly *Poroplast*®)

Uses: compression for chronic leg ulcers; continuous pressure and support in patients hypersensitive to rubber and zinc oxide.

Elastic Adhesive Bandage, BP. Woven fabric, elastic in warp (crepe-twisted cotton threads), weft of cotton and/or viscose threads spread with adhesive mass containing zinc oxide. 4.5 m stretched (all): 5 cm, net price = £2.84; 7.5 cm = £4.10; 10 cm = £5.46 (Robinsons—*Flexoplast*®; S&N—*Elastoplast*®Bandage). 7.5 cm width supplied when size not stated

Uses: compression for chronic leg ulcers; compression and support for fractured ribs, clavicles, swollen or sprained joints

NHS **Half-spread Elastic Adhesive Bandage, BP 1988.** Fabric as for elastic adhesive bandage but only partially spread with adhesive. (S&N)

Uses: compression for leg ulcers; compression and support for fractured ribs, clavicles, swollen/sprained joints

NHS **Ventilated Elastic Adhesive Bandage, BP.**
Fabric as for elastic adhesive bandage but adhesive spread such that there are regular strips of unspread fabric along length. (S&N)

Uses: compression for leg ulcers; compression and support for fractured ribs, clavicles, swollen/sprained joints

NHS **Extension strapping, BP.** Woven fabric, elastic in weft, spread with adhesive mass containing zinc oxide, warp threads cotton and/or viscose, weft threads crepe-twisted cotton. (S&N)

Uses: support of light strains, joints and limbs removed from plaster casts, fractured ribs; traction bandaging

NHS **Cohesive extensible bandages**
These elastic bandages adhere to themselves and not to the patient's skin, which prevents slipping during use. 3M—*Coban*®, 4.5 m stretched (2.5, 5, 7.5, 10 and 15 cm); J&J—*Secure*® *Forte*, 4.5 m stretched (6, 8 and 10 cm); S&N—*Coplus*®, 6.3 m stretched (2.5, 3.8, 5, 7.5, 10 and 15 cm)

Uses: support of sprained joints

MEDICATED BANDAGES

Zinc Paste Bandage, BP. Cotton fabric, plain weave, impregnated with suitable paste containing zinc oxide; requires additional bandaging. Net price 6 m × 7.5 cm = £2.70 (Seton—*Zincaband*® (15%)); £2.88 (S&N—*Viscopaste PB7*® (10%), *additives:* include hydroxybenzoates)

Zinc Paste and Calamine Bandage (Drug Tariff specification 5). Cotton fabric, plain weave, impregnated with suitable paste containing calamine and zinc oxide; requires additional bandaging. Net price 6 m × 7.5 cm = £2.79 (Seton—*Calaband*®)

Zinc Paste, Calamine, and Clioquinol Bandage, BP.
Cotton fabric, plain weave, impregnated with suitable paste containing calamine, clioquinol, and zinc oxide; requires additional bandaging. Net price 6 m × 7.5 cm = £2.79 (Seton—*Quinaband*®, *additives:* include hydroxybenzoates)

Zinc Paste and Coal Tar Bandage, BP. Cotton fabric, plain weave, impregnated with a suitable paste containing coal tar and zinc oxide; requires additional bandaging. Net price 6 m × 7.5 cm = £2.70 (Seton—*Tarband*®, *additives:* include hydroxybenzoates; S&N—*Coltapaste*®, *additives:* include wool fat)

Uses: see section 13.5

Zinc Paste and Ichthammol Bandage, BP. Cotton fabric, plain weave, impregnated with suitable paste containing zinc oxide and ichthammol; requires additional bandaging. Net price 6 m × 7.5 cm = £2.70 (Seton—*Icthaband*®(15/2%), *additives:* include hydroxybenzoates; S&N—*Ichthopaste*®(6/2%), *additives:*none as listed in section 13.1)

Uses: see section 13.5

13.13.2   Surgical adhesive tapes

PERMEABLE ADHESIVE TAPES

Zinc Oxide Adhesive Tape, BP 1988. (Zinc Oxide Plaster). Fabric, plain weave, warp and weft of cotton and/or viscose, spread with an adhesive containing zinc oxide. 1.25 cm, net price 3 m = 52p, 5 m = 72p; 2.5 cm, 1 m = 33p, 3 m = 78p, 5 m = £1.05; 5 cm × 5 m = £1.79; 7.5 cm × 5 m = £2.66 (most suppliers)

Drug Tariff specifies 1 m × 2.5 cm supplied when size not stated

Uses: securing dressings and immobilising small areas

Permeable Woven Synthetic Adhesive Tape, BP 1988. Non-extensible closely woven fabric, spread with a polymeric adhesive. 5 m (all): 1.25 cm, net price = 61p; 2.5 cm = 89p; 5 cm = £1.57 (Beiersdorf—*Leukosilk*®)

Uses: securing dressings

For patients with skin reaction to other plasters and strapping, requiring use for long periods

Elastic Adhesive Tape, BP 1988 (Elastic Adhesive Plaster). Woven fabric, elastic in warp (crepe-twisted cotton threads), weft of cotton and/or viscose threads, spread with adhesive mass containing zinc oxide. 1.5 m stretched × 2.5 cm, net price = 69p; 4.5 m stretched × 2.5 cm = £1.30 (Robinsons—*Flexoplast*®; S&N—*Elastoplast*®).

Uses: securing dressings

For 5 cm width, see Elastic Adhesive Bandage, section 13.13.1

Permeable Non-woven Synthetic Adhesive Tape, BP 1988. Backing of paper-based or non-woven textile material spread with a polymeric adhesive mass. 5 m (all): BioDiagnostics—*Scanpor*® (net price 1.25 cm = 39p, 2.5 cm = 63p, 5 cm = £1.09); Beiersdorf—*Leukopor*® (1.25 cm = 42p, 2.5 cm = 66p, 5 cm = £1.16); 3M—*Micropore*® (1.25 cm = 52p, 2.5 cm = 80p, 5 cm = £1.44); S&N—*Hypal 2*® (1.25 cm = 56p, 2.5 cm = 85p, 5 cm = £1.57). Where no brand stated by prescriber, net price of tape supplied not to exceed 39p (1.25 cm), 63p (2.5 cm), £1.09 (5 cm)

Uses: securing dressings; skin closures for small incisions

For patients with skin reaction to other plasters and strapping, requiring use for long periods

---

OCCLUSIVE ADHESIVE TAPES

Impermeable Plastic Adhesive Tape, BP 1988.
Extensible water-impermeable plastic film spread with an adhesive mass. 2.5 cm × 3 m, net price = £1.00; 5 m = £1.50; 5 cm × 5 m = £1.91; 7.5 cm × 5 m = £2.76 (Robinsons; Seton; S&N)
Uses: securing dressings; covering site of infection where exclusion of air, water, and water vapour is required
Impermeable Plastic Synthetic Adhesive Tape, BP 1988. Extensible water-impermeable plastic film spread with a polymeric adhesive mass. 5 m (both): net price, 2.5 cm = £1.37; 5 cm = £2.61 (3M—*Blenderm®*)
Uses: isolating wounds from external environment; covering sites where total exclusion of water and water vapour required; securing dressings and appliances

13.13.3   Adhesive dressings
(also termed Island dressings)

PERMEABLE ADHESIVE DRESSINGS

NHS Elastic Adhesive Dressing, BP. Wound dressing or dressing strip, pad attached to piece of extension plaster, leaving suitable adhesive margin; both pad and margin covered with suitable protector; pad may be dyed yellow and may be impregnated with suitable antiseptic (see below); extension plaster may be perforated or ventilated
Uses: general purpose wound dressing
Note. Permitted antiseptics are aminacrine hydrochloride, chlorhexidine hydrochloride (both 0.07–0.13%), chlorhexidine gluconate (0.11–0.20%); domiphen bromide (0.05–0.25%)
NHS Permeable Plastic Wound Dressing, BP. Consisting of an absorbent pad, which may be dyed and impregnated with a suitable antiseptic (see under Elastic Adhesive Dressing), attached to a piece of permeable plastic surgical adhesive tape, to leave a suitable adhesive margin; both pad and margin covered with suitable protector (most suppliers)
Uses: general purpose wound dressing, permeable to air and water

VAPOUR-PERMEABLE (SEMIPERMEABLE) ADHESIVE DRESSINGS

Vapour-permeable Waterproof Plastic Wound Dressing, BP (former Drug Tariff title: Semipermeable Waterproof Plastic Wound Dressing). Consists of absorbent pad, may be dyed and impregnated with suitable antiseptic (see under Elastic Adhesive Dressing), attached to piece of semipermeable waterproof surgical adhesive tape, to leave suitable adhesive margin; both pad and margin covered with suitable protector. 8.5 cm × 6 cm, net price = 29p (S&N—*Elastoplast Airstrip®*)
Uses: general purpose waterproof wound dressing, permeable to air and water vapour

OCCLUSIVE ADHESIVE DRESSINGS

NHS Impermeable Plastic Wound Dressing, BP.
Consists of absorbent pad, may be dyed and impregnated with suitable antiseptic (see under Elastic Adhesive Dressing), attached to piece of impermeable plastic surgical adhesive tape, to leave suitable adhesive margin;

both pad and margin covered with suitable protector (most suppliers)
Uses: protective covering for wounds requiring an occlusive dressing

13.13.4   Surgical absorbents

Absorbent Cotton, BP. Carded cotton fibres of not less than 10 mm average staple length, available in rolls and balls. 25 g, net price = 52p; 100 g = £1.20; 500 g = £4.15 (most suppliers). 25-g pack to be supplied when weight not stated
Uses: general purpose cleansing and swabbing, pre-operative skin preparation, application of medicaments; supplementary absorbent pad to absorb excess wound exudate
Absorbent Cotton, Hospital Quality. As for absorbent cotton but lower quality materials, shorter staple length etc. 100 g, net price = 86p; 500 g = £2.79 (most suppliers)
Drug Tariff specifies to be supplied only where specifically ordered
Uses: suitable only as general purpose absorbent, for swabbing, and routine cleansing of incontinent patients; not for wound cleansing
Gauze and Cotton Tissue, BP 1988. Consists of absorbent cotton enclosed in absorbent cotton gauze type 12 or absorbent cotton and viscose gauze type 2. 500 g, net price = £5.37 (most suppliers, including Robinsons—*Gamgee Tissue®* (blue label))
Uses: absorbent and protective pad, as burns dressing on non-adherent layer
Gauze and Cotton Tissue (Drug Tariff specification 14). Similar to above. 500 g, net price = £3.96 (most suppliers, including Robinsons—*Gamgee Tissue®* (pink label))
Drug Tariff specifies to be supplied only where specifically ordered
Uses: absorbent and protective pad, as burns dressing on non-adherent layer
Absorbent Lint, BPC. Cotton cloth of plain weave with nap raised on one side from warp yarns. 25 g, net price = 69p; 100 g = £2.10; 500 g = £8.82 (most suppliers). 25-g pack supplied where no quantity stated
Uses: external absorbent protective dressing
Absorbent Cotton Gauze, BP 1988. Cotton fabric of plain weave, in rolls and as swabs (see below), usually Type 13 light, sterile. 90 cm (all)×1 m, net price = 82p; 3 m = £1.73; 5 m = £2.70; 10 m = £5.23 (most suppliers). 1-m packet supplied when no size stated
Uses: pre-operative preparation, for cleansing and swabbing
Note. Drug Tariff also includes unsterilised absorbent cotton gauze, 25 m roll, net price = £11.73
Cellulose Wadding, BP 1988. Delignified wood pulp bleached white, in multiple laminate form. 500 g, net price = £2.22 (most suppliers, including Robinsons—*Cellosene®*)
Uses: absorbing large volumes of fluid
Gauze and Cellulose Wadding Tissue, BP 1988. Consists of thick layer of cellulose wadding enclosed in absorbent cotton gauze type 12 or absorbent cotton and viscose gauze type 2. 500 g, net price = £2.98 (most suppliers)
Uses: absorbing large volumes of fluid
NHS Absorbent Muslin, BP 1988. Fabric of plain weave, warp threads of cotton, weft threads of cotton and/or viscose
Uses: wet dressing, soaked in 0.9% sterile sodium chloride solution
NHS Absorbent Cotton Ribbon Gauze, BP. Cotton fabric of plain weave in ribbon form with fast selvedge edges
Uses: post-surgery cavity packing for sinus, dental, throat cavities etc.

Absorbent Cotton and Viscose Ribbon Gauze, BP. Woven fabric in ribbon form with fast selvedge edges, warp threads of cotton, weft threads of viscose or combined cotton and viscose yarn, sterile. 5 m (both) × 1.25 cm, net price = 62p; 2.5 cm = 69p

Uses: post-surgery cavity packing for sinus, dental, throat cavities etc.

Gauze Swab, BP 1988. Consists of absorbent cotton gauze type 13 light or absorbent cotton and viscose gauze type 1 folded into squares or rectangles of 8-ply with no cut edges exposed. Sterile, 7.5 cm square, net price 5-pad packet = 29p; non-sterile, 10 cm square 100-pad packet = £4.86 (most suppliers)

Filmated Gauze Swab, BP 1988. As for Gauze Swab, but with thin layer of Absorbent Cotton enclosed within. Non-sterile, 10 cm × 10 cm, net price 100-pad packet = £5.96 (Vernon-Carus—*Cotfil*®)

Uses: general swabbing and cleansing

Non-woven Fabric Swab (Drug Tariff specification 28). Consists of non-woven fabric folded 4-ply; alternative to gauze swabs, type 13 light. Sterile, 7.5 cm square, net price 5-pad packet = 26p; non-sterile, 10 cm square, 100-pad packet = £3.36 (J & J—*Topper 8*®); 100-pad pack = £3.36 (CliniMed)

Uses: general purpose swabbing and cleansing; absorbs more quickly than gauze

Filmated Non-woven Fabric Swab (Drug Tariff specification 29). Film of viscose fibres enclosed within non-woven viscose fabric folded 8-ply. Non-sterile, 10 cm square, net price 100-pad packet = £4.78 (J & J—*Regal*®)

Uses: general purpose swabbing and cleansing

13.13.5   Wound dressing pads

Perforated Film Absorbent Dressing (Drug Tariff specification 9). Low-adherence dressing consisting of 3 layers; wound-facing layer, film of poly-(ethylene terephthalate) perforated in regular pattern; absorbent middle layer of type 1 consists of non-woven bleached cotton and viscose fibres or mixture of these with poly-acrylonitrile fibres; in type 2 (**NHS**) middle layer consists of bleached cotton fibres; backing layer of type 1 is apertured non-woven cellulose material; in type 2, the backing layer is identical with wound-facing layer; in type 3 outer layer comprises sleeve of film of poly(ethylmethylacrylate) perforated in regular pattern, forming wound-facing layer on side without join and backing layer on side with join (absorbent middle layer consists of bleached cotton fibres or viscose fibres or mixture of these sandwiched between two layers of apertured non-woven cellulose material); in type 4 wound-facing layer is similar to that in type 1 (absorbent middle layer consists of bleached cotton fibres and backing layer identical with wound-facing layer).

Type 1, 5 cm × 5 cm, net price, each = 12p; 10 cm × 10 cm = 20p; 20 cm × 10 cm = 38p (S&N— *Melolin*® (type 1); Kendall—*Telfa*® (type 2)).

Type 3, 5 cm × 5 cm, net price, each = 10p; 10 cm × 10 cm = 18p; 20 cm × 10 cm = 35p (J&J— *Release* ®)

Type 4, 5 cm × 5 cm, net price, each = 9p; 10 cm × 10 cm = 16p; 20 cm × 10 cm = 32p (Robinson—*Skintact*®)

Where size not stated, 5 cm size supplied

Uses: dressing for post-operative and low exudate wounds; low adherence property and low absorption capacity

Knitted Viscose Primary Dressing, BP. Warp knitted fabric manufactured from a bright viscose monofilament. 9.5 cm × 9.5 cm (both): net price = 27p (J&J—*N-A Dressing*®); net price = 23p (S&N—*Tricotex*®)

Uses: low adherence wound contact layer for use on ulcerative and other granulating wounds with superimposed absorbent pad

Sterile Dressing Pack (Drug Tariff specification 10; Scottish, 16). Contains gauze and cotton tissue pad, gauze swabs, absorbent cotton balls, absorbent paper towel, water repellent inner wrapper. Net price per pack = 69p

Sterile Dressing Pack with Non-woven Pads (Drug Tariff specification 35). Contains non-woven fabric covered dressing pad (*Surgipad*®), non-woven fabric swabs (*Topper 8*®), absorbent cotton wool balls, absorbent paper towel, water repellent inner wrapper. Net price per pack = 71p

NHS Ete® . Wound pad of rayon wadding with rayon silk wound contact layer stitched in chequered pattern (Molnlycke)

Uses: leg wounds, decubitus ulcers, minor burns, donor sites

NHS Melolite® . Absorbent fabric pad covered on both sides by polyethylene net (S&N)

Uses: primary dressing over clean sutured wounds, lacerations, and abrasions

NHS Mesorb® . Cellulose wadding pad with gauze wound contact layer and non-woven repellent backing (Molnlycke)

Uses: post-operative dressing for heavily exuding wounds

NHS Perfron® . Absorbent pad consisting of alternate layers of absorbent cotton and crepe cellulose tissue, in sleeve of non-woven viscose fabric with coating of polypropylene (J&J)

Uses: low adherence pad for heavily exuding wounds; laminate structure delays strike through

NHS * Surgipad® . Absorbent pad of absorbent cotton and viscose in sleeve of non-woven viscose fabric (J&J)

Uses: for heavily exuding wounds requiring frequent dressing changes

* Except in Sterile Dressing Pack with Non-woven Pads

Charcoal cloth dressings

Uses: to deodorise discharging, infected, malodorous wounds and ulcers

NHS Actisorb Plus® . Knitted fabric of activated charcoal, with one-way stretch, with silver residues, within spun-bonded nylon sleeve. Net price (each) 10.5 cm × 10.5 cm = £1.37; 19 cm × 10.5 cm = £2.66 (J&J)

NHS Carbonet® . Activated charcoal dressing. 10 cm × 10 cm, net price, each = £1.36; 10 cm × 20 cm = £3.05 (S&N)

NHS Carbosorb® . Outer cover of non-woven polyester-nylon fabric, activated charcoal cloth layer bonded to outer cover and semipermeable polyurethane film contact layer (Seton)

NHS CliniSorb®**Odour Control Dressings** . Layer of activated charcoal cloth between viscose rayon with outer polyamide coating. Net price 10 cm × 10 cm, 10 = £13.20; 10 cm × 20 cm, 10 = £17.60; 15 cm × 25 cm, 10 = £28.60 (CliniMed)

NHS Lyofoam C® . Lyofoam sheet with layer of activated charcoal cloth and additional outer envelope of polyurethane foam. 10 cm × 10 cm, net price, each = £1.26; 15 cm × 20 cm = £2.80 (Ultra)

Medicated viscose dressing

Povidone-iodine Fabric Dressing (Drug Tariff specification 43). Knitted viscose primary dressing impregnated with povidone-iodine ointment 10%, 5 cm × 5 cm, net price, each = 23p; 9.5 cm × 9.5 cm = 37p (J&J—*Inadine*®)

Uses: wound contact layer for abrasions and superficial burns; max. 4 dressings at same time

---

13.13.6   Tulle dressings

Non-medicated tulle dressings
Paraffin Gauze Dressing, BP (Tulle Gras). Fabric of leno weave, weft and warp threads of cotton and/or viscose yarn, impregnated with white or yellow soft paraffin; sterile. 10 cm × 10 cm, net price, each = 29p; pack of 10 pieces = £2.02 (most suppliers including Seton—*Paratulle*®; Roussel—*Unitulle*®; S&N—*Jelonet*®)
Uses: treatment of abrasions, burns, and other injuries of skin, and ulcerative conditions; post-operatively as penile and vaginal dressing and for sinus packing; heavier loading for skin graft transfer

Medicated tulle dressings
Chlorhexidine Gauze Dressing, BP. Fabric of leno weave, weft and warp threads of cotton and/or viscose yarn, impregnated with ointment containing chlorhexidine acetate; sterile. 5 cm × 5 cm, net price each = 21p; 10 cm × 10 cm = 44p (Seton—*Serotulle*®; Roussel—*Clorhexitulle*®; S&N—*Bactigras*®)
PoM **Framycetin Gauze Dressing, BP.** Fabric of leno weave, weft and warp threads of cotton, impregnated with ointment containing framycetin sulphate 1% in white soft paraffin containing 10% wool fat; sterile. 10 cm × 10 cm, net price each =23p; NHS 10 cm × 30 cm, 10 = £8.45 (Roussel—*Sofra-Tulle*®)
Cautions: large areas (risk of ototoxicity); see also cautions in section 13.10.1
Uses: wide range of infected lesions
PoM **Sodium Fusidate Gauze Dressing, BP .** Leno weave cotton gauze impregnated with ointment containing sodium fusidate 2% in white soft paraffin and wool fat. 10 cm × 10 cm, net price = 22p (Leo—*Fucidin Intertulle*®)

13.13.7   Vapour-permeable films and membranes

Vapour-permeable Adhesive Film Dressing, BP
(Semi-permeable Adhesive Dressing) . Sterile, extensible, waterproof, water vapour-permeable polyurethane film coated with synthetic adhesive mass; transparent. Supplied in single-use pieces. Type 1: 10 cm × 12 cm, net price = £1.12 (S&N—*Opsite*® *Flexigrid*), Type 2: 10 cm × 12 cm, net price = £1.17 (3M—*Tegaderm*®). Type 3: 10.2 cm × 12.7 cm, net price = £1.20 (J&J—*Bioclusive*®); Type 4, 7.5 cm × 10 cm, net price each = 62p; 10 cm × 14 cm, each = £1.06 (Beiersdorf—*Cutifilm*®)
Uses: post-operative dressing, donor sites, IV sites, superficial decubitus ulcers, amputation stumps, stoma care; protective cover to prevent skin breakdown
NHS **Omiderm**® . Sterile, water-vapour permeable polyurethane film. Net price 5 cm × 7 cm, 20 = £26.09; 8 cm × 10 cm, 20 = £46.12; 18 cm × 10 cm, 10 = £46.12; 60 cm × 10 cm, 10 = £154.96; 21 cm × 31 cm, 5 = £79.33 (IATRO)
Uses: ulcers; donor sites; superficial and partial thickness burns
NHS **Spyroflex**® (formerly Flexipore 6000) . Sterile, semipermeable, polyurethane membrane with hydrophilic adhesive. Net price 10 cm × 10 cm, 25 = £46.25; 20 cm × 20 cm, 10 = £68.40; 10 cm × 30 cm, 15 cm × 20 cm, 10 = £51.50; 20 cm × 30 cm, 5 = £51.50 (BritCair)
Uses: minor trauma, skin closure (alternative to skin sutures)
NHS **Spyrosorb**® . Sterile, semipermeable, absorbent polyurethane membrane with polyurethane film and hydrophilic adhesive. Net price 10 cm × 10 cm, 25 = £51.50; 20 cm × 20 cm, 10 = £68.70 (BritCair).
Uses: leg ulcers, pressure sores

13.13.8   Gel and colloid dressings

Occlusive or semi-occlusive dressings which adhere to dry skin and interact with moisture in the wound to form a gel; may remain on a wound for up to 7 days.

Hydrogels
NHS **Bard Absorption Dressing**® . A dry polysaccharide derivative in flake form which is mixed with water and applied directly into the wound. 60-g pack
Uses: treatment of wounds and ulcers.
Debrisan® (DrugTariff title: Dextranomer Paste Pad Dressing (Sterile), Drug Tariff specification 49). Spherical beads of dextranomer packed in plastic castors, single-use sachets, paste or pads. Beads sprinkled onto cleansed wound and covered with a suitable non-woven, adhesive, semi-occlusive covering, or sterile dressing. Alternatively paste or pad is applied and covered in similar manner. Beads, net price 4-g sachet = £1.94, 60 g = £29.01; paste in sachets, 4 × 10 g = £19.89; pads, 3 g sachet = £2.36 (Pharmacia)
Uses: debriding agent to remove necrotic tissue
NHS **Fibracol**® . Calcium alginate with collagen matrix. Net price 5 cm × 5 cm each = 98p; 9.5 cm × 9.5 cm = £1.30; 10 cm × 20 cm = £3.60 (J & J)
Uses: small size for foot ulcers, pressure sores and toe nail beds; large size for moderate to heavily exuding wounds, leg ulcers, pressure sores
NHS **Geliperm**® . Gel sheets, dry and wet forms; tubed granulated gel. Dry, 11 cm × 25 cm, net price 6 sheets = £51.23; granulate, 20 g, 6 tubes = £19.92, 50 g, 6 tubes = £49.80. Wet, 10 cm × 10 cm, net price, 20 sheets = £44.85, 12 cm × 13 cm, 6 sheets = £25.62; 12 cm × 26 cm, 6 sheets = £51.23 (Geistlich)
Uses: wound and ulcer dressing, burns, donor sites
Intrasite® **Gel** (formerly Scherisorb®) Drug Tariff specification 50. A ready-mixed hydrogel containing modified carboxymethylcellulose polymer applied directly into the wound. 15-g sachet, net price = £1.75 (S&N)
PoM **Iodosorb**® . Powder, microbeads of cadexomer iodine (modified starch gel containing iodine 0.9%). Net price 3-g sachet = £1.93; also Iodosorb® Ointment, 4 × 10 g = £18.05; 2 × 20 g = £18.05; also Iodoflex® Paste, 5 × 5-g units = £20.40; 3 × 10-g units = £24.50 (Perstorp)
Uses: for venous leg ulcers and pressure sores apply 3 mm layer to wound surface and renew daily (3 times weekly for ointment or paste) or when saturated with exudate; *caution:* thyroid disorders
NHS **Kaltocarb**® . Dressing in 3 layers: wound-facing layer of calcium alginate fibre; absorbent middle layer of activated charcoal cloth; backing layer of bonded polyester and viscose non-woven material. Net price 7.5 cm × 12 cm, 25 = £51.48; 15 cm × 15 cm, 15 = £67.80 (BritCair)
Uses. discharging infected malodorous wounds and ulcers
NHS **Kaltoclude**® . Calcium alginate fibre bonded to semi-permeable copolymer adhesive film. Pack of 25 (both); 10 cm × 10 cm, net price per pack = £44.75; 15 cm × 20 cm = £133.25 (BritCair)
Uses: light to moderately exuding wounds such as leg ulcers and pressure sores
Kaltogel®
Calcium sodium alginate fibre, highly absorbent, quick gelling dressing, net price 10 cm ×10 cm = £1.48 (BritCair)
Uses: moderate to heavily exudating wounds including leg ulcers, pressure sores, fungating lesions
Kaltostat® (Drug Tariff title: Calcium Alginate Dressing, Drug Tariff specification 41, type 2). Calcium alginate fibre, flat non-woven pads, 5 cm × 5 cm, net price each = 72p; 7.5 cm × 12 cm = £1.57; other sizes (NHS) 10 cm × 20 cm, 25 = £92.75; 15 cm × 25 cm, 25 = £160.00;

30 cm × 60 cm, 5 = £123.40; wound packing, 2 g, 25 = £82.00; also (**NHS**) Kaltostat Fortex®, 10 cm × 10 cm, 10 = £31.50 (BritCair)
Uses: haemostatic

Sorbsan® (Drug Tariff title: Calcium Alginate Dressing, type 1 Drug Tariff specification 41). Calcium alginate fibre, highly absorbent, flat non-woven pads, 5 cm × 5 cm, net price, each = 84p; 10 cm × 10 cm = £1.49; other sizes (**NHS**) 10 cm × 20 cm, 5 = £21.50; surgical packing 30 cm, 5 = £23.75; ribbon, 40 cm (+12.5-cm probe), 5 = £16.00; also (bonded to a secondary absorbent viscose pad) Sorbsan® Plus (**NHS**), 7.5 cm × 10 cm, 5 = £11.00; 10 cm × 15 cm, 5 = £22.00 (Steriseal)
Uses: heavily to moderately exudating wounds

NHS Sorbsan® SA . Calcium alginate fibre, highly absorbent flat non-woven pads for wound contact bonded to adhesive semipermeable polyurethane foam. Net price 9 cm × 11 cm, 5 = £11.00 (Steriseal)
Uses: moderately to lightly exudating shallow wounds

Tegagel® (Drug Tariff title: Calcium Alginate Dressing, Drug Tariff specification 41, type 1b). Net price each 5 cm × 5 cm = 70p; 10 cm × 10 cm = £1.45
Uses: for leg ulcers, pressure sores, second degree burns, post-operative wounds, fungating carcinomas

NHS Tielle® . Semi-permeable, foamed gel with non-woven wicking layer and polyurethane backing layer. Net price 11 cm × 11 cm, 10 = £22.50 (J&J)
Uses: light to moderately exuding wounds, leg ulcers

NHS Vigilon® . Semi-permeable hydrogel sheets on a polyethylene mesh support. Sterile, 3 in × 6 in, net price 10 = £35.50, 4 in × 4 in, 10 = £35.50; non-sterile, 4 in × 4 in, 10 = £24.75, 13 in × 24 in, 2 = £43.00 (Seton)

Hydrocolloids

NHS Biofilm® . Hydrocolloid dressing with non-woven fibre backing; also in powder form for direct application into wound: 10 cm × 10 cm, net price 10 = £16.50; 20 cm × 20 cm, 5 = £28.50; powder, 10 sachets = £18.20 (CliniMed)

Comfeel® . (Drug Tariff specification 42, type 2). Soft elastic pad consisting of carmellose (carboxymethylcellulose) sodium particles embedded in adhesive mass; smooth outer layer and polyurethane film backing; available as sheets, powder in plastic blister units and paste for direct application into the wound: ulcer dressing, 10 cm × 10 cm, net price each = £2.04; 15 cm × 15 cm − £4.07; 20 cm × 20 cm = £6.10; other sizes (NHS) 4 cm × 6 cm, 30 = £22.20; transparent dressing, 5 cm × 7 cm, 10 = £9.70; 9 cm × 14 cm, 10 = £28.60; 15 cm × 20 cm, 5 − £31.20; powder 6 g, 10 = £24.80; paste 12-g sachet, 10 = £12.00 (Coloplast)

NHS Dermiflex® . Hydrocolloid dressing bonded to PVC foam 10.2 cm × 10.2 cm, net price, each= £1.95 (J&J)

Granuflex® (formerly Granuflex® E) Drug Tariff specification 42, Type 1b. Hydrocolloid wound contact layer bonded to plastic foam layer, with outer semipermeable polyurethane film. 10 cm × 10 cm, net price each = £2.12; 15 cm × 15 cm = £3.99; 15 cm × 20 cm = £4.35; 20 cm × 20 cm, 1 = £5.99; **NHS** 20 cm × 30 cm, 5 = £55.75; also Granuflex® ExtraThin (**NHS**), 7.5 cm × 7.5 cm, 5 = £5.05; 10 cm × 10 cm, 5 = £6.26; 15 cm × 15 cm, 5 = £13.27; 5 cm × 10 cm, 5 = £6.92; 5 cm × 20 cm, 10 = £13.82; also Granuflex® Compression Bandage (**NHS**), 10 cm × 6.5 m (stretched), 6 = £32.64; also Granuflex® Paste (**NHS**), net price 30 g = £2.68; also (**NHS**), Granuflex® Bordered Dressing, 6 cm × 6 cm, 5 = £7.38; 10 cm × 10 cm, 5 = £15.61; 15 cm × 15 cm, 5 = £30.98; triangular dressing, 10 cm × 13 cm, 5 = £15.61; 15 cm × 18 cm, 5 = £26.55 (Convatec)
Uses: chronic ulcers, pressure sores, open wounds, debridement of wounds; powders and pastes used with sheet dressings to fill deep or heavily exudating wounds

Tegasorb® (Drug Tariff specification 42, Type 3). Hydrocolloid dressing 10 cm × 12 cm (oval), net price

each = £1.93; 13 cm × 15 cm (oval), 1 = £3.64; other sizes (**NHS**) 17 cm × 20 cm (oval), 5 = £17.50 (3M)
Uses: chronic wounds such as leg ulcers and pressure sores

13.13.9   Foam dressings

Polyurethane Foam Dressing, BP. Absorbent foam dressing of low adherence; sterile. 7.5 cm × 7.5 cm, net price, each = 77p; 10 cm × 10 cm, each = 92p; 10 cm × 17.5 cm, each = £1.44; 15 cm × 20 cm, each = £1.94; other sizes (**NHS**) 10 cm × 25 cm, 35 = £58.05; 25 cm × 30 cm, each = £3.91 (Ultra—*Lyofoam*®)
Uses: treatment of burns, decubitus ulcers, donor sites, granulating wounds

NHS Cavi-Care® Soft slightly absorbent wound dressing of low adherence prepared by mixing thoroughly for 15 seconds immediately before use and allowing to expand its volume within the wound. Conforming foam wound dressing, 20 g, net price = £8.03 (S&N)
Uses: in the management of open granulating wounds such as pressure sores, abdominal wall breakdown, pilonidal sinus excision

NHS Allevyn® . Hydrophilic polyurethane dressing; foam sheets with trilaminate structure, non-adherent wound contact layer, foam based central layer, bacteria and waterproof outer layer. 5 cm × 5 cm, each = 92p; 10 cm × 10 cm, each = £2.05; 10 cm × 20 cm, each = £3.31; 20 cm × 20 cm, each = £8.40; also Allevyn®Heel; Allevyn® Cavity, circular (5 and 10 cm), tubular (2.5 cm × 9 cm and 4 cm × 12 cm) (S&N)
Uses: treatment of heavily exuding wounds, specifically venous leg ulcers

13.13.10   Elastic hosiery

Before elastic hosiery can be dispensed, the quantity (single or pair), article (including accessories), and compression class (I, II or III) must be specified by the prescriber; all dispensed articles must state on the packaging that they conform with Drug Tariff technical specification No. 40, for further details see Drug Tariff

Graduated compression hosiery
Class 1 Light Support
Hosiery, compression at ankle 14–17 mm Hg, thigh length or below knee with knitted in heel. Net price per pair, circular knit (standard), thigh length = £5.64, below knee − £5 14; light weight elastic net (made-to-measure), thigh length = £14.90, below knee = £11.64
Uses: superficial or early varices, varicosis during pregnancy
Class 2 Medium Support
Hosiery, compression at ankle 18–24 mm Hg, thigh length or below knee with knitted in heel. Net price per pair, circular knit (standard), thigh length = £8.40, below knee = £7.50, (made-to-measure), thigh length = £28.16, below knee = £17.60; net (made-to-measure), thigh length = £14.90, below knee = £11.64; flat bed (made-to-measure, only with closed heel and open toe), thigh length = £28.16, below knee = £17.60
Uses: varices of medium severity, ulcer treatment and prophylaxis, mild oedema, varicosis during pregnancy
Class 3 Strong Support
Hosiery, compression at ankle 25–35 mm Hg, thigh length or below knee with open or knitted in heel. Net price per pair, circular knit (standard), thigh length = £9.94, below knee = £8.52, (made-to-measure) thigh length = £28.16, below knee = £17.60; one way stretch (made-to-measure, only with open heel and open toe), thigh length = £28.16, below knee = £17.60
Uses: gross varices, post thrombotic venous insufficiency, gross oedema, ulcer treatment and prophylaxis

Accessories
Suspender, for thigh stockings, net price = 50p, belt (specification 13), = £3.73, fitted (additional price) = 50p

Anklets
Class 2 Medium Support
Anklets, compression 18–24 mm Hg, circular knit (standard and made-to-measure), net price per pair = £4.92;
flat bed (standard and made-to-measure) = £10.32; net
(made-to-measure) = £9.58
Uses: soft tissue support
Class 3 Strong Support
Anklets, compression 25–35 mm Hg, circular knit (standard and made-to-measure), net price per pair = £6.86;
one way stretch (standard and made-to-measure) =
£6.86
Uses: soft tissue support

Kneecaps
Class 2 Medium Support
Kneecaps, circular knit (standard and made-to-measure),
net price per pair = £4.92; flat bed (standard and made-
to-measure) = £10.32; net (made-to-measure) = £7.96
Uses: soft tissue support
Class 3 Strong Support
Kneecaps, circular knit (standard and made-to-measure),
net price per pair = £6.58; one way stretch (standard and
made-to-measure) = £6.58
Uses: soft tissue support

13.14   Topical circulatory preparations

These preparations are used to improve circulation in conditions such as bruising, superficial thrombophlebitis, chilblains and varicose veins but are of little value. Chilblains
are best managed by avoidance of exposure to cold; neither systemic nor topical vasodilator therapy is established
as being effective. Sclerotherapy of varicose veins is
described in section 2.13.

Rubefacients are described in section 10.3.2.

Hirudoid® (Panpharma)
Cream, heparinoid 0.3% in a vanishing-cream basis. Net
price 50 g = £2.38
Additives: include hydroxybenzoates (parabens)
Gel, heparinoid 0.3%. Net price 50 g = £2.38
Additives: include propylene glycol, fragrance
Apply up to 4 times daily in superficial soft-tissue inju-
ries and superficial thrombophlebitis

Lasonil® (Bayer)
Ointment, heparinoid 50 units, hyaluronidase 150 units/g.
Net price 14 g = 38p; 40 g = £1.90
Additives: include wool fat derivative
Apply 2–3 times daily in superficial soft-tissue injuries

Secaderm® (Fisons)
Salve (= ointment), colophony 26%, melaleuca oil 5.6%,
phenol 2.4%, terebene 5.25%, turpentine oil 6%. For
boils and chilblains. Net price 15 g = 87p
Additives: include beeswax
Apply 1–2 times daily and cover with dressing

14:Immunological products and
VACCINES

In this chapter, immunisation is discussed under the following headings:

14.1	Active immunity
14.2	Passive immunity
14.3	Storage and use
14.4	Vaccines and antisera
14.5	Immunoglobulins
14.6	International travel

14.1 Active immunity

Vaccines may consist of:

1. a *live attenuated* form of an infective agent, as in the vaccines which are used against virus diseases such as rubella and measles, or BCG used against tuberculosis,
2. *inactivated* preparations of the virus (e.g. influenza vaccine) or bacteria (e.g. whole cell typhoid vaccine), or
3. *extracts of* or *detoxified exotoxins* produced by a micro-organism (e.g. tetanus vaccine).

They stimulate production of antibodies and other components of the immune mechanism.

For **live attenuated** vaccines, immunisation is generally achieved with a single dose (but 3 doses are required with oral poliomyelitis and oral typhoid vaccines). Live virus multiplies in the body and usually produces a durable immunity but not always as long as that of the natural infection. When two live virus vaccines are required (and are not available as a combined preparation) they should be given either simultaneously at different sites or with an interval of at least 3 weeks.

Inactivated vaccines may require a primary series of injections of vaccine to produce an adequate antibody response and in most cases reinforcing or 'booster' injections are required. The duration of immunity following the use of inactivated vaccines varies from months to many years.

Extracts of or **detoxified exotoxins** are more immunogenic if adsorbed onto an adjuvant (such as aluminium hydroxide). As in the case of inactivated vaccines they require a primary series of injections followed by reinforcing doses.

The health departments of the UK have issued a memorandum, *Immunisation against Infectious Disease 1994* which describes the vaccines, immunoglobulins, and antisera in routine use in the UK; recommended schemes for immunisation in childhood are included and advice is given on storage, technique, and record keeping. It can be obtained from:

HMSO Publications Centre
PO Box 276, London SW8 5DT
Telephone orders, 071-873 9090.

SIDE-EFFECTS. Some vaccines (e.g. poliomyelitis vaccines) produce very few reactions, while others (e.g. measles and rubella vaccines) may produce a very mild form of the disease. Some vaccines may produce discomfort at the site of injection and mild fever and malaise. Occasionally there are more seri-ous untoward reactions and these should always be reported in the usual way to the CSM. Anaphylactic reactions are very rare but can be fatal (see section 3.4.3 for management).

CONTRA-INDICATIONS. Most vaccines have some basic contra-indication to their use, and the manufacturer's leaflet should always be consulted. In general, vaccination should be postponed if the subject is suffering from an *acute illness*. Minor infections without fever or systemic upset are not contra-indications.

Some viral vaccines contain small quantities of antibiotics such as neomycin or polymyxin (or both); such vaccines may need to be withheld from individuals who are *sensitive to the antibiotic*. *Hypersensitivity to egg* contra-indicates influenza vaccine (residual egg protein present) and, if evidence of previous anaphylactic reaction, also MMR and yellow fever vaccines.

Live vaccines should not be routinely administered to *pregnant women* because of possible harm to the fetus but where there is a significant risk of exposure (e.g. to poliomyelitis or yellow fever), the need for vaccination outweighs any possible risk to the fetus. Live vaccines should not be given to individuals with *impaired immune responsiveness*, whether caused by disease (for special reference to *AIDS*, see below) or as a result of radiotherapy or treatment with high doses of corticosteroids or other immunosuppressive drugs[1,2]. They should not be given to those suffering from *malignant conditions* or other tumours of the reticulo-endothelial system[2].

VACCINES AND AIDS. The Department of Health has advised that HIV-positive subjects with or without symptoms can receive the following live vaccines:

measles[2] (or MMR), mumps, poliomyelitis[3], rubella;

and the following inactivated vaccines:

cholera, diphtheria, haemophilus influenzae type b, hepatitis A, hepatitis B, influenza, meningococcal, pertussis, pneumococcal, poliomyelitis[3], tetanus, typhoid (injection).

HIV-positive subjects should **not** receive:

BCG, yellow fever[4], typhoid (oral)

Note. The above advice differs from that for other immunocompromised patients.

---

1. Live vaccines should be postponed until at least 3 months after stopping corticosteroids and 6 months after stopping chemotherapy.
2. Consideration should be given to use of normal immunoglobulin after exposure to measles (see p.481) and to varicella-zoster immunoglobulin after exposure to chickenpox or herpes zoster (see p.482).
3. Virus may be excreted for longer periods than in normal subjects; contacts should be warned of this and of need for washing hands after changing a vaccinated infant's nappies; HIV-positive contacts are at greater risk than normal contacts. For HIV-positive symptomatic subjects inactivated poliomyelitis vaccine can be used at discretion of clinician.
4. Because insufficient evidence of safety.

Immunisation programmes

There is no contra-indication to administration of pertussis vaccine to unimmunised older children in order to protect infants and siblings. Since a course of 3 injections is required to protect against pertussis, vaccine cannot be used to control an outbreak.

If the pertussis component has been omitted from earlier immunisations 3 doses of pertussis vaccine can be given at monthly intervals to provide protection.

Where the basic course against diphtheria and tetanus is incomplete triple vaccine may be used to begin or complete the course against whooping-cough so that the infant is not given more injections than necessary.

Measles/mumps/rubella (MMR) vaccine can be given at the time of the reinforcing dose of diphtheria/tetanus vaccine and poliomyelitis vaccine; because the diphtheria/tetanus vaccine can be more painful, measles/mumps/rubella vaccine should be injected first; the diphtheria/tetanus should then be given with a separate syringe and needle in the opposite limb (or a second appointment can be made).

Vaccines for the childhood immunisation programme should be obtained via local Health Authorities or (in England only) direct from Farillon rather than by FP10 prescription.

Age	Vaccine	Interval	Notes
During the first year of life	DTPer/Vac/Ads *and* Haemophilus influenzae b *and* Pol/Vac (Oral)	3 doses at intervals of 4 weeks	The first doses should be given at 2 months of age
During the second year of life	Meas/Mump/Rub (MMR) Vac (Live)		At 12–15 months of age
	Haemophilus influenzae b		One dose at 13 months–4 years of age if not previously immunised
At school entry or entry to nursery school	DT/Vac/Ads *and* Pol/Vac (Oral)	Preferable to allow an interval of at least 3 years after completing basic course	
	Meas/Mump/Rub (MMR) Vac (Live)		Unless documented history of measles/mumps/rubella immunisation *or* valid contra-indication *or* laboratory evidence of immunity to measles, mumps, and rubella
Between 10th and 14th birthdays	BCG	Leave an interval of not less than 3 weeks between BCG and rubella immunisation	For tuberculin-negative children. For tuberculin-negative contacts at any age
Between 10th and 14th birthdays (girls only)	Rub/Vac (Live)		See MR vaccine (both sexes), p.475
On leaving school or before employment or further education	Pol/Vac (Oral) *and* DT/Vac/Ads (Adult)		
Adult life	Pol/Vac (Oral) if previously unimmunised	3 doses at intervals of 4 weeks	No adult should remain unimmunised; reinforcing doses for travellers to countries where polio endemic and for health care workers in possible contact with polio
	Rub/Vac (Live) for susceptible women of child-bearing age		Women of child-bearing age should be tested for rubella antibodies and if sero-negative offered rubella immunisation. Pregnancy must be excluded and patient warned not to become pregnant for 1 month after
	Tet/Vac/Ads if previously unimmunised	For previously unimmunised adults: 2 doses at an interval of 4 weeks followed by a third dose 4 weeks later	A reinforcing dose 10 years after primary course and again 10 years later maintains a satisfactory level of protection; give DT/Vac/Ads (Adult) if diphtheria cover also needed
	Hepatitis A and B, Influenza, Pneumococcal		All for individuals (adults or children) in high-risk groups, see under individual vaccines

14.2 Passive immunity

Immunity with immediate protection against certain infective organisms can be obtained by injecting preparations made from the plasma of immune individuals with adequate levels of antibody to the disease for which protection is sought (see under Immunoglobulins, section 14.5). This passive immunity lasts only a few weeks; where necessary passive immunisation can be repeated.

Antibodies of human origin are usually termed *immunoglobulins*. The term *antiserum* is applied to material prepared in animals. Because of serum sickness and other allergic-type reactions that may follow injections of antisera, this therapy has been replaced wherever possible by the use of immunoglobulins. Reactions are theoretically possible after injection of human immunoglobulins but reports of such reactions are very rare.

14.3 Storage and use

Care must be taken to store all vaccines and other immunological products under the conditions recommended in the manufacturer's leaflet, otherwise the preparation may become denatured and totally ineffective. **Refrigerated storage** is usually necessary; many vaccines need to be stored at 2–8°C and not allowed to freeze. Opened multidose vials which have not been fully used should be discarded *within one hour* if no preservative is present (most live virus vaccines) or *within 3 hours* or at the end of a session (when vaccines containing a preservative are used but also including oral poliomyelitis vaccine).

Particular attention must be paid to the instructions on the use of diluents and ampoules of vaccine should always be *adequately shaken* before use to ensure uniformity of the material to be injected.

Note. The Department of Health has advised against the use of jet guns for vaccination owing to the risk of transmitting blood-borne infections, such as HIV.

14.4 Vaccines and antisera

AVAILABILITY. Anthrax, rabies, smallpox, and yellow fever vaccines, botulism antitoxin, and snake venom antitoxin are available from local designated holding centres. Details of names, addresses, and telephone numbers of holding centres are given in:
The Health Service Supply Purchasing Guide, section D pp. 1101–1199, and
The Pharmaceutical Supplies Bulletin, volume 8, no. 5, Oct. 1985, 63/85.

For antivenom, see Emergency Treatment of Poisoning p.25.

Enquiries for vaccines not available commercially can also be made to

Department of Health
Room 715
133–155 Waterloo Road
London SE1 8UG
telephone 071-972 4476/7

In Scotland information about availability of vaccines can be obtained from the Chief Administrative Pharmaceutical Officer of the local Health Board. In Wales enquiries should be directed to the Welsh Office, Cathays Park, Cardiff CF1 3NQ, telephone 0222 825111, extn 4658 and in Northern Ireland to the Department of Health and Social Services, Dundonald House, Belfast BT4 3FS, telephone 0232 520000.

For further details of availability, see under individual vaccines.

ANTHRAX VACCINE
Anthrax vaccine is available for anyone subject to heavy exposure to anthrax, such as those exposed to infected hides and carcasses and to imported bonemeal, fishmeal, and feeding stuffs. The vaccine is the alum precipitate of an antigen from *Bacillus anthracis* and, following the primary course of injections, reinforcing doses should be given at about yearly intervals.

PoM Anthrax Vaccine
Dose: initial course 3 doses of 0.5 mL by intramuscular injection at intervals of 3 weeks followed by a 4th dose after an interval of 6 months
Reinforcing doses: 0.5 mL annually
Available from Public Health Laboratory Service

BCG VACCINES
BCG (Bacillus Calmette-Guérin) is a live attenuated strain derived from *Mycobacterium bovis* which stimulates the development of hypersensitivity to *M. tuberculosis*. BCG vaccine should be given intradermally by operators skilled in the technique (see below); the percutaneous multiple puncture technique is an acceptable alternative **only** for young infants in whom the technique of intradermal injection may be difficult (18–20 puncture points are required).

Within 2–6 weeks a small swelling appears at the injection site which progresses to a papule or to a benign ulcer about 10 mm in diameter and heals in 6–12 weeks. A dry dressing may be used if the ulcer discharges, but the air should **not** be excluded.

The CSM has reported that serious reactions with BCG are uncommon and most often consist of prolonged ulceration or subcutaneous abscess formation due to faulty injection technique.

BCG is recommended for the following groups if **successful** BCG immunisation has not previously been carried out and they are negative for tuberculoprotein hypersensitivity:

contacts of those with active respiratory tuberculosis (immigrants in whose communities there is a high incidence of tuberculosis may be regarded as contacts—newborn infants need not be tested for sensitivity but should be immunised without delay);

health service staff (including medical students, hospital medical staff, nurses, and anybody who comes into contact with patients, including physiotherapists and radiographers, technical staff in pathology departments and any others considered to be at special risk because of the likelihood of contact with infective patients or their sputum; particularly important to test staff in maternity and paediatric departments);

children between their tenth and fourteenth birthdays (see schedule, section 14.1);

veterinary and other staff who handle animal species known to be susceptible to tuberculosis;

those travelling to countries with a high incidence of tuberculosis (section 14.6)

Apart from newborn infants any person being considered for BCG immunisation must first be given a skin test for hypersensitivity to tuberculoprotein (see under Diagnostic agents, below).

It is recommended that an interval of at least 3 weeks should be allowed between the administration of a live virus vaccine and BCG. However, when BCG is given to infants, there is no need to delay the primary immunisations, including poliomyelitis.

See section 14.1 for general contra-indications. BCG is also contra-indicated in subjects with generalised septic skin conditions (in the case of eczema, a vaccination site free from lesions should be chosen).

Intradermal

PoM **Bacillus Calmette-Guérin Vaccine.**
BCG Vaccine, Dried Tub/Vac/BCG. A freeze-dried preparation of live bacteria of a strain derived from the bacillus of Calmette and Guérin.

Dose: 0.1 mL (INFANT under 3 months 0.05 mL) by intradermal injection

Available from District Health Authorities or (in England only) direct from Farillon

INTRADERMAL INJECTION TECHNIQUE. After swabbing with spirit and allowing to dry, skin is stretched between thumb and forefinger and needle (size 25G or 26G) inserted (bevel upwards) for about 2 mm into superficial layers of dermis (almost parallel with surface). Needle should be short with short bevel (can usually be seen through epidermis during insertion). Raised blanched bleb showing tips of hair follicles is sign of correct injection; 7 mm bleb ≡ 0.1 mL injection; if considerable

resistance not felt, needle is removed and reinserted before giving more vaccine.

Injection site is at insertion of deltoid muscle onto humerus (sites higher on arm more likely to lead to keloid formation); tip of shoulder should be **avoided**; for cosmetic reasons, upper and lateral surface of thigh may be preferred and this is an acceptable alternative.

PoM **Bacillus Calmette-Guérin Vaccine, Isoniazid-Resistant.** A freeze-dried preparation of live bacteria of an isoniazid-resistant strain derived from the bacillus of Calmette and Guérin.

Dose: 0.1 mL (INFANT under 3 months 0.05 mL) by intradermal injection; for active immunisation of tuberculosis contacts receiving prophylactic treatment with isoniazid—but **no longer recommended.**

Available from Evans (special order)

Percutaneous

PoM **Bacillus Calmette-Guérin Vaccine, Percutaneous** Tub/Vac/BCG(Perc). A preparation of live bacteria of a strain derived from the bacillus of Calmette and Guérin.

Dose: 0.02 mL by percutaneous administration but only recommended as an alternative for infants, see notes on previous page.

Available from District Health Authorities or (in England only) direct from Farillon

DIAGNOSTIC AGENTS. In the *Mantoux test* the initial diagnostic dose in patients in whom tuberculosis is suspected (or who are known to be hypersensitive to tuberculin) is 1 unit of tuberculin PPD in 0.1 mL by intradermal injection and in subsequent tests 10 and finally 100 units in 0.1 mL may be given. For routine pre-BCG skin-testing the 10-unit dose of tuberculin PPD is used. In the *Heaf test* (multiple puncture) a solution containing 100 000 units in 1 mL is used.

PoM **Tuberculin PPD.** Prepared from the heat treated products of growth and lysis of the appropriate species of mycobacterium, and containing 100 000 units/mL. Net price 1-mL amp = £4.99. Also available diluted 1 in 100 (1000 units/mL), 1 in 1000 (100 units/mL), and 1 in 10 000 (10 units/mL). Net price 1 mL (all) = £2.22

Available from District Health Authorities or (in England only) direct from Farillon

BOTULISM ANTITOXIN

A trivalent botulism antitoxin is available for the post-exposure prophylaxis of botulism and for the treatment of persons thought to be suffering from botulism. It specifically neutralises the toxins produced by *Clostridium botulinum* types A, B, and E. It is not effective against infantile botulism as the toxin (type A) is seldom, if ever, found in the blood in this type of infection.

Hypersensitivity reactions are a problem. It is essential to read the contra-indications, warnings, and details of sensitivity tests on the package insert. Prior to treatment checks should be made regarding previous administration of any antitoxin and history of any allergic condition, e.g. asthma, hay fever, etc. All patients should be tested for sensitivity (diluting the antitoxin if history of allergy).

PoM **Botulism Antitoxin.** A preparation containing the specific antitoxic globulins that have the power of neutralising the toxins formed by types A, B, and E of *Clostridium botulinum.*

Note. The BP title Botulinum Antitoxin is not used because the preparation currently available has a higher phenol content (0.45% against 0.25%).

Dose: prophylaxis, 20 mL by intramuscular injection as soon as possible after exposure; treatment, 20 mL by slow intravenous infusion followed by 10 mL 2–4 hours later if necessary, and further doses at intervals of 12–24 hours.

Available from local designated centres. For supplies outside working hours apply to Department of Health Duty Officer, telephone 071-210 5371

CHOLERA VACCINE

Cholera vaccine contains heat-killed Inaba and Ogawa sub-types of *Vibrio cholerae,* Serovar O1. Cholera vaccine provides little protection and cannot control the spread of the disease. The Department of Health has therefore advised that:

immunisation against cholera is no longer a legal requirement for entry into any foreign country and should not be required of any traveller. However, border officials in some countries may still ask people travelling from endemic or epidemic areas for evidence of immunisation. Travellers who are likely to cross borders from such areas, especially overland, should therefore be advised to have the vaccine here before travel rather than risk injections abroad. For this purpose one injection is sufficient.

Travellers to a country where cholera exists should be warned that attention to food and water and personal hygiene is **essential,** even after vaccination.

PoM **Cholera Vaccine** Cho/Vac. Net price 1.5-mL vial = £4.51

Dose: first dose, as specified on the label, usually 0.5 mL by deep subcutaneous or intramuscular injection; second dose, after at least a week and preferably 4 weeks, 1 mL; reinforcing dose every 6 months on continued exposure; CHILD 1–5 years 0.1 mL, second dose 0.3 mL, 5–10 years 0.3 mL, second dose 0.5 mL

Note. For purposes of **providing a certificate for travellers** the Department of Health has recommended that **one injection is sufficient,** see notes above. If it is required to give the full course, adverse reactions can be minimised by giving the second and subsequent doses intradermally in a volume of 0.2 mL (0.1 mL at two separate sites) if the subcutaneous dose is more than 0.5 mL, and 0.1 mL if the subcutaneous dose is 0.5 mL or less.

Available from Evans

DIPHTHERIA VACCINES

Protection against diphtheria is essentially due to antitoxin, the production of which is stimulated by vaccines prepared from the toxin of *Corynebacterium diphtheriae.* These are more effective and cause fewer reactions if adsorbed onto a mineral carrier. Adsorbed diphtheria vaccines are recommended for the routine immunisation of babies and given in the form of a triple vaccine, **adsorbed diphtheria, tetanus, and pertussis vaccine.** A dose of poliomyelitis vaccine, live (oral) is generally given at the same time as each of the doses of

the triple vaccine (see schedule, section 14.1). Adsorbed diphtheria and tetanus vaccine is used in place of the triple vaccine when immunisation against pertussis is contra-indicated.

A reinforcing dose of **adsorbed diphtheria and tetanus vaccine** is recommended at school entry (4–5 years of age). This should preferably be given after an interval of at least 3 years from the last dose of the basic course. A further reinforcing dose is now recommended at school leaving; for this purpose **adsorbed diphtheria and tetanus vaccine for adults and adolescents** (a special low-dose version combined in a single injection with tetanus vaccine) has been developed.

Other reinforcing doses of diphtheria vaccine are not recommended as a routine except in the case of those who work in units where there is a potentially high risk of infection such as those employed in infectious disease units or microbiology laboratories. A low-dose vaccine, **adsorbed diphtheria vaccine for adults,** is available for this purpose.

The Chief Medical Officer has issued a warning on diphtheria in the former USSR. *Previously immunised* travellers require a booster dose if they are to live or work with local residents and their primary immunisation was more than 10 years ago. *Unimmunised travellers* require a full course of 3 doses at monthly intervals (**important:** adults and children over 10 years requiring either a primary course or a booster should be given a **low-dose** vaccine—those also requiring tetanus cover can be given the special low-dose version combined with tetanus vaccine).

See section 14.1 for general contra-indications.

FOR CHILDREN

With tetanus and pertussis (triple vaccine)

PoM **Adsorbed Diphtheria, Tetanus, and Pertussis Vaccine** DTPer/Vac/Ads.   Prepared from diphtheria formol toxoid, tetanus formol toxoid, and pertussis vaccine adsorbed on a mineral carrier (aluminium hydroxide).

Dose: primary immunisation of children, 0.5 mL by intramuscular or deep subcutaneous injection at 2 months followed by second dose after 4 weeks and third dose after another 4 weeks (see schedule, section 14.1)

Available from District Health Authorities or (in England only) direct from Farillon as Trivax-AD® (Evans).

With tetanus

PoM **Adsorbed Diphtheria and Tetanus Vaccine** DT/Vac/Ads. Prepared from diphtheria formol toxoid and tetanus formol toxoid adsorbed on a mineral carrier (aluminium hydroxide).

Dose: primary immunisation of children omitting pertussis component, 0.5 mL by intramuscular or deep subcutaneous injection at 2 months followed by second dose after 4 weeks and third dose after another 4 weeks (see schedule, section 14.1); reinforcement at school entry, 0.5 mL (see schedule, section 14.1)

Available from District Health Authorities or (in England only) direct from Farillon

Single antigen
PoM **Adsorbed Diphtheria Vaccine.** Dip/Vac/

Ads. Prepared from diphtheria formol toxoid adsorbed on a mineral carrier (aluminium hydroxide). Net price 0.5-mL amp = £1.12
Note. Used only for contacts of a diphtheria case or carrier; immunised children under 10 years are given one dose of 0.5 mL by intramuscular or by deep subcutaneous injection, unimmunised children under 10 years are given three doses of 0.5 mL with an interval of 4 weeks between first and second doses and another 4 weeks between second and third; adults and children over 10 years must be given diphtheria vaccine for adults, adsorbed (see below).
Available from District Health Authorities or (in England only) direct from Farillon

FOR ADULTS AND ADOLESCENTS

The small quantity of diphtheria toxoid present in the preparations below is sufficient to recall immunity in individuals previously immunised against diphtheria but whose immunity may have diminished with time; it is insufficient to cause the serious reactions that may occur when diphtheria vaccine of conventional formulation is used in an individual who is already immune. The dilute vaccine must be used when immunising adults and children over 10 years; for school leavers a low-dose version combined in a single injection with tetanus vaccine is available (see notes above).

With tetanus
PoM **Adsorbed Diphtheria and Tetanus Vaccine for Adults and Adolescents,** DT/

Vac/Ads for Adults. Prepared from diphtheria formol toxoid and tetanus formol toxoid adsorbed on a mineral carrier (aluminium hydroxide).
Dose: primary immunisation in patients over 10 years, three doses each of 0.5 mL by intramuscular or deep subcutaneous injection separated by intervals of 4 weeks; reinforcement, 0.5 mL after 10 years
Available from District Health Authorities or (in England only) direct from Farillon as Diftavax® (Merieux)

Single antigen
PoM **Adsorbed Diphtheria Vaccine for Adults.** Dip/Vac/Ads for Adults. Net price 0.5-mL

amp = £3.80
Dose: primary immunisation in patients over 10 years, three doses each of 0.5 mL by intramuscular or deep subcutaneous injection separated by intervals of 1 month; reinforcement, 0.5 mL
Note. Unimmunised adults and children over 10 years who are contacts of a diphtheria case or carrier are given the primary immunisation course; immunised adults and children over 10 years are given the reinforcement dose.
Available from distributor (Regent)

PASSIVE IMMUNISATION

Diphtheria antitoxin is used for passive immunisation; it is prepared in horses therefore reactions are common after administration.
It is now only used in suspected cases of diphtheria (without waiting for bacteriological confirmation); tests for hypersensitivity should be first carried out.
It is no longer used for prophylaxis because of the risk of hypersensitivity; unimmunised contacts should be promptly investigated and given erythromycin prophylaxis (see section 5.1, table 2) and vaccine (see notes above).

PoM **Diphtheria Antitoxin** Dip/Ser.

Dose: prophylactic 500 to 2000 units by intramuscular injection (but **not** used, see notes above); therapeutic 10 000 to 30 000 units increased to 40 000 to 100 000 units in severe cases; doses of up to 30 000 units should be given intramuscularly but for those over 40 000 units a portion is given intramuscularly followed by the bulk of the dose intravenously after an interval of ½–2 hours
Note. Children require the same dose as adults, depending on the severity of the case.
Available from Merieux on a named patient basis or stocks may be held by hospital pharmacies

HAEMOPHILUS INFLUENZAE TYPE B VACCINE

Haemophilus influenzae type b vaccine (Hib) is given in a course of 3 doses at monthly intervals usually at the same time as routine childhood immunisation against diphtheria, tetanus, pertussis and poliomyelitis (see schedule, section 14.1) in infants from 2 months of age. Children under 13 months of age who have already commenced or completed their primary routine immunisation should still receive 3 doses of Hib vaccine at monthly intervals. Children between 13 months and 4 years of age are at lower risk of infection, and the vaccine is effective after a single dose. The risk of infection falls sharply after the age of 4 years therefore the vaccine is not recommended for adults and children over 4 years except for those with immunodeficiency such as splenectomy.
See section 14.1 for general contra-indications

▼ PoM **Haemophilus influenzae type b**

(Hib)
Capsular conjugated polysaccharide vaccine
Dose: 0.5 mL by intramuscular or deep subcutaneous injection in a different limb from other concurrently administered vaccines; for primary immunisation 3 doses are required at intervals of 1 month (see schedule, section 14.1)
Available from District Health Authorities or (in England only) direct from Farillon—Merieux (Act-HIB®) brand; Lederle (HibTITER®) brand may be supplied in Wales. Each company's vaccine is prepared by conjugation to a different type of protein therefore the different brands are not interchangeable. If it is necessary to change brands during a primary immunisation course the entire course should be repeated

HEPATITIS A VACCINE

Hepatitis A vaccine is a formaldehyde inactivated hepatitis A virus (HAV) vaccine prepared from HM 175 strain grown in human diploid cells. The vaccine is an alternative to human normal immunoglobulin for frequent travellers to moderate to high risk areas or those who stay for more than 3 months.
Protection against hepatitis A should be considered for those travelling to destinations outside Northern and Western Europe, North America, Australia and New Zealand. A single-dose vaccine (Havrix Monodose®) is now available. Travellers to high-risk areas who require immunisation less than

two weeks before departure may be given the single-dose vaccine plus normal immunoglobulin at a different injection site. Administration of human normal immunoglobulin at the same time as the vaccine, at different injection sites, does not affect rate of seroconversion but the level of antibody may be reduced. In the UK some occupational groups such as sewage workers may be at risk from infection.

Side-effects, usually mild, include transient soreness, erythema, and induration at the injection site. Less common effects include fever, malaise, fatigue, headache, nausea, and loss of appetite.

See section 14.1 for general contra-indications

▼ **PoM Havrix®** (SmithKline Beecham)
A suspension of formaldehyde-inactivated hepatitis A virus (HM 175 grown in human diploid cells) 720 ELISA units/mL adsorbed onto aluminium hydroxide. Net price 1-mL pre-filled syringe = £13.60; 0.5 mL paediatric prefilled syringe (Havrix Junior®) = £9.83
Dose: by intramuscular injection (see note below), 2 doses of 1 mL, the second 2–4 weeks after the first dose; booster dose, 1 mL 6–12 months following the initial dose. CHILD 1–15 years, 0.5 mL
Note. The deltoid region is the preferred site of injection in adults. The subcutaneous route may be used for patients with haemophilia

▼ **PoM Havrix Monodose®** (SmithKline Beecham)
A suspension of formaldehyde-inactivated hepatitis A virus (HM 175 grown in human diploid cells) 1440 ELISA units/mL adsorbed onto aluminium hydroxide. Net price 1-mL prefilled syringe = £21.60
Dose: by intramuscular injection (see note below), 1 mL as a single dose; booster dose, 1 mL 6–12 months following the initial dose; CHILD under 15 years, use Havrix Junior®
Note. Patients who have already started a course of Havrix® (720 ELISA units/mL) vaccine (above) should continue to receive it, both to complete the primary course and booster. The deltoid region is the preferred site of injection in adults. The subcutaneous route may be used for patients with haemophilia

HEPATITIS B VACCINE

Hepatitis B vaccine contains inactivated hepatitis B virus surface antigen (HBsAg) adsorbed on aluminium hydroxide adjuvant. It is made biosynthetically using recombinant DNA technology. The vaccine is used in individuals at high risk of contracting hepatitis B.

In the UK, high-risk groups include:
  parenteral drug abusers;
  individuals who frequently change sexual partners;
  close family contacts of a case or carrier;
  Infants born to mothers who have had acute hepatitis B during pregnancy or who are hepatitis B carriers. Active immunisation is started immediately after delivery; if the hepatitis B occurred during pregnancy or the mother is a carrier who is e antigen positive or without anti-e antibody, *hepatitis B immunoglobulin* (see p.482) is given at the same time as the vaccine;
  haemophiliacs, those receiving regular blood transfusions or blood products, and relatives responsible for the administration of such products;

  patients with chronic renal failure;
  health care personnel who have direct contact with blood or blood-stained body fluids or with patients' tissues;
  trainee health care workers;
  other occupational risk groups such as morticians and embalmers;
  staff and clients of residential accommodation for the mentally handicapped;
  inmates of custodial institutions, who will be in custody for at least 6 months and those in custody for shorter periods who belong to other risk groups;
  those travelling to areas of high prevalence who intend to seek employment as health care workers or who plan to remain there for lengthy periods and who may therefore be at increased risk of acquiring infection as the result of medical or dental procedures carried out in those countries.

Short-term tourists or business travellers are not generally at increased risk of infection but may place themselves at risk by their sexual behaviour when abroad.

It should be borne in mind that immunisation takes up to 6 months to confer adequate protection; the duration of immunity is thought to last for 3 to 5 years.

More detailed guidance is given in the memorandum *Immunisation against Infectious Disease 1994*. Immunisation does not eliminate the need for commonsense precautions for avoiding the risk of infection from known carriers by the routes of infection which have been clearly established, see *Guidance for Clinical Health Care Workers: Protection against Infection with HIV and Hepatitis Viruses* and *Protecting Health Care Workers* and *Patients from Hepatitis B*. Accidental inoculation of hepatitis B virus-infected blood into a wound, incision, needle-prick, or abrasion may lead to infection, whereas it is unlikely that indirect exposure to a carrier will do so.

Specific **hepatitis B immunoglobulin** ('HBIG') is available for use with the vaccine in those accidentally infected and in infants (section 14.5).

See section 14.1 for general contra-indications.

PoM Engerix B® (SmithKline Beecham)
A suspension of hepatitis B surface antigen (rby, prepared from yeast cells by recombinant DNA technique) 20 micrograms/mL adsorbed onto aluminium hydroxide. Net price 0.5 mL (paediatric) vial = £8.66; 1-mL vial = £11.55; 1-mL prefilled syringe = £12.13
Dose: by intramuscular injection (see note below), 3 doses of 1 mL (20 micrograms), the second 1 month and the third 6 months after the first dose; more rapid (e.g. for travellers), third dose 2 months after first dose with booster at 12 months; CHILD birth to 12 years 3 doses of 0.5 mL (10 micrograms); INFANTS born to HBsAg-positive mothers, 3 doses of 0.5 mL (10 micrograms), first dose at birth with hepatitis B immunoglobulin injection (separate site)
Note. The deltoid muscle is the preferred site of injection in adults; the anterolateral thigh is the preferred site in infants and children; the buttock must not be used because vaccine efficacy may be reduced. The subcutaneous route is used for patients with haemophilia.

▼ PoM **H-B-Vax® II** (MSD)

A suspension of hepatitis B surface antigen (prepared from yeast cells by recombinant DNA technique) 10 micrograms/mL adsorbed onto aluminium hydroxide. Net price 1-mL vial = £11.95

Dose: by intramuscular injection (see note below) 3 doses of 1 mL (10 micrograms), the second 1 month and the third 6 months after the first dose; CHILD birth to 10 years 3 doses of 0.5 mL (5 micrograms); INFANTS born to HBsAg-positive mothers, 3 doses of 0.5 mL (5 micrograms), first dose at birth with hepatitis B immunoglobulin injection (separate site)

Note. The deltoid muscle is preferred site of injection in adults; the anterolateral thigh is the preferred site in infants and children; the buttock must not be used because vaccine efficacy may be reduced. The subcutaneous route is used for patients with haemophilia.

INFLUENZA VACCINES

While most viruses are antigenically stable, the influenza viruses A and B (especially A) are constantly altering their antigenic structure as indicated by changes in the haemagglutinins (H) and neuraminidases (N) on the surface of the viruses. It is essential that influenza vaccines in use contain the H and N components of the prevalent strain or strains. Every year the World Health Organization recommends which strains should be included.

The recommended strains are grown in the allantoic cavity of chick embryos (therefore **contraindicated** in those hypersensitive to eggs).

Since **influenza vaccines** will not control epidemics they are recommended *only for persons at high risk.* Immunisation is strongly recommended for those of all ages, especially the elderly, with the following conditions:

chronic respiratory disease, including asthma;
chronic heart disease;
chronic renal failure;
diabetes mellitus, and other endocrine disorders;
immunosuppression due to disease or treatment.

Influenza vaccination is also recommended for residents of nursing homes, old peoples homes, and other long-stay facilities.

In non-pandemic years immunisation is not recommended for Health Service staff, except for those at high risk (owing to medical disorders).

Interactions: Appendix 1 (influenza vaccine).

See section 14.1 for general contra-indications.

PoM **Inactivated influenza Vaccine (Split Virion)** (Merieux)

Inactivated influenza vaccine (split virion vaccine). Net price 0.5-mL disposable syringe = £5.10

Dose: 0.5 mL by deep subcutaneous or intramuscular injection; CHILD 6–35 months, 0.25 mL repeated once after 4–6 weeks; 3–12 years, 0.5 mL repeated once after 4–6 weeks

PoM **Fluarix®** (SmithKline Beecham)

Inactivated influenza vaccine (split virion vaccine). Net price 0.5-mL disposable syringe = £5.18

Dose: 0.5 mL by deep subcutaneous or intramuscular injection; CHILD 6 months to 6 years, 0.25 mL repeated once after 4-6 weeks; 0.25 mL as a single dose if previously vaccinated

PoM **Fluvirin®** (Evans)

Inactivated influenza vaccine, surface antigen. Net price 0.5-mL disposable syringe = £5.09

Dose: 0.5 mL by deep subcutaneous or intramuscular injection; CHILD 4–13 years, 0.5 mL repeated once after 4–6 weeks

PoM **Fluzone®** (Servier)

Inactivated influenza vaccine (split virion vaccine). Net price 0.5-mL disposable syringe = £5.18

Dose: 0.5 mL by deep subcutaneous or intramuscular injection; CHILD 6 months to 3 years, 0.25 mL repeated once after 4–6 weeks; 4–13 years, 0.5 mL repeated once after 4–6 weeks

PoM **Influvac Sub-unit®** (Duphar)

Inactivated influenza vaccine, surface antigen. Net price 0.5-mL disposable syringe = £5.08

Dose: 0.5 mL by deep subcutaneous or intramuscular injection; CHILD 4–13 years, 0.5 mL repeated once after 4–6 weeks

MEASLES VACCINE

Measles vaccine has been replaced by a combined measles/mumps/rubella vaccine (MMR vaccine) for all eligible children.

Administration of a measles-containing vaccine to children may be associated with a mild measles-like syndrome with a measles-like rash and pyrexia about a week after injection. Much less commonly, convulsions and, very rarely, encephalitis have been reported. Convulsions in infants are much less frequently associated with measles vaccines than with other conditions leading to febrile episodes.

MMR vaccine may be used in the control of outbreaks of measles (see under MMR vaccine, below).

Single antigen vaccine
  Available from Evans and Merieux on a named patient basis

Combined vaccines, see under MMR and MR vaccines

MMR VACCINE

A combined **measles/mumps/rubella vaccine** (MMR vaccine) has been introduced with the aim of eliminating rubella (and congenital rubella syndrome), measles, and mumps. Health authorities have an obligation to ensure that every child has received MMR vaccine by entry to primary school, unless there is a valid contra-indication, parental refusal, or laboratory evidence of previous infection. Immunisation records should be checked; where there is no record of MMR immunisation or where the child has received single-antigen measles vaccine, parents should be advised that their children should receive MMR.

MMR vaccine has replaced measles vaccine for children of both sexes aged 12 to 15 months (or after this age if appointments have been missed).

MMR vaccine should be given to children of both sexes aged 4 to 5 years before starting primary school (irrespective of previous measles vaccine or of a history of measles, mumps, or rubella) unless there is:

a documented history of MMR vaccination;
a valid contra-indication (see below);
laboratory evidence of immunity to measles, mumps, and rubella.

MMR vaccine may also be used in the control of outbreaks of measles and should be offered to susceptible children within 3 days of exposure to infection (**important:** MMR vaccine is not suitable for prophylaxis following exposure to mumps or rubella since the antibody response to the mumps and rubella components is too slow for effective prophylaxis).

Children with partially or totally impaired immune responsiveness should not receive live vaccines (for advice on AIDS see section 14.1). If they have been exposed to measles infection they should be given immunoglobulin (section 14.5).

As with measles vaccine, malaise, fever and/or a rash may occur with MMR vaccine, most commonly about a week after immunisation and lasting about 2 to 3 days. Parents should be given written information and advice for reducing fever (including the use of paracetamol). Parotid swelling occasionally occurs, usually in the third week. Postvaccination meningoencephalitis was reported (rarely and with complete recovery) following immunisation with MMR vaccine containing Urabe mumps vaccine, which has now been discontinued; the rate using Jeryl Lynn mumps vaccine is very much lower. Children with post-vaccination symptoms are not infectious.

Contra-indications to MMR include:

children with untreated malignant disease or altered immunity, and those receiving immunosuppressive drugs or radiotherapy, or high-dose corticosteroids;
children who have received another live vaccine by injection within 3 weeks;
children with allergies to neomycin or kanamycin, or a history of anaphylaxis due to any cause;
children with acute febrile illness (vaccination should be deferred);
if given to adult women, pregnancy should be avoided for 1 month (as for rubella vaccine);
should not be given within 3 months of an immunoglobulin injection.

It should be noted that:

children with a personal or close family history of convulsions should be given MMR vaccine, provided the parents understand that there may be a febrile response;
immunoglobulin must not be given with MMR vaccine since the immune response to rubella and mumps may be inhibited; doctors should seek specialist paediatric advice rather than refuse vaccination;
allergy to egg is only a contra-indication if the child has had an anaphylactic reaction to food containing egg (dislike of egg or refusal to eat is not a contra-indication).

PoM MMR Vaccine

Live, measles, mumps, and rubella vaccine

Dose: 0.5 mL by deep subcutaneous or by intramuscular injection

Available from District Health Authorities or (in England only) direct from Farillon as MMR II® (MSD)

MR VACCINE

The Joint Committee on Vaccination and Immunisation has recommended that all school children in school forms aged 5 up to 16 years should be immunised in a school-based campaign. The vaccine recommended is measles/rubella (MR) vaccine. During November 1994, school based immunisation programmes will be set up to provide the highest possible levels of coverage with MR vaccine. All children will be invited for immunisation, irrespective of history of measles, rubella disease, previous measles or rubella immunisation, or previous MMR immunisation. For those that are already immune, re-immunisation will provide a booster; for those that are still susceptible, it will provide protection. The provision of rubella vaccine in this campaign will allow the discontinuation of the present school rubella immunisation programme. Therefore, from September 1994, single antigen rubella vaccine need no longer be given to girls at around 11 years of age.

PoM MR Vaccine

Live, measles and rubella vaccine

Dose: 0.5 mL by deep subcutaneous or by intramuscular injection

Available from Farillon (to District Health Authorities only) as Merieux brand or SmithKline Beecham (Eolarix®) brand

MENINGOCOCCAL POLYSACCHARIDE VACCINE

Meningococcal polysaccharide vaccine is indicated for areas of the world where the risk of acquiring meningococcal infection is much higher than in the UK, particularly for travellers proposing to travel 'rough'.

These areas include New Delhi, Nepal, Mecca (see below), and the meningitis belt of Africa, which encompasses southern sub-Saharan parts of Senegal, Mali, Niger, Chad, and Sudan; all of Gambia, Guinea, Togo, and Benin; South-west Ethiopia; northern parts of Sierra Leone, Liberia, Ivory Coast, Nigeria, Cameroon, Central African Republic, Uganda, and Kenya.

Saudi Arabia requires vaccination of pilgrims to Mecca during the Haj annual pilgrimage; this may apply to others visiting Saudi Arabia in the months leading up to August.

For advice on the immunisation of *close contacts* of disease cases of Group A and Group C meningococcal meningitis in the UK and on the role of the vaccine in the control of *local outbreaks*, see the memorandum *Immunisation against Infectious Disease, 1994.*

PoM AC Vax® (SmithKline Beecham)

Meningococcal polysaccharide vaccine prepared from *Neisseria meningitidis* (meningococcus) groups A and C. Net price single-dose vial (with diluent) = £6.86

Dose: ADULT and CHILD aged 2 months and over, 0.5 mL by deep subcutaneous or intramuscular injection

PoM **Mengivac (A+C)®** (Merieux)

Meningococcal polysaccharide vaccine prepared from *Neisseria meningitidis* (meningococcus) groups A and C. Net price single-dose vial (with syringe containing diluent) = £6.69

Dose: ADULT and CHILD aged over 18 months, 0.5 mL by deep subcutaneous or intramuscular injection

Note. The lower age range for AC Vax® and Mengivac (A+C)® differ; in the case of Mengivac (A+C)® the data sheet states that young children and infants respond less well to the vaccine than older children and adults, with little response to the Group C polysaccharide under 18 months of age and a poor response to Group A polysaccharide under 3 months of age. Additionally, protection in infants under 18 months of age is of shorter duration

MUMPS VACCINE

Mumps vaccine consists of a live attenuated strain of virus grown in chick-embryo tissue culture.

See under MMR vaccine and section 14.1 for contra-indications.

PoM **Mumpsvax®** (Morson)

Mumps vaccine (Jeryl Lynn strain). Net price single-dose vial (with diluent) = £4.00

Dose: ADULT and CHILD over 1 year, 0.5 mL by subcutaneous injection

Combined vaccines
With measles and rubella
See MMR Vaccine

PERTUSSIS VACCINE
(Whooping-cough vaccine)

Pertussis vaccine is usually given combined with diphtheria and tetanus vaccine (in triple vaccine) starting at 2 months of age (see section 14.1).

With some vaccines available in the early 1960s persistent screaming and collapse were reported but these reactions are rarely observed with the vaccines now available.

Convulsions and encephalopathy have been reported as rare complications, but such conditions may arise from other causes and be falsely attributed to the vaccine. Neurological complications after whooping cough itself are considerably more common than after the vaccine.

As with any other elective immunisation procedure it is advisable to postpone vaccination if the child is suffering from any acute illness, until fully recovered. Minor infections without fever or systemic upset are not reasons to delay immunisation. Immunisation should not be carried out in children who have a history of severe local or general reaction to a preceding dose; the following reactions should be regarded as severe:

Local—an extensive area of redness and swelling which becomes indurated and involves most of the antero-lateral surface of the thigh or a major part of the circumference of the upper arm.

General—fever equal to or more than 39.5°C within 48 hours of vaccine, anaphylaxis, bronchospasm, laryngeal oedema, generalised collapse, prolonged unresponsiveness, prolonged inconsolable screaming, and convulsions occurring within 72 hours.

A personal or family history of allergy is **not** a contra-indication to immunisation against whooping cough; nor are stable neurological conditions such as cerebral palsy or spina bifida.

Children with problem histories. When there is a personal or family history of *febrile* convulsions, there is an increased risk of these occurring after pertussis immunisation. In such children, immunisation is *recommended* but advice on the *prevention of fever* (see p.469) should be given at the time of immunisation.

In a recent British study, children with a family history of epilepsy were immunised with pertussis vaccine without any significant adverse events. These childrens' developmental progress has been normal. In children with a close family history (first degree relatives) of *idiopathic epilepsy*, there may be a risk of developing a similar condition, irrespective of vaccine. Immunisation is *recommended* for these children.

Where there is a *still evolving neurological problem*, immunisation should be *deferred* until the condition is stable. When there has been a documented history of *cerebral damage in the neonatal period*, immunisation should be *carried out unless there is evidence of an evolving neurological abnormality.* If immunisation is to be deferred, this should be stated on the neonatal discharge summary. Where there is doubt, appropriate advice should be sought from a consultant paediatrician, district immunisation co-ordinator or consultant in public health medicine *rather than withholding vaccine.*

▼ PoM **Acellular Pertussis Vaccine, AVP** (Lederle)

Unlicensed single-antigen acellular pertussis vaccine (APV) has been made available by the Department of Health under Crown Immunity only for completion of immunisation against pertussis in those children whose course of pertussis vaccine was not given (or not completed) as part of their triple vaccine course

Dose: 0.5 mL by intramuscular or deep subcutaneous injection, 3 doses at intervals of 1 month

Available from Farillon on a named-patient basis

Note. Should be ordered only when required for use

Combined vaccine (*pertussis, tetanus*, and *diphtheria*), see under Diphtheria vaccines

PNEUMOCOCCAL VACCINE

A polyvalent pneumococcal vaccine is available for the immunisation of persons (over the age of 2 years) for whom the risk of contracting pneumococcal pneumonia is unusually high or dangerous. For example in patients with:

Homozygous sickle cell disease;
Asplenia or severe dysfunction of the spleen;
Chronic renal disease or nephrotic syndrome;
Immunodeficiency or immunosuppression due to disease or treatment, including HIV infection;
Chronic heart disease;
Chronic lung disease;
Chronic liver disease including cirrhosis;
Diabetes mellitus.

Where possible, the vaccine should be given at least two weeks before splenectomy (together with advice about increased risk of pneumococcal infec-

---

tion) and before chemotherapy. Prophylactic antibiotic therapy against pneumococcal infection should not be stopped after immunisation. The vaccine is effective in a single dose if the types of pneumonia in the community are reflected in the polysaccharides contained in the vaccine. It should not be given in pregnancy, or when breast-feeding, or when there is infection. Hypersensitivity reactions may occur.

REVACCINATION. Routine revaccination of adults is not recommended owing to the possibility of an increased incidence of adverse reactions; nor should those who have previously received the 14-valent vaccine (Pneumovax®) be routinely revaccinated with the 23-valent vaccine (Pneumovax®II). Revaccination is however recommended for *adults with chronic conditions which increase the risk of fatal pneumococcal infection* (and who did not have a serious or severe reaction to the previous vaccination) and those shown to have *a rapid decline in pneumococcal antibody levels* (e.g. those with nephrotic syndrome, renal failure or who are transplant recipients); the revaccination is recommended 4 or more years after the 14-valent vaccine (Pneumovax®) and 6 or more years after the 23-valent vaccine (Pneumovax®II).

Revaccination after 3–5 years (not sooner) should be considered for children at highest risk of pneumococcal infection (e.g. with asplenia, sickle-cell disease, or nephrotic syndrome) who would be 10 years or less at revaccination.

IMPORTANT. Not for intradermal injection which may cause severe local reactions
See section 14.1 for general contra-indications.

PoM **Pneumovax® II** (Morson)
Polysaccharide from each of 23 capsular types of pneumococcus. Net price 0.5-mL vial = £9.94
Dose: 0.5 mL by subcutaneous or intramuscular injection; CHILD under 2 years, not recommended (suboptimal response and also safety and efficacy not established)

POLIOMYELITIS VACCINES
There are two types of poliomyelitis vaccine, poliomyelitis vaccine, live (oral) (Sabin) and poliomyelitis vaccine, inactivated (Salk). The oral vaccine, consisting of a mixture of attenuated strains of virus types 1, 2, and 3 is at present generally used in the UK.

INITIAL COURSE. **Poliomyelitis vaccine, live (oral)** is given on 3 occasions, usually at the same time as routine immunisation against diphtheria, tetanus, pertussis, and haemophilus influenzae b (see schedule, section 14.1). The initial course of 3 doses should also be given to all unimmunised adults.

REINFORCEMENT. A reinforcing dose of oral poliomyelitis vaccine is recommended at school entry at which time children should also receive a reinforcing dose of diphtheria and tetanus vaccine, and a dose of MMR vaccine if this has not already been given. Oral poliomyelitis vaccine is also recommended at school leaving.

Vaccine-associated poliomyelitis and poliomyelitis in contacts of vaccinees are both rare. In England and Wales there is an annual average of 1

recipient and 1 contact case in relation to over 2 million doses of oral vaccine. The need for strict personal hygiene must be stressed; the contacts of a recently vaccinated baby should be advised of the necessity for personal hygiene, particularly of the need to wash their hands after changing the baby's napkins.

Contra-indications to the use of oral poliomyelitis vaccine include vomiting and diarrhoea, and immunodeficiency disorders (or household contacts of patients with immunodeficiency disorders). See section 14.1 for further contra-indications.

Poliomyelitis vaccine (inactivated) may be used for those in whom poliomyelitis vaccine (oral) is contra-indicated because of immunosuppressive disorders (for advice on AIDS see section 14.1).

TRAVELLERS. Travellers to areas other than Australia, New Zealand, Northern and Western Europe, and North America should be given a full course of oral poliomyelitis vaccine if they have not been immunised in the past. Those who have not received immunisation within the last 10 years should be given a booster dose of oral poliomyelitis vaccine.

Live (oral) (Sabin)
PoM **Poliomyelitis Vaccine, Live (Oral)** Pol/
Vac (Oral)[1]. A suspension of suitable live attenuated strains of poliomyelitis virus, types 1, 2, and 3. Available in single-dose and 10-dose containers
Dose: 3 drops from a multidose container or the total contents of a single-dose container; for primary immunisation 3 doses are required (see schedule, section 14.1)
Available from District Health Authorities or (in England only) direct from Farillon
1. BP permits code OPV for vaccine in single doses provided it also appears on pack.
Note. Poliomyelitis vaccine loses potency once the container has been opened, therefore any vaccine remaining at the end of an immunisation session should be discarded; whenever possible sessions should be arranged to avoid undue wastage.

Inactivated (Salk)
PoM **Poliomyelitis Vaccine, Inactivated** Pol/
Vac (Inact). An inactivated suspension of suitable strains of poliomyelitis virus, types 1, 2, and 3.
Dose: 0.5 mL or as stated on the label by deep subcutaneous or intramuscular injection; for primary immunisation 3 doses are required (see schedule, section 14.1)
Available (in England only) direct from Farillon *and* from Scottish Common Services Agency, telephone 031-552 6255, extn 2283 *and* Welsh Health Common Services Authority, telephone 0222 471234 *and* Central Services Agency, Belfast, telephone 0232 324431
Note. Should be ordered one dose at a time (on a named patient basis) and only when required for use

RABIES VACCINE
A human diploid cell **rabies vaccine** is now in use. It should be offered prophylactically to those at high risk—those working in quarantine stations, animal handlers, veterinary surgeons, and field workers who may be exposed to bites of possibly infected wild animals.

The Department of Health has advised that for *prophylactic use* the vaccine produces a good antibody response when given in a 3-dose schedule on days 0, 7, and 28, with a reinforcing dose every 2–3 years to those at continued risk.

For *post-exposure treatment of previously immunised patients* two reinforcing doses are needed (one on day 0 and one on day 3–7). Rabies immunoglobulin is not needed for those who have been fully immunised.

For *post-exposure treatment of previously unimmunised patients* (or those whose prophylaxis is possibly inadequate) a course of injections should be started as soon as possible after exposure (days 0, 3, 7, 14, 30, and 90). The course may be discontinued if it is proved that the patient was not at risk. There are no specific contra-indications to this diploid cell vaccine and its use should be considered whenever a patient has been attacked by an animal in a country where rabies is endemic, even if there is no direct evidence of rabies in the attacking animal. **Rabies immunoglobulin** (section 14.5) should also be considered on day 0.

Staff in attendance on a patient who is highly suspected of, or known to be suffering from, rabies should be offered immunisation. Four intradermal doses of 0.1 mL of human diploid cell vaccine (Merieux) given on the same day at different sites (ensuring correct intradermal technique) has been suggested for this purpose [unlicensed route].

Advice on post-exposure immunisation and treatment of rabies is available from the Virus Reference Laboratory, Central Public Health Laboratory, Colindale, London NW9 5HT, tel 081-200 4400.

PoM **Rabies Vaccine BP Pasteur Merieux**
(Merieux)

Freeze-dried inactivated Wistar rabies virus strain PM/WI 38 1503-3M cultivated in human diploid cells. Single-dose vial with syringe containing diluent

IMPORTANT. Studies have shown that when this vaccine is injected into the gluteal region there is a poor response. Concomitant administration of chloroquine may also affect the antibody response. Because of the potential consequences of inadequately treated rabies exposure and because there is no indication that fetal abnormalities have been associated with rabies vaccination, pregnancy is **not** considered a contra-indication to post-exposure prophylaxis. If there is substantial risk of exposure to rabies, pre-exposure prophylaxis may also be indicated during pregnancy

Dose: prophylactic, 1 mL by deep subcutaneous or intramuscular injection in the deltoid region, on days 0, 7, and 28; also further reinforcing doses every 2–3 years to those at continued risk

Note. This replaces the previous schedule which involved giving a second dose after 1 month and a third after 6–12 months. If this full course was not given it is still probable that in most cases 2 doses conferred protection provided they were given *1 month apart*. Subjects who have received 2 injections 1 month apart and also remain at continued risk should receive a reinforcing dose 6–12 months later, followed by further reinforcing doses at intervals of 2–3 years

Post-exposure, see notes above

Staff in attendance, see notes above

Also available from local designated centres (special workers and post-exposure treatment)

RUBELLA VACCINE
The selective policy of protecting women of childbearing age from the risks of rubella (German measles) in pregnancy has been extended to a policy of eliminating the circulation of rubella among young children. The existing rubella immunisation policy is therefore being reinforced by the mass immunisation of children of both sexes, using combined measles, mumps, and rubella vaccine (MMR vaccine).

Rubella vaccine is recommended for *prepubertal girls between their tenth and fourteenth birthdays* (unless there is documented evidence that they have received MMR) [**Important:** but see also MR vaccine, p.475] and for *seronegative women of child-bearing age* (see schedule, section 14.1) as well as those who might put pregnant women at risk of infection (e.g. nurses and doctors in obstetric units).

Rubella vaccine may conveniently be offered to previously *unimmunised and seronegative post-partum women.* Immunising susceptible post-partum women a few days after delivery is important as far as the overall reduction of congenital abnormalities in the UK is concerned, for about 60% of these abnormalities occur in the babies of multiparous women.

PREGNANCY. Rubella immunisation should be avoided in early pregnancy, and women of child-bearing age should be advised not to become pregnant within 1 month of immunisation. However, despite active surveillance in the UK, the USA, and Germany, no case of congenital rubella syndrome has been reported following inadvertent immunisation shortly before or during pregnancy. There is thus no evidence that the vaccine is teratogenic, and termination of pregnancy following inadvertent immunisation should not be routinely recommended; potential parents should be given this information before making a decision about termination.

Susceptible pregnant women who are exposed to rubella and who do not want therapeutic abortion may be offered normal immunoglobulin injection (section 14.5).

See section 14.1 for general contra-indications.

PoM **Rubella Vaccine, Live** Rub/Vac (Live).

Prepared from Wistar RA 27/3 strain propagated in human diploid cells

Dose: 0.5 mL by deep subcutaneous or by intramuscular injection (see schedule, section 14.1 and notes above)

Available from District Health Authorities or (in England only) direct from Farillon as *Almevax®* (Evans), *Ervevax®* (SmithKline Beecham), *Rubavax®* (Merieux)

Combined vaccines, see under MMR and MR vaccines

SMALLPOX VACCINE
Smallpox vaccination is no longer required routinely in the UK and other countries because global eradication of smallpox has now been achieved. Workers in laboratories where pox viruses (such as vaccinia) are handled, and others whose work involves an identifiable risk of exposure to pox virus, should be advised of the possible risk and

vaccination should be considered. Detailed guidance for laboratory staff has been prepared by the Advisory Committee on Dangerous Pathogens and the Advisory Committee on Genetic Manipulation. There is no requirement for smallpox vaccination of travellers.

PoM **Smallpox Vaccine** Var/Vac. Consists of a suspension of live vaccinia virus grown in the skin of living animals, supplied in freeze-dried form with diluent

Advice on the need for vaccination and on contra-indications should be obtained from the Virus Reference Laboratory, Central Public Health Laboratory, Colindale (081-200 4400) who will also supply the vaccine on a named-patient basis (free of charge)

TETANUS VACCINES

(Tetanus toxoids)

Tetanus vaccines stimulate the production of the protective antitoxin. In general, adsorption on aluminium hydroxide, aluminium phosphate, or calcium phosphate improves antigenicity. Adsorbed tetanus vaccine is offered routinely to babies in combination with adsorbed diphtheria vaccine (DT/ Vac/Ads) and more usually also combined with killed *Bordetella pertussis* organisms as a triple vaccine, adsorbed diphtheria, tetanus, and pertussis vaccine (DT Per/Vac/Ads), see schedule, section 14.1.

Of the single antigen tetanus vaccines adsorbed tetanus vaccine is again preferred to the plain vaccine. Adsorbed vaccine must not be given intradermally.

In children, the triple vaccine not only gives protection against tetanus in childhood but also gives the basic immunity for subsequent reinforcing doses of tetanus vaccine at school entry and at school leaving (combined with low-dose adsorbed diphtheria vaccine) and also when a potentially tetanus-contaminated injury has been received. Normally, tetanus vaccine should not be given unless more than 10 years have elapsed since the last reinforcing dose because of the possibility that hypersensitivity reactions may develop.

Active immunisation is important for persons in older age groups who may never have had a routine or complete course of immunisation when younger. In these persons a course of adsorbed tetanus vaccine may be given. Very rarely, tetanus has developed after abdominal surgery; patients awaiting elective surgery should be asked about tetanus immunisation and immunised if necessary.

See section 14.1 for general contra-indications.

For serious, potentially contaminated wounds tetanus immunoglobulin injection (section 14.5) should be selectively used in addition to wound toilet, adsorbed tetanus vaccine, and benzylpenicillin or another appropriate antibiotic.

Single antigen vaccines
The BP directs that when Tetanus Vaccine is prescribed or demanded and the form is not stated, Adsorbed Tetanus Vaccine may be dispensed or supplied.

PoM **Adsorbed Tetanus Vaccine** Tet/Vac/Ads.
Prepared from tetanus formol toxoid with a mineral carrier (aluminium hydroxide).
Dose: 0.5 mL or as stated on the label, by intramuscular or deep subcutaneous injection followed after 4 weeks by a second dose and after a further 4 weeks by a third
Note. This dose reflects the guidelines of the Joint Committee on Vaccination and Immunisation, see *Immunisation against Infectious Disease* 1994
Available from Evans (net price 0.5-mL amp = 71p, and as **Clostet®**, net price 0.5-mL single-dose syringe = £1.40), Merieux (net price 0.5-mL amp = 55p; 0.5-mL single-dose syringe = £1.20; 5-mL vial = £2.80), and from Servier (net price 0.5-mL amp = 62p; 0.5-mL syringe = £1.36)
PoM **Tetanus Vaccine** Tet/Vac/FT. Tetanus formol toxoid
Dose: as for Adsorbed Tetanus Vaccine which is preferred (see notes above)
Available from Evans (net price 0.5-mL amp = 71p)

Combined vaccines, see Diphtheria Vaccines

TYPHOID VACCINES

There are now three types of typhoid vaccine available, two given by injection and a third given by mouth. **None** of these typhoid vaccines is a substitute for personal hygiene (see section 14.6).

The original **typhoid vaccine, a whole cell** vaccine is normally given in 2 doses at intervals of 4–6 weeks for primary immunisation, with reinforcing doses about every 3 years on continued exposure. Local reactions to this vaccine, which consist of swelling, pain, and tenderness appear about 2–3 hours after *intramuscular or deep subcutaneous injection*. Systemic reactions, which consist of fever, malaise, and headache, may also occur and usually last for about 36 hours after injection. If severe reactions are experienced after the first dose *intradermal injection* may be preferred for the second dose and for subsequent boosters, as these reactions are virtually absent when the intradermal route is used.

A capsular **polysaccharide typhoid vaccine** is now available for single dose administration by *intramuscular or deep subcutaneous injection* with a reinforcing dose every 3 years on continued exposure. Local reactions, including pain, swelling or erythema, may appear 48–72 hours after administration.

An **oral typhoid vaccine** is now also available. It is a **live attenuated** vaccine contained in an enteric-coated capsule. It is taken *by mouth* as three doses of one capsule on alternate days, providing protection 7–10 days after the last dose. Protection may persist for up to 3 years in those constantly (or repeatedly) exposed to *S. typhi*, but occasional travellers require a repeat course at intervals of 1 year. Oral typhoid vaccine is **contra-indicated** in individuals who are immunosuppressed (whether due to disease or its treatment) and is inactivated by concomitant administration of antibiotics or sulphonamides, administration of a dose should be coordinated so that mefloquine is not taken for at least 12 hours before or after a dose.

For general contra-indications to vaccines, see section 14.1.

Whole cell vaccine for injection

PoM Typhoid Vaccine Typhoid/Vac. A suspension of killed *Salmonella typhi* organisms. Net price 1.5-mL vial = £4.11

Dose: 0.5 mL by deep subcutaneous or intramuscular injection, second dose 0.5 mL after 4–6 weeks; CHILD 1–10 years, 0.25 mL; under 12 months, not recommended

Note. The Department of Health recommends that second dose and subsequent boosters can be given intradermally, in a volume of 0.1 mL, to reduce adverse reactions

Available from Evans

Polysaccharide vaccine for injection

PoM Typhim Vi® (Merieux)

Vi capsular polysaccharide typhoid vaccine, 50 micrograms/mL virulence polysaccharide antigen of *Salmonella typhi*. Net price 0.5-mL single-dose prefilled syringe = £10.68

Dose: 0.5 mL by deep subcutaneous or intramuscular injection; CHILD under 18 months, may show suboptimal response

Live oral vaccine

▼ **PoM Vivotif®** (Evans)

Capsules, e/c, live attenuated *Salmonella typhi* (Ty 21a). Net price 3-cap pack = £14.85. Label: 23, 25, C, administration

Dose: ADULT and CHILD over 6 years, 1 capsule on days 1, 3, and 5; under 6 years, not recommended

COUNSELLING. Swallow as soon as possible after placing in mouth with a cold or lukewarm drink; it is important to store in refrigerator

YELLOW FEVER VACCINE

Yellow fever vaccine consists of a live attenuated yellow fever virus (17D strain) grown in developing chick embryos. Infants under 9 months of age should only be vaccinated if the risk of yellow fever is unavoidable since there is a small risk of encephalitis. The vaccine should not be given to those with impaired immune responsiveness, or who have had an anaphylactic reaction to egg; it should not be given during pregnancy (but where there is a significant risk of exposure the need for immunisation outweighs any risk to the fetus). See section 14.1 for further contra-indications. Reactions are few. The immunity which probably lasts for life is officially accepted for 10 years starting from 10 days after primary immunisation and for a further 10 years immediately after revaccination.

PoM Yellow Fever Vaccine, Live Yel/Vac. A suspension of chick embryo proteins containing attenuated 17D strain virus

Dose: 0.5 mL by subcutaneous injection

Available (only to designated Yellow Fever Vaccination centres) as Arilvax® (Evans)

14.5   Immunoglobulins

Human immunoglobulins have replaced immunoglobulins of animal origin (antisera) which were frequently associated with hypersensitivity. Injection of immunoglobulins produces immediate protection lasting for several weeks.

The two types of human immunoglobulin preparation are **normal immunoglobulin** and **specific immunoglobulins**.

Further information about immunoglobulins is included in *Immunisation against Infectious Disease* (see section 14.1).

AVAILABILITY. **Normal immunoglobulin** is now only available from the *Public Health Laboratory Service* laboratories for contacts and the control of outbreaks. It is available commercially for other purposes.

Specific immunoglobulins are available from the *Public Health Laboratory Service* laboratories and *Regional Blood Transfusion Centres* in England and Wales with the exception of **tetanus immunoglobulin** which is distributed through *Regional Blood Transfusion Centres* to hospital pharmacies or blood transfusion departments and is also available to general medical practitioners. **Rabies immunoglobulin** is available from the *Central Public Health Laboratory, London.* The large amounts of **hepatitis B immunoglobulin** required by transplant centres should be obtained commercially.

In Scotland all immunoglobulins are available from the *Blood Transfusion Service.* **Tetanus immunoglobulin** is distributed by the *Blood Transfusion Service* to hospitals and general medical practitioners on demand.

NORMAL IMMUNOGLOBULIN
(Gamma Globulin)

Human **normal immunoglobulin** ('HNIG') is prepared from pools of at least 1000 donations of human plasma; it contains antibody to measles, mumps, varicella, hepatitis A, and other viruses that are currently prevalent in the general population.

CAUTIONS and SIDE-EFFECTS. Side-effects of immunoglobulins include malaise, chills, fever, and rarely anaphylaxis. Human normal immunoglobulin is **contra-indicated** in patients with known class specific antibody to immunoglobulin A (IgA).

Normal immunoglobulin may **interfere with the immune response to live virus vaccines** which should therefore only be given **at least 3 weeks before or 3 months after** an injection of normal immunoglobulin (this does not apply to yellow fever vaccine since normal immunoglobulin does not contain antibody to this virus). For travellers, if there is insufficient time, the recommended interval may have to be ignored.

INTRAMUSCULAR

Normal immunoglobulin is administered by intramuscular injection for the protection of susceptible contacts against **hepatitis A** virus (infectious hepatitis), **measles** and, to a lesser extent, **rubella**.

HEPATITIS A. Control of hepatitis A depends on good hygiene and many studies have also shown the value of normal immunoglobulin in the prevention and control of outbreaks of this disease. It is recommended for controlling infection in contacts in closed institutions and also, under certain conditions, in school and home contacts and for travellers going to areas where the disease is highly endemic (all countries excluding Northern and Western Europe, North America, Australia, and New Zealand). Alternatively, **hepatitis A vaccine** (see p.472) may be used for those aged 16 years or over visiting such countries frequently or who stay for longer than 3 months.

MEASLES. Normal immunoglobulin may be given for prophylaxis in children with compromised immunity (and in adults with compromised immunity who have no measles antibodies); it should be given as soon as possible after contact with measles. It should also be given to children under 12 months with recent severe illness for whom measles should be avoided; MMR vaccine should then be given (after an interval of **at least** 3 months) at around the usual age.

RUBELLA. Immunoglobulin after exposure does **not** prevent infection in non-immune contacts and is **not** recommended for protection of pregnant women exposed to rubella. It may however reduce the likelihood of a clinical attack which may possibly reduce the risk to the fetus. It should only be used when termination of pregnancy would be unacceptable when it should be given as soon as possible after exposure. Serological follow-up of recipients is essential. For routine prophylaxis, see **Rubella Vaccine** (p.478).

REPLACEMENT THERAPY. Normal immunoglobulin may also be given intramuscularly for replacement therapy, but intravenous formulations (see next column) are normally preferred.

For intramuscular use

PoM Human Normal Immunoglobulin Human normal immunoglobulin injection. 250-mg vial; 750-mg vial

Dose: by deep intramuscular injection, Hepatitis A travel prophylaxis (2 months or less abroad), 250 mg; CHILD under 10 years 125 mg; longer travel prophylaxis (3–5 months abroad) and to control outbreaks, 500 mg; CHILD under 10 years 250 mg

Measles prophylaxis, CHILD under 1 year 250 mg, 1–2 years 500 mg, 3 years and over 750 mg; to allow attenuated attack, CHILD under 1 year 100 mg, 1 year and over 250 mg

Rubella in pregnancy, prevention of clinical attack, 750 mg

Available from BPL and SNBTS and from Public Health Laboratory Service (for contacts and control of outbreaks only, see p.480)

PoM Gammabulin® (Immuno)

Human normal immunoglobulin injection. Net price 2-mL vial = £3.12; 5-mL vial = £6.35; 10-mL vial = £10.70
Dose: see below

PoM Kabiglobulin® (Pharmacia)

Human normal immunoglobulin injection 16%. Net price 2-mL amp = £2.78; 5-mL amp = £6.00
Dose: see below
Note. Doses for Gammabulin® and Kabiglobulin® are expressed in terms of volume:
Dose: by intramuscular injection,
Hepatitis A prophylaxis, ADULT and CHILD 0.02–0.04 mL/kg; greater exposure risk, 0.06–0.12 mL/kg
Measles prophylaxis, 0.2 mL/kg; to allow attenuated attack, 0.04 mL/kg
Rubella in pregnancy, prevention of clinical attack, 20 mL
Antibody deficiency syndromes, see data sheet

INTRAVENOUS

Special formulations for intravenous administration are available for replacement therapy for patients with congenital agammaglobulinaemia and hypogammaglobulinaemia, for the treatment of idiopathic thrombocytopenic purpura and Kawasaki syndrome, and for the prophylaxis of infection following bone marrow transplantation.

For intravenous use
Available as: *Alphaglobin®* (2.5 g, 5 g, 10 g—Alpha), *Endobulin®* (500 mg, 1 g, 2.5 g, 5 g, 7.5 g, 10 g—Immuno); *Gamimune-N®* (500 mg, 2.5 g, 5 g—Cutter); Human Immunoglobulin (3 g—SNBTS); *Sandoglobulin®* (1 g, 3 g, 6 g—Sandoz); *Venoglobulin®* (2.5 g, 5 g, 10 g—Alpha); *Vigam®* (2.5 g, 5 g—BPL)

SPECIFIC IMMUNOGLOBULINS

Specific immunoglobulins are prepared by pooling the plasma of selected donors with high levels of the specific antibody required.

Although a hepatitis B vaccine is now available for those at high risk of infection, specific **hepatitis B immunoglobulin** ('HBIG') is available for use in association with the vaccine for the prevention of infection in laboratory and other personnel who have accidentally become contaminated with hepatitis B virus, and in infants born to mothers who have become infected with this virus in pregnancy or who are high-risk carriers.

Following exposure to a rabid animal, specific **rabies immunoglobulin** of human origin should be injected at the site of the bite and also given intramuscularly. Rabies vaccine should also be given.

Rubella immunoglobulin of human origin is indicated in early pregnancy where the immunity status is in doubt and termination of pregnancy is unacceptable where it should be given within 5 days of significant exposure. Serological follow-up of recipients is essential for 12 weeks following administration. For routine prophylaxis, see Rubella vaccine.

Tetanus immunoglobulin of human origin ('HTIG') should be used selectively in addition to wound toilet, vaccine, and benzylpenicillin (or another appropriate antibiotic) for the more seriously contaminated wounds; it is rarely required for those with an established immunity in whom protection may be achieved by a reinforcing dose of vaccine if considered advisable. The administration of tetanus immunoglobulin should be considered for patients not known to have received active immunisation (a) whose wound was sustained more than 6 hours before treatment was received and (b) with puncture wounds or wounds potentially heavily contaminated with tetanus spores, septic, or with much devitalised tissue. A dose of adsorbed tetanus vaccine should be given at the same time as the tetanus immunoglobulin and the course of vaccine subsequently completed.

Varicella-zoster immunoglobulin (VZIG) is indicated in *immunosuppressed patients at risk*, including those who within 3 months of contact have been on high-dose corticosteroid therapy (e.g. prednisolone 2 mg/kg daily for more than one week), *infants at risk*, and in *pregnant women at risk*. (**Important:** for full details consult *Immunisation against Infectious Diseases 1994*. It should also be noted that **varicella vaccine** is available on a named-patient basis from *SmithKline Beecham* or *Merieux*.)

Hepatitis B
PoM Hepatitis B Immunoglobulin (Antihepatitis B Immunoglobulin). See notes above
 Dose: by intramuscular injection (as soon as possible after exposure), ADULT 500 units; CHILD under 4 years 200 units, 5–9 years 300 units;NEONATE 200 units as soon as possible after birth; for full details see *Immunisation against Infectious Diseases*
 Available from Public Health Laboratory Service (except for Transplant Centres, see p.480), also available from BPL and SNBTS

Rabies
PoM Rabies Immunoglobulin (Antirabies Immunoglobulin Injection). See notes above
 Dose: 20 units/kg, half by intramuscular injection and half by infiltration around wound
 Available from Public Health Laboratory Service (also from BPL and SNBTS)

Rubella
PoM Rubella Immunoglobulin (Antirubella Immunoglobulin Injection). See notes above
 Dose: by deep intramuscular injection, prophylaxis in early pregnancy (within 5 days of exposure) 125 000 units
 Available from SNBTS (25 000 unit vial)

Tetanus
PoM Tetanus Immunoglobulin (Antitetanus Immunoglobulin Injection). See notes above
 Dose: by intramuscular injection, prophylactic 250 units, increased to 500 units if more than 24 hours have elapsed or there is risk of heavy contamination
 Therapeutic, 150 units/kg (multiple sites)
 Available from BPL and SNBTS
PoM Tetabulin® (Immuno)
 Tetanus immunoglobulin injection. Net price 250 unit prefilled syringe = £15.50
 Dose: by intramuscular injection, prophylactic, 250 units, increased to 500 units if wound older than 12 hours or if risk of heavy contamination or if patient weighs more than 90 kg; second dose of 250 units given after 3–4 weeks if patient immunosuppressed or if active immunisation with tetanus vaccine contra-indicated
 Therapeutic, 30–300 units/kg

PoM Tetanus Immunoglobulin for Intravenous Use. Used for proven or suspected clinical tetanus
 Dose: by intravenous infusion, 5000–10 000 units
 Available from SNBTS (2500-unit vial) on a named patient basis

Varicella-Zoster
PoM Varicella-Zoster Immunoglobulin (Anti-varicella-zoster Immunoglobulin) See notes above
 Dose: by deep intramuscular injection, prophylaxis (as soon as possible—not later than 10 days after exposure), CHILD up to 5 years 250 mg, 6–10 years 500 mg, 11–14 years 750 mg, over 15 years 1 g; second dose required if further exposure occurs after 3 weeks
 Note. No evidence that effective in treatment of severe disease—**acyclovir** (see section 5.3) should be used. An *intravenous preparation* of **normal immunoglobulin** (see Intravenous Therapy p.481) may be used to provide an immediate source of antibody.
 Available from Public Health Laboratory Service (also from BPL and SNBTS)

ANTI-D (Rh₀) IMMUNOGLOBULIN

Anti-D immunoglobulin is available to prevent a rhesus-negative mother from forming antibodies to fetal rhesus-positive cells which may pass into the maternal circulation during childbirth or abortion. It should be injected within 72 hours of the birth or abortion but even if a longer period has elapsed it may still give protection and should be administered. The objective is to protect any subsequent child from the hazard of haemolytic disease of the newborn.

Joint Committee on Vaccination and Immunisation recommendation on live vaccines.
Rubella vaccine may be administered in the postpartum period simultaneously with anti-D (Rh₀) immunoglobulin injection providing separate syringes are used and the products are administered into contralateral limbs. A blood test should be done not sooner than 8 weeks later to ensure that rubella antibodies have been produced. If blood transfusion was necessary vaccination should be delayed for 3 months.
MMR vaccine should not be given within 3 months of an injection of anti-D (Rh₀) immunoglobulin injection.

PoM Anti-D (Rh₀) Immunoglobulin Injection.
 Available from Regional Blood Transfusion Centres and from BPL and SNBTS
 Dose: by deep intramuscular injection, to rhesus-negative woman for prevention of D (Rh₀) sensitisation:
 Following abortion or birth of rhesus-positive infant, 500 units immediately or within 72 hours; for transplacental bleed in excess of 5 mL fetal red cells, extra 100–125 units per mL fetal red cells
 Following any potentially sensitising episode (e.g. stillbirth, amniocentesis) up to 20 weeks' gestation 250 units per episode (after 20 weeks, 500 units) immediately or within 72 hours
 Following Rh₀(D) incompatible blood transfusion, 125 units per mL transfused rhesus-positive red cells
 *Note.*These doses reflect recommendations of the Standing Medical Advisory Committee on Haemolytic Disease of the Newborn.

PoM **Partobulin®** (Immuno)

Anti-D (Rh$_0$) immunoglobulin injection 1250 units/mL, net price 1-mL vial = £15.50; 1-mL prefilled syringe = £16.48

Dose: by intramuscular injection, to rhesus-negative woman for prevention of D (Rh$_0$) sensitisation:

Following abortion, miscarriage or birth of rhesus-positive infant, 1250 units immediately or within 72 hours; for transplacental bleed in excess of 25 mL fetal blood (1% of fetal erythrocytes), 5000 units (*or* 50 units per mL fetal blood)

Antenatal prophylaxis, 1250 units may be given at weeks 28 and 34 of pregnancy; a dose of 1250 units is still needed immediately or within 72 hours of delivery (see above)

Following any potentially sensitising episode (e.g. amniocentesis) 1250 units immediately or within 72 hours

Following Rh$_0$(D) incompatible blood transfusion, at least 50–100 units per mL transfused rhesus-positive red cells

---

INTERFERONS

INTERFERON ALFA

See section 8.2.4

INTERFERON GAMMA-1b

(Immune interferon)

Indications: adjunct to antibiotics to reduce frequency of serious infection in patients with chronic granulomatous disease

Cautions: severe hepatic or renal impairment; seizure disorders or compromised central nervous system function; pre-existing cardiac disease (including ischaemia, congestive heart failure, and arrhythmias); monitor before and during treatment: haematological tests (including full blood count, differential white cell count, and platelet count), blood chemistry tests (including renal and liver function tests) and urinalysis

DRIVING. May impair ability to drive or operate machinery; effects may be enhanced by alcohol

Side-effects: fever, headache, chills, myalgia, fatigue; nausea, vomiting, arthralgia, rashes and injection-site reactions reported

▼ PoM **Immukin®** (Boehringer Ingelheim)

Injection, recombinant human interferon gamma-1b 200 micrograms/mL. Net price 0.5-mL vial = £88.00

Dose: by subcutaneous injection, 50 micrograms/m^2 3 times a week; patients with body surface area of 0.5 m^2 or less, 1.5 micrograms/kg 3 times a week; not yet recommended for children under 6 months

14.6 International travel

Note. For advice on **malaria chemoprophylaxis**, see section 5.4.1.

No particular immunisation is required for travellers to the United States, Europe, Australia, or New Zealand although all travellers should have immunity to tetanus and poliomyelitis (and childhood immunisations should be up to date). In Non-European areas surrounding the Mediterranean, in Africa, the Middle East, Asia, and South America, certain special precautions are required.

Long-term travellers to areas that have a high incidence of **poliomyelitis** or **tuberculosis** should be immunised with the appropriate vaccine; in the case of poliomyelitis previously immunised adults may be given a reinforcing dose of oral poliomyelitis vaccine. BCG immunisation is recommended for travellers proposing to stay for longer than one month (or in close contact with the local population) in Asia, Africa, or Central and South America; it should preferably be given three months or more before departure.

International Certificates of vaccination against **yellow fever** (section 14.4) are still required for travel to much of Africa and South America.

Immunisation against **meningococcal meningitis** is recommended for a number of areas of the world (for details, see section 14.4).

Overland travellers to Asia and Africa and others at high risk may be given **normal immunoglobulin injection** (section 14.5) for protection against hepatitis A; **hepatitis A vaccine** (section 14.2) is preferable for frequent travellers and those planning to go for more than 3–5 months. If immunoglobulin is to be given, it is preferable to complete any active immunisation 4 weeks beforehand; an interval of 2 weeks is acceptable provided the immunoglobulin is given just before departure. If time is short, it can be given with any vaccine (including polio).

Typhoid vaccine is indicated for travellers to those countries where typhoid is endemic but is no substitute for personal precautions. Food should be freshly prepared and hot, avoiding uncooked vegetables (including green salads); only fruits which can be peeled should be eaten. Only suitable bottled water, or water that has been boiled, or treated with sterilising tablets should be used for drinking purposes. This advice also applies to cholera and other diarrhoeal diseases (including travellers' diarrhoea).

Cholera vaccine is no substitute for personal hygiene and has little value in preventing infections. For current advice, see p.471.

For advice on **diphtheria vaccine** and the former USSR, see p.471.

The Department of Health has issued a booklet, *Health Advice For Travellers* (code: T5) which can be obtained from travel agents, post offices, or by telephoning 0800 555 777 (24-hour service).

It provides details of immunisation requirements or recommendations country-by-country, health insurance, and reciprocal agreements. Further advice (including details of requirements in relation to **Japanese** and **tick-borne encephalitis**) may be obtained from the Department of Health memorandum, *Immunisation against Infectious Disease* (for details, section 14.1).

Immunisation requirements change from time to time, and information on the current requirements for any particular country may be obtained from:

Communicable Disease Surveillance Centre Travel Unit, 61 Colindale Avenue, London NW9 5EQ, telephone 081-200 6868

Communicable Diseases (Scotland) Unit, Ruchill Hospital, Bilslend Drive, Glasgow G20 9NB, telephone 041-946 7120

Scottish Home and Health Department, St. Andrew's House, Edinburgh EH1 3DE, telephone 031-556 8400

Welsh Office, Cathays Park, Cardiff CF1 3NQ, telephone 0222 825111

Department of Health and Social Services, Dundonald House, Upper Newtownards Road, Belfast BT4 3FS, telephone 0232 520000

or from the embassy or legation of the appropriate country.

15:Drugs used in
ANAESTHESIA

This chapter describes briefly drugs used in anaesthesia; the reader is referred to other sources for more detailed information. The chapter is divided into two sections:

15.1 General anaesthesia
15.2 Local anaesthesia

15.1 General anaesthesia

15.1.1 Intravenous anaesthetics
15.1.2 Inhalational anaesthetics
15.1.3 Antimuscarinic premedication drugs
15.1.4 Sedative and analgesic peri-operative drugs
15.1.5 Muscle relaxants
15.1.6 Anticholinesterases used in surgery
15.1.7 Antagonists for central and respiratory depression
15.1.8 Antagonists for malignant hyperthermia

Note. The drugs in section 15.1 should be used only by experienced personnel and where adequate resuscitative equipment is available.

ANAESTHESIA AND DRIVING. Patients given sedatives and analgesics during minor outpatient procedures should be very carefully warned about the risk of driving afterwards. For intravenous benzodiazepines and for a short general anaesthetic the risk extends to **at least 24 hours** after administration. Responsible persons should be available to take patients home. The dangers of taking **alcohol** should also be emphasised.

MODERN ANAESTHETIC TECHNIQUE. It is now common practice to administer several drugs with different actions to produce a state of surgical anaesthesia with minimal risk of toxic effects. An intravenous anaesthetic is frequently used for induction, followed by maintenance with inhalational anaesthetics, perhaps supplemented by other drugs administered intravenously. Specific drugs are often used to produce muscular relaxation. Many of the drugs used interfere with the reflex maintenance of spontaneous respiration and intermittent positive pressure ventilation by manual or mechanical means is commonly employed.

For certain procedures controlled hypotension may be required. Labetalol (see section 2.4), sodium nitroprusside (see section 2.5.1), and trimetaphan camsylate (see section 2.5.6) are used.

Beta-blockers (see section 2.4) or verapamil (see section 2.6.2) may be used to control arrhythmias during anaesthesia.

Prazosin (see section 2.5.4) is also used to control hypertension, particularly postoperatively.

GAS CYLINDERS

Each gas cylinder bears a label with the name of the gas contained in the cylinder. The name or chemical symbol of the gas is stencilled in paint on the shoulder of the cylinder; the letters are not less than 9 mm high on cylinders up to and including 80 mm diameter, not less than 12 mm high on cylinders over 80 mm and up to and including 105 mm diameter, and 19 mm high on cylinders above 105 mm diameter. The name or chemical symbol of the gas is also clearly and indelibly stamped on the cylinder valve.

The colours applied to the valve end of the cylinder extend down the cylinder to the shoulder; in the case of mixed gases the colours for the individual gases are applied in four segments, two for each colour. See table below.

Gas cylinders should be stored in a cool well-ventilated room, free from materials of a flammable nature.

No lubricant of any description should be used.

Name of gas	Symbol	Colour of cylinder body	Colour of valve end where different from body
Oxygen	O_2	Black	White
Nitrous oxide	N_2O	Blue	—
Cyclopropane[1]	C_3H_6	Orange	—
Carbon dioxide	CO_2	Grey	—
Ethylene	C_2H_4	Violet	—
Helium	He	Brown	—
Nitrogen	N_2	Grey	Black
Oxygen and carbon dioxide mixture	$O_2 + CO_2$	Black	White and Grey
Oxygen and helium mixture	$O_2 + He$	Black	White and Brown
Oxygen and nitrous oxide mixture	$O_2 + N_2O$	Blue	Blue and White
Air (medical)	AIR	Grey	White and Black

British Standard 1319:1976; Medical gas cylinders, valves and yoke connections. The colours used for gas cylinders comply with specifications in British Standards 4800 and 5252.
1. Cyclopropane is no longer manufactured in the UK.

SURGERY AND LONG-TERM MEDICATION. The risk of stopping long-term medication before surgery is often greater than the risk of continuing it during surgery. This applies particularly to corticosteroids, since patients with adrenal atrophy (see section 6.3.3) may experience a precipitous fall in blood pressure unless corticosteroid cover is provided during anaesthesia or in the immediate postoperative period. Anaesthetists must therefore know whether a patient is, or has been, taking corticosteroids. Other drugs that should not normally be stopped before surgery include analgesics, antiepileptics, antiparkinsonian drugs, bronchodilators, cardiovascular drugs, glaucoma drugs, and thyroid or antithyroid drugs. Although it is preferable to discontinue oral anticoagulants electively before operation, this is not possible in patients requiring long-term treatment (e.g. for valve prostheses). The haematologist or physician should be consulted for further advice.

Drugs that should be stopped before surgery include combined oral contraceptives (discontinue 4 weeks before major elective surgery with adequate alternative contraceptive arrangements—see Surgery, section 7.3.1 for details); hormone replacement therapy, however, does not normally need to be stopped (see section 6.4.1.1). In view of their hazardous interactions MAOIs should normally be stopped 2 weeks before surgery. Tricyclic antidepressants need not be stopped, but there may be an increased risk of arrhythmias and hypotension, therefore the anaesthetist should be informed if they are not. Lithium should be stopped 2 days before major surgery but the normal dose can be continued for minor surgery (with careful monitoring of fluids and electrolytes). To avoid withdrawal symptoms antidepressants need to be withdrawn gradually (see section 4.3.1).

It is vital that the anaesthetist should know of **all** drugs that a patient is (or has been) taking.

Patients with a full stomach present a hazard during induction since there is a danger of regurgitation and pulmonary aspiration. This may cause Mendelson's syndrome, particularly in the pregnant patient. Cricoid pressure is applied until the lungs have been protected by a cuffed endotracheal tube.

15.1.1   Intravenous anaesthetics

Intravenous anaesthetics may be used alone to produce anaesthesia for short surgical procedures but are more commonly used for induction only. Intravenous anaesthetics are potent drugs which nearly all produce their effect in one arm-brain circulation time and can cause apnoea and hypotension, and so adequate resuscitative facilities **must** be available. Large doses should be avoided in obstetrics, as the drug may cross the placental barrier. They are **contra-indicated** if the anaesthetist is not confident of being able to maintain the airway (e.g. in the presence of a tumour in the pharynx or larynx). Extreme care is required in surgery of the mouth, pharynx, or larynx and in patients with acute cardiovascular failure (shock) or fixed cardiac output.

Individual requirements vary considerably and the recommended dosage is only a guide. Smaller dosage is indicated in ill, shocked, or debilitated patients, while robust individuals may require more. For tracheal intubation, induction is followed by inhalational anaesthesia (section 15.1.2) or by a neuromuscular blocking drug (section 15.1.5).

TOTAL INTRAVENOUS ANAESTHESIA. This is a technique in which major surgery is carried out with all anaesthetic drugs given intravenously. Respiration is controlled, the lungs being inflated with oxygen-enriched air. Muscle relaxants are used to provide relaxation and prevent reflex muscle movements. The main problem to be overcome is the assessment of depth of anaesthesia.

ANAESTHESIA AND DRIVING. See previous page.

BARBITURATES

Thiopentone sodium is the most widely used intravenous anaesthetic, but has no analgesic properties. Induction is generally smooth and rapid, but owing to its potency, overdosage with cardiorespiratory depression may occur. It is alkaline and therefore irritant on misplaced injection outside the vein; arterial injection is particularly dangerous.

Awakening from a moderate dose of thiopentone is rapid due to redistribution of the drug in the whole body tissues. Metabolism is, however, slow and some sedative effects may persist for 24 hours. Repeated doses have a cumulative effect.

Methohexitone sodium is less irritant to tissues than thiopentone. Recovery is marginally more rapid than in the case of thiopentone, but induction is less smooth with an incidence of hiccup, tremor, involuntary movements, and pain on injection.

Both thiopentone and methohexitone are **contra-indicated** in porphyria (see section 9.8.2).

METHOHEXITONE SODIUM
(Methohexital)

Indications: induction and maintenance of anaesthesia for short procedures; with other anaesthetics for more prolonged anaesthesia

Cautions; Contra-indications; Side-effects: avoid or reduce dose in liver disease; see also under Thiopentone Sodium and notes above

Dose: by intravenous injection, usually as a 1% solution, 50–120 mg according to response at rate of 10 mg in 5 seconds; maintenance, 20–40 mg (2–4 mL of 1% solution) every 4–7 minutes; CHILD induction approx. 1 mg/kg

PoM **Brietal Sodium**® (Lilly)
Injection, powder for reconstitution, methohexitone sodium, net price 100 mg in 10-mL vial = £1.14; 500 mg in 50-mL vial = £2.95

THIOPENTONE SODIUM
(Thiopental Sodium)

Indications: induction of general anaesthesia; anaesthesia of short duration

Cautions; Contra-indications; Side-effects: see notes above; reduce induction dose in severe liver disease; avoid in porphyria (see section 9.8.2); **interactions:** Appendix 1 (anaesthetics)

Dose: by intravenous injection, in fit premedicated adults, initially 100–150 mg (4–6 mL of 2.5% solution) over 10–15 seconds, followed by futher quantity if necessary according to response after 30–60 seconds; *or* up to 4 mg/kg; CHILD induction 2–7 mg/kg

PoM Thiopentone Sodium (IMS)
Dispensing kit, thiopentone sodium with physiological saline to provide 2.5% solution, net price 2.5 g = 65p; 5 g = £1.08

PoM Intraval Sodium® (Rhône-Poulenc Rorer)
Injection 2.5%, powder for reconstitution, thiopentone sodium. Net price 500-mg amp = £1.07 (with water for injections £1.45); 2.5-g vial = £3.99 (with water for injections £4.68)

OTHER INTRAVENOUS ANAESTHETICS

Etomidate is an induction agent associated with rapid recovery without hangover effect. It causes less hypotension than other drugs used for induction. There is a high incidence of extraneous muscle movement and of pain on injection; these effects can be minimised by premedication with an opioid analgesic and the use of larger veins. There is evidence that repeated doses of etomidate have an undesirable suppressant effect on adrenocortical function.

Propofol is associated with rapid recovery without hangover effect. There is sometimes pain on intravenous injection, but significant extraneous muscle movements do not occur. The CSM have received reports of convulsions, anaphylaxis, and delayed recovery from anaesthesia after propofol administration; since some of the convulsions are delayed the CSM has advised special caution after day surgery. Propofol has been associated with bradycardia, occasionally profound; intravenous administration of an antimuscarinic may be necessary to prevent this.

Ketamine can be given by the intravenous or the intramuscular route, and has good analgesic properties when used in sub-anaesthetic dosage. The maximum effect occurs in more than one arm-brain circulation time. Muscle tone is increased and the airway is usually well maintained. There is cardiovascular stimulation and arterial pressure may rise with tachycardia. The main disadvantage is the high incidence of hallucinations and other transient psychotic sequelae, though it is believed that these are much less significant in children. The incidence can be reduced when drugs such as diazepam are also used. Ketamine is **contra-indicated** in patients with hypertension and is best avoided in those

prone to hallucinations. It is used mainly for paediatric anaesthesia, particularly when repeated administrations are required. Recovery is relatively slow.

Midazolam (section 15.1.4.1) is in increasing use as an induction agent.

ETOMIDATE

Indications: induction of anaesthesia

Cautions; Contra-indications; Side-effects: see notes above; porphyria (see section 9.8.2); **interactions:** Appendix 1 (anaesthetics)

Dose: by slow intravenous injection, 300 micrograms/kg; high-risk patients, 100 micrograms/kg/minute until anaesthetised (about 3 minutes)

PoM Hypnomidate® (Janssen)
Injection, etomidate 2 mg/mL in propylene glycol 35%. Net price 10-mL amp = £1.58
Concentrate injection, etomidate 125 mg (as hydrochloride)/mL. To be diluted before use. Net price 1-mL amp = £5.33
Note. With the concentrate use only glass syringes, avoid contact with plastics

---

KETAMINE

Indications: induction and maintenance of anaesthesia

Cautions; Contra-indications; Side-effects: see notes above; **interactions:** Appendix 1 (anaesthetics)

Dose: by intramuscular injection, short procedures, initially 6.5–13 mg/kg (10 mg/kg usually produces 12–25 minutes of surgical anaesthesia) Diagnostic manoeuvres and procedures not involving intense pain, initially 4 mg/kg

By intravenous injection over at least 60 seconds, short procedures, initially 1–4.5 mg/kg (2 mg/kg usually produces 5–10 minutes of surgical anaesthesia)

By intravenous infusion of a solution containing 1 mg/mL, longer procedures, induction, total dose of 0.5–2 mg/kg; maintenance (using microdrip infusion), 10–45 micrograms/kg/minute, rate adjusted according to response

PoM Ketalar® (P-D)
Injection, ketamine (as hydrochloride) 10 mg/mL, net price 20-mL vial = £3.52; 50 mg/mL, 10-mL vial = £7.31; 100 mg/mL, 5-mL vial = £6.71

PROPOFOL

Indications: induction and maintenance of general anaesthesia; sedation of ventilated patients receiving intensive care, for up to 3 days

Cautions; Contra-indications; Side-effects: see notes above; monitor blood lipid concentrations in patients at risk of fat overload; contra-indicated

---

if history of propofol allergy (see CSM warning above); **interactions:** Appendix 1 (anaesthetics)

Dose: induction, *by intravenous injection*, 2–2.5 mg/kg (less in elderly) at a rate of 20–40 mg every 10 seconds; CHILD over 3 years 2.5 mg/kg adjusted as necessary

Maintenance, *by intravenous infusion*, 4–12 mg/kg/hour; CHILD over 3 years 9–15 mg/kg/hour

Sedation during intensive care (with assisted ventilation), *by intravenous infusion*, 1–4 mg/kg/hour for up to 3 days; CHILD not recommended

PoM **Diprivan**® (Zeneca)

Injection (emulsion), propofol 10 mg/mL, net price 20-mL amp = £3.88, 50-mL vial = £9.70, 100-mL vial = £19.40

15.1.2   Inhalational anaesthetics

Inhalational anaesthetics may be gases or volatile liquids. They can be used both for induction and maintenance of anaesthesia and may also be used following induction with an intravenous anaesthetic (section 15.1.1).

Gaseous anaesthetics require suitable equipment for storage and administration. They may be supplied via hospital pipelines or from metal cylinders. *Volatile liquid anaesthetics* are usually administered using calibrated vaporisers, using air, oxygen, or nitrous oxide–oxygen mixtures as the carrier gas.

To prevent hypoxia inhalational anaesthetics must be given with adequate concentrations of oxygen.

ANAESTHESIA AND DRIVING. See section 15.1.

VOLATILE LIQUID ANAESTHETICS

Halothane is a volatile liquid anaesthetic. Its advantages are that it is potent, induction is smooth, the vapour is non-irritant, pleasant to inhale, and seldom induces coughing or breath-holding; the incidence of postoperative vomiting is low. Despite these advantages, however, halothane is much less widely used than previously owing to its association with *severe hepatotoxicity* (**important:** see CSM advice, below).

Halothane causes cardiorespiratory depression and because of its potency is administered from calibrated vaporisers. Respiratory depression results in elevation of arterial carbon dioxide tension and perhaps ventricular arrhythmias. Intermittent positive-pressure ventilation must be carried out with care as myocardial depression may follow increase in blood concentrations. Halothane depresses the cardiac muscle fibres and may cause bradycardia. The result is diminished cardiac output and fall of arterial pressure. There is also peripheral vasodilatation. Adrenaline infiltrations should be used with care as ventricular dysrhythmias may result.

Halothane produces moderate muscle relaxation, but this may be inadequate for major abdominal surgery and specific muscle relaxants are then used.

CSM advice (halothane hepatotoxicity). In a publication on findings confirming that *severe hepatotoxicity* can follow halothane anaesthesia the CSM has reported that this occurs more frequently after repeated exposures to halothane and has a high mortality. The risk of severe hepatotoxicity appears to be increased by repeated exposures within a short time interval, but even after a long interval (sometimes of several years) susceptible patients have been reported to develop jaundice. Since there is no reliable way of identifying susceptible patients the CSM recommends the following precautions prior to use of halothane:

1. a careful anaesthetic history should be taken to determine previous exposure and previous reactions to halothane;
2. repeated exposure to halothane within a period of **at least** 3 months should be **avoided** unless there are **overriding** clinical circumstances;
3. a history of unexplained jaundice or pyrexia in a patient following exposure to halothane is an absolute **contra-indication** to its future use in that patient.

Enflurane is a volatile anaesthetic similar to halothane, but less potent, about twice the concentration being necessary for induction and maintenance.

Enflurane is a powerful cardiorespiratory depressant. Shallow respiration is likely to result in a rise of arterial carbon dioxide tension, but ventricular arrhythmias are uncommon and it is probably safe to use adrenaline infiltrations. Myocardial depression may result in a fall in cardiac output and in arterial hypotension.

Enflurane is usually given to supplement nitrous oxide–oxygen mixtures.

Isoflurane is an isomer of enflurane. It has a potency intermediate between that of halothane and enflurane, and even less of an inhaled dose is metabolised than with enflurane. Heart rhythm is generally stable during isoflurane anaesthesia, but heart-rate may rise, particularly in younger patients. Systemic arterial pressure may fall, due to a decrease in systemic vascular resistance and with less decrease in cardiac output than occurs with halothane. Respiration is depressed. Muscle relaxation is produced and muscle relaxant drugs potentiated.

Desflurane is a newly introduced rapid acting volatile liquid anaesthetic. It is reported to have about one-fifth the potency of isoflurane. Owing to limited experience it is not recommended in neurosurgical patients; owing to frequent occurrence of cough, breath-holding, apnoea, laryngospasm and increased secretions it is not recommended for induction in children.

DESFLURANE

Indications; Cautions; Contra-indications; Side-effects: see notes above; **interactions:** Appendix 1 (anaesthetics)

Dose: using a specifically designed calibrated vaporiser, *induction*, 4–11%; CHILD not recommended for induction

Maintenance, 2–6% in nitrous oxide; 2.5–8.5% in oxygen or oxygen-enriched air

---

Abbreviations and symbols, see inside front cover

▼ PoM **Suprane**® (Pharmacia)
Desflurane. Net price 240 mL = £46.50

ENFLURANE

Indications; Cautions; Side-effects: see notes above, porphyria (see section 9.8.2); **Interactions:** Appendix 1 (anaesthetics)
Dose: using a specifically calibrated vaporiser, *induction*, increased gradually from 0.4% to max. of 4.5% in air, oxygen, or nitrous oxide–oxygen, according to response
Maintenance, 0.5–3% in nitrous oxide–oxygen

Enflurane (Abbott)
Enflurane. Net price 250 mL = £49.50

HALOTHANE

Indications; Cautions; Contra-indications; Side-effects: see notes above (**important:** CSM advice see also notes above); porphyria (see section 9.8.2); **interactions:** Appendix 1 (anaesthetics)
Dose: using a specifically calibrated vaporiser, *induction*, increased gradually to 2–4% in oxygen or nitrous oxide–oxygen; CHILD 1.5–2%
Maintenance, 0.5–2%

Halothane (Rhône-Poulenc Rorer)
Halothane. Net price 250 mL = £10.23
Fluothane® (Zeneca)
Halothane. Net price 250 mL = £16.36

ISOFLURANE

Indications; Cautions; Side-effects: see notes above, **interactions:** Appendix 1 (anaesthetics)
Dose: using a specifically calibrated vaporiser, *induction*, increased gradually from 0.5% to 3%, in oxygen or nitrous oxide–oxygen
Maintenance, 1–2.5% in nitrous oxide–oxygen; an additional 0.5–1% may be required when given with oxygen alone; caesarean section, 0.5–0.75% in nitrous oxide–oxygen

Isoflurane (Abbott)
Isoflurane. Net price 100 mL = £41.00

NITROUS OXIDE

Nitrous oxide is used for induction and maintenance of anaesthesia and, in sub-anaesthetic concentrations, for analgesia. For *anaesthesia* it is commonly used in a concentration of 50 to 70% in oxygen as part of a balanced technique in association with other inhalational or intravenous agents. Nitrous oxide is unsatisfactory as a sole anaesthetic owing to lack of potency, but is useful as part of a sequence of drugs since it allows a significant reduction in dosage.

A mixture of nitrous oxide and oxygen containing 50% of each gas (Entonox®) is used to produce *analgesia without loss of consciousness*. Self-administration using a demand valve is popular and may be appropriate in obstetric practice, for changing painful dressings, as an aid to postoperative physiotherapy, and in emergency ambulances.

Nitrous oxide may have a deleterious effect if used in patients with an air-containing closed space since nitrous oxide diffuses into such a space with a resulting build up of pressure. This effect may be dangerous in the presence of a pneumothorax which may enlarge to compromise respiration.

Exposure of patients to nitrous oxide for prolonged periods, either by continuous or by intermittent administration, may result in megaloblastic anaemia due to interference with the action of vitamin B_{12}. For the same reason, exposure of anaesthetists and theatre staff to nitrous oxide should be minimised. Depression of white cell formation may also occur.

NITROUS OXIDE

Indications; Cautions; Side-effects: see notes above; **interactions:** Appendix 1 (anaesthetics)

Dose: using a suitable anaesthetic apparatus, a mixture with 20–30% oxygen for *induction* and *maintenance* of light anaesthesia

Analgesic, as a mixture with 50% oxygen, according to the patient's needs

15.1.3 Antimuscarinic premedication drugs

Antimuscarinic premedication drugs are used (less commonly nowadays) to dry bronchial and salivary secretions which are increased by intubation and some inhalational anaesthetics. They are also used before or with neostigmine (section 15.1.6) to prevent bradycardia, excessive salivation, and other muscarinic actions of neostigmine. They are also used to prevent bradycardia and hypotension associated with agents such as halothane, propofol, and suxamethonium.

Atropine is the most commonly used. Intravenous administration immediately before anaesthesia or intramuscular injection (which should be given 30–60 minutes before the operation) is satisfactory. For its role in acute arrhythmias after myocardial infarction, see section 2.3.1; see also cardiopulmonary resuscitation algorithm, section 2.7.

Hyoscine effectively reduces secretions and also provides a degree of amnesia. It produces less tachycardia than atropine. In some patients, especially the elderly, hyoscine may cause the central anticholinergic syndrome (excitement, ataxia, hallucinations, behavioural abnormalities, and drowsiness).

Glycopyrronium bromide produces good drying of salivary secretions. When given intravenously it produces less tachycardia than atropine.

Phenothiazines have too little drying activity to be effective when used alone.

ATROPINE SULPHATE

Indications: drying secretions, reversal of excessive bradycardia; with neostigmine for reversal of competitive neuromuscular block; other indications, see sections 1.2, 2.3.1, 11.5

Cautions: cardiovascular disease; see also section 1.2; **interactions:** Appendix 1 (antimuscarinics)

Side-effects: tachycardia; see also section 1.2

Dose: premedication, *by intravenous injection,* 300–600 micrograms immediately before induction of anaesthesia, and in incremental doses of 100 micrograms for the treatment of bradycardia

By intramuscular injection, 300–600 micrograms 30–60 minutes before induction; CHILD 20 micrograms/kg

For control of muscarinic side-effects of neostigmine in reversal of competitive neuromuscular block, *by intravenous injection,* 0.6–1.2 mg

Acute arrhythmias after myocardial infarction, see section 2.3.1; see also cardiopulmonary resuscitation algorithm, section 2.7

PoM **Atropine** (Non-proprietary)

Injection, atropine sulphate 600 micrograms/mL. Net price 1-mL amp = 33p

Note. Other strengths also available

PoM **Min-I-Jet ® Atropine Sulphate** (IMS)

Injection, atropine sulphate 100 micrograms/mL, net price 5-mL disposable syringe = £3.78; 10-mL disposable syringe = £4.24

CD **Morphine and Atropine Injection,** see under Morphine Salts (section 15.1.4.3)

GLYCOPYRRONIUM BROMIDE

Indications; Cautions; Side-effects: see under Atropine Sulphate

Dose: premedication, *by intramuscular or intravenous injection,* 200–400 micrograms, *or* 4–5 micrograms/kg to a max. of 400 micrograms; CHILD, *by intramuscular or intravenous injection,* 4–8 micrograms/kg to a max. of 200 micrograms; intra-operative use, *by intravenous injection,* as for premedication

For control of muscarinic side-effects of neostigmine in reversal of competitive neuromuscular block, *by intravenous injection,* 10–15 micrograms/kg with 50 micrograms/kg neostigmine; CHILD, 10 micrograms/kg with 50 micrograms/kg neostigmine

PoM **Robinul®** (Wyeth)

Injection, glycopyrronium bromide 200 micrograms/mL. Net price 1-mL amp = 32p; 3-mL amp = 53p

PoM **Robinul-Neostigmine®,** see under Neostigmine Methylsulphate (section 15.1.6)

HYOSCINE HYDROBROMIDE

(Scopolamine Hydrobromide)

Indications: drying secretions, amnesia; other indications, see sections 4.6, 11.5

Cautions; Side-effects: see under Atropine Sulphate; may slow heart; avoid in the elderly (see notes above); porphyria (see section 9.8.2)

Dose: premedication, *by subcutaneous or intramuscular injection,* 200–600 micrograms 30–60 minutes before induction of anaesthesia, usually with papaveretum; CHILD 15 micrograms/kg

PoM **Hyoscine** (Non-proprietary)

Injection, hyoscine hydrobromide 400 micrograms/mL, net price 1-mL amp = £2.21; 600 micrograms/mL, 1-mL amp = £1.28

CD **Papaveretum and Hyoscine Injection,** see under Papaveretum (section 15.1.4.3)

15.1.4   Sedative and analgesic perioperative drugs

15.1.4.1 Anxiolytics and neuroleptics

15.1.4.2 Non-opioid analgesics

15.1.4.3 Opioid analgesics

These drugs are given to allay the apprehension of the patient in the pre-operative period (including the night before operation), to relieve pain and discomfort when present, and to augment the action of subsequent anaesthetic agents. A number of the drugs used also provide some degree of pre-operative amnesia. The choice will vary with the individual patient, the nature of the operative procedure, the anaesthetic to be used and other prevailing circumstances such as outpatients, obstetrics, recovery facilities etc. The choice would also vary in elective and emergency operations.

For many procedures, particularly minor operations, premedication is omitted completely and in these circumstances antisialogogues will usually be given intravenously, if indicated, either with or just before the induction agent.

PREMEDICATION IN CHILDREN. Oral or rectal administration is preferred to injections where possible but is not altogether satisfactory. Oral **trimeprazine** is still used but when given alone it may cause postoperative restlessness when pain is present. An alternative is **diazepam**. Some anaesthetists prefer the use of adult regimens, with dosage on a weight basis. (For guidelines on dose calculation in children, see Prescribing for Children, p. 11.)

Atropine or hyoscine is often given orally to children, but may be given intravenously immediately before induction.

ANAESTHESIA AND DRIVING. See section 15.1.

15.1.4.1 ANXIOLYTICS AND NEUROLEPTICS

Anxiolytic benzodiazepines are widely used whereas neuroleptics (e.g. chlorpromazine) are now rarely used.

BENZODIAZEPINES

Oral premedication with benzodiazepines is increasing in popularity; a short-acting oral benzodiazepine now being the most common premedicant.

Benzodiazepines are also of particular value for the production of light sedation during unpleasant procedures or during operations under local anaesthesia (including dentistry). The resultant amnesia is such that the patient is unlikely to have any unpleasant memories of the procedure (however, benzodiazepines, particularly when used for deep sedation, can sometimes induce sexual fantasies).

Diazepam is relatively insoluble in water and preparations formulated in organic solvents are painful on intravenous injection and followed by a high incidence of venous thrombosis (which may not be noticed until a week after the injection); they are also painful on intramuscular injection, and absorption from the injection site is erratic. An emulsion preparation for intravenous injection (Diazemuls®) is less irritant and is followed by a negligible incidence of venous thrombosis; it is not suitable for intramuscular injection. Diazepam is also available as a rectal solution (e.g. Stesolid®).

Benzodiazepines are also of particular value for sedation of patients in intensive care units, particularly those on ventilators. Since they have no analgesic action they are often given in conjunction with small doses of opioid analgesics.

Benzodiazepines may on occasions cause marked respiratory depression and facilities for treatment of this are essential.

Diazepam is used to produce light sedation with amnesia. The 'sleep' dose shows too great an individual variation to recommend it for induction of anaesthesia. It is a long-acting drug, and a second period of drowsiness can occur 4–6 hours after its administration.

Temazepam has a shorter action and a relatively more rapid onset than diazepam. Used orally as a premedicant, anxiolytic and sedative effects are produced which continue for one and a half hours. After this period patients are usually fully alert but there may be residual drowsiness. It has proved useful as a premedicant in inpatient and day-case surgery.

Lorazepam produces more prolonged sedation than temazepam. In addition amnesia is commonplace. It is used as a premedicant the night prior to major surgery. A further, smaller, dose may be required the following morning if any delay in the commencement of surgery is anticipated. Alternatively the first dose may be given in the early morning of the day of operation.

Midazolam is a water-soluble benzodiazepine which is often used in preference to diazepam. Recovery is faster than with diazepam. The incidence of side-effects is low but the CSM has received reports of respiratory depression (sometimes associated with severe hypotension) following intravenous administration.

DIAZEPAM

Indications: premedication; sedation with amnesia, and in conjunction with local anaesthesia; other indications, see sections 4.1.2, 4.8.2, 10.2.2
Cautions; Contra-indications; Side-effects: see notes above and sections 4.1.2, 4.8.2
Dose: by mouth, 5 mg at night, 5 mg on waking, and 5 mg 2 hours before minor or dental surgery
By intravenous injection, into a large vein 10–20 mg over 2–4 minutes as sedative cover for minor surgical and medical procedures; premedication 100–200 micrograms/kg
By rectum in solution, ADULT and CHILD over 3 years 10 mg; CHILD 1–3 years and elderly 5 mg

Preparations
See section 4.1.2

LORAZEPAM

Indications: sedation with amnesia; as pre-medication; other indications, see sections 4.1.2, 4.8.2
Cautions; Contra-indications; Side-effects: see under Diazepam
Dose: by mouth, 2–3 mg the night before operation; 2–4 mg 1–2 hours before operation
By slow intravenous injection, preferably diluted with an equal volume of sodium chloride intravenous infusion 0.9% or water for injections, 50 micrograms/kg 30–45 minutes before operation
By intramuscular injection, diluted as above, 50 micrograms/kg 1–1½ hours before operation

PoM **Ativan®** (Wyeth)
Injection, lorazepam 4 mg/mL. Net price 1-mL amp = 40p
Tablets, see section 4.1.2

MIDAZOLAM

Indications: sedation with amnesia, and in conjunction with local anaesthesia; premedication, induction
Cautions; Contra-indications; Side-effects: see under Diazepam; see notes above for CSM warning; **important:** plasma concentration increased by erythromycin—profound sedation reported with oral midazolam (not on UK market); other **interactions:** Appendix 1 (benzodiazepines)
Dose: sedation, *by intravenous injection* over 30 seconds, 2 mg (elderly 1–1.5 mg) followed after 2 minutes by increments of 0.5–1 mg if sedation not adequate; usual range 2.5–7.5 mg (about 70 micrograms/kg), elderly 1–2 mg

Premedication, *by intramuscular injection*, 70–100 micrograms/kg 30–60 minutes before surgery; usual dose 5 mg (2.5 mg in elderly)

Induction, *by slow intravenous injection*, 200–300 micrograms/kg (elderly 100–200 micrograms/kg)

Sedation of patients receiving intensive care, *by intravenous infusion*, initially 30–300 micrograms/kg given over 5 minutes, then 30–200 micrograms/kg/hour; reduce dose (or omit initial dose) in hypovolaemia, vasoconstriction, or hypothermia; low doses may be adequate if opioid analgesic also used; avoid abrupt withdrawal after prolonged administration (safety after more than 14 days not established)

PoM **Hypnovel®** (Roche)

Injection, midazolam (as hydrochloride) 2 mg/mL, net price 5-mL amp = £1.01; 5 mg/mL, 2-mL amp = 85p

TEMAZEPAM

Indications: premedication before minor surgery; anxiety before investigatory procedures; hypnotic, see section 4.1.1

Cautions; Contra-indications; Side-effects: see under Diazepam

Dose: by mouth, premedication, 20–40 mg (elderly, 10–20 mg) 1 hour before operation; CHILD 1 mg/kg (max. 30 mg)

Preparations

See section 4.1.1

CHLORMETHIAZOLE

Chlormethiazole has been used as an intravenous infusion to maintain sleep during surgery carried out under regional anaesthesia, including extradural block. It has no analgesic effect, little cardiac and respiratory depression, and may be used in elderly patients.

CHLORMETHIAZOLE

(Clomethiazole)

Indications: sedative during regional anaesthesia; other indications, see sections 4.1.1, 4.8.2, 4.10

Cautions; Contra-indications; Side-effects: see section 4.10

Dose: by intravenous infusion, as a 0.8% solution of chlormethiazole edisylate, induction 25 mL (200 mg)/minute for 1–2 minutes; maintenance 1–4 mL (8–32 mg)/minute

IMPORTANT. See special cautions for intravenous infusion, section 4.10

Preparations

See section 4.10

PHENOTHIAZINES AND RELATED

Neuroleptics such as chlorpromazine and droperidol are rarely used in the UK for premedication. Trimeprazine is used as a premedicant for children.

CHLORPROMAZINE HYDROCHLORIDE

Indications: see under Dose; other indications, see section 4.2.1

Cautions; Contra-indications; Side-effects: see section 4.2.1

Dose: induction of hypothermia (to prevent shivering), *by deep intramuscular injection*, 25–50 mg every 6–8 hours; CHILD 1–12 years, initially 0.5–1 mg/kg, followed by maintenance 500 micrograms/kg every 4–6 hours

Preparations

See section 4.2.1

DROPERIDOL

Indications: anti-emetic, pre-operative sedation; neuroleptanalgesia; other indications, see section 4.2.1

Cautions; Contra-indications; Side-effects: see section 4.2.1

Dose: premedication, *by intramuscular injection*, up to 10 mg 60 minutes before operation; CHILD 200–500 micrograms/kg

Neuroleptanalgesia, *by intravenous injection*, 5–15 mg at induction with an opioid analgesic; CHILD 200–300 micrograms/kg

PoM **Droleptan®** (Janssen)

Injection, droperidol 5 mg/mL. Net price 2-mL amp = 90p

PROMETHAZINE HYDROCHLORIDE

Indications: pre-operative sedative and antimuscarinic; anti-emetic, see section 4.6; other indications, see sections 3.4.1, 3.4.3

Cautions; Side-effects: see section 4.6

Dose: premedication, *by mouth*, CHILD 2–5 years 15–20 mg, 6–10 years 20–25 mg

By deep intramuscular injection, 25–50 mg 1 hour before operation; CHILD 5–10 years, 6.25–12.5 mg

Preparations

See sections 3.4.1 and 15.1.4.3 (with pethidine)

TRIMEPRAZINE TARTRATE

(Alimemazine Tartrate)

Indications: pre-operative sedation, anti-emetic; other indications, see section 3.4.1

Cautions; Side-effects: see notes above and section 3.4.1

Dose: by mouth, premedication; CHILD 2–7 years up to 2 mg/kg 1–2 hours before operation

Preparations

See section 3.4.1

15.1.4.2 NON-OPIOID ANALGESICS

As NSAIDs do not depress respiration, do not impair gastro-intestinal motility, and do not cause dependence, they may be useful alternatives (or adjuncts) to the use of opioids for the relief of post-operative pain; they may also be useful alternatives to the use of local anaesthetic techniques. They may be inadequate for the relief of severe pain.

Diclofenac, ketoprofen (both section 10.1.1), and **ketorolac** can be given by injection as well as by mouth. Injections of diclofenac and ketoprofen are given by the intramuscular route deep into the gluteal muscle to minimise pain and tissue damage. Ketorolac is less irritant but pain has been reported on intramuscular injection; it can also be given by intravenous injection.

KETOROLAC TROMETAMOL

Indications: short-term management of moderate to severe acute postoperative pain

Cautions: reduce dose in elderly and in those weighing less than 50 kg; reduce dose and monitor in mild renal impairment (avoid if moderate or severe, see also Appendix 3 and section 10.1.1); heart failure, hepatic impairment and other conditions leading to reduction in blood volume or in renal blood flow (including those taking diuretics); cardiac decompensation, hypertension or similar conditions (fluid retention and oedema reported); do not give with anticoagulants (including low-dose heparin), oxpentifylline, probenecid, lithium salts, or other NSAIDs; other **interactions:** Appendix 1 (NSAIDs) GASTRO-INTESTINAL EFFECTS. Elderly and debilitated more prone to risk of gastro-intestinal effects (risk increasing with increased dose and duration); see also under Contra-indications and Side-effects below

Contra-indications: history of hypersensitivity to aspirin or any other NSAID (severe anaphylactic reactions reported), history of asthma; complete or partial syndrome of nasal polyps, angioedema or bronchospasm; history of peptic ulceration or gastro-intestinal bleeding; haemorrhagic diatheses (including coagulation disorders) and operations with high risk of haemorrhage or incomplete haemostasis; confirmed or suspected cerebrovascular bleeding; moderate or severe renal impairment; hypovolaemia or dehydration; pregnancy (including labour and delivery) and breast-feeding

Side-effects: side-effects reported include anaphylaxis (with rash, bronchospasm, laryngeal oedema and hypotension), fluid retention (see Cautions), nausea, dyspepsia, abdominal discomfort, bowel changes, peptic ulceration, gastro-intestinal bleeding (elderly at greater risk), pancreatitis, drowsiness, dizziness, headache, sweating, dry mouth, excessive thirst, mental and sensory changes, convulsions, myalgia, aseptic meningitis, hyponatraemia, hyperkalaemia, raised blood urea and creatinine, urinary symptoms and acute renal failure, flushing or pallor, bradycardia, hypertension, purpura, thrombocytopenia, dyspnoea and pulmonary oedema, skin reactions (some severe, including Stevens-Johnson and Lyell's syndromes), postoperative wound haemorrhage, haematoma, epistaxis, oedema, liver function changes (discontinue if clinical symptoms); pain at injection site; for general side-effects of NSAIDs, see also section 10.1.1

Dose: by mouth, PATIENT over 16 years, 10 mg every 4–6 hours (ELDERLY every 6–8 hours); max. 40 mg daily; max. duration of treatment 7 days; CHILD under 16 years, not recommended

By intramuscular injection or by intravenous injection over not less than 15 seconds, PATIENT over 16 years, initially 10 mg, then 10–30 mg every 4–6 hours when required (every 2 hours in initial postoperative period); max. 90 mg daily (ELDERLY max. 60 mg daily); max. duration of treatment 2 days by either route

Note. Pain relief may not occur upwards of 30 minutes after intravenous or intramuscular injection. When converting from parenteral to oral administration, total combined dose on the day of converting should not exceed 90 mg (60 mg in the elderly) of which the oral component should not exceed 40 mg; patients should be converted to oral route as soon as possible

▼ PoM **Toradol**® (Syntex)
Tablets, ivory, f/c, ketorolac trometamol 10 mg, net price 20 = £6.52. Label: 17, 21
Injection, ketorolac trometamol 10 mg/mL, net price 1-mL amp = £1.06; 30 mg/mL, 1-mL amp = £1.28

15.1.4.3 OPIOID ANALGESICS

Opioid analgesics were formerly commonly used as premedicants given intramuscularly about an hour before operation, usually combined with an antisialogogue. Sometimes they were combined with a phenothiazine or droperidol. The main side-effects of opioid analgesics are respiratory depression, cardiovascular depression, and nausea and vomiting. The principal advantages were that opioid analgesics provided analgesia persisting into the operative period giving a reduced chance of awareness during anaesthesia with full doses of muscle relaxants. Nowadays anaesthetists are more likely to give potent opioids by the intravenous route at induction.

INTRA-OPERATIVE ANALGESIA. Many of the conventional opioid analgesics are used to supplement general anaesthesia, usually in combination with nitrous oxide–oxygen and a muscle relaxant. Pethidine was the first to be used for this purpose but other drugs now available include alfentanil, fentanyl, meptazinol, nalbuphine, and phenoperidine. The longer-acting drugs morphine and papaveretum, although equally effective for this purpose, are not commonly used because of the problems of respiratory depression in the postoperative period.

Small doses of opioids given immediately before or with thiopentone will reduce the induction dose of the barbiturate and this is a popular technique in poor-risk patients. **Alfentanil** and **fentanyl** are particularly useful in this respect because of their short duration of action although there may be some cumulation with large doses. Alfentanil may be preferable for short operations because of its very brief duration of action; for long procedures it can be given as a continuous infusion.

Repeated doses of intra-operative analgesics should be given with care, since not only may the respiratory depression persist into the post-operative period but it may become apparent for the first time postoperatively when the patient is away from immediate nursing attention. The specific opioid antagonist, naloxone (section 15.1.7), will immediately reverse this respiratory depression but the dose may have to be repeated. In clinical doses it will also reverse most of the analgesia. An alternative and equally acceptable approach is to use the specific respiratory stimulant, doxapram (see section 3.5.1), which can be given in an infusion and which will not affect the opioid analgesia. The use of intra-operative opioids should be borne in mind when prescribing postoperative analgesics. In many instances they will delay the need for the first dose but caution is necessary since there may be some residual respiratory depression potentiated by the postoperative analgesic.

Fentanyl may produce severe respiratory depression, especially in patients with decreased respiratory function or when other respiratory depressant drugs have been given. Respiratory depression may be treated by artificial ventilation or be reversed by naloxone or doxapram (see above). Alfentanil may also cause severe respiratory depression, especially when other respiratory depressant drugs have already been given; this may be reversed with naloxone.

Meptazinol can be used for analgesia during or after operation. It is associated with nausea and vomiting, but is claimed to have a reduced incidence of respiratory depression.

For general notes on analgesics, see section 4.7.

ALFENTANIL

Indications: analgesia especially during short operative procedure and outpatient surgery; enhancement of anaesthesia; analgesia and suppression of respiratory activity in patients receiving intensive care with assisted ventilation, for up to 4 days

Cautions; Contra-indications; Side-effects: see section 4.7.2 and notes above

Dose: by intravenous injection, spontaneous respiration, ADULT, initially up to 500 micrograms over 30 seconds; supplemental, 250 micrograms

With assisted ventilation, ADULT and CHILD, initially 30–50 micrograms/kg; supplemental, 15 micrograms/kg

By intravenous infusion, with assisted ventilation, ADULT and CHILD, initially 50–100 micrograms/kg over 10 minutes *or* as a bolus, followed by maintenance of 0.5–1 micrograms/kg/minute

Analgesia and suppression of respiratory activity during intensive care, with assisted ventilation, *by intravenous infusion*, initially 2 mg/hour (approx. 30 micrograms/kg/hour) subsequently adjusted according to response (usual range 0.5–10 mg/hour); more rapid initial control may be obtained with an intravenous dose of 5 mg given in divided portions over 10 minutes (slowing if hypotension or bradycardia occur); additional doses of 0.5–1 mg may be given by intravenous injection during short painful procedures

CD Rapifen® (Janssen)

Injection, alfentanil 500 micrograms (as hydrochloride)/mL. Net price 2-mL amp = 72p; 10-mL amp = £3.31

Intensive care injection, alfentanil 5 mg (as hydrochloride)/mL. To be diluted before use. Net price 1-mL amp = £2.65

BUPRENORPHINE

Indications: peri-operative analgesia; premedication; analgesia in other situations, see section 4.7.2

Cautions; Contra-indications; Side-effects: see section 4.7.2; effects only partially reversed by naloxone

Dose: pain, *by slow intravenous injection*, 300–450 micrograms

Premedication, *by sublingual administration*, 400 micrograms

By intramuscular injection, 300 micrograms

Preparations
See section 4.7.2

FENTANYL

Indications: analgesia during operation, neuroleptanalgesia, enhancement of anaesthesia; respiratory depressant in assisted respiration

Cautions; Contra-indications; Side-effects: see section 4.7.2 and notes above

Dose: by intravenous injection, with spontaneous respiration, 50–200 micrograms, then 50 micrograms as required; CHILD 3–5 micrograms/kg, then 1 microgram/kg as required

With assisted ventilation, 0.3–3.5 mg, then 100–200 micrograms as required; CHILD 15 micrograms/kg, then 1–3 micrograms/kg as required

CD Sublimaze® (Janssen)

Injection, fentanyl 50 micrograms (as citrate)/mL. Net price 2-mL amp = 24p; 10-mL amp = £1.17
Available as a generic from David Bull, Evans

MEPTAZINOL

See section 4.7.2

MORPHINE SALTS

Indications: analgesia during and after operation; enhancement of anaesthesia; pre-operative sedation; analgesia in other situations, see section 4.7.2

Cautions; Contra-indications; Side-effects: see section 4.7.2 and notes above

Dose: by subcutaneous or intramuscular injection, up to 10 mg 1–1½ hours before operation; CHILD, *by intramuscular injection*, 150 micrograms/kg. See also section 4.7.2 for analgesia

CD Morphine Sulphate Injection, morphine sulphate, 10 mg/mL. Net price 1-mL amp = 51p; other strengths see section 4.7.2

CD Morphine and Atropine Injection, morphine sulphate 10 mg, atropine sulphate 600 micrograms/mL. Net price 1-mL amp = 73p
Dose: premedication, by subcutaneous injection, 0.5–1 mL

NALBUPHINE HYDROCHLORIDE

Indications: peri-operative analgesia; premedication; analgesia in other situations, see section 4.7.2

Cautions; Contra-indications; Side-effects: see section 4.7.2 and notes above; also caution in ambulant patients (impairment of mental and physical ability)

Dose: acute pain, *by subcutaneous, intramuscular, or intravenous injection,* 10–20 mg, adjusted according to response; CHILD up to 300 micrograms/kg repeated once or twice as necessary. See also section 4.7.2. for analgesia

Premedication, *by subcutaneous, intramuscular, or intravenous injection,* 100–200 micrograms/kg

Induction, *by intravenous injection,* 0.3–1 mg/kg over 10–15 minutes

Intra-operative analgesia, *by intravenous injection,* 250–500 micrograms /kg at 30-minute intervals

PoM Nubain® (Du Pont)
Injection, nalbuphine hydrochloride 10 mg/mL. Net price 1-mL amp = 73p; 2-mL amp = £1.13

PAPAVERETUM

IMPORTANT. Do not confuse with papaverine (see section 7.4.5)

A mixture of 253 parts of morphine hydrochloride, 23 parts of papaverine hydrochloride and 20 parts of codeine hydrochloride

REFORMULATION. *BP 1993, Amendments No. 1,* includes the following explanation concerning the reformulation of papaveretum: *papaveretum injection* contains the three alkaloids *morphine, papaverine* and *codeine;* in reformulating the injection to remove *noscapine,* the amounts of the other three alkaloids have been maintained; thus the total amount of material per mL has decreased. Before reformulation the *lower strength injection* (which provides *the equivalent of 5 mg of the major component, morphine*) contained 10 mg per mL of the four-component material; it now contains 7.7 mg of papaveretum per mL. Likewise, before reformulation the *higher strength injection* (which provides *the equivalent of 10 mg of morphine*) contained 20 mg per mL of the four-component material; it now contains 15.4 mg of papaveretum per mL. The CSM has advised that to avoid confusion the figures of 7.7 mg/mL or 15.4 mg/mL should be used for prescribing purposes.

Indications: postoperative analgesia; premedication

Cautions; Contra-indications; Side-effects: see section 4.7.2 and notes above

Dose: by subcutaneous, intramuscular, or intravenous injection, 7.7–15.4 mg repeated every 4 hours if necessary (ELDERLY initially 7.7 mg); CHILD up to 1 month 115.5 micrograms/kg, 1–12 months 115.5–154 micrograms/kg, 1–12 years 154–231 micrograms/kg

INTRAVENOUS DOSE. In general the intravenous dose should be quarter to half corresponding subcutaneous or intramuscular dose.

CD Papaveretum (Non-proprietary)
Injection, papaveretum 7.7 mg/mL (providing the equivalent of 5 mg of anhydrous morphine/mL). Net price 1-mL amp = 71p
Available from Martindale
Injection, papaveretum 15.4 mg/mL (providing the equivalent of 10 mg of anhydrous morphine/mL). Net price 1-mL amp = 13p
Available from Martindale, Roche (Omnopon®)

With hyoscine
CD Papaveretum and Hyoscine Injection,
papaveretum 15.4 mg (providing the equivalent of 10 mg of anhydrous morphine), hyoscine hydrobromide 400 micrograms/mL. Net price 1-mL amp = 83p
Dose: premedication, by subcutaneous or intramuscular injection, 0.5–1 mL

PETHIDINE HYDROCHLORIDE

Indications: peri-operative analgesia, enhancement of anaesthesia, for basal narcosis with phenothiazines; premedication; analgesia in other situations, see section 4.7.2

Cautions; Contra-indications; Side-effects: convulsions may occur with excessive doses; see section 4.7.2 and notes above

Dose: premedication, *by intramuscular injection,* 25–100 mg 1 hour before operation; CHILD 0.5–2 mg/kg

Adjunct to nitrous oxide–oxygen, *by slow intravenous injection,* 10–25 mg repeated when required

See also section 4.7.2 for analgesia

CD Pethidine (Non-proprietary)
Injection, pethidine hydrochloride 50 mg/mL, net price 1-mL amp = 11p; 2-mL amp = 14p; 10 mg/mL, 5-mL amp = 75p; 10-mL amp = 79p
Various strengths available from Martindale, Roche
Tablets, see section 4.7.2

With promethazine
CD Pamergan P100® (Martindale)
Injection, pethidine hydrochloride 50 mg, promethazine hydrochloride 25 mg/mL. Net price 2mL amp = 69p
Dose: premedication, 2 mL by intramuscular injection 1–1½ hours before operation; CHILD, by intramuscular injection, 8–12 years 0.75 mL, 13–16 years 1 mL

PHENOPERIDINE HYDROCHLORIDE

Indications: analgesia during operation, neuroleptanalgesia, enhancement of anaesthetics; respiratory depressant in prolonged assisted respiration

Cautions; Contra-indications; Side-effects: see under Pethidine Hydrochloride and Fentanyl. Doses above 1 mg cause respiratory depression and require assisted ventilation (effects may be terminated with naloxone)

Dose: by intravenous injection, with spontaneous respiration, up to 1 mg, then 500 micrograms every 40–60 minutes as required; CHILD 30–50 micrograms/kg

With assisted ventilation, 2–5 mg, then 1 mg as required; CHILD 100–150 micrograms/kg

CD Operidine® (Janssen)
Injection, phenoperidine hydrochloride 1 mg/mL. Net price 2-mL amp = 76p; 10-mL amp = £3.95

TRAMADOL HYDROCHLORIDE

See section 4.7.2

15.1.5   Muscle relaxants

Muscle relaxants used in anaesthesia are also known as **neuromuscular blocking drugs** or **myoneural blocking drugs**. By specific blockade of the neuromuscular junction they enable light levels of anaesthesia to be employed with adequate relaxation of the muscles of the abdomen and diaphragm. They also relax the vocal cords and allow the passage of a tracheal tube. Their action differs from the muscle relaxants acting on the spinal cord or brain which are used in musculoskeletal disorders (see section 10.2.2).

Patients who have received a muscle relaxant should **always** have their respiration assisted or controlled until the drug has been inactivated or antagonised (section 15.1.6).

NON-DEPOLARISING MUSCLE RELAXANTS

Drugs of this group (also known as competitive muscle relaxants) cause blockade by competing with acetylcholine at the receptor site at the neuromuscular junction. These drugs are best suited to the production of paralysis of long duration. They have a slower, less complete action than the depolarising muscle relaxants and should be avoided in myasthenia gravis.

These drugs may be used during surgical operations and for patients receiving long-term ventilation in intensive care units, when larger total doses will be appropriate.

The action of the competitive muscle relaxants may be reversed with anticholinesterases such as neostigmine (section 15.1.6).

Atracurium and **vecuronium** are much more widely employed than the other muscle relaxants, atracurium because of its non-enzymatic elimination and vecuronium because it has the fewest side-effects.

Atracurium has a duration of action of 15 to 35 minutes. Histamine release may occur. The drug is without vagolytic or sympatholytic properties. It has an advantage over other non-depolarising muscle relaxants in patients with renal or hepatic impairment, as it is degraded by non-enzymatic Hofmann elimination, which is independent of liver and kidney function. It is non-cumulative on repeated dosage. Its action is reversed by neostigmine. Duration of action may be prolonged in hypothermia.

Vecuronium has a duration of action of 20 to 30 minutes. Large doses may have a cumulative effect. The drug does not generally cause histamine release, sympathetic blockade, or vagolytic effects.

Pancuronium does not cause ganglionic blockade or significant changes in blood pressure and may therefore be favoured when it is important to maintain cardiac output.

Tubocurarine starts to act between 3–5 minutes and lasts for about 30 minutes after injection. It may cause an erythematous rash on the chest and neck and this is probably due to histamine release. Onset of blockade may be associated with hypotension and this, though transient, may be important in poor-risk patients.

Gallamine has a more rapid onset of action and recovery than tubocurarine or pancuronium. It causes undesirable tachycardia by its vagolytic action. It should be avoided in patients with severe renal disease.

Mivacurium is a new competitive muscle relaxant with a duration of action of about 15 minutes. Histamine release may occur particularly on rapid injection. It does not cause significant vagolytic effects. More prolonged muscle paralysis may occur in patients with low or atypical plasma pseudocholinesterase enzymes.

Rocuronium is a new competitive muscle relaxant reported to act within 1–2 minutes and to have a duration of action of 30 to 40 minutes. It is reported to be virtually free of cardiovascular effects.

ATRACURIUM BESYLATE

(Atracurium Besilate)

Indications: non-depolarising muscle relaxant of short to medium duration

Cautions; Contra-indications; Side-effects: see notes above; **interactions:** Appendix 1 (muscle relaxants)

Dose: by intravenous injection, ADULT and CHILD over 1 month initially 300–600 micrograms/kg, then 100–200 micrograms/kg as required

By intravenous infusion, 5–10 micrograms/kg/minute (300–600 micrograms/kg/hour)

PoM Tracrium® (Wellcome)
Injection, atracurium besylate 10 mg/mL. Net price 2.5-mL amp = £1.86; 5-mL amp = £3.38; 25-mL amp = £14.53

GALLAMINE TRIETHIODIDE

Indications: non-depolarising muscle relaxant of medium duration

Cautions; Contra-indications; Side-effects: see notes above; reduce dose in renal impairment (avoid if severe); **interactions:** Appendix 1 (muscle relaxants)

Dose: by intravenous injection, 80–120 mg, then 20–40 mg as required; NEONATE, 600 micrograms/kg; CHILD, 1.5 mg/kg

PoM **Flaxedil®** (Rhône-Poulenc Rorer)
Injection, gallamine triethiodide 40 mg/mL. Net price 2-mL amp = 72p

MIVACURIUM CHLORIDE

Indications: non-depolarising muscle relaxant of short duration

Cautions; Contra-indications; Side-effects: see notes above; **interactions:** Appendix 1 (muscle relaxants)

Dose: by intravenous injection, initially 70–150 micrograms/kg, then 100 micrograms/kg every 15 minutes; CHILD 2–12 years, initially, 100–200 micrograms/kg, then followed by 100 micrograms/kg every 6–7 minutes

Note. Recommended speed of injection is 5–15 seconds (up to 60 seconds in those with asthma or heart disease)

By intravenous infusion, maintenance of block, 8–10 micrograms/kg/minute, adjusted. if necessary every 3 minutes by 1 microgram/kg/minute to usual dose of 6–7 micrograms/kg/minute; CHILD 2–12 years, usual dose 10–15 micrograms/kg/minute

▼ PoM **Mivacron®** (Wellcome)
Injection, mivacurium 2 mg/mL (as chloride), net price 5-mL amp = £2.86; 10-mL amp = £4.62

PANCURONIUM BROMIDE

Indications: non-depolarising muscle relaxant of medium duration

Cautions; Contra-indications; Side-effects: see notes above; caution in hepatic impairment; reduce dose in renal impairment; **interactions:** Appendix 1 (muscle relaxants)

Dose: by intravenous injection, initially for intubation 50–100 micrograms/kg then 10–20 micrograms/kg as required; CHILD initially 60–100 micrograms/kg, then 10–20 micrograms/kg, NEONATE 30–40 micrograms/kg initially then 10–20 micrograms/kg

Intensive care, *by intravenous injection,* 60 micrograms/kg every 1–1½ hours

PoM **Pavulon®** (Organon-Teknika)
Injection, pancuronium bromide 2 mg/mL. Net price 2-mL amp = 66p
Available as a generic from David Bull

ROCURONIUM BROMIDE

Indications: non-depolarising muscle relaxant of medium duration

Cautions; Contra-indications; Side-effects: see notes above; caution in hepatic and renal impairment; **Interactions:** Appendix 1 (muscle relaxants)

Dose: by intravenous injection, intubation, 600 micrograms/kg; maintenance, 150 micrograms/kg

By intravenous infusion, 300–600 micrograms/kg/hour (after initial intravenous injection of 600 micrograms/kg)

▼ PoM **Esmeron®** (Organon-Teknika)
Injection, rocuronium bromide 10 mg/mL, net price 5-mL amp = £5.33, 10-mL amp = £10.67

TUBOCURARINE CHLORIDE

Indications: non-depolarising muscle relaxant of medium to long duration

Cautions; Contra-indications; Side-effects: see notes above. Reduce dose in renal impairment; **interactions:** Appendix 1 (muscle relaxants)

Dose: by intravenous injection, initially 15–30 mg according to circumstances then 5–10 mg as required; CHILD, initially 300–500 micrograms/kg then 60–100 micrograms/kg as required; NEONATE initially 200–250 micrograms/kg then 40–50 micrograms/kg as required

PoM **Jexin®** (Evans)
Injection, tubocurarine chloride 10 mg/mL. Net price 1.5-mL amp = 71p

VECURONIUM BROMIDE

Indications: non-depolarising muscle relaxant of short to medium duration

Cautions; Contra-indications; Side-effects: see notes above; reduce dose in renal impairment; **Interactions:** Appendix 1 (muscle relaxants)

Dose: by intravenous injection, intubation, 80–100 micrograms/kg; maintenance 20–30 micrograms/kg according to response; NEONATE and INFANT up to 4 months, initially 10–20 micrograms/kg then incremental doses to achieve response; CHILD over 5 months, as adult dose (up to 1 year onset more rapid and high intubation dose may not be required)

By intravenous infusion, 50–80 micrograms/kg/hour (after initial intravenous injection of 40–100 micrograms/kg)

PoM **Norcuron®** (Organon-Teknika)
Injection, powder for reconstitution, vecuronium bromide. Net price 10-mg vial = £4.23 (with water for injections)

Cautionary label wordings, see inside back cover   Prices are **net**, see p.1

DEPOLARISING MUSCLE RELAXANTS

Suxamethonium is the only commonly used drug of this group. With a 5-minute duration of action it is ideal for passage of a tracheal tube but may be used in repeated dosage for longer procedures.

It acts by mimicking acetylcholine at the neuromuscular junction but disengagement from the receptor site and subsequent breakdown is slower than for acetylcholine; depolarisation is therefore prolonged and neuromuscular blockade results.

It produces rapid, complete, and predictable paralysis, and recovery is spontaneous. Unlike the non-depolarising muscle relaxants its action cannot be reversed and clinical application is therefore limited.

Suxamethonium should be given after induction of anaesthesia because paralysis is usually preceded by painful muscle fasciculation. There is a transient rise in plasma potassium and creatine phosphokinase and there may be muscle pains postoperatively. Suxamethonium is **contra-indicated** in severe liver disease and in burned patients. Premedication with atropine is desirable.

Prolonged muscle paralysis may occur in patients with low or atypical plasma pseudocholinesterase enzymes. Prolonged paralysis may also occur in **dual block**, which occurs after repeated doses of suxamethonium have been used and is caused by the development of a non-depolarising block following the primary depolarising block. Artificial ventilation should be continued until muscle function is restored. Dual block is diagnosed by giving a short-acting anticholinesterase such as edrophonium; if an improvement occurs the block is treated with neostigmine (section 15.1.6).

SUXAMETHONIUM CHLORIDE

Indications: depolarising muscle relaxant of short duration

Cautions; Contra-indications; Side-effects: see notes above; **interactions:** Appendix 1 (muscle relaxants)

Dose: by intravenous injection, 600 micrograms/kg (range 0.3–1.1 mg/kg depending on degree of relaxation required); usual range 20–100 mg

By intravenous infusion, as a 0.1% solution, 2–5 mg/minute (2–5 mL/minute)

PoM **Anectine**® (Wellcome)
Injection, suxamethonium chloride 50 mg/mL. Net price 2-mL amp = 73p
PoM **Scoline**® (Evans)
Injection, suxamethonium chloride 50 mg/mL. Net price 2-mL amp = 31p

15.1.6   Anticholinesterases used in surgery

Anticholinesterases reverse the effects of the non-depolarising (competitive) muscle relaxant drugs such as tubocurarine but they prolong the action of the depolarising muscle relaxant drug suxamethonium.

Edrophonium has a transient action and is used to diagnose dual block caused by suxamethonium (section 15.1.5).

Neostigmine has a longer duration of action than edrophonium. It is the specific drug for reversal of non-depolarising (competitive) blockade. It acts within one minute of intravenous injection and lasts for 20 to 30 minutes; a second dose may then be necessary. It is also used in the treatment of dual block. Atropine or glycopyrronium (section 15.1.3) should be given before or with neostigmine in order to prevent bradycardia, excessive salivation, and other muscarinic actions of neostigmine.

EDROPHONIUM CHLORIDE

Indications: see under Dose

Cautions; Contra-indications; Side-effects: see section 10.2.1 and notes above. Atropine should also be given

Dose: brief reversal of non-depolarising neuromuscular blockade, *by intravenous injection* over several minutes, 500–700 micrograms/kg (after or with atropine sulphate 600 micrograms)

Diagnosis of dual block, *by intravenous injection,* 10 mg (with atropine)

Diagnosis of myasthenia gravis, section 10.2.1

PoM **Camsilon**[1]® (Cambridge)
Injection, edrophonium chloride 10 mg/mL. Net price 1-mL amp = £1.01
1. Formerly Tensilon®

NEOSTIGMINE METHYLSULPHATE

Indications: see under Dose

Cautions; Contra-indications; Side-effects: see section 10.2.1 and notes above. Atropine should also be given

Dose: reversal of non-depolarising neuromuscular blockade, *by intravenous injection* over 1 minute, 50–70 micrograms/kg (max. 5 mg) after or with atropine sulphate 0.6–1.2 mg

Myasthenia gravis, see section 10.2.1

PoM **Prostigmin**® (Roche)
Injection, neostigmine methylsulphate 500 micrograms/mL, net price 1-mL amp = 16p; 2.5 mg/mL, 1-mL amp = 16p

With glycopyrronium
PoM **Robinul-Neostigmine**® (Wyeth)
Injection, neostigmine methylsulphate 2.5 mg, glycopyrronium bromide 500 micrograms/mL. Net price 1-mL amp = 53p
Dose: by intravenous injection over 10–30 seconds, 1–2 mL *or* 0.02 mL/kg; CHILD 0.02 mL/kg (*or* 0.2 mL/kg of a 1 in 10 dilution using water for injections or sodium chloride injection 0.9%)

15.1.7   Antagonists for central and respiratory depression

The opioid antagonist **naloxone** can be used to reverse respiratory depression caused by opioid analgesics. Unless the dosage is carefully adjusted, analgesia may also be reversed. **Doxapram** is a respiratory stimulant which does not reverse the other effects of opioid analgesics.

Flumazenil is a benzodiazepine antagonist for the reversal of the central sedative effects of benzodiazepines in anaesthetic and similar procedures. It is important to recognize that the half-life of flumazenil is shorter than those of diazepam and midazolam, in order to avoid the risk of patients becoming resedated.

DOXAPRAM HYDROCHLORIDE

Indications: see under Dose

Cautions; Contra-indications; Side-effects: see section 3.5.1

Dose: postoperative respiratory depression, *by intravenous injection* over at least 30 seconds, 1–1.5 mg/kg repeated if necessary after intervals of 1 hour

By intravenous infusion, 2–3 mg/minute adjusted according to response

Ventilatory failure, see section 3.5.1

PoM **Dopram**® (Wyeth)
Injection, doxapram hydrochloride 20 mg/mL. Net price 5-mL amp = £1.07
Intravenous infusion: see section 3.5.1

FLUMAZENIL

Indications: reversal of sedative effects of benzodiazepines in anaesthetic, intensive care, and diagnostic procedures

Cautions: short-acting (repeat doses may be necessary—benzodiazepine effects may persist for at least 24 hours); benzodiazepine dependence (may precipitate withdrawal symptoms); ensure neuromuscular blockade cleared before giving; avoid rapid injection in high-risk or anxious patients and following major surgery; hepatic impairment; severe head injury (rapid reversal of benzodiazepine sedation may increase risk of raised intracranial pressure); elderly, children, pregnancy and breast-feeding

Contra-indications: epileptics who have received prolonged benzodiazepine therapy

Side-effects: nausea, vomiting, and flushing; if wakening too rapid, agitation, anxiety, and fear; transient increase in blood pressure and heart-rate in intensive care patients; very rarely convulsions (particularly in epileptics)

Dose: by intravenous injection, 200 micrograms over 15 seconds, then 100 micrograms at 60-second intervals if required; usual dose range, 300–600 micrograms; max. total dose 1 mg (2 mg in intensive care); question aetiology if no response to repeated doses

By intravenous infusion, if drowsiness recurs after injection, 100–400 micrograms/hour, adjusted according to level of arousal

PoM **Anexate**® (Roche)
Injection, flumazenil 100 micrograms/mL. Net price 5-mL amp = £16.32

NALOXONE HYDROCHLORIDE

Indications: reversal of opioid-induced respiratory depression

Cautions: cardiovascular disease or those receiving cardiotoxic drugs (serious adverse cardiovascular effects); physical dependence on opioids (precipitates withdrawal); has short duration of action

Dose: by intravenous injection, 100–200 micrograms (1.5–3 micrograms/kg); if response inadequate, increments of 100 micrograms every 2 minutes; further doses *by intramuscular injection* after 1–2 hours if required

CHILD, *by intravenous injection,* 10 micrograms/kg; subsequent dose of 100 micrograms/kg if no response; if intravenous route not possible, may be given in divided doses by *intramuscular or subcutaneous injection*

NEONATE, *by subcutaneous, intramuscular, or intravenous injection,* 10 micrograms/kg, repeated every 2 to 3 minutes *or* 200 micrograms (60 micrograms/kg) *by intramuscular injection* as a single dose at birth (onset of action slower)

PoM **Naloxone Hydrochloride** (Non-proprietary)
Injection, naloxone hydrochloride 20 micrograms/mL. Net price 2-mL amp = £3.57

Injection, naloxone hydrochloride 400 micrograms/mL—see under Emergency Treatment of Poisoning p.21

PoM **Narcan**®—see under Emergency Treatment of Poisoning p.21

PoM **Narcan Neonatal**® (Du Pont)
Injection, naloxone hydrochloride 20 micrograms/mL. Net price 2-mL amp = £3.48

15.1.8 Antagonists for malignant hyperthermia

Dantrolene is used in the treatment of malignant hyperthermia which is a rare but lethal complication of anaesthesia. It is characterised by a rapid rise in temperature, increasing muscle rigidity, tachycardia, and acidosis and can be triggered off by volatile anaesthetics, especially halothane, and suxamethonium. Dantrolene acts on skeletal muscle by interfering with calcium efflux in the muscle cell and stopping the contractile process. Known trigger agents should be avoided during anaesthesia.

DANTROLENE SODIUM

Indications: malignant hyperthermia

Cautions: avoid extravasation; **interactions:** Appendix 1 (muscle relaxants)

Dose: by rapid intravenous injection, 1 mg/kg, repeated as required to a cumulative max. of 10 mg/kg

PoM **Dantrium Intravenous**® (Procter & Gamble Pharm.)
Injection, powder for reconstitution, dantrolene sodium. Net price 20-mg vial = £22.52 (hosp. only)

15.2   Local anaesthesia

The use of local anaesthetics by injection or by application to mucous membranes to produce local analgesia is discussed in this section.

See also section 1.7 (colon and rectum), section 11.7 (eye), section 12.3 (oropharynx), and section 13.3 (skin).

USE OF LOCAL ANAESTHETICS. Local anaesthetic drugs act by causing a reversible block to conduction along nerve fibres. The smaller the nerve fibre the more sensitive it is so that a differential block may occur where the smaller fibres carrying pain sensation and automatic impulses are blocked, sparing coarse touch and movement. The drugs used vary widely in their potency, toxicity, duration of action, stability, solubility in water, and ability to penetrate mucous membranes. These variations determine their suitability for use by various routes, e.g. topical (surface), infiltration, plexus, epidural (extradural) or spinal block.

ADMINISTRATION. In estimating the safe dosage of these drugs it is important to take account of the rate at which they are absorbed and excreted as well as their potency. The patient's age, weight, physique, and clinical condition, the degree of vascularity of the area to which the drug is to be applied, and the duration of administration are other factors which must be taken into account.

Local anaesthetics do not rely on the circulation to transport them to their sites of action, but uptake into the general circulation is important in terminating their action. Following most regional anaesthetic procedures, maximum arterial plasma concentrations of anaesthetic develop within about 10 to 25 minutes, so careful surveillance for toxic effects is necessary during the first 30 minutes after injection.

Epidural anaesthesia is commonly used during surgery, often combined with general anaesthesia, because of its protective effect against the stress response of surgery. It is often used when good postoperative pain relief is essential (e.g. aortic aneurysm surgery or major gut surgery).

TOXICITY. Toxic effects associated with the local anaesthetics are usually a result of excessively high plasma concentrations. The main effects are excitation of the central nervous system (nervousness, nausea, and convulsions) followed by depression. Less commonly the cardiovascular system is depressed. Hypersensitivity reactions occur mainly with the ester-type local anaesthetics such as amethocaine, benzocaine, cocaine, and procaine; reactions are less frequent with the amide types such as lignocaine, bupivacaine, and prilocaine.

USE OF VASOCONSTRICTORS. Toxicity may occur with repeated dosages due to accumulation of the drug, and reducing doses should therefore be given. Toxic effects may also occur if the injection is too rapid. Local anaesthetics should **not** be injected into inflamed or infected tissues nor should they be

applied to the traumatised urethra. Under these conditions the drug may be so rapidly absorbed that a systemic rather than a local reaction is produced.

Most local anaesthetics, with the exception of cocaine, cause dilatation of blood vessels. The addition of a vasoconstrictor such as **adrenaline** diminishes local blood flow, slows the rate of absorption of the local anaesthetic, and prolongs its local effect. Care is necessary when using adrenaline for this purpose because, in excess, it may produce ischaemic necrosis.

Adrenaline should **not** be added to injections used in digits and appendages. When adrenaline is included in an injection of lignocaine or procaine the final concentration should be 1 in 200 000. In dental surgery, up to 1 in 80 000 of adrenaline is used with local anaesthetics. There is no justification for using higher concentrations.

The total dose of adrenaline should **not** exceed 500 micrograms and it is essential not to exceed a concentration of 1 in 200 000 if more than 50 mL of the mixture is to be injected. For general cautions associated with the use of adrenaline, see section 2.7. For drug interactions, see Appendix 1 (sympathomimetics).

LIGNOCAINE

Lignocaine is the most widely used local anaesthetic drug. It acts more rapidly and is more stable than most other local anaesthetics. It is effectively absorbed from mucous membranes and is a useful surface anaesthetic in concentrations of 2 to 4%. Except for surface anaesthesia, solutions should not usually exceed 1% in strength. The duration of the block (with adrenaline) is about 1½ hours.

LIGNOCAINE HYDROCHLORIDE
(Lidocaine Hydrochloride)

Indications: see under Dose; also dental anaesthesia; ventricular arrhythmias (section 2.3.2)

Cautions: epilepsy, hepatic or respiratory impairment, impaired cardiac conduction, bradycardia; porphyria (see section 9.8.2); reduce dose in elderly or debilitated; resuscitative equipment should be available; see section 2.3.2 for effects on heart; **interactions:** Appendix 1 (lignocaine)

Contra-indications: hypovolaemia, complete heart block; do not use solutions containing adrenaline for anaesthesia in appendages

Side-effects: CNS effects include confusion, respiratory depression and convulsions; hypotension and bradycardia (may lead to cardiac arrest); hypersensitivity reported; see also notes above

Dose: adjusted according to site of operation and response of patient

By injection, max. dose 200 mg, or 500 mg with solutions which also contain adrenaline. Max. dose of adrenaline 500 micrograms (see also notes above)

Infiltration anaesthesia, 0.25–0.5%, with adrenaline 1 in 200 000, using 2–50 mL of a 0.5% solution in minor surgery and up to 60 mL in more extensive surgery

---

Nerve blocks, with adrenaline 1 in 200 000, 1% to a max. of 50 mL, 2% to a max. of 25 mL

Epidural and caudal block, with adrenaline 1 in 200 000, 1% to a max. of 50 mL, 2% to a max. of 25 mL

Surface anaesthesia, usual strengths 2–4%. Mouth, throat, and upper gastro-intestinal tract, max. 200 mg

Lignocaine hydrochloride injections

PoM Lignocaine (Non-proprietary)

Injection 0.5%, lignocaine hydrochloride 5 mg/mL, net price 10-mL amp = 22p

Injection 1%, lignocaine hydrochloride 10 mg/mL, net price 2-mL amp = 11p; 5-mL amp = 16p; 10-mL amp = 29p; 20-mL amp = 40p

Injection 2%, lignocaine hydrochloride 20 mg/mL, net price 2-mL amp = 17p; 5-mL amp = 19p

PoM Min-I-Jet® Lignocaine Hydrochloride with Adrenaline (IMS)

Injection, lignocaine hydrochloride 5 mg/mL, adrenaline 1 in 200 000 (5 micrograms/mL). Net price 5-mL disposable syringe = £3.88

PoM Xylocaine® (Astra)

Injection 0.5%, anhydrous lignocaine hydrochloride 5 mg/mL. Net price 20-mL vial = 67p

Injection 0.5% with adrenaline 1 in 200 000, anhydrous lignocaine hydrochloride 5 mg/mL, adrenaline 1 in 200 000. Net price 20-mL vial = 69p

Injection 1%, anhydrous lignocaine hydrochloride 10 mg/mL. Net price 20-mL vial = 69p

Injection 1% with adrenaline 1 in 200 000, anhydrous lignocaine hydrochloride 10 mg/mL, adrenaline 1 in 200 000. Net price 20-mL vial = 71p

Injection 2%, anhydrous lignocaine hydrochloride 20 mg/mL. Net price 20-mL vial = 73p

Injection 2% with adrenaline 1 in 200 000, anhydrous lignocaine hydrochloride 20 mg/mL, adrenaline 1 in 200 000. Net price 20-mL vial = 75p

Lignocaine injections for dental use

A large variety of lignocaine injections, plain or with adrenaline or noradrenaline, is also available in dental cartridges under the names **Lignostab®**, **Xylocaine®**, and **Xylotox®**.

Lignocaine for surface anaesthesia

Note. Local anaesthetic ointments can be absorbed through the rectal mucosa therefore excessive application should be avoided, particularly in infants and children

PoM Emla® (Astra)

Drug Tariff cream, lignocaine 2.5%, prilocaine 2.5%. Net price 5-g tube = £1.73

Surgical pack cream, lignocaine 2.5%, prilocaine 2.5%. Net price 30-g tube = £10.25

Premedication pack cream, lignocaine 2.5%, prilocaine 2.5%. Net price 10 × 5-g tube with 25 occlusive dressings = £19.50

Anaesthesia before e.g. venepuncture (not for infants), apply a thick layer under an occlusive dressing 1–5 hours before procedure; split skin grafting, apply a thick layer under an occlusive dressing 2–5 hours before procedure; genital warts (not for children), apply up to 10 g 5–10 minutes before removal

Cautions: not for wounds, mucous membranes (except genital warts in adults) or atopic dermatitis; avoid use near eyes or middle ear; side-effects include transient paleness, redness, and oedema

Instillagel® (CliniFlex)

Gel, lignocaine hydrochloride 2%, chlorhexidine gluconate solution 0.25%, in a sterile lubricant basis in disposable syringe. Net price 6-mL syringe = £1.24; 11-mL syringe = £1.39

Dose: 6–11 mL into urethra

Xylocaine® (Astra)

Antiseptic gel, anhydrous lignocaine hydrochloride 2%, chlorhexidine gluconate solution 0.25% in a sterile lubricant basis. Net price 20 g = £1.09; 20-g single-use syringe (Accordion®) = 98p

Dose: into urethra, men 10 mL followed by 3–5 mL; women 5–10 mL

Gel, anhydrous lignocaine hydrochloride 2%, in a sterile lubricant water-miscible basis. Net price 20 g = 78p; 20-g single-use syringe (Accordion®) = 98p

Dose:

Into urethra, men 10 mL, followed by further 10 mL (total of up to 40 mL for cystoscopy); women 5–10 mL

Endoscopy, 10–20 mL

Endotracheal intubation, 5 mL applied to surface of tube (avoid introducing gel into lumen)

Ointment, lignocaine 5% in a water-miscible basis. Net price 15 g = 83p

Dose: max. 35 g in 24 hours

Spray (= pump spray), lignocaine 10% (100 mg/g) supplying 10 mg lignocaine/dose; 500 spray doses per container. Net price 50-mL bottle = £3.21

Dose: dental practice, 1–5 doses; maxillary sinus puncture, 3 doses; during delivery in obstetrics, up to 20 doses; procedures in pharynx, larynx, and trachea, up to 20 doses

Topical 4%, anhydrous lignocaine hydrochloride 40 mg/mL. Net price 30-mL bottle = £1.24

Dose: bronchoscopy, 2–3 mL with suitable spray; biopsy in mouth, 3–4 mL with suitable spray *or* swab (with adrenaline if necessary); max. 7.5 mL

BUPIVACAINE

The great advantage of bupivacaine over other local anaesthetics is its duration of action of up to 8 hours when used for nerve blocks. It has a slow onset of action, taking up to 30 minutes for full effect. It is often used in lumbar epidural blockade and is particularly suitable for continuous epidural analgesia in labour; it then has a 2- to 3-hour duration of action. It is **contra-indicated** in intravenous regional anaesthesia (Bier's block). It is the principal drug for spinal anaesthesia in the UK.

BUPIVACAINE HYDROCHLORIDE

Indications: see under Dose

Cautions; Contra-indications; Side-effects: see under Lignocaine Hydrochloride and notes above; myocardial depression may be more severe and more resistant to treatment; contra-indicated in intravenous regional anaesthesia (Bier's block); **interactions:** Appendix 1 (bupivacaine)

Dose: adjusted according to site of operation and response of patient

Local infiltration, 0.25% (up to 60 mL)

Peripheral nerve block, 0.25% (max. 60 mL), 0.5% (max. 30 mL)

Epidural block,

 Surgery, *lumbar,* 0.5–0.75% (max. 20 mL of either)

  caudal, 0.5% (max. 30 mL)

 Labour, *lumbar,* 0.25–0.5% (max. 12 mL of either)

  caudal, 0.25% (max. 30 mL), 0.5% (max. 20 mL)

Note. 0.75% **contra-indicated** for epidural use in obstetrics.

PoM Marcain Heavy® (Astra)

Injection, anhydrous bupivacaine hydrochloride 5 mg, glucose 80 mg/mL. Net price 4-ml amp = £1.00

Dose: spinal anaesthesia, 2–4 mL

PoM Marcain® (Astra)

Injection, anhydrous bupivacaine hydrochloride 2.5 mg/mL (*Marcain®* 0.25%), net price 10-mL amp = £1.13; 5 mg/mL (*Marcain®* 0.5%), 10-mL amp = £1.30; 7.5 mg/mL (*Marcain®* 0.75%), 10-mL amp = £1.95. Marcain® 0.25, 0.5 and 0.75% also available as 10-mL polyamps

Note. Bupivacaine hydrochloride injection 0.25% and 0.5% also available from David Bull

PoM Marcain with Adrenaline® (Astra)

Injection 0.25%, bupivacaine hydrochloride 2.5 mg/mL, adrenaline 1 in 200 000. Net price 10-mL amp = £1.27

Injection 0.5%, bupivacaine hydrochloride 5 mg/mL, adrenaline 1 in 200 000. Net price 10-mL amp = £1.43

PRILOCAINE

Prilocaine is a local anaesthetic of low toxicity which is similar to lignocaine. If used in high doses, methaemoglobinaemia may occur which can be treated with intravenous injection of methylene blue 1% using a dose of 1 mg/kg.

PRILOCAINE HYDROCHLORIDE

Indications: infiltration, intravenous regional anaesthesia, nerve block; also dental anaesthesia

Cautions; Contra-indications; Side-effects: see under Lignocaine Hydrochloride and notes above; avoid in anaemia or congenital or acquired methaemoglobinaemia

Dose: adjusted according to site of operation and response of patient, to max. 400 mg used alone, or 600 mg if used with felypressin

PoM Citanest® (Astra)

Injection 0.5%, prilocaine hydrochloride 5 mg/mL. Net price 20-mL multidose vial = 73p; 50-mL multidose vial = £1.02; 50-mL single dose vial = £1.30

Injection 1%, prilocaine hydrochloride 10 mg/mL. Net price 20-mL multidose vial = 75p; 50-mL multidose vial = £1.06

Injection 2%, prilocaine hydrochloride 20 mg/mL. Net price 10-mL single dose vial = 75p

Injection 4%, prilocaine hydrochloride 40 mg/mL. Net price 2-mL cartridge = 13p

PoM Citanest with Octapressin® (Astra)

Injection 3%, prilocaine hydrochloride 30 mg/mL, felypressin 0.03 unit/mL. For dental use. Net price 2-mL cartridge and self-aspirating cartridge (both) = 13p

PROCAINE

Procaine is now seldom used. It is as potent an anaesthetic as lignocaine but has a shorter duration of action. It provides less intense analgesia because it has less tendency to spread through the tissues. It is poorly absorbed from mucous membranes and is of no value as a surface anaesthetic. When used for infiltration or regional anaesthesia, adrenaline 1 in 200 000 is generally added. Its metabolite para-aminobenzoic acid inhibits the action of the sulphonamides.

PROCAINE HYDROCHLORIDE

Indications: local anaesthesia by infiltration and regional routes (but see notes above)

Cautions; Side-effects: see notes above

Dose: adjusted according to site of operation and patient's response

By injection, up to 1 g (200 mL of 0.5% solution or 100 mL of 1%) with adrenaline 1 in 200 000

PoM Procaine Injection, procaine hydrochloride 2% (20 mg/mL) in sodium chloride intravenous infusion. Net price 2-mL amp = 57p

OTHER LOCAL ANAESTHETICS

Amethocaine is an effective local anaesthetic for topical application. It is rapidly absorbed from mucous membranes and should **never** be applied to inflamed, traumatised, or highly vascular surfaces. It should **never** be used to provide anaesthesia for bronchoscopy or cystoscopy, as lignocaine is a safer alternative. It is used in ophthalmology (see section 11.7) and in skin preparations (see section 13.3). Hypersensitivity to amethocaine has been reported.

Benzocaine is a local anaesthetic of low potency and toxicity. It is an ingredient of some proprietary throat lozenges (see section 12.3.3).

Cocaine readily penetrates mucous membranes and is an effective surface anaesthetic with an intense vasoconstrictor action. However, apart from its use in otolaryngology (see below), it has now been replaced by less toxic alternatives. It has marked sympathomimetic activity and should

---

never be given by injection because of its toxicity. As a result of its intense stimulant effect on the central nervous system it is a drug of addiction. Cocaine is still used in otolaryngology and is applied to the nasal mucosa in concentrations of 4 to 10% (40–100 mg/mL). The maximum total dose recommended for application to the nasal mucosa in fit adults is a total of 1.5 mg/kg, which is equivalent to a total topical dose of approximately 100 mg for an adult male. It should be used only by those skilled in the precautions needed to *minimise absorption*

and the *consequent risk of arrhythmias*. Although cocaine interacts with other drugs liable to induce arrhythmias, including adrenaline, some otolaryngologists consider that combined use of topical cocaine with topical adrenaline (in the form of a paste or a solution), improves the operative field and may possibly reduce absorption. Cocaine is a mydriatic as well as a local anaesthetic but owing to corneal toxicity it is now little used in ophthalmology (see section 11.7). Cocaine should be avoided in porphyria (see section 9.8.2).

Appendix 1: Interactions

Two or more drugs given at the same time may exert their effects independently or may interact. The interaction may be potentiation or antagonism of one drug by another, or occasionally some other effect. Adverse drug interactions should be reported to the CSM as for other adverse drug reactions.

Drug interactions may be **pharmacodynamic** or **pharmacokinetic**.

PHARMACODYNAMIC INTERACTIONS

These are interactions between drugs which have similar or antagonistic pharmacological effects or side-effects. They may be due to competition at receptor sites, or occur between drugs acting on the same physiological system. They are usually predictable from a knowledge of the pharmacology of the interacting drugs; in general, those demonstrated with one drug are likely to occur with related drugs. They occur to a greater or lesser extent in most patients who receive the interacting drugs.

PHARMACOKINETIC INTERACTIONS

These occur when one drug alters the absorption, distribution, metabolism, or excretion of another, thus increasing or reducing the amount of drug available to produce its pharmacological effects. They are not easily predicted and many of them affect only a small proportion of patients taking the combination of drugs. Pharmacokinetic interactions occurring with one drug cannot be assumed to occur with related drugs unless their pharmacokinetic properties are known to be similar.

Pharmacokinetic interactions are of several types:

AFFECTING ABSORPTION. The rate of absorption or the total amount absorbed can both be altered by drug interactions. Delayed absorption is rarely of clinical importance unless high peak plasma concentrations are required (e.g. when giving an analgesic). Reduction in the total amount absorbed, however, may result in ineffective therapy.

DUE TO CHANGES IN PROTEIN BINDING. To a variable extent most drugs are loosely bound to plasma proteins. Protein-binding sites are non-specific and one drug can displace another thereby increasing its proportion free to diffuse from plasma to its site of action. This only produces a detectable increase in effect if it is an extensively bound drug (more than 90%) that is not widely distributed throughout the body. Even so displacement rarely produces more than transient potentiation because this increased concentration of free drug results in an increased rate of elimination.

Displacement from protein binding plays a part in the potentiation of warfarin by phenylbutazone, sulphonamides, and tolbutamide but the importance of these interactions is due mainly to the fact that warfarin metabolism is also inhibited.

AFFECTING METABOLISM. Many drugs are metabolised in the liver. Induction of the hepatic microsomal enzyme system by one drug can gradually increase the rate of metabolism of another, resulting in lower plasma concentrations and a reduced effect. On withdrawal of the inducer plasma concentrations increase and toxicity may occur. Barbiturates, griseofulvin, most antiepileptics, and rifampicin are the most important enzyme inducers in man. Drugs affected include warfarin and the oral contraceptives.

Conversely when one drug inhibits the metabolism of another higher plasma concentrations are produced, rapidly resulting in an increased effect with risk of toxicity. Some drugs which potentiate warfarin and phenytoin do so by this mechanism.

AFFECTING RENAL EXCRETION. Drugs are eliminated through the kidney both by glomerular filtration and by active tubular secretion. Competition occurs between those which share active transport mechanisms in the proximal tubule. Thus probenecid delays the excretion of many drugs including penicillins, some cephalosporins, indomethacin, and dapsone; aspirin may increase the toxicity of methotrexate by a similar mechanism.

RELATIVE IMPORTANCE OF INTERACTIONS

Many drug interactions are harmless and many of those which are potentially harmful only occur in a small proportion of patients; moreover, the severity of an interaction varies from one patient to another. Drugs with a small therapeutic ratio (e.g. phenytoin) and those which require careful control of dosage (e.g. anticoagulants, antihypertensives, and antidiabetics) are most often involved.

Patients at increased risk from drug interactions include the elderly and those with impaired renal or liver function.

HAZARDOUS INTERACTIONS. The symbol • has been placed against interactions that are **potentially hazardous** and where combined administration of the drugs involved should be **avoided** (or only undertaken with caution and appropriate monitoring).

Interactions that have no symbol do not usually have serious consequences.

List of drug interactions

The following is an alphabetical list of drugs and their interactions; to avoid excessive cross-referencing each drug or group is listed twice: in the alphabetical list and also against the drug or group with which it interacts; changes in the interactions lists since BNF No. 27 (March 1994) are <u>underlined</u>.

For explanation of symbol • see previous page

Acarbose
  Anion-exchange Resins: *cholestyramine* enhances hypoglycaemic effect of *acarbose*
  Pancreatin: hypoglycaemic effect of *acarbose* reduced by *pancreatin*

ACE Inhibitors
  Alcohol: enhanced hypotensive effect
  Aldesleukin: enhanced hypotensive effect
  <u>Allopurinol</u>: increased risk of toxicity with *captopril*, especially in renal impairment
• Anaesthetics: enhanced hypotensive effect
• Analgesics: antagonism of hypotensive effect and increased risk of renal failure with *NSAIDs*; hyperkalaemia with *indomethacin and possibly other NSAIDs*
  Antacids: absorption of *fosinopril* reduced
  <u>Anti-arrhythmics</u>: *procainamide* increases risk of toxicity with *captopril*, especially in renal impairment
  Antibacterials: absorption of *tetracyclines* reduced by *quinapril* (tablets contain magnesium carbonate excipient)
  Antidepressants: enhanced hypotensive effect
  <u>Antidiabetics</u>: hypoglycaemic effect possibly enhanced
  other Antihypertensives: enhanced hypotensive effect
  Antipsychotics: severe postural hypotension with *chlorpromazine and possibly other phenothiazines*
  Anxiolytics and Hypnotics: enhanced hypotensive effect
  Beta-blockers: enhanced hypotensive effect
  Calcium-channel Blockers: enhanced hypotensive effect
  Cardiac Glycosides: plasma concentration of *digoxin* possibly increased by *captopril*
  Corticosteroids: antagonism of hypotensive effect
• Cyclosporin: increased risk of hyperkalaemia
• Diuretics: enhanced hypotensive effect (can be extreme); hyperkalaemia with *potassium-sparing diuretics*
  Dopaminergics: *levodopa* enhances hypotensive effect
• Lithium: *ACE inhibitors* reduce excretion of *lithium* (increased plasma-lithium concentration)
  Muscle Relaxants: *baclofen* enhances hypotensive effect
  Nitrates: enhance hypotensive effect
  Oestrogens and Progestogens: *oestrogens and combined oral contraceptives* antagonise hypotensive effect
• Potassium Salts: hyperkalaemia
  Sympathomimetics: *see* Sympathomimetics (main list)
  Ulcer-healing Drugs: *carbenoxolone* antagonises hypotensive effect
  Uricosurics: *probenecid* reduces excretion of *captopril*

Acebutolol *see* Beta-blockers
Acemetacin *see* NSAIDs
Acetazolamide (general hypokalaemic interactions *as for* Diuretics)
  Analgesics: *aspirin* reduces excretion of *acetazolamide* (risk of toxicity)
  Anti-arrhythmics: excretion of *quinidine* reduced in alkaline urine (occasionally increased plasma concentrations)
  Antiepileptics: *phenytoin* possibly increases risk of osteomalacia
  Lithium: *lithium* excretion increased

Acitretin
  Alcohol: etretinate formed in presence of *alcohol*
• Anticoagulants: possible antagonism of anticoagulant effect of *warfarin*
• Cytotoxics: increased plasma concentration of *methotrexate* (also increased risk of hepatotoxicity)

Acrivastine *see* Antihistamines
Acrosoxacin *see* 4-Quinolones
Acyclovir and Famciclovir
  other Antivirals: extreme lethargy reported on administration of *zidovudine* with *intravenous acyclovir*
  Uricosurics: *probenecid* reduces *acyclovir* and possibly *famciclovir* excretion (increased plasma concentrations and risk of toxicity)

Adenosine
  Note. Possibility of interaction with drugs tending to impair cardiac conduction
• Antiplatelet Drugs: effect enhanced and extended by *dipyridamole* (**important** risk of toxicity)
  Theophylline: antagonism of anti-arrhythmic effect

Adrenaline *see* Sympathomimetics
Adrenergic Neurone Blockers (*see also* Bretylium)
  Alcohol: enhanced hypotensive effect
• Anaesthetics: enhanced hypotensive effect
  Analgesics: *NSAIDs* antagonise hypotensive effect
  Antidepressants: *tricyclics* antagonise hypotensive effect
  other Antihypertensives: enhanced hypotensive effect
  Antipsychotics: *phenothiazines* enhance hypotensive effect (antagonism of hypotensive effect with higher doses of *chlorpromazine*)
  Anxiolytics and Hypnotics: enhanced hypotensive effect
  Beta-blockers: enhanced hypotensive effect
  Calcium-channel Blockers: enhanced hypotensive effect
  Corticosteroids: antagonism of hypotensive effect
  Diuretics: enhanced hypotensive effect
  Dopaminergics: *levodopa* enhances hypotensive effect
  Nitrates: enhance hypotensive effect
  Oestrogens and Progestogens: *oestrogens and combined oral contraceptives* antagonise hypotensive effect
  Pizotifen: antagonism of hypotensive effect
• Sympathomimetics: *some anorectics and some cough and cold remedies (e.g. ephedrine)* antagonise hypotensive effect
  Ulcer-healing Drugs: *carbenoxolone* antagonises hypotensive effect

Alcohol
  ACE Inhibitors: enhanced hypotensive effect
  Analgesics: sedative and hypotensive effect of *opioid analgesics* enhanced
  Antibacterials: disulfiram-like reaction with *cephamandole, metronidazole, nimorazole and tinidazole*
• Anticoagulants: anticoagulant effects of *warfarin and nicoumalone* enhanced
• Antidepressants: sedative effect of *tricyclic and related antidepressants* enhanced; *tyramine contained in some alcoholic and dealcoholised beverages* interacts with *MAOIs* (hypertensive crisis)—but if no tyramine, enhanced hypotensive effect

Alcohol (*continued*)
Antidiabetics: enhanced hypoglycaemic effect; flushing with *chlorpropamide* (in susceptible subjects); increased risk of lactic acidosis with *metformin*
Antiepileptics: CNS side-effects of *carbamazepine* possibly enhanced
Antihistamines: enhanced sedative effect
Antihypertensives: enhanced hypotensive effect; sedative effect of *indoramin* enhanced
Antimuscarinics: sedative effect of *hyoscine* enhanced
Antipsychotics: enhanced sedative effect
Anxiolytics and Hypnotics: enhanced sedative effect
Beta-blockers: enhanced hypotensive effect
Cytotoxics: disulfiram-like reaction with *procarbazine*
Dopaminergics: reduced tolerance to *bromocriptine*
Lofexidine: enhanced sedative effect
Monosulfiram: disulfiram-like reaction
Muscle Relaxants: *baclofen* enhances sedative effect
Nabilone: enhanced sedative effect
Nitrates: enhanced hypotensive effect
Retinoids: *etretinate* formed from *acitretin* in presence of *alcohol*
Alcuronium *see* Muscle Relaxants (non-depolarising)
Aldesleukin
Antihypertensives: enhanced hypotensive effect
Alfentanil *see* Opioid Analgesics
Alfuzosin *see* Alpha-blockers
Allopurinol
ACE Inhibitors: increased risk of toxicity with *captopril*, especially in renal impairment
Anticoagulants: effects of *nicoumalone and warfarin* possibly enhanced
Cyclosporin: plasma-cyclosporin concentration possibly increased (risk of nephrotoxicity)
• Cytotoxics: effects of *azathioprine, cyclophosphamide, and mercaptopurine* enhanced with increased toxicity
Allyloestrenol *see* Progestogens
Alpha-blockers
ACE Inhibitors: enhanced hypotensive effect
Alcohol: enhanced hypotensive effect; sedative effect of *indoramin* enhanced
Aldesleukin: enhanced hypotensive effect
• Anaesthetics: enhanced hypotensive effect
Analgesics: *NSAIDs* antagonise hypotensive effect
other Antihypertensives: additive hypotensive effect
Antidepressants: enhanced hypotensive effect
Antipsychotics: enhanced hypotensive effect
Anxiolytics and Hypnotics: enhanced hypotensive and sedative effect
• Beta-blockers: enhanced hypotensive effect; increased risk of first-dose hypotensive effect of *post-synaptic alpha-blockers such as prazosin*
• Calcium-channel Blockers: enhanced hypotensive effect; increased risk of first-dose hypotensive effect of *post-synaptic alpha-blockers such as prazosin*
Corticosteroids : antagonism of hypotensive effect
• Diuretics: enhanced hypotensive effect; increased risk of first-dose hypotensive effect of *post-synaptic alpha-blockers such as prazosin*
Dopaminergics: *levodopa* enhances hypotensive effect
Muscle Relaxants: *baclofen* enhances hypotensive effect
Nitrates: enhanced hypotensive effect
Oestrogens and Progestogens: *oestrogens and combined oral contraceptives* antagonise hypotensive effect
Ulcer-healing Drugs: *carbenoxolone* antagonises hypotensive effect

Alprazolam *see* Benzodiazepines and other Anxiolytics and Hypnotics
Aluminium Hydroxide *see* Antacids and Adsorbents
Amantadine
Antihypertensives: *methyldopa* and *metirosine* have extrapyramidal side-effects
Antimuscarinics: increased antimuscarinic side-effects
Antipsychotics: all have extrapyramidal side-effects
Domperidone and Metoclopramide: have extrapyramidal side-effects
Tetrabenazine: has extrapyramidal side-effects
Ambutonium *see* Antimuscarinics
Amikacin *see* Aminoglycosides
Amiloride *see* Diuretics (potassium-sparing)
Aminoglutethimide
• Anticoagulants: metabolism of *nicoumalone and warfarin* accelerated (reduced anticoagulant effect)
Antidiabetics: manufacturer advises metabolism of *oral antidiabetics* possibly accelerated
Cardiac Glycosides: metabolism of *digitoxin only* accelerated (reduced effect)
Corticosteroids: metabolism of *dexamethasone* accelerated (reduced effect)
other Hormone Antagonists: plasma concentration of *tamoxifen* reduced
Theophylline: metabolism of *theophylline* accelerated (reduced effect)
Aminoglycosides
other Antibacterials: increased risk of nephrotoxicity with *colistin*; increased risk of ototoxicity and nephrotoxicity with *capreomycin* and *vancomycin*
Anticoagulants: *see* Phenindione and Warfarin
Antifungals: increased risk of nephrotoxicity with *amphotericin*
Bisphosphonates: severe hypocalcaemia
• Botulinum Toxin: neuromuscular block enhanced (risk of toxicity)
• Cholinergics: antagonism of effect of *neostigmine and pyridostigmine*
• Cyclosporin: increased risk of nephrotoxicity
• Cytotoxics: increased risk of nephrotoxicity and possibly of ototoxicity with *cisplatin*
• Diuretics: increased risk of ototoxicity with *loop diuretics*
• Muscle Relaxants: effect of *non-depolarising muscle relaxants such as tubocurarine* enhanced
Aminophylline *see* Theophylline
Amiodarone
• *other* Anti-arrhythmics: additive effect with *disopyramide, flecainide, procainamide, and quinidine* (increased risk of ventricular arrhythmias); increased plasma concentrations of *flecainide and procainamide*; increased myocardial depression with any anti-arrhythmic
• Anticoagulants: metabolism of *nicoumalone and warfarin* inhibited (enhanced anticoagulant effect)
• Antiepileptics: metabolism of *phenytoin* inhibited (increased plasma concentration)
• Antihistamines: increased risk of ventricular arrhythmias with *astemizole* and *terfenadine*
• Antimalarials: increased risk of ventricular arrhythmias with *halofantrine*
• Antipsychotics: increased risk of ventricular arrhythmias with *phenothiazines*
• Beta-blockers: increased risk of bradycardia, AV block, and myocardial depression
• Calcium-channel Blockers: *diltiazem and verapamil* increase risk of bradycardia, AV block, and myocardial depression
• Cardiac Glycosides: increased plasma concentration of *digoxin* (halve digoxin maintenance dose)

Amiodarone (*continued*)

Cyclosporin: plasma concentration of cyclosporin possibly increased

Diuretics: toxicity increased if hypokalaemia occurs with *acetazolamide, loop diuretics, and thiazides*

Ulcer-healing Drugs: *cimetidine* increases plasma concentrations of *amiodarone*

Amitriptyline *see* Antidepressants, Tricyclic

Amlodipine *see* Calcium-channel Blockers

Amoxapine *see* Antidepressants, Tricyclic

Amoxycillin *see* Penicillins

Amphetamines *see* Sympathomimetics

Amphotericin

Antibacterials: increased risk of nephrotoxicity with *aminoglycosides*

other Antifungals: antagonises *miconazole*

• Cyclosporin: increased risk of nephrotoxicity

Diuretics: increased risk of hypokalaemia with *loop diuretics* and *thiazides*

Ampicillin *see* Penicillins

Amylobarbitone *see* Barbiturates and Primidone

Anabolic Steroids

• Anticoagulants: anticoagulant effect of *nicoumalone, phenindione, and warfarin* enhanced

Anaesthetics (*see also* Surgery and Long-term Medication, section 15.1)

• ACE Inhibitors: enhanced hypotensive effect

Antibacterials: effect of *thiopentone* enhanced by *sulphonamides*

Antidepressants: risk of arrhythmias and hypotension increased with *tricyclics*

• Antihypertensives: enhanced hypotensive effect

• Antipsychotics: enhanced hypotensive effect

Anxiolytics and Hypnotics: enhanced sedative effect

• Beta-blockers: enhanced hypotensive effect

• Calcium-channel Blockers: enhanced hypotensive effect and AV delay with *verapamil*

• Dopaminergics: risk of arrhythmias if *volatile liquid anaesthetics such as halothane* given with *levodopa*

• Sympathomimetics: risk of arrhythmias if *adrenaline or isoprenaline* given with *volatile liquid anaesthetics such as halothane*

Theophylline: increased risk of arrhythmias with *halothane*

Analgesics *see* Aspirin, Nefopam, NSAIDs, Opioid Analgesics, and Paracetamol

Anion-exchange Resins *see* Cholestyramine and Colestipol

Antacids and Adsorbents

ACE Inhibitors: *antacids* reduce absorption of *fosinopril*

Analgesics: excretion of *aspirin* increased in alkaline urine; *antacids* reduce absorption of *diflunisal*

Anti-arrhythmics: excretion of *quinidine* reduced in alkaline urine (may occasionally increase plasma concentrations)

Antibacterials: *antacids* reduce absorption of *azithromycin, cefpodoxime, ciprofloxacin, isoniazid, norfloxacin, ofloxacin, pivampicillin, rifampicin, and most tetracyclines*

Antiepileptics: *antacids* reduce absorption of *gabapentin* and *phenytoin*

Antifungals: *antacids* reduce absorption of *itraconazole* and *ketoconazole*

Antiplatelet Drugs: *dipyridamole* patient information leaflet advises avoidance of *antacids*

Antimalarials: *antacids* reduce absorption of *chloroquine and hydroxychloroquine*

Antipsychotics: *antacids* reduce absorption of *phenothiazines*

Antacids and Adsorbents (*continued*)

Bisphosphonates: *antacids* reduce absorption (give at least 2 hours apart)

Iron: *magnesium trisilicate* reduces absorption of *oral iron*

Lithium: *sodium bicarbonate* increases excretion (reduced plasma-lithium concentration)

Penicillamine: *antacids* reduce absorption

Antazoline *see* Antihistamines

Anti-arrhythmics *see* individual drugs

Anticholinergics *see* Antimuscarinics

Anticoagulants *see* Heparin, Phenindione, and Warfarin

Antidepressants *see* individual entries for Antidepressants, Serotonin-uptake Inhibitor; Antidepressants, Tricyclic; MAOIs; Mianserin; Moclobemide; Trazodone; Tryptophan; and Viloxazine

Antidepressants, Serotonin-uptake Inhibitor

Alcohol: effects possibly enhanced

Anti-arrhythmics: plasma-flecainide concentration increased by *fluoxetine*

• Anticoagulants: effect of *nicoumalone and warfarin* possibly enhanced

• *other* Antidepressants: CNS effects of *MAOIs* increased (risk of toxicity); *serotonin-uptake inhibitor* should not be started until 2 weeks after stopping *MAOI;* conversely, *MAOI* should not be started until at least 1 week after *serotonin-uptake inhibitor* has been stopped (at least 5 weeks for *fluoxetine*, at least 2 weeks for *paroxetine*); *moclobemide see* p.169; *fluoxetine, fluvoxamine* and *paroxetine* increase plasma concentrations of some *tricyclics*; agitation and nausea with *tryptophan*

Antiepileptics: antagonism (convulsive threshold lowered); plasma concentration of *carbamazepine* increased by *fluoxetine* and *fluvoxamine*; plasma concentration of *phenytoin* increased by *fluoxetine*; *phenytoin and possibly other antiepileptics* reduce plasma concentration of *paroxetine*

Antipsychotics: plasma concentration of *haloperidol* increased by *fluoxetine*

Beta-blockers: plasma concentration of *propranolol* increased by *fluvoxamine*

• Dopaminergics: hypertension and CNS excitation with *fluoxetine* and *selegiline*

• Lithium: increased risk of CNS toxicity

• Sumatriptan: risk of CNS toxicity

• Theophylline: plasma-theophylline concentration increased by *fluvoxamine* (**important:** see p.120)

Antidepressants, Tricyclic

• Alcohol: enhanced sedative effect

Anaesthetics: risk of arrhythmias and hypotension increased

• Anti-arrhythmics: increased risk of arrhythmias with drugs which prolong QT interval

Antibacterials: plasma concentrations of some *tricyclics* reduced by *rifampicin* (reduced antidepressant effect)

• *other* Antidepressants: CNS excitation and hypertension with *MAOIs; tricyclic or related antidepressant* should not be started until 2 weeks after stopping *MAOI;* conversely, *MAOI* should not be started until at least 1 week after *tricyclic or related antidepressant* has been stopped; *moclobemide see* p.169; *fluoxetine, fluvoxamine* and *paroxetine* increase plasma concentrations of some *tricyclics*

• Antiepileptics: antagonism (convulsive threshold lowered); plasma concentrations of some *tricyclics* reduced (reduced antidepressant effect)

Antidepressants, Tricyclic (*continued*)
- Antihistamines: increased antimuscarinic and sedative effects; increased risk of ventricular arrhythmias with *astemizole* and *terfenadine*

  Antihypertensives: in general, hypotensive effect enhanced, but antagonism of effect of *adrenergic neurone blockers* and of *clonidine* (and increased risk of hypertension on clonidine withdrawal); possible risk of hypotension with *tricyclics* and *apraclonidine*
- Antimalarials: increased risk of ventricular arrhythmias with *halofantrine*

  Antimuscarinics: increased antimuscarinic side-effects

  Antipsychotics: increased plasma concentrations of *tricyclic antidepressants* and increased antimuscarinic side-effects with *phenothiazines*

  Anxiolytics and Hypnotics: enhanced sedative effect

  Barbiturates: *see under* Antiepileptics, above

  Calcium-channel Blockers: *diltiazem* and *verapamil* increase plasma concentration of *imipramine* and possibly *other tricyclics*

  Disulfiram: inhibition of metabolism of *tricyclics* (increased plasma concentrations and increased disulfiram reaction reported with *alcohol with amitriptyline*)

  Diuretics: increased risk of postural hypotension

  Muscle Relaxants: enhanced muscle relaxant effect of *baclofen*

  Nitrates: reduced effect of *sublingual nitrates* (owing to dry mouth)

  Oestrogens and Progestogens: *oral contraceptives* antagonise antidepressant effect (but side-effects may be increased due to increased plasma concentrations of *tricyclics*)
- Sympathomimetics: hypertension and arrhythmias with *adrenaline* (but local anaesthetics with adrenaline appear to be safe); hypertension with *noradrenaline*

  Ulcer-healing Drugs: plasma concentrations of *amitriptyline, desipramine, doxepin, imipramine, nortriptyline, and probably other tricyclics* increased by *cimetidine* (inhibition of metabolism)

Antidiabetics (includes Insulin, Metformin, and Sulphonylureas)

ACE Inhibitors: possibly enhance hypoglycaemic effect

Alcohol: enhanced hypoglycaemic effect; flushing with *chlorpropamide* (in susceptible subjects); risk of lactic acidosis with *metformin*
- Analgesics: *azapropazone, phenylbutazone* and possibly *other NSAIDs* enhance effect of *sulphonylureas*
- Antibacterials: *chloramphenicol, co-trimoxazole, 4-quinolones, sulphonamides,* and *trimethoprim* enhance effect of *sulphonylureas; rifamycins* reduce effect of *sulphonylureas* (accelerates metabolism)

  Antidepressants: *MAOIs* enhance hypoglycaemic effect

  Antiepileptics: *plasma-phenytoin* concentration transiently increased by *tolbutamide* (possibility of toxicity)
- Antifungals: *miconazole* and possibly *fluconazole* enhance effect of *sulphonylureas*
- Antihistamines: depressed thrombocyte count with concomitant use of *oral antidiabetics* and *ketotifen* (avoid combination)

  Antihypertensives: hypoglycaemic effect antagonised by *diazoxide*

  Antipsychotics: *phenothiazines* possibly antagonise hypoglycaemic effect of *sulphonylureas*

Antidiabetics (*continued*)

Beta-blockers: enhanced hypoglycaemic effect (and masking of warning signs such as tremor)

Calcium-channel Blockers: *nifedipine* may occasionally impair glucose tolerance

Clofibrate Group: may improve glucose tolerance and have an additive effect

Corticosteroids: antagonism of hypoglycaemic effect

Diuretics: hypoglycaemic effect antagonised by *loop and thiazide diuretics; chlorpropamide* increases risk of hyponatraemia with *thiazides in combination with potassium-sparing diuretics*

Hormone Antagonists: manufacturer advises metabolism of *oral antidiabetics* possibly accelerated by *aminoglutethimide; octreotide* may reduce *insulin and antidiabetic drug* requirements in diabetes mellitus

Lithium: may occasionally impair glucose tolerance

Oestrogens and Progestogens: *oral contraceptives* antagonise hypoglycaemic effect

Ulcer-healing Drugs: *cimetidine* inhibits renal excretion of *metformin* (increased plasma-metformin concentrations); *cimetidine* and *ranitidine* enhance hypoglycaemic effect of *sulphonylureas*
- Uricosurics: *sulphinpyrazone* enhances effect of *sulphonylureas*

Antiepileptics *see* individual drugs and p. 193

Antifungals, imidazole and triazole (*see* individual entries for other antifungals)

Antacids and Adsorbents: *antacids* reduce absorption of *itraconazole* and *ketoconazole*

Antibacterials: *rifampicin* accelerates metabolism of *fluconazole, itraconazole* and *ketoconazole* (reduced plasma concentration); **important:** *rifabutin* and **CSM advice, see** p. 526
- Anticoagulants: effect of *nicoumalone* and *warfarin* enhanced by *fluconazole, itraconazole, ketoconazole,* and *miconazole* (note: oral gel absorbed)
- Antidiabetics: effect of *sulphonylureas* enhanced by *miconazole* and possibly *fluconazole*
- Antiepileptics: effect of *phenytoin* enhanced by *fluconazole* and *miconazole;* plasma concentrations of *itraconazole* and *ketoconazole* reduced by *phenytoin*

  other Antifungals: *amphotericin* antagonises effect of *miconazole*
- Antihistamines: *itraconazole, ketoconazole* and possibly *other imidazoles* (and *triazoles*) inhibit *astemizole* and *terfenadine* metabolism (cardiac toxicity reported)

  Antimuscarinics: reduced absorption of *ketoconazole*
- Cardiac Glycosides: plasma concentration of *digoxin* increased by *itraconazole*
- Cyclosporin: metabolism inhibited by *itraconazole, ketoconazole,* and possibly *fluconazole* (increased plasma-cyclosporin concentration)

  Theophylline: plasma-theophylline concentration possibly increased by *fluconazole*

  Ulcer-healing Drugs: *histamine H$_2$- antagonists* reduce absorption of *itraconazole* and *ketoconazole; omeprazole* reduces absorption of *ketoconazole* and possibly *itraconazole; sucralfate* reduces absorption of *ketoconazole*

Antihistamines

Note. Sedative interactions apply to a lesser extent to the non-sedative antihistamines, and they do not appear to potentiate the effects of alcohol

Alcohol: enhanced sedative effect
- Anti-arrhythmics: increased risk of ventricular arrhythmias with *astemizole* and *terfenadine*

Antihistamines (*continued*)
- Antibacterials: metabolism of *astemizole* and *terfenadine* inhibited by *erythromycin* and other *macrolides*
- Antidepressants: *MAOIs* and *tricyclics* increase antimuscarinic and sedative effects; *tricyclics* increase risk of ventricular arrhythmias with *astemizole* and *terfenadine*
- Antidiabetics: depressed thrombocyte count with concomitant use of *oral antidiabetics* and *ketotifen* (avoid combination)
- Antiepileptics: plasma concentration of *carbamazepine* increased by *terfenadine* (increased toxicity)
- Antifungals: *itraconazole, ketoconazole* and possibly *other imidazoles* (and *triazoles*) inhibit *astemizole* and *terfenadine* metabolism (cardiac toxicity reported)
- Antimalarials: *halofantrine* increases risk of ventricular arrhythmias with *astemizole* and *terfenadine*

  Antimuscarinics: increased antimuscarinic side-effects
- Antipsychotics: increased risk of ventricular arrhythmias with *astemizole* and *terfenadine*

  Anxiolytics and Hypnotics: enhanced sedative effect
- Beta-blockers: *sotalol* increases risk of ventricular arrhythmias with *astemizole* and *terfenadine*

  Betahistine: antagonism (theoretical)
- Diuretics: hypokalaemia increases risk of ventricular arrhythmias with *astemizole* and *terfenadine*

Antihypertensives *see* individual drugs or groups

Antimalarials *see* individual drugs

Antimuscarinics

Note. Many drugs have antimuscarinic effects; concomitant use of two or three such drugs can increase side-effects such as dry mouth, urine retention, and constipation; concomitant use can also lead to confusion in the elderly; interactions do not generally apply to antimuscarinics used by inhalation

  Alcohol: sedative effect of *hyoscine* enhanced

  Analgesics: increased antimuscarinic effects with *nefopam*

  Anti-arrhythmics: increased antimuscarinic effects with *disopyramide; atropine* delays absorption of *mexiletine*

  Antidepressants: increased antimuscarinic side-effects with *tricyclics* and *MAOIs*

  Antifungals: reduced absorption of *ketoconazole*

  Antihistamines: increased antimuscarinic side-effects

  Antipsychotics: increased antimuscarinic side-effects of *phenothiazines* (but reduced plasma concentrations)

  Cisapride: antagonism of gastro-intestinal effect

  Domperidone and Metoclopramide: *antimuscarinics such as propantheline* antagonise gastro-intestinal effects

  Dopaminergics: increased antimuscarinic side-effects with *amantadine*

  Nitrates: reduced effect of *sublingual nitrates* (failure to dissolve under tongue owing to dry mouth)

Antiplatelet Drugs *see* Aspirin and Dipyridamole

Antipsychotics *see* Phenothiazines and other Antipsychotics

Antivirals *see* individual drugs

Anxiolytics *see* Benzodiazepines and other Anxiolytics and Hypnotics

Apomorphine

  Antipsychotics: antagonism of effects

Appetite Suppressants *see* Sympathomimetics

Apraclonidine

  Antidepressants: possible risk of hypertension with *tricyclics*

  Sympathomimetics: possible risk of hypertension with *adrenaline* and *noradrenaline*

Aspirin

  other Analgesics: avoid concomitant administration of other *NSAIDs* (increased side-effects)

  Antacids and Adsorbents: excretion of *aspirin* increased in alkaline urine
- Anticoagulants: increased risk of bleeding due to antiplatelet effect

  Antiepileptics: enhancement of effect of *phenytoin* and *valproate*

  Corticosteroids: increased risk of gastro-intestinal bleeding and ulceration
- Cytotoxics: reduced excretion of *methotrexate* (increased toxicity)

  Diuretics: antagonism of diuretic effect of *spironolactone;* reduced excretion of *acetazolamide* (risk of toxicity)

  Domperidone and Metoclopramide: *metoclopramide* enhances effect of *aspirin* (increased rate of absorption)

  Mifepristone: manufacturer recommends avoid *aspirin* until 8–12 days after *mifepristone*

  Uricosurics: effect of *probenecid and sulphinpyrazone* reduced

Astemizole *see* Antihistamines

Atenolol *see* Beta-blockers

Atracurium *see* Muscle Relaxants (non-depolarising)

Atropine *see* Antimuscarinics

Auranofin *see* Gold

Azapropazone *see* NSAIDs

Azatadine *see* Antihistamines

Azathioprine
- Allopurinol: enhancement of effect with increased toxicity
- Antibacterials: manufacturer reports interaction with *rifampicin* (transplants possibly rejected)

Azithromycin *see* Erythromycin and other Macrolides

Azlocillin *see* Penicillins

Aztreonam
- Anticoagulants: anticoagulant effect of *nicoumalone* and *warfarin* enhanced

Baclofen *see* Muscle Relaxants

Bambuterol *see* Sympathomimetics, Beta$_2$

Barbiturates and Primidone

  Alcohol: enhanced sedative effect

  Anti-arrhythmics: metabolism of *disopyramide and quinidine* increased (reduced plasma concentrations)

  Antibacterials: metabolism of *chloramphenicol, doxycycline, and metronidazole* accelerated (reduced effect); *sulphonamides* enhance effect of *thiopentone*
- Anticoagulants: metabolism of *nicoumalone and warfarin* accelerated (reduced anticoagulant effect)
- Antidepressants: antagonism of anticonvulsant effect (convulsive threshold lowered); metabolism of *mianserin* and *tricyclics* accelerated (reduced plasma concentrations)
- Antiepileptics: concomitant administration of *phenobarbitone or primidone* with other antiepileptics may enhance toxicity without a corresponding increase in antiepileptic effect; moreover interactions can complicate monitoring of treatment; interactions include enhanced effects, increased sedation, and reductions in plasma concentrations; for further details see p.193

Barbiturates and Primidone (*continued*)

Antifungals: *phenobarbitone* accelerates metabolism of *griseofulvin* (reduced effect)

- Antipsychotics: antagonism of anticonvulsant effect (convulsive threshold lowered)
- Calcium-channel Blockers: effect of *diltiazem, felodipine, isradipine, verapamil* and probably *nicardipine* and *nifedipine* reduced

Cardiac Glycosides: metabolism of *digitoxin only* accelerated (reduced effect)

- Corticosteroids: metabolism of *corticosteroids* accelerated (reduced effect)
- Cyclosporin: metabolism of *cyclosporin* accelerated (reduced effect)
- Oestrogens and Progestogens: metabolism of *gestrinone, tibolone,* and *oral contraceptives* accelerated (reduced contraceptive effect, **important:** see p.313)

Theophylline: metabolism of *theophylline* accelerated (reduced effect)

Thyroxine: metabolism of thyroxine accelerated (may increase thyroxine requirements in hypothyroidism)

Vitamins: vitamin D requirements possibly increased

Beclomethasone *see* Corticosteroids

Bendrofluazide *see* Diuretics (thiazide)

Benorylate *see* Aspirin *and* Paracetamol

Benperidol *see* Phenothiazines and other Antipsychotics

Benzhexol *see* Antimuscarinics

Benzodiazepines and other Anxiolytics and Hypnotics

Alcohol: enhanced sedative effect

Anaesthetics: enhanced sedative effect

Analgesics: *opioid analgesics* enhance sedative effect

Antibacterials: *erythromycin* inhibits metabolism of *midazolam* (increased plasma-midazolam concentration, **important** see also p.491); *isoniazid* inhibits metabolism of *diazepam; rifampicin* increases metabolism of *diazepam* and possibly *other benzodiazepines*

Anticoagulants: *chloral hydrate* may transiently enhance effect of *nicoumalone and warfarin*

Antidepressants: enhanced sedative effect; manufacturer contra-indicates *buspirone* with *MAOIs*

Antiepileptics: metabolism of *clonazepam* accelerated (reduced effect); plasma-phenytoin concentrations increased or decreased by *diazepam* and possibly *other benzodiazepines*

Antihistamines: enhanced sedative effect

Antihypertensives: enhanced hypotensive effect; enhanced sedative effect with *alpha-blockers*

Antipsychotics: enhanced sedative effect

Disulfiram: metabolism of *diazepam and chlordiazepoxide* inhibited (enhanced sedative effect)

Dopaminergics: *benzodiazepines* occasionally antagonise effect of *levodopa*

Lofexidine: enhanced sedative effect

Muscle Relaxants: *baclofen* enhances sedative effect

Nabilone: enhanced sedative effect

Ulcer-healing Drugs: *cimetidine* inhibits metabolism of *benzodiazepines and chlormethiazole* (increased plasma concentrations); *omeprazole* inhibits metabolism of *diazepam* (increased plasma concentrations)

Benzthiazide *see* Diuretics (thiazide)

Benztropine *see* Antimuscarinics

Beta-blockers

Note. Since systemic absorption may follow topical application of beta-blockers to the eye the possibility of interactions, in particular, with drugs such as verapamil should be borne in mind

ACE Inhibitors: enhanced hypotensive effect

Alcohol: enhanced hypotensive effect

Aldesleukin: enhanced hypotensive effect

- Anaesthetics: enhanced hypotensive effect; increased risk of *bupivacaine* toxicity with *propranolol*

Analgesics: *NSAIDs* antagonise hypotensive effect

- Anti-arrhythmics: increased risk of myocardial depression and bradycardia; with *amiodarone* increased risk of bradycardia and AV block; increased risk of *lignocaine* toxicity with *propranolol; propafenone* increases plasma concentration of *metoprolol* and *propranolol*

Antibacterials: *rifampicin* accelerates metabolism of *bisoprolol* and *propranolol* (reduced plasma concentration)

Antidepressants: *fluvoxamine* increases plasma concentration of *propranolol*

Antidiabetics: enhanced hypoglycaemic effect (and masking of warning signs such as tremor)

- Antihistamines: risk of ventricular arrhythmias associated with *sotalol* increased by *astemizole* and *terfenadine*
- Antihypertensives: enhanced hypotensive effect; increased risk of withdrawal hypertension with *clonidine*; increased risk of first-dose hypotensive effect with *post-synaptic alpha-blockers such as prazosin*
- Antimalarials: risk of ventricular arrhythmias associated with *sotalol* increased by *halofantrine*; increased risk of bradycardia with *mefloquine*
- Antipsychotics: risk of ventricular arrhythmias associated with *sotalol* increased by *phenothiazines*; plasma concentration of *chlorpromazine* increased by *propranolol*

Anxiolytics and Hypnotics: enhanced hypotensive effect

- Calcium-channel Blockers: increased risk of bradycardia and AV block with *diltiazem*; severe hypotension and heart failure occasionally with *nifedipine* (but useful combination, see p.90); asystole, severe hypotension, and heart failure with *verapamil* (see p.93)

Cardiac Glycosides: increased AV block and bradycardia

Cholinergics: *propranolol* antagonises effect of *neostigmine and pyridostigmine*

Corticosteroids: antagonism of hypotensive effect

Diuretics: enhanced hypotensive effect; risk of ventricular arrhythmias associated with *sotalol* increased by hypokalaemia

Ergotamine: increased peripheral vasoconstriction

Muscle Relaxants: *propranolol* enhances effect

Oestrogens and Progestogens: *oestrogens* and *combined oral contraceptives* antagonise hypotensive effect

- Sympathomimetics: severe hypertension with *adrenaline and noradrenaline* (especially with *non-selective beta-blockers*); severe hypertension also possible with *sympathomimetics in anorectics and cough and cold remedies*

Theophylline: *beta-blockers* should be avoided on pharmacological grounds (bronchospasm)

Thyroxine: metabolism of *propranolol* accelerated (reduced effect)

Ulcer-healing Drugs: plasma concentrations of *labetalol and propranolol* increased by *cimetidine;* hypotensive effect antagonised by *carbenoxolone*

Xamoterol: antagonism of effect of xamoterol and reduction in beta-blockade

Betahistine
Antihistamines: antagonism (theoretical)
Betamethasone see Corticosteroids
Betaxolol see Beta-blockers
Bethanechol see Cholinergics
Bethanidine see Adrenergic Neurone Blockers
Bezafibrate see Clofibrate Group
Biperiden see Antimuscarinics
Bismuth Chelate
Antibacterials: reduced absorption of *tetracyclines*
Bisoprolol see Beta-blockers
Bisphosphonates
Antacids: reduced absorption (give at least 2 hours apart)
Antibacterials: severe hypocalcaemia reported with *aminoglycosides*
Calcium Salts: reduced absorption (give at least 2 hours apart)
Iron: reduced absorption (give at least 2 hours apart)
Botulinum Toxin
• Antibacterials: effects enhanced by *aminoglycosides* and *spectinomycin* (risk of toxicity)
• Muscle Relaxants: effects enhanced by *non-depolarising muscle relaxants such as tubocurarine*
Bretylium (*see also* Adrenergic Neurone Blockers)
other Anti-arrhythmics: increased myocardial depression with any combination of two or more anti-arrhythmics
Bromazepam see Benzodiazepines and other Anxiolytics and Hypnotics
Bromocriptine
Alcohol: reduced tolerance to *bromocriptine*
Antibacterials: *erythromycin* increases plasma concentration
Antipsychotics: antagonism of hypoprolactinaemic and antiparkinsonian effects
Domperidone and Metoclopramide: antagonise hypoprolactinaemic effect
Budesonide see Corticosteroids
Bumetanide see Diuretics (loop)
Bupivacaine
Anti-arrhythmics: increased myocardial depression
Beta-blockers: increased risk of *bupivacaine* toxicity with *propranolol*
Buprenorphine see Opioid Analgesics
Buspirone (general sedative interactions as for Benzodiazepines and other Anxiolytics and Hypnotics)
Antidepressants: *MAOIs* contra-indicated by manufacturer
Butobarbitone see Barbiturates
Cabergoline
Antibacterials: increased risk of toxicity with *erythromycin and other macrolides*
Antipsychotics: antagonism of hypoprolactinaemic effect
Domperidone and Metoclopramide: antagonism of hypoprolactinaemic effect
Calcium Salts
Antibacterials: reduced absorption of *tetracyclines*
Bisphosphonates: reduce absorption (give at least 2 hours apart)
Cardiac Glycosides: large intravenous doses of *calcium* can precipitate arrhythmias
Diuretics: increased risk of hypercalcaemia with *thiazides*
Calcium-channel Blockers
ACE Inhibitors: enhanced hypotensive effect
Aldesleukin: enhanced hypotensive effect
• Anaesthetics: *verapamil* increases hypotensive effect of *general anaesthetics* and risk of AV delay

Calcium-channel Blockers (*continued*)
• Anti-arrhythmics: *amiodarone-induced* risk of bradycardia, AV block, and myocardial depression increased by *diltiazem and verapamil*; plasma-concentration of *quinidine* reduced by *nifedipine*; increased risk of myocardial depression and asystole if *verapamil* given with *flecainide*; with *verapamil* raised plasma concentration of *quinidine* (extreme hypotension may occur)
Antibacterials: *rifampicin* increases metabolism of *diltiazem and verapamil and possibly isradipine and nifedipine* (reduced plasma concentrations)
Antidepressants: *diltiazem* and *verapamil* increase plasma concentration of *imipramine and possibly other tricyclics*
Antidiabetics: *nifedipine* may occasionally impair glucose tolerance
• Antiepileptics: effect of *carbamazepine* enhanced by *diltiazem and verapamil; diltiazem* and *nifedipine* increase plasma concentration of *phenytoin*; effect of *felodipine* and *isradipine* and probably *nicardipine and nifedipine* reduced by *carbamazepine, phenobarbitone, phenytoin, and primidone*; effect of *diltiazem* and *verapamil* reduced by *phenobarbitone* and *phenytoin*
Antihypertensives: enhanced hypotensive effect
Antimalarials: possible increased risk of bradycardia with some *calcium-channel blockers* and *mefloquine*
Antipsychotics: enhanced hypotensive effect
Barbiturates: see *under* Antiepileptics, above
• Beta-blockers: increased risk of bradycardia and AV block with *diltiazem;* occasionally severe hypotension and heart failure with *nifedipine* (but useful combination, see p.90); asystole, severe hypotension, and heart failure with *verapamil* (see p.93)
• Cardiac Glycosides: plasma concentration of *digoxin* increased by *diltiazem, nicardipine, verapamil* and possibly *nifedipine*; increased AV block and bradycardia with *verapamil*
Cyclosporin: plasma-cyclosporin concentrations increased by *diltiazem, nicardipine, and verapamil;* possibly increases plasma concentration of *nifedipine*
Lithium: neurotoxicity may occur without increased plasma-lithium concentrations in patients given *diltiazem and verapamil*
Muscle Relaxants: *nifedipine* and *verapamil* enhance effect of *non-depolarising muscle relaxants such as tubocurarine*; hypotension, myocardial depression, and hyperkalaemia with *verapamil* and intravenous *dantrolene*
Sympathomimetics: see Sympathomimetics (main list)
• Theophylline: *diltiazem and verapamil* enhance effect
Ulcer-healing Drugs: *cimetidine* inhibits metabolism of *some calcium-channel blockers* (increased plasma concentrations)
Canrenoate see Diuretics (*as for* spironolactone)
Capreomycin
other Antibacterials: increased risk of nephrotoxicity with *colistin*; increased risk of nephrotoxicity and ototoxicity with *aminoglycosides and vancomycin*
Cytotoxics: increased risk of nephrotoxicity and ototoxicity with *cisplatin*
Captopril see ACE Inhibitors
Carbachol see Cholinergics
Carbamazepine
Alcohol: CNS side-effects of *carbamazepine* possibly enhanced
• Analgesics: *dextropropoxyphene* enhances effect of *carbamazepine;* effect of *tramadol* decreased by *carbamazepine*

Carbamazepine (*continued*)
- Antibacterials: metabolism of *doxycycline* accelerated (reduced effect); plasma-carbamazepine concentration increased by *clarithromycin, erythromycin and isoniazid* (also isoniazid hepatotoxicity possibly increased)
- Anticoagulants: metabolism of *nicoumalone and warfarin* accelerated (reduced anticoagulant effect)
- Antidepressants: antagonism of anticonvulsant effect (convulsive threshold lowered); plasma concentration of *carbamazepine* increased by *fluoxetine, fluvoxamine,* and *viloxazine*; metabolism of *mianserin* and *tricyclics* accelerated (reduced plasma concentrations); manufacturer advises avoid with *MAOIs* or within 2 weeks of *MAOIs*
- *other* Antiepileptics: concomitant administration of *two or more antiepileptics* may enhance toxicity without a corresponding increase in antiepileptic effect; moreover interactions between individual antiepileptics can complicate monitoring of treatment; interactions include enhanced effects, increased sedation, and reductions in plasma concentrations; for further details, see p.193
- Antihistamines: plasma concentration increased by *terfenadine* (increased toxicity)
  Antimalarials: antagonism of anticonvulsant effect
- Antipsychotics: antagonism of anticonvulsant effect (convulsive threshold lowered); metabolism of *haloperidol* accelerated (reduced plasma-haloperidol concentration)
- Calcium-channel Blockers: *diltiazem and verapamil* enhance effect of *carbamazepine*; effect of *felodipine, isradipine* and probably *nicardipine* and *nifedipine* reduced
  Cardiac Glycosides: metabolism of *digitoxin only* accelerated (reduced effect)
- Corticosteroids: metabolism accelerated (reduced effect)
- Cyclosporin: metabolism accelerated (reduced plasma-cyclosporin concentration)
- Hormone Antagonists: *danazol* inhibits metabolism of *carbamazepine* (enhanced effect)
  Lithium: neurotoxicity may occur without increased plasma-lithium concentration
  Muscle Relaxants: effect of *non-depolarising muscle relaxants* antagonised (recovery from neuromuscular blockade accelerated)
- Oestrogens and Progestogens: *carbamazepine* accelerates metabolism of *oral contraceptives* (reduced contraceptive effect, **important:** see p.313) and of *gestrinone and tibolone*
  Theophylline: metabolism of *theophylline* accelerated (reduced effect)
  Thyroxine: metabolism accelerated (may increase thyroxine requirements in hypothyroidism)
- Ulcer-healing Drugs: metabolism inhibited by *cimetidine* (increased plasma-carbamazepine concentration)
  Vitamins: *carbamazepine* possibly increases *vitamin D* requirements

Carbenicillin *see* Penicillins

Carbenoxolone
Note. Do not apply to small amounts used topically on oral mucosa
  Antihypertensives: antagonism of hypotensive effect
  Cardiac Glycosides: toxicity increased if hypokalaemia occurs
  Corticosteroids: increased risk of hypokalaemia
  Diuretics: antagonism of diuretic effect; increased risk of hypokalaemia with *acetazolamide, thiazides, and loop diuretics*; inhibition of ulcer healing with *amiloride and spironolactone*

Cardiac Glycosides
  ACE Inhibitors: *captopril* possibly increases plasma concentration of *digoxin*

Cardiac Glycosides (*continued*)
  Analgesics: *NSAIDs* may exacerbate heart failure, reduce GFR and increase plasma-cardiac glycoside concentrations
  Anion-exchange Resins: absorption reduced by *cholestyramine and colestipol*
- Anti-arrhythmics: plasma concentration of *digoxin* increased by *amiodarone, propafenone, and quinidine* (halve maintenance dose of digoxin)
  Antibacterials: *erythromycin* and possibly *other macrolides* enhance effect of *digoxin*; *rifamycins* accelerate metabolism of *digitoxin only* (reduced effect)
  Antiepileptics: metabolism of *digitoxin only* accelerated (reduced effect)
- Antifungals: plasma concentration of *digoxin* increased by *itraconazole*
- Antimalarials: *quinine* (includes use of quinine for cramp) and possibly *chloroquine* and *hydroxychloroquine* raises plasma concentration of *digoxin* (halve maintenance dose of digoxin); possible increased risk of bradycardia with *mefloquine*
  Barbiturates: *see under* Antiepileptics, above
  Beta-blockers: increased AV block and bradycardia
  Calcium Salts: large intravenous doses of *calcium* can precipitate arrhythmias
- Calcium-channel Blockers: plasma concentration of *digoxin* increased by *diltiazem, nicardipine, verapamil* and possibly *nifedipine*; increased AV block and bradycardia with *verapamil*
  Corticosteroids: increased risk of hypokalaemia
- Diuretics: increased toxicity if hypokalaemia occurs with *acetazolamide, loop diuretics, and thiazides*; effects of *digoxin* enhanced by *spironolactone*
  Hormone Antagonists: *aminoglutethimide* accelerates metabolism of *digitoxin only* (reduced effect)
  Muscle Relaxants: arrhythmias with *suxamethonium*
  Ulcer-healing Drugs: increased toxicity if hypokalaemia occurs with *carbenoxolone*; absorption possibly reduced by *sucralfate*

Carfecillin *see* Penicillins

Carteolol *see* Beta-blockers

Celiprolol *see* Beta-blockers

Cephalosporins
  Alcohol: disulfiram-like reaction with *cephamandole*
  Antacids and Adsorbents: *antacids* reduce absorption of *cefpodoxime*
- Anticoagulants: anticoagulant effect of *warfarin and nicoumalone* enhanced by *cephamandole* and possibly others
  Probenecid: reduced excretion of *cephalosporins* (increased plasma concentrations)
  Ulcer-healing Drugs: *histamine H$_2$-antagonists* reduce absorption of *cefpodoxime*

Cetirizine *see* Antihistamines

Chloral (general sedative interactions *as for* Benzodiazepines and other Anxiolytics and Hypnotics)
  Anticoagulants: may transiently enhance anticoagulant effect of *nicoumalone and warfarin*

Chloramphenicol
  other Antibacterials: *rifampicin* accelerates metabolism (reduced chloramphenicol-plasma concentration)
- Anticoagulants: anticoagulant effect of *nicoumalone and warfarin* enhanced
- Antidiabetics: effect of *sulphonylureas* enhanced
- Antiepileptics: metabolism accelerated by *phenobarbitone* (reduced chloramphenicol-plasma concentration); increased plasma concentration of *phenytoin* (risk of toxicity)
  Barbiturates: *see under* Antiepileptics, above

Chlordiazepoxide *see* Benzodiazepines

Chlormethiazole (for general sedative interactions *see also* Benzodiazepines and other Anxiolytics and Hypnotics)
Ulcer-healing Drugs: *cimetidine* inhibits metabolism (increased plasma-chlormethiazole concentration)
Chlormezanone *see* Benzodiazepines and other Anxiolytics and Hypnotics
Chloroquine and Hydroxychloroquine
Antacids: reduced absorption
Antiepileptics: antagonism of anticonvulsant effect
other Antimalarials: increased risk of convulsions with *mefloquine;* increased risk of arrhythmias with *halofantrine* (**important:** see also CSM advice under Halofantrine, p.259)
• Cardiac Glycosides: *chloroquine* and *hydroxychloroquine* possibly increase plasma concentration of *digoxin*
Cholinergics: *chloroquine* and *hydroxychloroquine* have potential to increase symptoms of myasthenia gravis and thus diminish effect of *neostigmine* and *pyridostigmine*
Ulcer-healing Drugs: *cimetidine* inhibits metabolism of *chloroquine* (increased plasma concentration)
Vaccines: *see* Rabies Vaccine p.477
Chlorothiazide *see* Diuretics (thiazide)
Chlorpheniramine *see* Antihistamines
Chlorpromazine *see* Phenothiazines and other Antipsychotics
Chlorpropamide *see* Antidiabetics (sulphonylurea)
Chlorprothixene *see* Phenothiazines and other Antipsychotics
Chlorthalidone *see* Diuretics (thiazide-related)
Cholestyramine and Colestipol
Analgesics: reduced absorption of *paracetamol* and *phenylbutazone*
Antibacterials: antagonism of effect of oral *vancomycin*
• Anticoagulants: anticoagulant effect of *nicoumalone, phenindione, and warfarin* may be enhanced or reduced
Antidiabetics: hypoglycaemic effect of *acarbose* enhanced by *cholestyramine*
Cardiac Glycosides: reduced absorption
Diuretics: reduced absorption of *thiazides* (give at least 2 hours apart)
Thyroxine: reduced absorption
Cholinergics
Anti-arrhythmics: *procainamide, quinidine* and possibly *propafenone* antagonise effect of *neostigmine and pyridostigmine*
• Antibacterials: *aminoglycosides, clindamycin and colistin* antagonise effect of *neostigmine and pyridostigmine*
Antimalarials; *chloroquine* and *hydroxychloroquine* have potential to increase symptoms of myasthenia gravis and thus diminish effect of *neostigmine* and *pyridostigmine*
Beta-blockers: *propranolol* antagonises effect of *neostigmine and pyridostigmine*
Lithium: antagonism of effect of *neostigmine and pyridostigmine*
Muscle Relaxants: *demecarium and ecothiopate eye-drops, and neostigmine and pyridostigmine* enhance effect of *suxamethonium,* but antagonise effect of *non-depolarising muscle relaxants such as tubocurarine*
Cilazapril *see* ACE Inhibitors
Cimetidine *see* Histamine H2-antagonists
Cinnarizine *see* Antihistamines
Cinoxacin *see* 4-Quinolones
Ciprofibrate *see* Clofibrate Group
Ciprofloxacin *see* 4-Quinolones
Cisapride
Analgesics: *opioid analgesics* possibly antagonise effect on gastro-intestinal motility
Anticoagulants: effect of *oral anticoagulants* possibly enhanced

Cisapride (*continued*)
Antimuscarinics: antagonism of effect on gastro-intestinal motility
Cisplatin
• Antibacterials: *aminoglycosides and capreomycin* increase risk of nephrotoxicity and possibly of ototoxicity
Diuretics: increased risk of nephrotoxicity and ototoxicity
Clarithromycin *see* Erythromycin and other Macrolides
Clemastine *see* Antihistamines
Clindamycin
Cholinergics: antagonism of effect of *neostigmine and pyridostigmine*
Muscle relaxants: enhancement of effect of *non-depolarising muscle relaxants such as tubocurarine*
Clobazam *see* Benzodiazepines and other Anxiolytics and Hypnotics
Clodronate Sodium *see* Bisphosphonates
Clofibrate Group
• Anticoagulants: enhancement of effect of *nicoumalone, phenindione, and warfarin*
Antidiabetics: may improve glucose tolerance and have additive effect
other Lipid-lowering Drugs: increased risk of myopathy with *pravastatin and simvastatin*
Clomipramine *see* Antidepressants, Tricyclic
Clomocycline *see* Tetracyclines
Clonazepam (general sedative interactions *as for* Benzodiazepines and other Anxiolytics and Hypnotics)
• *other* Antiepileptics: concomitant administration of two or more antiepileptics may enhance toxicity without a corresponding increase in antiepileptic effect; moreover interactions between individual antiepileptics can complicate monitoring of treatment; interactions include enhanced effects, increased sedation, and reductions in plasma concentrations; for further details, see p.193
Clonidine (for general hypotensive interactions *see also* Hydralazine)
• Antidepressants: *tricyclics* antagonise hypotensive effect and also increase risk of rebound hypertension on *clonidine* withdrawal
• Beta-blockers: increased risk of hypertension on *clonidine* withdrawal
Clopamide *see* Diuretics (thiazide)
Clorazepate *see* Benzodiazepines and other Anxiolytics and Hypnotics
Cloxacillin *see* Penicillins
Clozapine
Note. Clozapine should not be used concurrently with drugs associated with a substantial potential for causing agranulocytosis, such as co-trimoxazole, chloramphenicol, sulphonamides, penicillamine, or cytotoxics
see also Phenothiazines and other Antipsychotics
Codeine *see* Opioid Analgesics
Colchicine
Cyclosporin: possibly increases risk of nephrotoxicity (increased plasma-cyclosporin concentration)
Cold and Cough Remedies *see* Antihistamines and Sympathomimetics
Colestipol *see* Cholestyramine and Colestipol
Colistin (other interactions *as for* Aminoglycosides)
Muscle Relaxants: enhanced muscle relaxant effect
Contraceptives, Oral
Note. Also covers oestrogens taken alone; in case of hormone replacement therapy low dose unlikely to induce interactions
ACE Inhibitors: *oestrogens* and *combined oral contraceptives* antagonise hypotensive effect

Contraceptives, Oral (*continued*)
- Antibacterials: *rifamycins* accelerate metabolism of both *combined and progestogen-only oral contraceptives* (reduced contraceptive effect, important: see p.313); when *broad-spectrum antibiotics such as ampicillin and tetracycline* given with *combined oral contraceptives* possibility of reduced contraceptive effect (risk probably small, but see p.313)
- Anticoagulants: antagonism of anticoagulant effect of *nicoumalone, phenindione, and warfarin*
  Antidepressants: antagonism of antidepressant effect has been reported, and side-effects of *tricyclics* may be increased due to higher plasma concentrations
  Antidiabetics: antagonism of hypoglycaemic effect
- Antiepileptics: *carbamazepine, phenobarbitone, phenytoin, and primidone* accelerate metabolism (reduced contraceptive effect, important: see p.313)
- Antifungals: *griseofulvin* accelerates metabolism (reduced contraceptive effect, important: see p.313)
  Antihypertensives: *combined oral contraceptives* antagonise hypotensive effect
  Barbiturates: *see under* Antiepileptics, above
  Beta-blockers: *oestrogens* and *combined oral contraceptives* antagonise hypotensive effect
- Cyclosporin: increased plasma-cyclosporin concentration
  Diuretics: *combined oral contraceptives* antagonise diuretic effect
  Theophylline: *combined oral contraceptives* delay excretion (increased plasma-theophylline concentration)

Corticosteroids
Note. Do not generally apply to corticosteroids used for topical action (including inhalation)
  Analgesics: increased risk of gastro-intestinal bleeding and ulceration with *aspirin* and *NSAIDs*
- Antibacterials: *rifampicin* accelerates metabolism of *corticosteroids* (reduced effect)
  Antidiabetics: antagonism of hypoglycaemic effect
- Antiepileptics: *carbamazepine, phenobarbitone, phenytoin, and primidone* accelerate metabolism of *corticosteroids* (reduced effect)
  Antihypertensives: antagonism of hypotensive effect
  Barbiturates: *see under* Antiepileptics, above
  Cardiac Glycosides: increased toxicity if hypokalaemia occurs with *corticosteroids*
- Cyclosporin: plasma-cyclosporin concentration increased by high-dose *methylprednisolone*; *cyclosporin* increases plasma concentration of *prednisolone*
  Diuretics: antagonism of diuretic effect; *acetazolamide, loop diuretics, and thiazides* increase risk of hypokalaemia
  Hormone Antagonists: *aminoglutethimide* accelerates metabolism of *dexamethasone* (reduced effect)
  Sympathomimetics *see* Sympathomimetics, Beta$_2$ (main list)
  Ulcer-healing Drugs: *carbenoxolone* increases risk of hypokalaemia
  Vaccines: see p.467

Co-trimoxazole and Sulphonamides
  Anaesthetics: effect of *thiopentone* enhanced
- Anticoagulants: effect of *nicoumalone and warfarin* enhanced
- Antidiabetics: effect of *sulphonylureas* enhanced
- Antiepileptics: antifolate effect and plasma concentration of *phenytoin* increased by *co-trimoxazole*
  Antimalarials: increased risk of antifolate effect with *pyrimethamine* (includes *Fansidar*® and *Maloprim*®)
- Cyclosporin: increased risk of nephrotoxicity

Co-trimoxazole and Sulphonamides (*continued*)
  Cytotoxics: antifolate effect of *methotrexate* increased by *co-trimoxazole*
  Potassium Aminobenzoate: inhibits effect of *sulphonamides*

Cyclizine *see* Antihistamines
Cyclobarbitone *see* Barbiturates
Cyclopenthiazide *see* Diuretics (thiazide)
Cyclopentolate *see* Antimuscarinics
Cyclophosphamide and Ifosfamide
- Allopurinol: toxicity of *cyclophosphamide* increased
- Anticoagulants: *ifosfamide* possibly enhances effect of *warfarin*
  Muscle Relaxants: *cyclophosphamide* enhances effect of *suxamethonium*
Cycloserine
  other Antibacterials: increased CNS toxicity with *isoniazid*
- Antiepileptics: increased plasma concentration of *phenytoin* (risk of toxicity)
Cyclosporin
- ACE Inhibitors: increased risk of hyperkalaemia
  Allopurinol: possibly increases plasma-cyclosporin concentration (risk of toxicity)
- Analgesics: increased risk of nephrotoxicity with *NSAIDs*; *cyclosporin* increases plasma concentration of *diclofenac* (halve diclofenac dose)
  Anti-arrhythmics: *amiodarone* and *propafenone* possibly increase plasma-cyclosporin concentration
- Antibacterials: *aminoglycosides, co-trimoxazole (and trimethoprim alone),* and *4-quinolones* increase risk of nephrotoxicity; *doxycycline* and *erythromycin* and possibly *other macrolides* increase plasma-cyclosporin concentration; *rifampicin, intravenous sulphadimidine, intravenous trimethoprim* (and possibly *sulphadiazine*) reduce plasma-cyclosporin concentration
- Antiepileptics: *carbamazepine, phenobarbitone, phenytoin, and primidone* accelerate metabolism (reduced plasma-cyclosporin concentration)
- Antifungals: *amphotericin* increases risk of nephrotoxicity; *griseofulvin* possibly reduces plasma-cyclosporin concentration; *itraconazole, ketoconazole* and possibly *fluconazole* inhibit metabolism (increased plasma-cyclosporin concentration)
  Barbiturates: *see under* Antiepileptics, above
- Calcium-channel Blockers: *diltiazem, nicardipine, and verapamil* increase plasma-cyclosporin concentration; *cyclosporin* possibly increases plasma concentration of *nifedipine*
- Colchicine: possibly increases risk of nephrotoxicity (increased plasma-cyclosporin concentration)
- Corticosteroids: *high-dose methylprednisolone* increases plasma-cyclosporin concentration; *cyclosporin* increases plasma concentration of *prednisolone*
- Cytotoxics: increased risk of neurotoxicity with *doxorubicin*; increased risk of nephrotoxicity with *melphalan*; increased toxicity with *methotrexate*
- Diuretics: *potassium-sparing diuretics* increase risk of hyperkalaemia
- Hormone Antagonists: *danazol* inhibits metabolism (increased plasma-cyclosporin concentration); *octreotide* reduces absorption (reduced plasma-cyclosporin concentration)
  Lipid-lowering Drugs: increased risk of myopathy with *pravastatin, simvastatin* and possibly *fluvastatin*
- Oestrogens and Progestogens: *progestogens* inhibit metabolism (increased plasma-cyclosporin concentration)
- Potassium Salts: increased risk of hyperkalaemia

Cyclosporin (*continued*)
* Ulcer-healing Drugs: *cimetidine* possibly increases plasma-cyclosporin concentration
  Vaccines: *see* Vaccines (main list)
Cyproheptadine *see* Antihistamines
Cytotoxics *see under* individual drugs
Dalteparin *see* Heparin
Danazol
* Anticoagulants: effect of *nicoumalone and warfarin* enhanced (inhibits metabolism)
* Antiepileptics: inhibits metabolism of *carbamazepine* (increased plasma-carbamazepine concentration)
* Cyclosporin: inhibits metabolism (increased plasma-cyclosporin concentration)
Dantrolene *see* Muscle Relaxants
Dapsone
  Antibacterials: plasma concentration reduced by *rifamycins*
  Probenecid: *dapsone* excretion reduced (increased risk of side-effects)
Debrisoquine *see* Adrenergic Neurone Blockers
Demecarium *see* Cholinergics
Demeclocycline *see* Tetracyclines
Desferrioxamine
  Antipsychotics: manufacturer advises avoid *prochlorperazine*
Desflurane *see* Anaesthetics (volatile liquid)
Desipramine *see* Antidepressants, Tricyclic
Desogestrel *see* Progestogens
Dexamethasone *see* Corticosteroids
Dexamphetamine *see* Sympathomimetics
Dexfenfluramine *see* Sympathomimetics
Dextromoramide *see* Opioid Analgesics
Dextropropoxyphene *see* Opioid Analgesics
Diamorphine *see* Opioid Analgesics
Diazepam *see* Benzodiazepines and other Anxiolytics and Hypnotics
Diazoxide (general hypotensive interactions *as for* Hydralazine)
  Antidiabetics: antagonism of hypoglycaemic effect
Dichlorphenamide *see* Acetazolamide
Diclofenac *see* NSAIDs
Dicyclomine *see* Antimuscarinics
Diethylpropion *see* Sympathomimetics
Diflunisal *see* NSAIDs
Digitoxin *see* Cardiac Glycosides
Digoxin *see* Cardiac Glycosides
Dihydrocodeine *see* Opioid Analgesics
Dihydroergotamine *see* Ergotamine
Diltiazem *see* Calcium-channel Blockers
Dimenhydrinate *see* Antihistamines
Diphenhydramine *see* Antihistamines
Diphenylpyraline *see* Antihistamines
Diphenoxylate *see* Opioid Analgesics
Dipipanone *see* Opioid Analgesics
Dipivefrine *see* Sympathomimetics (*as for* adrenaline)
Dipyridamole
  Antacids: patient information leaflet advises avoidance of *antacids*
* Anti-arrhythmics: effect of *adenosine* enhanced and extended (**important** risk of toxicity)
* Anticoagulants: enhanced effect due to antiplatelet action of *dipyridamole*
Disodium Etidronate *see* Bisphosphonates
Disodium Pamidronate *see* Bisphosphonates
Disopyramide
* *other* Anti-arrhythmics: *amiodarone* increases risk of ventricular arrhythmias; increased myocardial depression with any *anti-arrhythmic*
* Antibacterials: plasma concentration of *disopyramide* reduced by *rifampicin* but increased by *erythromycin* (risk of toxicity)
  Antiepileptics: plasma concentration of *disopyramide* reduced by *phenobarbitone, phenytoin, and primidone*

Disopyramide (*continued*)
* Antihistamines: increased risk of ventricular arrhythmias with *astemizole* and *terfenadine*
* Antimalarials: increased risk of ventricular arrhythmias with *halofantrine*
  Antimuscarinics: increased antimuscarinic side-effects
* Antipsychotics: increased risk of ventricular arrhythmias with *phenothiazines*
  Barbiturates: *see under* Antiepileptics, above
* Diuretics: toxicity of *disopyramide* increased if hypokalaemia occurs with *acetazolamide, loop diuretics, and thiazides*
  Nitrates: reduced effect of *sublingual nitrates* (failure to dissolve under tongue owing to dry mouth)
Distigmine *see* Cholinergics
Disulfiram
  Alcohol: disulfiram reaction (*see* section 4.10)
  Antibacterials: psychotic reaction with *metronidazole* reported
* Anticoagulants: effect of *nicoumalone and warfarin* enhanced
  Antidepressants: inhibition of metabolism of *tricyclic antidepressants* (increased plasma concentrations); increased disulfiram reaction with alcohol reported if *amitriptyline* also taken
* Antiepileptics: inhibition of metabolism of *phenytoin* (increased risk of toxicity)
  Anxiolytics and Hypnotics: inhibition of metabolism of *chlordiazepoxide and diazepam* (enhanced sedative effect)
  Theophylline: inhibition of metabolism (increased risk of toxicity)
Diuretics
* ACE Inhibitors: enhanced hypotensive effect (can be extreme); risk of hyperkalaemia with *potassium-sparing diuretics*
  Analgesics: *diuretics* increase risk of nephrotoxicity of *NSAIDs*; *NSAIDs* notably indomethacin antagonise diuretic effect; *indomethacin and possibly other NSAIDs* increase risk of hyperkalaemia with *potassium-sparing diuretics*; occasional reports of decreased renal function when *indomethacin* given with *triamterene*; diuretic effect of *spironolactone* antagonised by *aspirin*; *aspirin* reduces excretion of *acetazolamide* (risk of toxicity)
  Anion-exchange Resins: *cholestyramine and colestipol* reduce absorption of *thiazides* (give at least 2 hours apart)
* Anti-arrhythmics: toxicity of *amiodarone, disopyramide, flecainide, and quinidine* increased if hypokalaemia occurs; action of *lignocaine, mexiletine, and tocainide* antagonised by hypokalaemia; *acetazolamide* reduces excretion of *quinidine* (increased plasma concentration)
* Antibacterials: *loop diuretics* increase ototoxicity of *aminoglycosides, colistin, and vancomycin*
  Antidepressants: increased risk of postural hypotension with *tricyclics*
  Antidiabetics: hypoglycaemic effect antagonised by *loop and thiazide diuretics; chlorpropamide* increases risk of hyponatraemia associated with *thiazides in combination with potassium-sparing diuretics*
  Antifungals: increased risk of hypokalaemia if *loop diuretics* and *thiazides* given with *amphotericin*
* Antihistamines: hypokalaemia increases risk of ventricular arrhythmias with *astemizole* and *terfenadine*
  Antihypertensives: enhanced hypotensive effect; increased risk of first-dose hypotensive effect of post-synaptic *alpha-blockers such as prazosin*; increased risk of hypokalaemia with *indapamide*

Diuretics (*continued*)
- Antimalarials: electrolyte disturbances increase risk of ventricular arrhythmias with *halofantrine*
  Antipsychotics: in hypokalaemia increased risk of ventricular arrhythmias with *pimozide*
  Beta-blockers: in hypokalaemia increased risk of ventricular arrhythmias with *sotalol*
  Calcium Salts: risk of hypercalcaemia with *thiazides*
- Cardiac Glycosides: increased toxicity if hypokalaemia occurs with *acetazolamide, loop diuretics, and thiazides;* effect enhanced by *spironolactone*
  Corticosteroids: increased risk of hypokalaemia with *acetazolamide, loop diuretics, and thiazides;* antagonism of diuretic effect
- Cyclosporin: increased risk of hyperkalaemia with *potassium-sparing diuretics*
  Cytotoxics: increased risk of nephrotoxicity and ototoxicity with *cisplatin*
  other Diuretics: increased risk of hypokalaemia if *acetazolamide, loop diuretics or thiazides* given together; profound diuresis possible if *metolazone* given with *frusemide* (p.59)
  Hormone Antagonists: *trilostane* increases risk of hyperkalaemia with *potassium-sparing diuretics*
- Lithium: lithium excretion reduced by *loop diuretics and thiazides* (increased plasma-lithium concentration and risk of toxicity—*loop diuretics* safer than *thiazides*); lithium excretion increased by *acetazolamide*
  Oestrogens and Progestogens: *oestrogens and combined oral contraceptives* antagonise diuretic effect
- Potassium Salts: hyperkalaemia with *potassium-sparing diuretics*
  Ulcer-healing Drugs: increased risk of hypokalaemia if *acetazolamide, loop diuretics, and thiazides* given with *carbenoxolone; carbenoxolone* antagonises diuretic effect; *amiloride and spironolactone* antagonise ulcer-healing effect of *carbenoxolone*
  Vitamins: increased risk of hypercalcaemia if *thiazides* given with *vitamin D*

Domperidone
  Analgesics: *opioid analgesics* antagonise effect on gastro-intestinal activity
  Antimuscarinics: antagonism of effect on gastro-intestinal activity
  Dopaminergics: antagonism of hypoprolactinaemic effect of *bromocriptine*

Dopamine *see* Sympathomimetics
Dopaminergics *see* Amantadine, Bromocriptine, Levodopa, and Lysuride
Dopexamine *see* Sympathomimetics
Dothiepin *see* Antidepressants, Tricyclic
Doxapram
  Sympathomimetics: risk of hypertension
  Theophylline: increased CNS stimulation
Doxazosin *see* Alpha-blockers (post-synaptic)
Doxepin *see* Antidepressants, Tricyclic
Doxorubicin
- Cyclosporin: increased risk of neurotoxicity
Doxycycline *see* Tetracyclines
Droperidol *see* Phenothiazines and other Antipsychotics
Dydrogesterone *see* Progestogens
Ecothiopate *see* Cholinergics
Edrophonium *see* Cholinergics
Enalapril *see* ACE Inhibitors
Enflurane *see* Anaesthetics (volatile liquid)
Enoxaparin *see* Heparin
Ephedrine *see* Sympathomimetics
Ergotamine
  Antibacterials: ergotism with *erythromycin* and possibly *azithromycin*
  Beta-blockers: increased peripheral vasoconstriction
- Sumatriptan: increased risk of vasospasm (see section 4.7.4.1)

Erythromycin and other Macrolides
  Note. Do not apply to small amounts used topically
  Analgesics: plasma concentration of *alfentanil* increased by *erythromycin*
  Antacids and Adsorbents: *antacids* reduce absorption of *azithromycin*
- Anti-arrhythmics: plasma concentration of *disopyramide* increased by *erythromycin* (risk of toxicity)
- *other* Antibiotics: **important:** *rifabutin* and **CSM advice,** see p.526
- Anticoagulants: effect of *nicoumalone and warfarin* enhanced by *erythromycin* and possibly enhanced by *other macrolides*
- Antiepileptics: *clarithromycin* and *erythromycin* inhibit metabolism of *carbamazepine* (increased plasma-carbamazepine concentration)
- Antihistamines: *erythromycin* and *other macrolides* inhibit metabolism of *astemizole* and *terfenadine* (see p.130)
  Anxiolytics and Hypnotics: *erythromycin* inhibits metabolism of *midazolam* (increased plasma-midazolam concentration, **important** see also p.491)
  Cardiac Glycosides: effect of *digoxin* enhanced by *erythromycin* and possibly enhanced by *other macrolides*
- Cyclosporin: *erythromycin* and possibly *other macrolides* inhibit metabolism (increased plasma-cyclosporin concentration)
  Dopaminergics: plasma concentration of *bromocriptine* increased by *erythromycin*
  Ergotamine: ergotism reported
- Theophylline: *clarithromycin* and *erythromycin* inhibit metabolism (increased plasma-theophylline concentration)

Esmolol *see* Beta-blockers
Ethacrynic Acid *see* Diuretics (loop)
Ethinyloestradiol *see* Contraceptives, Oral
Ethosuximide
- Antibacterials: *isoniazid* increases plasma concentrations (increased risk of toxicity)
- Antidepressants: antagonism (convulsive threshold lowered)
- *other* Antiepileptics: concomitant administration of two or more antiepileptics may enhance toxicity without a corresponding increase in antiepileptic effect; moreover interactions between individual antiepileptics can complicate monitoring of treatment; interactions include enhanced effects, increased sedation, and reductions in plasma concentrations; for further details, see p.193
- Antipsychotics: antagonism (convulsive threshold lowered)

Ethynodiol *see* Progestogens
Etidronate Disodium *see* Bisphosphonates
Etodolac *see* NSAIDs
Famciclovir *see* Acyclovir and Famciclovir
Famotidine *see* Histamine H₂-antagonists
Fansidar® contains Sulfadoxine and Pyrimethamine
Felodipine *see* Calcium-channel Blockers
Fenbufen *see* NSAIDs
Fenfluramine *see* Sympathomimetics
Fenofibrate *see* Clofibrate Group
Fenoprofen *see* NSAIDs
Fenoterol *see* Sympathomimetics, Beta₂
Fentanyl *see* Opioid Analgesics
Ferrous Salts *see* Iron
Flavoxate *see* Antimuscarinics
Flecainide
- *other* Anti-arrhythmics: *amiodarone* increases plasma-flecainide concentration (and increases risk of ventricular arrhythmias); increased myocardial depression with any *anti-arrhythmic*

Flecainide (*continued*)

Antidepressants: *fluoxetine* increases plasma-flecainide concentration

* Antihistamines: increased risk of ventricular arrhythmias with *astemizole* and *terfenadine*

Antimalarials: *quinine* increases plasma concentration of *flecainide*

* Beta-blockers: increased myocardial depression and bradycardia
* Calcium-channel Blockers: increased myocardial depression and asystole with *verapamil*
* Diuretics: toxicity increased if hypokalaemia occurs

Ulcer-healing Drugs: *cimetidine* inhibits metabolism of *flecainide* (increased plasma-flecainide concentration)

Flucloxacillin *see* Penicillins

Fluconazole *see* Antifungals, Imidazole and Triazole

Fludrocortisone *see* Corticosteroids

Flunitrazepam *see* Benzodiazepines and other Anxiolytics and Hypnotics

Fluorouracil

Antibacterials: *metronidazole* inhibits metabolism (increased toxicity)

Ulcer-healing Drugs: *cimetidine* inhibits metabolism (increased plasma-fluorouracil concentration)

Fluoxetine *see* Antidepressants, Serotonin-uptake Inhibitor

Flupenthixol *see* Phenothiazines and other Antipsychotics

Fluphenazine *see* Phenothiazines and other Antipsychotics

Flurazepam *see* Benzodiazepines and other Anxiolytics and Hypnotics

Flurbiprofen *see* NSAIDs

Fluspirilene *see* Phenothiazines and other Antipsychotics

Flutamide

* Anticoagulants: effect of *warfarin* enhanced

Fluticasone *see* Corticosteroids

Fluvastatin

Antibacterials: metabolism accelerated by *rifampicin* (reduced effect)

Cyclosporin: possibly increased risk of myopathy

Fluvoxamine *see* Antidepressants, Serotonin-uptake Inhibitor

Folic Acid *see* Vitamins

Fosfomycin

Domperidone and Metoclopramide: reduced plasma and urine concentrations with *metoclopramide*

Fosinopril *see* ACE Inhibitors

Framycetin *see* Aminoglycosides

Frusemide *see* Diuretics (loop)

Gabapentin

Antacids and Adsorbents: *antacids* reduce absorption

other Antiepileptics: none demonstrated with *carbamazepine, phenobarbitone, phenytoin,* or *valproate*

Gallamine *see* Muscle Relaxants (non-depolarising)

Ganciclovir

Note: Increased risk of myelosuppression with other *myelosuppressive drugs*—consult data sheet

other Antivirals: profound myelosuppression with *zidovudine*

Gemfibrozil *see* Clofibrate Group

Gentamicin *see* Aminoglycosides

Gestodene *see* Progestogens

Gestrinone

Antibacterials: *rifampicin* accelerates metabolism (reduced plasma concentration)

Antiepileptics: *carbamazepine, phenobarbitone, phenytoin, and primidone* accelerate metabolism (reduced plasma concentration)

Glibenclamide *see* Antidiabetics (sulphonylurea)

Gliclazide *see* Antidiabetics (sulphonylurea)

Glipizide *see* Antidiabetics (sulphonylurea)

Gliquidone *see* Antidiabetics (sulphonylurea)

Glyceryl Trinitrate (general hypotensive interactions *as for* Hydralazine)

Anti-arrhythmics: *disopyramide* may reduce effect of *sublingual nitrates* (owing to dry mouth)

* Anticoagulants: excretion of *heparin* increased by *glyceryl trinitrate infusion* (reduced anticoagulant effect)

Antidepressants: *tricyclics* may reduce effect of *sublingual nitrates* (owing to dry mouth)

Antimuscarinics: *antimuscarinics such as atropine and propantheline* may reduce effect of *sublingual nitrates* (owing to dry mouth)

Gold

Note. Increased risk of toxicity with other nephrotoxic and myelosuppressive drugs

Griseofulvin

* Anticoagulants: metabolism of *nicoumalone and warfarin* accelerated (reduced anticoagulant effect)

Antiepileptics: metabolism accelerated by *phenobarbitone* (reduced effect)

Cyclosporin: plasma-cyclosporin concentration possibly reduced

* Oestrogens and Progestogens:: metabolism of *oral contraceptives* accelerated (reduced contraceptive effect, **important:** see p.313)

Guanethidine *see* Adrenergic Neurone Blockers

Guar Gum

Antibacterials: absorption of *phenoxymethylpenicillin* reduced

Halofantrine

* Anti-arrhythmics: increased risk of ventricular arrhythmias with drugs which prolong QT interval
* Antidepressants: increased risk of ventricular arrhythmias with *tricyclics*
* Antihistamines: increased risk of ventricular arrhythmias with *astemizole* and *terfenadine*
* *other* Antimalarials: increased risk of arrhythmias with *chloroquine, mefloquine* and *quinine* (**important:** see also CSM advice under Halofantrine, p.259)
* Antipsychotics: increased risk of of ventricular arrhythmias with *phenothiazines*
* Beta-blockers: increased risk of ventricular arrhythmias with *sotalol*
* Diuretics: increased risk of ventricular arrhythmias if electrolyte disturbances occur

Haloperidol *see* Phenothiazines and other Antipsychotics

Halothane *see* Anaesthetics (volatile liquid)

Heparin

* Analgesics: *aspirin* enhances anticoagulant effect; increased risk of haemorrhage with *ketorolac*, see p.493

Antiplatelet Drugs: *aspirin and dipyridamole* enhance anticoagulant effect

* Nitrates: *glyceryl trinitrate infusion* increases excretion (reduced anticoagulant effect)

Hexamine

Potassium Citrate: urine should be acid

Histamine H1-antagonists *see* Antihistamines

Histamine H2-antagonists

Analgesics: *cimetidine* inhibits metabolism of *opioid analgesics notably pethidine* (increased plasma concentrations)

Anthelmintics: *cimetidine* possibly inhibits metabolism of *mebendazole* (increased plasma concentration)

* Anti-arrhythmics: *cimetidine* increases plasma concentrations of *amiodarone, flecainide, lignocaine, procainamide, propafenone, quinidine,* and possibly *moracizine*

Histamine H2-Antagonists (*continued*)

Antibacterials: absorption of *cefpodoxime* reduced; *rifampicin* accelerates metabolism of *cimetidine* (reduced plasma-cimetidine concentration); *cimetidine* inhibits metabolism of *metronidazole* (increased plasma-metronidazole concentration)

• Anticoagulants: *cimetidine* enhances anticoagulant effect of *nicoumalone and warfarin* (inhibits metabolism)

Antidepressants: *cimetidine* inhibits metabolism of *amitriptyline, desipramine, doxepin, imipramine, moclobemide, and nortriptyline* (increased plasma concentrations)

Antidiabetics: *cimetidine* inhibits renal excretion of *metformin* (increased plasma concentration); *cimetidine* and *ranitidine* enhance hypoglycaemic effect of *sulphonylureas*

• Antiepileptics: *cimetidine* inhibits metabolism of *carbamazepine and phenytoin* (increased plasma concentrations)

Antifungals: absorption of *itraconazole and ketoconazole* reduced; plasma concentration of *terbinafine* increased by *cimetidine*

Antimalarials: *cimetidine* inhibits metabolism of *chloroquine and quinine* (increased plasma concentrations)

Antipsychotics: *cimetidine* may enhance effect of *chlorpromazine, clozapine, and possibly other antipsychotics*

Anxiolytics and Hypnotics: *cimetidine* inhibits metabolism of *benzodiazepines and chlormethiazole* (increased plasma concentrations)

Beta-blockers: *cimetidine* inhibits metabolism of *beta-blockers such as labetalol and propranolol* (increased plasma concentrations)

Calcium-channel Blockers: *cimetidine* inhibits metabolism of *some calcium-channel blockers* (increased plasma concentrations)

• Cyclosporin: *cimetidine* possibly increases plasma-cyclosporin concentration

Cytotoxics: *cimetidine* increases plasma concentration of *fluorouracil*

• Theophylline: *cimetidine* inhibits metabolism (increased plasma-theophylline concentration)

Homatropine *see* Antimuscarinics

Hydralazine

ACE Inhibitors: enhanced hypotensive effect

Alcohol: enhanced hypotensive effect

Aldesleukin: enhanced hypotensive effect

• Anaesthetics: enhanced hypotensive effect

Analgesics: *NSAIDs* antagonise hypotensive effect

Antidepressants: enhanced hypotensive effect

other Antihypertensives: additive hypotensive effect

Antipsychotics: enhanced hypotensive effect

Anxiolytics and Hypnotics: enhanced hypotensive effect

Beta-blockers: enhanced hypotensive effect

Calcium-channel Blockers: enhanced hypotensive effect

Corticosteroids: antagonism of hypotensive effect

Diuretics: enhanced hypotensive effect

Dopaminergics: *levodopa* enhances hypotensive effect

Muscle Relaxants: *baclofen* enhances hypotensive effect

Nitrates: enhanced hypotensive effect

Oestrogens and Progestogens: *oestrogens and combined oral contraceptives* antagonise hypotensive effect

Ulcer-healing Drugs: *carbenoxolone* antagonises hypotensive effect

Hydrochlorothiazide *see* Diuretics (thiazide)

Hydrocortisone *see* Corticosteroids

Hydroflumethiazide *see* Diuretics (thiazide)

Hydroxychloroquine   *see*   Chloroquine   and Hydroxychloroquine

Hydroxyprogesterone *see* Progestogens

Hydroxyzine *see* Antihistamines

Hyoscine *see* Antimuscarinics (for general sedative interactions *see also* Antihistamines)

Hypnotics *see* Benzodiazepines and other Anxiolytics and Hypnotics

Ibuprofen *see* NSAIDs

Ifosfamide *see* Cyclophosphamide and Ifosfamide

Imipramine *see* Antidepressants, Tricyclic

Indapamide *see* Diuretics (thiazide-related)

Indomethacin *see* NSAIDs

Indoramin *see* Alpha-blockers

Influenza Vaccine

Anticoagulants: effect of *warfarin* occasionally enhanced

Antiepileptics: effect of *phenytoin* enhanced

Theophylline: effect occasionally enhanced

Insulin *see* Antidiabetics

Interferons

Note. Consult data sheet for interactions of interferon gamma

Theophylline: *interferon alfa* inhibits metabolism of *theophylline* (enhanced effect)

Ipratropium *see* Antimuscarinics

Iprindole *see* Antidepressants, Tricyclic

Iron

Antacids: *magnesium trisilicate* reduces absorption of *oral iron*

Antibacterials: *tetracyclines* reduce absorption of *oral iron* (and *vice versa*); absorption of *ciprofloxacin, norfloxacin,* and *ofloxacin* reduced by *oral iron*

Bisphosphonates: reduced absorption (give at least 2 hours apart)

Dopaminergics: absorption of *levodopa* may be reduced

Penicillamine: reduced absorption of *penicillamine*

Trientine: reduced absorption of *oral iron*

Zinc: reduced absorption of *oral iron* (and *vice versa*)

Isocarboxazid *see* MAOIs

Isoflurane *see* Anaesthetics (volatile liquid)

Isometheptene *see* Sympathomimetics

Isoniazid

Antacids and Adsorbents: *antacids* reduce absorption

other Antibacterials: increased CNS toxicity with *cycloserine*

• Antiepileptics: metabolism of *carbamazepine, ethosuximide, and phenytoin* inhibited (enhanced effect); also, with *carbamazepine*, isoniazid hepatotoxicity possibly increased

Anxiolytics and Hypnotics: metabolism of *diazepam* inhibited

Theophylline: *isoniazid* possibly increases plasma theophylline concentration

Isoprenaline *see* Sympathomimetics

Isosorbide Dinitrate *see* Glyceryl Trinitrate

Isosorbide Mononitrate *see* Glyceryl Trinitrate

Isradipine *see* Calcium-channel Blockers

Itraconazole *see* Antifungals, Imidazole and Triazole

Kanamycin *see* Aminoglycosides

Kaolin *see* Antacids and Adsorbents

Ketoconazole *see* Antifungals, Imidazole and Triazole

Ketoprofen *see* NSAIDs

Ketorolac *see* NSAIDs and p.493

Ketotifen *see* Antihistamines

Labetalol *see* Beta-blockers

Lacidipine *see* Calcium-channel Blockers

Lamotrigine
- *other* Antiepileptics: concomitant administration of *two or more antiepileptics* may enhance toxicity without a corresponding increase in antiepileptic effect; moreover interactions between individual antiepileptics can complicate monitoring of treatment; interactions include enhanced effects, increased sedation, and reductions in plasma concentrations; for further details, see p.193

Lansoprazole *see* Proton Pump Inhibitors

Levobunolol *see* Beta-blockers

Levodopa
- Anaesthetics: risk of arrhythmias with *volatile liquid anaesthetics such as halothane*
- Antidepressants: hypertensive crisis with *MAOIs* (including *moclobemide*)—avoid for at least 2 weeks after stopping MAOI

  Antihypertensives: enhanced hypotensive effect

  Antipsychotics: antagonism of effect

  Anxiolytics and Hypnotics: occasional antagonism of effect by *chlordiazepoxide, diazepam, lorazepam and possibly other benzodiazepines*

  Domperidone and Metoclopramide: levodopa-plasma concentrations increased by *metoclopramide*

  Iron: absorption of *levodopa* may be reduced

  Vitamins: effect of *levodopa* antagonised by *pyridoxine* unless a *dopa decarboxylase inhibitor* also given

Levonorgestrel *see* Progestogens

Lignocaine
  other Anti-arrhythmics: increased myocardial depression

  Beta-blockers: increased risk of myocardial depression; increased risk of *lignocaine* toxicity with *propranolol*

  Diuretics: effect of *lignocaine* antagonised by hypokalaemia with *acetazolamide, loop diuretics, and thiazides*

  Ulcer-healing Drugs: *cimetidine* inhibits metabolism of *lignocaine* (increased risk of toxicity)

Lisinopril *see* ACE Inhibitors

Lithium
- ACE Inhibitors: *lithium* excretion reduced (increased plasma-lithium concentration)
- Analgesics: *NSAIDs* reduce excretion of *lithium* (possibility of toxicity)—*ketorolac*, see p.493

  Antacids and Adsorbents: *sodium bicarbonate* increases excretion of *lithium* (reduced plasma-lithium concentrations)

  Antibacterials: *lithium* toxicity reported with *metronidazole* and *spectinomycin*
- Antidepressants: *fluoxetine, fluvoxamine, paroxetine, and sertraline* increase risk of CNS toxicity

  Antidiabetics: *lithium* may occasionally impair glucose tolerance

  Antiepileptics: neurotoxicity may occur with *carbamazepine and phenytoin* without increased plasma-lithium concentration

  Antihypertensives: neurotoxicity may occur with *methyldopa* without increased plasma-lithium concentration

  Antipsychotics: increased risk of extrapyramidal effects and possibility of neurotoxicity (notably with *haloperidol*)

  Calcium-channel Blockers: neurotoxicity may occur with *diltiazem and verapamil* without increased plasma-lithium concentration

  Cholinergics: *lithium* antagonises effect of *neostigmine and pyridostigmine*

Lithium (*continued*)
- Diuretics: *lithium* excretion reduced by *loop diuretics and thiazides* (increased plasma-lithium concentration and risk of toxicity—*loop diuretics* safer than *thiazides*); *lithium* excretion increased by *acetazolamide*

  Domperidone and Metoclopramide: increased risk of extrapyramidal effects and possibility of neurotoxicity with *metoclopramide*

  Muscle Relaxants: muscle relaxant effect enhanced; *baclofen* possibly aggravates hyperkinesis
- Sumatriptan: risk of CNS toxicity

  Theophylline: *lithium* excretion increased (reduced plasma-lithium concentration)

Lofepramine *see* Antidepressants, Tricyclic

Lofexidine
  Alcohol: enhanced sedative effect

  Anxiolytics and Hypnotics: enhanced sedative effect

Loprazolam *see* Benzodiazepines and other Anxiolytics and Hypnotics

Loratadine *see* Antihistamines

Lorazepam *see* Benzodiazepines and other Anxiolytics and Hypnotics

Lormetazepam *see* Benzodiazepines and other Anxiolytics and Hypnotics

Loxapine *see* Phenothiazines and other Antipsychotics

Lymecycline *see* Tetracyclines

Lysuride
  Antipsychotics: antagonism of effect

Macrolides *see* Erythromycin and other Macrolides

Magnesium Salts (*see also* Antacids and Adsorbents)
  Muscle Relaxants: effect of *non-depolarising muscle relaxants such as tubocurarine* enhanced by *parenteral magnesium salts*

Magnesium Trisilicate *see* Antacids and Adsorbents

Maloprim® contains Dapsone and Pyrimethamine

MAOIs
  Note. For interactions of reversible MAO-A inhibitors (RIMAs) see Moclobemide, and for interactions of MAO-B inhibitors see Selegiline
- Alcohol: some *alcoholic and dealcoholised beverages contain tyramine* which interacts with *MAOIs* (hypertensive crisis)—but if no tyramine, enhanced hypotensive effect; foods, *see* MAOI card, section 4.3.2
- Analgesics: CNS excitation or depression (hypertension or hypotension) with *pethidine and possibly other opioid analgesics*; manufacturer advises avoid *nefopam*

  Anorectics: *see* Sympathomimetics, below
- *other* Antidepressants: enhancement of CNS effects and toxicity with *other MAOIs* (avoid for at least a week after stopping *previous MAOIs* then start with reduced dose); CNS excitation and hypertension with most *tricyclics and related antidepressants* (avoid for at least 2 weeeks after stopping MAOI, and avoid MAOI for at least 1 week after stopping tricyclic); enhancement of CNS effects and toxicity possible with *serotonin-uptake inhibitors* (avoid for at least 2 weeks after stopping MAOI, and avoid MAOI for at least 1 week after stopping serotonin-uptake inhibitor—*fluoxetine* for at least 5 weeks and *paroxetine* for at least 2 weeks); CNS excitation and confusion with *tryptophan* (reduce tryptophan dose)

  Antidiabetics: effect of *insulin, metformin, and sulphonylureas* enhanced
- Antiepileptics: antagonism of anticonvulsant effect (convulsive threshold lowered); manufacturer advises avoid *carbamazepine* with or within 2 weeks of *MAOIs*
- Antihypertensives: hypotensive effect enhanced

  Antihistamines: increased antimuscarinic and sedative effects

  Antimuscarinics: increased side-effects

MAOIs (*continued*)

- Antipsychotics: CNS excitation and hypertension with *oxypertine*

  Anxiolytics and Hypnotics: manufacturer advises avoidance of *buspirone*

- Dopaminergics: hypertensive crisis with *levodopa* (avoid for at least 2 weeks after stopping MAOI)

- Sumatriptan: risk of CNS toxicity

- Sympathomimetics: hypertensive crisis with *sympathomimetics such as dexamphetamine and other amphetamines, dexfenfluramine, diethylpropion, dopamine, dopexamine, ephedrine, fenfluramine, isometheptene, pemoline, phentermine, phenylephrine, phenylpropanolamine, and pseudoephedrine*

- Tetrabenazine: CNS excitation and hypertension

Maprotiline *see* Antidepressants, Tricyclic

Mebendazole

Ulcer-healing Drugs: metabolism possibly inhibited by *cimetidine* (increased plasma-mebendazole concentration)

Medroxyprogesterone *see* Progestogens

Mefenamic Acid *see* NSAIDs

Mefloquine

Antiepileptics: antagonism of anticonvulsant effect

other Antimalarials: increased risk of convulsions with *chloroquine* and *quinine*, but should not prevent use of intravenous quinine in severe cases; for full precautions see footnote on p. 256 (also applies to *quinidine*); increased risk of ventricular arrhythmias with *halofantrine* (**important**: see also CSM advice under Halofantrine, p. 259)

Beta-blockers: possible increased risk of bradycardia

Calcium-channel Blockers: possible increased risk of bradycardia with some *calcium-channel blockers*

Cardiac Glycosides: possible increased risk of bradycardia with *digoxin*

Vaccines: *see* Typhoid Vaccine, p. 479

Mefruside *see* Diuretics (thiazide)

Melphalan

Antibacterials: increased toxicity with *nalidixic acid*

- Cyclosporin: increased risk of nephrotoxicity

Mepacrine

other Antimalarials: increased plasma concentration of *primaquine* (risk of toxicity)

Mepenzolate *see* Antimuscarinics

Meprobamate *see* Benzodiazepines and other Anxiolytics and Hypnotics

Meptazinol *see* Opioid Analgesics

Mequitazine *see* Antihistamines

Mercaptopurine

- Allopurinol: enhancement of effect (increased toxicity)

Mestranol *see* Contraceptives, Oral

Metaraminol *see* Sympathomimetics (*as* noradrenaline)

Metformin *see* Antidiabetics

Methadone *see* Opioid Analgesics

Methocarbamol *see* Muscle Relaxants

Methohexitone *see* Barbiturates and Primidone

Methotrexate

- Analgesics: excretion reduced by *aspirin, azapropazone, diclofenac, indomethacin, ketoprofen, naproxen, phenylbutazone, and probably other NSAIDs* (increased risk of toxicity)

Methotrexate (*continued*)

- Antibacterials: antifolate effect increased by *co-trimoxazole and trimethoprim*; excretion reduced by penicillins (increased risk of toxicity)

  Antiepileptics: *phenytoin* increases antifolate effect

  Antimalarials: antifolate effect increased by *pyrimethamine* (ingredient of *Fansidar®* and *Maloprim®*)

- Cyclosporin: increased toxicity

- Retinoids: plasma concentration of *methotrexate* increased by *acitretin* (also increased risk of hepatotoxicity)

- Uricosurics: excretion reduced by *probenecid* (increased risk of toxicity)

Methotrimeprazine *see* Phenothiazines and other Antipsychotics

Methoxamine *see* Sympathomimetics (*as* noradrenaline)

Methyclothiazide *see* Diuretics (thiazide)

Methyldopa

Alcohol: enhanced hypotensive effect

- Anaesthetics: enhanced hypotensive effect

  Analgesics: *NSAIDs* antagonise hypotensive effect

  Antidepressants: enhanced hypotensive effect

  other Antihypertensives: enhanced hypotensive effect

  Antipsychotics: increased risk of extrapyramidal effects; enhanced hypotensive effect

  Anxiolytics and Hypnotics: enhanced hypotensive effect

  Beta-blockers: enhanced hypotensive effect

  Calcium-channel Blockers: enhanced hypotensive effect

  Corticosteroids: antagonism of hypotensive effect

  Diuretics: enhanced hypotensive effect

  Dopaminergics: antagonism of antiparkinsonian effect; *levodopa* enhances hypotensive effect

  Lithium: neurotoxicity may occur without increased plasma-lithium concentration

  Nitrates: enhance hypotensive effect

  Oestrogens and Progestogens: *oestrogens and combined oral contraceptives* antagonise hypotensive effect

  Sympathomimetics: *see* Sympathomimetics (main list)

  Ulcer-healing Drugs: *carbenoxolone* antagonises hypotensive effect

Methylphenobarbitone *see* Barbiturates

Methylprednisolone *see* Corticosteroids

Metipranolol *see* Beta-blockers

Metirosine

Antipsychotics: increased risk of extrapyramidal effects

Dopaminergics: antagonism

Metoclopramide

Analgesics: increased absorption of *aspirin and paracetamol* (enhanced effect); *opioid analgesics* antagonise effect on gastro-intestinal activity

Antibacterials: reduced plasma and urine concentrations of *fosfomycin*

Antimuscarinics: antagonism of effect on gastro-intestinal activity

Antipsychotics: increased risk of extrapyramidal effects

Dopaminergics: antagonism of hypoprolactinaemic effect of *bromocriptine*; increased plasma concentration of *levodopa*

Lithium: increased risk of extrapyramidal effects and possibility of neurotoxicity

Tetrabenazine: increased risk of extrapyramidal effects

Metolazone *see* Diuretics (thiazide-related)

Metoprolol *see* Beta-blockers

Metronidazole
Alcohol: disulfiram-like reaction
- Anticoagulants: effect of *nicoumalone and warfarin* enhanced
- Antiepileptics: *metronidazole* inhibits metabolism of *phenytoin* (increased plasma-phenytoin concentration); *phenobarbitone* accelerates metabolism of *metronidazole* (reduced plasma-metronidazole concentration)
Cytotoxics: *metronidazole* inhibits metabolism of *fluorouracil* (increased toxicity)
Disulfiram: psychotic reactions reported
Lithium: increased toxicity reported
Ulcer-healing Drugs: *cimetidine* inhibits metabolism (increased plasma-metronidazole concentration)

Mexiletine
Analgesics: *opioid analgesics* delay absorption
- *other* Anti-arrhythmics: increased myocardial depression with any combination of *anti-arrhythmics*
Antibacterials: *rifampicin* accelerates metabolism (reduced plasma-mexiletine concentration)
Antiepileptics: *phenytoin* accelerates metabolism (reduced plasma-mexiletine concentration)
Antimuscarinics: *atropine* delays absorption
Diuretics: action of *mexiletine* antagonised by hypokalaemia due to *acetazolamide, loop diuretics, and thiazides*
Theophylline: plasma-theophylline concentration increased

Mianserin
Alcohol: enhanced effect
other Antidepressants: as for Antidepressants, Tricyclic
Antiepileptics: antagonism (convulsive threshold lowered); reduced antidepressant effect (reduced plasma-mianserin concentration)
Anxiolytics and Hypnotics: enhanced effect

Miconazole *see* Antifungals, Imidazole and Triazole
Midazolam *see* Benzodiazepines and other Anxiolytics and Hypnotics
Mifepristone
Analgesics: manufacturer recommends avoid *aspirin* and *NSAIDs* until 8–12 days after *mifepristone* administration

Minocycline *see* Tetracyclines
Minoxidil *see* Hydralazine for general hypotensive interactions
Mivacurium *see* Muscle Relaxants (non-depolarising)
Moclobemide
Note. Moclobemide is a reversible MAO-A inhibitor (RIMA), see also p.169
- Analgesics: CNS excitation or depression (hypertension or hypotension) with *codeine , pethidine,* and possibly *fentanyl , morphine,* and *other opioid analgesics*; effects of *ibuprofen* and possibly *other NSAIDs* enhanced
- Anorectics: as for MAOIs (see main list)
- *other* Antidepressants: see p.169
- Dopaminergics: hypertensive crisis with *levodopa*
- Sumatriptan: risk of CNS toxicity
- Sympathomimetics: as for MAOIs (see main list)
Ulcer-healing Drugs: *cimetidine* inhibits metabolism (increased plasma-moclobemide concentration)

Monoamine-oxidase Inhibitors *see* MAOIs, Moclobemide, and Selegiline
Monosulfiram
Alcohol: disulfiram-like reaction
Moracizine
other Anti-arrhythmics: increased myocardial depression with any *anti-arrhythmic*
Theophylline: metabolism of *theophylline* accelerated (reduced effect)
Ulcer-healing Drugs: *cimetidine* possibly increases plasma-moracizine concentration
Morphine *see* Opioid Analgesics

Muscle Relaxants
ACE Inhibitors: enhanced hypotensive effect with *baclofen*
Alcohol: enhanced sedative effect with *baclofen*
- Anti-arrhythmics: *procainamide* and *quinidine* enhance muscle relaxant effect
- Antibacterials: effect of *non-depolarising muscle relaxants* such as *tubocurarine* enhanced by *aminoglycosides, azlocillin, clindamycin and colistin*
Antidepressants: *tricyclics* enhance muscle relaxant effect of *baclofen*
Antiepileptics: effect of *non-depolarising muscle relaxants* antagonised by *carbamazepine* (recovery from neuromuscular blockade accelerated)
Antihypertensives: enhanced hypotensive effect with *baclofen*
Anxiolytics and Hypnotics: enhanced sedative effect with *baclofen*
Beta-blockers: *propranolol* enhances muscle relaxant effect
- Botulinum Toxin: neuromuscular block enhanced by *non-depolarising muscle relaxants* such as *tubocurarine* (risk of toxicity)
Calcium-channel Blockers: *nifedipine* and *verapamil* enhance effect of *non-depolarising muscle relaxants* such as *tubocurarine*; hypotension, myocardial depression, and hyperkalaemia reported with intravenous *dantrolene* and *verapamil*
Cardiac Glycosides: arrhythmias if *suxamethonium* given with *digoxin*
Cholinergics: *demecarium* and *ecothiopate* eye-drops, and *neostigmine,* and *pyridostigmine* enhance effect of *suxamethonium* but antagonise effect of *non-depolarising muscle relaxants* such as *tubocurarine*
Cytotoxics: *cyclophosphamide and thiotepa* enhance effect of *suxamethonium*
Lithium: *lithium* enhances muscle relaxant effect; *baclofen* possibly aggravates hyperkinesis
Magnesium Salts: *parenteral magnesium* enhances effect of *non-depolarising muscle relaxants* such as *tubocurarine*
Sympathomimetics: *bambuterol* enhances effect of *suxamethonium*

Nabilone
Alcohol: sedative effect of *nabilone* enhanced
Anxiolytics and Hypnotics: enhanced sedative effect
Nabumetone *see* NSAIDs
Nadolol *see* Beta-blockers
Nalbuphine *see* Opioid Analgesics
Nalidixic Acid *see* 4-Quinolones
Nandrolone *see* Anabolic Steroids
Naproxen *see* NSAIDs
Nefopam
- Antidepressants: manufacturer recommends avoid *MAOIs*
Antimuscarinics: increased side-effects
Neomycin *see* Aminoglycosides
Neostigmine *see* Cholinergics
Netilmicin *see* Aminoglycosides
Nicardipine *see* Calcium-channel Blockers
Nicotine and Tobacco
Theophylline: *tobacco smoking* increases metabolism (reduced plasma-theophylline concentration)
Nicoumalone *see* Warfarin and other Coumarins
Nifedipine *see* Calcium-channel Blockers
Nimodipine *see* Calcium-channel Blockers
Nimorazole alcohol interaction *as for* Metronidazole
Nitrates *see* Glyceryl Trinitrate
Nitrazepam *see* Benzodiazepines and other Anxiolytics and Hypnotics

Nitrofurantoin

Uricosurics: *probenecid* reduces excretion of *nitrofurantoin* (risk of toxicity)

Nitroprusside *as for* Hydralazine

Nizatidine *see* Histamine H2-antagonists

Noradrenaline *see* Sympathomimetics

Norethisterone *see* Progestogens

Norfloxacin *see* 4-Quinolones

Norgestimate *see* Progestogens

Norgestrel *see* Progestogens

Nortriptyline *see* Antidepressants, Tricyclic

NSAIDs (*see also* Aspirin)

Note. Do not generally apply to NSAIDS used for topical action

- ACE Inhibitors: antagonism of hypotensive effect; increased risk of renal failure and increased risk of hyperkalaemia on administration with *indomethacin* and possibly *other NSAIDs*
- *other* Analgesics: avoid concomitant administration of two or more *NSAIDs* (increased side-effects)

Anion-exchange Resins: *cholestyramine* reduces absorption of *phenylbutazone*

Antacids and Adsorbents: *antacids* reduce absorption of *diflunisal*

- Antibacterials: *NSAIDs* increase risk of convulsions with *4-quinolones*

Anticoagulants: *see* Warfarin; increased risk of haemorrhage with *ketorolac* and all *anticoagulants* (including low-dose heparin), see p.493

Antidepressants: *moclobemide* enhances effect of *ibuprofen* and possibly *other NSAIDs*

- Antidiabetics: effect of *sulphonylureas* enhanced by *azapropazone*, *phenylbutazone* and possibly *other NSAIDs*
- Antiepileptics: effect of *phenytoin* enhanced by *azapropazone and phenylbutazone*

Antihypertensives: antagonism of hypotensive effect

Beta-blockers: antagonism of hypotensive effect

Cardiac Glycosides: *NSAIDs* may exacerbate heart failure, reduce GFR, and increase plasma-cardiac glycoside concentration

Corticosteroids: increased risk of gastro-intestinal bleeding and ulceration

- Cyclosporin: increased risk of nephrotoxicity
- Cytotoxics: excretion of *methotrexate* reduced by *aspirin, azapropazone, diclofenac, indomethacin, ketoprofen, naproxen, phenylbutazone and probably other NSAIDs* (increased risk of toxicity)

Diuretics: risk of nephrotoxicity of *NSAIDs* increased; *NSAIDs* notably indomethacin antagonise diuretic effect; *indomethacin and possibly other NSAIDs* increase risk of hyperkalaemia with *potassium-sparing diuretics*; occasional reports of decreased renal function when *indomethacin* given with *triamterene*

- Lithium: excretion of *lithium* reduced by *diclofenac, ibuprofen, indomethacin, ketorolac* (see p.493), *mefenamic acid, naproxen, phenylbutazone, piroxicam, and probably other NSAIDs* (possibility of toxicity)

Mifepristone: manufacturer recommends avoid *aspirin* and *NSAIDs* until 8-12 days after *mifepristone* administration

Thyroxine: false low total plasma-thyroxine concentration with *phenylbutazone*

- Uricosurics: *probenecid* delays excretion of *indomethacin, ketoprofen, ketorolac* (see p.493), *and naproxen* (raised plasma concentrations)
- Vasodilators: risk of ketorolac-associated bleeding increased by *oxpentifylline*, see p.493

Octreotide

Antidiabetics: reduces *insulin and antidiabetic drug* requirements in diabetes mellitus

Cyclosporin: absorption of *cyclosporin* reduced (reduced plasma concentration)

Oestradiol *see* Contraceptives, Oral

Oestriol *see* Contraceptives, Oral

Oestrogens *see* Contraceptives, Oral

Ofloxacin *see* 4-Quinolones

Omeprazole *see* Proton Pump Inhibitors

Opioid Analgesics

Alcohol: enhanced sedative and hypotensive effect

Anti-arrhythmics: delayed absorption of *mexiletine*

Antibacterials: *rifampicin* accelerates metabolism of *methadone* (reduced effect); *erythromycin* increases plasma concentration of *alfentanil*

- Anticoagulants: *dextropropoxyphene* may enhance effect of *nicoumalone and warfarin*
- Antidepressants: CNS excitation or depression (hypertension or hypotension) if *pethidine and possibly other opioid analgesics* given to patients receiving *MAOIs* (including *moclobemide*)
- Antiepileptics: *dextropropoxyphene* enhances effect of *carbamazepine*; effect of *tramadol* decreased by *carbamazepine*

Antivirals: *methadone* possibly increases plasma concentration of *zidovudine*

Anxiolytics and Hypnotics: enhanced sedative effect

Cisapride: possible antagonism of gastro-intestinal effect

Domperidone and Metoclopramide: antagonism of gastro-intestinal effects

- Dopaminergics: hyperpyrexia and CNS toxicity reported with *selegiline*

Ulcer-healing Drugs: *cimetidine* inhibits metabolism of opioid analgesics notably *pethidine* (increased plasma concentration)

Orciprenaline *see* Sympathomimetics

Orphenadrine *see* Antimuscarinics

Oxatomide *see* Antihistamines

Oxazepam *see* Benzodiazepines and other Anxiolytics and Hypnotics

Oxitropium *see* Antimuscarinics

Oxpentifylline

- Analgesics: increased risk of bleeding with *ketorolac*, see p.493

Oxprenolol *see* Beta-blockers

Oxybutynin *see* Antimuscarinics

Oxymetazoline *see* Sympathomimetics

Oxymetholone *see* Anabolic Steroids

Oxypertine *see* Phenothiazines and other Antipsychotics

Oxytetracycline *see* Tetracyclines

Pamidronate Sodium *see* Bisphosphonates

Pancreatin

Antidiabetics: hypoglycaemic effect of *acarbose* reduced

Pancuronium *see* Muscle Relaxants (non-depolarising)

Papaveretum *see* Opioid Analgesics

Paracetamol

Anion-exchange Resins: *cholestyramine* reduces absorption of *paracetamol*

Anticoagulants: prolonged regular use of *paracetamol* possibly enhances *warfarin*

Domperidone and Metoclopramide: *metoclopramide* accelerates absorption of *paracetamol* (enhanced effect)

Paroxetine *see* Antidepressants, Serotonin-uptake Inhibitor

Pemoline *see* Sympathomimetics

Penbutolol *see* Beta-blockers

Penicillamine

  Antacids: reduced absorption of *penicillamine*

  Iron: reduced absorption of *penicillamine*

  Zinc: reduced absorption of *penicillamine*

Penicillins

  Antacids: reduced absorption of *pivampicillin*

  Anticoagulants: *see* Phenindione and Warfarin

- Cytotoxics: reduced excretion of *methotrexate* (increased risk of toxicity)

  Guar Gum: reduced absorption of *phenoxymethylpenicillin*

  Muscle Relaxants: effects of *non-depolarising muscle relaxants* such as *tubocurarine* enhanced by *azlocillin*

  Oestrogens and Progestogens: *see* Contraceptives, Oral

  Probenecid: reduced excretion of *penicillins*

Pentaerythritol Tetranitrate *see* Glyceryl Trinitrate

Pentazocine *see* Opioid Analgesics

Pergolide

  Antipsychotics: antagonism of effect

Pericyazine *see* Phenothiazines and other Antipsychotics

Perindopril *see* ACE Inhibitors

Perphenazine *see* Phenothiazines and other Antipsychotics

Pethidine *see* Opioid Analgesics

Phenazocine *see* Opioid Analgesics

Phenelzine *see* MAOIs

Phenindamine *see* Antihistamines

Phenindione

  Note. Change in patient's clinical condition, particularly associated with liver disease, intercurrent illness, or drug administration, necessitates more frequent testing. Major changes in diet (especially involving vegetables) may also affect anticoagulant control

- Anabolic Steroids: anticoagulant effect enhanced by *oxymetholone, stanozolol and others*
- Analgesics: anticoagulant effect enhanced by *aspirin*; increased risk of haemorrhage with *ketorolac*, see p.493

  Anion exchange Resins: anticoagulant effect enhanced or reduced by *cholestyramine*

  Antibacterials: although studies have failed to demonstrate interaction common experience in anticoagulant clinics is that INR can be altered by course of *oral broad-spectrum antibiotic such as ampicillin* (may also apply to antibiotics given for local action on gut such as *neomycin*)

- Antiplatelet Drugs: anticoagulant effect enhanced by *aspirin and dipyridamole*
- Clofibrate Group: enhanced anticoagulant effect
- Oestrogens and Progestogens: : anticoagulant effect antagonised by *oral contraceptives*
- Thyroxine: enhanced anticoagulant effect
- Vitamins: anticoagulant effect antagonised by vitamin K (present in some enteral feeds)

Pheniramine *see* Antihistamines

Phenobarbitone *see* Barbiturates

Phenoperidine *see* Opioid Analgesics

Phenothiazines and other Antipsychotics

  ACE Inhibitors: severe postural hypotension with *chlorpromazine* and possibly *other phenothiazines*

  Alcohol: enhanced sedative effect

- Anaesthetics: enhanced hypotensive effect

  Antacids: reduced absorption of *phenothiazines*

- Anti-arrhythmics: increased risk of ventricular arrhythmias with drugs which prolong QT interval

  Antibacterials: *rifampicin* accelerates metabolism of *haloperidol* (reduced plasma-haloperidol concentration)

Phenothiazines and other Antipsychotics (*continued*)

- Antidepressants: increased plasma concentrations and increased antimuscarinic effects notably on administration of *tricyclics* with *phenothiazines; fluoxetine* increases plasma concentration of *haloperidol; oxypertine* causes CNS excitation and hypertension with *MAOIs*

  Antidiabetics: hypoglycaemic effect of *sulphonylureas* possibly antagonised

- Antiepileptics: antagonism (convulsive threshold lowered); *carbamazepine* accelerates metabolism of *haloperidol* (reduced plasma concentration); *phenytoin* accelerates metabolism of *clozapine*
- Antihistamines: increased risk of ventricular arrhythmias with *astemizole* and *terfenadine*

  Antihypertensives: enhanced hypotensive effect; higher doses of *chlorpromazine* antagonise hypotensive effect of *adrenergic neurone blockers*; increased risk of extrapyramidal effects on administration of *methyldopa* and *metirosine*

- Antimalarials: increased risk of ventricular arrhythmias with *halofantrine*
- Antimuscarinics: antimuscarinic side-effects of *phenothiazines* increased (but reduced plasma concentrations)

  Anxiolytics and Hypnotics. enhanced sedative effect

- Beta-blockers: *phenothiazines* increase risk of ventricular arrhythmias with *sotalol; propranolol* increases plasma concentration of *chlorpromazine*

  Calcium-channel Blockers: enhanced hypotensive effect

  Desferrioxamine: manufacturer advises avoid *prochlorperazine*

  Diuretics: hypokalaemia increases risk of ventricular arrhythmias with *pimozide*

  Domperidone and Metoclopramide: increased risk of extrapyramidal effects with *metoclopramide*

  Dopaminergics: antagonism of hypoprolactinaemic and antiparkinsonian effects of *bromocriptine*; antagonism of effect of *apomorphine, levodopa, lysuride,* and *pergolide*

  Lithium: increased risk of extrapyramidal effects and possibility of neurotoxicity with *clozapine, haloperidol and phenothiazines*

  Tetrabenazine: increased risk of extrapyramidal effects

  Ulcer-healing Drugs: *cimetidine* may enhance effects of *chlorpromazine, clozapine,* and possibly *other antipsychotics*

Phenoxymethylpenicillin *see* Penicillins

Phentermine *see* Sympathomimetics

Phentolamine *see* Alpha-blockers

Phenylbutazone *see* NSAIDs

Phenylephrine *see* Sympathomimetics

Phenylpropanolamine *see* Sympathomimetics

Phenytoin

- Analgesics: plasma-phenytoin concentration increased by *aspirin, azapropazone, and phenylbutazone*

  Antacids: reduced *phenytoin* absorption

- Anti-arrhythmics: *amiodarone* increases plasma-phenytoin concentration; *phenytoin* reduces plasma concentrations of *disopyramide, mexiletine, and quinidine*

Phenytoin (*continued*)
- Antibacterials: plasma-phenytoin concentration increased by *chloramphenicol, cycloserine, isoniazid, and metronidazole*; plasma-phenytoin concentration and antifolate effect increased by *co-trimoxazole* and *trimethoprim*; plasma phenytoin concentration reduced by *rifamycins*; plasma concentration of *doxycycline* reduced by *phenytoin*
- Anticoagulants: metabolism of *nicoumalone and warfarin* accelerated (possibility of reduced anticoagulant effect, but enhancement also reported)
- Antidepressants: antagonism of anticonvulsant effect (convulsive threshold lowered); *fluoxetine* and *viloxazine* increase plasma-phenytoin concentration; *phenytoin* reduces plasma concentrations of *mianserin, paroxetine, and tricyclics*

  Antidiabetics: plasma-phenytoin concentration transiently increased by *tolbutamide* (possibility of toxicity)
- *other* Antiepileptics: concomitant administration of *two or more antiepileptics* may enhance toxicity without a corresponding increase in antiepileptic effect; moreover interactions between individual antiepileptics can complicate monitoring of treatment; interactions include enhanced effects, increased sedation, and reductions in plasma concentrations; for further details see p.193
- Antifungals: plasma-phenytoin concentration increased by *fluconazole and miconazole*; plasma concentration of *itraconazole* and *ketoconazole* reduced

  Antimalarials: antagonism of anticonvulsant effect; increased risk of antifolate effect with *pyrimethamine* (includes *Fansidar®* and *Maloprim®*)

  Antiplatelet Drugs: plasma-phenytoin concentration increased by *aspirin*
- Antipsychotics: antagonism of anticonvulsant effect (convulsive threshold lowered); *phenytoin* accelerates metabolism of *clozapine*

  Anxiolytics and Hypnotics: *diazepam* and possibly *other benzodiazepines* increase or decrease plasma-phenytoin concentration
- Calcium-channel Blockers: *diltiazem* and *nifedipine* increase plasma concentration of *phenytoin*; effect of *felodipine, isradipine* and probably *diltiazem, nicardipine, nifedipine,* and *verapamil* reduced

  Cardiac Glycosides: metabolism of *digitoxin only* accelerated (reduced effect)
- Corticosteroids: metabolism of *corticosteroids* accelerated (reduced effect)
- Cyclosporin: metabolism of *cyclosporin* accelerated (reduced plasma concentration)

  Cytotoxics: reduced absorption of *phenytoin*; increased antifolate effect with *methotrexate*
- Disulfiram: plasma-phenytoin concentration increased

  Diuretics: increased risk of osteomalacia with *carbonic anhydrase inhibitors*

  Food: some *enteral foods* may interfere with absorption of *phenytoin*

  Lithium: neurotoxicity may occur without increased plasma-lithium concentration
- Oestrogens and Progestogens: metabolism of *gestrinone, tibolone, and oral contraceptives* accelerated (reduced contraceptive effect, **important:** see p.313)

  Theophylline: metabolism of *theophylline* accelerated (reduced plasma-theophylline concentration)

  Thyroxine: metabolism of *thyroxine* accelerated (may increase thyroxine requirements in hypothyroidism)

Phenytoin (*continued*)
- Ulcer-healing Drugs: *cimetidine* inhibits metabolism (increased plasma-phenytoin concentration); *sucralfate* reduces absorption; *omeprazole* enhances effect of *phenytoin*
- Uricosurics: plasma-phenytoin concentration increased by *sulphinpyrazone*

  Vaccines: effect enhanced by *influenza vaccine*

  Vitamins: plasma-phenytoin concentration occasionally reduced by *folic acid*; *vitamin D* requirements possibly increased

Physostigmine *see* Cholinergics
Phytomenadione *see* Vitamins (Vitamin K)
Pimozide *see* Phenothiazines and other Antipsychotics (**CSM**: *see also* p.156)
Pindolol *see* Beta-blockers
Pipenzolate *see* Antimuscarinics
Piperazine
   other Anthelmintics: antagonism of *pyrantel*
Piperazine Oestrone Sulphate *see* Contraceptives, Oral
Pipothiazine *see* Phenothiazines and other Antipsychotics
Pirbuterol *see* Sympathomimetics, Beta$_2$
Piretanide *see* Diuretics (loop)
Piroxicam *see* NSAIDs
Pivampicillin *see* Penicillins
Pizotifen
   Antihypertensives: hypotensive effect of *adrenergic neurone blockers* antagonised
Poldine *see* Antimuscarinics
Polymyxins *see* Colistin
Polythiazide *see* Diuretics (thiazides)
Potassium Aminobenzoate
   Antibacterials: effect of *sulphonamides* inhibited
Potassium Salts (includes Salt Substitutes)
- ACE Inhibitors: hyperkalaemia
- Cyclosporin: increased risk of hyperkalaemia
- Diuretics: hyperkalaemia with *potassium-sparing diuretics*
Pravastatin
   Cyclosporin: increased risk of myopathy
   other Lipid-lowering Drugs: increased risk of myopathy with *clofibrate group*
Prazosin *see* Alpha-blockers (post-synaptic)
Prednisolone *see* Corticosteroids
Prednisone *see* Corticosteroids
Primaquine
   other Antimalarials: *mepacrine* increases plasma concentration of *primaquine* (risk of toxicity)
Primidone *see* Barbiturates and Primidone
Probenecid
   ACE Inhibitors: reduced excretion of *captopril*
- Analgesics: *aspirin* antagonises effect; excretion of *indomethacin, ketoprofen, ketorolac* (see p.493), *and naproxen* delayed (increased plasma concentrations)

  Antibacterials: reduced excretion of *cephalosporins, cinoxacin, dapsone, nalidixic acid, nitrofurantoin, and penicillins* (increased plasma-concentrations); antagonism by *pyrazinamide*

  Antivirals: reduced excretion of *acyclovir, zidovudine,* and possibly *famciclovir* (increased plasma concentrations and risk of toxicity)
- Cytotoxics: reduced excretion of *methotrexate* (increased risk of toxicity)
Procainamide
   ACE Inhibitors: increased risk of toxicity with *captopril*, especially in renal impairment
- *other* Anti-arrhythmics: *amiodarone* increases procainamide-plasma concentrations; increased myocardial depression with *any anti-arrhythmic*

  Antibacterials: *trimethoprim* increases plasma concentration of *procainamide*
- Antihistamines: increased risk of ventricular arrhythmias with *astemizole* and *terfenadine*

Procainamide (*continued*)
- Antimalarials: increased risk of ventricular arrhythmias with *halofantrine*
- Antipsychotics: increased risk of ventricular arrhythmias with *phenothiazines*

  Cholinergics: antagonism of effect of *neostigmine* and *pyridostigmine*
- Muscle Relaxants: muscle relaxant effect enhanced
- Ulcer-healing Drugs: *cimetidine* inhibits excretion (increased plasma-procainamide concentration)

Procarbazine
  Alcohol: disulfiram-like reaction

Prochlorperazine *see* Phenothiazines and other Antipsychotics

Procyclidine *see* Antimuscarinics

Progesterone *see* Progestogens

Progestogens (*see also* Contraceptives, Oral)
- Cyclosporin: increased plasma-cyclosporin concentration (inhibition of metabolism)

Proguanil
- Anticoagulants: effect of *warfarin* possibly enhanced

Promazine *see* Phenothiazines and other Antipsychotics

Promethazine *see* Antihistamines

Propafenone
  other Anti-arrhythmics: *quinidine* increases plasma concentration of *propafenone*; increased myocardial depression with any *anti-arrhythmic*
  Antibacterials: *rifampicin* reduces plasma concentration of *propafenone*
- Anticoagulants: increased plasma concentration of *warfarin and nicoumalone* (enhanced effect)
- Antihistamines: increased risk of ventricular arrhythmias with *astemizole* and *terfenadine*
  Beta-blockers: increased plasma concentration of *metoprolol* and *propranolol*
- Cardiac Glycosides: increased plasma concentrations of *digoxin* (halve maintenance dose of digoxin)
  Cholinergics: possible antagonism of effect of *neostigmine* and *pyridostigmine*
  Cyclosporin: plasma-cyclosporin concentration possibly increased
  Theophylline: increased plasma-theophylline concentration
- Ulcer-healing Drugs: *cimetidine* increases plasma-propafenone concentration

Propantheline *see* Antimuscarinics

Propranolol *see* Beta-Blockers

Proton Pump Inhibitors
- Anticoagulants: effects of *warfarin* enhanced by *omeprazole*; interaction with *lansoprazole* possibly differs
- Antiepileptics: effects of *phenytoin* enhanced
  Antifungals: absorption of *ketoconazole* and possibly *itraconazole* reduced
  Anxiolytics and Hypnotics: metabolism of *diazepam* inhibited by *omeprazole* (increased effect possible)

Protriptyline *see* Antidepressants, Tricyclic

Pseudoephedrine *see* Sympathomimetics

Pyrantel
  other Anthelmintics: antagonism of *piperazine*

Pyrazinamide
  Uricosurics: antagonism of effect of *probenecid and sulphinpyrazone*

Pyridostigmine *see* Cholinergics

Pyridoxine *see* Vitamins

Pyrimethamine
  Antibacterials: increased antifolate effect with *co-trimoxazole* and *trimethoprim*
  Antiepileptics: increased antifolate effect with *phenytoin*
  Cytotoxics: increased antifolate effect with *methotrexate*

Quinalbarbitone *see* Barbiturates and Primidone

Quinapril *see* ACE Inhibitors

Quinidine
  Antacids: reduced excretion in alkaline urine (plasma-quinidine concentration occasionally increased)
- *other* Anti-arrhythmics: *amiodarone* increases plasma-quinidine concentrations (and increases risk of ventricular arrhythmias); plasma concentration of *propafenone* increased; increased myocardial depression with *any anti-arrhythmic*
  Antibacterials: *rifamycins* accelerate metabolism (reduced plasma-quinidine concentration)
  Anticoagulants: effect of *nicoumalone and warfarin* may be enhanced
  Antiepileptics: *phenobarbitone, phenytoin, and primidone* accelerate metabolism (reduced plasma-quinidine concentration)
- Antihistamines: increased risk of ventricular arrhythmias with *astemizole* and *terfenadine*
- Antimalarials: increased risk of ventricular arrhythmias with *halofantrine*
- Antipsychotics: increased risk of ventricular arrhythmias with *phenothiazines*
  Barbiturates: *see under* Antiepileptics, above
- Calcium-channel Blockers: *nifedipine* reduces plasma-quinidine concentration; *verapamil* increases plasma-quinidine concentration (possibility of extreme hypotension)
- Cardiac Glycosides: plasma concentration of *digoxin* increased (halve digoxin maintenance dose)
  Cholinergics: antagonism of effect of *neostigmine* and *pyridostigmine*
- Diuretics: *acetazolamide* reduces excretion (plasma-quinidine concentration occasionally increased); quinidine toxicity increased if hypokalaemia occurs with *acetazolamide, loop diuretics, and thiazides*
- Muscle Relaxants: muscle relaxant effect enhanced
- Ulcer-healing Drugs: *cimetidine* inhibits metabolism (increased plasma-quinidine concentration)

Quinine
  Anti-arrhythmics: plasma concentration of *flecainide* increased
- *other* Antimalarials: *see* Halofantrine, Mefloquine
- Cardiac Glycosides: plasma concentration of *digoxin* increased (halve digoxin maintenance dose); includes use of quinine for cramps
  Ulcer-healing Drugs: *cimetidine* inhibits metabolism (increased plasma-quinine concentration)

4-Quinolones
- Analgesics: increased risk of convulsions with *NSAIDs*
  Antacids and Adsorbents: *antacids* reduce absorption of *ciprofloxacin, norfloxacin* and *ofloxacin*
- Anticoagulants: anticoagulant effect of *nicoumalone and warfarin* enhanced by *ciprofloxacin, nalidixic acid, norfloxacin* and *ofloxacin*
- Antidiabetics: effect of *sulphonylureas* enhanced
  Cyclosporin: increased risk of nephrotoxicity
  Cytotoxics: toxicity of *melphalan* increased by *nalidixic acid*
  Iron: absorption of *ciprofloxacin, norfloxacin,* and *ofloxacin* reduced by *oral iron*
- Theophylline: *ciprofloxacin* and *norfloxacin* increase plasma-theophylline concentration
  Ulcer-healing Drugs: *sucralfate* reduces absorption of *ciprofloxacin, norfloxacin,* and *ofloxacin*
  Uricosurics: *probenecid* reduces excretion of *cinoxacin* and *nalidixic acid* (increased side-effects)
  Zinc Salts: *zinc* reduces absorption of *ciprofloxacin*

Rabies Vaccine *see* p.477

Ramipril *see* ACE Inhibitors

Ranitidine *see* Histamine H2-antagonists
Remoxipride *see* Phenothiazines and other Antipsychotics
Reproterol *see* Sympathomimetics, Beta$_2$
Rifabutin *see* Rifamycins
Rifampicin *see* Rifamycins
Rifamycins

Analgesics: metabolism of *methadone* accelerated (reduced effect)

Antacids: reduced absorption of *rifampicin*

Anti-arrhythmics: metabolism accelerated—reduced plasma concentrations of *disopyramide, mexiletine, propafenone, and quinidine*

• *other* Antibacterials: metabolism of *chloramphenicol* accelerated by *rifampicin* (reduced plasma concentration); plasma concentration of *dapsone* reduced; **CSM advice:** plasma concentration of *rifabutin* increased by *clarithromycin* (risk of uveitis)

• Anticoagulants: metabolism of *nicoumalone and warfarin* accelerated (reduced anticoagulant effect)

Antidepressants: metabolism of some *tricyclics* accelerated by *rifampicin* (reduced plasma concentration)

• Antidiabetics: metabolism of *chlorpropamide, tolbutamide and possibly other sulphonylureas* accelerated (reduced effect)

• Antiepileptics: metabolism of *phenytoin* accelerated (reduced plasma concentration)

• Antifungals: metabolism of *fluconazole, itraconazole and ketoconazole* accelerated by *rifampicin* (reduced plasma concentration); plasma concentration of *terbinafine* reduced by *rifampicin*; **CSM advice:** plasma concentration of *rifabutin* increased by *fluconazole* (risk of uveitis)

Antipsychotics: metabolism of *haloperidol* accelerated by *rifampicin* (reduced plasma concentration)

Anxiolytics and Hypnotics: metabolism of *diazepam* and possibly *other benzodiazepines* accelerated (reduced plasma concentration)

Beta-blockers: metabolism of *bisoprolol* and *propranolol* accelerated by *rifampicin* (reduced plasma concentration)

Calcium-channel Blockers: metabolism of *diltiazem* and *verapamil and possibly isradipine* and *nifedipine* accelerated by *rifampicin* (reduced plasma concentration)

Cardiac Glycosides: metabolism of *digitoxin only* accelerated (reduced effect)

• Corticosteroids: metabolism of *corticosteroids* accelerated (reduced effect)

• Cyclosporin: metabolism accelerated (reduced plasma-cyclosporin concentration)

• Cytotoxics: manufacturer reports interaction with *azathioprine* (transplants possibly rejected)

Lipid-lowering Drugs: metabolism of *fluvastatin* accelerated (reduced effect)

• Oestrogens and Progestogens: : metabolism accelerated (contraceptive effect of *both combined and progestogen-only oral contraceptives* reduced, **important:** see p. 313)

Theophylline: metabolism accelerated by *rifampicin* (reduced plasma-theophylline concentration)

Thyroxine: metabolism of *thyroxine* accelerated by *rifampicin* (may increase requirements in hypothyroidism)

Ulcer-healing Drugs: metabolism of *cimetidine* accelerated by *rifampicin* (reduced plasma concentration)

Rimiterol *see* Sympathomimetics, Beta$_2$
Risperidone *see* Phenothiazines and other Antipsychotics
Ritodrine *see* Sympathomimetics, Beta$_2$, and p. 308
Rocuronium *see* Muscle Relaxants (non-depolarising)
Rowachol®

Anticoagulants: effect of *nicoumalone and warfarin* may be reduced
Salbutamol *see* Sympathomimetics, Beta$_2$
Salmeterol *see* Sympathomimetics, Beta$_2$
Salt Substitutes *see* Potassium Salts
Selegiline

Note. Selegiline is an MAO-B inhibitor, see also p. 202

• Analgesics: hyperpyrexia and CNS toxicity with *pethidine*

• Antidepressants: hypertension and CNS excitation with *fluoxetine*
Sermorelin

Avoid preparations which affect release of growth hormone, see p. 297
Sertraline *see* Antidepressants, Serotonin-uptake Inhibitor
Simvastatin

• Anticoagulants: effect of *nicoumalone and warfarin* may be enhanced

Cyclosporin: increased risk of myopathy
other Lipid-lowering Drugs: increased risk of myopathy with *clofibrate group*
Sodium Aurothiomalate *see* Gold
Sodium Bicarbonate *see* Antacids and Adsorbents
Sodium Clodronate *see* Bisphosphonates
Sodium Valproate *see* Valproate
Sotalol *see* Beta-blockers
Spectinomycin

Botulinum Toxin: neuromuscular block enhanced (risk of toxicity)

Lithium: increased toxicity reported
Spironolactone *see* Diuretics (potassium-sparing)
Stanozolol *see* Anabolic Steroids
Streptomycin *see* Aminoglycosides
Sucralfate

Antibacterials: reduced absorption of *ciprofloxacin, norfloxacin, ofloxacin,* and *tetracycline*

• Anticoagulants: absorption of *warfarin* possibly reduced

• Antiepileptics: reduced absorption of *phenytoin*
Antifungals: reduced absorption of *ketoconazole*
Cardiac Glycosides: absorption of *cardiac glycosides* possibly reduced
Thyroxine: reduced absorption of *thyroxine*
Sulfadoxine *see* Co-trimoxazole and Sulphonamides
Sulfametopyrazine *see* Co-trimoxazole and Sulphonamides
Sulindac *see* NSAIDs
Sulphadiazine *see* Co-trimoxazole and Sulphonamides
Sulphadimidine *see* Co-trimoxazole and Sulphonamides
Sulphinpyrazone

Analgesics: *aspirin* antagonises uricosuric effect
Antibacterials: *pyrazinamide* antagonises effect

• Anticoagulants: anticoagulant effect of *nicoumalone and warfarin* enhanced

• Antidiabetics: effect of *sulphonylureas* enhanced

• Antiepileptics: plasma concentration of *phenytoin* increased
Theophylline: plasma-theophylline concentration reduced
Sulphonamides *see* Co-trimoxazole and Sulphonamides
Sulphonylureas *see* Antidiabetics
Sulpiride *see* Phenothiazines and other Antipsychotics
Sumatriptan

• Antidepressants: risk of CNS toxicity with *MAOIs* (including *moclobemide*) and *serotonin-uptake inhibitors*

Sumatriptan (*continued*)
- Ergotamine: increased risk of vasospasm (see section 4.7.4.1)
- Lithium: risk of CNS toxicity

Suxamethonium *see* Muscle Relaxants

Sympathomimetics (*see below* for Beta$_2$-Sympathomimetics)
- Anaesthetics: risk of arrhythmias if *adrenaline and isoprenaline* given with *volatile liquid anaesthetics*
- Antidepressants: with *tricyclics* administration of *adrenaline and noradrenaline* may cause hypertension and arrhythmias (but local anaesthetics with adrenaline appear to be safe); with *MAOIs* administration of inotropics such as *dopamine* and *dopexamine* may cause hypertensive crisis; also with *MAOIs* administration of *dexamphetamine and other amphetamines, dexfenfluramine, diethylpropion, ephedrine, fenfluramine, isometheptene, pemoline, phentermine, phenylephrine, phenylpropanolamine, and pseudoephedrine* may cause hypertensive crisis (these drugs are contained in anorectics or cold and cough remedies)

  Antihypertensives: sympathomimetics in *anorectics and cold and cough remedies (see* above) antagonise hypotensive effect of *adrenergic neurone blockers;* possible risk of hypertension with *apraclonidine* and *adrenaline* or *noradrenaline;* hypotensive effect of some other antihypertensives may be enhanced by *dexfenfluramine and fenfluramine*
- Beta-blockers: severe hypertension with *adrenaline and noradrenaline* (especially with non-selective beta-blockers); severe hypertension also possible with sympathomimetics in *anorectics and cold and cough remedies, see* above

  Respiratory Stimulants: risk of hypertension with *doxapram*

  other Sympathomimetics: *dopexamine* possibly potentiates effect of *adrenaline* and *noradrenaline*

Sympathomimetics, Beta$_2$
  Corticosteroids: increased risk of hypokalaemia if high doses of *corticosteroids* given with high doses of *bambuterol, fenoterol, pirbuterol, reproterol, rimiterol, ritodrine, salbutamol, salmeterol, terbutaline* and *tulobuterol*
  Muscle Relaxants: effect of *suxamethonium* enhanced by *bambuterol*
  Theophylline: increased risk of hypokalaemia if given with high doses of *bambuterol, fenoterol, pirbuterol, reproterol, rimiterol, ritodrine, salbutamol, salmeterol, terbutaline, and tulobuterol*

Tamoxifen
- Anticoagulants: anticoagulant effect of *nicoumalone and warfarin* enhanced
  other Hormone Antagonists: *aminoglutethimide* reduces plasma-tamoxifen concentration

Temazepam *see* Benzodiazepines and other Anxiolytics and Hypnotics

Tenoxicam *see* NSAIDs

Terazosin *see* Alpha-blockers (post-synaptic)

Terbinafine
  Antibacterials: plasma concentration reduced by *rifampicin*
  Ulcer-healing Drugs: plasma concentration increased by *cimetidine*

Terbutaline *see* Sympathomimetics, Beta$_2$

Terfenadine *see* Antihistamines

Tetrabenazine (general extrapyramidal interactions *as for* phenothiazines)
- Antidepressants: CNS excitation and hypertension with *MAOIs*

Tetracyclines
  ACE Inhibitors: *quinapril* reduces absorption (tablets contain magnesium carbonate excipient)
  Antacids: reduced absorption
  Anticoagulants: *see* Phenindione and Warfarin
  Antiepileptics: *carbamazepine, phenobarbitone, phenytoin, and primidone* increase metabolism of *doxycycline* (reduced plasma concentration)
  Barbiturates: *see under* Antiepileptics, above
  Calcium Salts: reduced absorption of *tetracyclines*
- Cyclosporin: *doxycycline* increases plasma-cyclosporin concentration
  Dairy products: reduced absorption (except *doxycycline* and *minocycline*)
  Iron: absorption of *oral iron* reduced by *tetracyclines* and *vice versa*
  Oestrogens and Progestogens: *see* Contraceptives, Oral (main list)
  Ulcer-healing Drugs: *bismuth chelate* and *sucralfate* reduce absorption
  Zinc Salts: reduced absorption (and *vice versa*)

Theophylline
  Anaesthetics: increased risk of arrhythmias with *halothane*
  Anthelmintics: *thiabendazole* may increase plasma-theophylline concentration
  Anti-arrhythmics: antagonism of anti-arrhythmic effect of *adenosine*; plasma-theophylline concentration increased by *mexiletine* and *propafenone*; plasma-theophylline concentration reduced by *moracizine*
- Antibacterials: plasma-theophylline concentration increased by *ciprofloxacin, clarithromycin, erythromycin,* and *norfloxacin* and possibly increased by *isoniazid*; plasma-theophylline concentration reduced by *rifampicin*
- Antidepressants: plasma-theophylline concentration increased by *fluvoxamine* (**important:** see p.120) and *viloxazine*
  Antiepileptics: plasma-theophylline concentration reduced by *carbamazepine, phenobarbitone, phenytoin,* and *primidone*
  Antifungals: plasma-theophylline concentration possibly increased by *fluconazole*
  Barbiturates: *see under* Antiepileptics, above
  Beta-blockers: should be avoided on pharmacological grounds (bronchospasm)
- Calcium channel Blockers: plasma-theophylline concentration increased by *diltiazem and verapamil*
  Disulfiram: increases plasma-theophylline concentration
  Hormone Antagonists: plasma-theophylline concentration reduced by *aminoglutethimide*
  Interferons: plasma-theophylline concentration increased by *interferon alfa*
  Lithium: *lithium* excretion accelerated (reduced plasma-lithium concentration)
  Nicotine and Tobacco: plasma-theophylline concentration reduced by *tobacco smoking*
  Oestrogens and Progestogens: plasma-theophylline concentration increased by *combined oral contraceptives*
  Respiratory Stimulants: increased CNS stimulation
  Sympathomimetics: increased risk of hypokalaemia if *theophylline* given with high doses of *bambuterol, fenoterol, pirbuterol, reproterol, rimiterol, ritodrine, salbutamol, salmeterol, terbutaline, and tulobuterol*
- Ulcer-healing Drugs: plasma-theophylline concentration increased by *cimetidine*
  Uricosurics: plasma-theophylline concentration reduced by *sulphinpyrazone*
  Vaccines: plasma-theophylline concentration occasionally increased by *influenza vaccine*

Thiabendazole

Theophylline: plasma concentration may be increased

Thiazides *see* Diuretics

Thiopentone *see* Barbiturates and Primidone

Thioridazine *see* Phenothiazines and other Antipsychotics

Thiotepa

Muscle Relaxants: effect of *suxamethonium* enhanced

Thyroxine

Analgesics: false low total plasma-thyroxine concentration with *phenylbutazone*

Anion-exchange Resins: *cholestyramine* reduces absorption of *thyroxine*

Antibacterials: *rifampicin* accelerates metabolism of thyroxine (may increase requirements in hypothyroidism)

• Anticoagulants: effect of *nicoumalone, phenindione, and warfarin* enhanced

Antiepileptics: *carbamazepine, phenobarbitone, phenytoin, and primidone* accelerate metabolism of *thyroxine* (may increase requirements in hypothyroidism)

Barbiturates: *see under* Antiepileptics, above

Beta-blockers: metabolism of *propranolol* accelerated (reduced effect)

Ulcer-healing Drugs: *sucralfate* reduces absorption of *thyroxine*

Tiaprofenic Acid *see* NSAIDs

Tibolone

Antibacterials: *rifampicin* accelerates metabolism (reduced plasma concentration)

Antiepileptics: *carbamazepine, phenobarbitone, phenytoin, and primidone* accelerate metabolism (reduced plasma concentration)

Timolol *see* Beta-blockers

Tinidazole alcohol interaction *as for* Metronidazole

Tinzaparin *see* Heparin

Tobramycin *see* Aminoglycosides

Tocainide

other Anti-arrhythmics: increased myocardial depression with any anti-arrhythmic

Beta-blockers: increased risk of bradycardia and myocardial depression

Diuretics: effect of *tocainide* antagonised by hypokalaemia with *acetazolamide, loop diuretics, and thiazides*

Tolazamide *see* Antidiabetics (sulphonylurea)

Tolbutamide *see* Antidiabetics (sulphonylurea)

Tolmetin *see* NSAIDs

Torasemide *see* Diuretics (loop)

Tramadol *see* Opioid Analgesics

Trandolapril *see* ACE Inhibitors

Tranylcypromine *see* MAOIs

Trazodone

Alcohol: enhanced sedative effect

• other Antidepressants: as for Antidepressants, Tricyclic

Antiepileptics: antagonism of anticonvulsant effect

Anxiolytics and Hypnotics: enhanced sedative effect

Triamcinolone *see* Corticosteroids

Triamterene *see* Diuretics (potassium-sparing)

Triclofos *see* Chloral

Trientine

Iron: absorption of *oral iron* reduced

Trifluoperazine *see* Phenothiazines and other Antipsychotics

Trifluperidol *see* Phenothiazines and other Antipsychotics

Trilostane

Diuretics: increased risk of hyperkalaemia with *potassium-sparing diuretics*

Trimeprazine *see* Antihistamines

Trimethoprim

Anti-arrhythmics: plasma concentration of *procainamide* increased

Anticoagulants: effect of *nicoumalone* and *warfarin* possibly enhanced

Antidiabetics: effect of *sulphonylureas* enhanced

Antiepileptics: antifolate effect of *phenytoin* increased

Antimalarials: increased risk of antifolate effect with *pyrimethamine* (ingredient of *Fansidar®* and *Maloprim®*)

• Cyclosporin: increased risk of nephrotoxicity

Cytotoxics: antifolate effect of *methotrexate* increased

Trimipramine *see* Antidepressants, Tricyclic

Tripotassium Dicitratobismuthate *see* Bismuth Chelate

Triprolidine *see* Antihistamines

Tropicamide *see* Antimuscarinics

Tryptophan

• *other* Antidepressants: CNS excitation and confusion with *MAOIs* (reduce tryptophan dose); agitation and nausea with *fluoxetine, fluvoxamine, paroxetine, and sertraline*

Tubocurarine *see* Muscle Relaxants (non-depolarising)

Tulobuterol *see* Sympathomimetics, Beta$_2$

Typhoid Vaccine *see* p.479

Ulcer-healing Drugs *see* individual drugs

Uricosurics *see* individual drugs

Vaccines *see* Influenza Vaccine (p.474), Rabies Vaccine (p.477), Typhoid Vaccine (p.479)

Note. For a general warning on *live vaccines* and *high doses of corticosteroids* or *other immunosuppressive drugs*, see section 14.1

Valproate

Analgesics: *aspirin* enhances effect

• Antidepressants: antagonism of anticonvulsant effect (convulsive threshold lowered)

• *other* Antiepileptics: concomitant administration of *two or more antiepileptics* may enhance toxicity without a corresponding increase in antiepileptic effect; moreover, interactions between individual antiepileptics can complicate monitoring of treatment; interactions include enhanced effects, increased sedation, and reductions in plasma concentrations; for further details, see p.193

• Antimalarials: antagonism of anticonvulsant effect

• Antipsychotics: antagonism of anticonvulsant effect (convulsive threshold lowered)

Vancomycin

Anion-exchange Resins: antagonism of *oral vancomycin* by *cholestyramine*

other Antibacterials: increased risk of ototoxicity and nephrotoxicity with *aminoglycosides and capreomycin*

Diuretics: increased risk of ototoxicity with *loop diuretics*

Vecuronium *see* Muscle Relaxants (non-depolarising)

Verapamil *see* Calcium-channel Blockers

Vigabatrin

• *other* Antiepileptics: concomitant administration of *two or more antiepileptics* may enhance toxicity without a corresponding increase in antiepileptic effect; moreover, interactions between individual antiepileptics can complicate monitoring of treatment; interactions include enhanced effects, increased sedation, and reductions in plasma concentrations; for further details, see p.193

Viloxazine

- *other* Antidepressants: as for Antidepressants, Tricyclic
- Antiepileptics: increased plasma concentrations of *carbamazepine* and *phenytoin*

  Theophylline: increased plasma-theophylline concentration

Vitamins

- Anticoagulants: anticoagulant effect of *nicoumalone, phenindione, and warfarin* antagonised by *vitamin K* (present in some enteral feeds)

  Antiepileptics: *folic acid* occasionally reduces plasma-phenytoin concentration; *vitamin D* requirements possibly increased by *carbamazepine, phenobarbitone, phenytoin,* and *primidone*

  Diuretics: increased risk of hypercalcaemia if *thiazides* given with *vitamin D*

  Dopaminergics: effect of *levodopa* antagonised by *pyridoxine* (unless a dopa decarboxylase inhibitor also given)

Warfarin and other Coumarins

Note. Change in patient's clinical condition, particularly associated with liver disease, intercurrent illness, or drug administration, necessitates more frequent testing. Major changes in diet (especially involving vegetables) may also affect warfarin control.

- Alcohol: enhanced anticoagulant effect

  Allopurinol: anticoagulant effect possibly enhanced

- Anabolic Steroids: *oxymetholone, stanozolol and others* enhance anticoagulant effect

- Analgesics: *aspirin* increases risk of bleeding due to antiplatelet effect; anticoagulant effect seriously enhanced by *azapropazone (see also* p.380) and *phenylbutazone,* and possibly enhanced by *diflunisal, flurbiprofen, mefenamic acid, piroxicam, sulindac, and possibly other NSAIDs*; anticoagulant effect possibly also enhanced by *dextropropoxyphene* and by prolonged regular use of *paracetamol*; increased risk of haemorrhage with *ketorolac,* see p.493

- Anion-exchange Resins: *cholestyramine* may enhance or reduce anticoagulant effect

- Anti-arrhythmics: *amiodarone and propafenone* enhance anticoagulant effect; *quinidine* may enhance anticoagulant effect

- Antibacterials: anticoagulant effect reduced by *rifamycins*; anticoagulant effect enhanced by *aztreonam, cephamandole, chloramphenicol, ciprofloxacin, co-trimoxazole, erythromycin, metronidazole, ofloxacin,* and *sulphonamides*; anticoagulant effect possibly also enhanced by *azithromycin, clarithromycin, nalidixic acid, neomycin, norfloxacin, tetracyclines,* and *trimethoprim*; although studies have failed to demonstrate interaction, common experience in anticoagulant clinics is that INR can be altered following course of oral *broad-spectrum antibiotic,* such as *ampicillin* (may also apply to antibiotics given for local action on gut such as *neomycin*)

- Antidepressants: *serotonin-uptake inhibitors* may enhance anticoagulant effect

- Antiepileptics: reduced anticoagulant effect with *carbamazepine, phenobarbitone, and primidone*; both reduced and enhanced effects reported with *phenytoin*

- Antifungals: anticoagulant effect reduced by *griseofulvin;* anticoagulant effect enhanced by *fluconazole, itraconazole, ketoconazole, and miconazole* (note: oral gel absorbed)

Warfarin and other Coumarins (*continued*)

- Antimalarials: anticoagulant effect possibly enhanced by *proguanil*
- Antiplatelet Drugs: *aspirin and dipyridamole* increase risk of bleeding due to antiplatelet effect

  Anxiolytics and Hypnotics: *chloral* may transiently enhance anticoagulant effect

- Barbiturates: anticoagulant effect reduced

  Cisapride: effect of *oral anticoagulants* possibly enhanced

- Clofibrate Group: enhanced anticoagulant effect
- Cytotoxics: anticoagulant effect possibly enhanced by *ifosfamide*
- Disulfiram: enhanced anticoagulant effect
- Hormone Antagonists: *aminoglutethimide* reduces anticoagulant effect; *danazol, flutamide, and tamoxifen* enhance anticoagulant effect
- Oestrogens and Progestogens: *oral contraceptives* reduce anticoagulant effect
- Retinoids: *acitretin* possibly reduces anticoagulant effect

  Rowachol®: may reduce anticoagulant effect

- Simvastatin: may enhance anticoagulant effect
- Thyroxine: enhanced anticoagulant effect
- Ulcer-healing Drugs: *sucralfate* possibly reduces anticoagulant effect (reduced absorption); *cimetidine and omeprazole* enhance anticoagulant effect
- Uricosurics: *sulphinpyrazone* enhances anticoagulant effect

  Vaccines: *influenza vaccine* occasionally enhances anticoagulant effect

- Vitamins: *vitamin K* reduces anticoagulant effect; major changes in diet (especially involving vegetables) may affect control, vitamin K also present in some enteral feeds

Xamoterol

  Beta-blockers: antagonism of effect of *xamoterol* and reduction in beta-blockade

Xipamide *see* Diuretics (thiazide-related)

Xylometazoline *see* Sympathomimetics

Zidovudine

Note. Increased risk of toxicity with other nephrotoxic and myelosuppressive drugs—for further details consult data sheet

  Analgesics: *methadone* possibly increases plasma zidovudine concentration

  other Antivirals: extreme lethargy reported on administration of *intravenous acyclovir*; profound myelosuppression with *ganciclovir*

  Uricosurics: *probenecid* increases plasma-zidovudine concentration and risk of toxicity

Zinc

  Antibacterials: reduced absorption of *ciprofloxacin*; *tetracyclines* reduce absorption of *zinc* (and *vice versa*)

  Iron: reduced absorption of *oral iron* (and *vice versa*)

  Penicillamine: reduced absorption of *penicillamine*

Zolpidem *see* Benzodiazepines and other Anxiolytics and Hypnotics

Zopiclone (general sedative interactions *as for* Benzodiazepines and other Anxiolytics and Hypnotics)

Zuclopenthixol *see* Phenothiazines and other Antipsychotics

Appendix 2: Liver Disease

Liver disease may alter the response to drugs in several ways as indicated below, and drug prescribing should be kept to a minimum in all patients with severe liver disease. The main problems occur in patients with jaundice, ascites, or evidence of encephalopathy.

IMPAIRED DRUG METABOLISM. Metabolism by the liver is the main route of elimination for many drugs, but the hepatic reserve appears to be large and liver disease has to be severe before important changes in drug metabolism occur. Routine liver-function tests are a poor guide to the capacity of the liver to metabolise drugs, and in the individual patient it is not possible to predict the extent to which the metabolism of a particular drug may be impaired.

A few drugs, e.g. rifampicin and fusidic acid, are excreted in the bile unchanged and may accumulate in patients with intrahepatic or extrahepatic obstructive jaundice.

HYPOPROTEINAEMIA. The hypoalbuminaemia in severe liver disease is associated with reduced protein binding and increased toxicity of some highly-protein-bound drugs such as phenytoin and prednisolone.

REDUCED CLOTTING. Reduced hepatic synthesis of blood-clotting factors, indicated by a prolonged prothrombin time, increases the sensitivity to oral anticoagulants such as warfarin and phenindione.

HEPATIC ENCEPHALOPATHY. In severe liver disease many drugs can further impair cerebral function and may precipitate hepatic encephalopathy. These include all sedative drugs, opioid analgesics, those diuretics that produce hypokalaemia, and drugs that cause constipation.

FLUID OVERLOAD. Oedema and ascites in chronic liver disease may be exacerbated by drugs that give rise to fluid retention, e.g. NSAIDs, corticosteroids, and carbenoxolone.

HEPATOTOXIC DRUGS. Hepatotoxicity is either dose-related or unpredictable (idiosyncratic). Drugs causing dose-related toxicity may do so at lower doses than in patients with normal liver function, and some drugs producing reactions of the idiosyncratic kind do so more frequently in patients with liver disease. These drugs should be avoided.

Table of drugs to be avoided or used with caution in liver disease

The list of drugs given below is not comprehensive and is based on current information concerning the use of these drugs in therapeutic dosage. Products introduced or amended since publication of BNF No. 27 (March 1994) are underlined.

Drug	Comment	Drug	Comment
Acarbose	Avoid	Antacids	In patients with fluid retention, avoid those containing large amounts of sodium, e.g. magnesium trisilicate mixture, Gaviscon® Avoid those causing constipation—can precipitate coma
ACE Inhibitors	Use of prodrugs such as cilazapril, enalapril, fosinopril, perindopril, quinapril, ramipril, and trandolapril requires close monitoring in patients with impaired liver function		
Acemetacin see NSAIDs		Anticoagulants, Oral	Avoid, especially if prothrombin time is already prolonged
Acitretin	Avoid—further impairment of liver function may occur		
Acrivastine see Antihistamines		Antidepressants, MAOI see MAOIs	
Acrosoxacin see 4-Quinolones		Antidepressants, Serotonin-uptake Inhibitor	Reduce dose or avoid in severe liver disease
Alfentanil see Opioid Analgesics			
Alfuzosin	Reduce dose in mild to moderate liver disease; avoid if severe	Antidepressants, Tricyclic (and related)	Tricyclics preferable to MAOIs but sedative effects increased (avoid in severe liver disease); iprindole may cause idiosyncratic hepatotoxicity
Allyloestrenol see Progestogens			
Aminophylline see Theophylline			
Amitriptyline see Antidepressants, Tricyclic		Antihistamines	Avoid—may precipitate coma; astemizole and terfenadine, see also p.130
Amlodipine	Reduce dose		
Amoxapine see Antidepressants, Tricyclic			
Anabolic Steroids	Preferably avoid—dose-related toxicity	Antipsychotics	All can precipitate coma; phenothiazines are hepatotoxic
Analgesics see NSAIDs and Opioid Analgesics			
Androgens	Preferably avoid—dose-related toxicity with some, and produce fluid retention		

Table of drugs to be avoided or used with caution in liver disease (*continued*)

Drug	Comment
Anxiolytics and Hypnotics	All can precipitate coma; small dose of oxazepam or temazepam probably safest; reduce oral dose of chlormethiazole
Aspirin	Avoid—increased risk of gastro-intestinal bleeding
Astemizole *see* Antihistamines	
Auranofin *see* Gold	
Aurothiomalate *see* Gold	
Azapropazone *see* NSAIDs	
Azatadine *see* Antihistamines	
Azathioprine	May need dose reduction
Bambuterol	Avoid in severe liver disease
Bendrofluazide *see* Thiazides	
Benorylate [aspirin-paracetamol ester] *see* Aspirin	
Benperidol *see* Antipsychotics	
Benzodiazepines *see* Anxiolytics and Hypnotics	
Beta-blockers *see* individual drugs	
Bezafibrate	Avoid in severe liver disease
Bromazepam *see* Anxiolytics and Hypnotics	
Brompheniramine *see* Antihistamines	
Bumetanide *see* Loop Diuretics	
Bupivacaine *see* Lignocaine	
Buprenorphine *see* Opioid Analgesics	
Carbamazepine	For advice on patient counselling, see p.194
Carbenoxolone	Produces sodium and water retention and hypokalaemia
Cetirizine *see* Antihistamines	
Chenodeoxycholic Acid	Avoid in chronic liver disease; patients with non-functioning gall-bladder do not respond
Chloral Hydrate *see* Anxiolytics and Hypnotics	
Chloramphenicol	Avoid—increased risk of bone-marrow depression
Chlordiazepoxide *see* Anxiolytics and Hypnotics	
Chlormethiazole	Reduce oral dose; *see* Anxiolytics and Hypnotics
Chlormezanone *see* Anxiolytics and Hypnotics	
Chlorothiazide *see* Thiazides	
Chlorpheniramine *see* Antihistamines	
Chlorpromazine *see* Antipsychotics	
Chlorpropamide *see* Sulphonylureas	
Chlorthalidone *see* Thiazides	
Cholestyramine	Interferes with absorption of fat-soluble vitamins and may aggravate malabsorption in primary biliary cirrhosis
Choline Theophyllinate *see* Theophylline	
Cilazapril *see* ACE Inhibitors	
Cimetidine	Increased risk of confusion; reduce dose
Cinnarizine *see* Antihistamines	
Cinoxacin *see* 4-Quinolones	
Ciprofibrate	Avoid in severe liver disease
Ciprofloxacin *see* 4-Quinolones	
Cisapride	Halve dose initially
Clavulanic Acid [ingredient] *see* Co-amoxiclav and Timentin®	
Clemastine *see* Antihistamines	
Clindamycin	Reduce dose
Clobazam *see* Anxiolytics and Hypnotics	
Clofibrate	Avoid in severe liver disease

Drug	Comment
Clomiphene	Avoid in severe liver disease
Clomipramine *see* Antidepressants, Tricyclic	
Clopamide *see* Thiazides	
Clorazepate *see* Anxiolytics and Hypnotics	
Clozapine *see* Antipsychotics	
Co-amoxiclav	Cholestatic jaundice, see p.221
Codeine *see* Opioid Analgesics	
Contraceptives, Oral	Avoid in active liver disease and in patients with a history of pruritus or cholestasis during pregnancy
Cyclizine *see* Antihistamines	
Cyclofenil	Avoid in severe liver disease
Cyclopenthiazide *see* Thiazides	
Cyclosporin	May need dose adjustment
Cyproheptadine *see* Antihistamines	
Cyproterone Acetate	Avoid—dose-related toxicity
Dalteparin *see* Heparin	
Danaparoid *see* Heparin	
Dantrolene	Avoid—may cause severe liver damage
Demeclocycline *see* Tetracyclines	
Desipramine *see* Antidepressants, Tricyclic	
Desogestrel *see* Progestogens	
Dexfenfluramine	Manufacturer advises avoid
Dextromethorphan *see* Opioid Analgesics	
Dextromoramide *see* Opioid Analgesics	
Dextropropoxyphene *see* Opioid Analgesics	
Diamorphine *see* Opioid Analgesics	
Diazepam *see* Anxiolytics and Hypnotics	
Diclofenac *see* NSAIDs	
Didanosine	Reduce initial dose
Diflunisal *see* NSAIDs	
Dihydrocodeine *see* Opioid Analgesics	
Diltiazem	Reduce dose
Dimenhydrinate *see* Antihistamines	
Diphenoxylate *see* Opioid Analgesics	
Diphenylpyraline *see* Antihistamines	
Dipipanone *see* Opioid Analgesics	
Dothiepin *see* Antidepressants, Tricyclic	
Doxepin *see* Antidepressants, Tricyclic	
Doxorubicin	Reduce dose according to bilirubin concentration
Doxycycline *see* Tetracyclines	
Droperidol *see* Antipsychotics	
Dydrogesterone *see* Progestogens	
Enalapril *see* ACE Inhibitors	
Enoxaparin *see* Heparin	
Epirubicin	Reduce dose according to bilirubin concentration
Ergometrine	Avoid in severe liver disease
Ergotamine	Avoid in severe liver disease—risk of toxicity increased
Erythromycin	May cause idiosyncratic hepatotoxicity
Ethacrynic Acid *see* Loop Diuretics	
Ethinyloestradiol *see* Oestrogens	
Ethynodiol Diacetate *see* Progestogens	
Etodolac *see* NSAIDs	
Felodipine	Reduce dose
Fenbufen *see* NSAIDs	
Fenofibrate *see* Clofibrate	

Table of drugs to be avoided or used with caution in liver disease (*continued*)

Drug	Comment
Fenoprofen *see* NSAIDs	
Fentanyl *see* Opioid Analgesics	
Flecainide	Avoid (or reduce dose) in severe liver disease
Flucloxacillin	Cholestatic jaundice, see p.218
Fluconazole	Toxicity with related drugs
Flunitrazepam *see* Anxiolytics and Hypnotics	
Fluoxetine *see* Antidepressants, Serotonin-uptake Inhibitor	
Flupenthixol *see* Antipsychotics	
Fluphenazine *see* Antipsychotics	
Flurazepam *see* Anxiolytics and Hypnotics	
Flurbiprofen *see* NSAIDs	
Fluspirilene *see* Antipsychotics	
Fluvastatin	Avoid
Fluvoxamine *see* Antidepressants, Serotonin-uptake Inhibitor	
Fosfestrol *see* Oestrogens	
Fosinopril *see* ACE Inhibitors	
Frusemide *see* Loop Diuretics	
Fusidic Acid	Impaired biliary excretion; may be increased risk of hepatotoxicity; avoid or reduce dose
Gemfibrozil	Avoid in severe liver disease
Gestodene *see* Progestogens	
Gestronol *see* Progestogens	
Glibenclamide *see* Sulphonylureas	
Gliclazide *see* Sulphonylureas	
Glipizide *see* Sulphonylureas	
Gliquidone *see* Sulphonylureas	
Gold (auranofin, aurothiomalate)	Avoid in severe liver disease—hepatotoxicity may occur
Haloperidol *see* Antipsychotics	
Halothane *see* p.488	
Heparin	Reduce dose in severe liver disease
Hydrochlorothiazide *see* Thiazides	
Hydroflumethiazide *see* Thiazides	
Hydroxyprogesterone Hexanoate *see* Progestogens	
Hydroxyzine *see* Antihistamines	
Hypnotics *see* Anxiolytics and Hypnotics	
Ibuprofen *see* NSAIDs	
Idarubicin	Reduce dose according to bilirubin concentration
Imipramine *see* Antidepressants, Tricyclic	
Indapamide *see* Thiazides	
Indomethacin *see* NSAIDs	
Iprindole *see* Antidepressants, Tricyclic (and related)	
Isocarboxazid *see* MAOIs	
Isoniazid	Avoid if possible—idiosyncratic hepatotoxicity more common
Isotretinoin	Avoid—further impairment of liver function may occur
Isradipine	Reduce dose
Itraconazole	Avoid—toxicity with related drugs
Ketoconazole	Induces hepatitis-like reaction; may accumulate in severe liver disease; contra-indicated unless no alternative; see also p.250

Drug	Comment
Ketoprofen *see* NSAIDs	
Ketorolac *see* NSAIDs	
Ketotifen *see* Antihistamines	
Labetalol	Avoid—severe hepatocellular injury reported
Lacidipine	Reduce dose
Lamotrigine	Manufacturer advises avoid
Lansoprazole	In severe liver disease dose should not exceed 30 mg daily
Levonorgestrel *see* Progestogens	
Lignocaine	Avoid (or reduce dose) in severe liver disease
Lofepramine *see* Antidepressants, Tricyclic	
Loop Diuretics	Hypokalaemia may precipitate coma; potassium-sparing diuretic should be used to prevent this; increased risk of hypomagnesaemia in alcoholic cirrhosis
Loprazolam *see* Anxiolytics and Hypnotics	
Lorazepam *see* Anxiolytics and Hypnotics	
Lormetazepam *see* Anxiolytics and Hypnotics	
Loxapine *see* Antipsychotics	
Lymecycline *see* Tetracyclines	
Magnesium Salts	Avoid in hepatic coma if risk of renal failure
MAOIs	May cause idiosyncratic hepatotoxicity
Maprotiline *see* Antidepressants, Tricyclic (and related)	
Medroxyprogesterone Acetate *see* Progestogens	
Mefenamic Acid see NSAIDs	
Mefloquine	Avoid for prophylaxis in severe liver disease
Mefruside *see* Thiazides	
Megestrol Acetate *see* Progestogens	
Meprobamate *see* Anxiolytics and Hypnotics	
Meptazinol *see* Opioid Analgesics	
Mequitazine *see* Antihistamines	
Mesterolone *see* Androgens	
Mestranol *see* Oestrogens	
Metformin	Avoid—increased risk of lactic acidosis
Methadone *see* Opioid Analgesics	
Methohexitone	Avoid or reduce dose
Methotrexate	Dose-related toxicity—avoid in non-malignant conditions (e.g. psoriasis)
Methotrimeprazine *see* Antipsychotics	
Methoxsalen	Avoid or reduce dose
Methyclothiazide *see* Thiazides	
Methyldopa	Avoid—increased risk of hepatotoxicity
Metoclopramide	Reduce dose in severe liver disease
Metolazone *see* Thiazides	
Metoprolol	Reduce oral dose
Metronidazole	Reduce dose in severe liver disease
Mexiletine	Avoid (or reduce dose) in severe liver disease
Mianserin *see* Antidepressants, Tricyclic (and related)	
Minocycline *see* Tetracyclines	

Table of drugs to be avoided or used with caution in liver disease (*continued*)

Drug	Comment	Drug	Comment
Mivacurium	Reduce dose	Phenoperidine *see* Opioid Analgesics	
Moclobemide	Reduce dose in severe liver disease	Phenothiazines *see* Antipsychotics	
Monoamine-oxidase Inhibitors *see* MAOIs		Phenylbutazone *see* NSAIDs	
Morphine *see* Opioid Analgesics		Phenytoin	Reduce dose to avoid toxicity
Nabumetone *see* NSAIDs		Pholcodine *see* Opioid Analgesics	
Nalbuphine *see* Opioid Analgesics		Pimozide *see* Antipsychotics	
Nalidixic Acid *see* 4-Quinolones		Piperazine	Manufacturer advises avoid
Nandrolone *see* Anabolic Steroids		Piperazine Oestrone Sulphate *see* Oestrogens	
Naproxen *see* NSAIDs		Pipothiazine *see* Antipsychotics	
Narcotic Analgesics *see* Opioid Analgesics		Piracetam	Avoid
Nicardipine	Reduce dose	Piretanide *see* Loop Diuretics	
Nifedipine	Reduce dose	Piroxicam *see* NSAIDs	
Niridazole	Increased CNS toxicity in patients with cirrhosis or portal-systemic shunts	Plicamycin	Avoid if possible (increased risk of toxicity)
		Polyoestradiol *see* Oestrogens	
Nitrazepam *see* Anxiolytics and Hypnotics		Polythiazide *see* Thiazides	
Nitrofurantoin	Cholestatic jaundice and chronic active hepatitis reported	Pravastatin	Avoid in active liver disease or unexplained persistent elevations in liver-function tests
Nitroprusside	Avoid in severe liver disease	Prednisolone	Side-effects more common
Norethisterone *see* Progestogens		Prednisone	Prednisolone is preferable (prednisone needs conversion to prednisolone by liver before active)
Norfloxacin *see* 4-Quinolones			
Norgestimate *see* Progestogens			
Norgestrel *see* Progestogens			
Nortriptyline *see* Antidepressants, Tricyclic		Primidone	May precipitate coma
NSAIDs	Increased risk of gastro-intestinal bleeding and can cause fluid retention	Procainamide	Avoid or reduce dose
		Prochlorperazine *see* Antipsychotics	
		Progesterone *see* Progestogens	
Oestradiol *see* Oestrogens		Progestogens	Avoid; *see also* Contraceptives, Oral
Oestriol *see* Oestrogens			
Oestrogens	Avoid; *see also* Contraceptives, Oral	Promazine *see* Antipsychotics	
		Promethazine *see* Antihistamines	
Ofloxacin *see* 4-Quinolones		Propafenone	Reduce dose
Omeprazole	In severe liver disease not more than 20 mg daily should be needed	Propranolol	Reduce oral dose
		Protriptyline *see* Antidepressants, Tricyclic	
		Pyrazinamide	Avoid—idiosyncratic hepatotoxicity more common
Ondansetron	Reduce dose; not more than 8 mg daily in severe liver disease	Quinapril *see* ACE Inhibitors	
		4-Quinolones	See section 5.1.12; hepatitis with necrosis reported with *ciprofloxacin; nalidixic acid* partially conjugated in liver; reduce dose of *ofloxacin* in severe liver disease
Opioid Analgesics	Avoid or reduce dose—may precipitate coma		
Oral Contraceptives *see* Contraceptives, Oral			
Oxatomide *see* Antihistamines			
Oxazepam *see* Anxiolytics and Hypnotics			
Oxprenolol	Reduce oral dose	Ramipril *see* ACE Inhibitors	
Oxymetholone *see* Anabolic Steroids		Ranitidine	Increased risk of confusion; reduce dose
Oxypertine *see* Antipsychotics			
Oxytetracycline *see* Tetracyclines		Rifabutin	Avoid if possible (or reduce dose) in severe hepatic impairment
Paclitaxel	Avoid in severe liver disease		
Papaveretum *see* Opioid Analgesics			
Paracetamol	Dose-related toxicity—avoid large doses	Rifampicin	Impaired elimination; may be increased risk of hepatotoxicity; avoid or do not exceed 8mg/kg daily
Paroxetine *see* Antidepressants, Serotonin-uptake Inhibitor			
Pentazocine *see* Opioid Analgesics		Risperidone *see* Antipsychotics	
Pericyazine *see* Antipsychotics		Rocuronium	Reduce dose
Perindopril *see* ACE Inhibitors		Salsalate *see* Aspirin	
Perphenazine *see* Antipsychotics		Sertraline *see* Antidepressants, Serotonin-uptake Inhibitor	
Pethidine *see* Opioid Analgesics			
Phenazocine *see* Opioid Analgesics		Simvastatin	Avoid—hepatotoxic
Phenelzine *see* MAOIs		Sodium Aurothiomalate *see* Gold	
Phenindamine *see* Antihistamines		Sodium Bicarbonate *see* Antacids	
Pheniramine *see* Antihistamines		Sodium Fusidate *see* Fusidic Acid	
Phenobarbitone	May precipitate coma	Sodium Nitroprusside *see* Nitroprusside	

Table of drugs to be avoided or used with caution in liver disease (*continued*)

Drug	Comment	Drug	Comment
Sodium Valproate *see* Valproate		*Timentin*®	Cholestatic jaundice, see p. 223
Stanozolol *see* Anabolic Steroids			
Stilboestrol *see* Oestrogens		Tinzaparin *see* Heparin	
Sulindac *see* NSAIDs		Tocainide	Avoid (or reduce dose) in severe liver disease
Sulphonylureas	Increased risk of hypoglycaemia in severe liver disease; avoid or use small dose; can produce jaundice	Tolazamide *see* Sulphonylureas	
		Tolbutamide *see* Sulphonylureas	
		Tolmetin *see* NSAIDs	
Suxamethonium	Prolonged apnoea may occur in severe liver disease due to reduced hepatic synthesis of pseudocholinesterase	Torasemide *see* Loop Diuretics	
		Tramadol *see* Opioid Analgesics	
		Trandolapril *see* ACE Inhibitors	
		Tranylcypromine *see* MAOIs	
Temazepam *see* Anxiolytics and Hypnotics		Trazodone *see* Antidepressants, Tricyclic (and related)	
Tenoxicam *see* NSAIDs		Triclofos *see* Anxiolytics and Hypnotics	
Terbinafine	Reduce dose	Trifluoperazine *see* Antipsychotics	
Terfenadine *see* Antihistamines		Trifluperidol *see* Antipsychotics	
Testosterone *see* Androgens		Trimeprazine *see* Antihistamines	
<u>Tetracyclines</u>	Avoid (or use with caution)—dose-related toxicity by i/v route	Trimipramine *see* Antidepressants, Tricyclic	
		Triprolidine *see* Antihistamines	
Theophylline	Reduce dose	<u>Tulobuterol</u>	Avoid
Thiazides	Hypokalaemia may precipitate coma (potassium-sparing diuretic can prevent); increased risk of hypomagnesaemia in alcoholic cirrhosis	Valproate	Avoid if possible—hepatotoxicity and liver failure may occasionally occur (usually in first 6 months); see also p. 197
		Verapamil	Reduce oral dose
		Zidovudine	Accumulation may occur
Thiopentone	Reduce dose for induction in severe liver disease	Zolpidem *see* Anxiolytics and Hypnotics	
		Zopiclone	Reduce dose
Thioridazine *see* Antipsychotics		Zuclopenthixol *see* Antipsychotics	
Tiaprofenic acid *see* NSAIDs			
Tibolone	Avoid in severe liver disease		

Appendix 3: Renal Impairment

The use of drugs in patients with reduced renal function can give rise to problems for several reasons:

failure to excrete a drug or its metabolites may produce toxicity;

sensitivity to some drugs is increased even if elimination is unimpaired;

many side-effects are tolerated poorly by patients in renal failure;

some drugs cease to be effective when renal function is reduced.

Many of these problems can be avoided by reducing the dose or by using alternative drugs.

Principles of dose adjustment in renal impairment

The level of renal function below which the dose of a drug must be reduced depends on whether the drug is eliminated entirely by renal excretion or is partly metabolised, and on how toxic it is.

For many drugs with only minor or no dose-related side-effects very precise modification of the dose regimen is unnecessary and a simple scheme for dose reduction is sufficient.

For more toxic drugs with a small safety margin dose regimens based on glomerular filtration rate should be used. For those where both efficacy and toxicity are closely related to plasma concentrations recommended regimens should be seen only as a guide to initial treatment; subsequent treatment must be adjusted according to clinical response and plasma concentration.

The total daily maintenance dose of a drug can be reduced either by reducing the size of the individual doses or by increasing the interval between doses. For some drugs, if the size of the maintenance dose is reduced it will be important to give a loading dose if an immediate effect is required. This is because when a patient is given a regular dose of any drug it takes more than five times the half-life to achieve steady-state plasma concentrations. As the plasma half-life of drugs excreted by the kidney is prolonged in renal failure it may take many days for the reduced dosage to achieve a therapeutic plasma concentration. The loading dose should usually be the same size as the initial dose for a patient with normal renal function.

Nephrotoxic drugs should, if possible, be avoided in patients with renal disease because the consequences of nephrotoxicity are likely to be more serious when the renal reserve is already reduced.

Use of dosage table

Dose recommendations are based on the severity of renal impairment. This is expressed in terms of glomerular filtration rate (GFR), usually measured by the **creatinine clearance**. The serum-creatinine concentration can be used instead as a measure of renal function but is only a rough guide unless corrected for age, weight, and sex. Nomograms are available for making the correction and should be used where accuracy is important.

Renal impairment is arbitrarily divided into 3 grades:

Grade	GFR	Serum creatinine (approx.)
Mild	20–50 mL/min	150–300 µmol/litre
Moderate	10–20 mL/min	300–700 µmol/litre
Severe	<10 mL/min	> 700µmol/litre

Note. Conversion factors are:
Litres/24 hours = mL/minute × 1.44
mL/minute = Litres/24 hours × 0.69

Renal function declines with age; many elderly patients have a glomerular filtration rate below 50 mL/minute which, because of reduced muscle mass, may not be indicated by a raised serum creatinine. It is wise to assume at least mild impairment of renal function when prescribing for the elderly.

The following table may be used as a guide to drugs which are known to require a reduction in dose in renal impairment, and to those which are potentially harmful or are ineffective. Drug prescribing should be kept to the minimum in all patients with severe renal disease.

If renal impairment is considered likely on clinical grounds renal function should be checked before prescribing **any** drug which requires dose modification even when renal impairment is mild.

Table of drugs to be avoided or used with caution in renal impairment

Products introduced or amended since publication of BNF No. 27 (March 1994) are <u>underlined</u>.

Drug and Degree of impairment	Comment	Drug and Degree of impairment	Comment

<u>Acarbose</u>
  Moderate to severe
	Manufacturer advises avoid
	—no information available
		Acetazolamide
		  Mild
		Acipimox
		  Mild
			Avoid; metabolic acidosis
			
			Reduce dose

Acebutolol *see* Beta-blockers Acemetacin *see* NSAIDs			

Table of drugs to be avoided or used with caution in renal impairment (*continued*)

Drug and Degree of impairment	Comment
Acitretin	
Mild	Avoid; increased risk of toxicity
Acrivastine	
Moderate	Avoid; excreted by kidney
Acyclovir	
Moderate to severe	Reduce dose; possible transient increase in plasma urea
Alcuronium see Tubocurarine	
Alfentanil see Opioid Analgesics	
Alfuzosin	
Moderate	Reduce dose
Allopurinol	
Moderate	100 mg daily; increased toxicity; rashes
Severe	100 mg on alternate days
Alprazolam see Anxiolytics and Hypnotics	
Alteplase	
Moderate	Risk of hyperkalaemia
Aluminium Salts	
Severe	Aluminium is absorbed and may accumulate
Note. Absorption of aluminium from aluminium salts is increased by citrates, which are contained in many effervescent preparations (such as effervescent analgesics)	
Amantadine	
Mild to moderate	Reduce dose; excreted by kidney
Severe	Avoid
Amikacin see Aminoglycosides	
Amiloride see Potassium-sparing Diuretics	
Aminoglycosides	
Mild	Reduce dose; monitor plasma concentrations; ototoxic; nephrotoxic; *see also* p.231
Amiodarone	
Moderate	Accumulation of iodine may increase risk of thyroid dysfunction
Amoxycillin	
Severe	Reduce dose; rashes more common
Amphotericin	
Mild	Use only if no alternative; nephrotoxicity may be reduced with use of complexes (see also p.248)
Ampicillin	
Severe	Reduce dose; rashes more common
Amylobarbitone	
Severe	Reduce dose; active metabolite accumulates
Analgesics see Opioid Analgesics and NSAIDs	
Antipsychotics	
Severe	Start with small doses; increased cerebral sensitivity; *see also* Sulpiride
Anxiolytics and Hypnotics	
Severe	Start with small doses; increased cerebral sensitivity
Aspirin	
Severe	Avoid; sodium and water retention; deterioration in renal function; increased risk of gastro-intestinal bleeding
Atenolol see Beta-blockers	
Auranofin see Gold	
Aurothiomalate see Gold	
Azapropazone see NSAIDs (excreted by kidney)	

Drug and Degree of impairment	Comment
Azathioprine	
Severe	Reduce dose
Azlocillin	
Moderate	Reduce dose
Aztreonam	
Moderate	Reduce dose
Bacampicillin	
Severe	Reduce dose; rashes more common
Baclofen	
Mild	Use smaller doses; excreted by kidney
Bambuterol	
Mild	Reduce dose
Bendrofluazide see Thiazides	
Benorylate [aspirin-paracetamol ester] see Aspirin	
Benperidol see Antipsychotics	
Benzodiazepines see Anxiolytics and Hypnotics	
Benzylpenicillin	
Severe	Max. 6 g daily; neurotoxicity—high doses may cause convulsions
Beta-blockers	
Moderate	Start with small dose of acebutolol (active metabolite accumulates); reduce dose of atenolol, nadolol, pindolol, sotalol (all excreted unchanged)
Severe	Start with small dose; higher plasma concentrations after oral administration; may reduce renal blood flow and adversely affect renal function in severe impairment; manufacturer advises avoid celiprolol
Betaxolol see Beta-blockers	
Bethanidine	
Moderate	Avoid; increased postural hypotension; decrease in renal blood flow
Bezafibrate	
Mild to moderate	Reduce dose; further deterioration in renal function
Severe	Avoid
Bicarbonate see Sodium Bicarbonate	
Bismuth Chelate	
Severe	Avoid
Bisoprolol see Beta-blockers	
Bleomycin	
Moderate	Reduce dose
Bromazepam see Anxiolytics and Hypnotics	
Bumetanide	
Moderate	May need high doses
Buprenorphine see Opioid Analgesics	
Calcitonin	
Moderate	Reduce dose
Capreomycin	
Mild	Reduce dose; nephrotoxic; ototoxic
Captopril	
Mild	Reduce dose and monitor response; avoid if possible; excreted by kidney; hyperkalaemia and other side-effects more common (but specialised role in some forms of renal disease), *see also* p.83
Carbamazepine	Manufacturer advises caution

Table of drugs to be avoided or used with caution in renal impairment (*continued*)

Drug and Degree of impairment	Comment
Carbenicillin	
Moderate	Reduce dose; neurotoxic; may produce bleeding diathesis; 1 g contains 5.4 mmol sodium
Carbenoxolone	
Moderate	Avoid; fluid retention
Carboplatin *see* Cisplatin	
Cefadroxil	
Moderate	Reduce dose
Cefixime	
Moderate	Reduce dose
Cefodizime	
Moderate	Reduce dose
Cefotaxime	
Severe	Use half dose
Cefoxitin	
Mild	Reduce dose
Cefpodoxime	
Moderate	Reduce dose
Cefsulodin	
Moderate	Reduce dose
Ceftazidime	
Mild	Reduce dose
Ceftizoxime	
Mild	Reduce dose
Ceftriaxone	
Severe	Monitor plasma concentration
Cefuroxime	
Moderate to severe	Reduce parenteral dose
Celiprolol *see* Beta-blockers	
Cephalexin	
Severe	Max. 500 mg daily
Cephamandole	
Mild	Reduce dose
Cephazolin	
Mild	Reduce dose
Cephradine	
Mild	Reduce dose
Cetirizine	
Moderate	Use half dose
Chloral Hydrate *see* Anxiolytics and Hypnotics	
Chloramphenicol	
Severe	Avoid unless no alternative; dose-related depression of haematopoiesis
Chlordiazepoxide *see* Anxiolytics and Hypnotics	
Chlormethiazole *see* Anxiolytics and Hypnotics	
Chlormezanone *see* Anxiolytics and Hypnotics	
Chloroquine	
Mild to moderate	Reduce dose; only on prolonged use
Severe	Avoid
Chlorothiazide *see* Thiazides	
Chlorpromazine *see* Antipsychotics	
Chlorpropamide	
Mild	Avoid; tolbutamide and gliquidone suitable alternatives
Chlorthalidone *see* Thiazides	
Cilazapril	
Mild	Reduce dose and monitor response; avoid if possible; *see also* Captopril
Cimetidine	
Mild to moderate	600–800 mg daily; occasional risk of confusion
Severe	400 mg daily
Cinoxacin	
Moderate	Avoid; nausea, rashes
Ciprofibrate	
Moderate	100 mg on alternate days
Severe	Avoid

Drug and Degree of impairment	Comment
Ciprofloxacin	
Moderate	Use half dose
Cisapride	
Moderate	Start with half dose
Cisplatin	
Mild	Avoid if possible; nephrotoxic and neurotoxic
Citrates	Absorption of aluminium from aluminium salts is increased by citrates, which are contained in many effervescent preparations (such as effervescent analgesics)
Clarithromycin	
Moderate	Reduce dose
Clavulanic acid [ingredient] *see* Co-amoxiclav, Timentin®	
Clobazam *see* Anxiolytics and Hypnotics	
Clodronate sodium	
Mild to moderate	Use half dose and monitor serum creatinine
Severe	Avoid
Clofibrate	
Mild to moderate	Reduce dose; further deterioration in renal function; myopathy
Severe	Avoid
Clopamide *see* Thiazides	
Clorazepate *see* Anxiolytics and Hypnotics	
Clozapine *see* Antipsychotics	
Co-amoxiclav	
Moderate	Reduce dose
Codeine	
Moderate	Avoid; increased and prolonged effect; *see also* Opioid Analgesics
Colchicine	
Severe	Avoid or reduce dose if no alternative
Colistin	
Mild	Reduce dose; nephrotoxic; neurotoxic
Co-trimoxazole	
Moderate	Reduce dose; rashes and blood disorders; may cause further deterioration in renal function
Cyclopenthiazide *see* Thiazides	
Cyclophosphamide	
Moderate	Reduce dose
Cycloserine	
Mild to moderate	Reduce dose
Severe	Avoid
Cyclosporin *see* p.337 (*see also* p.438 if used in atopic dermatitis or psoriasis and p.391 if used in rheumatoid arthritis)	
Debrisoquine	
Moderate	Avoid; increased postural hypotension; decrease in renal blood flow
Demeclocycline *see* Tetracyclines	
De-Nol®, De-Noltab®	
Severe	Avoid
Desmopressin	Antidiuretic effect may be reduced; **important:** see also p.298
Dexfenfluramine	Manufacturer advises avoid
Dextromethorphan *see* Opioid Analgesics	
Dextromoramide *see* Opioid Analgesics	
Dextropropoxyphene	
Severe	Avoid; increased CNS toxicity

Table of drugs to be avoided or used with caution in renal impairment (*continued*)

Drug and Degree of impairment	Comment	Drug and Degree of impairment	Comment
Diamorphine *see* Opioid Analgesics		Fenofibrate	
Diazepam *see* Anxiolytics and Hypnotics		Mild	200mg daily
Diazoxide		Moderate	100mg daily
Severe	75–150 mg i/v; increased sensitivity to hypotensive effect	Severe	Avoid
		Fenoprofen *see* NSAIDs	
Diclofenac *see* NSAIDs		Fentanyl *see* Opioid Analgesics	
Didanosine		Flecainide	
Mild to moderate	Reduce dose; excreted by kidney	Mild	Max. initial dose 100mg daily
Diflunisal *see* NSAIDs (excreted by kidney)		Fluconazole	
Digitoxin		Mild	Reduce dose for multiple dose therapy
Severe	Max. 100micrograms daily; *see also* Digoxin	Flucytosine	
Digoxin		Mild	Reduce dose
Mild	Reduce dose; toxicity increased by electrolyte disturbances; *see also* p.55	Flunitrazepam *see* Anxiolytics and Hypnotics	
		Fluoxetine	
		Mild to moderate	Start with smaller dose
Dihydrocodeine		Severe	Avoid
Moderate	Avoid; increased and prolonged effect; *see also* Opioid Analgesics	Flupenthixol *see* Antipsychotics	
		Fluphenazine *see* Antipsychotics	
		Flurazepam *see* Anxiolytics and Hypnotics	
Diltiazem	Start with smaller dose	Flurbiprofen *see* NSAIDs	
Dimenhydrinate		Fluspirilene *see* Antipsychotics	
Severe	Manufacturer advises may accumulate	Fluvastatin	
		Severe	Avoid
Diphenoxylate *see* Opioid Analgesics		Fluvoxamine	
Dipipanone *see* Opioid Analgesics		Moderate	Start with smaller dose
Disodium Etidronate *see* Etidronate Disodium		Foscarnet	
Disodium Pamidronate *see* Pamidronate Disodium		Mild	Reduce dose; consult data sheet
Disopyramide		Fosfomycin	
Mild	100mg every 8 hours *or* 150mg every 12 hours	Severe	Avoid—therapeutic urinary concentrations not achieved
Moderate	100mg every 12 hours	Fosinopril	
Severe	150mg every 24 hours	Mild	Start with 10mg daily; *see also* Captopril
Domperidone		Frusemide	
Severe	Reduce dose by 30–50%	Moderate	May need high doses; deafness may follow rapid i/v injection
Doxycycline *see* Tetracyclines			
Droperidol *see* Antipsychotics			
Effervescent preparations *see* Citrates		*Fybogel Mebeverine*®	
Enalapril		Severe	Avoid; contains 7mmol potassium per sachet
Mild	Reduce dose and monitor response; avoid if possible; *see also* Captopril	Gabapentin	
		Mild	Reduce dose; consult data sheet
Ephedrine		Gallamine	
Severe	Avoid; increased CNS toxicity	Moderate	Avoid; prolonged paralysis
Ergometrine		Ganciclovir	
Severe	Manufacturer advises avoid	Mild	Reduce dose; consult data sheet
Ergotamine		Gaviscon®	
Moderate	Avoid; nausea and vomiting; risk of renal vasoconstriction	Severe	Avoid; high sodium content
		Gemfibrozil	
Erythromycin		Severe	Start with 900mg daily
Severe	Max. 1.5g daily (ototoxicity)	Gentamicin *see* Aminoglycosides	
Esmolol *see* Beta-blockers		Glibenclamide	
Ethacrynic Acid		Severe	Avoid; increased risk of prolonged hypoglycaemia
Severe	Avoid; ototoxic	Gliclazide	
Ethambutol		Severe	Start with small dose; increased risk of hypoglycaemia
Mild	Reduce dose; optic nerve damage		
Etidronate Disodium		Glipizide	
Mild	Max. 5mg/kg daily; excreted by kidney	Severe	Start with small dose; increased risk of hypoglycaemia
Moderate	Avoid		
Etodolac *see* NSAIDs		Gliquidone	
Etoposide		Severe	May need dose reduction; increased risk of hypoglycaemia
Mild	Reduce dose		
Famciclovir			
Moderate to severe	Reduce dose		
Famotidine			
Severe	Reduce dose		
Fenbufen *see* NSAIDs			

Table of drugs to be avoided or used with caution in renal impairment (*continued*)

Drug and Degree of impairment	Comment
Gold (auranofin, aurothiomalate)	
Mild	Avoid; nephrotoxic
Guanethidine	
Moderate	Avoid; increased postural hypotension and decrease in renal blood flow
Haloperidol *see* Antipsychotics	
Heparin	
Severe	Risk of bleeding increased
Hexamine	
Mild	Avoid; ineffective
Hydralazine	
Moderate	Start with small dose; increased hypotensive effect
Hydrochlorothiazide *see* Thiazides	
Hydroflumethiazide *see* Thiazides	
Hydroxychloroquine	
Mild to moderate	Reduce dose; only on prolonged use
Severe	Avoid
Hypnotics *see* Anxiolytics and Hypnotics	
Ibuprofen *see* NSAIDs	
Idarubicin	
Mild	Reduce dose
Ifosfamide	
Moderate	Reduce dose
Indapamide *see* Thiazides	
Indomethacin *see* NSAIDs	
Inosine Pranobex	
Mild	Avoid; metabolised to uric acid
Insulin	
Severe	May need dose reduction; insulin requirements fall; compensatory response to hypoglycaemia is impaired
Isoniazid	
Severe	Max. 200 mg daily; peripheral neuropathy
Isotretinoin	
Mild	Avoid; increased risk of toxicity
Kanamycin *see* Aminoglycosides	
Ketoprofen *see* NSAIDs	
Ketorolac *see* NSAIDs and p. 493	
Lamotrigine	Manufacturer advises avoid
Lisinopril	
Mild	Reduce dose and monitor response; *see also* Captopril
Lithium	
Mild	Avoid if possible or reduce dose and monitor plasma concentration carefully
Moderate	Avoid
Loprazolam *see* Anxiolytics and Hypnotics	
Lorazepam *see* Anxiolytics and Hypnotics	
Lormetazepam *see* Anxiolytics and Hypnotics	
Loxapine *see* Antipsychotics	
Lymecycline *see* Tetracyclines	
Magnesium Salts	
Moderate	Avoid or reduce dose; increased risk of toxicity; magnesium carbonate mixture and magnesium trisilicate mixture also have high sodium content
Mefenamic Acid *see* NSAIDs	
Mefloquine	
Mild	Avoid prophylactic use
Mefruside *see* Thiazides	
Melphalan	
Moderate	Reduce dose
Severe	Avoid high intravenous doses
Meprobamate *see* Anxiolytics and Hypnotics	

Drug and Degree of impairment	Comment
Meptazinol *see* Opioid Analgesics	
Mercaptopurine	
Moderate	Reduce dose
Mesalazine	
Mild	Avoid; nephrotoxic
Metformin	
Mild	Avoid; increased risk of lactic acidosis
Methadone *see* Opioid Analgesics	
Methocarbamol	
Mild	Avoid; increased plasma urea and acidosis due to solvent in injection
Methotrexate	
Mild	Reduce dose; accumulates; nephrotoxic
Moderate	Avoid
Methotrimeprazine *see* Antipsychotics	
Methyclothiazide *see* Thiazides	
Methyldopa	
Moderate	Start with small dose; increased sensitivity to hypotensive and sedative effect
Metoclopramide	
Severe	Avoid or use small dose; increased risk of extrapyramidal reactions
Metolazone *see* Thiazides	
Metoprolol *see* Beta-blockers	
Milrinone	
Mild	Reduce dose and monitor response
Minocycline *see* Tetracyclines	
Mivacurium	
Severe	Reduce dose; prolonged paralysis
Morphine	
Moderate	Avoid; increased and prolonged effect; *see also* Opioid Analgesics
Nabumetone *see* NSAIDs	
Nadolol *see* Beta-blockers	
Nalbuphine *see* Opioid Analgesics	
Nalidixic Acid	
Moderate	Avoid; increased risk of nausea, vomiting, rashes, photosensitivity; ineffective because of inadequate urine concentration
Naproxen *see* NSAIDs	
Narcotic Analgesics *see* Opioid Analgesics	
Neomycin	
Mild	Avoid; ototoxic; nephrotoxic
Neostigmine	
Moderate	May need dose reduction
Netilmicin *see* Aminoglycosides	
Nicardipine	
Moderate	Start with small dose
Nifedipine	
Moderate	Start with small dose; reversible deterioration in renal function has been reported
Nitrazepam *see* Anxiolytics and Hypnotics	
Nitrofurantoin	
Mild	Avoid; peripheral neuropathy; ineffective because of inadequate urine concentrations
Nitroprusside	
Moderate	Avoid prolonged use
Nizatidine	
Mild	Use half dose
Moderate	Use one-quarter dose

Table of drugs to be avoided or used with caution in renal impairment (*continued*)

Drug and Degree of impairment	Comment	Drug and Degree of impairment	Comment
Norfloxacin		**Pirenzepine**	
Moderate	Use half dose	Moderate	Reduce dose
Severe	Avoid	**Piroxicam** *see* NSAIDs	
NSAIDs		**Pivampicillin**	
Mild	Avoid if possible; deterioration in renal function (**important**: see p. 379); sodium and water retention; deterioration also reported after topical use	Severe	Reduce dose; rashes more common
		Plicamycin	
		Moderate	Avoid if possible
		Polythiazide *see* Thiazides	
		Potassium Salts	
Ofloxacin		Moderate	Avoid routine use; high risk of hyperkalaemia
Mild	Usual initial dose, then use half dose	**Potassium-sparing Diuretics**	
Moderate	Usual initial dose, then 100 mg every 24 hours	Mild	Monitor plasma K⁺; high risk of hyperkalaemia in renal impairment; amiloride excreted by kidney unchanged
Olsalazine			
Mild	Manufacturer advises avoid if significant renal impairment		
		Moderate	Avoid
Opioid Analgesics		**Povidone-iodine**	
Moderate	Use small doses—avoid codeine, dihydrocodeine, morphine; increased cerebral sensitivity; *see also* individual entries	Severe	Avoid regular application to inflamed or broken mucosa
		Prazosin	
		Severe	Start with small dose; increased sensitivity to hypotensive effect and possible CNS toxicity
Severe	Avoid dextropropoxyphene, pethidine, tramadol		
Oxazepam *see* Anxiolytics and Hypnotics		**Primaxin®**	
Oxprenolol *see* Beta-blockers		Mild	Reduce dose
Oxypertine *see* Antipsychotics		**Primidone**	
Oxytetracycline *see* Tetracyclines		Severe	Avoid large doses
Pamidronate Disodium		**Probenecid**	
Severe	Divide daily dose	Moderate	Avoid; ineffective and toxicity increased
Pancuronium *see* Tubocurarine			
Papaveretum *see* Opioid Analgesics		**Procainamide**	
Paroxetine		Mild	Avoid or reduce dose
Moderate	Start with smaller dose	**Procarbazine**	
Penbutolol *see* Beta-blockers		Moderate	Reduce dose
Penicillamine		**Prochlorperazine** *see* Antipsychotics	
Mild	Avoid if possible or reduce dose; nephrotoxic	**Proguanil**	
		Severe	Avoid or reduce dose; increased risk of haematological toxicity
Pentamidine			
Mild	Reduce dose; consult data sheet		
Pentazocine *see* Opioid Analgesics		**Promazine** *see* Antipsychotics	
Pericyazine *see* Antipsychotics		**Propranolol** *see* Beta-blockers	
Perindopril		**Propylthiouracil**	
Mild	Reduce dose frequency and monitor response; *see also* Captopril	Mild	Reduce dose
		Pseudoephedrine	
		Severe	Avoid; increased CNS toxicity
Perphenazine *see* Antipsychotics			
Pethidine		**Pyridostigmine**	
Severe	Avoid; increased CNS toxicity; *see also* Opioid Analgesics	Moderate	Reduce dose; excreted by kidney
		Quinapril	
Phenazocine *see* Opioid Analgesics		Mild	Start with 2.5 mg daily; *see also* Captopril
Phenobarbitone			
Severe	Avoid large doses	**Ramipril**	
Phenoperidine *see* Opioid Analgesics		Mild	Start with 1.25 mg daily; *see also* Captopril
Phenothiazines *see* Antipsychotics			
Phenylbutazone *see* NSAIDs		**Ranitidine**	
Pholcodine *see* Opioid Analgesics		Severe	Use half normal dose; occasional risk of confusion
Pimozide *see* Antipsychotics			
Pindolol *see* Beta-blockers		**Regulan®**	
Piperacillin		Severe	Avoid; contains 6.4 mmol potassium per sachet
Moderate	Reduce dose		
Piperazine		**Remoxipride** *see* Antipsychotics	
Severe	Reduce dose; neurotoxic	**Rifabutin**	
Pipothiazine *see* Antipsychotics		Moderate	Reduce dose
Piracetam		**Risperidone** *see* Antipsychotics	
Mild	Use half dose	**Rocuronium**	
Moderate	Use one-quarter dose	Moderate	Reduce dose; prolonged paralysis
Severe	Avoid	**Salcatonin** *see* Calcitonin	

Table of drugs to be avoided or used with caution in renal impairment (*continued*)

Drug and Degree of impairment	Comment	Drug and Degree of impairment	Comment
Salicylates *see* Aspirin		Thiazides and Related Diuretics	
Salsalate *see* Aspirin		Moderate	Avoid; ineffective
Salt Substitutes			(metolazone remains
Moderate	Avoid routine use; high risk of hyperkalaemia (*see* section 9.2.1.1)		effective but risk of excessive diuresis)
Sertraline	Manufacturer recommends avoid	Thioguanine	
		Moderate	Reduce dose
Simvastatin		Thioridazine *see* Antipsychotics	
Moderate to severe	Reduce dose	Tiaprofenic Acid *see* NSAIDs	
Sodium Aurothiomalate *see* Gold		Ticarcillin	
Sodium Bicarbonate		Moderate	Reduce dose; 1 g contains 5.3 mmol sodium
Severe	Avoid; specialised role in some forms of renal disease	*Timentin*®	
Sodium Cellulose Phosphate		Moderate	Reduce dose
Mild to moderate	Reduce dose	Timolol *see* Beta-blockers	
Severe	Avoid	Tobramycin *see* Aminoglycosides	
Sodium Clodronate *see* Clodronate Sodium		Tocainide	
Sodium Nitroprusside *see* Nitroprusside		Mild	Reduce dose
Sodium Salts		Tolazamide	
Severe	Avoid	Severe	May need dose reduction; increased risk of hypoglycaemia
Solpadeine®			
Severe	Avoid; contains 18.5 mmol sodium per tablet		
Solpadol®		Tolbutamide	
Severe	Avoid; contains 18.6 mmol sodium per tablet	Severe	May need dose reduction; increased risk of hypoglycaemia
Sotalol *see* Beta-blockers		Tolmetin *see* NSAIDs (excreted by kidney)	
Spironolactone *see* Potassium-sparing Diuretics		Torasemide	
Streptomycin *see* Aminoglycosides		Moderate	May need high doses
Sucralfate		Tramadol *see* Opioid Analgesics	
Severe	Avoid; aluminium is absorbed and may accumulate	Trandolapril	
		Mild	Start with 500 micrograms daily and monitor response; *see also* Captopril
Sulfametopyrazine *see* Sulphonamides			
Sulindac *see* NSAIDs (excreted by kidney)		Triamterene *see* Potassium-sparing Diuretics	
Sulphadiazine		Triclofos *see* Anxiolytics and Hypnotics	
Severe	Avoid; high risk of crystalluria	Trifluoperazine *see* Antipsychotics	
		Trifluperidol *see* Antipsychotics	
Sulphadimidine *see* Sulphonamides		Trimeprazine	
Sulphasalazine		Severe	Avoid
Severe	Ensure high fluid intake; rashes and blood disorders; crystalluria a risk	Trimethoprim	
		Moderate	Reduce dose
Sulphinpyrazone		Tripotassium Dicitratobismuthate *see* Bismuth Chelate	
Moderate	Avoid; ineffective as uricosuric	Tubocurarine	
Sulphonamides		Moderate	Reduce dose; prolonged paralysis with large or repeated doses
Moderate	Ensure high fluid intake; rashes and blood disorders; crystalluria a risk		
		Tulobuterol	
Sulphonylureas *see under* individual drugs		Mild	May need dose reduction; excreted by kidney
Sulpiride		Moderate to severe	Avoid
Moderate	Avoid if possible, or reduce dose	Vancomycin	
		Mild	Avoid parenteral use if possible; ototoxic; nephrotoxic
Teicoplanin			
Mild	Reduce dose after 4 days; consult data sheet	Vecuronium *see* Tubocurarine	
		Vigabatrin	
Temazepam *see* Anxiolytics and Hypnotics		Mild	Reduce dose; excreted by kidney
Temocillin			
Moderate	Reduce dose	Xamoterol	
Tenoxicam *see* NSAIDs		Moderate	Reduce dose; excreted by kidney
Terbinafine			
Mild	Use half normal dose	Xipamide *see* Thiazides	
Tetracyclines (except doxycycline and minocycline)		Zidovudine	
Mild	Avoid—use doxycycline or minocycline if necessary; anti-anabolic effect, increased plasma urea, further deterioration in renal function	Mild	Excreted by kidney; increased risk of toxicity
		Zuclopenthixol *see* Antipsychotics	

Appendix 4: Pregnancy

Drugs can have harmful effects on the fetus at any time during pregnancy. Experience with many drugs in pregnancy is limited.

During the *first trimester* they may produce congenital malformations (teratogenesis), and the period of greatest risk is from the third to the eleventh week of pregnancy.

During the *second* and *third trimesters* drugs may affect the growth and functional development of the fetus or have toxic effects on fetal tissues; and drugs given shortly before term or during labour may have adverse effects on labour or on the neonate after delivery.

The following table lists drugs which may have harmful effects in pregnancy and indicates the trimester of risk.

The table is based on human data but information on *animal* studies has been included for some newer drugs when its omission might be misleading.

Drugs should be prescribed in pregnancy only if the expected benefit to the mother is thought to be greater than the risk to the fetus, and all drugs should be avoided if possible during the first trimester. Drugs which have been extensively used in pregnancy and appear to be usually safe should be prescribed in preference to new or untried drugs; and the smallest effective dose should be used.

Few drugs have been shown conclusively to be teratogenic in man but no drug is safe beyond all doubt in early pregnancy. Screening procedures are available where there is a known risk of certain defects.

It should be noted that the BNF provides independent advice and may not always agree with the data sheets.

Absence of a drug from the list does not imply safety.

Table of drugs to be avoided or used with caution in pregnancy

Products introduced or amended since publication of BNF No. 27 (March 1994) are underlined.

Drug (Trimester of risk)	Comment
Acarbose	Manufacturer advises avoid
ACE Inhibitors (1, 2, 3)	Avoid; may adversely affect fetal and neonatal blood pressure control and renal function; also possible skull defects and oligohydramnios; toxicity in *animal* studies
Acebutolol *see* Beta-blockers	
Acemetacin *see* NSAIDs	
Acetazolamide *see* Diuretics	
Acetohexamide *see* Sulphonylureas	
Acitretin (1,2,3)	Teratogenic; effective contraception must be used for at least 1 month before treatment, during treatment, and for at least 2 years after stopping
Acrivastine *see* Antihistamines	
Acyclovir	Experience limited—manufacturer advises use only when potential benefits outweigh possibility of unknown risks
Albendazole	Manufacturer advises teratogenic in *animal* studies
Alclometasone *see* Corticosteroids	
Alcohol	
(1, 2)	Regular daily drinking is teratogenic (`fetal alcohol syndrome') and may cause growth retardation; occasional single drinks are probably safe
(3)	Withdrawal syndrome may occur in babies of alcoholic mothers
Alfentanil *see* Opioid Analgesics	
Allyloestrenol *see* Progestogens	
Alprazolam *see* Anxiolytics and Hypnotics	

Drug (Trimester of risk)	Comment
Alteplase *see* Streptokinase	
Amantadine	Toxicity in *animal* studies
Amikacin *see* Aminoglycosides	
Amiloride *see* Diuretics	
Aminoglutethimide	Avoid; toxicity in *animal* studies and may affect fetal sexual development
Aminoglycosides (2, 3)	Auditory or vestibular nerve damage; risk greatest with streptomycin; probably very small with gentamicin and tobramycin, but avoid unless essential
Aminophylline *see* Theophylline	
Amiodarone (2, 3)	Possible risk of neonatal goitre; use only if no alternative
Amitriptyline *see* Antidepressants, Tricyclic	
Amlodipine *see* Calcium-channel Blockers	
Amoxapine *see* Antidepressants, Tricyclic	
Amphotericin	Not known to be harmful but manufacturer advises avoid unless expected benefit outweighs potential risk
Amylobarbitone *see* Barbiturates	
Anabolic Steroids (1, 2, 3)	Masculinisation of female fetus
Anaesthetics, General (3)	Depress neonatal respiration
Anaesthetics, Local (3)	With large doses, neonatal respiratory depression, hypotonia, and bradycardia after paracervical or epidural block; neonatal methaemoglobinaemia with prilocaine and procaine
Analgesics *see* Opioid Analgesics and NSAIDs	
Androgens (1, 2, 3)	Masculinisation of female fetus
Anistreplase *see* Streptokinase	

Table of drugs to be avoided or used with caution in pregnancy (*continued*)

Drug (Trimester of risk)	Comment	Drug (Trimester of risk)	Comment
Anticoagulants		Aurothiomalate *see* Gold	
Heparin (1, 2, 3)	Osteoporosis has been reported after prolonged use	Azapropazone *see* NSAIDs	
Oral Anticoagulants (1, 2, 3)	Congenital malformations; fetal and neonatal haemorrhage *See also* section 2.8	Azatadine *see* Antihistamines	
		Azathioprine *see* p.336	
		Azelastine *see* Antihistamines	
Antidepressants		Aztreonam	Manufacturer advises avoid (but no evidence of teratogenicity)
MAOIs (including moclobemide), Serotonin-uptake Inhibitor (1, 2, 3)	No evidence of harm but manufacturers advise avoid unless compelling reasons	Baclofen	Manufacturer advises toxicity in *animal* studies
		Bambuterol *see* section 3.1.1 [text]	
		Barbiturates (3)	Withdrawal effects in neonate; *see also* Phenobarbitone
Tricyclic (and related) (3)	Tachycardia, irritability, and muscle spasms in neonate reported with imipramine	Beclomethasone *see* Corticosteroids	
		Bendrofluazide *see* Diuretics	
Antiepileptics	Benefit of treatment outweighs risk to fetus; risk of teratogenicity greater if more than one drug used; **important**: *see also* carbamazepine, ethosuximide, phenobarbitone, phenytoin, valproate, and p.193	Benorylate [aspirin-paracetamol ester] *see* Aspirin	
		Benperidol *see* Antipsychotics	
		Benserazide [ingredient] *see Madopar*®	
		Benzodiazepines *see* Anxiolytics and Hypnotics	
		Beta-blockers (3)	May cause intra-uterine growth retardation, neonatal hypoglycaemia, and bradycardia; risk greater in severe hypertension
Antihistamines	No evidence of teratogenicity; some packs of antihistamines sold to the public carry warning to avoid in pregnancy; manufacturer of astemizole advises avoid (see p.129)		
		Betamethasone *see* Corticosteroids	
		Betaxolol *see* Beta-blockers	
		Bethanidine *see* Guanethidine	
		Bezafibrate *see* Clofibrate	
Antimalarials (1, 3)	Benefit of prophylaxis and treatment in malaria outweighs risk; **important**: *see also* individual drugs and p.256	Bismuth Chelate	Manufacturer advises avoid on theoretical grounds
		Bisoprolol *see* Beta-blockers	
		Bisphosphonates	Manufacturers advise avoid
Antipsychotics (3)	Extrapyramidal effects in neonate occasionally reported	Bromazepam *see* Anxiolytics and Hypnotics	
		Brompheniramine *see* Antihistamines	
		Budesonide *see* Corticosteroids	
Anxiolytics and Hypnotics (3)	Depress neonatal respiration. Benzodiazepines cause neonatal drowsiness, hypotonia, and withdrawal symptoms; avoid large doses and regular use; short-acting benzodiazepines preferable to long-acting	Bumetanide *see* Diuretics	
		Bupivacaine *see* Anaesthetics, Local	
		Buprenorphine *see* Opioid Analgesics	
		Buserelin	Avoid
		Cabergoline	Once regular ovulatory cycles have been achieved manufacturer advises discontinuation for one month before intended conception (but no evidence of teratogenicity)
Aspirin (3)	Impaired platelet function and risk of haemorrhage; delayed onset and increased duration of labour with increased blood loss; avoid analgesic doses if possible in last few weeks (low doses probably not harmful); with high doses, closure of fetal ductus arteriosus *in utero* and possibly persistent pulmonary hypertension of newborn; kernicterus in jaundiced neonates		
		Calcipotriol	Manufacturer advises avoid if possible
		Calcitonin	Information not available
		Calcium-channel Blockers	May inhibit labour and manufacturers advise that diltiazem and some dihydropyridines are teratogenic in *animals*
Astemizole *see* Antihistamines			
Atenolol *see* Beta-blockers		Capreomycin	Manufacturer advises teratogenic in *animal* studies
Auranofin *see* Gold		Captopril *see* ACE Inhibitors	

Table of drugs to be avoided or used with caution in pregnancy (*continued*)

Drug (Trimester of risk)	Comment	Drug (Trimester of risk)	Comment
Carbamazepine (1)	Risk of teratogenesis including increased risk of neural tube defects (counselling and screening and adequate folate supplements advised); *see also* Antiepileptics and **CSM advice**, p.193	Clomiphene	Possible effects on fetal development
		Clomipramine *see* Antidepressants, Tricyclic	
		Clomocycline *see* Tetracyclines	
		Clonazepam *see* Antiepileptics	
		Clorazepate *see* Anxiolytics and Hypnotics	
		Clozapine	Manufacturer advises avoid
(3)	Because of neonatal bleeding tendency associated with some antiepileptics, manufacturer advises prophylactic vitamin K₁ for mother before delivery (as well as for neonate)	Codeine *see* Opioid Analgesics	
		Colistin (2, 3)	Avoid—possible risk of fetal toxicity
		Contraceptives, Oral	Epidemiological evidence suggests no harmful effects on fetus
Carbenoxolone (3)	Avoid; causes sodium retention with oedema	Corticosteroids (2, 3)	Benefit of treatment, e.g. in asthma, outweighs risk; high doses (>10 mg prednisolone daily) may produce fetal and neonatal adrenal suppression; corticosteroid cover required by mother during labour
Carbimazole (2, 3)	Neonatal goitre and hypothyroidism; has been associated with aplasia cutis of the neonate		
Celiprolol *see* Beta-blockers			
Cephalosporins	Not known to be harmful	Co-trimoxazole	
Cetirizine *see* Antihistamines		(1)	Theoretical teratogenic risk (trimethoprim a folate antagonist)
Chenodeoxycholic Acid (1, 2, 3)	Theoretical risk of effects on fetal metabolism	(3)	Neonatal haemolysis and methaemoglobinaemia; fear of increased risk of kernicterus in neonates appears to be unfounded
Chloral hydrate *see* Anxiolytics and Hypnotics			
Chloramphenicol (3)	Neonatal 'grey syndrome'	Cromoglycate	Not known to be harmful; *see also* section 3.1.1 [text]
Chlordiazepoxide *see* Anxiolytics and Hypnotics		Cyclizine *see* Antihistamines	
Chlormethiazole *see* Anxiolytics and Hypnotics		Cyclopenthiazide *see* Diuretics	
Chlormezanone *see* Anxiolytics and Hypnotics		Cyclosporin *see* p.327	
Chloroquine *see* Antimalarials		Cyproheptadine *see* Antihistamines	
Chlorothiazide *see* Diuretics		Cyproterone [ingredient] *see* *Dianette*®	
Chlorpheniramine *see* Antihistamines		Cytotoxic Drugs (1)	Most are teratogenic; *see* section 8.1
Chlorpromazine *see* Antipsychotics			
Chlorpropamide *see* Sulphonylureas		Dalteparin *see* Anticoagulants (Heparin)	
Chlorprothixene *see* Antipsychotics		Danaparoid	Insufficient information available
Chlortetracycline *see* Tetracyclines			
Chlorthalidone *see* Diuretics		Danazol (1, 2, 3)	Has weak androgenic effects and virilisation of female fetus reported
Cilazapril *see* ACE Inhibitors			
Cinnarizine *see* Antihistamines		Dapsone (3)	Neonatal haemolysis and methaemoglobinaemia; adequate folate supplements should be given to mother
Ciprofibrate *see* Clofibrate			
Ciprofloxacin *see* 4-Quinolones			
Cisapride	Manufacturer advises avoid	Debrisoquine *see* Guanethidine	
Clarithromycin	Not known to be harmful but manufacturer advises avoid unless expected benefit outweighs potential risk	Demeclocycline *see* Tetracyclines	
		Desferrioxamine	Manufacturer advises toxicity in *animal* studies
Clemastine *see* Antihistamines		Desflurane *see* Anaesthetics, General	
Clindamycin	Not known to be harmful	Desipramine *see* Antidepressants, Tricyclic	
Clobazam *see* Anxiolytics and Hypnotics		Desogestrel *see* Contraceptives, Oral	
Clobetasol *see* Corticosteroids		Desonide *see* Corticosteroids	
Clobetasone *see* Corticosteroids		Desoxymethasone *see* Corticosteroids	
Clodronate sodium *see* Bisphosphonates		Dexamethasone *see* Corticosteroids	
Clofibrate (1, 2, 3)	Avoid—theoretical possibility of interference with embryonic growth and development due to anticholesterol effect	Dexfenfluramine (1,2,3)	No evidence of teratogenicity but not recommended

Table of drugs to be avoided or used with caution in pregnancy *(continued)*

Drug (Trimester of risk)	Comment
Dextromethorphan *see* Opioid Analgesics	
Dextromoramide *see* Opioid Analgesics	
Dextropropoxyphene *see* Opioid Analgesics	
Diamorphine *see* Opioid Analgesics	
Dianette® (1, 2, 3)	Feminisation of male fetus (due to cyproterone)
Diazepam *see* Anxiolytics and Hypnotics	
Diazoxide (2, 3)	Prolonged use may produce alopecia and impaired glucose tolerance in neonate; inhibits uterine activity during labour
Diclofenac *see* NSAIDs	
Diethylpropion	Avoid—congenital malformations reported to CSM
Diflucortolone *see* Corticosteroids	
Diflunisal *see* NSAIDs	
Digoxin	May need dosage adjustment
Dihydrocodeine *see* Opioid Analgesics	
Dihydroergotamine *see* Ergotamine	
Diltiazem *see* Calcium-channel Blockers	
Dimenhydrinate *see* Antihistamines	
Diphenhydramine *see* Antihistamines	
Diphenoxylate *see* Opioid Analgesics	
Diphenylpyraline *see* Antihistamines	
Dipipanone *see* Opioid Analgesics	
Disodium Etidronate *see* Bisphosphonates	
Disodium Pamidronate *see* Bisphosphonates	
Disopyramide (3)	May induce labour
Distigmine	Manufacturer advises avoid (may stimulate uterine contractions)
Disulfiram (1)	High concentrations of acetaldehyde which occur in presence of alcohol may be teratogenic
Diuretics	Not used to treat hypertension in pregnancy
(1)	Manufacturers advise avoid acetazolamide and torasemide (toxicity in *animal* studies)
(3)	Thiazides may cause neonatal thrombocytopenia
Domperidone	Manufacturer advises avoid
Dothiepin *see* Antidepressants, Tricyclic	
Doxepin *see* Antidepressants, Tricyclic	
Doxycycline *see* Tetracyclines	
Droperidol *see* Antipsychotics	
Dydrogesterone *see* Progestogens	
Enalapril *see* ACE Inhibitors	
Enflurane *see* Anaesthetics, General	
Enoxaparin *see* Anticoagulants (Heparin)	
Ephedrine	Not known to be harmful
Ergotamine (1, 2, 3)	Oxytocic effects on the pregnant uterus
Erythromycin	Not known to be harmful

Drug (Trimester of risk)	Comment
Esmolol *see* Beta-blockers	
Ethacrynic acid *see* Diuretics	
Ether *see* Anaesthetics, General	
Ethinyloestradiol *see* Contraceptives, Oral	
Ethionamide (1)	May be teratogenic
Ethosuximide (1)	May possibly be teratogenic; *see* Antiepileptics
Ethynodiol *see* Contraceptives, Oral	
Etidronate Disodium *see* Bisphosphonates	
Etodolac *see* NSAIDs	
Etomidate *see* Anaesthetics, General	
Etretinate (1, 2, 3)	Teratogenic; effective contraception must be used for at least 1 month before treatment, during treatment, and for at least two years after stopping
Famciclovir *see* Acyclovir	
Fansidar®	
(1)	Possible teratogenic risk (pyrimethamine a folate antagonist)
(3)	Neonatal haemolysis and methaemoglobinaemia; fear of increased risk of kernicterus in neonates appears to be unfounded *see also* Antimalarials
Felodipine *see* Calcium-channel Blockers	
Fenbufen *see* NSAIDs	
Fenofibrate (1, 2, 3)	Manufacturer advises toxicity in *animal* studies; *see also* Clofibrate
Fenoprofen *see* NSAIDs	
Fenoterol *see* section 3.1.1 [text]	
Fentanyl *see* Opioid Analgesics	
Finasteride (1, 2, 3)	Avoid unprotected intercourse (see section 6.4.2). May cause feminisation of male fetus
Flecainide	Manufacturer advises toxicity in *animal* studies
Fluclorolone *see* Corticosteroids	
Fluconazole	Manufacturer advises toxicity at high doses in *animal* studies
Flucytosine (1)	Possible teratogenic risk
Flunitrazepam *see* Anxiolytics and Hypnotics	
Fluocinolone *see* Corticosteroids	
Fluocinonide *see* Corticosteroids	
Fluocortolone *see* Corticosteroids	
Fluoxetine *see* Antidepressants, Serotonin-uptake Inhibitor	
Flupenthixol *see* Antipsychotics	
Fluphenazine *see* Antipsychotics	
Flurandrenolone *see* Corticosteroids	
Flurazepam *see* Anxiolytics and Hypnotics	
Flurbiprofen *see* NSAIDs	
Fluspirilene *see* Antipsychotics	

Table of drugs to be avoided or used with caution in pregnancy (*continued*)

Drug (Trimester of risk)	Comment
Fluticasone *see* Corticosteroids	
Fluvastatin *see* Clofibrate	
Fluvoxamine *see* Antidepressants, Serotonin-uptake Inhibitor	
Foscarnet	Manufacturer advises avoid
Fosfomycin	Not known to be harmful, but manufacturer advises avoid unless expected benefit outweighs potential risk
Fosinopril *see* ACE Inhibitors	
Framycetin *see* Aminoglycosides	
Frusemide *see* Diuretics	
Gabapentin *see* Antiepileptics	
Ganciclovir	Avoid—teratogenic risk
Gemfibrozil *see* Clofibrate	
Gentamicin *see* Aminoglycosides	
Gestodene *see* Contraceptives, Oral	
Gestrinone (1, 2, 3)	Avoid
Glibenclamide *see* Sulphonylureas	
Gliclazide *see* Sulphonylureas	
Glipizide *see* Sulphonylureas	
Gliquidone *see* Sulphonylureas	
Gold	
Auranofin	Manufacturer advises teratogenicity in *animal* studies; effective contraception should be used during and for at least 6 months after treatment
Aurothiomalate (1, 2, 3)	No good evidence of harm but avoid if possible
Granisetron	Information not available
Griseofulvin	Avoid (fetotoxicity and teratogenicity in *animals*)
Growth Hormone	Avoid on theoretical grounds
Guanethidine (3)	Postural hypotension and reduced uteroplacental perfusion; should not be used to treat hypertension in pregnancy
Halcinonide *see* Corticosteroids	
Halofantrine (1)	Manufacturer advises toxicity in *animal* studies
Haloperidol *see* Antipsychotics	
Halothane *see* Anaesthetics, General	
Heparin *see* Anticoagulants	
Hydralazine (1)	Manufacturer advises toxicity in *animal* studies
Hydrochlorothiazide *see* Diuretics	
Hydrocortisone *see* Corticosteroids	
Hydroflumethiazide *see* Diuretics	
Hydroxychloroquine	Avoid for rheumatic disease (but for malaria *see* Antimalarials)
Hydroxyprogesterone *see* Progestogens	
Hydroxyzine *see* Antihistamines	
Hypnotics *see* Anxiolytics and Hypnotics	
Ibuprofen *see* NSAIDs	

Drug (Trimester of risk)	Comment
Idoxuridine	Manufacturers advise toxicity in *animal* studies
Imipramine *see* Antidepressants, Tricyclic	
Immunosuppressants *see* section 8.1	
Indapamide *see* Diuretics	
Indomethacin *see* NSAIDs	
Insulin (1,2,3)	Insulin requirements should be assessed frequently by an experienced diabetic physician
Interferons	Manufacturers recommend avoid unless compelling reasons
Iodine and Iodides (2, 3)	Neonatal goitre and hypothyroidism
Radioactive iodine (1, 2, 3)	Permanent hypothyroidism—avoid
Iprindole *see* Antidepressants, Tricyclic (and related)	
Isocarboxazid *see* Antidepressants, MAOI	
Isoflurane *see* Anaesthetics, General	
Isotretinoin (1, 2, 3)	Teratogenic; effective contraception must be used for at least 1 month before oral treatment, during treatment and for at least 1 month after stopping; also avoid topical treatment
Isradipine *see* Calcium-channel Blockers	
Itraconazole	Manufacturer advises toxicity at high doses in *animal* studies
Kanamycin *see* Aminoglycosides	
Ketamine *see* Anaesthetics, General	
Ketoconazole	Manufacturer advises teratogenicity in *animal* studies; packs carry a warning to avoid in pregnancy
Ketoprofen *see* NSAIDs	
Ketorolac *see* NSAIDs and p.493	
Ketotifen *see* Antihistamines	
Labetalol *see* Beta-blockers	
Lacidipine *see* Calcium-channel Blockers	
Lamotrigine *see* Antiepileptics	
Lansoprazole	Manufacturer advises avoid
Lenograstim	Manufacturer advises insufficient information
Levodopa	Manufacturers advise toxicity in *animal* studies
Levonorgestrel *see* Contraceptives, Oral	
Lignocaine *see* Anaesthetics, Local	
Lindane	Manufacturer advises toxicity in *animal* studies
Lisinopril *see* ACE Inhibitors	
Lithium (1, 2, 3)	Dose requirements increased; congenital malformations; neonatal goitre reported; lithium toxicity (hypotonia and cyanosis) in neonate if maternal therapy poorly controlled

Table of drugs to be avoided or used with caution in pregnancy (*continued*)

Drug (Trimester of risk)	Comment
Lofepramine *see* Antidepressants, Tricyclic	
Loprazolam *see* Anxiolytics and Hypnotics	
Loratadine *see* Antihistamines	
Lorazepam *see* Anxiolytics and Hypnotics	
Lormetazepam *see* Anxiolytics and Hypnotics	
Lymecycline *see* Tetracyclines	
Madopar® *see* Levodopa	
Maloprim®	
(1)	Possible teratogenic risk (pyrimethamine a folate antagonist)
(3)	Neonatal haemolysis and methaemoglobinaemia (due to dapsone); adequate folate supplements should be given to mother; *see also* Antimalarials
Maprotiline *see* Antidepressants, Tricyclic (and related)	
Mebendazole	Manufacturer advises toxicity in *animal* studies
Mefenamic Acid *see* NSAIDs	
Mefloquine (1)	Manufacturer advises teratogenicity in *animal* studies; avoid for prophylaxis, *see* p. 260
Mefruside *see* Diuretics	
Melphalan *see* Cytotoxic Drugs	
Menadiol (3)	Neonatal haemolytic anaemia, hyperbilirubinaemia and increased risk of kernicterus in jaundiced infants
Meprobamate *see* Anxiolytics and Hypnotics	
Meptazinol *see* Opioid Analgesics	
Mesalazine	Negligible quantities cross placenta
Mesterolone *see* Androgens	
Mestranol *see* Contraceptives, Oral	
Metaraminol (1, 2, 3)	Avoid—may reduce placental perfusion
Metformin (1, 2, 3)	Avoid
Methadone *see* Opioid Analgesics	
Methohexitone *see* Anaesthetics, General	
Methotrexate *see* Cytotoxic Drugs	
Methotrimeprazine *see* Antipsychotics	
Methyclothiazide *see* Diuretics	
Methylphenobarbitone *see* Antiepileptics	
Methylprednisolone *see* Corticosteroids	
Metolazone *see* Diuretics	
Metoprolol *see* Beta-blockers	
Metronidazole	Manufacturer advises avoidance of high-dose regimens
Metyrapone	Avoid (may impair biosynthesis of fetal-placental steroids)
Mianserin *see* Antidepressants, Tricyclic (and related)	

Drug (Trimester of risk)	Comment
Mifepristone	Manufacturer advises that if treatment fails, essential that pregnancy be terminated by another method
Minocycline *see* Tetracyclines	
Minoxidil (3)	Neonatal hirsutism reported
Misoprostol (1, 2, 3)	Avoid; increases uterine tone
Mitomycin *see* Cytotoxic Drugs	
Moclobemide *see* Antidepressants, MAOI	
Molgramostim	Manufacturer advises toxicity in *animal* studies
Moracizine	Information not available
Morphine *see* Opioid Analgesics	
Nabumetone *see* NSAIDs	
Nadolol *see* Beta-blockers	
Nafarelin	Avoid
Nalbuphine *see* Opioid Analgesics	
Nalidixic acid *see* 4-Quinolones	
Naloxone	Manufacturer advises use only if expected benefit outweighs potential risk
Nandrolone *see* Anabolic Steroids	
Naproxen *see* NSAIDs	
Narcotic Analgesics *see* Opioid Analgesics	
Nedocromil *see* section 3.1.1 [text]	
Neomycin *see* Aminoglycosides	
Neostigmine (3)	Neonatal myasthenia with large doses
Netilmicin *see* Aminoglycosides	
Nicardipine *see* Calcium-channel Blockers	
Nicotine (1,2,3)	Avoid
Nicoumalone *see* Anticoagulants, Oral	
Nifedipine *see* Calcium-channel Blockers	
Nimodipine *see* Calcium-channel Blockers	
Nitrazepam *see* Anxiolytics and Hypnotics	
Nitrofurantoin (3)	May produce neonatal haemolysis if used at term
Nitrous oxide *see* Anaesthetics, General	
Nizatidine	Manufacturer advises toxicity at high doses in *animal* studies
Noradrenaline (1, 2, 3)	Avoid—may reduce placental perfusion
Norethisterone *see* Contraceptives, Oral	
Norfloxacin *see* 4-Quinolones	
Norgestimate *see* Contraceptives, Oral	
Nortriptyline *see* Antidepressants, Tricyclic	
NSAIDs	
(1)	Some manufacturers advise toxicity in *animal* studies
(3)	With regular use closure of fetal ductus arteriosus *in utero* and possibly persistent pulmonary hypertension of the newborn. Delayed onset and increased duration of labour

Table of drugs to be avoided or used with caution in pregnancy (*continued*)

Drug (Trimester of risk)	Comment
Octreotide (1, 2, 3)	Avoid; possible effect on fetal growth
Oestrogens *see* Contraceptives, Oral	
Ofloxacin *see* 4-Quinolones	
Omeprazole	Manufacturer advises toxicity in *animal* studies
Opioid Analgesics (3)	Depress neonatal respiration; withdrawal effects in neonates of dependent mothers; gastric stasis and risk of inhalation pneumonia in mother during labour
Orphenadrine	Information not available
Oxatomide *see* Antihistamines	
Oxazepam *see* Anxiolytics and Hypnotics	
Oxprenolol *see* Beta-blockers	
Oxybutynin	Manufacturer advises toxicity at high doses in *animal* studies
Oxymetholone *see* Anabolic Steroids	
Oxypertine *see* Antipsychotics	
Oxytetracycline *see* Tetracyclines	
Paclitaxel *see* Cytotoxic Drugs	
Pamidronate Disodium *see* Bisphosphonates	
Pancreatin	Not known to be harmful
Papaveretum *see* Opioid Analgesics	
Paroxetine *see* Antidepressants, Serotonin-uptake Inhibitor	
Penbutolol *see* Beta-blockers	
Penicillamine (1, 2, 3)	Fetal abnormalities reported rarely; avoid if possible
Penicillins	Not known to be harmful
Pentazocine *see* Opioid Analgesics	
Pericyazine *see* Antipsychotics	
Perindopril *see* ACE Inhibitors	
Perphenazine *see* Antipsychotics	
Pethidine *see* Opioid Analgesics	
Phenelzine *see* Antidepressants, MAOI	
Phenindamine *see* Antihistamines	
Phenindione *see* Anticoagulants, Oral	
Pheniramine *see* Antihistamines	
Phenobarbitone (1, 3)	Congenital malformations. Neonatal bleeding tendency—prophylactic vitamin K_1 for mother before delivery (as well as for neonate); *see also* Antiepileptics
Phenoperidine *see* Opioid Analgesics	
Phenothiazines *see* Antipsychotics	
Phentolamine	Information not available

Drug (Trimester of risk)	Comment
Phenytoin (1, 3)	Congenital malformations (screening advised); adequate folate supplements should be given to mother. Neonatal bleeding tendency—prophylactic vitamin K_1 for mother before delivery (as well as for neonate). Caution in interpreting plasma concentrations—bound may be reduced but free (i.e. effective) unchanged; *see also* Antiepileptics
Pholcodine *see* Opioid Analgesics	
Pimozide *see* Antipsychotics	
Pindolol *see* Beta-blockers	
Piperazine	No clinical evidence of harm but packs sold to the general public carry a warning to avoid in pregnancy except on medical advice
Pipothiazine *see* Antipsychotics	
Piracetam	Manufacturer advises avoid
Pirbuterol *see* section 3.1.1 [text]	
Piroxicam *see* NSAIDs	
Podophyllum resin (1, 2, 3)	Avoid—neonatal death and teratogenesis have been reported
Polythiazide *see* Diuretics	
Povidone-iodine (2, 3)	Sufficient iodine may be absorbed to affect the fetal thyroid
Pravastatin *see* Clofibrate	
Prednisolone *see* Corticosteroids	
Prednisone *see* Corticosteroids	
Prilocaine (3)	Neonatal methaemoglobinaemia; *see also* Anaesthetics, Local
Primaquine (3)	Neonatal haemolysis and methaemoglobinaemia; *see also* Antimalarials
Primidone *see* Phenobarbitone	
Probucol *see* Clofibrate	
Procaine (3)	Neonatal methaemoglobinaemia; *see also* Anaesthetics, Local
Prochlorperazine *see* Antipsychotics	
Progestogens (1)	High doses may possibly be teratogenic
Proguanil	Adequate folate supplements should be given to mother; *see also* Antimalarials
Promazine *see* Antipsychotics	
Promethazine *see* Antihistamines	
Propofol *see* Anaesthetics, General	
Propranolol *see* Beta-blockers	
Propylthiouracil (2, 3)	Neonatal goitre and hypothyroidism
Prothionamide (1)	May be teratogenic
Protriptyline *see* Antidepressants, Tricyclic	

Table of drugs to be avoided or used with caution in pregnancy (*continued*)

Drug (Trimester of risk)	Comment
Pseudoephedrine	Not known to be harmful
Pyridostigmine (3)	Neonatal myasthenia with large doses
Pyrimethamine (1)	Possible teratogenic risk (folate antagonist); adequate folate supplements should be given to mother; *see also* Antimalarials
Quinapril *see* ACE Inhibitors	
Quinine (1)	High doses are teratogenic; but in malaria benefit of treatment outweighs risk
4-Quinolones (1, 2, 3)	Arthropathy in *animal* studies
Ramipril *see* ACE Inhibitors	
Remoxipride *see* Antipsychotics	
Reproterol *see* section 3.1.1 [text]	
Rifabutin	Information not available
Rifampicin (1)	Manufacturers advise very high doses teratogenic in *animal* studies; *see also* p.239
(3)	Risk of neonatal bleeding may be increased
Rimiterol *see* section 3.1.1 [text]	
Risperidone *see* Antipsychotics	
Ritodrine	For use in premature labour see section 7.1.3
Salbutamol	For use in asthma *see* section 3.1.1 [text]
(3)	For use in premature labour see section 7.1.3
Salcatonin *see* Calcitonin	
Salicylates *see* Aspirin	
Salmeterol *see* section 3.1.1 [text]	
Salsalate *see* Aspirin	
Sertraline *see* Antidepressants, Serotonin-uptake Inhibitor	
Simvastatin	Manufacturer advises toxicity in *animal* studies
Sodium Aurothiomalate *see* Gold	
Sodium Clodronate *see* Bisphosphonates	
Sodium Cromoglycate *see* Cromoglycate	
Sodium Valproate *see* Valproate	
Sotalol *see* Beta-blockers	
Spironolactone	Manufacturers advise toxicity in *animal* studies
Stanozolol *see* Anabolic Steroids	
Stilboestrol (1)	High doses associated with vaginal carcinoma, urogenital abnormalities, and reduced fertility in female offspring
Streptokinase (1, 2, 3)	Possibility of premature separation of placenta in first 18 weeks; theoretical possibility of fetal haemorrhage throughout pregnancy; avoid postpartum use—maternal haemorrhage

Drug (Trimester of risk)	Comment
Streptomycin *see* Aminoglycosides	
Sulfadoxine *see* Sulphonamides	
Sulfametopyrazine *see* Sulphonamides	
Sulindac *see* NSAIDs	
Sulphadiazine *see* Sulphonamides	
Sulphadimidine *see* Sulphonamides	
Sulphasalazine (3)	Theoretical risk of neonatal haemolysis; adequate folate supplements should be given to mother
Sulphonamides (3)	Neonatal haemolysis and methaemoglobinaemia; fear of increased risk of kernicterus in neonates appears to be unfounded
Sulphonylureas (3)	Neonatal hypoglycaemia; insulin is normally substituted in all diabetics; if oral drugs are used therapy should be stopped at least 2 days before delivery
Sulpiride *see* Antipsychotics	
Tamoxifen	Possible effects on fetal development
Temazepam *see* Anxiolytics and Hypnotics	
Tenoxicam *see* NSAIDS	
Terbinafine	Information not available
Terbutaline	For use in asthma *see* section 3.1.1 [text]
(3)	For use in premature labour *see* section 7.1.3
Terfenadine *see* Antihistamines	
Testosterone *see* Androgens	
Tetracyclines (2, 3)	Dental discoloration; maternal hepatotoxicity with large parenteral doses
Theophylline (3)	Neonatal irritability and apnoea have been reported
Thiabendazole (1)	Teratogenic in *animal* studies
Thiazides (3)	May cause neonatal thrombocytopenia; *see also* Diuretics
Thiopentone *see* Anaesthetics, General	
Thioridazine *see* Antipsychotics	
Thymoxamine	Manufacturer advises avoid
Tiaprofenic Acid *see* NSAIDs	
Timolol *see* Beta-blockers	
Tinidazole	Manufacturer advises avoid in first trimester
Tinzaparin *see* Anticoagulants (Heparin)	
Tobramycin *see* Aminoglycosides	
Tocainide	Manufacturer advises toxicity in *animal* studies
Tolbutamide *see* Sulphonylureas	
Tolmetin *see* NSAIDs	
Torasemide *see* Diuretics	
Tramadol *see* Opioid Analgesics	
Trandolapril *see* ACE Inhibitors	
Tranylcypromine *see* Antidepressants, MAOI	

Table of drugs to be avoided or used with caution in pregnancy (*continued*)

Drug (Trimester of risk)	Comment	Drug (Trimester of risk)	Comment
Trazodone *see* Antidepressants, Tricyclic (and related)		Vaccines (live) (1)	Theoretical risk of congenital malformations, but need for vaccination may outweigh possible risk to fetus (*see also* p.467)
Tretinoin	Avoid; other retinoids teratogenic		
Triamcinolone *see* Corticosteroids		Valproate (1, 3)	Increased risk of neural tube defects (counselling and screening advised— **important**: see also **CSM** advice, p.193); neonatal bleeding and neonatal hepatotoxicity also reported; *see also* Antiepileptics
Triamterene *see* Diuretics			
Tribavirin	Manufacturer advises avoid		
Triclofos *see* Anxiolytics and Hypnotics			
Trifluoperazine *see* Antipsychotics			
Trifluperidol *see* Antipsychotics			
Trilostane (1, 2, 3)	Interferes with placental sex hormone production	Verapamil *see* Calcium-channel Blockers	
Trimeprazine *see* Antihistamines		Vigabatrin	Manufacturer advises toxicity in *animal* studies; *see also* Antiepileptics
Trimetaphan (3)	Avoid. Risk of paralytic ileus in newborn		
Trimethoprim (1)	Theoretical teratogenic risk (folate antagonist)	Viloxazine *see* Antidepressants, Tricyclic (and related)	
Trimipramine *see* Antidepressants, Tricyclic		Vitamin A (1)	Excessive doses may be teratogenic; *see also* p.369
Tripotassium Dicitratobismuthate *see* Bismuth Chelate		Warfarin *see* Anticoagulants, Oral	
Triprolidine *see* Antihistamines		Xamoterol	Manufacturer advises toxicity in *animal* studies
Tropisetron	Manufacturer advises toxicity in *animal* studies		
Tulobuterol *see* section 3.1.1 [text]		Xipamide *see* Diuretics	
Urokinase (1, 2, 3)	Possibility of premature separation of placenta in first 18 weeks; theoretical possibility of fetal haemorrhage throughout pregnancy; avoid postpartum use—maternal haemorrhage	Zidovudine	Limited information available; manufacturer advises use only if clearly indicated
		Zolpidem *see* Anxiolytics and Hypnotics	
		Zuclopenthixol *see* Antipsychotics	

Appendix 5: Breast-feeding

Administration of some drugs to nursing mothers may cause toxicity in the infant (e.g. ergotamine), whereas administration of others (e.g. digoxin), has little effect on the neonate. Some drugs inhibit lactation (e.g. bromocriptine).

Toxicity to the infant can occur if the drug enters the milk in pharmacologically significant quantities. Milk concentrations of some drugs (e.g. iodides), may exceed those in the maternal plasma so that therapeutic doses in the mother may cause toxicity to the infant. Some drugs inhibit the infant's sucking reflex (e.g. phenobarbitone). Drugs in breast milk may, at least theoretically, cause hypersensitivity in the infant even when concentrations are too low for a pharmacological effect.

The following table lists drugs:

which should be used with caution or which are contra-indicated in breast-feeding for the reasons given above;

which, on present evidence, may be given to the mother during breast-feeding, because they are excreted in milk in amounts which are too small to be harmful to the infant;

which are not known to be harmful to the infant although they are present in milk in significant amounts.

For many drugs there is insufficient evidence available to provide guidance and it is advisable only to administer essential drugs to a mother during breast-feeding. Because of the inadequacy of currently available information on drugs in breast milk the following table should be used only as a guide; absence from the table does not imply safety.

Table of drugs excreted in breast milk

Products introduced or amended since publication of BNF No. 27 (March 1994) are underlined.

Drug	Comment
Acarbose	Manufacturer advises avoid
Acebutolol see Beta-blockers	
Acemetacin	Manufacturer advises avoid
Acetazolamide	Amount too small to be harmful
Acetohexamide see Sulphonylureas	
Acitretin	Avoid
Acrivastine see Antihistamines	
Acyclovir	Significant amount in milk
Alcohol	Large amounts may affect infant and reduce milk consumption
Alfacalcidol see Vitamin D	
Alprazolam see Benzodiazepines	
Aminoglutethimide	Avoid
Aminophylline see Theophylline	
Amiodarone	Avoid; present in milk in significant amounts; theoretical risk from release of iodine; see also Iodine
Amitriptyline see Antidepressants, Tricyclic	
Amoxapine see Antidepressants, Tricyclic	
Amphetamines	Significant amount in milk. Avoid
Amphotericin	No information available
Amylobarbitone see Barbiturates	
Androgens	Avoid; may cause masculinisation in the female infant or precocious development in the male infant; high doses suppress lactation
Anthraquinones	Avoid; large doses may cause increased gastric motility and diarrhoea (particularly cascara and danthron)

Drug	Comment
Anticoagulants, Oral	Risk of haemorrhage; increased by vitamin-K deficiency; warfarin appears safe but phenindione should be avoided
Antidepressants, Serotonin-uptake Inhibitor see individual entries	
Antidepressants, Tricyclic (and related)	Amount of tricyclic antidepressants (including related drugs such as mianserin and trazodone) too small to be harmful but most manufacturers advise avoid; accumulation of doxepin metabolite may cause sedation and respiratory depression
Antihistamines	Significant amount of some antihistamines; although not known to be harmful some manufacturers advise avoid; drowsiness in infant reported with clemastine
Antipsychotics	Although amount excreted in milk probably too small to be harmful, animal studies indicate possible adverse effects of these drugs on developing nervous system therefore avoid unless absolutely necessary; drowsiness in infant reported with chlorpromazine; significant amount of sulpiride excreted in milk (best avoided); also avoid clozapine

Table of drugs excreted in breast milk (*continued*)

Drug	Comment
Aspirin	Avoid—possible risk of Reye's syndrome; regular use of high doses could impair platelet function and produce hypoprothrombinaemia in infant if neonatal vitamin K stores low
Astemizole *see* Antihistamines	
Atenolol *see* Beta-blockers	
Atropine	May possibly have antimuscarinic effects in infants
Auranofin *see* Gold	
Aurothiomalate *see* Gold	
Azatadine *see* Antihistamines	
Baclofen	Amount too small to be harmful
Barbiturates	Avoid if possible (*see also* phenobarbitone); large doses may produce drowsiness
Beclomethasone *see* Corticosteroids	
Bendrofluazide *see* Thiazides	
Benperidol *see* Antipsychotics	
Benzodiazepines	Avoid repeated doses; lethargy and weight loss may occur in infant
Beta-blockers and Labetalol	Monitor infant; possible toxicity due to beta-blockade but amount of most beta-blockers excreted in milk too small to affect infant; acebutolol, atenolol, nadolol, and sotalol are present in greater amounts than other beta-blockers; manufacturer advises avoid celiprolol
Betamethasone *see* Corticosteroids	
Betaxolol *see* Beta-blockers	
Bezafibrate	Manufacturer advises avoid
Bisoprolol *see* Beta-blockers	
Bromazepam *see* Benzodiazepines	
Bromide salts	Avoid; sedation and rash in infant
Bromocriptine	Suppresses lactation
Brompheniramine *see* Antihistamines	
Bupivacaine	Amount too small to be harmful
Buprenorphine	Amount too small to be harmful
Butobarbitone *see* Barbiturates	
Cabergoline	Suppresses lactation
Caffeine	Regular intake of large amounts can affect infant
Calciferol *see* Vitamin D	
Calcipotriol	No information available
Calcitonin	Avoid; inhibits lactation in *animals*
Calcitriol *see* Vitamin D	
Captopril	Amount probably too small to be harmful, but manufacturer advises avoid

Drug	Comment
Carbamazepine	Amount probably too small to be harmful but severe skin reaction reported in 1 infant
Carbimazole	Amounts in milk may be sufficient to affect neonatal thyroid function therefore lowest effective dose should be used (*see also* section 6.2.2)
Carisoprodol	Concentrated in milk; no adverse effects reported but best avoided
Cascara *see* Anthraquinones	
Ceftazidime	Excreted in low concentration
Celiprolol *see* Beta-blockers	
Cetirizine *see* Antihistamines	
Chloral Hydrate	Sedation in infant
Chloramphenicol	Use another antibiotic; may cause bone-marrow toxicity in infant; concentration in milk usually insufficient to cause `grey syndrome'
Chlordiazepoxide *see* Benzodiazepines	
Chlormethiazole	Amount too small to be harmful
Chloroquine	Amount too small to be harmful; inadequate for reliable protection against malaria, see section 5.4.1
Chlorothiazide *see* Thiazides	
Chlorpheniramine *see* Antihistamines	
Chlorpromazine	Drowsiness in infant reported; *see* Antipsychotics
Chlorpropamide *see* Sulphonylureas	
Chlortetracycline *see* Tetracyclines	
Chlorthalidone *see* Thiazides	
Cholecalciferol *see* Vitamin D	
Cimetidine	Significant amount—not known to be harmful but manufacturer advises avoid
Ciprofibrate	No information available
Ciprofloxacin	Avoid—high concentrations in breast milk
Cisapride	Amount too small to be harmful
Clavulanic acid (in co-amoxiclav, *Timentin*®)	Amount too small to be harmful
Clemastine *see* Antihistamines	
Clindamycin	Amount probably too small to be harmful but bloody diarrhoea reported in 1 infant
Clobazam *see* Benzodiazepines	
Clodronate Sodium	No information available
Clomipramine *see* Antidepressants, Tricyclic	
Clomocycline *see* Tetracyclines	
Clorazepate *see* Benzodiazepines	
Clozapine	Avoid
Codeine	Amount too small to be harmful

Table of drugs excreted in breast milk (*continued*)

Drug	Comment
Colchicine	Caution because of its cytotoxicity
Contraceptives, Oral	Avoid combined oral contraceptives until weaning or for 6 months after birth (adverse effects on lactation); progestogen-only contraceptives do not affect lactation (start 3 weeks after birth or later)
Corticosteroids	Continuous therapy with high doses (>10 mg prednisolone daily) could possibly affect infant's adrenal function—monitor carefully
Cortisone Acetate *see* Corticosteroids	
Co-trimoxazole	Small risk of kernicterus in jaundiced infants and of haemolysis in G6PD-deficient infants (due to sulphamethoxazole)
Cough mixtures containing iodides	Use alternative cough mixtures; *see* Iodine
Cromoglycate	Unlikely to be excreted in milk
Cyclopenthiazide *see* Thiazides	
Cycloserine	Amount too small to be harmful
Cyclosporin	Excreted in milk—manufacturer advises avoid
Cyproheptadine *see* Antihistamines	
Cyproterone Acetate	Caution; possibility of anti androgen effects in neonate
Cytotoxics	Discontinue breast-feeding
Danaparoid	No information available
Danazol	No data available but avoid because of possible androgenic effects in infant
Dantron *see* Anthraquinones	
Dapsone	Haemolytic anaemia; although significant amount in milk risk to infant very small
Demeclocycline *see* Tetracyclines	
Desipramine *see* Antidepressants, Tricyclic	
Desogestrel *see* Contraceptives, Oral	
Dexamethasone *see* Corticosteroids	
Dexamphetamine *see* Amphetamines	
Dexfenfluramine	Avoid
Dextropropoxyphene	Amount too small to be harmful
Diamorphine	Therapeutic doses unlikely to affect infant; withdrawal symptoms in infants of dependent mothers; breast-feeding no longer considered best method of treating dependence in offspring of dependent mothers and should be stopped
Diazepam *see* Benzodiazepines	

Drug	Comment
Diclofenac	Amount too small to be harmful
Digoxin	Amount too small to be harmful
Dihydrotachysterol *see* Vitamin D	
Diltiazem	Significant amount—manufacturer advises avoid
Diphenhydramine *see* Antihistamines	
Diphenylpyraline *see* Antihistamines	
Disopyramide	Amount probably too small to be harmful—monitor infant for antimuscarinic effects
Domperidone	Amount probably too small to be harmful
Dothiepin *see* Antidepressants, Tricyclic	
Doxepin *see* Antidepressants, Tricyclic	
Doxycycline *see* Tetracyclines	
Droperidol *see* Antipsychotics	
Enalapril	Amount probably too small to be harmful
Ephedrine	Irritability and disturbed sleep reported
Ergocalciferol *see* Vitamin D	
Ergotamine	Avoid where possible; ergotism may occur in infant; repeated doses may inhibit lactation
Erythromycin	Only small amounts in milk
Esmolol *see* Beta-blockers	
Ethambutol	Amount too small to be harmful
Ethamsylate	Significant amount but not known to be harmful
Ethinyloestradiol *see* Contraceptives, Oral	
Ethosuximide	Significant amount; hyperexcitability and poor suckling reported
Ethynodiol *see* Contraceptives, Oral	
Etodolac	Manufacturer advises avoid
Etretinate	Avoid
Famciclovir	No information available
Famotidine	Amount too small to be harmful
Fansidar®	Small risk of kernicterus in jaundiced infants and of haemolysis in G6PD-deficient infants (due to sulfadoxine)
Fenbufen	Amount too small to be harmful
Fenoprofen	Amount too small to be harmful
Fentanyl	Manufacturer advises avoid
Filgrastim	No information available
Flecainide	Significant amount but not known to be harmful
Flunitrazepam *see* Benzodiazepines	
Fluoxetine	Only small amounts in milk but could accumulate in infant—manufacturer advises avoid
Flupenthixol *see* Antipsychotics	

Table of drugs excreted in breast milk (*continued*)

Drug	Comment	Drug	Comment
Fluphenazine *see* Antipsychotics		Isoniazid	Monitor infant for possible toxicity; theoretical risk of convulsions and neuropathy; prophylactic pyridoxine advisable in mother and infant
Flurazepam *see* Benzodiazepines			
Flurbiprofen	Amount too small to be harmful		
Fluticasone *see* Corticosteroids			
Fluvastatin	Manufacturer advises avoid	Isotretinoin	Avoid
Fluvoxamine	Amount too small to be harmful	Ketoprofen	Amount probably too small to be harmful but manufacturer advises avoid unless essential
Fosfomycin	Excreted in milk—manufacturer advises avoid unless real need		
		Ketorolac	Avoid
Frusemide	Amount too small to be harmful	Ketotifen *see* Antihistamines	
		Labetalol *see* Beta-blockers	
Gabapentin	No information available	Lamotrigine	No information available
Ganciclovir	Avoid	Lansoprazole	No information available
Gestodene *see* Contraceptives, Oral		Lenograstim	No information available
Glibenclamide *see* Sulphonylureas		Levodopa	No information available
Gliclazide *see* Sulphonylureas		Levonorgestrel *see* Contraceptives, Oral	
Glipizide *see* Sulphonylureas		Lignocaine	Amount too small to be harmful
Gliquidone *see* Sulphonylureas			
Glymidine *see* Sulphonylureas		Lindane *see* section 13.10.4	
Gold (auranofin, aurothiomalate)	Caution—excreted in milk; theoretical possibility of rashes and idiosyncratic reactions	Liothyronine	May interfere with neonatal screening for hypothyroidism
		Lisinopril	No information available
Granisetron	No information available	Lithium salts	Monitor infant for possible intoxication; low incidence of adverse effects but increased by continuous ingestion; good control of maternal plasma concentrations minimises the risk
Halofantrine	Avoid		
Haloperidol *see* Antipsychotics			
Heparin	Amount too small to be harmful		
Hydrochlorothiazide *see* Thiazides			
Hydrocortisone *see* Corticosteroids			
Hydroflumethiazide *see* Thiazides		Lofepramine *see* Antidepressants, Tricyclic	
Hydroxychloroquine	Amount too small to be harmful	Loprazolam *see* Benzodiazepines	
		Lorazepam *see* Benzodiazepines	
Hydroxyzine *see* Antihistamines		Lormetazepam *see* Benzodiazepines	
Hyoscine	Amount too small to be harmful	Lymecycline *see* Tetracyclines	
		Lysuride	May suppress lactation
Ibuprofen	Amount too small to be harmful	*Maloprim*®	Haemolytic anaemia (due to dapsone); risk to infant very small
Idoxuridine	May possibly make milk taste unpleasant		
		Maprotiline *see* Antidepressants, Tricyclic (and related)	
Imipramine *see* Antidepressants, Tricyclic		Mebendazole	No information available
Indapamide *see* Thiazides		Mebeverine	Amount too small to be harmful
Indomethacin	Amount probably too small to be harmful but convulsions reported in one infant		
		Medroxyprogesterone Acetate *see* Progestogens	
Insulin	Amount too small to be harmful	Mefenamic Acid	Amount too small to be harmful
		Mefloquine	Avoid—excreted in milk
Interferons	No information available	Mefruside *see* Thiazides	
Iodine	Stop breast-feeding; danger of neonatal hypothyroidism or goitre; appears to be concentrated in milk	Meprobamate	Avoid; concentration in milk may exceed maternal plasma concentrations fourfold and may cause drowsiness in infant
Radioactive iodine	Breast-feeding contra-indicated after therapeutic doses. With diagnostic doses withhold breast-feeding for at least 24 hours	Mequitazine *see* Antihistamines	
		Mesalazine	Diarrhoea reported but manufacturer advises none detected in breast milk
Iprindole *see* Antidepressants, Tricyclic (and related)		Mestranol *see* Contraceptives, Oral	

Table of drugs excreted in breast milk (*continued*)

Drug	Comment
Methadone	Withdrawal symptoms in infant; breast-feeding permissible during maintenance but dose should be as low as possible and baby monitored to avoid sedation
Methotrimeprazine *see* Antipsychotics	
Methyclothiazide *see* Thiazides	
Methyldopa	Amount too small to be harmful
Methylprednisolone *see* Corticosteroids	
Metoclopramide	Amount probably too small to be harmful
Metolazone *see* Thiazides	
Metoprolol *see* Beta-blockers	
Metronidazole	Significant amount in milk; manufacturer advises avoid large single doses
Mexiletine	Amount too small to be harmful
Mianserin *see* Antidepressants, Tricyclic (and related)	
Minocycline *see* Tetracyclines	
Minoxidil	Significant amount but not known to be harmful
Moclobemide	Amount too small to be harmful, but patient leaflet advises avoid
Moracizine	Excreted in milk—manufacturer advises avoid
Morphine	Therapeutic doses unlikely to affect infant; withdrawal symptoms in infants of dependent mothers; breast-feeding not best method of treating dependence in offspring and should be stopped
Nadolol *see* Beta-blockers	
Nafarelin	No information available
Nalidixic Acid	Risk to infant very small but one case of haemolytic anaemia reported
Naloxone	No information available
Naproxen	Amount too small to be harmful
Nefopam	Amount too small to be harmful
Neostigmine	Amount probably too small to be harmful; monitor infant
Nicoumalone *see* Anticoagulants, Oral	
Nifedipine	Amount too small to be harmful but manufacturer advises avoid
Nitrazepam *see* Benzodiazepines	
Nitrofurantoin	Only small amounts in milk but could be enough to produce haemolysis in G6PD-deficient infants
Nizatidine	Amount too small to be harmful
Norethisterone *see* Contraceptives, Oral	
Norgestimate *see* Contraceptives, Oral	

Drug	Comment
Nortriptyline *see* Antidepressants, Tricyclic	
NSAIDs *see* individual entries	
Octreotide	Avoid
Oestrogens	Avoid; adverse effects on lactation; *see also* Contraceptives, Oral
Ofloxacin	Manufacturer advises avoid
Omeprazole	No information available
Opioid Analgesics *see* individual entries	
Orphenadrine	Excreted in milk—manufacturer advises avoid
Oxatomide *see* Antihistamines	
Oxazepam *see* Benzodiazepines	
Oxitropium	No information available
Oxprenolol *see* Beta-blockers	
Oxypertine *see* Antipsychotics	
Oxytetracycline *see* Tetracyclines	
Papaveretum *see* Morphine	
Paracetamol	Amount too small to be harmful
Penbutolol *see* Beta-blockers	
Pergolide	May suppress lactation
Pericyazine *see* Antipsychotics	
Perphenazine *see* Antipsychotics	
Phenindamine *see* Antihistamines	
Phenindione *see* Anticoagulants, Oral	
Pheniramine *see* Antihistamines	
Phenobarbitone	Avoid when possible; drowsiness may occur but risk probably small; one report of methaemoglobinaemia with phenobarbitone and phenytoin
Phenolphthalein	Avoid; increased gastric motility, diarrhoea, and possibly rash
Phentolamine	No information available
Phenytoin	Amount too small to be harmful
Pimozide *see* Antipsychotics	
Pindolol *see* Beta-blockers	
Piracetam	Manufacturer advises avoid
Pirenzepine	Amount too small to be harmful
Piroxicam	Amount too small to be harmful
Pizotifen	Amount probably too small to be harmful, but patient information leaflet advises avoid
Polythiazide *see* Thiazides	
Povidone-iodine	Avoid; iodine absorbed from vaginal preparations is concentrated in milk
Pravastatin	Small amount excreted in milk—manufacturer advises avoid
Prednisolone *see* Corticosteroids	
Prednisone *see* Corticosteroids	
Primidone *see* Phenobarbitone	
Prochlorperazine *see* Antipsychotics	

Table of drugs excreted in breast milk (*continued*)

Drug	Comment	Drug	Comment
Progestogens	High doses suppress lactation but *see also* Contraceptives, Oral	Terbinafine	Excreted in milk—manufacturer advises avoid
Proguanil *see* Chloroquine		Terbutaline	Amount too small to be harmful
Promazine *see* Antipsychotics		Terfenadine *see* Antihistamines	
Promethazine *see* Antihistamines		Tetracyclines	Avoid (although absorption and therefore discoloration of teeth in infant probably usually prevented by chelation with calcium in milk)
Propranolol *see* Beta-blockers			
Propylthiouracil	Monitor infant's thyroid status but amounts in milk probably too small to affect infant; high doses might affect neonatal thyroid function		
		Theophylline	Irritability in infant reported; modified-release preparations probably safe
Protriptyline *see* Antidepressants, Tricyclic		Thiamine	Severely thiamine-deficient mothers should avoid breast-feeding as toxic methylglyoxal excreted in milk
Pseudoephedrine	Amount too small to be harmful		
Pyrazinamide	Amount too small to be harmful	Thiazides	Amount too small to be harmful; large doses may suppress lactation
Pyridostigmine	Amount probably too small to be harmful	Thioridazine *see* Antipsychotics	
Pyrimethamine	Significant amount but not known to be harmful	Thyroxine	May interfere with neonatal screening for hypothyroidism
Quinalbarbitone *see* Barbiturates		Tiaprofenic acid	Amount too small to be harmful
Quinidine	Significant amount but not known to be harmful	Timolol *see* Beta-blockers	
Ramipril	Manufacturer advises avoid	Tolazamide *see* Sulphonylureas	
Ranitidine	Significant amount but not known to be harmful	Tolbutamide *see* Sulphonylureas	
Rifabutin	No information available	Tolmetin	Amount too small to be harmful
Rifampicin	Amount too small to be harmful	Trazodone	Amount too small to be harmful
Risperidone *see* Antipsychotics		Triamcinolone *see* Corticosteroids	
Senna *see* Anthraquinones		Trifluoperazine *see* Antipsychotics	
Sodium Cromoglycate *see* Cromoglycate		Trifluperidol *see* Antipsychotics	
Sodium Valproate *see* Valproate		Trimeprazine *see* Antihistamines	
Sotalol *see* Beta-blockers		Trimipramine *see* Antidepressants, Tricyclic	
Sulfametopyrazine *see* Sulphonamides		Triprolidine *see* Antihistamines	
Sulphadiazine *see* Sulphonamides		Tropisetron	No information available
Sulphadimidine *see* Sulphonamides		Tulobuterol	No information available
Sulphasalazine	Small amounts in milk but bloody diarrhoea and rashes have been reported; theoretical risk of neonatal haemolysis especially in G6PD-deficient infants	Valproate	Amount too small to be harmful
		Vancomycin	Excreted in milk—manufacturer advises avoid
		Verapamil	Amount too small to be harmful
Sulphinpyrazone	No information available	Vigabatrin	No information available—manufacturer advises avoid
Sulphonamides	Small risk of kernicterus in jaundiced infants particularly with long-acting sulphonamides, and of haemolysis in G6PD-deficient infants	Viloxazine *see* Antidepressants, Tricyclic (and related)	
		Vitamin A	Theoretical risk of toxicity in infants of mothers taking large doses
Sulphonylureas	Caution; theoretical possibility of hypoglycaemia in infant	Vitamin D (and related compounds)	Caution with high doses; may cause hypercalcaemia in infant
Sulpiride	Best avoided; significant amounts in milk; *see also* Antipsychotics	Warfarin *see* Anticoagulants, Oral	
		Xipamide *see* Thiazides	
Teicoplanin	No information available	Zidovudine	No information available
Temazepam *see* Benzodiazepines		Zopiclone	Amount too small to be harmful
Tenoxicam	No information available	Zuclopenthixol *see* Antipsychotics	

Appendix 6: Intravenous Additives

INTRAVENOUS ADDITIVE POLICIES. A local policy on the addition of drugs to intravenous fluids should be drawn up by a multi-disciplinary team in each Health Authority and issued as a document to the members of staff concerned.

Centralised additive services are provided in a number of hospital pharmacy departments and should be used in preference to making additions on wards.

The information that follows should be read in conjunction with local policy documents.

Guidelines

1. Drugs should only be added to infusion containers when constant plasma concentrations are needed or when the administration of a more concentrated solution would be harmful.
2. In general, only one drug should be added to any infusion container and the components should be compatible. Ready-prepared solutions should be used whenever possible. Drugs should not normally be added to blood products, mannitol, or sodium bicarbonate. Only specially formulated additives should be used with fat emulsions or amino-acid solutions (see section 9.3).
3. Solutions should be thoroughly mixed by shaking and checked for absence of particulate matter before use.
4. Strict asepsis should be maintained throughout and in general the giving set should not be used for more than 24 hours.
5. The infusion container should be labelled with the patient's name, the name and quantity of additives, and the date and time of addition (and the new expiry date or time). Such additional labelling should not interfere with information on the manufacturer's label that is still valid. When possible, containers should be retained for a period after use in case they are needed for investigation.
6. It is good practice to examine intravenous infusions from time to time while they are running. If cloudiness, crystallisation, change of colour, or any other sign of interaction or contamination is observed the infusion should be discontinued.

Problems

MICROBIAL CONTAMINATION. The accidental entry and subsequent growth of micro-organisms converts the infusion fluid pathway into a potential vehicle for infection with micro-organisms, particularly species of Candida, Enterobacter, and Klebsiella. Ready-prepared infusions containing the additional drugs, or infusions prepared by an additive service (when available) should therefore be used in preference to making extemporaneous additions to infusion containers on wards etc. However, when this is necessary strict aseptic procedure should be followed.

INCOMPATIBILITY. Physical and chemical incompatibilities may occur with loss of potency, increase in toxicity, or other adverse effect. The solutions may become opalescent or precipitation may occur, but in many instances there is no visual indication of incompatibility. Interaction may take place at any point in the infusion fluid pathway, and the potential for incompatibility is increased when more than one substance is added to the infusion fluid.

Common incompatibilities. Precipitation reactions are numerous and varied and may occur as a result of pH, concentration changes, 'salting-out' effects, complexation or other chemical changes. Precipitation or other particle formation must be avoided since, apart from lack of control of dosage on administration, it may initiate or exacerbate adverse effects. This is particularly important in the case of drugs which have been implicated in either thrombophlebitis (e.g. diazepam) or in skin sloughing or necrosis caused by extravasation (e.g. sodium bicarbonate and certain cytotoxic drugs). It is also especially important to effect solution of colloidal drugs and to prevent their subsequent precipitation in order to avoid a pyrogenic reaction (e.g. amphotericin).

It is considered undesirable to mix beta-lactam antibiotics, such as semi-synthetic penicillins and cephalosporins, with proteinaceous materials on the grounds that immunogenic and allergenic conjugates could be formed.

A number of preparations undergo significant loss of potency when added singly or in combination to large volume infusions. Examples include ampicillin in infusions that contain glucose or lactates, mustine hydrochloride in isotonic saline and gentamicin/carbenicillin combinations. The breakdown products of dacarbazine have been implicated in adverse effects.

Blood. Because of the large number of incompatibilities, drugs should not normally be added to blood and blood products for infusion purposes. Examples of incompatibility with blood include hypertonic mannitol solutions (irreversible crenation of red cells), dextrans (rouleaux formation and interference with cross-matching), glucose (clumping of red cells), and oxytocin (inactivated).

If the giving set is not changed after the administration of blood, but used for other infusion fluids, a fibrin clot may form which, apart from blocking the set, increases the likelihood of microbial growth.

Intravenous fat emulsions may break down with coalescence of fat globules and separation of phases when additions such as antibiotics or electrolytes are made, thus increasing the possibility of embolism. Only specially formulated products such as Vitlipid N® (see section 9.3) may be added to appropriate intravenous fat emulsions.

Other infusions that frequently give rise to incompatibility include amino acids, mannitol, and sodium bicarbonate.

Bactericides such as chlorocresol 0.1% or phenylmercuric nitrate 0.001% are present in some injection solutions. The total volume of such solutions added to a container for infusion on one occasion should not exceed 15 mL.

Method

Ready-prepared infusions should be used whenever available. **Potassium chloride** is usually available in concentrations of 20, 27, and 40 mmol/litre in sodium chloride intravenous infusion (0.9%), glucose intravenous infusion (5%) or sodium chloride and glucose intravenous infusion. **Lignocaine hydrochloride** is usually available in concentrations of 0.1 or 0.2% in glucose intravenous infusion (5%).

When addition is required to be made extemporaneously, any product reconstitution instructions such as those relating to concentration, vehicle, mixing, and handling precautions should be strictly followed using an aseptic technique throughout. Once the product has been reconstituted, addition to the infusion fluid should be made immediately in order to minimise microbial contamination and, with certain products, to prevent degradation or other formulation change which may occur; e.g. reconstituted ampicillin injection degrades rapidly on standing, and also may form polymers which could cause sensitivity reactions.

It is also important in certain instances that an infusion fluid of specific pH be used. **Amphotericin** injection requires dilution in glucose injection of pH greater than 4.2 and **frusemide** injection should be added to infusions of pH greater than 5.5.

When drug additions are made it is important to mix thoroughly; additions should not be made to an infusion container that has been connected to a giving set, as mixing is hampered. If the solutions are not thoroughly mixed a concentrated layer of the additive may form owing to differences in density. **Potassium chloride** is particularly prone to this 'layering' effect when added without adequate mixing to infusions packed in non-rigid infusion containers; if such a mixture is administered it may have a serious effect on the heart.

A time limit between addition and completion of administration must be imposed for certain admixtures to guarantee satisfactory drug potency and compatibility. For admixtures in which degradation occurs without the formation of toxic substances, an acceptable limit is the time taken for 10% decomposition of the drug. When toxic substances are produced stricter limits may be imposed. Because of the risk of microbial contamination a maximum time limit of 12 hours should be imposed for additions made elsewhere than in hospital pharmacies offering central additive service.

Certain injections must be protected from light during continuous infusion to minimise oxidation, e.g. amphotericin, dacarbazine, and sodium nitroprusside.

Dilution with a small volume of an appropriate vehicle and administration using a motorised infusion pump is advocated for preparations such as heparin where strict control over administration is required. In this case the appropriate dose may be dissolved in a convenient volume (e.g. 24 to 48 mL) of sodium chloride intravenous infusion (0.9%).

Use of table

The table lists preparations given by three methods:

continuous infusion,

intermittent infusion, and

addition *via* the drip tubing.

Drugs for **continuous infusion** must be diluted in a large volume infusion. Penicillins and cephalosporins are not usually given by continuous infusion because of stability problems and because adequate plasma and tissue concentrations are best obtained by intermittent infusion. Where it is necessary to administer them by continuous infusion, detailed literature should be consulted.

Drugs that are both compatible and clinically suitable may be given by **intermittent infusion** in a relatively small volume of infusion over a short period of time, e.g. 100 mL in 30 minutes. The method is used if the product is incompatible or unstable over the period necessary for continuous infusion; the limited stability of ampicillin or amoxycillin in large volume glucose or lactate infusions may be overcome in this way.

Intermittent infusion is also used if adequate plasma and tissue concentrations are not produced by continuous infusion as in the case of drugs such as carbenicillin, dacarbazine, gentamicin, and ticarcillin.

An in-line burette may be used for intermittent infusion techniques in order to achieve strict control over the time and rate of administration, especially for infants and children and in intensive care units. Intermittent infusion may also make use of the 'piggy-back' technique provided that no additions are made to the primary infusion. In this method the drug is added to a small secondary container connected to a Y-type injection site on the primary infusion giving set; the secondary solution is usually infused within 30 minutes.

Addition *via* the drip tubing is indicated for a number of cytotoxic drugs in order to minimise extravasation. The preparation is added aseptically *via* the rubber septum of the injection site of a fast-running infusion. In general, drug preparations intended for a bolus effect should be given directly into a separate vein where possible. Failing this, administration may be made *via* the drip tubing provided that the preparation is compatible with the infusion fluid when given in this manner.

Table of drugs given by intravenous infusion

Covers addition to Glucose 5 and 10%, Sodium chloride 0.9%, Compound sodium chloride (Ringer's solution), and Compound sodium lactate (Hartmann's solution). Compatibility with glucose 5% and with sodium chloride 0.9% indicates compatibility with any strength of sodium chloride and glucose infusion. Infusion of a large volume of hypotonic solution should be avoided therefore care should be taken if water for injections is used. The information in the Table relates to the proprietary preparations indicated; for other preparations suitability should be checked with the manufacturer

Acetylcysteine (*Parvolex®*)

Continuous *in* Glucose 5%

See Emergency Treatment of Poisoning

Aclarubicin hydrochloride (*Aclacin®*)

Intermittent *in* Glucose 5% *or* Sodium chloride 0.9%

Dissolve initially in 10 mL water for injections or sodium chloride 0.9% then dilute with 200–500 mL infusion fluid to a concentration of 200–500 micrograms/ mL; give over 30–60 minutes and protect from light during administration; pH of glucose infusion should be between 5 and 6

Acyclovir sodium (*Zovirax IV®*)

Intermittent *in* Sodium chloride 0.9% *or* Sodium chloride and glucose *or* Compound sodium lactate

Initially reconstitute to 25 mg/mL in water for injections or sodium chloride 0.9% then dilute to not more than 5 mg/mL with the infusion fluid; minimum volume 50 mL; to be given over 1 hour; alternatively, may be administered in a concentration of 25 mg/mL using a suitable infusion pump and given over 1 hour

Aldesleukin (*Proleukin®*)

Continuous *in* Glucose 5%

Reconstitute each vial with 1.2 mL water for injections (do not shake or allow to foam); dilute in up to 500 mL glucose 5% containing albumin 0.1% (albumin added and thoroughly mixed in glucose 5% solution before adding aldesleukin); polypropylene, PVC, polyolefin, or glass containers with polyethylene or PVC giving sets may be used; do not use in-line filter

Alfentanil hydrochloride (*Rapifen® preparations*)

Continuous *or* intermittent *in* Glucose 5% *or* Sodium chloride 0.9% *or* Compound sodium lactate

Alprostadil (*Prostin VR®*)

Continuous *in* Glucose 5% *or* Sodium chloride 0.9%

Amikacin sulphate (*Amikin®*)

Intermittent *in* Glucose 5% *or* Sodium chloride 0.9% *or* Compound sodium lactate

To be given over 30 minutes

Aminophylline

Continuous *in* Glucose 5% *or* Sodium chloride 0.9% *or* Compound sodium lactate

Amiodarone hydrochloride (*Cordarone X®*)

Continuous *or* intermittent *in* Glucose 5%

Suggested initial infusion volume 250 mL given over 20–120 minutes; for repeat infusions up to 1.2 g in max. 500 mL; infusion in extreme emergency see section 2.3.2; should not be diluted to less than 600 micrograms/mL; incompatible with sodium chloride infusion

Amoxicillin sodium (*Amoxil®*)

[1]Intermittent *in* Glucose 5% *or* Sodium chloride 0.9%

Reconstituted solutions diluted and given without delay; suggested volume 100 mL given over 30–60 minutes

via drip tubing *in* Glucose 5% *or* Sodium chloride 0.9% *or* Ringer's solution *or* Compound sodium lactate

Amphotericin (colloidal) (*Amphocil®*)

Intermittent *in* Glucose 5%

Initially reconstitute with water for injections (50 mg in 10 mL, 100 mg in 20 mL), shaking gently to dissolve (fluid may be opalescent) then dilute to a concentration of 625 micrograms/mL (1 volume of reconstituted solution with 7 volumes of infusion fluid); give over 60–90 minutes (or longer if not tolerated over 90 minutes); incompatible with sodium chloride or other electrolyte solutions, flush existing intravenous line with glucose 5% or use separate line

Amphotericin (liposomal) (*AmBisome®*)

Intermittent *in* Glucose 5%

Reconstitute each vial with 12 mL water for injections (both vial and water for injections should be cooled to 2– 8°C before reconstitution) and shake vigorously; incubate reconstituted vial at 65°C for 10 minutes and allow to cool to room temperature; withdraw requisite dose from vial and introduce into infusion fluid through the 5 micron filter provided to produce a final concentration of 500 micrograms/mL; infuse over 30–60 minutes; incompatible with sodium chloride solutions, flush existing intravenous line with glucose 5% or use separate line

Amphotericin sodium deoxycholate complex (*Fungizone®*)

Continuous *in* Glucose 5%

Dissolve thoroughly at reconstitution stage; preparation must be diluted in a large volume infusion; pH of the glucose must not be below 4.2 (check each container); protect from light; suggested infusion time 6 hours

Ampicillin sodium (*Penbritin®*)

[1]Intermittent *in* Glucose 5% *or* Sodium chloride 0.9%

Reconstituted solutions diluted and given without delay; suggested volume 100 mL given over 30–60 minutes

via drip tubing *in* Glucose 5% *or* Sodium chloride 0.9% *or* Ringer's solution *or* Compound sodium lactate

Ampicillin/cloxacillin (sodium salts) (*Ampiclox®*)

Intermittent *or via* drip tubing *in* Glucose 5% *or* Sodium chloride 0.9%

Reconstituted solutions diluted and given without delay; suggested volume 100 mL given over 30–60 minutes

via drip tubing *in* Glucose 5% *or* Sodium chloride 0.9% *or* Ringer's solution *or* Compound sodium lactate

---

1. Continuous infusion not usually recommended

Table of drugs given by intravenous infusion (*continued*)

Amsacrine (*Amsidine*®)
Intermittent *in* Glucose 5%
Reconstitute with diluent provided and dilute to suggested volume 500 mL; give over 60–90 minutes; use glass syringes; incompatible with sodium chloride infusion

Atenolol (*Tenormin*®)
Intermittent *in* Glucose 5% *or* Sodium chloride 0.9%
Suggested infusion time 20 minutes

Atracurium besylate (*Tracrium*®)
Continuous *in* Glucose 5% *or* Sodium chloride 0.9% *or* Compound sodium lactate
Stability varies with diluent

Azathioprine (sodium salt) (*Imuran*®)
via drip tubing *in* Glucose 5% *or* Sodium chloride 0.9%

Azlocillin sodium (*Securopen*® (5 g)
Intermittent *in* Glucose 5 and 10% *or* Sodium chloride 0.9% *or* Ringer's solution
Intermittent infusion suggested for doses over 2 g; to be given over 20–30 minutes

Aztreonam (*Azactam*®)
Intermittent *in* Glucose 5% *or* Sodium chloride 0.9% *or* Ringer's solution *or* Compound sodium lactate
Dissolve initially in water for injections (1 g per 3 mL) then dilute to a concentration of less than 20 mg/mL; to be given over 20–60 minutes

Benzylpenicillin sodium (*Crystapen*®)
[1]Intermittent *in* Glucose 5% *or* Sodium chloride 0.9%
Suggested volume 100 mL given over 30–60 minutes

Betamethasone sodium phosphate (*Betnesol*®)
Continuous *or* intermittent *or* *via* drip tubing *in* Glucose 5% *or* Sodium chloride 0.9%

Bleomycin sulphate
Intermittent *in* Sodium chloride 0.9%
To be given slowly; suggested volume 200 mL

Bumetanide (*Burinex*®)
Intermittent *in* Glucose 5% *or* Sodium chloride 0.9%
Suggested volume 500 mL given over 30–60 minutes

Calcium gluconate
Continuous *in* Glucose 5% *or* Sodium chloride 0.9%
Avoid bicarbonates, phosphates, or sulphates

Carbenicillin sodium (*Pyopen*®)
Intermittent *in* Glucose 5% *or* Water for injections
Suggested volume 100 mL given over 30–40 minutes

Carboplatin (*Paraplatin*®)
Continuous *in* Glucose 5% *or* Sodium chloride 0.9%
Final concentration as low as 500 micrograms/mL; give over 15–60 minutes

Carmustine (*BiCNU*®)
Intermittent *in* Glucose 5% *or* Sodium chloride 0.9%
Reconstitute with diluent provided; give over 1–2 hours

Cefodizime sodium (*Timecef*®)
Intermittent *in* Glucose 5% *or* Sodium chloride 0.9% *or* Ringer's solution *or* Compound sodium lactate *or* Water for injections
Dissolve in 40 mL infusion fluid and give over up to 30 minutes

Cefotaxime sodium (*Claforan*®)
Intermittent *in* Glucose 5% *or* Sodium chloride 0.9% *or* Compound sodium lactate *or* Water for injections
Suggested volume 40–100 mL given over 20–60 minutes

Cefoxitin sodium (*Mefoxin*®)
[1]Intermittent *or* *via* drip tubing *in* Glucose 5 and 10% *or* Sodium chloride 0.9%

Cefsulodin sodium (*Monaspor*®)
[1]Intermittent *or* *via* drip tubing *in* Glucose 5% *or* Sodium chloride 0.9%
When giving by intermittent infusion over more than 30–60 minutes, give first dose as a slow bolus injection

Ceftazidime pentahydrate (*Fortum*®, *Kefadim*®)
Intermittent *or* *via* drip tubing *in* Glucose 5 and 10% *or* Sodium chloride 0.9% *or* Compound sodium lactate
Dissolve 2 g initially in 10 mL (3 g in 15 mL) infusion fluid; for *Fortum*® dilute further to a concentration of 40 mg/mL; for *Kefadim*® dilute further to a concentration of 20 mg/mL; give over up to 30 minutes

Ceftizoxime sodium (*Cefizox*®)
Continuous *or* intermittent *or* *via* drip tubing *in* Glucose 5 and 10% *or* Sodium chloride 0.9% *or* Ringer's solution *or* Compound sodium lactate
Suggested volume 50–100 mL

Ceftriaxone (sodium salt) (*Rocephin*®)
Intermittent *or* *via* drip tubing *in* Glucose 5% and 10% *or* Sodium chloride 0.9%
Give intermittent infusion of 2 g (50 mg/kg or more for children) over at least 30 minutes; not to be given with infusion fluids containing calcium

Cefuroxime sodium (*Zinacef*®)
Intermittent *or* *via* drip tubing *in* Glucose 5% *or* Sodium chloride 0.9% *or* Compound sodium lactate
Dissolve initially in water for injections (at least 2 mL for each 250 mg, 15 mL for 1.5 g); suggested volume 50–100 mL given over 30 minutes

Cephamandole nafate (*Kefadol*®)
[1]Intermittent *or* *via* drip tubing *in* Glucose 5 and 10% *or* Sodium chloride 0.9%

Cephazolin sodium (*Kefzol*®)
[1]Intermittent *or* *via* drip tubing *in* Glucose 5 and 10% *or* Sodium chloride 0.9% *or* Compound sodium lactate

Cephradine (*Velosef*®)
Continuous *or* intermittent *in* Glucose 5 and 10% *or* Sodium chloride 0.9% *or* Ringer's solution *or* Compound sodium lactate

Chloramphenicol sodium succinate (*Kemicetine*®)
Intermittent *or* *via* drip tubing *in* Glucose 5% *or* Sodium chloride 0.9%

Chloroquine sulphate (*Nivaquine*®)
Continuous *in* Sodium chloride 0.9%
See also section 5.4.1

Cimetidine (*Tagamet*®)
Continuous *or* intermittent *in* Glucose 5% *or* Sodium chloride 0.9%
For intermittent infusion suggested volume 100 mL given over 30–60 minutes

Table of drugs given by intravenous infusion (*continued*)

Cisplatin *Cisplatin* (Lederle), *Cisplatin powder for injection* (Lederle)
Continuous *in* Sodium chloride 0.9% *or* Sodium chloride and glucose
Reconstitute cisplatin powder for injection with water for injections (10 mg in 10 mL, 50 mg in 50 mL); suggested volume 2 litres given over 6–8 hours

Clarithromycin (*Klaricid® I.V.*)
Intermittent *in* Glucose 5% *or* Sodium chloride 0.9% *or* Ringer's solution *or* Compound sodium lactate
Dissolve initially in water for injections (500 mg in 10 mL) then dilute to a concentration of 2 mg/mL; give over 60 minutes

Clindamycin phosphate (*Dalacin C®*)
Continuous *or* intermittent *in* Glucose 5% *or* Sodium chloride 0.9%
Dilute to a concentration of 300 mg in 50 mL; give each 300 mg over at least 10 minutes (1.2 g over at least 45 minutes)

Clomipramine hydrochloride (*Anafranil®*)
Intermittent *in* Glucose 5% *or* Sodium chloride 0.9%
Suggested volume 125–500 mL given over 45–120 minutes

Clonazepam (*Rivotril®*)
Intermittent *in* Glucose 5 and 10% *or* Sodium chloride 0.9%
Suggested volume 250 mL

Cloxacillin sodium (*Orbenin®*)
[1]Intermittent *in* Glucose 5% *or* Sodium chloride 0.9%
Suggested volume 100 mL given over 30–60 minutes
via drip tubing *in* Glucose 5% *or* Sodium chloride 0.9% *or* Ringer's solution *or* Compound sodium lactate

Co-amoxiclav (*Augmentin®*)
Intermittent *in* Sodium chloride 0.9% *or* Water for injections; see also package leaflet
Suggested volume 50–100 mL given over 30–40 minutes and completed within 4 hours of reconstitution
via drip tubing *in* Glucose 5% *or* Sodium chloride 0.9%

Co-fluampicil (sodium salts) (*Magnapen®*)
Intermittent *in* Glucose 5% *or* Sodium chloride 0.9%
Reconstituted solutions diluted and given without delay; suggested volume 100 mL given over 30–60 minutes
via drip tubing *in* Glucose 5% *or* Sodium chloride 0.9% *or* Ringer's solution *or* Compound sodium lactate

Colistin sulphomethate sodium (*Colomycin®*)
Continuous or intermittent *in* Glucose 5% *or* Sodium chloride 0.9% *or* Ringer's solution
Max. 6 hours between addition and completion of administration

Co-trimoxazole (*Septrin® for infusion*)
Intermittent *in* Glucose 5 and 10% *or* Sodium chloride 0.9% *or* Ringer's solution
Dilute contents of 1 ampoule (5 mL) to 125 mL, 2 ampoules (10 mL) to 250 mL or 3 ampoules (15 mL) to 500 mL; suggested duration of infusion 90 minutes (but may be adjusted according to fluid requirements); if fluid restriction necessary, 1 ampoule may be diluted with 75 mL glucose 5%

Cyclophosphamide (*Endoxana®*)
Intermittent *or via* drip tubing *in* Glucose 5% *or* Sodium chloride 0.9% *or* Water for injections
For intermittent infusion suggested volume 50–100 mL given over 5–15 minutes
via drip tubing *in* Glucose 5%

Cyclosporin (*Sandimmun®*)
Continuous *in* Glucose 5% *or* Sodium chloride 0.9%
Dilute to a concentration of 50 mg in 20–100 mL; give over 2–6 hours; not to be used with PVC equipment

Cytarabine (*Alexan®*, *Cytosar®*)
Continuous *or* intermittent *or via* drip tubing *in* Glucose 5% *or* Sodium chloride 0.9%
Reconstitute *Cytosar®* with the diluent provided; check container for haze or precipitate during administration

Dacarbazine (*DTIC-Dome®*)
Intermittent *in* Glucose 5% *or* Sodium chloride 0.9%
Suggested volume 125–250 mL given over 15–30 minutes; protect infusion from light

Dactinomycin (*Cosmegen Lyovac®*)
Intermittent *or via* drip tubing *in* Glucose 5% *or* Sodium chloride 0.9%
Reconstitute with water for injections

Desferrioxamine mesylate (*Desferal®*)
Continuous *or* intermittent *in* Glucose 5% *or* Sodium chloride 0.9%

Desmopressin (*DDAVP®*)
Intermittent *in* Sodium chloride 0.9%
Dilute with 50 mL and give over 20 minutes

Dexamethasone sodium phosphate (*Decadron®*, *Dexamethasone* (Organon))
Continuous *or* intermittent *or via* drip tubing *in* Glucose 5% *or* Sodium chloride 0.9%
Dexamethasone (Organon) can also be infused in Ringer's solution or Compound sodium lactate

Diazepam (solution) (*Valium®*)
Continuous *in* Glucose 5% *or* Sodium chloride 0.9%
Dilute to a concentration of not more than 40 mg in 500 mL; max. 6 hours between addition and completion of administration; adsorbed to some extent by the plastics of the infusion set

Diazepam (emulsion) (*Diazemuls®*)
Continuous *in* Glucose 5 and 10%
May be diluted to a max. concentration of 200 mg in 500 mL; max. 6 hours between addition and completion of administration; adsorbed to some extent by the plastics of the infusion set
via drip tubing *in* Glucose 5 and 10% *or* Sodium chloride 0.9%
Adsorbed to some extent by the plastics of the infusion set

---

1. Continuous infusion not usually recommended

Table of drugs given by intravenous infusion (*continued*)

Digoxin (*Lanoxin®*)
Continuous *in* Glucose 5% *or* Sodium chloride 0.9%
To be given slowly; see also section 2.1.1

Digoxin-specific antibody fragments (*Digibind®*)
Intermittent *in* Sodium chloride 0.9%
Dissolve initially in water for injections (4 mL/vial) then dilute with the sodium chloride 0.9% and give through a 0.22 micronsterile, disposable filter over 20 minutes

Dinoprostone (*Prostin E2®*)
Continuous *or* intermittent *in* Glucose 5% *or* Sodium chloride 0.9%

Disodium etidronate (*Didronel IV®*)
Continuous *in* Sodium chloride 0.9%
Dilute in large-volume infusion, suggested minimum volume 250 mL; minimum period of infusion 2 hours

Disodium pamidronate (*Aredia®*)
Continuous *in* Sodium chloride 0.9%
Reconstitute each 15 mg with 5 mL water for injections and dilute to a concentration of 15 mg in 125 mL; give each 15 mg over at least 1 hour; not to be given with infusion fluids containing calcium

Disopyramide phosphate (*Rythmodan®*)
Continuous *or* intermittent *in* Glucose 5% *or* Sodium chloride 0.9% *or* Ringer's solution *or* Compound sodium lactate
Max. rate by continuous infusion 20–30 mg/hour (or 400 micrograms/kg/hour)

Dobutamine hydrochloride (*Dobutrex®*)
Continuous *in* Glucose 5% *or* Sodium chloride 0.9%
Dilute to a concentration of 0.5–1 mg/mL and give *via* a controlled infusion device; give higher concentration (max. 5 mg/mL) with infusion pump; incompatible with bicarbonate

Dopamine hydrochloride (*Intropin®*)
Continuous *in* Glucose 5% *or* Sodium chloride 0.9% *or* Compound sodium lactate
Dilute to a concentration of 1.6 mg/mL; incompatible with bicarbonate

Dopexamine hydrochloride (*Dopacard®*)
Continuous *in* Glucose 5% *or* Sodium chloride 0.9%
Dilute to a concentration of 400 or 800 micrograms/mL; give *via* infusion pump or other device which provides accurate control of rate; contact with metal should be minimised; incompatible with bicarbonate

Doxorubicin hydrochloride (*Doxorubicin Rapid Dissolution, Doxorubicin Solution*) (both Farmitalia Carlo Erba)
via drip tubing *in* Glucose 5% *or* Sodium chloride 0.9%
Reconstitute *Doxorubicin Rapid Dissolution* with water for injections or sodium chloride 0.9% (10 mg in 5 mL, 50 mg in 25 mL); give over 2–3 minutes

Electrolytes (*Addiphos®*)
Continuous *in* Glucose 5 and 10%
Suggested volume 500 mL

Enoximone (*Perfan®*)
Continuous *or* intermittent *in* Sodium chloride 0.9% *or* Water for injections
Dilute to a concentration of 2.5 mg/mL; incompatible with glucose solutions; use only plastic containers or syringes

Epirubicin hydrochloride (*Pharmorubicin® Rapid Dissolution, Pharmorubicin® Solution*)
via drip tubing *in* Sodium chloride 0.9%
Reconstitute *Pharmorubicin® Rapid Dissolution* with sodium chloride 0.9% or with water for injections (10 mg in 5 mL, 20 mg in 10 mL, 50 mg in 25 mL); give over 3–5 minutes

Epoprostenol (*Flolan®*)
Continuous *in* Sodium chloride 0.9%
Reconstitute with the diluent provided (pH 10.5) to make a concentrate; use this concentrate within 12 hours and store at 2–8°C; dilute with not more than 6 times the volume of sodium chloride 0.9% before use

Erythromycin lactobionate
Continuous *or* intermittent *in* Glucose 5% (neutralised with sodium bicarbonate) *or* Sodium chloride 0.9% *or* Compound sodium lactate
Dissolve initially in water for injections (1 g in 20 mL) then dilute to a concentration of 1 mg/mL for continuous infusion and 1–5 mg/mL for intermittent infusion

Esmolol hydrochloride (*Brevibloc®*)
Continuous *or* intermittent *in* Glucose 5% *or* Sodium chloride 0.9%
Dilute to a concentration of 10 mg/mL; for continuous infusion use a suitable infusion control device; incompatible with bicarbonate

Ethacrynic acid (sodium salt) (*Edecrin®*)
via drip tubing *in* Glucose 5% *or* Sodium chloride 0.9%
pH of glucose infusion should be adjusted to above 5

Ethanol
Continuous *in* Glucose 5% *or* Sodium chloride 0.9% *or* Ringer's solution *or* Compound sodium lactate
Dilute to a concentration of 5–10%

Etoposide (*Vepesid®*)
Intermittent *in* Sodium chloride 0.9%
Dilute to a concentration of not more than 250 micrograms/mL and give over not less than 30 minutes and not more than 6 hours; check container for haze or precipitate during administration; may dissolve certain types of filter

Filgrastim (*Neupogen®*)
Continuous *or* intermittent *in* Glucose 5%
For a filgrastim concentration of less than 1 500 000 units/mL (15 micrograms/mL) albumin solution (human serum albumin) is added to produce a final albumin concentration of 2 mg/mL; should not be diluted to a filgrastim concentration of less than 200 000 units/mL (2 micrograms/mL) and should not be diluted with sodium chloride solution

Flecainide acetate (*Tambocor®*)
Continuous *or* intermittent *in* Glucose 5% *or* Sodium chloride 0.9% *or* Compound sodium lactate
Minimum volume in infusion fluids containing chlorides 500 mL

Table of drugs given by intravenous infusion (*continued*)

Flucloxacillin sodium (*Floxapen®*)
[1]Intermittent *in* Glucose 5% *or* Sodium chloride 0.9%
Suggested volume 100 mL given over 30–60 minutes
via drip tubing *in* Glucose 5% *or* Sodium chloride 0.9% *or* Ringer's solution *or* Compound sodium lactate

Flumazenil (*Anexate®*)
Continuous *in* Glucose 5% *or* Sodium chloride 0.9%

Fluorouracil sodium
Continuous *or via* drip tubing *in* Glucose 5%
For continuous infusion suggested volume 500 mL given over 4 hours

Folinic acid (calcium salt) (*Calcium Leucovorin®, Refolinon®*)
Continuous *in* Sodium chloride 0.9%
Calcium Leucovorin® can also be infused in Glucose 5 and 10% *or* Compound sodium lactate

Foscarnet trisodium (*Foscavir®*)
Continuous *in* Glucose 5%
Dilute to a concentration of 12 mg/mL or less for infusion into peripheral vein (undiluted solution *via* central venous line only)

Frusemide (sodium salt) (*Lasix®*)
Continuous *in* Sodium chloride 0.9% *or* Ringer's solution
Infusion pH must be above 5.5 and rate should not exceed 4 mg/minute; glucose solutions are unsuitable

Fusidic acid (diethanolamine salt) (*Fucidin®*)
Continuous *in* Glucose 5% (but see below) *or* Sodium chloride 0.9%
Reconstitute with the buffer solution provided and dilute to a max. concentration of diethanolamine fusidate 1.16 mg/mL (= sodium fusidate 1 mg/mL); to be given over not less than 6 hours; incompatible if glucose solution too acidic

Ganciclovir (sodium salt) (*Cymevene®*)
Intermittent *in* Glucose 5% *or* Sodium chloride 0.9% *or* Ringer's solution *or* Compound sodium lactate
Reconstitute initially in water for injections (500 mg/10 mL) then dilute to not more than 10 mg/mL with infusion fluid (usually 100 mL); give over 1 hour through an in-line filter provided

Gentamicin sulphate (*Cidomycin®*)
Intermittent *or via* drip tubing *in* Glucose 5% *or* Sodium chloride 0.9%
Suggested volume for intermittent infusion 50–100 mL given over 20 minutes

Glyceryl trinitrate (*Nitrocine®, Nitronal®, Tridil®*)
Continuous *in* Glucose 5% *or* Sodium chloride 0.9%
For *Tridil®* dilute to a concentration of not more than 400 micrograms/mL; for *Nitrocine®* suggested infusion concentration 100 micrograms/mL; incompatible with polyvinyl chloride infusion containers such as Viaflex® or Steriflex®; use glass or polyethylene containers or give *via* a syringe pump

Granisetron hydrochloride (*Kytril®*)
Intermittent *in* Glucose 5% *or* Sodium chloride 0.9% *or* Compound sodium lactate
Dilute 3 mL in 20–50 mL infusion fluid and give over 5 minutes

Heparin sodium
Continuous *in* Glucose 5% *or* Sodium chloride 0.9%
Administration with a motorised pump advisable

Hydralazine hydrochloride (*Apresoline®*)
Continuous *in* Sodium chloride 0.9% *or* Ringer's solution
Suggested infusion volume 500 mL

Hydrocortisone sodium phosphate (*Efcortesol®*)
Continuous *or* intermittent *or via* drip tubing *in* Glucose 5% *or* Sodium chloride 0.9%

Hydrocortisone sodium succinate (*Efcortelan Soluble®, Solu-Cortef®*)
Continuous *or* intermittent *or via* drip tubing *in* Glucose 5% *or* Sodium chloride 0.9%

Idarubicin hydrochloride (*Zavedos®*)
via drip tubing *in* Sodium chloride 0.9%
Reconstitute with water for injections; give over 5–10 minutes

Ifosfamide (*Mitoxana®*)
Continuous *or* intermittent *or via* drip tubing *in* Glucose 5% *or* Sodium chloride 0.9%
For continuous infusion, suggested volume 3 litres given over 24 hours; for intermittent infusion, give over 30–120 minutes

Imipenem/cilastatin (sodium salt) (*Primaxin®*)
[1]Intermittent *in* Glucose 5% *or* Sodium chloride 0.9%
Dilute to a concentration of 5 mg (as imipenem)/mL; infuse 250–500 mg (as imipenem) over 20–30 minutes, 1 g over 40–60 minutes

Insulin (soluble)
Continuous *in* Sodium chloride 0.9% *or* Compound sodium lactate
Adsorbed to some extent by plastics of infusion set; see also section 6.1.3; ensure insulin is not injected into 'dead space' of injection port of the infusion bag

Isoprenaline hydrochloride (*Saventrine IV®*)
Continuous *in* Glucose 5% *or* Sodium chloride and glucose
Dilute in a large-volume infusion; suggested minimum volume 500 mL; pH of the infusion must be below 5.

Isosorbide dinitrate (*Cedocard IV®, Isoket 0.05®, Isoket 0.1%®*)
Continuous *in* Glucose 5% *or* Sodium chloride 0.9%
Adsorbed to some extent by polyvinyl chloride infusion containers; preferably use glass or polyethylene containers or give *via* a syringe pump; *Isoket 0.05%®* can alternatively be administered undiluted using a syringe pump with a glass or rigid plastic syringe

Kanamycin sulphate (*Kannasyn®*)
Intermittent *in* Glucose 5% *or* Sodium chloride 0.9%
Dilute to 2.5 mg/mL and give at a rate of 3–4 mL/minute

Ketamine hydrochloride (*Ketalar®*)
Continuous *in* Glucose 5% *or* Sodium chloride 0.9%
Dilute to 1 mg/mL; microdrip infusion for maintenance of anaesthesia

1. Continuous infusion not usually recommended

Table of drugs given by intravenous infusion (*continued*)

Labetalol hydrochloride (*Trandate®*)
Intermittent *in* Glucose 5% *or* Sodium chloride and glucose
Dilute to a concentration of 1 mg/mL; suggested volume 200 mL; adjust rate with in-line burette

Lenograstim (*Granocyte®*)
Intermittent *in* Sodium chloride 0.9%
Initially reconstitute with 1 mL water for injection provided (do not shake vigorously) then dilute content of each vial with 100 mL infusion fluid; give over 30 minutes

Lignocaine hydrochloride (*Xylocard 20%®*)
Continuous *in* Glucose 5% *or* Sodium chloride 0.9% *or* Ringer's solution
Suggested infusion concentration 0.2%; use ready-prepared solution when available

Melphalan (*Alkeran®*)
Continuous *or via* drip tubing *in* Sodium chloride 0.9%
Reconstitute with the solvent and diluent provided then dilute with infusion fluid; max. 2 hours between addition and completion of administration

Mesna (*Uromitexan®*)
Continuous *or via* drip tubing *in* Glucose 5% *or* Sodium chloride 0.9%

Metaraminol tartrate (*Aramine®*)
Continuous *or via* drip tubing *in* Glucose 5% *or* Sodium chloride 0.9% *or* Ringer's solution *or* Compound sodium lactate
Suggested infusion volume 500 mL

Methocarbamol (*Robaxin®*)
Intermittent *in* Glucose 5% *or* Sodium chloride 0.9%
Dilute to a concentration of not less than 1 g in 250 mL

Methotrexate sodium (*Methotrexate*) (Lederle)
Continuous *or via* drip tubing *in* Glucose 5% *or* Sodium chloride 0.9% *or* Compound sodium lactate *or* Ringer's solution
Dilute in a large-volume infusion; max. 24 hours between addition and completion of administration

Methyldopate hydrochloride (*Aldomet®*)
Intermittent *in* Glucose 5%
Suggested volume 100 mL given over 30–60 minutes

Methylprednisolone sodium succinate (*Solu-Medrone®*)
Continuous *or* intermittent *or via* drip tubing *in* Glucose 5% *or* Sodium chloride 0.9%
Reconstitute initially with water for injections

Metoclopramide hydrochloride (*Maxolon HighDose®*)
Continuous *or* intermittent *in* Glucose 5% *or* Sodium chloride 0.9% *or* Compound sodium lactate
Loading dose, dilute with 50–100 mL and give over 15–30 minutes; maintenance dose, dilute with 500 mL and give over 8–12 hours; for intermittent infusion dilute with at least 50 mL and give over at least 15 minutes

Mexiletine hydrochloride (*Mexitil®*)
Continuous *in* Glucose 5% *or* Sodium chloride 0.9%

Miconazole (*Daktarin®*)
Continuous *or* intermittent *in* Glucose 5% *or* Sodium chloride 0.9%
Minimum period of infusion 30 minutes; for intermittent infusion suggested volume 200–500 mL

Milrinone (*Primacor®*)
Continuous *in* Glucose 5% *or* Sodium chloride 0.9%
Dilute to a suggested concentration of 200 micrograms/mL

Mitozantrone hydrochloride (*Novantrone®*)
via drip tubing *in* Glucose 5% *or* Sodium chloride 0.9%
Suggested volume at least 50 mL given over at least 3–5 minutes

Molgramostim (*Leucomax®*)
Intermittent *in* Glucose 5% *or* Sodium chloride 0.9%
Reconstitute each vial with 1 mL water for injections; dilute with 25–100 mL infusion fluid to a concentration of not less than 80000 units/mL; give over 4–6 hours; infusion through low protein binding 0.2 or 0.22 micron filter recommended; some infusion sets (e.g. Port-A-Cath®) adsorb molgramostim and should not be used

Mustine hydrochloride (Boots)
via drip tubing *in* Glucose 5% *or* Sodium chloride 0.9%

Naftidrofuryl oxalate (*Praxilene Forte®*)
Intermittent *in* Glucose 5 and 10% *or* Sodium chloride 0.9%
Suggested volume 250–500 mL given over 90–120 minutes

Naloxone (*Min-I-Jet® Naloxone Hydrochloride, Narcan®*)
Continuous *in* Glucose 5% *or* Sodium chloride 0.9%
Dilute to a concentration of 4 micrograms/mL

Netilmicin sulphate (*Netillin®*)
Intermittent *or via* drip tubing *in* Glucose 5 and 10% *or* Sodium chloride 0.9%
For intermittent infusion suggested volume 50–200 mL given over 90–120 minutes

Nimodipine (*Nimotop®*)
via drip tubing *in* Glucose 5% *or* Sodium chloride 0.9% *or* Ringer's solution
Not to be added to infusion container; administer *via* an infusion pump through a Y-piece into a central catheter; incompatible with polyvinyl chloride giving sets or containers; protect infusion from light

Nizatidine (*Axid®*)
Continuous *or* intermittent *in* Glucose 5% *or* Sodium chloride 0.9% *or* Compound sodium lactate
For continuous infusion, dilute 300 mg in 150 mL and give at a rate of 10 mg/hour; for intermittent infusion, dilute 100 mg in 50 mL and give over 15 minutes

Noradrenaline solution strong sterile (*Levophed®*)
Continuous *in* Glucose 5% *or* Sodium chloride and glucose
Dilute in a large-volume infusion; pH of the infusion solution must be below 6

Ondansetron hydrochloride (*Zofran®*)
Continuous *or* intermittent *in* Glucose 5% *or* Sodium chloride 0.9% *or* Ringer's solution

Table of drugs given by intravenous infusion (*continued*)

Oxytocin (*Syntocinon®*)
Continuous *in* Glucose 5%
For *induction or stimulation of labour* dilute 1 unit with
1 litre glucose 5% (preferable to use lower volume given
via controlled infusion device); for *missed abortion* dilute
10–20 units with 500 mL glucose 5%; sodium chloride
0.9% or Ringer's solution may only be used if glucose
clinically inappropriate; close attention to patient's fluid
and electrolyte status essential

Paclitaxel (*Taxol®*)
Continuous *in* Glucose 5% *or* Sodium chloride 0.9%
Begin infusion within 3 hours of dilution; dilute to a
concentration of 0.3–1.2 mg/mL and give through a
0.22 micron in-line filter over 3 hours; not to be used with
PVC equipment (short PVC inlet or outlet on filter may be
acceptable)

Pentamidine isethionate (*Pentacarinat®*)
Intermittent *in* Glucose 5% *or* Sodium chloride 0.9%
Dissolve initially in water for injections (300 mg in 3–5
mL) then dilute in 50–250 mL; give over at least 60
minutes

Pentostatin (*Nipent®*)
Intermittent *in* Glucose 5% *or* Sodium chloride 0.9%
Dilute with 25–50 mL and give over 20–30 minutes

Phenoxybenzamine hydrochloride (*Dibenyline®*)
Intermittent *in* Sodium chloride 0.9%
Dilute in 200–500 mL infusion; give over at least 2
hours; max. 4 hours between dilution and completion of
administration

Phentolamine mesylate (*Rogitine®*)
Intermittent *in* Glucose 5% *or* Sodium chloride 0.9%

Phenylephrine hydrochloride
Intermittent *in* Glucose 5% *or* Sodium chloride 0.9%

Piperacillin sodium (*Pipril®*)
Intermittent *in* Glucose 5% *or* Sodium chloride 0.9%
or Compound sodium lactate *or* Water for injections
Minimum volume 50 mL given over 20–40 minutes

Piperacillin/tazobactam (sodium salts) (*Tazocin®*)
Intermittent *in* Glucose 5% *or* Sodium chloride 0.9%
or Water for injections
Reconstitute initially with water for injections or
sodium chloride infusion 0.9% (2.25 g in 10 mL, 4.5 g in
20 mL) then dilute with 50 mL infusion fluid; give over
20–30 minutes

Plicamycin (*Mithracin®*)
Continuous *in* Glucose 5% *or* Sodium chloride 0.9%
Reconstitute 2.5 mg with 4.9 mL water for injections
then dilute appropriate dose to suggested volume of
1000 mL given over 4–6 hours

Potassium canrenoate (*Spiroctan-M®*)
Intermittent *in* Glucose 5% *or* Sodium chloride 0.9%
Suggested volume 250 mL

Potassium chloride
Continuous *in* Glucose 5% *or* Sodium chloride 0.9%
Dilute in a large-volume infusion; mix thoroughly to
avoid 'layering', especially in non-rigid infusion
containers; use ready-prepared solutions when possible

Procainamide hydrochloride (*Pronestyl®*)
Continuous *or* intermittent *in* Glucose 5%
For maintenance, dilute to a concentration of *either*
2 mg/mL and give at a rate of 1–3 mL/minute *or* 4 mg/
mL and give at a rate of 0.5–1.5 mL/minute

Propofol (emulsion) (*Diprivan®*)
via drip tubing *in* Glucose 5% *or* Sodium chloride
0.9%
Not to be mixed with other therapeutic agents or
infusion fluids; to be administered *via* a Y-piece close to
injection site
Continuous *in* Glucose 5%
Dilute to a concentration not less than 2 mg/mL;
administer using suitable device to control infusion rate;
use glass or PVC containers (if PVC bag used it should be
full—withdraw volume of infusion fluid equal to that of
propofol to be added); give within 6 hours of preparation;
propofol may alternatively be infused undiluted using a
suitable infusion pump

Quinine dihydrochloride
Continuous *in* Sodium chloride 0.9%
To be given over 4 hours; see also section 5.4.1

Ranitidine hydrochloride (*Zantac®*)
Intermittent *in* Glucose 5% *or* Sodium chloride 0.9%
or Compound sodium lactate

Rifampicin (*Rifadin®*, *Rimactane®*)
Intermittent *in* Glucose 5 and 10% *or* Sodium
chloride 0.9% *or* Ringer's solution
Reconstitute with solvent provided then dilute with
250 mL (*Rimactane®*) or 500 mL (*Rifadin®*) infusion
fluid; give over 2–3 hours

Ritodrine hydrochloride (*Yutopar®*)
Continuous *in* Glucose 5%
Give *via* controlled infusion device, preferably a
syringe pump; if syringe pump available dilute to a
concentration of 3 mg/mL; if syringe pump not available
dilute to a concentration of 300 micrograms/mL; close
attention to patient's fluid and electrolyte status essential

Rocuronium bromide (*Esmeron®*)
Continuous *or via* drip tubing *in* Glucose 5% *or*
Sodium chloride 0.9%

Salbutamol sulphate (*Ventolin® For Intravenous
Infusion*)
Continuous *in* Glucose 5%
For *bronchodilatation* dilute 5 mg with 500 mL glucose
5% or sodium chloride 0.9%; for *premature labour* dilute
with glucose 5% to a concentration not exceeding
500 micrograms/mL (preferable to use low volume); give
via controlled infusion device; close attention to patient's
fluid and electrolyte status essential

Salcatonin (*Miacalcic®*)
Continuous *in* Sodium chloride 0.9%
Diluted solution given without delay; dilute in 500 mL
and give over at least 6 hours; glass or hard plastic
containers should not be used; approx. 20% loss of
potency on dilution (take into account when calculating
dose)

Sodium calciumedetate (*Ledclair®*)
Continuous *in* Glucose 5% *or* Sodium chloride 0.9%
Dilute to a concentration of not more than 3%;
suggested volume 250–500 mL given over at least 1 hour

---

1. Continuous infusion not usually recommended

Table of drugs given by intravenous infusion (continued)

Sodium clodronate (*Bonefos® Concentrate, Loron®*)
Continuous *in* Sodium chloride 0.9%
Dilute 300 mg in 500 mL and give over at least 2 hours (*or* 1.5 g in 500 mL and give over 4 hours—*Bonefos® Concentrate* only); *Bonefos® Concentrate* can also be diluted in Glucose 5%

Sodium nitroprusside (*Nipride®*)
Continuous *in* Glucose 5% *or* Sodium chloride 0.9% *or* Ringer's solution *or* Compound sodium lactate
Reconstitute with solvent provided then dilute immediately with 250–1000 mL infusion fluid; preferably infuse *via* infusion device to allow precise control; protect infusion from light

Sodium valproate (*Epilim®*)
Continuous *or* intermittent *in* Glucose 5% *or* Sodium chloride 0.9%
Reconstitute with solvent provided then dilute with infusion fluid

Streptokinase (*Kabikinase®, Streptase®*)
Continuous *in* Sodium chloride 0.9%
Kabikinase® can also be infused in Glucose 5%

Sulphadiazine sodium
Continuous *in* Sodium chloride 0.9%
Suggested volume 500 mL; ampoule solution has a pH of over 10

Suxamethonium chloride (*Anectine®, Scoline®*)
Continuous *in* Glucose 5% *or* Sodium chloride 0.9%

Teicoplanin (*Targocid®*)
[1]Intermittent *in* Glucose 5% *or* Sodium chloride 0.9% *or* Compound sodium lactate
Reconstitute initially with water for injections provided; infuse over 30 minutes

Temocillin sodium (*Temopen®*)
Intermittent *in* Glucose 5% *or* Sodium chloride 0.9% *or* Ringer's solution *or* Compound sodium lactate
Dissolve initially in water for injections (500 mg in 10 mL; 1–2 g in 20 mL) then dilute with infusion fluid and give over 30–40 minutes

Terbutaline sulphate (*Bricanyl®*)
Continuous *in* Glucose 5%
For *bronchodilatation* dilute 1.5–2.5 mg with 500 mL glucose 5% or sodium chloride 0.9% and give over 8–10 hours; for *premature labour* dilute in glucose 5% and give *via* controlled infusion device preferably a syringe pump; if syringe pump available dilute to a concentration of 100 micrograms/mL; if syringe pump not available dilute to a concentration of 10 micrograms/mL; close attention to patient's fluid and electrolyte status essential

Tetracycline hydrochloride (*Achromycin Intravenous®*)
Continuous *in* Glucose 5% *or* Sodium chloride 0.9% *or* Compound sodium lactate
Reconstitute initially with water for injections (250 mg in 5 mL, 500 mg in 10 mL) then dilute to at least 100 mL (max. 1 litre) and give at a rate not exceeding 100 mL in 5 minutes preferably through a 0.22 micron filter

Theophylline (solubilised with lysine) (*Labophylline®*)
Continuous *in* Glucose 5% *or* Sodium chloride 0.9%

Ticarcillin sodium (*Ticar®*)
Intermittent *in* Glucose 5% *or* Water for injections
Suggested volume 100–150 mL given over 30–40 minutes

Ticarcillin sodium/clavulanic acid (*Timentin®*)
Intermittent *in* Glucose 5% *or* Water for injections
Suggested volume glucose 5%, 50–150 mL (depending on dose) or water for injections, 25–100 mL; given over 30–40 minutes

Tobramycin sulphate (*Nebcin®*)
Intermittent *or via* drip tubing *in* Glucose 5% *or* Sodium chloride 0.9%
For adult intermittent infusion suggested volume 50–100 mL (children proportionately smaller volume) given over 20–60 minutes

Tocainide hydrochloride (*Tonocard®*)
Intermittent *in* Glucose 5% *or* Sodium chloride 0.9%
Suggested volume 50–100 mL given over 15–30 minutes

Tramadol hydrochloride (*Zydol®*)
Continuous *or* intermittent *in* Glucose 5% *or* Sodium chloride 0.9%

Treosulfan (*Treosulfan*) (Medac)
Intermittent *in* Water for injections
Infusion suggested for doses above 5 g; dilute to a concentration of 5 g in 100 mL

Trimetaphan camsylate (*Arfonad®*)
Intermittent *in* Sodium chloride 0.9% *or* Sodium chloride and glucose
Dilute to a concentration of 0.05–0.1% (0.25% if fluid restriction necessary)

Trimethoprim lactate (*Monotrim®*)
via drip tubing *in* Glucose 5% *or* Sodium chloride 0.9% *or* Compound sodium lactate

Trisodium edetate (*Limclair®*)
Continuous *in* Glucose 5% *or* Sodium chloride 0.9%
Suggested volume 500 mL given over 2–3 hours

Tropisetron hydrochloride (*Navoban®*)
Intermittent *or via* drip tubing *in* Glucose 5% *or* Sodium chloride 0.9% *or* Ringer's solution
Suggested volume for infusion 100 mL

Urokinase (*Urokinase*) (Leo)
Continuous *in* Sodium chloride 0.9%

Vancomycin hydrochloride (*Vancocin®*)
[1]Intermittent *in* Glucose 5% *or* Sodium chloride 0.9%
Reconstitute 500 mg with 10 mL water for injections and dilute to 100–200 mL with infusion fluid; give over at least 60 minutes (rate not to exceed 10 mg/minute for doses over 500mg); use continuous infusion only if intermittent not feasible

Vasopressin, synthetic (*Pitressin®*)
Intermittent *in* Glucose 5%
Suggested concentration 20 units/100 mL given over 15 minutes

Vecuronium bromide (*Norcuron®*)
Continuous *in* Glucose 5% *or* Sodium chloride 0.9% *or* Ringer's solution
Reconstitute with the solvent provided

Vinblastine sulphate (*Velbe®*)
via drip tubing *in* Sodium chloride 0.9%
Reconstitute with the diluent provided; give within approx. 1 minute

Table of drugs given by intravenous infusion (*continued*)

Vincristine sulphate (*Oncovin®*)
via drip tubing *in* Glucose 5% *or* Sodium chloride 0.9%

Vindesine sulphate (*Eldisine®*)
via drip tubing *in* Glucose 5% *or* Sodium chloride 0.9%
Reconstitute with the diluent provided

Vitamins B & C (*Pabrinex® I/V High potency*)
Intermittent *or via* drip tubing *in* Glucose 5% *or* Sodium chloride 0.9%
Ampoule contents should be mixed, diluted, and administered without delay; give over 10 minutes (see CSM advice, section 9.6.2)

Vitamins, multiple
(*Multibionta®*)
Intermittent *in* Glucose 5% *or* Sodium chloride 0.9%
Dilute 10 mL in not less than 250 mL of infusion fluid (adults); see also section 9.3
(*Solivito N®*)
Intermittent *in* Glucose 5 and 10%
Suggested volume 500–1000 mL given over 2–3 hours; see also section 9.3

Zidovudine (*Retrovir®*)
Intermittent *in* Glucose 5%
Dilute to a concentration of 2 mg/mL or 4 mg/mL and give over 1 hour

---

1. Continuous infusion not usually recommended

Appendix 7: Borderline Substances

In certain conditions some foods (and toilet preparations) have characteristics of drugs and the Advisory Committee on Borderline Substances advises as to the circumstances in which such substances may be regarded as drugs. Prescriptions issued in accordance with the Committee's advice and endorsed 'ACBS' will normally not be investigated.

General Practitioners are reminded that the ACBS recommends products on the basis that they may be regarded as drugs for the management of specified conditions. Doctors should satisfy themselves that the products can safely be prescribed, that patients are adequately monitored and that, where necessary, expert hospital supervision is available.

FOODS WHICH MAY BE PRESCRIBED ON FP10

Note. This is a list of food products which the ACBS has approved. The clinical condition for which the product has approval follows each entry.

Advera® (Abbott)

Liquid, providing protein 14.2 g, carbohydrate 51.1 g, fat 5.4 g, energy 1262 kJ (299 kcal)/237 mL, with vitamins and minerals. Gluten-free. Orange and chocolate flavours. Net price 237-mL can = £2.26. For use as a necessary nutritional supplement prescribed on medical grounds for: short-bowel syndrome, intractable malabsorption, pre-operative preparation of patients who are undernourished, proven inflammatory bowel disease, following total gastrectomy, bowel fistulas, disease-related malnutrition. Not to be prescribed for any child under 5 years of age

Aglutella® (Ultrapharm)

Rice, low protein. Net price 500 g = £3.95. For phenylketonuria, similar amino acid abnormalities, renal failure, liver failure and liver cirrhosis

AL 110® (Nestlé)

Powder, protein 14 g, fat 25 g, carbohydrate 55.3 g, energy 2100 kJ (502 kcal)/100 g with vitamins and minerals. Net price 400 g = £7.27. For proven lactose intolerance in pre-school children, galactosaemia, and galactokinase deficiency

Albumaid® (Scientific Hospital Supplies)

Albumaid XP, powder, amino acids 40%, carbohydrate 50%, fat nil, phenylalanine not more than 10 mg per 100 g, with vitamins, minerals, and trace elements. Net price 200 g = £20.87. For phenylketonuria

Albumaid XP Concentrate, powder, amino acids 85%, carbohydrate and fat nil, phenylalanine not more than 25 mg per 100 g, with vitamins, minerals, and trace elements. Net price 200 g = £36.54. For phenylketonuria

Alcoholic Beverages see under Rectified Spirit

Alembicol D® (Alembic Products)

Fractionated coconut oil. Net price 5 kg = £123.00. For steatorrhoea associated with cystic fibrosis of the pancreas, intestinal lymphangiectasia, surgery of the intestine, chronic liver disease, liver cirrhosis, other proven malabsorption syndromes; and in a ketogenic diet in the management of epilepsy

Alfare® (Nestlé)

Powder, protein 16.5 g, fat 24 g, carbohydrate 51.7 g, energy 2010 kJ (480 kcal) /100 g with vitamins and minerals. Net price 400 g = £5.49. For disaccharide and whole protein intolerance, or where amino acids or peptides are indicated in conjunction with medium chain triglycerides

Amino Acid Modules (Scientific Hospital Supplies)

Leucine-Free Amino Acid Mix, powder, essential and non-essential amino acids 93%, except leucine. Net price 200 g = £45.08. For isovaleric acidaemia.

Methionine, Threonine, Valine-Free and Isoleucine-Low Amino Acid Mix, powder, essential and non-essential amino acids 93%, except methionine, threonine, and valine, with trace amounts of isoleucine. Net price 200 g = £45.08. For methylmalonic or propionic acidaemia.

Phenylalanine, Tyrosine, and Methionine-Free Amino Acid Mix, powder, essential and non-essential amino acids 93%, except methionine, phenylalanine, and tyrosine. Net price 200 g = £45.08. For tyrosinaemia type I where plasma concentrations are above normal

Tyrosine and Phenylalanine-Free Amino Acid Mix, powder, essential and non-essential amino acids 93%, except phenylalanine and tyrosine. Net price 200 g = £45.08. For tyrosinaemia where plasma concentrations are normal

Aminogran® (UCB Pharma)

Food Supplement, powder, containing all essential amino acids except phenylalanine, for use with mineral mixture (see below). Net price 500 g = £42.77. For phenylketonuria

Mineral Mixture, powder, containing all appropriate minerals for use with the above food supplement and other synthetic diets. Net price 250 g = £7.24. For phenylketonuria and as a mineral supplement in synthetic diets

Analog® (Scientific Hospital Supplies)

Note. Analog products are generally intended for use in children up to 1 year

Analog MSUD, powder, essential and non-essential amino acids 15.5% except isoleucine, leucine and valine, with carbohydrate, fat, vitamins, minerals, and trace elements. Net price 400 g = £20.78. For maple syrup urine disease

Analog RVHB, powder, essential and non-essential amino acids 15.5% except methionine, with carbohydrate, fat, vitamins, minerals, and trace elements. Net price 400 g = £20.78. For hypermethioninaemia; homocystinuria

Analog XLeu, powder, essential and non-essential amino acids 15.5% except leucine, with carbohydrate, fat, vitamins, minerals, and trace elements. Net price 400 g = £20.78. For isovaleric acidaemia

Analog XLys, powder, essential and non-essential amino acids 15.5% except lysine, with carbohydrate, fat, vitamins, minerals, and trace elements. Net price 400 g = £20.78. For hyperlysinaemia

Analog XMet, Thre, Val, Isoleu, powder, essential and non-essential amino acids 15.5% except methionine, threonine, valine and low isoleucine, with carbohydrate, fat, vitamins, minerals, and trace elements. Net price 400 g = £20.78. For methylmalonic or propionic acidaemia

Analog XP, powder, essential and non-essential amino acids 15.5% except phenylalanine, with carbohydrate, fat, vitamins, minerals, and trace elements. Net price 400 g = £15.54. For phenylketonuria

Analog XPhen, Tyr, powder, essential and non-essential amino acids 15.5% except phenylalanine and tyrosine, with carbohydrate, fat, vitamins, minerals and trace elements. Net price 400 g = £20.78. For tyrosinaemia

Aproten® (Ultrapharm)

Various products, gluten-free, low protein, low Na^+ and K^+. Net prices: anellini 500 g = £3.95; biscuits 180 g (36) = £2.80; bread mix 250 g = £2.00; cake mix 300 g = £2.10; crispbread 240 g = £3.95; ditalini 500 g = £3.95; flour 300 g = £1.84; rigatini 500 g = £3.95; spaghetti 500 g = £3.95; tagliatelle 250 g = £2.10. For phenylketonuria; similar amino acid abnormalities; renal failure; liver failure and liver cirrhosis; gluten-sensitive enteropathies including steatorrhoea due to gluten sensitivity, coeliac disease, and dermatitis herpetiformis

Arnott ® (Ultrapharm)

Rice Cookies, gluten-free. Net price 200 g = £1.68. For gluten-sensitive enteropathies including steatorrhoea due to gluten sensitivity, coeliac disease, and dermatitis herpetiformis

Barkat® (Gluten Free Foods)

Bread mix, gluten-free. Net price 500g = £3.60. For gluten-sensitive enteropathies including steatorrhoea due to gluten sensitivity, coeliac disease, and dermatitis herpetiformis

Bi-Aglut® (Ultrapharm)

Biscuits, gluten-free. Net price 180 g (36) = £2.60

Cracker toast, gluten-, lactose-, and milk-protein-free. Net price 240 g (40) = £3.60. For gluten-sensitive enteropathies including steatorrhoea due to gluten sensitivity, coeliac disease, dermatitis herpetiformis

Calogen® (Scientific Hospital Supplies)

Emulsion, arachis oil 50% in water. Net price 250 mL = £3.18; 1 litre = £11.49. For renal failure and other conditions requiring a high-energy, low-fluid, low-electrolyte diet, disorders of amino acid metabolism or carbohydrate absorption; in a ketogenic diet in the management of epilepsy

Caloreen® (Clintec)

Powder, water-soluble dextrins, with less than 1.8 mmol of Na^+ and 0.3 mmol of $K^+/100$ g. Net price 250 g = £1.51; 5 kg = £24.79. For renal failure; liver cirrhosis; disaccharide intolerance (without isomaltose intolerance), disorders of amino acid metabolism (and other similar disorders) and /or whole protein intolerance; malabsorption states and other conditions (including proven hypoglycaemia) requiring a high energy, low fluid intake, whether or not sodium and /or potassium restriction is essential

Caprilon Formula® (Cow & Gate)

Powder, protein 11.8%, carbohydrate 55.1%, fat 28.3% (medium chain triglycerides 21.3%). Low in lactose, gluten- and sucrose-free. Used as a 12.7% solution. Net price 420 g = £10.10. For disorders in which a high intake of MCT is beneficial

Note. Caprilon Formula replaces MCT (1) powder

Carobel, Instant® (Cow & Gate)

Powder, carob seed flour. Net price 45 g = £2.63. For thickening feeds in the treatment of vomiting

Casilan® (Crookes)

Powder, whole protein, containing all essential amino acids, 90% with less than 0.1% Na^+. Net price 250 g = £4.40. For biochemically proven hypoproteinaemia

Clinifeed® (Clintec)

Clinifeed 400, protein 15 g, carbohydrate 55 g, fat 13.4 g, energy 1674 kJ (400 kcal)/375 mL, with vitamins and minerals, vanilla flavour. Fructose free. Net price 375-mL can = £1.20

Clinifeed Protein Rich, protein 30 g, carbohydrate 70 g, fat 11 g, energy 2092 kJ (500 kcal)/375 mL, with vitamins and minerals, vanilla flavour. Fructose- and lactose-free. Net price 375-mL can = £1.40

Both for use as necessary nutritional supplements prescribed on medical grounds for: short bowel syndrome, intractable malabsorption, pre-operative preparation of patients who are undernourished, proven inflammatory bowel disease, following total gastrectomy, dysphagia, bowel fistulas, disease-related malnutrition, continuous ambulatory peritoneal dialysis (CAPD), and haemodialysis. Not to be prescribed for any child under one year; use with caution for young children up to 5 years of age

Clinifeed Favour, protein 14.1 g, carbohydrate 49.9 g, fat 14.6 g, energy 1575 kJ (375 kcal)/375 mL, with vitamins and minerals, neutral flavour. Lactose-, fructose-, and sucrose-free. Net price 375-mL can = 97p; 500-mL Dripac = £1.90

Clinifeed Iso, protein 10.5 g, carbohydrate 49.2 g, fat 15.4 g, energy 1575 kJ (375 kcal)/375 mL, with vitamins and minerals, vanilla flavour. Fructose- and sucrose-free, and low sodium. Net price 375-mL can = £1.36

Both for use as the sole source of nutrition or as necessary nutritional supplements prescribed on medical grounds for: short bowel syndrome, intractable malabsorption, pre-operative preparation of patients who are undernourished, proven inflammatory bowel disease, following total gastrectomy, dysphagia, bowel fistulas, disease-related malnutrition. Not to be prescribed for any child under one year; use with caution for young children up to 5 years of age

Comminuted Chicken Meat (Cow & Gate)

Suspension (aqueous). Net price 150 g = £2.01. For carbohydrate intolerance in association with possible or proven intolerance of milk; glucose and galactose intolerance

Corn flour and corn starch. For hypoglycaemia associated with glycogen-storage disease

Corn oil (maize oil). Net price 100 mL = 25p. For familial hypercholesterolaemia

Dialamine® (Scientific Hospital Supplies)

Powder, essential amino acids 30%, with carbohydrate 62%, energy 1500 kJ (360 kcal)/100 g, with ascorbic acid, minerals, and trace elements. Flavour: orange. Net price 200 g = £17.43. For oral feeding where essential amino acid supplements are required; e.g. chronic renal failure, hypoproteinaemia, wound fistula leakage with excessive protein loss, conditions requiring a controlled nitrogen intake, and haemodialysis

dp® (Nutricia)

Cookies, low-protein, butterscotch- or chocolate-flavoured chip cookies. Net price 170 g = £5.64. For phenylketonuria; similar amino acid abnormalities; renal failure; liver failure and liver cirrhosis

Duobar® (Scientific Hospital Supplies)

Bar, protein-free (phenylalanine nil added), carbohydrate 56 g, fat 42 g, energy 2450 kJ (600 kcal)/100 g. Low sodium and potassium.

Strawberry and vanilla flavours. Net price 100-g bar = £1.75. For children and adults on protein-restricted diets and for conditions where there is a need for energy fortification and where fluid intake is restricted, such as renal disease, disorders of amino-acid metabolism, and liver disease

Duocal® (Scientific Hospital Supplies)

Liquid, emulsion providing carbohydrate 23.4 g, fat 7.1 g, energy 628 kJ (150 kcal)/100 mL. Low-electrolyte, gluten-, lactose-, and protein-free. Net price 250 mL = £1.70; 1 litre = £6.05

Super Soluble Powder, carbohydrate 72.7 g, fat 22.3 g, energy 1988 kJ (473 kcal)/100 g. Low electrolyte, gluten-, protein-, and lactose-free. Net price 400 g = £10.72.

Both for renal failure; liver cirrhosis; disaccharide intolerance (without isomaltose intolerance), disorders of amino acid metabolism (and other similar disorders), and /or whole protein intolerance; malabsorption states and other conditions requiring a high energy, low fluid intake, whether or not sodium and /or potassium restriction is essential

Elemental 028® (Scientific Hospital Supplies)

Powder, amino acids 12%, carbohydrate 70.5−72%, fat 6.64%, energy 1544−1568 kJ (364−370 kcal)/100 g with vitamins and minerals. For preparation with water before use. Net price 100-g box (orange flavoured or plain) = £3.82. For use as the sole source of nutrition or as a necessary nutritional supplement prescribed on medical grounds for: short-bowel syndrome, intractable malabsorption, proven inflammatory bowel disease, bowel fistulas. Not to be prescribed for any child under one year; use with caution for young children up to 5 years of age

Ener-G® (General Designs)

Gluten-free. Rice bread (sliced), brown, net price 200 g = £1.80, 400 g = £3.45; white, 200 g = £1.80. Tapioca bread (sliced), 200 g = £1.80. Rice pasta (macaroni, shells, small shells, and lasagna), 454 g = £3.45; spaghetti, 447 g = £3.45; tagliatelle and vermicelli, 300g = £3.45; cannelloni, 284 g = £3.45. Brown rice pasta: lasagne, 454 g = £3.45; macaroni, 454 g = £3.45; spaghetti, 447 g = £3.45. For gluten-sensitive enteropathies including steatorrhoea due to gluten sensitivity, coeliac disease, and dermatitis herpetiformis

Enrich® (Abbott)

Liquid with dietary fibre, providing protein 9.4 g, carbohydrate 38.3 g (including 5 g as dietary fibre), fat 8.8 g, energy 1090 kJ (260 kcal)/250 mL with vitamins and minerals. Lactose- and gluten-free. Vanilla and chocolate flavours. Net price 250-mL can = £1.74. For use as the sole source of nutrition or as a necessary nutritional supplement prescribed on medical grounds for: short-bowel syndrome, intractable malabsorption, pre-operative preparation of patients who are undernourished, proven inflammatory bowel disease, following total gastrectomy, dysphagia, disease-related malnutrition. Not to be prescribed for any child under one year; use with caution for young children up to 5 years of age

Ensure® (Abbott)

Liquid, protein 3.7%, fat 3.7%, carbohydrate 14.5%, with minerals and vitamins, lactose- and gluten-free, energy 1050 kJ (253 kcal)/250 mL. Vanilla flavour. Net price 237-mL bottle = £1.59; 250-mL can = £1.47. Chocolate, coffee, eggnog, nut, chicken, mushroom, and asparagus flavours. Net price 250-mL can = £1.47.

Powder, same composition as Ensure liquid when reconstituted. Net price 400 g = £6.23

Both for use as the sole source of nutrition or as a necessary nutritional supplement prescribed on medical grounds for: short bowel syndrome, intractable malabsorption, pre-operative preparation of patients who are undernourished, proven inflammatory bowel disease, following total gastrectomy, dysphagia, bowel fistulas, disease-related malnutrition. Neither to be prescribed for any child under one year; use with caution for young children up to 5 years of age

Ensure Plus® (Abbott)

Liquid, protein 6.3%, fat 5%, carbohydrate 20%, with vitamins and minerals, lactose- and gluten-free, energy 1570 kJ (375 kcal)/250 mL. Vanilla flavour. Net price 250-mL can = £1.84; 500-mL bottle = £3.68. Caramel, chocolate, strawberry, banana, fruit of the forest, raspberry, orange and vanilla flavours. Net price 200-mL Tetrapak = £1.37. As a necessary nutritional supplement prescribed on medical grounds for: short bowel syndrome, intractable malabsorption, pre-operative preparation of patients who are undernourished, proven inflammatory bowel disease, following total gastrectomy, dysphagia, bowel fistulas, disease-related malnutrition, continuous ambulatory peritoneal dialysis (CAPD), and haemodialysis. Not to be prescribed for any child under one year; use with caution for young children up to 5 years of age

Entera® (Fresenius)

Liquid, protein 11.3 g, carbohydrate 37.6 g, fat 11.66 g, energy 1260 kJ (300 kcal)/200 mL, with vitamins and minerals. Vanilla, strawberry, butterscotch, blackcurrant, chocolate-mint, vegetable cream, and neutral flavours. Net price 200-mL Tetrabrik = £1.35. For use as sole source of nutrition or as a necessary nutritional supplement prescribed on medical grounds for: short-bowel syndrome, intractable malabsorption, pre-operative preparation of patients who are undernourished, proven inflammatory bowel disease, following total gastrectomy, dysphagia, bowel fistulas, disease-related malnutrition. Not to be prescribed for any child under one year; use with caution for young children up to 5 years of age

Note. Entera replaces Fresubin High Energy 236-mL Tetrabrik

Farley's Gluten-free biscuits (Farley)

Biscuits. Net price 200 g = £1.38. For gluten-sensitive enteropathies including steatorrhoea due to gluten sensitivity, coeliac disease and dermatitis herpetiformis

Flexical® (Bristol-Myers)

Powder, protein 9.9%, carbohydrate 67%, fat 15% with vitamins and minerals. Gluten- and lactose-free. Net price 454 g = £9.36. For use as the sole source of nutrition or as a necessary nutritional supplement prescribed on medical grounds for: short-bowel syndrome, intractable malabsorption, proven inflammatory bowel disease, bowel fistulas. Not to be prescribed for any child under one year; use with caution for young children up to 5 years of age

Forceval Protein® (Unigreg)

Powder, calcium caseinate 60%, carbohydrate 30%, with vitamins and minerals, providing not less than 55% protein, not more than 1% of fat, not more than 0.12% of Na^+. Lactose- and gluten-free. Neutral flavour. Net price 300 g = £12.00; 8 × 15g-sachets = £5.12. For biochemically proven hypoproteinaemia

Formance® (Abbott)

Semi-solid, protein 6.8 g, carbohydrate 34.0 g, fat 9.7 g, energy 1050 KJ (250 kcal)/142 g with vitamins and minerals. Gluten-free. Vanilla, chocolate, and butterscotch flavours. Net price 142-g can = £1.66. As a necessary nutritional supplement prescribed on medical grounds for: short bowel syndrome, intractable malabsorption, pre-operative preparation of patients who are undernourished, proven inflammatory bowel disease, following total gastrectomy, dysphagia, bowel fistulas, disease-related malnutrition, continuous ambulatory peritoneal dialysis (CAPD), and haemodialysis. Not to be prescribed for any child under one year; use with caution for young children up to 5 years of age

Fortical® see **Polycal® Liquid**

Fortimel® (Cow & Gate)

Liquid, protein 19.4 g, carbohydrate 20.8 g, fat 4.2 g, energy 840 kJ (200 kcal)/200 mL with vitamins and minerals. Vanilla, strawberry, chocolate, coffee, apricot, and forest fruits flavours. Net price 200-mL carton = £1.05. As a necessary nutritional supplement prescribed on medical grounds for: short bowel syndrome, intractable malabsorption, pre-operative preparation of patients who are undernourished, proven inflammatory bowel disease, following total gastrectomy, dysphagia, bowel fistulas, disease-related malnutrition. Not to be prescribed for any child under one year; use with caution for young children up to 5 years of age

Fortipudding® (Cow & Gate)

Semi-solid, protein 15.3 g, carbohydrate 24 g, fat 4.5 g, energy 825 kJ (196 kcal)/150 g with vitamins and minerals. Vanilla, chocolate, and coffee flavours. Net price 150-g tub = £1.09. As a necessary nutritional supplement prescribed on medical grounds for: short bowel syndrome, intractable malabsorption, pre-operative preparation of patients who are undernourished, proven inflammatory bowel disease, following total gastrectomy, dysphagia, bowel fistulas, disease-related malnutrition or growth failure, continuous ambulatory peritoneal dialysis (CAPD) and haemodialysis. Not to be prescribed for any child under one year; use with caution for young children up to 5 years of age

Fortisip® (Cow & Gate)

Liquid, protein 10 g, carbohydrate 35.8 g, fat 13 g, energy 1260 kJ (300 kcal)/200 mL, with vitamins and minerals. Gluten-free and low lactose. Vanilla, banana, orange, strawberry, tropical fruits, mushroom, and neutral flavours. Net price 200 mL = £1.37. As a necessary nutritional supplement prescribed on medical grounds for: short-bowel syndrome, intractable malabsorption, pre-operative preparation of patients who are undernourished, proven inflammatory bowel disease, following total gastrectomy, dysphagia, disease-related malnutrition. Not to be prescribed for any child under one year; use with caution for young children up to 5 years of age

Fortison® see **Nutrison®**

Fresenius OPD® (Fresenius)

Liquid, protein 22.5 g, carbohydrate 75 g, fat 13 g, energy 2100kJ (500 kcal)/500 mL, with vitamins, minerals, and trace elements. Gluten-free, and low lactose. Net price 500-mL bottle = £3.99. As a necessary nutritional supplement prescribed on medical grounds for: short bowel syndrome, intractable malabsorption, pre-operative preparation of patients who are undernourished, proven inflammatory bowel disease, following total gastrectomy, dysphagia, bowel fistulas, disease-related malnutrition. Not to be prescribed for any child under one year; use with caution for young children up to 5 years of age

Fresubin® (Fresenius)

Liquid, protein 7.6 g, carbohydrate 27.6 g, fat 6.8 g, energy 840 kJ (200 kcal) /200 mL with vitamins and minerals. Gluten-free, low lactose and cholesterol. Net price 200-mL carton (nut, peach, black currant, chocolate, mocha, and vanilla flavours) = £1.09; 500-mL bottle (nut, peach, and vanilla flavours) = £2.35. For use as the sole source of nutrition or as a necessary nutritional supplement prescribed on medical grounds for: short-bowel syndrome, intractable malabsorption, pre-operative preparation of patients who are undernourished, proven inflammatory bowel disease, following total gastrectomy, dysphagia, bowel fistulas, disease-related malnutrition, and Refsum's disease. Not to be prescribed for any child under one year; use with caution for young children up to 5 years of age

High Energy Liquid, protein 28 g, carbohydrate 94 g, fat 29 g, energy 3150 kJ (750 kcal)/500 mL with vitamins and minerals. Gluten-free, cholesterol-free and low lactose. Net price 500-mL bottle = £3.10. For indications, see under Fresubin liquid (except Refsum's disease). Not to be prescribed for any child under 2 years; use with caution for young children up to 5 years of age

Note. Fresubin High Energy 236-mL Tetrabrik replaced by Entera

Fresubin Isofibre® (Fresenius)

Liquid with dietary fibre, protein 19 g, carbohydrate 69 g, fat 17 g, energy 2100 kJ(500 kcal)/500 mL, with vitamins and minerals. Net price 500-mL bottle = £3.10. Neutral flavour. For use as sole source of nutrition or as a necessary nutritional supplement prescribed on medical grounds for: short-bowel syndrome, intractable malabsorption, pre-operative preparation of patients who are undernourished, proven inflammatory bowel disease, following total gastrectomy, dysphagia, disease-related malnutrition. Not to be prescribed for any child under 2 years; use with caution for young children up to 5 years of age

Fresubin Plus F® (Fresenius)

Liquid foods with dietary fibre in 2 formulations. For use as the sole source of nutrition or as a necessary nutritional supplement prescribed on medical grounds for: short-bowel syndrome, intractable malabsorption, pre-operative preparation of patients who are undernourished, proven inflammatory bowel disease, following total gastrectomy, dysphagia, disease-related malnutrition. Not to be prescribed for any child under 1 year; use with caution for young children up to 5 years of age

Muesli-flavour, milk protein, cereals, coconut, sunflower oil, vitamins and minerals providing protein 19g, fat 17g, carbohydrate 69g, fibre 5g, energy 2100 kJ (500kcal)/500mL. Low sodium, lactose, and cholesterol. Net price 200 mL carton = £1.15; 500 mL bottle = £2.65

Vegetable soup-flavour, milk protein, beef fat and protein, sunflower oil, maize starch, vitamins and minerals providing protein 19 g, fat 17 g, carbohydrate 69 g, fibre 3 g, energy 2100 kJ (500 kcal)/500 mL. Gluten-free, low sodium, lactose, and cholesterol. Net price 200-mL bottle = £1.30

Fresubin 750® (Fresenius)

Liquid, protein 37.5 g, carbohydrate 85 g, fat 30 g, energy 3150 kJ (750 kcal)/500 mL with vitamins, minerals, and trace elements. Gluten-free and low lactose. Vanilla flavour. Net price 500-mL bottle = £2.75. As a necessary nutritional supplement prescribed on medical grounds for: short bowel syndrome, intractable malabsorption, pre-operative preparation of patients who are undernourished, proven inflammatory bowel disease, following total gastrectomy, dysphagia, bowel fistulas, disease-related malnutrition, continuous ambulatory peritoneal dialysis (CAPD), and haemodialysis. Not to be prescribed for any child under one year; use with caution for young children up to 5 years of age

Fructose (laevulose). For proven glucose/galactose intolerance

Galactomin® (Cow & Gate)

Formula 17 (new formula), powder, protein 14.5 g, fat 25.9 g, carbohydrate 56.9 g, mineral salts 3.4 g/100 g. Used as a 13.1% solution with additional vitamins in place of milk. Net price 400 g = £9.30. For proven lactose intolerance in preschool children, galactosaemia and galactokinase deficiency

Formula 19 (new formula), powder, protein 14.6 g, fat 30.8 g, carbohydrate 49.7 g (fructose as carbohydrate source), mineral salts 2.1 g/100 g, with vitamins. Used as a 12.9% solution in place of milk. Net price 400 g = £24.50. For glucose plus galactose intolerance

Generaid® (Scientific Hospital Supplies)

Powder, whey protein and additional branched-chain amino acids (protein equivalent 81%). Net price 200g (unflavoured) = £20.39. For patients with chronic liver disease and /or porto-hepatic encephalopathy

Plus Powder, whey protein and additional branched-chain amino acids (protein equivalent 11%) carbohydrate 62%, fat 19% with vitamins, minerals and trace elements. Net price 400 g = £11.90. For children over one year of age with hepatic disorders

Glucose (dextrose monohydrate). Net price 100g = 18p. For glycogen storage disease and sucrose/isomaltose intolerance

Glutafin® (Nutricia)

Gluten-free. Bread (whole or sliced), net price 400-g loaf = £2.30. Fibre bread (whole or sliced), 400-g loaf = £2.30. Bread with soya bran (dispensed in tin), 280 g = £1.56. Wheat-free white loaf (sliced or unsliced), 400 g = £2.59. Wheat-free white rolls, 400 g = £2.59. Mix, 500 g = £4.83. Baking mix, 500 g = £4.83. Fibre mix, 500 g = £4.83. Biscuits, savoury or tea, 125 g = £1.43. Biscuits, digestive or sweet, 150 g = £1.43. Biscuits, 200 g = £3.21. Crackers, 200 g = £2.34. High fibre crackers, 200 g = £1.96. Pasta (macaroni, pasta spirals, spaghetti short cut), 250 g = £2.56. For gluten-sensitive enteropathies including steatorrhoea due to gluten sensitivity, coeliac disease, and dermatitis herpetiformis

Gluten-free biscuits, see under Farley

Hepatic-Aid II® (Fresenius)

Powder, amino acids 4.4%, carbohydrate 16.8%, fat 3.6% when reconstituted. Low sodium and electrolytes; mineral and vitamin supplementation is required. Flavours: chocolate, chocolate mint, custard, and eggnog. Net price per packet = £7.95. For patients with chronic liver disease and/or porto-hepatic encephalopathy

Hycal® (SmithKline Beecham Brands)

Liquid, protein-free, low-electrolyte, glucose syrup solids 49.5%. Flavours: blackcurrant, lemon, orange, and raspberry. Net price 171 mL = 73p. For renal failure; liver cirrhosis or other conditions requiring a high-energy, low-fluid, low-electrolyte diet

InfaSoy® (Cow and Gate)[formerly Nutrilon Soya]

Powder, carbohydrate 7.1%, fat 3.6%, and protein 1.8% with vitamins and minerals when used as a 12.7% solution. Net price 450 g = £3.40; 900 g = £6.53. For proven lactose and associated sucrose intolerance in preschool children, galactokinase deficiency, galactosaemia, and proven whole cow's milk sensitivity

Instant Carobel see **Carobel, Instant**

Isomil® (Abbott)

Powder, protein 1.8%, carbohydrate 6.9%, fat 3.69% with vitamins and minerals when reconstituted. Lactose-free. Net price 400 g = £3.36. For proven lactose intolerance in preschool children, galactokinase deficiency, galactosaemia, and proven whole cow's milk sensitivity

Jevity® (Abbott)

Liquid, protein 4.2%, fat 3.5%, carbohydrate 13.4%, dietary fibre 1.36%, with vitamins and minerals. Gluten-, lactose-, and sucrose-free. Net price 500-mL bottle = £3.50. For use as the sole source of nutrition or as a necessary nutritional supplement prescribed on medical grounds for: short bowel syndrome, intractable malabsorption, pre-operative preparation of patients who are undernourished, proven inflammatory bowel disease, following total gastrectomy, dysphagia, disease-related malnutrition. Not to be prescribed for any child under 1 year; use with caution for young children up to 5 years of age

Juvela® (Scientific Hospital Supplies)

Gluten-free. Corn mix, fibre mix, and flour mix, net price 500 g = £4.80. Bread (whole or sliced), 400-g loaf = £2.28. Fibre bread (sliced and unsliced), 400-g loaf = £2.28. Bread rolls, 3 × 5 = £7.74, fibre bread rolls, 3 × 5 = £7.74. Digestive biscuits, 160 g = £1.69. Tea biscuits, 160 g = £1.69. For gluten-sensitive enteropathies including steatorrhoea due to gluten sensitivity, coeliac disease, and dermatitis herpetiformis

Low Protein/gluten-free. Mix, net price 500 g = £4.80. Bread, (whole or sliced) 400-g loaf = £2.28. Bread rolls, 3 × 5 rolls = £7.55. Biscuits, orange and cinnamon flavour, 150 g = £4.48; chocolate chip, 130 g = £4.48. For phenylketonuria and similar amino-acid abnormalities; renal failure; liver failure and liver cirrhosis; gluten-sensitive enteropathies, including steatorrhoea due to gluten sensitivity, coeliac disease and dermatitis herpetiformis

Kindergen® P R O D (Scientific Hospital Supplies)

Powder, protein 7.6 g, carbohydrate 60.6 g, fat 26.1 g, energy 2060 kJ (492 kcal)/100 g with vitamins and minerals. Net price 400 g = £12.18. For complete nutritional support or supplementary feeding for infants and children with chronic renal failure who are receiving peritoneal rapid overnight dialysis

Leucine-Free Amino Acid Mix see **Amino Acid Modules**

Lifestyle® (Ultrapharm)

Gluten-free. Brown bread (sliced and unsliced). Net price 400-g loaf = £1.96. White bread (sliced and unsliced), 400-g loaf = £1.96. Bread rolls, 400 g = £1.96. For gluten-sensitive enteropathies including steatorrhoea due to gluten sensitivity, coeliac disease, and dermatitis herpetiformis

Liga® (Jacobs Bakery)

Rusks, gluten-free, low sugar. Net price 6 = 57p. For gluten-sensitive enteropathies including steatorrhoea due to gluten sensitivity, coeliac disease, and dermatitis herpetiformis

Liquigen® (Scientific Hospital Supplies)

Emulsion, medium chain triglycerides 52%. Net price 250mL = £4.83; 1 litre = £17.84. For steatorrhoea associated with cystic fibrosis of the pancreas; intestinal lymphangiectasia, surgery of the intestine; chronic liver disease and liver cirrhosis; other proven malabsorption syndromes; ketogenic diet in the management of epilepsy; type I hyperlipoproteinaemia

Liquisorbon MCT® (Cow & Gate)

Liquid, protein 25 g, carbohydrate 61.5 g, fat 16.5 g, energy 2095 kJ (500 kcal)/500 mL with vitamins and minerals. Gluten- and fructose-free, low lactose. Strawberry, vanilla, and neutral flavours. Net price 500 mL = £2.80. As a necessary nutritional supplement prescribed on medical grounds for: short bowel syndrome, intractable malabsorption, pre-operative preparation of patients who are undernourished, proven inflammatory bowel disease, following total

gastrectomy, dysphagia, bowel fistulas, disease-related malnutrition. Not to be prescribed for any child under one year; use with caution for young children up to 5 years of age

Locasol New Formula® (Cow & Gate)

Powder, protein 14.6 g, carbohydrate 56.5 g, fat 26.1 g, mineral salts 1.9 g, not more than 55 mg of Ca^{2+}/100 g and vitamins. Used as a 13.1% solution in place of milk. Net price 400 g = £12.93. For calcium intolerance

Lofenalac® (Bristol-Myers)

Powder, protein 15%, carbohydrate 60%, fat 18%, phenylalanine not more than 0.1% with vitamins and minerals. Gluten-, sucrose-, and lactose-free. Net price 450 g = £8.00. For phenylketonuria

Loprofin® (Nutricia)

Low protein. Sweet biscuits, 150 g = £1.43; chocolate cream-filled biscuits, 125 g = £1.43; cookies (chocolate chip or cinnamon), 100 g = £4.70; wafers (orange, vanilla, or chocolate), 100 g = £1.40. Egg replacer, 250 g = £4.01. For phenylketonuria and similar amino acid abnormalities; renal failure; liver failure and liver cirrhosis

Low protein/gluten-free. Bread (sliced or whole), net price 400-g loaf = £2.30. Bread (white, with or without salt), 227 g = £1.56. Mix, 500 g = £4.83. Crackers, 150 g = £1.96. Pasta (macaroni, pasta spirals or spaghetti short-cut), 250 g = £2.56. For phenylketonuria and similar amino-acid abnormalities; renal failure; liver failure and liver cirrhosis; gluten-sensitive enteropathies including steatorrhoea due to gluten sensitivity, coeliac disease, and dermatitis herpetiformis

PKU Drink, protein 1 g (phenylalanine 30 mg), lactose 9.4 g, fat 4 g, energy 300 kJ (72 kcal)/200 mL. Net price 200-mL bottle = 47p. For phenylketonuria

Lorenzo's Oil (Scientific Hospital Supplies)

Liquid, glycerol trioleate oil 4 parts, glycerol trierucate oil 1 part. Net price 710 mL = £78.10. For biochemically proven and/or clinically manifest adrenoleukodystrophy

Low Protein Drink (Milupa)

Powder, protein 0.4%, carbohydrate 5.1%, fat 2% when reconstituted. Net price 400 g = £6.36. For inherited disorders of amino acid metabolism in childhood

Note. Termed Milupa lpd by manufacturer

Maxamaid® (Scientific Hospital Supplies)

Note. Maxamaid products are generally intended for use in children aged 2 to 8 years

MSUD, Maxamaid powder, essential and non-essential amino acids 30% except isoleucine, leucine, and valine, with carbohydrate, fat less than 0.5%, vitamins, minerals, and trace elements. Net price 575 g = £50.99. For maple syrup urine disease

RVHB, Maxamaid, powder, essential and non-essential amino acids 30% except methionine, with carbohydrate, fat less than 0.5%, vitamins, minerals, and trace elements. Net price 575 g = £50.99. For hypermethioninaemia, homocystinuria

XLys, Maxamaid, powder, essential and non-essential amino acids 30% except lysine, with carbohydrate, fat less than 0.5%, vitamins, minerals, and trace elements. Net price 575 g = £50.99. For hyperlysinaemia

Try, XLys, Maxamaid, powder, essential and non-essential amino acids 30% except lysine and tryptophan, with carbohydrate, fat less than 0.5%, vitamins, minerals, and trace elements. Net price 575 g = £50.99. For glutaric aciduria

XMet, Thre, Val, Isoleu, Maxamaid, powder, essential and non-essential amino acids 30% except methionine, threonine, valine and low isoleucine, with carbohydrate, fat less than 0.5%, vitamins, minerals, and trace elements. Net price 575 g = £50.99. For methylmalonic or propionic acidaemia

XP Maxamaid, essential and non-essential amino acids 30% except phenylalanine, with carbohydrate, vitamins, minerals, and trace elements. Net price 25-g bar = £1.35; powder (unflavoured), 500 g = £31.35; (orange-flavoured), 500 g = £31.35. For phenylketonuria. Not to be prescribed for children under 2 years of age

XP Maxamaid Concentrate, powder, essential and non-essential amino acids 65% except phenylalanine, with carbohydrate, fat less than 0.5%, vitamins, minerals, and trace elements. Unflavoured. Net price 200 g – £38.50. For phenylketonuria. Not to be prescribed for children under 2 years of age

XPhen, Tyr, Maxamaid, powder, essential and non-essential amino acids 30% except phenylalanine and tyrosine, with carbohydrate, fat less than 0.5%, vitamins, minerals, and trace elements. Net price 575 g = £50.99. For tyrosinaemia

Maxamum® (Scientific Hospital Supplies)

Note. Maxamum products are generally intended for use in children over 8 years

MSUD, Maxamum, powder, essential and non-essential amino acids 47% except isoleucine, leucine, and valine, with carbohydrate, fat less than 0.5%, vitamins, minerals, and trace elements. Orange-flavoured. Net price 200 g = £28.44. For maple syrup urine disease

RVHB, Maxamum, powder, essential and non-essential amino acids 47% except methionine, with carbohydrate, fat less than 0.5%, vitamins, minerals, and trace elements. Unflavoured. Net price 200 g = £28.44. For hypermethioninaemia, homocystinuria

XMet, Thre, Val, Isoleu, Maxamum, powder, essential and non-essential amino acids 47% except methionine, threonine, valine, and low isoleucine, with carbohydrate, fat less than 0.5%, vitamins, minerals, and trace elements. Unflavoured. Net price 200 g = £28.44. For methylmalonic or propionic acidaemia

XP Maxamum, powder, essential and non-essential amino acids 47% except phenylalanine, with carbohydrates, vitamins, minerals, and trace elements. Unflavoured. Net price 500 g = £48.45; orange-flavoured, 500 g = £48.45. For phenylketonuria. Not to be prescribed for children under 8 years

Maxijul® (Scientific Hospital Supplies)

Liquid, carbohydrate 50%, with potassium 0.004%, sodium 0.023%. Gluten-, lactose-, and fructose-free. Flavours: black currant, lemon and lime, orange, and natural. Net price 200 mL = 76p

Super Soluble Powder, glucose polymer, potassium 0.004%, sodium 0.046%. Gluten-, lactose-, and fructose-free. Net price 4 × 140-g sachet pack = £2.68, 200 g = £1.44, 2.5 kg = £12.00.

Both for renal failure; liver cirrhosis; disaccharide intolerance (without isomaltose intolerance); disorders of amino acid metabolism (and other similar disorders) and/or whole protein intolerance; malabsorption states and other conditions requiring a high-energy, low-fluid intake

Maxijul LE® (Scientific Hospital Supplies)

Powder, modification of Maxijul with lower concentrations of sodium and potassium. Net price 100 g = £1.23, 2 kg = £16.33. For indications, see under Maxijul where sodium and/or potassium restriction is also essential

Maxipro HBV® Super Soluble (Scientific Hospital Supplies)

Powder, whey protein and additional amino acids (protein equivalent 80%). Net price 200 g = £5.52; 1 kg = £22.07. For biochemically proven hypoproteinaemia. Not to be prescribed for any child under one year; unsuitable as a sole source of nutrition

Maxisorb® (Scientific Hospital Supplies)

Powder, protein 12 g, carbohydrate 9 g, fat 6 g, energy 565 kJ (135 kcal)/30 g with minerals. Vanilla, strawberry and chocolate flavours. Net price 5 × 30-g sachets = £2.37. As a necessary nutritional supplement prescribed on medical grounds for: short bowel syndrome, intractable malabsorption, pre-operative preparation of patients who are undernourished, proven inflammatory bowel disease, following total gastrectomy, dysphagia, bowel fistulas, disease-related malnutrition, continuous ambulatory peritoneal dialysis (CAPD) and haemodialysis.

Not to be prescribed for any child under one year; use with caution for young children up to 5 years of age

MCT Oil

Triglycerides from medium chain fatty acids. For steatorrhoea associated with cystic fibrosis of the pancreas; intestinal lymphangiectasia; surgery of the intestine; chronic liver disease and liver cirrhosis; other proven malabsorption syndromes; in a ketogenic diet in the management of epilepsy; in type I hyperlipoproteinaemia

Available from Bristol-Myers (net price 950 mL = £7.80); Cow & Gate (net price 1 litre = £14.54)

MCT (1) (Cow & Gate) replaced by Caprilon®

MCT Pepdite® (Scientific Hospital Supplies)

Powder, essential and non-essential amino acids, peptides, medium chain triglycerides, monoglyceride of sunflower oil, with carbohydrate, fat, vitamins, minerals, and trace elements.

MCT Pepdite 0–2. Net price 400 g = £11.43

MCT Pepdite 2+. Net price 400 g = £11.43

Both for disorders in which a high intake of medium chain triglyceride is beneficial

Metabolic Mineral Mixture® (Scientific Hospital Supplies)

Powder, essential mineral salts. Net price 100 g = £6.45. For mineral supplementation in synthetic diets

Methionine, Threonine, Valine-Free and Isoleucine-Low Amino Acid Mix see **Amino Acid Modules**

Milupa® Low Protein Drink see under **Low Protein Drink**

Milupa® PKU2 and PKU3 see under **PKU2** and **PKU3**

Minafen® (Cow & Gate)

Powder, equivalent of 12.5% protein, carbohydrate 48%, fat 31%, not more than 0.02% of phenylalanine. For use as 13.6% solution with additional vitamins. Net price 400 g = £16.41. For phenylketonuria

MSUD Aid III® (Scientific Hospital Supplies)

Powder, containing full range of amino acids except isoleucine, leucine, and valine, with vitamins, minerals, and trace elements. Net price 200 g = £49.59. For maple syrup urine disease and related conditions where it is necessary to limit the intake of branched chain amino acids

Neocate® (Scientific Hospital Supplies)

Powder, essential and non-essential amino acids, maltodextrin, fat, vitamins, minerals, and trace elements. Net price 400 g = £16.41. For proven whole protein intolerance, short bowel syndrome, intractable malabsorption, proven inflammatory bowel disease, and bowel fistulas

Nepro® (Abbott)

Liquid, protein 16.6 g, carbohydrate 51.1 g, fat 22.7 g, energy 1986 kJ (475 kcal)/237 mL with vitamins and minerals. Net price 237-mL can = £2.28. For patients with chronic renal failure who are on haemodialysis or continuous ambulatory peritoneal dialysis (CAPD), or patients with cirrhosis or other conditions requiring a high energy, low fluid, low electrolyte diet

Nestargel® (Nestlé)

Powder, carob seed flour 96.5%, calcium lactate 3.5%. Net price 125 g = £3.46. For thickening feeds in the treatment of vomiting

Nutramigen® (Bristol-Myers)

Powder, protein 13%, carbohydrate 62%, fat 18% with vitamins and minerals. Gluten-, sucrose-, and lactose-free. Net price 425 g = £7.00. For disaccharide and/or whole protein intolerance where additional medium chain triglyceride is not indicated

Nutrilon Soya® see **InfaSoy®**

Nutrison® (Cow & Gate) [formerly Fortison®]

Energy-plus, liquid, protein 30 g, carbohydrate 92 g, fat 29 g, energy 3200 kJ (755 kcal)/500 mL. Net price 500 mL = £2.71; 1 litre (Steriflo®) = £5.67. As a necessary nutritional supplement prescribed on medical grounds for: short bowel syndrome, intractable malabsorption, pre-operative preparation of patients who are undernourished, proven inflammatory bowel disease, following total gastrectomy, dysphagia, bowel fistulas, disease-related malnutrition. Not to be prescribed for any child under one year; use with caution for young children up to 5 years of age

Fibre, liquid, protein 20g, carbohydrate 61.5g, fat 19.5g, fibre 7.5g, energy 2125kJ (505kcal)/500mL. Net price 500-mL bottle = £2.62; 1 litre (Steriflo®) = £5.48. For use as the sole source of nutrition or as a necessary nutritional supplement prescribed on medical grounds for: short bowel syndrome, intractable malabsorption, pre-operative preparation of patients who are undernourished, proven inflammatory bowel disease, following total gastrectomy, dysphagia, disease-related malnutrition. Not to be prescribed for any child under two years; use with caution for young children up to 5 years of age

Paediatric, liquid, protein 5.4 g, carbohydrate 24.4 g, fat 9 g, energy 850 kJ (202 kcal)/200 mL. Net price 200-mL bottle = £1.82. For use as the sole source of nutrition or as a necessary nutritional supplement prescribed on medical grounds for: short bowel syndrome, intractable malabsorption, pre-operative preparation of patients who are undernourished, dysphagia, bowel fistulas, disease-related malnutrition or growth failure. Not to be prescribed for any child under one year

Soya, liquid, protein 20g, carbohydrate 61.5g, fat 19.5g, energy 2125 kJ (505 kcal)/500 mL, with vitamins and minerals. Gluten-free. Net price 500 mL = £2.81; 1 litre (Steriflo®) = £5.88. For milk intolerance and lactose intolerance. Not to be prescribed for any child under one year, unsuitable as a sole source of nutrition for young children up to 5 years of age

Standard, liquid, protein 20g, carbohydrate 61.5 g, fat 19.5g, energy 2125 kJ (505kcal)/500mL, with vitamins and minerals. Net price 500mL = £2.31; 1 litre (Steriflo®) = £4.83. For use as the sole source of nutrition or as a necessary nutritional supplement prescribed on medical grounds for: short bowel syndrome, intractable malabsorption, pre-operative preparation of patients who are undernourished, proven inflammatory bowel disease, following total gastrectomy, dysphagia, bowel fistulas, disease-related malnutrition. Not to be prescribed for any child under one year; use with caution for young children up to 5 years of age

Orgran® (FoodWatch)

Low protein/gluten-free. Pasta (annelini, ribbons, rigatini). Net price 500g = £3.71. For phenylketonuria, similar amino acid abnormalities; renal failure; liver failure and liver cirrhosis; gluten-sensitive enteropathies including steatorrhoea due to gluten sensitivity, coeliac disease, and dermatitis herpetiformis

Osmolite® (Abbott)

Liquid, protein 10.0 g, carbohydrate 33.9 g, fat 8.7 g, energy 1050 kJ (250 kcal)/250mL with vitamins and minerals. Gluten- and lactose-free. Net price 250-mL can = £1.49; 500-mL bottle = £2.98. For use as the sole source of nutrition or as a necessary nutritional supplement prescribed on medical grounds for: short-bowel syndrome, intractable malabsorption, pre-operative preparation of patients who are undernourished, for proven inflammatory bowel disease, following total gastrectomy, dysphagia, bowel fistulas, disease-related malnutrition. Not to be prescribed for any child under one year; use with caution for young children up to 5 years of age

OsterSoy® (Farley)

Powder, providing protein 2%, carbohydrate 7%, fat 3.8% with vitamins and minerals when reconstituted. Gluten-, sucrose-, and lactose-free. Net price 450 g = £3.45. For proven lactose and sucrose intolerance in pre-school children, galactokinase deficiency, galactosaemia, and proven whole cow's milk protein sensitivity

Paediasure® (Abbott)

Liquid, protein 3%, fat 5%, carbohydrate 11%, with minerals and vitamins, gluten-free, energy 1046kJ (250kcal)/250mL. Vanilla flavour. Net price 250-mL can = £2.13. For use as the sole source of nutrition or as a necessary nutritional supplement prescribed on medi-

cal grounds for: short-bowel syndrome, intractable malabsorption, pre-operative preparation of patients who are undernourished, dysphagia, bowel fistulas; and disease-related malnutrition or growth failure. Not to be prescribed for any child under one year

Paediatric Seravit® (Scientific Hospital Supplies)

Powder, vitamins, minerals, low sodium and potassium, and trace elements. Net price 100g (unflavoured) = £5.00; pineapple flavour, 100g = £5.33

For vitamin and mineral supplementation in restrictive therapeutic diets in infants and children

Pastariso® (General Designs)

Gluten-free. Brown rice pasta (spaghetti, elbow macaroni, fettucini, fusilli, mini elbows, and spirals). Net price 284g = £1.87; fettucini, 227g = £1.87. For gluten-sensitive enteropathies including steatorrhoea due to gluten sensitivity, coeliac disease and dermatitis herpetiformis

Pepdite® (Scientific Hospital Supplies)

Powder, essential and non-essential amino acids, peptides, with carbohydrate, fat, vitamins, minerals, and trace elements.

Pepdite 0–2. Providing 1925 kJ (460 kcal)/100 g. Net price 400 g = £10.39

Pepdite 2+. Providing 1787 kJ (425 kcal)/100 g. Net price 400 g = £10.39

Both for disaccharide and/or whole protein intolerance, or where amino acids or peptides are indicated in conjunction with medium chain triglycerides

Peptamen® (Clintec)

Liquid, protein 4%, carbohydrate 12.7%, fat 3.9%, energy 420 kJ (100 kcal)/100 mL, with vitamins and minerals. Lactose- and gluten-free. Vanilla, orange and strawberry flavours. Net price 250-mL can = £2.95; 1 litre (spike and hang) = £13.50. For use as the sole source of nutrition or as a necessary nutritional supplement prescribed on medical grounds for: short bowel syndrome, intractable malabsorption, proven inflammatory bowel disease, bowel fistulas. Not to be prescribed for any child under one year; use with caution for young children up to 5 years of age

Flavour sachets, citrus, chocolate, vanilla, strawberry, cappucino flavours. Net price 24-sachet pack = £7.50. For use with vanilla Peptamen

Pepti-2000 LF® (Cow & Gate)

Liquid, protein 20g, fat 5g, carbohydrate 94g, energy 2100kJ (500kcal)/500mL with vitamins and minerals. Gluten-free. Net price 500mL = £3.02; 1 litre (Steriflo®) = £6.28.

Powder, same composition as Pepti-2000 LF liquid when reconstituted. Net price 126-g sachet = £4.00.

For use as the sole source of nutrition or as a necessary nutritional supplement prescribed on medical grounds for: short bowel syndrome, intractable malabsorption, proven inflammatory bowel disease, bowel fistulas. Not to be prescribed for any child under one year; use with caution for young children up to 5 years of age

Pepti-Junior® (Cow & Gate)

Powder, protein 15.3 g, fat 28.3 g, carbohydrate 55.1 g, energy 2140 kJ (507 kcal)/100 g with vitamins and minerals. Used as a 13.1% solution in place of milk. Net price 450 g = £8.22. For disaccharide and/or whole protein intolerance or where amino acids and peptides are indicated in conjunction with medium chain triglycerides

Peptisorb® (Cow & Gate)

Liquid, amino acids and peptides 3.75%, carbohydrate 18.75%, fat 1.11%, with vitamins and minerals, low lactose, and fructose- and gluten-free, energy 2100 kJ (500 kcal)/500 mL. Net price 500mL = £4.83. For use as the sole source of nutrition or as a necessary nutritional supplement prescribed on medical grounds for: short bowel syndrome, intractable malabsorption, proven inflammatory bowel disease, bowel fistulas. Not to be prescribed for any child under one year; use with caution for young children up to 5 years of age

Peptisorbon® (Cow & Gate)

Powder, amino acids and peptides 18%, carbohydrate 70%, fat 5.3%, with vitamins and minerals, low lactose, and fructose- and gluten-free, energy 1393 kJ (333 kcal)/ sachet. Net price 83.3-g sachet = £2.17. As a necessary nutritional supplement prescribed on medical grounds for: short bowel syndrome, intractable malabsorption, pre-operative preparation of patients who are undernourished, proven inflammatory bowel disease, following total gastrectomy, dysphagia, bowel fistulas, disease-related malnutrition. Not to be prescribed for any child under one year; use with caution for young children up to 5 years of age

Perative® (Abbott)

Liquid, providing protein 15.8 g, carbohydrate 42.2 g, fat 8.82 g, energy 1313 kJ (310 kcal)/237 mL, with vitamins and minerals. Gluten-free, unflavoured. Net price 237-mL can = £2.70. For use as a necessary nutritional supplement prescribed on medical grounds for: short-bowel syndrome, intractable malabsorption, pre-operative preparation of patients who are undernourished, proven inflammatory bowel disease, following total gastrectomy, bowel fistulas, disease-related malnutrition. Not to be prescribed for any child under 5 years of age

Phenylalanine, Tyrosine and Methionine-Free Amino Acid Mix *see* **Amino Acid Modules**

Phlexy-10® (Scientific Hospital Supplies)

Powder, containing essential and non-essential amino acids except phenylalanine 10 g, carbohydrate 6.8 g/20-g sachet. Blackcurrant and apple flavour. Net price 20 x 20-g sachet = £46.00. For phenylketonuria

PK Aid 3® (Scientific Hospital Supplies)

Powder, containing essential and non-essential amino acids except phenylalanine. Net price 500 g = £81.84. For phenylketonuria

PKU 2® (Milupa)

Granules, containing essential and non-essential amino acids except phenylalanine; with vitamins, minerals, trace elements, 7.1% sucrose. Flavour: vanilla. Net price 500 g = £38.16. For phenylketonuria

PKU 3® (Milupa)

Granules, containing essential and non-essential amino acids except phenylalanine, vitamins, minerals, and trace elements, with 3.4% sucrose. Flavour vanilla. Net price 500 g = £38.16. For phenylketonuria, not recommended for child under 8 years

Pollal® (Ultrapharm)

Biscuits, Gluten- and lactose-free. Net price 200-g pack = £2.85. For gluten-sensitive enteropathies including steatorrhea due to gluten sensitivity, coeliac disease, and dermatitis herpetiformis

Polycal® (Cow & Gate)

Powder, glucose, maltose, and polysaccharides, providing 1610 kJ (380 kcal)/100 g. Net price 400 g = £2.73; 900 g = £4.86

For renal failure; liver cirrhosis; disaccharide intolerance (without isomaltose intolerance); disorders of amino acid metabolism (and other similar disorders) and/or whole protein intolerance; malabsorption states and other conditions, including proven hypoglycaemia, requiring a high-energy, low-fluid diet, whether or not sodium and/or potassium restriction is essential

Liquid [formerly Fortical® liquid], glucose polymers providing carbohydrate 61.5 g/100 mL. Low-electrolyte, protein-free. Flavours: apple, black currant, lemon, orange, and neutral. Net price 200 mL = £1.05. For renal failure; liver cirrhosis, disaccharide intolerance (without maltose intolerance); disorders of amino acid metabolism, and/or whole protein intolerance, malabsorption states, or other conditions including proven hypoglycaemia requiring a high-energy, low-fluid, low-electrolyte diet

Polycose® (Abbott)

Powder, glucose polymers, providing carbohydrate 94 g, energy 1600 kJ (380 kcal)/100 g. Net price 350-g can = £3.14. For renal failure; liver cirrhosis; disaccharide

intolerance (without isomaltose intolerance); disorders of amino acid metabolism (and other similar disorders) and/or whole protein intolerance; malabsorption states and other conditions, including proven hypoglycaemia, requiring a high-energy, low-fluid intake, whether or not sodium and/or potassium restriction is essential

Portagen® (Bristol-Myers)

Powder, protein 16.5%, carbohydrate 54%, fat 22% with vitamins and minerals. Gluten- and lactose-free. Net price 454 g = £6.23. For disorders in which a high intake of medium chain triglycerides is beneficial

Pregestimil® (Bristol-Myers)

Powder, protein 12.8%, carbohydrate 61.6%, fat 18.3% with vitamins and minerals. Gluten-, sucrose-, and lactose-free. Net price 450 g = £8.01. For disaccharide and/or whole protein intolerance or where amino acids or peptides are indicated in conjunction with medium chain triglycerides

Prejomin® (Milupa)

Granules, protein 13.3 g, carbohydrate 57 g, fat 24.2 g, energy 2090 kJ (499 kcal)/100 g, with vitamins and minerals. Gluten-free. For preparation with water before use. Net price 400 g = £8.47. For disaccharide and/or whole protein intolerance where additional medium chain triglyceride is not indicated

ProMod® (Abbott)

Powder, protein 75.8%, carbohydrate 10.2%, fat 9.1%. Gluten-free. Net price 275-g can = £8.40. For biochemically proven hypoproteinaemia

Prosobee® (Bristol-Myers)

Liquid concentrate, protein 4.1%, carbohydrate 13.7%, fat 7.2% with vitamins and minerals. Gluten-, sucrose-, and lactose-free. Net price 385 mL = £1.29

Powder, protein 15.6%, carbohydrate 51.4%, fat 27.9% with vitamins and minerals. Gluten-, sucrose-, and lactose-free. Net price 400 g = £3.22. For proven lactose and associated sucrose intolerance in pre-school children, galactokinase deficiency, galactosaemia, and proven whole cow's milk sensitivity

Protein Forte® (Fresenius)

Liquid, protein 20 g, carbohydrate 19 g, fat 5.2 g, energy 840 kJ (200 kcal)/200 mL, with vitamins, minerals, and trace elements. Gluten-free. Vanilla, strawberry, and chocolate flavours. Net price 200-mL Tetrabrik = £1.05. As a necessary nutritional supplement prescribed on medical grounds for: short bowel syndrome, intractable malabsorption, pre-operative preparation of patients who are undernourished, proven inflammatory bowel disease, following total gastrectomy, dysphagia, bowel fistulas, disease-related malnutrition, continuous ambulatory peritoneal dialysis (CAPD) and haemodialysis. Not to be prescribed for any child under one year; use with caution for young children up to 5 years of age

Protifar® (Cow & Gate)

Powder, protein 88.5%. Low lactose, gluten- and sucrose-free. Net price 225 g = £5.46. For biochemically proven hypoproteinaemia

Provide® (Fresenius)

Liquid, protein 9 g, carbohydrate 28 g, fat less than 1 g, energy 630 kJ (150 kcal)/250 mL with vitamins and minerals. Gluten- and lactose-free. Apple, blackcurrant, lemon and lime, and tropical fruit flavour. Net price 250-mL Tetrabrik = £1.20. As a necessary nutritional supplement prescribed on medical grounds for: short bowel syndrome, intractable malabsorption, pre-operative preparation of patients who are undernourished, proven inflammatory bowel disease, following total gastrectomy, dysphagia, bowel fistulas, disease-related malnutrition. Not to be prescribed for any child under one year; use with caution for young children up to 5 years of age

Reabilan® (Clintec)

Liquid, protein 11.8 g, carbohydrate 49.3 g, fat 14.6 g, energy 1575 kJ (375 kcal)/375 mL with vitamins and minerals. Gluten- and lactose-free. Net price 375-mL can = £3.08; 500-mL Dripac = £4.58. As a necessary nutritional supplement prescribed on medical grounds for: short bowel syndrome, intractable malabsorption, proven inflammatory bowel disease, bowel fistulas. Not to be prescribed for any child under 1 year; use with caution for young children up to 5 years of age

Rectified Spirit. Where the therapeutic qualities of alcohol are required rectified spirit (suitably flavoured and diluted) should be prescribed

Redwood® (JRJ)

Gluten-free. Corn pasta (spaghetti, shells, macaroni). Net price 250 g = £1.69. For gluten-sensitive enteropathies including steatorrhoea due to gluten sensitivity, coeliac disease and dermatitis herpetiformis

Rite-Diet® (Nutricia)

Gluten-free. Flour mix. Net price 500 g = £4.83. Bread mix. 500 g (brown) = £4.83; white, 500 g = £4.83. Bread (white). 400 g = £2.30. High-fibre bread (with soya bran). 400 g = £2.30. For gluten-sensitive enteropathies including steatorrhoea due to gluten sensitivity, coeliac disease, and dermatitis herpetiformis

Low protein/gluten-free. Baking mix. Net price 500 g = £4.83. Flour mix. 400 g = £4.83. White bread (with added fibre). 400 g = £2.30. For phenylketonuria and similar amino-acid abnormalities; renal failure; liver failure and liver cirrhosis; gluten-sensitive enteropathies including steatorrhoea due to gluten sensitivity, coeliac disease, and dermatitis herpetiformis

Schar ® (Ultrapharm)

Gluten-free, Bread. Net price 250 g = £1.41. Bread rolls, 200 g = £1.41. Bread mix, 500 g = £3.95. Cake mix, 500 g = £3.95. Crackers, 200 g = £2.15. Crispbread, 250 g = £2.82. Pasta (fusilli, penne, rigatoni, tagliatelle), 250 g = £1.90; lasagna, 250 g = £2.80; spaghetti, 500 g = £3.41. Pizza bases, 250 g = £4.12. Savoy biscuits, 200 g = £2.15. For gluten-sensitive enteropathies including steatorrhoea due to gluten sensitivity, coeliac disease, and dermatitis herpetiformis

SHS Modjul® Flavour System (Scientific Hospital Supplies)

Powder, blackcurrant, orange, pineapple, and savoury tomato flavours. Net price 100 g = £5.63

For use with any unflavoured products based on peptides or amino acids

Sno-Pro® (Scientific Hospital Supplies)

Drink, protein 220 mg (phenylalanine 12.5 mg), carbohydrate 8 g, fat 3.8 g, energy 272 kJ (65 kcal)/100 mL. Net price 200 mL = 57p. For phenylketonuria

Sunflower oil. Net price 100 mL = 32p. For familial hypercholesterolaemia (non-drug for multiple sclerosis)

Sunnyvale® (Everfresh)

Mixed grain bread, gluten-free. Net price 400 g = £1.19. For gluten-sensitive enteropathies including steatorrhoea due to gluten sensitivity, coeliac disease and dermatitis herpetiformis

Thick and Easy® (Fresenius)

Powder. Modified maize starch. Net price 225-g can = £3.75. For thickening of foods in dysphagia. Not to be prescribed for children under one year except in cases of failure to thrive

Thixo-D® (Cirrus)

Powder, modified maize starch, gluten-free. Net price 375-g pack = £5.30. For thickening of foods in dysphagia. Not to be prescribed for children under one year except in cases of failure to thrive

Triosorbon® (Cow & Gate)

Powder, protein 19%, carbohydrate 56%, fat 19%, with vitamins and minerals. Gluten-free. Net price 85-g sachet = £1.74. For use as the sole source of nutrition or as a necessary nutritional supplement prescribed on medical grounds for: short-bowel syndrome, intractable malabsorption, pre-operative preparation of patients who are undernourished, proven inflammatory bowel disease, following total gastrectomy, dysphagia, bowel fistulas, disease-related malnutrition. Not to be prescribed for any child under one year; use with caution for young children up to 5 years of age

Tritamyl® (Procea)

Flour, self-raising (starch-based), gluten- and lactose-free. Net price 2 kg = £5.10. For gluten-sensitive enteropathies including steatorrhoea due to gluten sensitivity, coeliac disease, and dermatitis herpetiformis

Trufree® (Cantassium)

Gluten-free, wheat-free flours. For gluten-sensitive enteropathies including steatorrhoea due to gluten sensitivity, coeliac disease, and dermatitis herpetiformis

No. 1. Net price 1 kg = £3.86

No. 2 with rice bran. Net price 1 kg = £4.65

No. 3 for Cantabread®. Net price 1 kg = £5.03

No. 4 white. Net price 1 kg = £3.86

No. 5 brown. Net price 1 kg = £3.86

No. 6 plain. Net price 1 kg = £3.71

No. 7 self-raising. Net price 500 g = £1.99, 1 kg = £3.94

Tyrosine and Phenylalanine-Free Amino Acid Mix: see Amino Acid Modules

Ultra® (Ultrapharm)

Gluten-free. High-fibre bread. Net price 500 g = £3.26. Crackerbread, 100 g = £1.72. For gluten-sensitive enteropathies including steatorrhoea due to gluten sensitivity, coeliac disease and dermatitis herpetiformis

Low protein/gluten-free. Brown bread (canned). Net price 500 g = £3.80. White bread (canned), 350 g = £2.75. PKU bread, 400 g = £2.10. PKU flour, 500 g = £2.98. PKU biscuits, 200 g = £2.15. PKU cookies, 250 g = £2.25. PKU pizza base, 400 g = £2.15. PKU savoy biscuits, 150 g = £2.00. For phenylketonuria (not canned brown bread) and similar amino-acid abnormalities; renal failure, liver failure, and liver cirrhosis; gluten-sensitive enteropathies including steatorrhoea due to gluten sensitivity, coeliac disease, and dermatitis herpetiformis

Valpiform® (General Designs)

Gluten-free. Bread mix (wheat free). Net price 1 kg = £5.18. Pastry mix, 1 kg = £5.18. For gluten-sensitive enteropathies including steatorrhoea due to gluten sensitivity, coeliac disease, and dermatitis herpetiformis

Vitaquick® (Vitaflo)

Powder. Modified maize starch. Net price 100 g = £1.85; 250 g = £3.16; 1 kg = £9.99. For thickening of foods in dysphagia. Not to be prescribed for children under one year old except in cases of failure to thrive

Wysoy® (Wyeth)

Powder, carbohydrate 6.9%, fat 3.6%, and protein 2.1% with vitamins and minerals when reconstituted. Net price 430 g = £3.16; 860 g = £6.05. For proven lactose and associated sucrose intolerance in pre-school children, galactokinase deficiency, galactosaemia and proven whole cow's milk sensitivity

---

CONDITIONS FOR WHICH FOODS MAY BE PRESCRIBED ON FP10

Note. This is a list of clinical conditions for which the ACBS has approved food products. It is essential to check the list of products (above) for availability.

Adrenoleukodystrophy: Lorenzo's Oil.

Amino acid metabolic disorders and similar protein disorders: low protein drink (Milupa); see also phenylketonuria; histidinaemia; homocystinuria; maple syrup urine disease; tyrosinaemia; synthetic diets; low-protein products.

Anorexia nervosa: see malnutrition (disease-related)

Bowel fistulas: Advera[1]; Clinifeed 400[1], Favour, Iso and Protein Rich[1]; Elemental 028; Enrich; Ensure; Ensure Plus[1]; Ensure Powder; Entera; Flexical; Formance[1]; Fortimel[1]; Fortipudding[1]; Fortisip[1]; Fresenius OPD[1]; Fresubin Liquid and Sip Feeds, High Energy, Plus F and 750[1]; Jevity; Liquisorb High Energy[1]; Liquisorb feed and drink; Liquisorbon MCT[1]; Maxisorb[1]; Nutrison Energy Plus[1], Fibre,

---

1. As a supplement only.

Paediatric and Standard; Osmolite; Paediasure; Peptamen; Pepti-2000 LF; Peptisorb; Peptisorbon; Perative1; Protein Forte1; Provide1; Reabilan1; Triosorbon.

Calcium intolerance: Locasol New Formula.

Carbohydrate malabsorption: Calogen. See also synthetic diets; malabsorption states.

Disaccharide intolerance (without isomaltose intolerance): Alfare; Caloreen; Duocal Super Soluble and Duocal Liquid; Maxijul LE, Liquid, Super Soluble; Nutramigen; Pepdite; Pepti-Junior; Polycal; Polycal Liquid; Polycose powder; Pregestimil; Prejomin. See also lactose intolerance; lactose with sucrose intolerance.

Glucose and galactose intolerance: Comminuted chicken meat (Cow & Gate); Fructose Galactomin Formula 19 (fructose formula).

Isomaltose intolerance: Glucose (dextrose).

Lactose intolerance[2]: AL110; Comminuted chicken meat (Cow & Gate); Galactomin Formula 17 (new formula); InfaSoy; Isomil powder; Nutramigen; Nutrison Soya; Ostersoy; Pepdite; Portagen; Pregestimil; Prejomin; Prosobee; Wysoy.

Lactose with sucrose intolerance[2]: Comminuted Chicken Meat (Cow & Gate); Galactomin Formula 17 (new formula); InfaSoy; Nutramigen; Ostersoy; Pepti-Junior; Pregestimil; Prejomin; Prosobee; Wysoy.

Sucrose intolerance[2]: Glucose (dextrose) and see also synthetic diets; malabsorption states; lactose with sucrose intolerance.

Cirrhosis of the liver and chronic liver disease: see liver disease.

Coeliac disease: see gluten-sensitive enteropathies.

Continuous Ambulatory Peritoneal Dialysis (CAPD): see dialysis.

Cystic fibrosis: see malabsorption states.

Dermatitis Herpetiformis: see gluten-sensitive enteropathies.

Dialysis: nutritional supplements for haemodialysis or continuous ambulatory peritoneal dialysis (CAPD) patients: Clinifeed 400, and Protein Rich; Ensure Plus; Formance; Fortipudding; Fresubin 750; Kindergen PROD; Maxisorb; Nepro; Protein Forte.

Disaccharide intolerance: see carbohydrate malabsorption.

Dysphagia[3]: Advera[1]; Clinifeed 400[1]; Favour, Iso and Protein Rich[1]; Enrich; Ensure; Ensure Plus[1]; Ensure Powder; Entera; Formance[1]; Fortimel[1]; Fortipudding[1]; Fortisip[1]; Fresubin OPD[1]; Fresubin Liquid and Sip Feeds, High Energy, Isofibre, Plus F and 750[1]; Jevity; Liquisorb High Energy[1]; Liquisorb feed and drink; Liquisorbon MCT[1]; Maxisorb[1]; Nutrison Energy Plus[1], Fibre, Paediatric and Standard; Osmolite; Paediasure; Peptisorbon; Perative[1]; Protein Forte[1]; Provide[1]; Thick & Easy (as a thickener); Thixo-D (as a thickener); Triosorbon; Vitaquick (as a thickener).

Epilepsy (ketogenic diet in): Alembicol D; Calogen; Liquigen; Medium Chain Triglyceride Oil (MCT).

Flavouring for use with any unflavoured product based on peptides or amino acids: SHS Flavour Modjul

Galactokinase deficiency and galactosaemia: AL 110; Galactomin Formula 17 (new formula); InfaSoy; Isomil powder; Ostersoy; Prosobee Liquid and Powder; Wysoy.

Gastrectomy (total): Advera[1]; Clinifeed 400[1], Favour, Iso and Protein Rich[1]; Enrich; Ensure; Ensure Plus[1]; Ensure Powder; Entera; Formance[1]; Fortimel[1]; Fortipudding[1]; Fortisip[1]; Fresenius OPD[1]; Fresubin Liquid and Sip Feeds, High Energy, Isofibre, Plus F and 750[1]; Jevity; Liquisorb High Energy[1]; Liquisorb Feed and Drink; Liquisorbon MCT[1]; Maxisorb[1]; Nutrison Energy Plus[1]; Fibre and Standard; Osmolite; Peptisorbon; Perative[1], Protein Forte[1]; Provide[1]; Triosorbon.

Glucose/galactose intolerance: Comminuted Chicken Meat (Cow & Gate); Galactomin Formula 19 (fructose formula); also see carbohydrate malabsorption.

Glutaric aciduria: XLys, Try Maxamaid

Gluten-sensitive enteropathies: Aproten products (anellini, biscuits, bread mix, cake mix, crispbread, ditalini, flour, rigatini, spaghetti, tagliatelle); Arnott gluten-free rice cookies; Barkat gluten-free bread mix; Bi-Aglut biscuits, flour, and gluten-free cracker toast; Ener-G brown and white rice bread, gluten-free tapioca bread, gluten-free rice pasta (cannelloni, lasagna, macaroni, shells, small shells, spaghetti, tagliatelli, vermicelli); brown rice pasta (lasagna, macaroni,

spaghetti); Glutafin bread, bread with soya bran (dispensed in tin), wheat-free white loaf (sliced or unsliced), wheat-free white rolls, fibre bread, baking mix, fibre mix, biscuits (digestive, savoury, sweet (without chocolate or sultanas), tea), crackers, high fibre crackers and pasta (spirals, macaroni, spaghetti vermicelli); Gluten-free biscuits (Farley); Gratis pasta and tricolour pasta; Juvela gluten-free corn mix, gluten-free loaf and high-fibre loaf (sliced and unsliced), bread rolls, gluten-free mix and fibre mix; Juvela low-protein loaf (sliced and unsliced), low-protein mix, and bread rolls; Juvela gluten-free digestive biscuits and tea biscuits; Juvela gluten-free, low-protein (chocolate chip, orange, and cinnamon flavour) cookies; Lifestyle gluten-free bread rolls; Lifestyle brown and white bread; Liga gluten-free rusks (Jacobs); Loprofin gluten-free low-protein bread (sliced and unsliced), bread (with or without salt), crackers, mix, pasta (macaroni, pasta spirals, spaghetti short-cut); Orgran gluten-free pasta (annelini, ribbons, rigatini); Pastariso gluten-free brown rice pasta (elbow macaroni, fettucini, fusilli, mini elbows, spaghetti, spirals, twists); Polial gluten-free biscuits; Promin pasta and tricolour pasta; Redwood gluten-free corn pasta (macaroni, shells, spaghetti); Rite-Diet gluten-free high-fibre bread (with added soya-bran); Rite-Diet gluten-free white bread 400 g; Rite-Diet gluten-free white bread mix; Rite-Diet gluten-free brown bread mix; Rite-Diet baking mix; Rite-Diet low-protein flour mix; Rite-Diet gluten-free flour mix; Rite-Diet low-protein white bread (with added fibre); Schar gluten-free bread, bread mix, bread rolls, cake mix, crackers, crispbread, pasta (fusilli, lasagna, penne, rigatoni, spaghetti, tagliatelli), pizza base savoy biscuits; Sunnyvale gluten-free bread; Trufree special dietary flours No. 1, No. 2 with rice bran, No. 3 for Cantabread, No. 4 white, No. 5 brown, No. 6 plain, No. 7 self-raising; Ultra gluten-free high-fibre bread; Ultra gluten-free crackerbread; Ultra low-protein, gluten-free canned bread (brown and white); Ultra PKU biscuits, PKU bread, PKU cookies, PKU flour, PKU pizza base, PKU savoy biscuits; Valpiform bread mix, pastry mix.

Glycogen storage disease: Caloreen; Corn Flour or Corn Starch; Glucose (dextrose); Maxijul LE, Liquid, and Super Soluble; Polycal; Polycal Liquid; Polycose.

Growth Failure (secondary to disease related anorexia): Fortipudding; Nutrison Paediatric; Paediasure.

Haemodialysis: see dialysis.

Histidinaemia: HF(2), and see also low-protein products; synthetic diets.

Homocystinuria: Analog RVHB; RVHB Maxamaid; RVHB Maxamum, and see also low-protein products; synthetic diets.

Hypercholesterolaemia (familial): Corn oil; Sunflower oil.

Hyperlipoproteinaemia type 1: Liquigen; Medium Chain Triglyceride Oil.

Hyperlysinaemia: Analog XLys; XLys Maxamaid

Hypermethioninaemia: Analog RVHB; Maxamaid RVHB; Maxamum RVHB.

---

1. As a supplement only.

2. Defined as a condition of intolerance to an intake of the relevant disaccharide confirmed by demonstrated clinical benefit of effectiveness of disaccharide free diet, and presence of reducing substances or excessive acid in stools, low concentration of corresponding disaccharidase enzyme on intestinal biopsy, or breath tests, or lactose tolerance tests.

3. Defined as that associated with intrinsic disease of the oesophagus, e.g. oesophagitis; neuromuscular disorders, e.g. multiple sclerosis and motor neurone disease; major surgery and/or radiotherapy for cancer of the upper digestive tract; protracted severe inflammatory disease of the upper digestive tract, e.g.Stevens-Johnson syndrome and epidermolysis bullosa.

Hypoglycaemia: Caloreen; Corn Flour or Corn Starch; Maxijul LE, Liquid, and Super Soluble; Polycal; Polycal Liquid; Polycose, and see also glycogen storage disease.

Hypoproteinaemia: Casilan; Dialamine; Forceval Protein; Maxipro HBV Super Soluble; ProMod; Protifar.

Inflammatory Bowel Disease: Advera[1]; Clinifeed 400[1], Favour, Iso and Protein Rich[1]; Elemental 028; Enrich; Ensure; Ensure Plus[1]; Ensure Powder; Entera; Flexical; Formance[1]; Fortimel[1]; Fortipudding[1]; Fortisip[1]; Fresenius OPD[1]; Fresubin Liquid and Sip Feeds, High energy, Isofibre; Plus F and 750[1]; Jevity; Liquisorb High Energy[1]; Liquisorb Feed and Drink; Liquisorbon MCT[1]; Maxisorb[1]; Nutrison Energy Plus[1], Fibre and Standard; Osmolite; Peptamen; Pepti-2000 LF; Peptisorb; Peptisorbon; Perative[1]; Protein Forte[1]; Provide[1]; Reabilan[1]; Triosorbon.

Intestinal lymphangiectasia: see malabsorption states.

Intestinal surgery: see malabsorption states.

Isomaltose intolerance: see carbohydrate malabsorption.

Isovaleric acidaemia: Leucine-Free Amino Acid Mix; X Leu Analog.

Lactose intolerance: see carbohydrate malabsorption.

Liver disease (i.e. chronic liver disease, cirrhosis): Aglutella low-protein rice; Alembicol D; Aproten products (anellini, biscuits, bread mix, cake mix, crispbread, ditalini, flour, rigatini, spaghetti, tagliatelle); Caloreen; dp Low-Protein butterscotch-flavoured or chocolate-flavoured chip cookies; Duobar; Duocal Super Soluble, and Duocal Liquid; Generaid; Generaid Plus; Hepatic Aid; Hycal; Juvela gluten-free low-protein (chocolate chip, orange, and cinnamon flavour) cookies; Juvela low-protein loaf (sliced and unsliced) and low-protein flour mix; Liquigen; Loprofin egg replacer; Loprofin gluten-free low-protein bread (sliced and unsliced), bread (with or without salt), mix, pasta (macaroni, spaghetti short-cut, pasta spirals); Loprofin low-protein sweet biscuits, chocolate cream-filled biscuits, crackers, cookies (chocolate chip, cinnamon), wafers (orange, chocolate, vanilla); Maxijul LE, Liquid, and Super Soluble; MCT (1) Powder; Medium Chain Triglyceride Oil; Nepro; Orgran low-protein pasta (anellini, ribbons, rigatini); Polycal; Polycal Liquid; Polycose; Portagen; Promin pasta and tricolour pasta; Rite-Diet low-protein white bread (with added fibre); Rite-Diet low-protein baking mix; Rite-Diet low-protein flour mix; Ultra Egg Replacer; Ultra low-protein, gluten-free canned bread (brown and white); Ultra PKU biscuits, PKU bread, PKU cookies, PKU flour, PKU pizza base, PKU savoy biscuits.

Low-protein products: Aglutella low-protein rice; Aproten products (anellini, biscuits, bread mix, cake mix, crispbread, ditalini, flour, rigatini, spaghetti, tagliatelle); dp Low-Protein butterscotch-flavoured or chocolate-flavoured chip cookies*; Juvela gluten-free low-protein (chocolate chip, orange, and cinnamon flavour) cookies; Juvela low-protein loaf (sliced and unsliced); Juvela low-protein mix; Juvela low-protein rolls; Loprofin egg replacer; Loprofin gluten-free low-protein bread (sliced and unsliced), bread (with or without salt), mix, pasta (macaroni, spaghetti short-cut, pasta spirals); Loprofin low-protein sweet biscuits*, chocolate cream-filled biscuits*, crackers, cookies* (chocolate chip, cinnamon), wafers* (orange, chocolate, vanilla); Orgran low-protein pasta (anellini, ribbons, rigatini); Promin pasta and tricolour pasta; Rite-Diet low-protein white bread (with added fibre); Rite-Diet low-protein flour mix; Rite-Diet low-protein baking mix; Ultra Egg Replacer; Ultra gluten-free, low-protein bread rolls; Ultra low-protein, gluten-free canned brown bread (except for phenylketonuria); Ultra low-protein, gluten-free canned white bread; Ultra white gluten-free, low-protein bread (sliced and unsliced); Ultra PKU biscuits, PKU bread, PKU cookies, PKU flour, PKU pizza base, PKU savoy biscuits.

*Not prescribable on ACBS for coeliac disease, dermatitis herpetiformis, steatorrhoea due to gluten sensitivity

Malabsorption states: (see also gluten-sensitive enteropathies; liver disease; carbohydrate malabsorption;

intestinal lymphangiectasia; milk intolerance and synthetic diets).

(a) Protein sources: Caprilon Formula; Comminuted Chicken Meat (Cow & Gate); Duocal Super Soluble and Liquid; Forceval Protein; Maxipro HBV; MCT Pepdite; Neocate; Pepdite.

(b) Fat: Alembicol D; Calogen; Caprilon Formula; Liquigen; Medium Chain Triglyceride Oil; MCT Pepdite.

(c) Carbohydrate: Caloreen; Fortical; Hycal; Maxijul LE, Liquid, and Super Soluble; Polycal; Polycal Liquid; Polycose.

(d) Complete Feeds. For use as the sole source of nutrition or as a necessary nutritional supplement prescribed on medical grounds: Caprilon Formula; Clinifeed Favour and Iso; Elemental 028; Enrich; Ensure; Ensure Powder; Entera; Fresubin Liquid and Sip Feeds, High Energy, Isofibre, and Plus F; Jevity; Liquisorb feed and drink, MCT (1) Powder (with appropriate vitamin and mineral supplements); MCT Pepdite; Nutrison Fibre, Paediatric and Standard; Osmolite; Paediasure; Pepdite; Peptamen; Pepti-2000 LF; Pepti-Junior; Peptisorb; Portagen; Pregestimil; Triosorbon.

(e) Nutritional supplements. Necessary nutritional supplements prescribed on medical grounds: Advera; Clinifeed 400, and Protein Rich; Ensure Plus; Formance; Fortimel; Fortipudding; Fortisip; Fresenius OPD; Fresubin 750; Liquisorb High Energy; Liquisorbon MCT; Maxisorb; Nutrison Energy Plus; Peptisorbon; Perative; Protein Forte; Provide; Reabilan.

(f) Minerals: Aminogran Mineral Mixture; Metabolic Mineral Mixture.

(g) Vitamins: As appropriate, and see synthetic diets.

(h) Vitamins and Minerals: Paediatric Seravit

Malnutrition (disease-related): Advera[1]; Clinifeed 400[1], Favour, Iso and Protein Rich; Clinutren 1.0 and 1.5[1]; Enrich; Ensure; Ensure Plus[1]; Ensure Powder; Entera; Formance[1]; Fortimel[1]; Fortipudding[1]; Fortisip[1]; Fresenius OPD[1]; Fresubin Liquid and Sip Feeds, High energy, Isofibre, Plus F and 750[1]; Jevity; Liquisorb High Energy[1]; Liquisorb Feed and Drink; Liquisorbon MCT[1]; Maxisorb[1]; Nutrison Energy Plus[1], Fibre, Paediatric and Standard; Osmolite; Paediasure; Peptisorbon; Perative[1]; Protein Forte[1]; Provide[1]; Triosorbon.

Maple syrup urine disease: Analog MSUD; MSUD Maxamaid; MSUD Maxamum; MSUD Aid III, and see also low-protein products; synthetic diets.

Methylmalonic or propionic acidaemia: Analog XMet, Thre, Val, Isoleu; XMet, Thre, Val, Isoleu Maxamaid; XMet, Thre, Val, Isoleu Maxamum; Methionine, Threonine, Valine-Free and Leucine-Low Amino Acid Mix.

Milk protein sensitivity: Comminuted Chicken Meat (Cow & Gate); InfaSoy; Isomil powder; Nutramigen; Nutrison Soya; Ostersoy; Prosobee Liquid and powder; Wysoy, and see also synthetic diets.

Neoplasia-related (associated) cachexia (anorexia): see Malnutrition (disease-related)

Nutritional support for adults (for precise conditions for which these products have ACBS approval, see products above):

A. **Nutritionally complete feeds.** For use as the sole source of nutrition or as a necessary nutritional supplement prescribed on medical grounds:
  (i) Gluten-Free: Clinifeed Iso; Entera; Fresubin Liquid, Sip Feeds, High Energy, and Plus F (vegetable soup flavour only); Liquisorb feed and drink; Nutrison Fibre and Standard; Triosorbon.
  (ii) Lactose-free: Clinifeed Favour.
  (iii)Lactose- and Gluten-Free: Enrich; Ensure, Ensure Powder; Fresubin Isofibre; Osmolite.
  (iv)Containing fibre: Enrich; Fresubin Isofibre; Fresubin Plus F; Jevity; Nutrison Fibre.
  (v) Elemental Feeds: Elemental 028; Flexical; Peptamen; Pepti-2000 LF; Peptisorb.

B. **Nutritional source supplements;** see synthetic diets; malabsorption states.
  (a) General supplements. Necessary nutritional supplements prescribed on medical grounds: Advera; Clinifeed 400, and Protein Rich; Ensure Plus; Formance; Fortimel; Fortipudding; Fortisip; Fresenius OPD; Fresubin 750;

Liquisorb High Energy; Liquisorbon MCT; Maxisorb; Nutrison Energy Plus; Peptisorbon; Perative; Protein Forte; Provide; Reabilan.

(b) Carbohydrates; lactose-free and gluten-free; Caloreen*; Super-Soluble Duocal, and Duocal Liquid*; Hycal*; Maxijul LE*, Liquid, and Super Soluble; Polycal; Polycal Liquid; Polycose.

*Have low electrolyte content.

(c) Fat: Alembicol D; Calogen; MCT Oil; Liquigen.

(d) Nitrogen: Casilan (whole protein based, low-sodium); Forceval Protein (whole protein based, low-sodium); Maxipro HBV (whole protein based, low-sodium); Pro-Mod (whey protein based, low-sodium).

(e) Minerals: Aminogran Mineral Mixture; Metabolic Mineral Mixture.

Phenylketonuria: Aglutella low-protein rice; Albumaid XP and XP Concentrate; Aminogran Food Supplement and Mineral Mixture; Analog XP; Aproten products (annellini, biscuits, bread mix, cake mix, crispbread, ditalini, flour, rigatini, spaghetti, tagliatelle); Calogen; Caloreen; dp Low-Protein butterscotch-flavoured or chocolate-flavoured chip cookies; Juvela low-protein loaf (sliced and unsliced); Juvela low-protein bread rolls; Juvela gluten-free low-protein (chocolate chip, orange, and cinnamon flavour) cookies; Juvela low-protein mix; Lofenalac; Loprofin egg replacer; Loprofin gluten-free, low-protein bread (sliced and unsliced), bread (with or without salt), mix and pasta (macaroni, spaghetti short-cut, pasta spirals); Loprofin low-protein sweet biscuits, chocolate cream-filled biscuits, crackers, cookies (chocolate chip, cinnamon), wafers (orange, chocolate, vanilla); Loprofin PKU drink; XP Maxamaid ; XP Bar Maxamaid; XP Concentrate Maxamaid; XP Maxamum; Metabolic Mineral Mixture; Milupa PKU2 and PKU3; Minafen; Orgran low-protein pasta (annelini, ribbons, rigatini); Phlexy-10 drink; PK Aid IV; PK Aid 3; Polycal; Polycose liquid and powder; Promin pasta and tricolour pasta; Rite-Diet low-protein white bread (with added fibre); Rite-Diet low-protein baking mix; Rite-Diet low-protein flour mix; Sno-Pro; Ultra Egg Replacer; Ultra low-protein, gluten-free canned white bread; and see low-protein products and synthetic diets; Ultra PKU biscuits, PKU bread; PKU cookies, PKU flour, PKU pizza base; PKU savoy biscuits.

Propionic acidaemia: Analog X Met, Thre, Val, Isoleu; X Met, Thre, Val, Isoleu Maxamaid; X Met Thre, Val, Isoleu Maxamum; Methionine, Threonine, Valine-Free and Isoleucine-Low Amino Acid Mix.

Protein intolerance: see milk protein sensitivity, whole protein sensitivity, low-protein products, synthetic diets, and amino acid metabolic disorders.

Refsum's Disease: Fresubin Liquid and Sip Feeds.

Renal dialysis: see dialysis.

Renal failure: Aglutella low-protein rice; Aproten products (annellini, biscuits, bread mix, cake mix, crispbread, ditalini, flour, rigatini, spaghetti, tagliatelle); Calogen; Caloreen; Dialamine; dp Low-Protein butterscotch-flavoured or chocolate-flavoured chip cookies; Duobar; Super-Soluble Duocal and Duocal Liquid; Fortical; Hycal; Juvela gluten-free low-protein (chocolate chip, orange, and cinnamon flavour) cookies; Juvela low-protein loaf (sliced and unsliced) and low-protein flour mix; Kindergen PROD; Loprofin gluten-free, low-protein bread (sliced and unsliced), bread (with or without salt), mix and pasta (macaroni, macaroni elbows, spaghetti short-cut, pasta spirals, tagliatelle, vermicelli); Loprofin egg replacer; Loprofin low-protein sweet biscuits, chocolate cream-filled biscuits, crackers, cookies (chocolate chip, cinnamon), wafers (orange, chocolate, vanilla); Maxijul LE, Liquid, and Super Soluble; Nepro; Orgran low-protein pasta (annelini, ribbons, rigatini); Polycal; Polycose liquid and powder; Promin pasta and tricolour pasta; Rite-Diet low-protein white bread (with added fibre); Rite-Diet low-protein flour mix; Rite-Diet low-protein baking mix; Rite-Diet low-sodium bread; Ultra Egg Replacer; Ultra low-protein, gluten-free canned bread (brown and white); Ultra PKU

biscuits, PKU cookies, PKU flour, PKU pizza base, PKU savoy biscuits.

Short bowel syndrome: see malabsorption states.

Sicca Syndrome: Glandosane; Luborant; Saliva Orthana; Salivace; Salivix.

Sodium dietary reduction: Rite-Diet low-sodium bread.

Sucrose intolerance: see carbohydrate malabsorption.

Synthetic diets:

(a) Fat: Alembicol D; Calogen; Liquigen; Medium Chain Triglyceride Oil.

(b) Carbohydrate: Caloreen; Hycal; Maxijul LE, Liquid, Super Soluble; Polycal; Polycal Liquid; Polycose powder.

(c) Minerals: Aminogran Mineral Mixture; Metabolic Mineral Mixture.

(d) Protein sources: see malabsorption states, complete feeds.

(e) Vitamins: as appropriate and see malabsorption states, nutritional support for adults.

(f) Vitamins and Minerals: Paediatric Seravit.

Tyrosinaemia: Analog XPhen, Tyr; XPhen, Tyr Maxamaid; Phenylalanine, Tyrosine and Methionine-Free Amino Acid Mix; Tyrosine and Phenylalanine-Free Amino Acid Mix.

Urea cycle disorders: L-Arginine Supplement for urea cycle disorders

Vomiting in infancy: Instant Carobel, Nestargel.

Whole protein sensitivity[2]**:** Alfare; Caprilon Formula; MCT Pepdite; Neocate; Nutramigen; Pepdite; Pepti-Junior; Pregestimil; Prejomin.

Xerostomia: Glandosane; Luborant; Saliva Orthana; Salivace; Salivix.

CONDITIONS FOR WHICH TOILET PREPARATIONS MAY BE PRESCRIBED ON FP10

Note. This is a list of clinical conditions for which the ACBS has approved toilet preparations. For details of the preparations see Chapter 13.

Birthmarks: see disfiguring skin lesions.

Dermatitis (includes contact, atopic and infective dermatoses, eczema and pruritic dermatoses): Aveeno Bath Oil; Aveeno Cream; Aveeno sachets (regular and oilated); Bath E45; Vaseline Dermacare Cream and Lotion; Wash E45.

Dermatitis herpetiformis: see gluten-sensitive enteropathies.

Disfiguring skin lesions (birthmarks, mutilating lesions and scars): Boots Covering Cream; Covermark products; Dermablend Cover Creme, Leg Cover, and Setting Powder; Dermacolor Camouflage cream and fixing powder; Keromask masking cream and finishing powder; Veil Cover cream and Finishing Powder. (Cleansing Creams, Cleansing Milks, and Cleansing Lotions are excluded.)

Disinfectants (antiseptics): drugs only when ordered in such quantities and with such directions as are appropriate for the treatment of patients. Not to be regarded as drugs if ordered for general hygienic purposes.

Eczema: see dermatitis.

Photodermatoses (skin protection in): Coppertone Supershade and Ultrashade 23; Piz Buin Sunblock Lotion 20; RoC Total Sunblock Cream SPF 16 (Colourless); RoC Total Sunblock Cream SPF 25 (Colourless and tinted); Spectraban 25; Spectraban Ultra 28; Sun E45 Cream 25; Sun E45 Lotion 15; Uvistat Babysun Cream 22; Uvistat Lipscreen 15; Uvistat Sun Block Cream 20; Uvistat Ultrablock Sun Cream 30.

Pruritus: see dermatitis.

---

1. As a supplement only

2. Defined as: intolerance to whole protein, proven by at least two withdrawal and challenge tests, as suggested by an accurate dietary history.

Appendix 8: Urinary and Stoma Appliances

This Appendix includes incontinence appliances, urethral catheters, and stoma products. Other products such as dressings, elastic hosiery, and glucose monitoring reagents are included in the relevant BNF chapters.

Incontinence appliances and urethral catheters

Incontinence appliances are listed in Part IXB of *Drug Tariff* or Part 5 of *Scottish Drug Tariff*; urethral catheters are included in Part IXA of *Drug Tariff* or Part 3 of Scottish *Drug Tariff*

DRAINABLE DRIBBLING APPLIANCES

Re-usable for at least 1 month (with exception of Alexa®)

Body's Care range
Bag (Body's Care)
 Dribbling bag with loops and tapes. Net price 1 = £14.46
Urinal (Body's Care)
 Drip male urinal with tap. Net price 1 = £38.72; 1 replacement belt = £9.56

Bullen range
Bags (Bullen)
 Net price 10 Dribblet® bags = £21.09; 10 Dribblet® sheath bags = £47.34

DePuy range
Aquadry® (DePuy)
 Male incontinence pouch. Net price 1 (with short or long tube) = £6.15
 Drip type urinal. Net price 1 = £46.25

Henleys range
Alexa® dribbler bag (Henleys)
 Plain bag, with draw strings. Net price 100 bags = £4.22; 100 bags with non-reflux valve = £16.25

Rüsch range
Peoplecare® (Rüsch)
Male drip urinal. Net price 1 = £45.07

Ward range
Bags (Ward)
 Male dribbling bag with diaphragm and belt. Net price 1 = £23.85

INCONTINENCE BELTS

Average life 6 months

Body's Care range
Waist belt for kipper bags (Body's Care)
 Net price 1 = £4.77; 1 (with webbing band) = £4.77

Rüsch range
Peoplecare® (Rüsch)
 Waist and support strap for kipper bag. Net price 1 = £6.06
 Rubber belt. Net price 1 = £3.33

Simcare range
Belts (Simcare)
 Rubber belt. Net price 1 = £5.03
 Web belt (small, medium, or large) = £10.43

Ward range
Belts (Ward)
 Waist belt for black kipper bag. Net price 1 = £4.37
 Rubber belt for PP (pubic pressure) urinal. Net price 1 = £3.78

INCONTINENCE SHEATHS

Unless otherwise indicated the incontinence sheaths (also known as penile sheaths or external catheters) listed below are of the soft, flexible, latex type. Each sheath may be left in place for 1 to 3 days between changes

Bard range
Integrity® (Bard)
 Incontinence sheath, self-adhesive. Net price 30 sheaths (25, 30, or 35 mm) = £36.25
Reliasheath® (Bard)
 Incontinence sheath with adhesive strip. Net price 30 sheaths (20, 25, 30, 35, or 40 mm) = £32.36
Uriplan® (Bard)
 Incontinence sheath. Net price 30 sheaths (20, 25, 30, 35, or 40 mm) = £21.67
 Uro sheath® (washable; may be used many times). Net price 1 (25, 35, or 40 mm) = £4.52

Camp range
Posey® (Camp)
 Incontinence sheath. 'Fastflow' incontinence sheath. Net price 10 sheaths (25, 30, or 35 mm) = £6.00

Coloplast range
Conveen® (Coloplast)
 Incontinence sheath, with anti-kink design and Uriliner® adhesive strip. Net price 30 sheaths (20, 25, 30, 35, or 40mm) = £38.88
Conveen self-sealing Urisheath® (Coloplast)
 Incontinence sheath. Net price 30 sheaths (25, 30, or 35mm) = £38.28

DePuy range
Aquadry® (DePuy)
 Incontinence sheath. Net price 10 sheaths (small, medium, large, or extra-large) = £9.22; 30 sheaths with bulbous end (small, medium, or large) = £26.59
Aquadry Freedom® (DePuy)
 Freedom® incontinence sheath, self-adhesive. Net price 30 sheaths (small, medium, or large) = £38.40
 Freedom Plus® incontinence sheath, self-adhesive. Net price 30 sheaths (small, medium, or large) = £38.40

EMS Medical range
Sheaths (EMS Medical)
 Incontinence sheath. Net price 100 sheaths (25, 30, or 35 mm) = £42.00; 30 sheaths (with liner; 25, 30, or 35mm) = £30.00

Fry Surgical range
Uridom® (Fry Surgical)
Incontinence sheath, with adhesive strip. Net price 30 sheaths = £27.07

Hospital Management and Supplies range
Macrodom® (Hospital Management and Supplies)
Incontinence sheath, including adhesive strip. Net price 30 sheaths (with 2-inch tube) = £21.50; 25 sheaths (with 5-inch tube) = £22.50
Macrodom Plus® (Hospital Management and Supplies)
Incontinence sheath, including adhesive strip. Net price 30 sheaths (small, medium, or large) = £23.00

Mediplus range
Medimates® (Mediplus)
Incontinence sheath with single-sided adhesive strip. Net price 30 sheaths (straight, 20, 25, 30, 35, or 40 mm; bulb, 25, 30, or 35 mm) = £28.30
Incontinence sheath with double-sided adhesive strip. Net price 30 sheaths (straight, 20, 25, 30, 35, or 40 mm; bulb, 25, 30, or 35 mm) = £30.20

North West Medical range
Uridrop® (North West Medical)
Incontinence sheath. Net price 30 sheaths (paediatric = 42 or 55 mm; sizes 1, 2, 3, or 4 = 70, 80, 100, or 107 mm) = £12.00; 100 = £40.00
Incontinence sheath, with Uristrip® adhesive strip. Net price 30 sheaths (paediatric = 42 or 55 mm; sizes 1, 2, 3, or 4 = 70, 80, 100, or 107 mm) = £24.00

Payne range
Incontiaid® (Payne)
Incontinence sheath. Net price 10 sheaths, with adhesive strip (sizes 20, 25, 30, 35 or 40 mm) = £11.92; 1 sheath, without adhesive strip (sizes 20, 25, 30, 35 or 40 mm) = 77p; 10 adhesive strips = £3.88

Rüsch range
Dryaid® (Rüsch)
Incontinence sheath. Net price 20 sheaths (with adhesive strip; small, medium, large, or extra-large) = £26.13; 20 sheaths (without adhesive strip; small, medium, large, or extra-large) = £15.14
Portasheath® (Rüsch)
Incontinence sheath. Net price 25 sheaths (25, 30, or 35 mm) = £21.25
Secure external catheter kit, with adhesive strip. Net price 10 sheaths (25, 30, or 35 mm) = £8.70

Salts range
Heritage Cohesive/Sheath Pack® (Salts)
Incontinence sheath, with adhesive. Net price 30 sheaths (17, 22, 25, 32, or 34 mm) = £30.88
Male continence sheath (Salts)
Incontinence sheath. Net price 10 sheaths (17, 22, 25, 32, or 34 mm) = £6.97

Seton range
Incontinence sheath (Seton)
Incontinence sheath. Net price 30 sheaths (small, medium, large, or extra-large) = £30.27; 30 sheaths with self-adhesive liner (small, medium, large, or extra-large) = £36.07

Sherwood range
Texas Catheter® (Sherwood)
Incontinence sheath, with adhesive strip. Net price 12 sheaths = £8.64
Uri Drain® (Sherwood)
Incontinence sheath, with double-sided adhesive strap (25, 30, or 35 mm). Net price 10 = £8.00

Simcare range
Continence sheath (Simcare)
Incontinence sheath. Net price 1 sheath (small, medium, large, or extra-large) = £1.30
Uro Flo® (Simcare)
Incontinence sheath, straight, including adhesive liner. Net price 30 sheaths (small, medium, or large) = £37.90
Uro Flo Mk2® (Simcare)
Incontinence sheath, bulbous, with adhesive liner. Net price 30 sheaths (small, medium or large) = £37.90.
Male incontinence sheath (Simcare)
Incontinence sheath. Net price 100 sheaths = £62.79

Simpla range
Bubble U® (Simpla)
Incontinence sheath, with adhesive foam strip. Net price 30 sheaths (small, medium, large, or extra-large) = £25.20
Incontinence sheath, with self-adhesive Uriseal® liner. Net price 30 sheaths (small, medium, large, or extra-large) = £36.25
Regard® (Simpla)
Incontinence sheath, with liners. Net price 30 sheaths (small, medium, large, or extra-large) = £32.67

FIXING STRIPS AND ADHESIVES

Bio Diagnostics
Urifix® tape. Net price 5 m = £4.90
Camp
Posey® sheath holder. Net price 12 (adult) = £12.45; 12 (paediatric) = £10.20
ConvaTec
Urihesive® strips. Net price 15 = £6.00
DePuy
Aquadry® penile liners. Net price 20 = £7.50
Dow Corning
Adhesive B (Silicone adhesive aerosol). Net price 207 g = £10.02
355 medical adhesive (brush-on silicone adhesive). Net price 1 = £3.03
EMS Medical
Urifix® tape. Net price 5 m = £4.90
North West Medical
Uristrip® adhesive strip. Net price 30 = £12.00; 100 = £40.00
Payne
Incontiaid® sheath holder. Net price 1 = 88p
Rüsch
Dryaid® strip. Net price 20 strips = £10.99
Salts
Heritage® sheath collar pack. Net price 30 = £3.55
NHS Cohesive® strips for use with sheaths. Net price 10 = £4.50

LEG BAGS

Most plastic bags suitable for use for 5–7 days; rubber bags re-usable for 4–6 months

Bard range
Uriplan® (Bard)
Leg bag, plastic, shaped, with tap outlet and elastic Velcro straps. Net price 10 bags (350 mL, direct inlet) = £22.43; 10 bags (350 mL, 12 inch inlet tube) = £22.11; 10 bags (500 mL, direct inlet) = £22.65; 10 bags (500 mL, 4 or 12 inch inlet tube) = £22.74; 10 bags (750 mL, direct inlet, or 4, 12, or 15 inch inlet tube) = £22.87
Seton Urisac® (Bard)
Leg bag, plastic. Net price 10 bags (350 mL, short tube) = £11.00; 10 bags (350 mL, long tube) = £11.32; 10 bags (500 mL, short tube) = £11.97; 10 bags (500 mL, long

tube) = £12.30; 10 bags (750 mL, short tube) = £12.62; 10 bags (750 mL, long tube) = £13.16

Body's Care range
Leg bags (Body's Care)
Kipper bag, black, white, or clear. Net price 1 bag = £21.94
Leg drainage bag, plastic, with tap outlet. Net price 10 bags (350 or 500 mL) = £18.97; 10 bags (750 mL) = £19.63

Coloplast range
Conveen® (Coloplast)
Standard leg bag, plastic. Net price, with 1 set Velcro bands, 10 bags (500 mL, 10 or 40 cm tube) = £18.05
Contour leg bag, plastic, shaped, sterile with sample port. Net price, with 1 set Velcro bands, 10 bags (600 mL, 5 or 30 cm tube; 800 mL, 45 cm tube) = £22.61; 10 non-sterile bags (600 mL, 45 cm adjustable tube) = £22.61

ConvaTec range
Accuseal® (ConvaTec)
Leg bag, plastic. Net price 10 bags (500 mL) = £17.22

DePuy range
Aquadry® (DePuy)
Catheter drainage bag, plastic. Net price 10 bags (small) = £20.65; 10 bags (large) = £21.20
Leg bag, plastic. Net price 10 bags (350, 500, or 750 mL, short or long tube) = £20.69

EMS Medical range
Leg drainage bags (EMS)
Leg bag, plastic. Net price 10 bags (500 mL, short or long tube) = £14.10

Incare range
Urinary leg bag (Incare)
Leg bag, plastic. Net price 10 bags (540 mL, 37 cm tube) = £22.75; 10 bags (540 mL, direct inlet) = £22.20

Payne range
Incontiaid® (Payne)
Leg bag, plastic. Net price 1 bag (500 or 750 mL) = £2.28
Single-chambered GU Black Kipper Bags (Payne)
Leg bag, single-chambered. Net price 1 bag (rubber, with box outlet tap) = £43.49; 1 rubber bag (for night use) = £47.49; 1 bag (for female use) = £35.28; 1 bag (rubber, kipper-style) = £35.28; 1 bag (rubber, Ross type) = £40.27
Leg bags (formerly Willis range)
Rubber bag, for catheter drainage, short neck leg strap. Net price 1 bag = £25.07; 1 bag with web belt and support strap) = £29.34
Rubber bag, female, drainage bag, with conical mount. Net price 1 bag = £23.80; 1 bag (with web belt and support strap) = £28.06

Pharma-Plast range
Careline® (Pharma-Plast)
Leg bag, plastic, with tap outlet and overnight connection tube. Net price, with 1 pair Velcro straps, 10 bags (350 mL, short or long tube) = £20.21; 10 bags (500 mL, short or long tube) = £20.75; 10 bags (750 mL, short or long tube) = £21.28

Rüsch range
Leg bag (Rüsch)
Leg bag, plastic. Net price 10 bags (short tube, 350 or 500 mL) = £13.48; 10 bags (long tube, 350 or 500 mL) = £14.41; 10 bags (750 mL) = £9.64
Kipper bags (Rüsch)
Leg bag. Net price 1 bag (clear/white plastic or all black plastic or rubber, with strap and buckle) = £25.30; 1 bag (clear/white plastic, without strap and buckle) = £20.74

Salts range
Heritage® (Salts)
Leg bag, plastic. Net price 10 bags (500 mL, short tube) = £12.86; 10 bags (500 mL, long tube) = £13.09; 10 bags (750 mL, short tube) = £14.33; 10 bags (750 mL, long tube) = £14.67; 5 leg bag packs = £9.18

Sherwood range
Argyle® (Sherwood)
Leg bag, plastic. Net price (350, 500 or 750 mL, short or long tube) = £21.30

Simcare range
NHS Meredith® (Simcare)
Top outlet bag. Net price 25 bags (2 litres) = £47.28
PVC drainage bag (Simcare)
Leg bag, plastic. Net price 1 bag (small or large) = £3.55
Rubber bags (Simcare)
Leg bag, rubber, with leg strap. Net price = £32.88
Uro-Flo® (Simcare)
Standard leg bag, plastic. Net price 10 bags (350, 500 or 750 mL, 5 or 30 cm tube) = £13.86

Simpla range
Regard® (Simpla)
Leg bag, plastic. Net price 10 bags (350 mL, short tube) = £22.50; 10 bags (500 mL, short tube or adjustable long tube) = £22.74; 10 bags (750 mL, adjustable long tube) = £22.85
Trident® (Simpla)
Leg bag, plastic. Net price 10 bags (350 mL, short tube) = £22.50; 10 bags (500 mL, short or long tube) = £22.74; 10 bags (750 mL, short, long, or adjustable long tube) = £22.85

Universal range
Unicorn® (Universal)
Leg bag, plastic. Net price 10 bags (350 mL, short tube) = £17.60; 10 bags (500 mL, short or long tube) = £17.80; 10 bags (750 mL, short or long tube) = £18.00

H G Wallace range
Leg bags (H G Wallace)
Leg bag, with valve outlet, natural latex straps, and plastic tube. Net price 10 bags (350 mL, short tube) = £21.79; 10 bags (350 mL, long tube) = £22.40; 1 bags (500 mL, short tube) = £22.27; 10 bags (500mL long tube) = £22.84; 10 bags (750 mL, short tube) = £22.60; 10 bags (750 mL, long tube) = £22.73
Leg bag, with twist tap, elastic straps, and plastic tube. Net price 10 bags (750 mL, short tube) = £22.64; 10 bags (750 mL, long tube, 30 cm) = £22.77
Tri-form® leg bag, plastic. Net price 10 bags (500 mL short tube) = £22.25; 10 bags (500 mL, medium tube) = £22.50; 10 bags (500 mL, long tube) = £22.70

Ward range
Kipper bag (Ward)
Leg bag, kipper type, rubber. Net price 1 bag (black, clear, or white) = £19.90
Leg drainage bag (Ward)
Leg bag, plastic. Net price 10 bags (350 mL) = £9.61; 1 bags (500 mL) = £9.90; 10 bags (750 mL) = £10.49
Comfort® (Ward)
Leg bag, plastic. Net price 10 bags (350 mL) = £9.65; 1 bags (500 mL) = £9.92; 10 bags (750 mL) = £10.44

NIGHT DRAINAGE BAGS

Suitable for night-time use for collection of urine from indwelling catheters or from incontinence sheaths; bag hangers normally supplied through community nursing service.
Drainage bags have life of 5–7 nights

Bard

Uriplan® drainage bag. Net price 10 bags = £10.13; Collection bag (non-drainable), 10 bags = £1.97

Body's Care

2 litre drainage bag with tap outlet. Net price 1 bag = £1.28

Coloplast

Conveen® 1.5 litre drainage bag with 90 cm tube. Net price 10 bags = £11.41

ConvaTec

Surgicare System® 2 litre drainage bag. Net price 5 bags (Accuseal®) = £7.10; 5 bags (night) = £7.10

DePuy

Aqua® range 2 litre urine drainage bag. Net price 10 bags (Aqua® 2, non-drainable) = £1.90; 10 bags (Aqua® 4) = £8.95

Pharma-Plast

Careline® range, 2 litre urine drainage bag with 90 cm inlet tube. Net price 10 bags (Careline® E1, non-drainable) = £1.76; 10 bags (Careline® E2, non-drainable, with non-reflux valve) = £1.88; 5 bags (Careline® E4, with non-reflux valve and tap outlet) = £4.61

Rand Rocket

Urine drainage bag (non-drainable, short or long tube). Net price 25 bags = £3.75

Rüsch

Drainage bags, 2 litre. Net price 10 bags (C) = £10.37; 10 bags with non-reflux valve and plug (CV) = £11.51; 10 bags with non-reflux valve and tap (CVT) = £11.93; 10 bags with non-reflux valve and wide bore tap (DVT) = £11.00

Salts

2 litre H2 urine drainage bag. Net price 10 bags with non-reflux valve and tap = £10.52

Sherwood

Argyle® 2 litre urinary drainage bag. Net price 10 bags = £9.60

Simcare

Uro-flo® night drainage bag. Net price 10 bags (female or male) = £13.51

Simpla

Regard® overnight drainage bag. Net price 10 bags = £9.45

Urine drainage bag. Net price 10 bags (S1, non-drainable) = £2.05; 10 bags (S2, non-drainable with non-reflux valve) = £2.19; 10 bags (night, short tube) = £10.23; 10 bags (S4, long tube) = £10.87

H G Wallace

Inbeds 2 litre drainage bag with twist tap. Net price 10 bags = £12.41

Ward

2 litre drainage bag with push/pull outlet. Net price 10 bags = £10.44

SUSPENSORY SYSTEMS

Drainage bag with support; bags may be used for 5–7 days

Bard

Urisac® Portabag® with belt. Net price 10 bags (plastic) = £10.25; 1 belt = £6.00

EMS Medical

Drainage bag with Shepheard Sporran belt. Net price 10 bags (plastic) = £14.10; 1 belt = £7.25

Rüsch

Portabag® with Portabelt®. Net price 10 bags (plastic) = £15.45; 1 belt = £8.63

H G Wallace

Holster bag with leg bag holster. Net price 10 bags (400 mL, plastic) = £17.48; 1 holster (24–30, 30–36, or 36–44 inch) = £8.17

TUBING AND ACCESSORIES

Bard

General purpose tubing. Net price 96 inch = £1.82
Urinary drainage economy tube. Net price 48 inch = £1.16
Adaptor for Uro sheath® (penile sheath to leg bag) 8 inch. Net price 1 = 92p
Uriplan® leg bag straps (washable). Net price 5 pairs = £10.63
Latex leg bag straps. Net price 10 pairs = £2.18
Seton range foam/Velcro leg bag straps. Net price 10 pairs = £4.14
Urisac® tapes. Net price 10 pairs = £4.58

Body's Care

Velcro leg straps. Net price 1 pair = £1.55
Leg bag connecting tube. Net price 1 = £1.21; 1 (with mount) = £2.05

Coloplast

Velcro bands (washable). Net price 10 pairs = £31.85

ConvaTec

Accuseal® leg bag extension tube. Net price 10 tubes = £6.36

DePuy

Leg bag connecting tube. Net price 10 = £6.55
Aquadry® leg straps. Net price 5 pairs = £8.75

EMS Medical

Velcro leg straps. Net price 10 = £5.00

Incare

Leg bag straps. Net price 1 pair (14 inch, calf or 23 inch, thigh) = £2.48

MMG

G-Strap. Net price 'adult' or 'short', 5 = £10.35; 'abdomen', 5 = £11.40

Payne

Rubber extension tube, 6 inch. Net price = £2.99
Rubber leg strap. Net price 1 = £1.05
Velcro leg strap. Net price 1 = 82p

Pharma-Plast

Careline® leg bag straps. Net price 10 = £11.25

Portex

Paul (Penrose) tubing. Net price 10 (6, 13, 19, or 25 mm) = £12.02; 10 (32, 38, 44, or 51 mm) = £12.02
Tapered adaptor (catheter to leg bag). Net price 1 = £5.46; 1 (stepped) = £7.94

Rüsch

Connecting tubes, net price 1 tube for kipper bag = £2.52; 14-inch connecting tube for drip urinal = £2.51; 1 connecting tube for all urinals with female connector = £3.83

Salts

Heritage® leg bag extension tube. Net price 2 tubes = £1.83

Sherwood

Argyle® foam and Velcro strap, washable. Net price 1 (75 cm, leg) = £1.69; 1 (150 cm, abdomen) = £3.17
Argyle Suregrip® general purpose tube, internal diameter 7 mm, length 2.7 m. Net price 50 tubes = £36.00
Argyle Penrose® tubing, internal diameter 6, 8, 10, 13, 16, 19, or 25 mm and length 44 cm. Net price 50 = £30.75

Simcare

Stopcock for Chiron plastic urinal bags (in place of screwcap). Net price 1 = £4.19
Rubber extension tube (with mounts). Net price = £4.19
Rubber tubing (length, 1.5 m). Net price 1 = £9.80
Plastic connector with tube. Net price 1 = £2.81
Female connector for Mitcham bag. Net price = £1.94
Night bag connector. Net price 1 = £1.18
Spare 'O' rings for pubic pressure urinal. Net price 5 = £1.11
Uro-Flo® elastic Velcro leg straps. Net price 5 pairs = £3.98

Simpla
Leg bag straps. Net price 20 pairs (foam) = £11.71; 5 pairs (elasticated, washable) = £11.54

H G Wallace
Leg bag extension tube. Net price 10 (30 cm) = £23.46; 10 (60 cm) = £25.80

Silgrip® leg straps. Net price 5 pairs (elasticated or Side-Fix thigh-fitting) = £11.51; 5 pairs (Side-Fix calf-fitting) = £10.94

URINAL SYSTEMS

Patients generally have two urinal systems (one to wash and one to wear). Each appliance should last for 6 months

Bard
Uriplan Maguire® urinal and adaptor. Net price (waist sizes 66–81 cm, 81–96 cm, or 96–112 cm) = £52.92

Male day and night urinal. Net price 1 (14 oz) = £38.10; 1 (20 oz) = £33.74

Mobile paraplegic day and night urinal. Net price 1 = £43.17

Uriplan Maguire® adaptor and tubing. Net price = £7.15

Bell and Croyden
Fridjohn male urinal. Net price 1 = £40.61

Male urinal, day and night use. Net price 1 (with long or short bag) = £37.35

Body's Care
Male day and night urinal with tap, covered bag, with band and suspensory, and leg strap with air vent. Net price 1 = £45.46

Male night urinal with tap, covered bag, with band and suspensory. Net price 1 = £55.31

Male day and night urinal with tap, long tube, covered bag, with band and suspensory with air vent. Net price 1 = £53.74

Male day and night urinal with tap, double bag, air vent, inflating rim, with band understraps. Net price 1 = £56.92

Male day and night urinal with tap, covered bag, diaphragm top, and air vent. Net price 1 = £49.19

Male day and night urinal with tap, improved pattern, inflating rim, short air vent, with band and understrap. Net price 1 = £53.98; 1 (with extension tube) = £56.98; 1 (with long bag) = £54.75

Male day and night urinal with tap, air vent, diaphragm top, with band and understrap. Net price 1 (with long bag) = £52.36; 1 (with short bag) = £48.52; 1 (with extension tube) = £52.19

Male day and night urinal with tap, air vent, with band and suspensory. Net price 1 (long bag) = £46.63

Male day urinal with tap, to contain penis and scrotum. Net price 1 (short bag, with band and understrap) = £43.96; 1 (with inner sheath and air vent) = £45.68

Male jockey appliance with tap. Net price 1 = £48.63

Spares

Replacement belt. Net price 1 = £9.56

Outer receiver. Net price 1 = £11.13

Inner sheath. Net price 5 = £11.13

Plastic bags. Net price 5 = £12.26

Rubber bag. Net price 1 = £20.42

Ring. Net price 1 = 82p

Stoke Mandeville male urinal with tap (specify sheath size). Net price 1 = £51.63; 1 (with double bag) = £61.99; 1 replacement sheath (specify size) = £5.11

Male pubic pressure urinal with tap (specify sheath size). Net price 1 (with rubber bag) = £55.21; 1 (with 5 plastic bags) = £51.97

Spares

Flange with sheaths. Net price 1 = £25.81

Cone. Net price (curved, small, medium, or large; straight,small, medium, large, or extra-large) = £10.23

Plastic bag. Net price 1 (small or large) = £12.26

Rubber bag. Net price 1 = £20.03

Rubber belt. Net price 1 = £3.67

Progress® long life plastic urinal. Net price 1 (inner sheath or scrotal) = £21.81

Fridjohn urinal. Net price 1 = £65.21

YB wet urinal. Net price 1 = £52.92

Essex appliance. Net price 1 = £44.18

One-piece belt. Net price 1 (rubber or plastic bag coverlet) = £44.31

Bullen
Child urinal. Net price 1 (with transverse bag = £67.16; 1 (with medium-size long bag) = £64.90

Male urinal. Net price 1 (with large-size long bag) = £72.01

DePuy
Aquadry® urinal. Net price 1 cross cut diaphragm and scrotal support; inner sheath and rubber understrap (1.125, 1.25, 1.375, 1.5, or 1.625 inch); pubic pressure; tapered inner sleeve trimmed to fit and rubber understrap; pressure ring, diaphragm and rubber understrap (1, 1.25, or 1.5 inch); pressure ring, diaphragm and scrotal support (1, 1.25, or 1.5 inch) = £49.67

Spares

Bag (for all standard urinals). Net price 5 (250 or 325 mL) = £10.85; rubber leg bag connecting tube with female attachment, net price 1 = £2.50

Flange (child: 0.5, 0.675, 0.75, 0.875, 1, 1.125, or 1.25 inch; adult: 1, 1.125, 1.25, 1.375, 1.5, 1.625, or 1.75 inch). Net price 1 = £24.47

Cones. Net price 1 (small, medium, or large; curved or straight) = £10.27

Rubber belt. Net price 1 (24, 28, 36, or 44 inch) = £2.85

Ellis
Hallam modular urinal. Net price 1 = £31.63; 1 spare bag = £1.68; 1 spare belt = £3.75

LRC
Dry sheaths. Net price 144 = £14.42

Payne
Male incontinence appliance with rubber belt. Net price 1 (MK1 with combined rubber flange and understraps) = £55.19; 1 (MK2 with rubber flange and fabric facepiece) = £59.35; 1 (MK3 with combined rubber flange, understraps, and coned top) = £48.98; 1 (MK9, with rubber flange and fabric facepiece) = £61.85

Lightweight male incontinence appliance. Net price 1 (MK4 with fabric facepiece and separate long flanged plastic bag with foam pad) = £34.99; 1 (MK5, with fabric facepiece, with belt combined, separate flange, and long flanged plastic bag) = £49.15; 1 (MK6 with combined flange and understraps and long flanged plastic bag with rubber belt) = £43.10; 1 (MK10, with fabric facepiece, with belt combined, separate flange, and long flanged plastic bag) = £51.65

Spares

Rubber flange. Net price 1 (with feathered diaphragm, MK2, MK5, MK9, MK10) = £15.98; 1 (MK1, MK6) = £24.74; 1 (with feathered diaphragm and combined reinforced top, MK3) = £28.07

Material facepiece. Net price 1 facepiece with belt and loop (MK2, MK4, MK5) = £18.53; 1 facepiece with support belt, loop and scrotal = £21.03

Flange support with wide belt and scrotal support (MK9, MK10). Net price 1 = £21.03

Reinforced cone top (MK1, MK2, MK9). Net price 1 = £10.76

Bag (MK1, MK2, MK3, MK9). Net price 1 plastic bag = £2.71; 1 rubber bag = £16.26

Bag, long flange plastic. Net price 1 MK4 bag = £4.15; 1 MK5, MK6, MK10 bag = £3.66

Belt (MK1, MK3, MK6). Net price 1 (elastic) = £7.38; 1 (web) = £5.16; 1 (rubber) = £3.49

Night connector (MK1, MK2, MK3, MK9). Net price 1 = £3.49

Payne's urine director. Net price 1 = £19.75

Stoke Mandeville condom urinal complete. Net price 1 = £45.54
Spares
Kipper bag. Net price 1 = £25.63
Belt. Net price 1 (38, 46, or 60 inch) = £5.43
Rubber tube and connector. Net price 1 = £2.00; rubber tubing = £4.10 per metre; nylon connector (GU or SM) 1 = £1.16
Dry incontinence sheath. Net price 144 = £13.26
Pubic pressure urinal complete with bag. Net price 1 (rubber or plastic bag) = £55.19
Spares
Pubic pressure flange with sheath (1-inch flange with 0.5, 0.625, 0.75, or 0.875 inch sheath; 1.25-inch flange with 0.875 or 1 inch sheath; 1.5-inch flange with 1.125 or 1.25 inch sheath; 1.75-inch flange with 1.375, 1.5, or 1.625 inch sheath). Net price 1 = £24.74
Coned top. Net price 1 (straight or curved: small, medium, or large; straight: extra-large) = £10.76
Replacements
Rubber bag with vent tube (MK1, MK2, MK3, MK9). Net price 1 = £19.52
Reinforced top with vent tube (MK1, MK2, MK3, MK9). Net price 1 = £14.14
Latex tubing, 8 or 10 mm bore. Net price per metre = £4.10
GU Condom set. Net price 1 = £47.49; 1 (with 40 oz bag) = £58.92
Urinal replacement parts
Nylon stud (GU or SM). Net price 1 = £1.16; 1 (with latex tube) = £2.00
Waist belt for single-chambered bag. Net price 1 (38, 46, or 60 inch) = £5.43
(formerly Willis range)
Male urinal, day and night, air tube to bag, inner sheath and diaphragm to receiver, web belt and cotton suspensory bag. Net price 1 = £46.33, 1 (long narrow Coutil®-covered bag, web belt and cotton suspensory bag) = £48.22
Male urinal, receiver to contain penis and scrotum, web waist band and tape understraps. Net price 1 (day, night, or small build) = £44.24
Male urinal, long rubber bag with 2 leg straps, loops and straps, flanged receiver, air tube, diaphragm and short conical inner sheath, web band and cotton suspensory bag. Net price 1 (day and night) = £45.77
Male urinal, short rubber bag, detachable bag and night tube, web belt and cotton suspensory bag. Net price 1 (day and night) = £36.88
Spares for above urinals
Suspension bag. Net price 1 (small, medium, or large) = £4.66

Rüsch

Thames urinal with bag and connecting tube. Net price 1 (standard or long bag) = £70.86
Severn urinal with bag and connecting tube. Net price 1 (standard, long, or 5 plastic bags) = £70.86; 5 Severn spare sheaths = £27.78
Mersey urinal with bag and connecting tube. Net price 1 (standard, long, or 5 plastic bags) = £70.86
Wye, male, MkII, light-weight urinal. Net price 1 (with separate connecting tube and on/off valve) = £22.90; 1 (with long night extension tube) = £26.69; 1 (with short or long bag) = £38.14
Arizona male urinal. Net price 1 = £70.86
'55' male urinal for paraplegic patients. Net price 1 = £69.80; 6 spare sheaths = £32.61
Stoke Mandeville pattern male urinal with double chamber rubber collection bag. Net price 1 (20, 24, 25, 28, 32, 35, 38, 42, 45, 48, 51, 54, 57, 60, or 63 mm sheath) = £70.86; 1 spare sheath = £6.54
Sahara one-piece top pubic pressure urinal with bag. Net price 1 paediatric (with small rubber collection bag or 5 small plastic collection bags) = £67.55; 1 standard or large (with standard or long rubber collection bag or 5 medium plastic collection bags, and connecting tube) = £67.55
Peoplecare® pubic pressure male urinal. Net price 1 paediatric (flange 25 mm and sheath 13, 16, 19, or 22 mm; or flange 29 mm and sheath 22 or 25 mm; or flange 32 mm and sheath 19, 22, or 25 mm) = £21.94; 1 adult (flange 38 mm and sheath 19, 22, 25, 29, or 32 mm; or flange 44 mm and sheath 35, 38, or 41 mm) = £21.94
Spares
Pubic pressure bag, standard. Net price 1 (medium) = £11.32; 1 (large) = £14.03; 1 (curved top, small, medium, or large) = £8.54; 1 (straight top, small, medium, large, or extra-large) = £8.54
Transverse rubber bag with tap. Net price 1 = £23.18
Pubic pressure flange for transverse rubber bag with tap. Net price 1 (double-based) = £21.94; 1 (adult, rubber) = £25.29
Kipper inco set with 1 black rubber kipper bag, 10 penile sheaths, waist and support strap, and connecting tube. Net price 1 = £37.96

Salts

Male pubic pressure urinal with rubber bag or 4 plastic bags. Net price 1 = £45.61
Spares
Pubic pressure flange with sheath (1-inch flange with 0.5, 0.625, 0.75, or 0.875 inch sheath; 1.25-inch flange with 0.75, 0.875, or 1 inch sheath; 1.5-inch flange with 0.75, 0.875, 1, 1.125 inch sheath; 1.75-inch flange with 1.375, 1.5, or 1.625 inch sheath). Net price 1 = £21.68
Cone. Net price 1 (small, medium, or large: straight or curved; extra-large: straight) = £9.65
Pubic pressure flange belt. Net price 1 = £19.05
Bags. Net price 4 (plastic, child or adult) = £10.61; 1 (rubber, child, adult, or transverse) = £10.61
Belt. Net price = £3.22

Simcare

Male pubic pressure urinal, child, with integral flange. Net price 1 (rubber bag, straight cone, medium) = £55.46; 1 (plastic bag, curved cone, small or medium) = £54.21
Spares
Pubic pressure flange with integral sheath for child. Net price 1 (25-mm flange with 13, 16, 19, or 22 mm sheath; 29-mm flange with 25 mm sheath; 32-mm flange with 25mm sheath) = £30.52
Cone. Net price 1 (small, medium, or large, straight or curved; extra-large, straight) = £12.91
Pubic pressure flange, double-based. Net price 1 (child, 32 mm, adult, 38 or 44 mm) = £27.29
Chailey male urinal. Net price 1 (child, plastic bag) = £57.07; 1 (adolescent or adult, rubber bag) = £57.17; 1 (adolescent or adult, plastic bag) = £64.81
Spares
Curved top with integral sheath and straps. Net price 1 (child: 22-mm sheath; adult: 22, 25, 29, 32, 35, 38, or 44 mm sheath) = £34.15
Belt, rubber. Net price 1 (61 or 91 cm) = £5.03
Bags, plastic (also suitable for pubic pressure and Chiron® urinals). Net price 1 (wide neck, adult, or child) = £3.36
Bags, rubber (also suitable for pubic pressure and Chiron® urinals). Net price 1 child size = £16.24; 1 adult size = £22.26
Male pubic pressure urinal, adult, with integral flange. Net price 1 (rubber bag, various sizes) = £64.25; 1 (plastic bag, various sizes) = £59.87
Replacement pubic pressure flange. Net price 1 = £30.52
Male pubic pressure urinal, adult, with double-based flange. Net price 1 (rubber bag, various sizes) = £64.25; 1 (plastic bag, various sizes) = £59.87
Replacement sheath. Net price 10 = £1.17
Bag, rubber, for pubic pressure urinals. Net price 1 (adult, with vent tube) = £26.63; 1 (adult, double) = £28.52
Stoke Mandeville urinal. Net price 1 (sheath type) = £58.54; 1 (double rubber bag) = £76.08

Spares

Sheath. Net price 1 = £7.98; 10 (for sheath type) = £3.51

Chiron male rubber urinal with webbing belt. Net price 1 = £52.69

Male one-piece urinal. Net price = £50.16

Surrey model lightweight urinal. Net price (MKI or MKII) = £47.66

Spares

Bag. Net price 10 = £29.91

Foam pad. Net price 5 (76 mm/32 mm) = £5.89

Chiron urinal. Net price 1 (male, plastic, rubber sheaths) = £27.26; 1 (geriatric, film-type sheaths) = £39.59; 1 (rubber sheaths) = £39.59

Spares

Sheath. Net price 1 (rubber) = £5.03; 10 (non-allerenic film type) = 93p

Net suspensory. Net price 1 = £11.83

Male urinal for bed use. Net price 1 = £44.47

Pubic flange, large opening. Net price 1 = £20.44

Transverse rubber bag and stopcock. Net price 1 (child) = £30.10

Steeper

Paraplegic male urinal for day and night use with porthole swan-neck top, adjustable elastic belt with linen front 4 buttonholes, and understraps suitable for sitting patients. Net price 1 = £54.36

Male rubber urinal for day use, porthole top, straight neck and inner sheath, adjustable elastic belt with linen front, 4 buttonholes, and understraps. Net price 1 = £40.15; 1 (with swan neck) = £43.41

Male urinal, rabbit eared, with inner sheath complete with waistband. Net price 1 = £38.50

Elastic waistband, adjustable with linen front, 4 buttonholes, and tape understraps for porthole type urinals. Net price 1 = £6.82

Adjustable waistband. Net price 1 = £3.77

Scrotal pouch for rabbit eared urinal. Net price 1 = £4.25

Male dribbling bag (rubber), curved with porthole diaphragm and adjustable webbing belt. Net price 1 = £19.61

Pubic pressure urinal with double-based flange, disposable film sheaths, and 4 plastic bags. Net price 1 = £35.86

Ward

Jockey male urinal. Net price 1 = £62.41

Varsity male urinal. Net price 1 = £48.17

Male urinal. Net price 1 (day use, covered bag, complete with belt suspensory and thigh strap) = £39.85; 1 (day and night, covered bag, air vent, belt suspensory) = £41.25; 1 (day and night, short bag and belt) = £42.70; 1 (day and night, short covered bag and belt) = £46.27; 1 (day and night, double chamber bag) = £48.10; 1 (day and night, long bag and belt) = £42.70

Paraplegic male urinal. Net price 1 = £58.35

Stoke Mandeville Pattern. Net price 1 = £56.06; 1 (removable rubber sheath, double chamber rubber bag, thigh strap and belt) = £50.35

Spare sheath. Net price 1 = £5.20

Male pubic pressure urinal. Net price 1 (rubber bag) = £52.24; 1 (plastic bag) = £46.28

Spares

Pubic pressure flange. Net price 1 = £23.96

Pubic pressure cone; Net price 1 = £9.47

Bags. Net price 1 (rubber) = £12.98; 1 (plastic) = £2.60

Male urinal. Net price 1 (day, covered bag complete with belt) = £37.93; 1 (day and night or night, covered bag complete with belt, suspensory, and thigh strap) = £50.12; 1 (day and night, long tube, air vent, rubber bag, complete with belt and thigh strap) = £45.49

Male urinal. Net price 1 (night, covered bag complete with belt, suspensory, and thigh strap) = £50.12

Male dribbling bag and tapes. Net price 1 = £18.51

Male urinal. Net price 1 (day and night, short covered bag or short bag and belt) = £42.70

Male urinal. Net price 1 (sheath and disc type with long rubber belt or sheath and suspensory with short or long covered bag) = £46.55

Male urinal. Net price 1 (conical top with short or long rubber bag) = £26.56

Night urinal. Net price 1 (with long tube) = £22.45

Stoke Mandeville sheath-type urinal, with 30 rubber film sheaths, rubber bag, and thigh strap and belt. Net price 1 = £44.58

St Peters pattern suprapubic bag. Net price 1 = £27.46

URETHRAL CATHETERS

Urethal catheter sizes are designated by the Charrière (Ch) gauge system; when the size is not stated by the prescriber the Drug Tariff recommends that size 14 or 16 be supplied. For the Foley catheter, if the balloon size is not stated, the 10 mL size should be supplied for adults, 5 mL for paediatric use (balloon sizes are defined as the amount of fluid required to fully inflate the volume of lumen).

Foley catheters for short-/medium-term use in adults

Bard

Uriplan®, teflon-coated latex, male or female. Net price, male (12-26 Ch: 10-mL balloon; 16-28 Ch: 30-mL balloon), 1 catheter = £1.98; female (Ch 12-26: 10-mL balloon), 1 catheter = £2.96; pre-filled with sterile water (Ch 12-26: 10-mL balloon), 1 catheter = £2.25

Rüsch

Soft Simplastic®, PVC, male or female. Net price, male (12-26 Ch: 10-mL balloon; 16-26 Ch: 30-mL balloon), 1 catheter = £4.26; female (12-22 Ch: 10-mL balloon; 16-22 Ch: 30-mL balloon), 1 catheter = £4.26

100 plus®, teflon-coated latex, male or female. Net price male (12-26 Ch: 10-mL balloon; 16-26 Ch: 30-mL balloon), 1 catheter = £1.91; female (12-22 Ch: 10-mL balloon; 16-32 Ch: 30-mL balloon), 1 catheter = £2.45

Simcare

Eschmann Folatex®, latex, male or female. Net price, male (12-28 Ch: 10- or 30-mL balloon), 1 catheter = £1.88; female (12-28 Ch: 10- or 30-mL balloon), 1 catheter = £3.30

Foley catheters for short-/medium-term use in children
All 8-10 Ch: 5-mL balloon

Bard

Uriplan®, teflon-coated latex. Net price 1 catheter = £5.45

Rüsch

100 plus®, teflon-coated latex. Net price 1 catheter = £4.10

Simcare

Eschmann Folatex®, latex. Net price 1 catheter = £3.44

Foley catheters for long-term use in adults

Bard

Biocath®, hydrogel-coated, male or female. Net price, male (12-26 Ch: 10- or 30-mL balloon), 1 catheter = £6.17; female (12-26 Ch: 10-mL balloon), 1 catheter = £6.17; pre-filled with sterile water, male or female (12-26 Ch: 10-mL balloon), 1 catheter = £6.43

Silastic®, silicone-coated. Net price (12-24 Ch: 10-mL balloon; 16-28 Ch: 30-mL balloon), 1 catheter = £6.99

Uriplan®, silicone elastomer-coated latex, male or female. Net price, male (12-26 Ch: 10-mL balloon; 16-28 Ch: 30-mL balloon), 1 catheter = £6.83; female (16-26 Ch: 30-mL balloon), 1 catheter = £6.83; pre-filled with sterile water, male or female (12-26 Ch: 10-mL balloon), 1 catheter = £7.39

Uriplan®, all silicone. Net price (12-24 Ch: 10-mL balloon; 16-24 Ch: 30-mL balloon), 1 catheter = £7.05

Medasil
All silicone, male or female. Net price, male (12-26 Ch: 10-mL balloon; 16-26 Ch: 30-mL balloon), 1 catheter = £4.62; female (12-26 Ch: 10-mL balloon; 16-26 Ch: 30-mL balloon), 1 catheter = £4.62

Rüsch
Silikon 100®, male or female. Net price, male (12-26 Ch: 10-mL balloon; 18-20 Ch: 20-mL balloon; 22-26 Ch: 30-mL balloon), 1 catheter = £6.07; female (12-22 Ch: 10-mL balloon; 18-20 Ch: 20-mL balloon; 22 Ch: 30-mL balloon), 1 catheter = £6.07

Ultrasil®, silicone elastomer-coated latex, male. Net price (12-26 Ch: 10-mL balloon; 16-26 Ch: 30-mL balloon), 1 catheter = £5.25

Sherwood
Argyle®, all silicone, male or female. Net price, male (12-24 Ch: 10-mL balloon; 16 Ch: 20-mL balloon; 18-26 Ch: 30-mL balloon), 1 catheter = £5.83; female (12-18 Ch: 10-mL balloon), 1 catheter = £5.83

Simpla
All silicone, male or female. Net price, male (12-26 Ch: 10-mL balloon; 16-18 Ch: 20-mL balloon; 20-26 Ch: 30-mL balloon), 1 catheter = £7.07; female (12-18 Ch: 10-mL balloon; 20-26 Ch: 30-mL balloon), 1 catheter = £7.02

Trident®, silicone elastomer coated latex, male. Net price (12-22 Ch: 10-mL balloon; 16-24 Ch: 30-mL balloon, 1 catheter = £4.50

Foley catheters for long-term use in children
All 8-10 Ch: 5-mL balloon
Bard
Biocath®, hydrogel-coated. Net price 1 catheter = £6.17
Medasil
All silicone. Net price 1 catheter = £4.62
Rüsch
Silikon 100®. Net price 1 catheter = £6.07
Sherwood
Argyle®, all silicone. Net price 1 catheter = £6.29
Simpla
All silicone. Net price 1 catheter = £7.25

Nélaton catheters ('ordinary' cylindrical catheter)
Bard
Reliacath®, teflon-coated latex, 14 Ch. Net price 5-catheter pack = £5.94
Reliacath®, plastic, male, female, or paediatric. Net price, male or female (12-18 Ch), 5-catheter pack = £5.65; paediatric (8-10 Ch), 5-catheter pack = £5.65
EMS
PVC, male, female or paediatric. Net price, male (10-18 Ch), 1 catheter = 95p, 5-catheter pack = £4.35; female (12-18 Ch), 1 catheter = 98p, 5-catheter pack = £4.68; paediatric (6-10 Ch), 1 catheter = 98p, 5-catheter pack = £4.65
Pennine
Male, female, or paediatric. Net price, male (12-16 Ch), 10-catheter pack = £3.23; female (10-14 Ch), 10-catheter pack = £2.94; paediatric (6-10 Ch), 10-catheter pack = £2.94
Portex
PVC, male or female, 8-14 Ch. Net price, male, 5-catheter pack = £6.77; female, 5-catheter pack = £6.46
Rüsch
Riplex Jacques®, PVC, male or female 8-18 Ch. Net price, male, 1 catheter = £1.47, 5-catheter pack = £6.30; female, 1 catheter = £1.31, 5-catheter pack = £5.73
Jacques®, soft red rubber, 8-18 Ch. Net price 1 catheter = £1.31, 5-catheter pack = £5.46
Simcare
PVC, male or female, 8-14 Ch. Net price, male, 5-catheter pack = £6.92; female, 5-catheter pack = £6.65
Uno Plast
PVC, male or female or paediatric. Net price, male (12-24 Ch), 5-catheter pack = £5.00; female (12-18 Ch),

5-catheter pack = £5.00; paediatric (6-10 Ch), 5-catheter pack = £5.00

Nelaton catheters (single use)
Astra Tech
Lofric®, PVC, single use, male, female, or paediatric. Net price, male (8-24 Ch); female (8-18 Ch); paediatric (6-10 Ch), 25-catheter pack (all) = £29.90

Scott catheters (short curved tubular catheter for women and girls)
Simcare
Polyethylene, female, 8-14 Ch. Net price 5-catheter pack = £10.85

STOMA APPLIANCES

Stoma appliances are listed in Part IXC of *Drug Tariff* or Part 6 of *Scottish Drug Tariff*.

It is not necessary to state an **order number** on a prescription for one of these products provided the **full details** as given in the BNF are included on the **prescription**.

CLOSED POUCHES AND COLOSTOMY SETS

Closed pouches are suitable for patients with a **colostomy** and well-formed stools

Body's Care range
Rubber bags screwcap (Body's Care)
Black butyl, one-piece closed pouch. Net price 1 day pouch = £24.41; 1 night pouch = £28.47
White rubber, one-piece closed pouch. Net price 1 day pouch = £13.56; 1 night pouch = £15.63
Rubber bags spout (Body's Care)
Black butyl, one-piece closed pouch. Net price 1 day pouch or night pouch = £25.77
White rubber, one-piece closed pouch. Net price 1 day pouch or night pouch = £12.20

CliniMed range
Biotrol® (CliniMed)
Biopore, one-piece with porous adhesive and filter, white. Net price 50 pouches (25, 30, 35, 40, 45, 50 mm holes) = £61.10
Colo S, one-piece pouch with skin protector adhesive, white. Net price 30 pouches (25, 30, 35, 40, 45, 50, or 60 mm holes) = £60.00
Elite Closed, covered one-piece pouch with skin protector adhesive and filter, white or beige. Net price 30 pouches (starter hole, 25, 30, 35, 40, 45, 50, 60, 70 mm or cut-to-fit holes) = £65.18; clear (25, 30, 35, 40, 45, 50, 60, 70 mm or cut-to-fit holes) 30 pouches = £58.80; starter hole, 30 = £59.60
Integrale, one-piece pouch with skin protector adhesive and filter, white. Net price 30 pouches (starter hole, 25, 30, 35, 40, 45, 50, 60, 70 mm or cut-to-fit holes) = £65.18
Preference Closed, fabric covered one-piece pouch with skin protector adhesive, porous adhesive collar, and filter, white or beige. Net price 30 pouches (starter hole, 25, 30, 35, 40, 45, 50, 60 mm or cut-to-fit holes) = £60.50

Coloplast range
Assura® (Coloplast)
Midi, closed pouches with flatus filter, opaque or clear. Net price 30 one-piece pouches (20, 25, 30, 35, 40, 45, or 50 mm holes) = £58.80; 30 two-piece pouches (to fit 40, 50, or 60 mm base plates) = £32.80; base plate (40, 50, or 60 mm), 5 = £13.00

Conseal® System (Coloplast)

Two-piece pouch. Net price 30 bags (to fit 40 or 50 mm base plates) = £33.06; base plate (40 or 50 mm) 5 = £12.27; colostomy plug (40×35 or 45 mm, 50×35 or 45 mm) 10 = £11.02; discharge bag (40 or 50 mm) 50 = £2.60

K-Flex® (Coloplast)

One-piece closed pouch with karaya skin protector and filter. Net price 30 pouches (clear: 10, 30, or 40 mm holes; opaque: 30 or 40 mm holes) = £60.30

Extra, one-piece closed pouch. Net price, No. 1 (24 mm hole), 100 pouches = £79.00; No. 2 (30 or 40 mm holes), 100 = £95.70; No. 3 (30 mm hole), 100 = £116.50, 50 mm hole, 100 = £116.50

Regular, one-piece closed pouch. Net price, No. 1 (24 mm hole), 100 pouches = £66.60; No. 2 (30 mm hole), 100 = £79.00; No. 3 (30 mm hole), 100 = £94.70; No. 5 (24 mm hole), 100 = £88.40

mc2000® (Coloplast)

One-piece pouch with double seal and filter, opaque or clear. Net price 30 pouches (25, 30, 35, 40, 45, 50, 55, or 60 mm holes) = £62.43

mc2002® (Coloplast)

Two-piece pouch with filter, opaque or clear. Net price 30 pouches (to fit 40 or 60 mm base plates) = £35.25; base plate (40 mm × 15 or 25 mm, 60 × 35 or 45 mm) 5 = £13.00; belt plate (40 or 60 mm) 10 = £5.20

pc3000® (Coloplast)

One-piece pouch, opaque or clear. Net price 30 pouches (25, 30, 35, 40, 45, 50, or 55 mm holes; 25 mm can be cut to fit up to 60 mm) = £58.68

ConvaTec range

Colodress® (ConvaTec)

Colodress, one-piece closed pouch with textured backing, opaque beige. Net price 30 pouches (19, 32, 38, 45, or 50 mm holes; 19 mm can be cut to fit) = £59.79

Colodress Plus, one-piece closed pouch with single-release paper and filter. Net price 30 pouches (opaque or clear: 19, 25, 32, 38, 45, 50, or 64 mm holes; opaque: 19 mm can be cut to fit) = £59.79; Mini pouches, 30 pouches (19, 25, 32, 38, or 45 mm holes) = £53.80

Surgicare System® 2 (ConvaTec)

System 2, two-piece closed pouch, white. Net price 30 pouches (to fit 38, 45, 57, or 70 mm flanges) = £29.86

System 2 Combihesive, two-piece closed pouch with textured backing, beige. Net price 30 pouches (to fit 38, 45, 57, or 70 mm flanges) = £29.86; with filter, 30 pouches (to fit 32, 38, 45, 57, or 70 mm flanges) = £30.84; Mini pouches, 20 pouches (to fit 32, 38, 45, or 57 mm flanges) = £16.90

Dansac range

Dansac® (Dansac)

Combi Colo F, one-piece pouch with filter, opaque or clear. Net price 100 pouches (standard pouch: 25, 30, 38, 44, 50, or 63 mm holes; small pouch: 25, 30, or 38 mm holes) = £151.10

CombiMicro C + S, one-piece pouch with porous adhesive, filter, skin barrier ring, and fabric backing, opaque or clear. Net price 30 pouches (25, 32, 38, 44, 50, 63 mm or cut-to-fit; 10-38mm; 38-63mm holes) = £63.32

Combi Micro Mini Petit C, one-piece pouch with porous adhesive skin protector, fabric backing, and filter, opaque. Net price 30 pouches (cut-to-fit) = £55.93

Standard Colo, one-piece pouch with filter, clear. Net price 100 pouches (22, 30, 32, or 38mm holes) = £135.71

Supersquare System, two-piece pouch with filter, opaque or clear. Net price 100 (standard or small) pouches to fit 50 mm base plate = £131.23; (small) pouches to fit 80 mm base plate = £166.43; base plate 10 (100 mm × 100 mm) = £27.57; 10 (125 mm × 125 mm) = £50.94

Unique, one-piece closed pouch, opaque or clear. Net price 30 pouches (25, 30, 35, 40, 45, 50, 60 mm or cut-to-fit holes) = £54.86; oval flange, opaque or clear, starter hole, net price 30 = £52.75

DePuy range

Schacht® (DePuy)

Colostomy bag (= pouch), one-piece closed pouch. Net price 100 pouches = £32.30

Colostomy appliance. Net price 1 appliance = £27.85

Slimline® (DePuy)

Colostomy appliance. Net price 1 appliance = £30.25

Hollister range

Classic® (Hollister)

All with 25, 32, 38, 44, 51, 64, or 76 mm holes

Adhesive (series 217), one-piece closed pouch with adhesive and filter, clear. Net price 50 pouches = £58.45

Karaya seal (series 716), one-piece pouch with karaya skin protector (without filter), must be worn with belt, clear. Net price 30 pouches = £49.71

Karaya seal with filter (series 211), one-piece closed pouch with karaya skin protector and filter, must be worn with belt, opaque. Net price 30 pouches = £49.71

Karaya 5® Seal (series 331 and 332), one-piece closed pouch with porous adhesive, karaya skin protector seal, and filter, may be worn with belt, opaque or clear. Net price 30 pouches = £60.27

Microporous adhesive (series 314), one-piece compact closed pouch with porous adhesive and filter, may be worn with belt, clear. Net price 50 pouches = £63.25

Guardian® (Hollister)

All with 38, 51, or 64 mm holes

Guardian (series 451 and 450), two-piece closed pouch with filter, opaque or clear. Net price 15 pouches = £14.28

Guardian mini-pouch (series 452), two-piece compact closed pouch with filter, opaque. Net price 15 pouches = £14.00

Flanges. Net price 'F floating flange (25, 38, 51, 64 mm) 5 = £11.62, (102 mm) 5 = £12.69; 'S' stationary flange (25, 38, 51, or 64 mm) 5 = £11.42

Stoma cap, with filter, opaque. Net price 30 (38, 51, or 64 mm) = £26.48

Belt adaptor. Net price 10 = £8.11.

HolliGard® (Hollister)

All with 25, 32, 38, 44, 51, 64, or 76 mm holes

Microporous adhesive (series 411), one-piece closed pouch with porous adhesive, HolliGard® seal, and filter, may be worn with belt, opaque. Net price 30 pouches = £63.30

Without adhesive (series 416), one-piece closed pouch with HolliGard® seal and filter, must be worn with belt, clear. Net price 30 pouches = £57.40

Premium® (Hollister)

All with 25, 32, 38, 44, 51, 64, or 76 mm holes

Karaya 5® Seal (series 355 and 353), one-piece closed pouch with porous adhesive, karaya skin protector and filter, may be worn with belt, opaque or clear. Net price 15 pouches = £30.47

Synthetic Seal (series 354 and 356), one-piece closed pouch with porous adhesive, synthetic skin protector seal and filter, opaque or clear. Net price 15 pouches = £31.77

Pelican range

Pelican® (Pelican)

Closed, one-piece pouch (formerly Simplaseel). Net price 30 pouches (26, 32, 40, 45, 50 mm or cut-to-fit holes) = £66.58; 30 casual pouches (32, 40, or 45 mm holes) = £61.94

Phoenix® (Pelican)

Closed, one-piece closed pouch. Net price (both 32, 40, or 45 mm holes) 100 pouches = £145.43; 100 casual pouches = £135.28

Sassco® (Pelican)

Closed, one-piece closed pouch. Net price 100 pouches (32, 40, or 45 mm holes) = £138.52

Rüsch range
Ostopore® (Rüsch)

Colo AV-opaque, one-piece closed pouch with adhesive and vent. Net price 30 pouches (25, 32, 38, or 45 mm holes) with 2 belt flanges = £40.56

Colo KAV-opaque, one-piece closed pouch with karaya seal skin protector, adhesive, and vent. Net price 30 pouches (25, 32, 38, 45, or 51 mm holes) with 5 belt flanges = £55.22

Colo KAV-transparent, one-piece closed pouch with karaya seal skin protector, adhesive, and vent. Net price 30 pouches (32, 38, 45, or 51 mm holes) with 30 belt flanges = £70.51

Rubber bags (Rüsch)

White rubber, one-piece closed pouch with spout outlet. Net price (both 19, 25, or 28 mm holes), 1 day pouch = £11.07; 1 night pouch = £11.94

Translet® (Rüsch)

Premier colostomy set, 1 adhesive ring with 6 bags. Net price 15 (27, 40, or 57 mm hole) = £61.62; spare bags 10 (18 or 28 cm length) = £4.72; adhesive rings or microporous spare adhesive rings (27, 40, or 57 mm) 5 = £6.32

Royal colostomy set, 1 adhesive ring and 6 odourproof bags. Net price 15 (27, 40, or 57 mm) = £85.80; spare bags (18 or 28 cm length) 10 = £7.50

Salts range
NHS Cohflex® (Salts)

Closed, one-piece pouch with single-release paper, wafer, and filter, fabric front and back, opaque. Net price 30 pouches (all may be cut to fit; 30, 40, 50, 60 mm or 10–60 mm cut-to-fit holes) = £60.34

Coloset® (Salts)

Closed, one-piece pouch. Net price 30 pouches (medium: 713655) = £13.82; (small: 713656) = £9.10; (large: 713658) = £11.46; (medium: 713659) = £10.46

Eakin® (Salts)

Closed, one-piece pouch, white or clear. 32, 45, or 64 mm holes, net price 20 pouches = £38.49; 90 mm hole, 20 pouches = £47.89

Kombo® (Salts)

Kombo closed, one-piece pouch with karaya skin protector seal and adhesive, clear. Net price (30, 40, 50, or 60 mm holes), 30 pouches = £55.65; with filter, 30 pouches = £66.35

Simplicity® (Salts)

Closed, two-piece closed pouch, clear or pink, medium. Net price, clear (40, 50, 60, or 70 mm) 30 = £14.64; pink (40, 50, or 60 mm holes) 30 = £14.50; flange, standard (30, 40, 50, or 60 mm hole) 5 = £2.65; flange with cohesive washer (30 or 40 mm) 5 = £11.90, (50 mm) 5 = £13.42

Simplicity 1® (Salts)

Anatomical, closed one-piece pouch. Net price, clear (cut-to-fit), 30 = £60.30; opaque (30, 40, 50, 60 mm, or cut-to-fit holes), 30 = £60.30

Closed, one-piece pouch with porous adhesive, skin protector seal, and filter, fabric front and back. Net price 30 pouches (all may be cut to fit; opaque: 30, 40, 50, or 60 mm holes; opaque or clear: cut-to-fit holes) = £62.75

Paediatric, closed one-piece pouch with single-release paper, porous adhesive, clear. Net price 30 pouches (13 mm cut-to-fit hole) = £40.86

Simplicity 2® (Salts)

Closed, two-piece closed pouch (may also be applied directly to skin). Net price 30 pouches (40, 50, 60, or 70 mm holes, also 30 mm only for direct application to skin) = £31.41; flange (30, 40, 50, or 60 mm) 5 = £13.12

Solo® (Salts)

Solo closed, one-piece pouch with single-release paper, and adhesive flange, clear. Net price (30, 40, 50, or 60 mm holes), 30 pouches = £16.78; with filter, 30 pouches = £25.34

Supasac® (Salts)

Closed, one-piece pouch. Net price 30 pouches (medium) = £21.56

Shannon range
Colostomy (Shannon)

Adhesive appliance. Net price, 1 appliance (TJS 948B) = £48.25

Appliance. Net price, 1 appliance (TJS 962) = £16.81

Day bag (= pouch). Net price 1 pouch, TJS 948f = £22.13; TJS 948j = £25.32

Disposable bag (= pouch). Net price TJS 948g, 100 pouches = £10.96

Night bag (= pouch). Net price 1 pouch, TJS 948e = £25.32; TJS 948k = £27.61

Outfit. Net price 1 TJS 948A = £74.72, 1 TJS 948NA = £72.36; 1 TJS 948T = £39.62

Easychange® (Shannon)

Appliance. Net price 1 appliance = £4.43

Spare bag (= pouch). Net price 100 pouches = £44.22

Shannon

Disposable bag (= pouch), closed pouches with plasters. Net price 12 pouches = £6.05

Elastic necks. Net price 50 pouches = £22.11

Shaw range
Hainsworth® (Shaw)

Hainsworth bag (= pouch), one-piece closed pouch. Net price (both 25, 32, 38, or 51 mm holes), 20 pouches with body mould adhesive = £37.45; 20 pouches with Healwell® adhesive = £19.65

Shaw (Shaw)

Colostomy outfit, comprising, 4-inch wide elastic belt with groinstrap (26- to 42-inch), 1 flange and 100 colostomy pouches. Net price one NSI 6 outfit with 11 × 6-inch pouches = £34.70; one NSI 7 outfit with 12 × 8-inch pouches = £35.40; one NSI 8 outfit with 11 × 6-inch pouches = £37.90

Double seal, one-piece closed pouch. Net price 100 11 × 6-inch pouches = £8.95; 100 12 × 8-inch pouches = £9.80

Stick-on bag (pouch), one-piece closed pouch with plasters. Net price 10 pouches = £7.45

Simcare range
Adhesive (Simcare)

Stomabag, one-piece closed pouch with adhesive, opaque. Net price (25, 32, 38, 44, 51, or 64 mm holes), 90 pouches = £114.99; with filter, 90 pouches = £129.24

Beta® (Simcare)

Closed, two-piece pouch with filter. Net price, 1 kit comprising 30 pouches and 8 Seel-a-peel sheets (100 × 100 mm) = £48.22; 90 spare pouches = £132.76

Chiron® (Simcare)

Adhesive appliance with spout bag. Net price 1 appliance (Mk I and Mk III) = £64.28

Clearseal bag (= pouch), one-piece closed pouch. Net price 10 pouches (305 × 127 mm: 22 mm hole) = £13.55

Closed bag, one-piece pouch. Net price 10 pouches (305 × 127 mm or 230 × 127 mm: 38 mm hole) = £13.55

Disposable bag (= pouch), one-piece closed pouch. Net price 10 pouches (305 × 102 mm or 305 × 127 mm: 19 mm hole) = £9.03

Reinforced, one-piece disposable pouch. Net price 10 pouches = £13.55

Chironseal® (Simcare)

Closed bag (= pouch), one-piece closed pouch. Net price 10 pouches (305 × 102, 305 × 127, 230 × 127, or 305 × 150 mm: 22 or 38 mm hole) = £10.16; 10 pouches (305 × 205 or 305 × 255 mm: 22 or 38 mm hole) = £11.67

Reinforced, one-piece disposable closed pouch. Net price 10 pouches (305 × 102 mm: 25 or 38 mm holes or 305 × 127 mm: 38 mm hole) = £13.55

EC1® (Simcare)

Colo Classic, one-piece closed pouch with wafer, comfort backing, and filter, opaque or clear. Net price 30 pouches (25, 32, 38, 44, 51, 64 mm or 15–64 mm cut-to-fit holes) = £63.92

Omni® (Simcare)

Closed, one-piece pouch with wafer, porous adhesive, filter. Net price 30 pouches (opaque: 25, 32, 38, 44, or 51 mm; opaque or clear: 15–44 mm cut-to-fit holes) = £64.85

Redifit® (Simcare)

Continuation bag (= pouch), one-piece closed pouch with karaya skin protector, may be worn with belt, opaque. Net price 20 pouches (32, 38, 44, 51, 64, or 75 mm holes) = £65.48

Non-adhesive bag (= pouch), one-piece closed pouch, must be worn with belt. Net price 20 pouches with karaya skin protector (opaque: 44 or 51 mm holes; clear: 44, 51, or 64 mm holes) = £65.48; without karaya, 20 pouches (opaque, 38 mm hole) = £49.69

Rediseal® (Simcare)

Small bag (= pouch), one-piece PVC compact closed pouch, opaque. Net price 10 pouches (38, 44, or 51 mm holes) = £12.79

Serenade® (Simcare)

WC Disposable, two-piece closed pouch. Net price 30 pouches (25, 32, 38, 44, or 51 mm holes) with filter = £31.20; 30 pouches (25, 32, 38, 44, or 51 mm holes) with soft-backing and filter = £32.78; Mini pouches, 30 pouches (15–51 mm) with soft backing and filter = £25.50; base plate (25, 32, 38, 44 or 51 mm), 10 = £26.00

Symphony® (Simcare)

WC Disposable, one-piece closed pouch with wafer and filter. Net price 30 pouches (opaque or clear: 25, 32, 38, 44, or 51 mm holes; opaque: 15–44 mm cut-to-fit holes) = £67.88

Ward range

Ward

Disposable bag (= pouch), one-piece closed pouch. Net price 10 pouches (12 × 4-inch) with 4 × 3-inch plasters = £7.53; 10 pouches (12 × 5-inch) with 4 × 4-inch plasters = £7.53

Celluloid colostomy cup, with sponge or solid rim. Net price 1 (small, medium, or large) cup = £31.24; with belt fitting, 1 cup = £35.65; 1 pouch with mount outlet = £12.98

Welland range

Vogue shorter closed bag® (Welland)

Colostomy bag (= pouch), one-piece pouch, opaque or clear. Net price 30 pouches (25, 32, 38, 44, 51 mm or 10 mm cut-to-fit holes) = £50.75

Welland (Welland)

Colostomy bag (= pouch), one-piece pouch with wafer and filter, opaque or clear. Net price 30 pouches (25, 32, 38, 44, 51, 60 mm, or 10 mm cut-to-fit holes) = £56.02

Softback colostomy bag, one-piece closed pouch with wafer, filter, and soft backing, opaque or clear. Net price 30 pouches (25, 32, 38, 44, 51, 60 mm or 10 mm cut-to-fit holes) = £51.53

Oval flange closed bag, one-piece pouch with oval shaped wafer, filter and soft backing, opaque or clear. Net price 30 pouches (10 mm cut-to-fit holes) = £57.20

DRAINABLE POUCHES AND ILEOSTOMY SETS

Drainable pouches are suitable for patients with an **ileostomy** or a **colostomy** with fluid effluent.

Body's Care range

Rubber bags screwcap (Body's Care)

Black butyl, one-piece pouch. Net price 1 day pouch = £24.41; 1 night pouch = £28.47

White rubber, one-piece pouch. Net price 1 day pouch = £13.56; 1 night pouch = £15.63

Rubber bags spout (Body's Care)

Black butyl, one-piece pouch. Net price 1 day or night pouch = £25.77

White rubber, one-piece pouch. Net price 1 day pouch = £12.20; 1 night pouch = £12.20

Bullen range

Lenbul® (Bullen)

Bag, with one-piece flange. Net price 1 pouch (25 or 51 mm holes) = £27.83; 1 lightweight pouch (25 or 51 mm holes) = £1.60

Day bag (= pouch), one-piece pouch. Net price 1 pouch with screwcap outlet = £12.13; 1 pouch with screwcap outlet and larger opening = £12.60; 1 pouch with metal strip = £14.56; 1 pouch with tap outlet = £14.09

Night bag (= pouch), one-piece pouch. Net price 1 pouch with screwcap outlet = £13.36; 1 pouch with screwcap outlet and larger opening = £13.87; 1 pouch with metal strip = £14.56; 1 pouch with tap outlet = £16.10

LOP-F7® (Bullen)

Ileostomy appliance. Net price 1 appliance = £38.68

OPR-F® (Bullen)

Ileostomy appliance. Net price 1 appliance = £80.69

SR-F® (Bullen)

Ileostomy set. Net price 1 set = £55.60

CliniMed range

Biotrol® (CliniMed)

Elite, fabric covered one-piece pouch with skin protector adhesive and clamp closure, white or beige. Net price 30 pouches (starter hole, 20, 25, 30, 35, 40, 45, 50, 60, 70 mm or cut-to-fit holes) = £66.70; 30 clear pouches (20, 25, 30, 35, 40, 45, 50, 60, 70 mm or cut-to-fit holes) = £59.40; starter hole, 30 = £61.10

Ileo S, one-piece pouch with skin protector adhesive, white. Net price 30 pouches (starter hole, 20, 25, 30, 35, 40, 45, 50, 60, 70 mm or cut-to-fit holes) = £66.70

Post-op, one-piece pouch with skin protector adhesive, for temporary or permanent colostomies or ileostomies, clear. Net price (cut-to-fit holes) small, 30 pouches = £67.48; large, 30 pouches = £95.25

Preference, fabric covered one-piece pouch with skin protector adhesive, porous adhesive collar, beige. Net price 30 pouches (starter hole, 20, 25, 30, 35, 40, 45, 50, 60 mm or cut-to-fit holes) = £66.70

Coloplast range

Ileo B® (Coloplast)

One-piece pouch with zinc oxide adhesive, clear or white. Net price 100 pouches (20 mm hole) = £143.60

Mini, one-piece compact pouch with zinc oxide adhesive, white. Net price 100 pouches (20 mm hole) = £142.50

K-Flex® (Coloplast)

One-piece pouch with karaya skin protector, clear. Net price 30 pouches (10 or 40 mm holes) = £66.78

mc2000® (Coloplast)

One-piece pouch with double seal, opaque or clear. Net price 30 pouches (20, 25, 30, 35, 40, 45, 50, 55, 60 mm holes or clear pouch with cut-to-fit hole) = £66.15

Mini, one-piece compact pouch, opaque. Net price 30 pouches (20, 25, 30, 35, or 40 mm holes) = £62.43

mc2002® (Coloplast)

Two-piece pouch, opaque or clear. Net price 30 open pouches (to fit 40 or 60 mm base plates) = £35.25; 30 closed pouches (to fit 40 or 60 mm base plates) = £39.00

pc3000® (Coloplast)

One-piece pouch, opaque or clear. Net price 30 pouches (20, 25, 30, 35, 40, 45, 50, 55, or 60 mm holes; 20 mm can be cut to fit up to 60 mm) = £58.98

Mini starter hole, one-piece pouch. Net price 30 pouches = £53.40

Sterile post-op bag, one-piece pouch. Net price 20 pouches (2200) = £44.80; (2202) = £29.20

ConvaTec range
Ileodress® (ConvaTec)

Ileodress, one-piece pouch with textured backing. Net price 10 standard pouches with clip (opaque or clear: 19, 38, 45, 50, or 64 mm holes; 19 mm can be cut to fit; opaque only: 25 and 32 mm holes) = £20.55; 10 small pouches with clip, opaque (19, 25, 32, 38, 45, 50, or 64 mm holes; 19 mm can be cut to fit) = £20.12

Ileodress Plus, one-piece pouch single-release paper. Net price 10 standard pouches with clip (opaque or clear: 19, 38, 45, 50, or 64 mm holes; 19 mm can be cut to fit; opaque only: 25 and 32 mm holes) = £20.55; 10 small pouches with clip, opaque (19, 25, 32, 38, 45, or 50 mm holes; 19 mm can be cut-to-fit) = £18.70

Little Ones® (ConvaTec)

Paediatric, one-piece pouch. Net price 15 pouches (8 mm cut-to-fit hole) = £28.28

Surgicare System® 2 (ConvaTec)

System 2, two-piece pouches, white. Net price 10 pouches with clip (to fit 32, 38, 45, 57, or 70 mm flanges) = £10.12

System 2 Combihesive, two-piece pouches with textured backing. Net price 10 standard or small pouches with clip, beige (to fit 32, 38, 45, 57, or 70 mm flanges) = £10.21; 10 standard pouches with clip, clear, to fit 45, 57, or 70 mm flanges = £10.21, to fit 100 mm flanges = £18.05

Dansac range
Dansac® (Dansac)

CombiMicro D + S, one-piece pouch with porous adhesive, skin barrier ring, and fabric backing. Net price 30 pouches (25, 32, 38, 44, 50, 63 mm or cut-to-fit holes), opaque = £64.81; clear, 30 pouches = £61.15

Mini Infant, one-piece pouch with skin barrier ring and fabric backing, clear. Net price 30 pouches (cut-to-fit holes) = £51.03; 30 pouches (cut-to-fit holes), opaque or clear = £62.32

Infant, one-piece pouch, opaque or clear. Net price 30 pouches (cut-to-fit holes) = £53.07

Mini Petit D, one-piece pouch with skin barrier ring and fabric backing, opaque or clear. Net price 30 pouches (cut-to-fit holes) = £55.91

Supersquare System, two piece pouch, opaque or clear. Net price 30 standard or small pouches to fit 50 mm base plate = £35.18; 30 standard pouches to fit 80 mm base plate = £52.85

Unique, one-piece pouch, opaque or clear. Net price 30 pouches (25, 30, 35, 40, 45, 50, 60 mm or cut-to-fit holes) = £52.75

DePuy range
Raymed® (DePuy)

Butyl day bag (= pouch), one-piece pouch. Net price 1 pouch with screwcap outlet = £22.60; 1 pouch with tap outlet = £23.75

Schacht® (DePuy)

Ileostomy, one-piece pouches. Net price 50 pouches = £19.80

Ileostomy appliance, odourproof. Net price 1 appliance = £29.25

Drew range
Drew

Ileostomy bag (= pouch), one-piece pouch. Net price 50 D1/1 pouches = £61.85; 50 D1/6 pouches = £44.15

Ileostomy appliance. Net price 1 appliance (D1/1) = £32.52; 1 appliance (D1/6) = £27.84

Hollister range
Classic® (Hollister)

Karaya seal (series 721), one-piece pouch with karaya skin protector seal, must be worn with belt, clear. Net price 30 pouches with 1 clamp (25, 32, 38, 44, 51, 64, or 76 mm hole) = £61.35

Karaya 5® transparent, one-piece pouch with karaya skin protector seal, may be worn with belt. 30- or 40-cm clear pouch with microporous adhesive (series 322 and 327), net price 30 pouches with 1 clamp (25, 32, 38, 44, 51, 64, or 76 mm hole) = £70.41; 30-cm pouches with regular adhesive (series 722) = £70.41

Karaya 5® opaque, one-piece pouch with karaya skin protector seal and porous adhesive, may be worn with belt. Net price 30 pouches with 1 clamp, 23-cm pouches (series 313: 25, 32, 38, 44, or 51 mm holes) = £70.41; 30-cm pouches (series 311: 25, 32, 38, 44, 51, 64, or 76 mm holes) = £67.80

Karaya 5® seal (series 360), one-piece pouch with porous adhesive and karaya skin protector seal, clear. Net price 15 pouches (25, 32, 38, 44, 51, 64, or 76 mm holes) with 1 clamp = £34.55

Loop ostomy bag (= pouch). Net price 20 pouches (3.5 or 4.5 inch) = £60.90

Loop ostomy gasket. Net price 10 (3.5 or 4.5 inch) = £60.90

Guardian® (Hollister)

All with 25, 38, 51, or 64 mm holes

Guardian (series 461 and 460), two-piece pouch, opaque or clear. Net price 10 pouches with 1 clamp = £9.52; larger pouch to fit 102-mm flange, 10 pouches (clear) with 1 clamp = £20.62

Guardian mini-pouch, two-piece compact pouch, opaque. Net price (series 464), 10 pouches = £9.36; NHS: with inner film and replaceable filter (series 463), 10 pouches with pack of filters and 1 clamp

NHS *With replaceable filter* (series 462), two-piece pouch with inner film and replaceable filter, clear. 10 pouches with pack of filters and 1 clamp

Impression® (Hollister)

One-piece pouch with Convex wafer, opaque or clear. Net price 10 pouches (19, 22, 25, 29, 32, 35, 38, 41, 44 or 51 mm holes) = £21.50

Premium® (Hollister)

Karaya 5® seal with filter (series 366), one-piece pouch with porous adhesive, karaya skin protector seal, and replaceable filter, may be worn with belt, clear. Net price 15 pouches (25, 32, 38, 44, 51, or 64 mm holes) with 1 clamp and filter elements = £38.44

Synthetic seal (series 364), one-piece pouch with porous adhesive and synthetic skin protector seal, clear. Net price 15 pouches (25, 32, 38, 44, 51, or 64 mm holes) with 1 clamp = £34.55

Marlen range
Ultra (Marlen)

All with 12, 16, 19, 22, 25, 29, 32, 34, 38, 41, 44, 48, 50, 54, 57, 60, 63, 67, 70, 73, 76 mm or cut-to-fit holes; opaque or clear; small or large

Drainable, one-piece pouch. Net price 15 pouches = £32.25; with convex flange, 15 pouches = £33.00

Pelican range
Sassco® (Pelican)

Ileostomy bag (= pouch), one-piece pouch. Net price 100 pouches (26 or 32 mm holes) = £159.03

Pelican® (Pelican)

Drainable bag (= pouch), formerly Simplaseel®, one-piece pouch, opaque. Net price 30 pouches (26, 32, 40, 45, or 50 mm holes) = £67.62

Post-op drainable bag (= pouch), one-piece pouch. Net price 10 pouches (20-80 mm cut-to-fit) = £36.66

Paediatric drainable bag (= pouch), one-piece pouch. Net price 30 pouches (7-40 mm cut-to-fit) = £58.81

Rüsch range
Birkbeck® (Rüsch)

Rubber, one-piece pouch, black or pink. Net price (both 19, 38, or 54 mm holes), 1 day pouch = £24.71; 1 night pouch = £28.26

Disposable, one-piece plastic pouch. Net price 100 pouches = £14.94

Ileostomy appliance. Net price 1 appliance "A" (19, 38, or 54 mm) = £86.26; 1 appliance "B" (19, 38, or 54 mm) = £55.66

Ostopore® (Rüsch)

Ileo KAV-opaque, one-piece pouch with karaya seal skin protector, adhesive, and vent, opaque. Net price 30 pouches (25, 32, or 38 mm holes) with 30 belt flanges and 10 clips = £61.78

Rubber bag (Rüsch)

White rubber, one-piece pouch. Net price, 1 day pouch (38, 44, or 51 mm holes) = £11.07; 1 screwcap pouch (38 mm hole) = £11.94; 1 pouch with vent (38 mm hole) = £13.23

White rubber child bag (= pouch), one-piece pouch. Net price (both 19, 25, or 28 mm holes), 1 day pouch = £10.66; 1 night pouch = £13.05

Salts range
Cohflex® (Salts)

NHS *Drainable,* one-piece pouch with single-release paper, wafer, and fabric front and back. Net price 30 pouches with integral closure clip (opaque: 30, 40, 50, or 60 mm, all may be cut to fit; clear: 10–60 mm cut-to-fit holes) = £59.94

Paediatric drainable, one-piece small pouch with single-release paper, wafer, and fabric backing, opaque/clear. Net price 30 pouches with integral closure clip (10–50 mm cut-to-fit holes) = £51.62

Eakin® (Salts)

Drainable, one-piece pouch, white or clear. Net price 20 small or large pouches (32, 45, or 64 mm holes) = £44.48; 20 wide pouches, clear (90 mm hole) = £94.42

Fistula, one-piece pouch. Net price 10 large pouches = £107.14; starter, 20 small pouches = £92.53, 20 medium pouches = £119.68

Light White (Salts)

Drainable, one-piece pouch, white. Net price 30 large, small, or medium pouches (all 25, 32, or 38 mm holes) = £44.47

Drainable self-adhesive, one-piece pouch with adhesive, white. Net price 30 pouches (large: 25, 32, 38, or 44 mm holes; small and medium: 25, 32, or 38 mm holes) = £50.46

Koenig Rutzen® screwcap (Salts)

All with screwcap outlet

Black butyl all rubber, one-piece pouch. Net price 1 pouch (large: 25, 29, 32, 35, 38, 44, or 51 mm holes; small: 25, 32, 38, 44, or 51 mm) = £27.30; with bridge (soft-face Maggie Bag), 1 pouch (large: 25, 32, 38, 44, or 51 mm holes; small: 25, 32, or 38 mm) = £36.62

Black butyl reinforced, one-piece pouch. Net price 1 large or small pouch (both 25, 32, or 38 mm holes) = £36.62; with bridge (hard-face Maggie Bag), 1 pouch (large: 25, 32, 38, 44, or 51 mm holes; small: 25, 32, or 38 mm) = £42.68

Koenig Rutzen® spout (Salts)

All with spout outlet

Black butyl all rubber, one-piece pouch. Net price 1 large or small pouch (both 25, 32, 38, 44, or 51 mm holes) = £20.61; with bridge, 1 pouch (large: 25, 32, 38, 44, or 51 mm holes; small: 25, 32, or 38 mm) = £26.72

Black butyl reinforced, one-piece pouch. Net price 1 large or small pouch (25, 32, or 38 mm holes) = £27.70; with bridge, 1 pouch (large: 25, 32, 38, 44, or 51 mm holes; small: 25, 32, or 38 mm) = £34.12

Kombo® (Salts)

Kombo drainable, one-piece pouch with karaya skin protector seal and adhesive, clear. Net price 30 pouches (30, 40, 50, 60, or 80 mm holes) = £53.31; with filter, 30 pouches = £64.01

Rubber bags (Salts)

All must be used with flange

Black butyl screw, one-piece bag with screwcap outlet. Net price 1 large or small pouch = £27.00

Black butyl spout, one-piece bag with spout outlet. Net price 1 large or small pouch = £19.48

White screw, one-piece bag with screwcap outlet. Net price 1 large or small pouch = £9.01

White spout, one-piece bag with spout outlet. Net price 1 large or small pouch = £7.62

Salger® (Salts)

Drainable, one-piece pouch. Net price 10 pouches (40 or 57 mm holes) = £10.38

Simplicity® (Salts)

Drainable, two-piece pouch, clear. Net price 30 230 × 137 mm pouches (40, 50, or 60 mm holes) = £16.69

Post-op, two-piece pouch, clear. Net price 30 300 × 125-mm pouches (40, 50, or 60 mm holes) = £14.50

Simplicity 1® (Salts)

Anatomical, one-piece pouch. Net price clear (cut-to-fit), 30 = £64.76; opaque (30, 40, 50, 60 mm or cut-to-fit holes), 30 = £64.76

Drainable, one-piece pouch with porous adhesive and skin protector seal, fabric front and back. Net price 30 pouches with integral closure clip (opaque: 30, 40, 50, or 60 mm, all may be cut to fit; opaque or clear: 10–60 mm cut-to-fit hole) = £65.45

Paediatric drainable, one-piece pouch with porous adhesive and skin protector seal, clear. Net price 30 pouches (cut-to-fit hole) = £40.86

Simplicity 2® (Salts)

Drainable, two-piece pouch (may also be applied directly to skin). Net price 15 pouches (40, 50, 60, or 70 mm holes, also 30 mm only for direct application to skin) = £17.43

Post-op, two-piece pouch (may also be applied directly to skin). Net price 30 pouches (40, 50, 60, or 70 mm holes, also 30 mm only for direct application to skin) = £34.42

Transverse, two-piece pouch (may also be applied directly to skin). Net price 10 pouches (cut-to-fit hole) = £39.13; 5 flanges = £19.14

Solo® (Salts)

Drainable, one-piece pouch with single-release paper and adhesive, clear. Net price 30 pouches (30, 40, 50, 60 or 80 mm holes) = £19.93; with filter, 30 pouches = £25.13

NHS United® (Salts)

Soft & Secure drainable, one-piece pouch, opaque or clear. Net price 10 pouches (38, 45, or 57 mm holes) = £8.47

Shaw range

Ileostomy outfit, with 5 inch wide elastic web belt. Net price 1 outfit (26–42 inch) = £53.10

Hainsworth® (Shaw)

Drainable bag, one-piece pouch with adhesive. Net price 20 pouches (0.875, 1, 1.25, or 1.5 inch holes) = £37.45

Rubber bags (Shaw)

Black screwcap, one-piece pouch with screwcap outlet. Net price (both 19, 38 or 54 mm holes), 1 day pouch = £21.05; 1 night pouch = £22.30

Simcare range

Adhesive (Simcare)

Stomabag, one-piece pouch with adhesive, opaque. Net price 60 pouches (19, 25, 32, 38, 51 mm or cut-to-fit holes) = £84.07

Cavendish® (Simcare)

Odourproof, one-piece pouch. Net price (all 25, 32, or 38 mm holes), 10 opaque pouches with non-adhesive flange = £29.17; 10 opaque pouches with adhesive flange = £35.13; 10 clear PVC pouches = £29.35

Chiron® screwcap (Simcare)

All with screwcap outlet

Butyl rubber day bag (= pouch), one-piece pouch, black. Net price 1 pouch (38, 44, or 51 mm hole) = £29.90

Butyl rubber night bag (= pouch), one-piece pouch, black. Net price 1 pouch (38 or 44 mm holes) =£35.88

Latex rubber day bag (= pouch), one-piece pouch. Net price 1 pouch (38 mm hole) = £14.97

Latex rubber night bag (= pouch), one-piece pouch. Net price 1 pouch (38 mm hole) = £19.81

White rubber day bag (= pouch), one-piece pouch. Net price 1 pouch (38, 44, or 51 mm) = £17.21, child-size pouch (38 mm hole) = £14.97; body-size outlet, 1 pouch (38 mm hole) = £17.21, child-size pouch (38 mm hole) = £13.60

White rubber night bag (= pouch), one-piece pouch. Net price 1 pouch (38 or 51 mm hole) = £19.81; body-size outlet, 1 pouch (38 mm hole) = £16.45

Chiron® spout (Simcare)

White rubber bag (= pouch), one-piece pouch. Net price 1 day pouch (38 mm hole) = £14.80; 1 night pouch (38 mm hole) = £16.08

EC1® (Simcare)

Ileo classic, one-piece pouch with wafer and comfort backing, opaque. Net price 30 pouches with 1 clamp (19, 25, 32, 38, 44 mm or 10–44 mm cut-to-fit holes) =£66.96

Mini classic, one-piece compact pouch with wafer and comfort backing, opaque or clear. Net price 30 pouches with 1 clamp (10–44 mm cut-to-fit holes) = £66.96

Post-op classic, one-piece pouch with wafer and comfort backing, clear. Net price 30 pouches with 1 clamp, 10–64 mm cut-to-fit holes = £69.06; 10–90 mm cut-to-fit holes = £97.72

Omni® (Simcare)

Drainable, one-piece pouch with porous adhesive wafer and replaceable filter. Net price 20 pouches (opaque: 25, 32, 38, 44 mm; opaque or clear: 10–44 mm cut-to-fit hole) = £44.61; NHS opaque (10–90 mm cut-to-fit hole) = £53.39

Redifit® (Simcare)

Opaque, one-piece pouch with karaya skin protector, may be worn with belt. Net price 20 pouches with 2 closure clips (25, 32, 38, 44, 51, or 64 mm holes) =£65.49; small outline pouches, 20 pouches with 2 closure clips (25, 32, or 38 mm) = £65.49

Clear fronted, one-piece pouch with karaya skin protector, may be worn with belt. Net price 20 pouches with 2 closure clips (25, 32, 44, 51, or 64 mm holes) = £65.49

Steeper range

Rubber bags (Steeper)

Bag, rubber. Net price 1 pouch, spring-in-neck, with vulcanite screw outlets (small) = £11.99, (medium) = £16.62, (large) = £17.02; 1 pouch, complete with collar = £19.69; 1 pouch, with tap outlet and skirt = £2.39

Night bag (= pouch), shaped rubber with long vertical spring vulcanite screw outlet. Net price 1 pouch = £18.63

Donald Rose (Steeper)

Bag (= pouch), with celluloid collars, solid, flat or fluid rims. Net price 1 pouch = £18.14

Ileostomy appliance. Net price 1 appliance (first stage) = £44.39; 1 appliance (second stage) = £43.90; 1 appliance (new improved) = £46.60

Ward range

Rubber bags (Ward)

Black rubber bag (= pouch), one-piece pouch with screwcap outlet. Net price (19, 35, or 54 mm hole), 1 day pouch = £15.69; 1 night pouch = £16.38

White rubber ileostomy bag (= pouch) with flange, pouch with St. Mark's flange. Net price 1 pouch = £23.78

White rubber ileostomy bag (= pouch), one-piece pouch. Net price 1 day pouch (screwcap or spout outlet) = £10.71; 1 night pouch (screwcap or spout outlet) = £12.06; tap outlet, 1 day pouch = £15.70; 1 night pouch = £17.47

White rubber transverse ileostomy bag (= pouch), one-piece pouch. Net price 1 pouch = £25.13

Welland range

Welland (Welland)

Ileostomy bag (= pouch), one-piece pouch with wafer, opaque or clear. Net price 30 pouches (25, 32, 38, 44, 51 mm, or 10 mm cut-to-fit holes) = £55.64

Softback ileostomy bag (= pouch), one-piece with wafer and soft backing, opaque or clear. Net price 30 pouches (25, 32, 38, 44, 51 mm, or 10 mm cut-to-fit holes) = £59.05

Mini-bag, one-piece with wafer, clear. Net price (both cut-to-fit holes), 30 pouches = £51.00; with soft backing, 30 pouches = £53.00

Oval drainable, one-piece pouch with wafer, opaque. Net price (both cut-to-fit holes), 30 pouches = £55.50; with soft backing, 30 pouches = £57.50

Oval post-op, one-piece pouch with wafer, clear. Net price (both cut-to-fit holes), 30 pouches = £55.50; with soft backing, 30 pouches = £57.50

UROSTOMY POUCHES

Body's Care range

Rubber bags (Body's Care)

Black butyl, one-piece pouch, odourless. Net price 1 day pouch (tap outlet) = £27.13; 1 night pouch (tap outlet) = £28.47

White rubber, one-piece pouch. Net price 1 day pouch (tap outlet) = £13.56; 1 night pouch (tap outlet) = £15.63

Bullen range

Lenbul® (Bullen)

Day bag (= pouch), one-piece pouch. Net price 1 pouch with tap outlet = £14.09; 1 pouch with large opening (for 4-inch flange with tap outlet) = £14.62; 1 pouch with metal strip = £15.77

Night bag (= pouch). Net price 1 pouch with tap outlet = £16.10; 1 pouch with large opening = £16.71

One-piece flange and bag (= pouch) with tap outlet. Net price 1 (1- or 2-inch hole) = £29.60

Baby's bag (= pouch) and flange with tap outlet. Net price 1 (1.25- or 2-inch hole, with or without night tube) = £40.75

Child's rubber cap and bag (= pouch) with non-reflux valve. Net price 1 small, 1 small with metal strip, or 1 large = £27.62; 1 large with metal strip = £29.70

Urostomy sets. Net price 1 LOP-U appliance (wire ring retainer with 1.5-inch elastic belt for small flange, 10 one-piece flanges and lightweight bags with 1-inch hole, 30 3.5 × 3.5-inch double-sided adhesive plasters) = £38.68; 1 OPR-U appliance (waterproof canvas retaining shield waistband, 2 one-piece flanges and bags with 1- or 2-inch hole and tap outlet, 30 3.5 × 3.5-inch double-sided adhesive plasters) = £80.69; 1 SR-U appliance (plastic retainer ring shield with 1-inch elastic belt for medium flange, Lenbul® 1.5-inch diameter flange, 1 Lenbul® day and 1 night bag with tap outlet, 30 3.5 × 3.5-inch double-sided adhesive plasters) = £60.60

Coloplast range

Stoma Urine (Coloplast)

Maxi, one-piece pouch with zinc oxide adhesive. Net price 30 pouches (13-mm hole) = £69.90

Midi, one-piece pouch with zinc oxide adhesive. Net price 30 pouches (13-mm hole) = £69.90

URO 2002® (Coloplast)

Two-piece pouch. Net price 20 small pouches (100 mL, to fit 40 mm base plate) = £50.60; 20 large pouches (375 mL, to fit 40 or 60 mm base plate) = £50.60

Base plate. Net price 5 plates (40 mm, to fit 10–35 mm stoma) or 5 plates (60 mm, to fit 10–55 mm stoma) = £13.31

Night drainage system. Net price 10 pouches (1.65 litre), 1 tube, and 2 connectors = £13.00; hospital pack, 10 pouches (1.65 litre), 5 tubes, and 10 connectors = £17.60

ConvaTec range
Surgicare System® 2 (ConvaTec)
Two-piece pouch, with non-reflux valve, clear. Net price 10 (small or standard) pouches (32, 38, 45, or 57 mm flange) = £22.04; 10 standard pouches (70 mm flange) = £23.87, (100 mm flange) = £35.94
Surgicare System® 2 Combihesive (ConvaTec)
Two-piece pouch with Accuseal® tap, and textured backing, clear. Net price 10 standard pouches (32, 38, 45, or 57 mm flange) = £22.59
Urodress® (ConvaTec)
One-piece pouch with Stomahesive® and tap. Net price 10 pouches (19, 25, 32, 38, or 45 mm holes) = £41.60

DePuy range
Raymed® (DePuy)
Butyl night bag (= pouch), one-piece pouch. Net price 1 pouch with screwcap outlet = £24.95; 1 pouch with tap outlet = £25.80

Drew range
Urostomy bags (Drew)
Urostomy bag (= pouch), one-piece pouch. Net price 50 pouches (D1/2, OSTO 06) = £76.34
Rubber bags (Drew)
Rubber bags (= pouch), one-piece pouch. Net price 1 pouch screwcap outlet (OSTO 16) = £13.03; 1 pouch (OSTO 17) tap outlet = £13.67
Ureterostomy appliance (Drew)
Ureterostomy appliance. Net price 1 appliance, 1–1.25 inch (D1/2, OSTO 05) = £38.83

Hollister range
Classic (Hollister)
Karaya 5® seal and regular adhesive with attachment for optional belt, one-piece pouch, clear. Net price 20 pouches (series 741, 23-cm pouch: 19, 25, 32, 38, 44, or 51 mm holes; series 746, 40-cm pouch and series 748, 30-cm pouch: 25, 32, 38, 44, or 51 mm holes) including 1 standard drain tube = £59.11
Regular adhesive with attachment for optional belt, one-piece pouch, clear. Net price 20 pouches (series 740, 23-cm pouch: 19, 25, 32, 38, 44, or 51 mm holes; series 745, 40-cm pouch and series 747, 30-cm pouch: 25, 32, 38, 44, or 51 mm holes) including 1 standard drain tube = £44.97
Regular adhesive only (beltless), one-piece pouch, clear. Net price 20 pouches (series 744, 23-cm pouch: 19, 25, 32, 38, 44, or 51 mm holes), including 1 standard drain tube = £44.97
First Choice® (Hollister)
Urostomy pouch with synthetic skin barrier and Microporous II adhesive (series 146). Net price 10 pouches (13–64 mm starter hole, 19, 25, 32, 38, 44, or 51 mm holes) = £41.60
Guardian® (Hollister)
Guardian, two-piece pouch with wide-bore tap and non-reflux valve (series 470). Net price 10 pouches (25-cm for max. 25, 38, or 51 mm stomas), including 1 drain tube adaptor = £21.88
Impression® (Hollister)
One-piece pouch with Convex wafer, synthetic seal and Microporous II adhesive, clear. Net price 10 pouches (13, 16, 19, 22, 25, 29, 32, 35, 38 or 44 mm holes) = £43.26
Lo-profile® (Hollister)
Karaya 5® seal and Microporous II adhesive with gasket for optional belt, one-piece pouch, with non-reflux valve, clear (series 143). Net price 10 pouches (25-cm pouch: 19, 25, 32, 38, 44, or 51 mm gasket), including 1 Lo-profile drain tube = £47.93

Microporous II adhesive only (beltless) one-piece pouch with non-reflux valve (series 142). Net price 10 pouches (25-cm pouch: 19, 25, 32, 38, 44, or 51 mm holes), including 1 Lo-profile drain tube = £37.86

Rüsch range
Rubber bags (Rüsch)
Black rubber (Birkbeck®), one-piece pouch with tap outlet. Net price 1 day pouch (19 mm hole) = £28.26; 1 night pouch (19 mm hole) = £30.83
Pink rubber, one-piece pouch with tap outlet. Net price 1 day pouch (19 mm hole) = £28.26; 1 night pouch (19 mm hole) = £30.83
White rubber, one-piece pouch with tap outlet. Net price 1 day pouch (19, 25, or 28 mm holes) = £15.35; 1 night pouch (19, 25, or 28 mm holes) = £15.77
White rubber (Glasgow), one-piece pouch. Net price 1 pouch (small or large tap) = £18.75
White rubber transverse, one-piece pouch. net price 1 left or right pouch (small, medium, or large) = £18.75

Salts range
Koenig Rutzen (Salts)
All rubber white rubber tap bag (= pouch), one-piece pouch with tap outlet. Net price 1 small or medium pouch (both 25, 32, or 38 mm holes) or 1 large pouch (25, 32, 38, 44, or 51 mm holes) = £14.81
All rubber black butyl bag (= pouch), one-piece pouch with tap outlet and non-reflux valve. Net price 1 medium or large pouch (both 19, 25, 32, or 38 mm holes) = £35.24; special size holes also available to order
All rubber MB black butyl bag (= pouch), one-piece pouch with tap outlet, bridge, and non-reflux valve. Net price 1 small, medium, or large pouch (all 19, 25, 32, or 38 mm holes) = £41.21; special size holes also available to order
Black butyl, reinforced bag (= pouch), one-piece pouch with tap outlet and non-reflux valve. Net price 1 medium or large pouch (both 19, 25, 32, or 38 mm holes) = £43.19; special size holes also available to order
MB black butyl, reinforced bag (= pouch), one-piece pouch with tap outlet and non-reflux valve. Net price 1 medium or large pouch (both 19, 25, 32, or 38 mm holes) = £49.48; special size holes also available to order
Rubber bags (Salts)
Black rubber bag (= pouch) (for use with flange), two-piece pouch with tap outlet. Net price 1 small, medium, or large pouch = £33.28; special size holes also available to order
White rubber bag (= pouch) for use with flange, two-piece pouch with tap outlet. Net price 1 small, medium, or large pouch = £9.74
Light White (Salts)
Urostomy pouch with Realistic® washer, one-piece pouch, white. Net price 20 large pouches (all 25, 32, or 38 mm holes) = £99.35
Urostomy pouch with Realistic® washer, one-piece pouch, clear. Net price 20 large or small pouches (all 25, 32, or 38 mm holes) = £99.35
Urostomy pouch, one-piece pouch, white. Net price 20 large pouches (25, 32, or 38 mm holes) = £74.66
Urostomy pouch, one-piece pouch, clear. Net price 20 large or small pouches (25, 32, or 38 mm holes) = £74.66
Urostomy pouch, one-piece pouch with adhesive, white. Net price 20 large pouches (25, 32, or 38 mm holes) = £78.84
Urostomy pouch, one-piece pouch with adhesive, clear. Net price 20 large or small pouches (both 25, 32, or 38 mm holes) = £78.84
Simplicity 1® (Salts)
Paediatric Uri-bag, one-piece pouch, 13 mm starter hole. Net price 15 pouches = £37.78

Simcare range
Carshalton (Simcare)

Bag (= pouch), one-piece pouch. Net price 10 oval or triangular pouches (both 25, 32, or 38 mm) with acrylic plaster = £17.97

Set, one-piece pouch. Net price 20 oval or triangular pouches with plasters, bodyplate, clamp, connector, and medium belt (both 25, 32, or 38 mm holes) = £61.15

Chiron Non-disposable (Simcare)

Butyl rubber bag (= pouch), one-piece pouch with stopcock outlet, odourless, black. Net price 1 day bag (22 mm) = £32.17

Latex rubber bag (= pouch), one-piece pouch with stopcock outlet. Net price (both 38 mm) 1 day bag = £22.28; 1 night bag = £25.27

Rubber child-size bag (= pouch), one-piece pouch with stopcock outlet, white. Net price 1 = £18.70

Rubber day bag (= pouch), one-piece pouch, white with stopcock outlet. Net price 1 (38 mm) = £22.28

Rubber night bag (= pouch), one-piece, white. Net price 1 (38, 44, or 51 mm) = £25.27

Chiron (Simcare)

Ileal bladder appliance, set comprises 1 web and elastic belt 25 mm wide, 1 wire pressure frame, 1 St Mark's pattern rubber flange (without diaphragm), 2 rubber day pouches with stopcock outlet, 30 double-sided plasters. Net price = £71.78

Mitcham (Simcare)

Maxi, one-piece pouch. Net price 10 pouches with adhesive flange (25, 32, or 38 mm) = £36.63, 10 pouches with nonadhesive flange (25, 32, or 38 mm) = £29.91

Mini, one-piece pouch. Net price 10 pouches with adhesive flange (19, 25, or 32 mm) = £36.63, 10 pouches with nonadhesive flange (25 mm or 32 mm) = £29.91

Standard, one-piece pouch. Net price 10 pouches with adhesive flange (19, 25, 32 or 38 mm) = £36.63, 10 pouches with nonadhesive flange (19, 25, 32, or 38 mm) = £29.91, 1 pouch with nonadhesive flange and foam pads (25, 32, or 38 mm) = £5.22

Rediflow (Simcare)

Adhesive set, may be worn with belt. Net price 20 pouches (19, 25, 32, 38, 44, or 51 mm) = £53.82

Ward range
Ward

Ureterostomy bag (= pouch) with tap outlet. Net price 1 night pouch = £17.14; 1 day pouch (19, 35, or 54 mm hole) = £16.04

ADHESIVE PREPARATIONS, ADHESIVE REMOVERS AND DEODORANTS

Adhesive preparations
Dow Corning DC 355® (Dow Corning)

Medical adhesive brushable. Net price 20-mL bottle (with brush) = £3.03

Hollister® (Hollister)

Medical adhesive spray (with silicones). Net price 170-g aerosol spray = £12.58

Latex adhesive solution (Salt)

Net price per tube = £1.77. Label: 15

Adhesive removers
Clear Peel® (CliniMed)

Adhesive remover. Net price 50 mL = £2.10

Hollister® (Hollister)

Adhesive remover spray. Net price 170-g spray = £10.54

Salts 'SPR' Plaster Remover (Rezolve®) (Salts)

Adhesive remover spray. Net price 70-g aerosol spray = £2.63. Label: 15

Deodorants
Atmocol® is used as a deodorising spray when emptying the appliance. The other deodorants listed are placed in the appliance.

Atmocol® (DePuy)

Aerosol deodorant. Net price 1 unit (400 sprays) = £1.90

Chironair Odour Control Liquid® (Simcare)

Deodorant solution. Net price 113 g = £5.23

Colostomy Plus® (Shannon)

Deodorant. Net price 1 unit = £2.68

Day-drop® (Loxley)

Deodorant solution. Net price 7.5 mL = 93p; 15 mL = £1.55; 30 mL = £2.65 (7.5 and 15 mL also available as Lemon Day-drop®)

Dor® (Pelican)

Deodorant solution. Net price 7 mL = £1.67

Forest Breeze® (Shaw)

Deodorant. Net price 1 unit = £2.97

LiMone® (CliniMed)

Deodorant spray. Net price 50 mL = £3.88

Ostobon® (Coloplast)

Deodorant powder. Net price 22 g = £3.53

Saltair No-Roma® (Salts)

Deodorant solution. Net price 30 mL = £2.10; 300 mL = £6.85

Stomogel® (DePuy)

Deodorant gel. Net price 50 g = £2.60

Sween® (Bullen & Smears)

Deodorant. Net price 15 mL = £3.95

Translet Plus One® (Rüsch)

Deodorant solution for men. Net price 7 mL = £2.88

Translet Plus Two® (Rüsch)

Deodorant solution for women. Net price 7 mL = £2.88

ADHESIVE DEVICES AND RINGS

Bullen range

Adhesive plaster, double-sided. Net price 10 zinc oxide plasters 3.5 × 3.5 inch = £3.91, 4 × 4 inch = £4.82, 5 × 5 inch = £8.15; 10 acrylic base plasters 3.5 × 3.5 inch = £3.62, 4 × 4 inch = £4.65, 5 × 5 inch = £7.83

Flange retention strips. Net price 50 strips 4 × 1 inch = £1.75, 4 × 2 inch = £2.37

3M range
Stomaseal® (3M)

Adhesive discs. Net price 12 discs (10 cm diameter) = £3.95

Rüsch range

Ostomy plasters, double sided. Net price 25 plasters (25 mm hole, or no hole) = £6.24

Salts range

Kidney seals. Net price 10 = £3.95

Reliaseal® (Salts)

Adhesive discs, double-sided, round, hypo-allergic. Net price 10 discs (13, 19, 22, 25, 29, 32, or 38 mm) = £15.12

Transacryl® (Salts)

Adhesive plasters, double-sided. Net price 10 plasters (25, 32, or 38 mm) = £5.02

Zopla® (Salts)

Adhesive plasters, double-sided. Net price (both 25, 32, or 38 mm) 10 square plasters = £3.77; 10 round plasters = £4.38

Shannon range

Adhesive plasters, double-sided. Net price 25 plasters = £14.91

Rings. Net price 5 rubber retaining rings = £5.96; 1 plastic locking ring = £2.22

Easychange® (Shannon)

Adhesive plasters, with rings (spare). Net price 5 plasters = £5.90

Shaw range

Adhesive plasters, double-sided, hole cut-to-size. Net price 10 plasters, 4 × 4 inch = £6.65; 5 × 5 inch = £6.90

Simcare range

Adhesive discs, double-sided. Net price 10 discs (76 mm diameter: 19 or 25 mm opening; 90 mm diameter: 32 or 38 mm opening) = £4.11

Rings, elastic, for use with spout bags. Net price 3 rings = £2.03

Carshalton® (Simcare)

Adhesive plasters. Net price both (25, 32, or 38 mm) 10 acrylic plasters = £4.36; 10 zinc oxide plasters = £6.90

Chiron® (Simcare)

Adhesive plasters, double-sided. Net price 10 plasters (90 mm square: 19 or 35 mm hole) = £5.58, (102 mm square: 19 or 35 mm hole) = £6.40, (127 mm square: 19 or 35 mm hole) = £7.06, (150 mm square and 102 × 76 mm: both 19 mm hole) = £7.88, (90 and 102 mm square: both 25 mm hole) = £7.88, (125 mm square: 25 mm hole) = £8.65

Clearseal plasters. Net price 10 plasters (100 mm square: 19 or 35 mm hole) = £6.40

Kidney seals, adhesive flange retaining strips. Net price 10 strips (small or large) = £4.48

Ward range

Adhesive plasters, double-sided with opening. Net price 10 plasters = £3.82

BAG CLOSURES

Clamps

Available from *CliniMed* (Biotrol® for post-op or for drainage pouches, 1 clamp = 95p), *Hollister* (for drainable pouches, 1 clamp = 95p, 20 = £15.32; for Premium® pouches, 1 clamp = 97p, 20 = £16.22), *Simcare* (10 clamps = £7.73; Carshalton®, 5 clamps = £9.16), *Simpla* (for Ileo® pouches, 20 clamps = £5.09)

Clips

Available from *ConvaTec* (10 beige clips = £2.65; for Surgicare System® 2, 10 white clips = £2.65; *Drew* (10 clips = 18p), *DePuy* (for Stomastar® drainable, 10 = £5.85), *Pelican* (drainable, 20 = £5.29, *Salts* (5 clips = £1.68), *Shaw* (1 clip = 60p), *Simcare* (for odourproof pouches, 10 = £5.91)

Closing Tape

Available from *Shannon* (1 reel = £1.44)

Fastening Ring

Rubber pouch fastening ring. Available from *Shaw* (1 ring = £1.00)

Ties

Available from *CliniMed* (30 soft-end ties = £2.32), *ConvaTec* (50 soft wire ties = £4.68)

BAG COVERS

Body's Care

Bag cover, cloth. Net price 1 cover = £3.78

Bullen

Bag cover, cloth, for day or night bags. Net price 1 cover = £7.86

CliniMed

Bag cover, cloth for closed or drainable Biotrol® pouches. Net price 5 covers = £7.55

Coloplast

Bag cover, cloth for closed or drainable MC2000® or MC2002® pouches (white or flesh), for MC2000® Mini pouches (decorated: white or flesh), for Ileo B® standard pouches, or for URO2002® pouches (white). Net price 5 covers = £19.76

ConvaTec

Bag cover, cloth for Surgicare System® 2. Net price 3 covers (for 32/38 mm Mini pouches or 45/57 mm pouches) = £6.16; 3 covers (for standard drainable pouches, urostomy pouches, large urostomy pouches, small closed 38/45 mm pouches: small drainable pouches, combihesive closed pouches, medium closed pouches: 57 and 70 mm) = £6.51

Drew

Bag cover, cotton. Net price 1 cover = £1.34

Hollister

Bag cover, non-woven. Net price 5 covers (for closed or non-drainable pouch) = £3.87

Nationwide Ostomy

Ostocover® bag cover, cloth, white or coloured. Net price 3 covers = £6.60

Pelican

Bag cover, cotton, for closed pouch. Net price 5 covers, normal = £9.59, casual = £9.53; for drainable pouch, 5 covers = £9.90

Rüsch

Bag cover, cloth for Ostopore® pouches. Net price 5 covers (small or large) = £17.06

Salts

Bag covers, cotton, appliance to be stated. Net price 1 cover = £3.28. Cloth, for Eakin® pouches, 1 cover small or large (both 32, 45 or 64 mm) = £3.99

Shaw

Bag covers, cloth. Net price 1 day pouch cover, cotton = £4.35; lycra = £4.60. 1 night cover, cotton = £4.60; lycra = £4.95

Simcare

Bag cover. Net price 1 day or night cotton pouch cover = £9.91; 5 stomabag covers (white or coloured) = £21.91; for Redifit® pouches, 1 cotton cover (25 and 32 mm, 38, 44, and 51 mm, 64, and 75 mm holes) = £7.08; for Symphony® pouches, 5 polyethylene covers = £4.06

Steeper

Bag cover, white linen. Net price 1 cover = £5.98

Welland

Bag shields, spunbonded polypropylene. Net price 10 shields (small: 25–44 mm; large: 10, 51, or 60 mm) = £2.80

BELTS

Body's Care

Belts. Net price 3-inch belt = £12.78: 3-inch one-piece belt, = £16.68; 4-inch one-piece belt = £16.85; 1-inch web and elastic with button and buckle fastening = £7.10; 2-inch belt = £8.40; 3-inch belt = £9.68; 1 girdle and panti-brief with hole for stoma and suspenders or understrap = £41.37; 1 St Mark's (male or female) = £49.29; 1 St Mark's Coutil ostomy = £33.41

Bullen

Belts. Net price 1.5-inch belt with aluminium retaining shield (small, medium, or large) = £9.31: 1.5-inch elastic belt with wire or plastic ring retainer (wire; small, medium, or large) = £9.50; 4-inch belt (wire; small, medium, or large) = £13.92; 1-inch elastic belt with plastic ring shield = £10.05: 1 waterproof canvas retaining shield (small, medium, or large) = £15.03; 1 St Mark's = £39.01

CliniMed

Waist belt for Biotrol® pouches. Net price 1 belt = £3.83

Coloplast

Belts. For Ileo B® pouches, net price 1 belt = £6.52 or for K-Flex® pouches, 1 belt = £4.97

ConvaTec

Belt, for Surgicare System® 2. Net price 1 belt = £2.65

Dansac

Belt with plates for Combi® pouches. Net price 1 belt plus 5 plates (19–44 mm or 50–63 mm) = £32.54

DePuy

Belts. Net price 1 ostomy girdle or panty girdle (white or pink colour) = £28.90; 1 4-inch nightbelt with waterproof backing = £9.25; for Schacht® pouches, 1 36-inch belt = £5.05; or for Slimline® pouches, 1 belt with belt-plate = £11.60

Drew

Belts. Net price 1 waistband with metal ends = £2.62, with plastic ends = £8.17; 1 day belt = £19.14; 1 night belt = £13.02; 1 ×4 inch belt (deep stoma hole) = £6.24; stoma/bones = £6.85

Hollister

Belt. Net price 1 adjustable ostomy belt (small, medium, or large) = £5.91; 10 = £49.19

Marlen

Belt. Net price 1 adjustable elastic waist belt = £2.65

Peacock

Belts. Net price 1 St Mark's belt = £38.15

Rüsch

Belts. Net price 5 elastic waistbands (Birkbeck®) = £32.54; 5 elastic waistbands with shields = £42.81; 5 retaining rings (19, 38, or 54 mm) = £8.12. 1 narrow or normal width belts (Ostopore®, waist: 17–34 inch or 28–56 inch) = £5.44. White rubber belting 28 mm = £3.56/metre, 72 mm = £7.35/metre. White sausage belt per metre = £7.32. 1 waist and support strap = £6.06

Sallis

Belts. Net price 1 night belt, 14a = £5.92; 14b = £9.40; 14c = £4.91; 1 day belt, 15a = £25.90; 15b = £7.23. 1 zipped pocket (to fit 15a, 15b and 16) = £4.40; 1 St Mark's = £23.74, 1 shield = £8.59; 1 ostomy girdle/pantie brief, with hole and suspenders,15c = £33.99

Salts

Belts. Net price 25 mm elastic belt (single), with 2 loops (standard 35 inch or extra-large 42 inch) = £3.03; with suspender ends = £3.03; double elastic with 4 loops = £4.22; with waterproof panel 102 mm = £12.26, 150 mm = £14.96; with 4 loops and retaining ring = £16.35. 1 rubber belt with straps and buckles = £5.08; with 2 fastening studs = £3.49. 25 mm button belt with or without loop = £3.03. 1 baby lycra belting = £12.07; with Velcro fastening (standard 35 inch or extra-large 42 inch) = £3.08. 1 colostomy belt = £63.68. 1 ileostomy girdle (Saltair®) = £40.67; 1 ileostomy elastic night belt (Saltair®) = £12.13. For Eakin® pouches, 1 elastic belt (small or large) = £3.13. For Salger® pouches, 1 elastic adjustable belt with or without Velcro fastening = £3.06

Shannon

Belt. Net price 1 elastic belt with shield and Velcro fastening = £7.39; with button and buckle fastening = £4.45

Shaw

Belts, colostomy, all made to measure. Net price 4 inch elastic web belt = £12.50; with under-strap or suspenders, 6 inch = £16.75, 8 inch = £24.05; with lace fastenings, 6 inch = £22.65; 8 inch = £28.70; 10 inch = £27.30; 12 inch = £30.00; 14 inch (made to measure) = £30.60; with zip panel, 10 inch = £34.45; 12 inch = £36.55; 14 inch = £38.25; elastic with nylon fronts, 10 inch = £32.05; 12 inch = £33.65; 14 inch = £35.80. 1 inch adjustable colostomy/ileostomy belt = £7.25; 4 inch (3 sections) = £18.35; 6 inch (3 sections) = £23.10. 1 colostomy night belt (net or rayon, no hole, for use with dressing pad), = £13.35. 4 inch ostomy belt with groin strap = £14.30; with lace fastenings = £15.20; with wire spring = £14.00; double zip panel = £7.25

Simcare

Belts. Net price 25 mm web and elastic belt (WL002 range) = £9.38; 51 mm = £10.94; 75 mm = £12.49; (WL008) 25 mm = £10.25; 1 belt, child (25 mm) = £7.88, 38 mm = £10.99. 1 web end belt with buckle (short) = £6.33. 1 narrow belt (flange diameter: 32, 38,

or 51 mm) = £19.50. 1 Leno belt (white with Velcro fastening, flange diameter: 38 mm) = £18.75. 1 Redifit adjustable belt (small, medium, or large) = £7.88. 1 non-slip belt = £16.08; 1 elastic non-slip belt = £10.99. 1 rubber belt ('sausage' or tubular) = £20.48; 1 narrow belt = £5.95. 1 two-way stretch night belt (small, medium, large, or extra-large) = £21.98. 1 stoma belt (small: 17–26 inch or medium: 26–43 inch) = £5.21. 1 Carshalton® belt (small, medium, or large) = £8.32

Steeper

Belts. Made to measure, all sizes. Net price 1 day belt = £37.76; 1 night belt = £27.80. 1 nylon elastic colostomy belt, with hook and eye fastening and 2 pairs of suspenders or understraps = £39.00. 1 two-way stretch pull-on elastic belt = £10.61; 1 adjustable belt with buckle fastening and celluloid hook ends = £8.04; 1 belt with double waistband and cellulosed hook ends = £8.04. 1 rubber adjustable belt with window = £10.72. 1 wide rubberised ileostomy belt with 2 straps and buttonholed ends for use with ileostomy boxes or with celluoid hook ends for use with ileostomy bags = £22.15. 1 belt with understraps or suspenders = £24.91. 1 window = £4.15. 1 colostomy belt, with 2 pairs of understraps or suspenders (Gabriel®) = £44.08

Ward

Belts. Net price 1 web and elastic belt with button and buckle fastening. Net price 1 belt (1 inch) = £6.67; 2 inch = £8.58; 3 inch = £9.76. 1 colostomy/ileostomy bath belt = £15.30. 1 plastic elastic belt with hook end = £9.29

FILTERS AND BRIDGES

Filters

Available from *CliniMed* (Biotrol®, 50 filters = £10.90), *Coloplast* (Filtrodor®, 50 filters = £17.15; Maclet®, 20 filter washers = £23.00), *ConvaTec* (Surgicare System® 2 for closed pouches, 30 filters = £7.66), *Cuxson* (50 patches = £2.86), *Hollister* (replacement filter elements for series 366 drainable bags, 20 = £2.62, 100 = £13.12), *Simcare* (for Beta® and mini bags, 20 = £6.64; Doublesure®, 10 filters = £3.15)

Bridges

Available from *Salts* (20 metal bridges ready fixed to lightweight and LWU disposable bags = £8.03; 30 bridges for use with other disposable bags = £12.05), *Simcare* (20 bridges = £2.82)

FLANGES

Body's Care

Flanges. Net price 1 St Mark's soft rubber = £11.53

Bullen

Flanges. Net price 1 lightweight, plastic flange (small, medium, or large) = £3.59. 1 flange for Lenbul® pouches (1 inch diameter, 2 inch base) = £8.84; 1.5 inch diameter, 3 inch base = £13.04; 2 inch diameter, 4 inch base = £15.22

ConvaTec

Flanges for Surgicare System® 2. Net price 10 Accordion flanges, 100 × 100 mm (70 mm hole) = £36.80; 127 × 127 mm (100 mm hole), 10 = £64.95. Combihesive flexible flanges, 100 × 100 mm (32, 38, or 45 mm hole), 5 = £12.74; 127 × 127 mm (57 or 70 mm hole), 5 = £13.87. Stomahesive flexible flanges, 100 × 100 mm (32, 38, 45, 57 or 70 mm holes), 5 = £11.23; Stomahesive flanges, 100 × 100 mm (32, 38, 45, 57 or 70 mm holes) 10 = £22.47; 127 ×127 mm (70 mm hole), 10 = £45.52; 152 × 152 mm (100 mm hole), 20 = £54.64

DePuy

Flanges. Net price 1 Ileo B® standard rubber flange (0.75, 1.0, 1.25, 1.375, 1.5 inch) = £8.00. For Schacht® pouches, 1 flange (with locking ring) = £5.10; 1 ileo flange (with locking ring) = £5.10. For Slimline® pouches, 1 padded flange = £4.00

Drew

Flange. Net price 1 kapok flange (1–1.5 inch) = £14.01

Hollister

Flanges for Impression® pouch. Net price 5 Convex flanges with synthetic seal and Microporous adhesive (13, 16, 19, 22, 25, 29, 32, 35, 38, 41, 44 or 51 mm holes) = £13.00

Rüsch

Flange. Net price 2 Birkbeck® white rubber flanges (75 mm base, 16 mm deep, 20 mm diameter); 90 mm base, 16 mm deep, 38 mm diameter; 110 mm base, 16 mm deep, 58 mm diameter = £20.72; St Mark's, in two rubbers with hard centre (76 mm base, 10 or 16 mm deep, 32 or 38 mm diameter), 2 flanges = £31.05; 76 mm base, 13 or 16 mm deep, 25 mm diameter, 2 flanges = £31.05; 102 mm base, 16 mm deep, 44 or 51 mm diameter, 2 flanges = £31.05; in soft honey coloured rubber (51 or 76 mm base, 13 mm deep, 25 mm diameter), 2 flanges = £18.11; (76 mm base, 10 or 16 mm deep, 32 or 38 mm diameter), 2 flanges = £18.11; 102 mm base, 16 mm deep, 44 or 51 mm diameter, 2 flanges = £18.11; with diaphragm, cowl, or dressing retainer at extra cost = £3.00: black, firm rubber (51 mm base, 13 mm deep, 25 mm diameter), 2 flanges = £20.72; 76 mm base, 10 or 16 mm deep, 32 or 38 mm diameter, 2 flanges = £20.72; 102 mm base, 16 mm deep, 44 or 51 mm diameter, 2 flanges = £20.72

Salts

Flange. Net price 1 flange (SF1, soft rubber, 25 mm) = £6.37; SF2, semi-rigid, 25 mm = £10.09; SF3, hard rubber, 25 mm = £7.28; SF4, soft rubber, 38 mm = £6.37; SF5, semi-rigid, 38 mm = £10.92; SF6, semi-rigid, hard rubber = £7.28; SF7, soft rubber, 51 mm = £8.02; SF8R, flexible, recessed, 32 mm = £10.09. 1 baby flange with diaphragm (19 mm) = £8.48. 1 Latex foam diaphragm flange = £35.70; 1 sheath for use with flange = £5.95. For Salger® pouches, 1 polythene flange (40 or 57 mm) = £1.80

Shannon

Flange ring. Net price 1 = £2.23

Shaw

Flange. Net price 1 rubber, adhesive = £5.25; rubber, non-stick = £6.35; with diaphragm = £8.25; non-stick inner diaphragm £2.45; 1 colostomy rubber foam facepiece (face hole diameter: 1.75, 2, 2.5, or 3 inch) = £9.60

Simcare

Flange. Net price 1 rubber flange (16 mm deep, 38 mm diameter) = £14.87; double base hole (38 mm diameter) = £19.71; blue rubber (51 mm base, 13 mm deep, 25 mm diameter or 76 mm base, 10 or 16 mm deep, 38 mm diameter) = £13.45; blue and brown, (76 mm base, 13 mm deep, 25 mm diameter; 10 or 16 mm deep, 38mm diameter) = £19.53. 1 belt flange (19, 25, 32, 38, 44, 51, or 64 mm) = 24p. For Chiron® pouches, 1 flange (10 or 16mm deep, 38mm diameter) = £14.87; 13mm deep, 25mm diameter = £14.87; 16 mm deep, 32 mm diameter = £14.87; plastic without diaphragm (13 mm deep, 32 or 38 mm diameter) = £7.44. For Redifit® pouches, 1 belt flange = 59p; St Mark's pattern, 1 flange (51 mm base: 13 mm deep, 25 mm diameter; 76 mm base, 13 mm deep, 25 mm diameter; 76 mm base, 10 or 16 mm deep, 32 or 38 mm diameter; 102 mm base, 16 mm deep, 44 or 51 mm diameter) = £12.67: with dressing retainer or with 16 mm canopy, 38 mm = £15.85

Ward

Flange. Net price 1 plastic/rubber air-filled flange = £15.17; 1 St Mark's standard = £9.96; 1 St Mark's with diaphragm = £12.16

IRRIGATION AND WASH-OUT APPLIANCES

Available from *Astra Tech* (Medena® 5 ileostomy catheters = £4.38), *CliniMed* (Biotrol®, 50 irrigation sleeves = £33.70 or 1 cone = £2.39), *Coloplast* (30 disposable sleeves (1540 or 1560) = £28.38; 1 colotip = £5.37; 1 irrigator bag = £10.15; 1 supporting plate = £5.10; 1 irrigation belt = £4.97), *Dansac* (1 water container = £15.72; 1 clamp = £6.81; 1 cone = £10.10; 1 brush = £1.71; 1 tube = £1.20; 1 belt = £32.54; Irri-drain® with ring holder for silicone ring, 20 = £20.10 or adhesive, 20 = £20.10; silicone ring, 1 = £4.04), *Hollister* (irrigator drain for use with Guardian® Two-Piece system/irrigator kit = £17.27; 20 irrigator drains = £24.17; 10 replacement cones = £61.27; 1 = £7.49; 1 stoma cone/irrigator kit = £17.27; 20 irrigator drains = £24.17; 10 replacement cones = £61.27; 1 = £7.49; 1 stoma lubricant = £4.24), *Ward* (1 wash-out cup = £24.57; 1 cap = £1.31; 1 belt = £7.11; 1 tube = £4.62)

PRESSURE PLATES, SHIELDS

Coloplast (1 supporting plate = £5.10), *ConvaTec* (5 System 2® convex inserts for Combihesive®, Stomahesive®, and flexible flanges, 38, 45, or 57 mm) = £1.25, *DePuy* (5 slimline rubber retaining rings = £2.75), *Drew* pressure plate (oval or round) = £2.68; pressure plate (4 slot) = £4.02; *Salts* (plastic retaining shield, single = £2.84, double = £4.38, large = £3.47; S S Wire retaining ring, large = £2.84, medium = £2.70, small = £2.63; light white anti-sag ring = £1.13, for belt use = £1.28, for velcro belt fastening = £1.46; convex plate for light white bag (32, 38, or 44 mm), 5 = £12.19; pressure plate for Kombo®, Simplicity®, or Solo® pouches (30, 40, 50, or 60 mm) = £1.77; Eakin® support frame (32, 45, 64, or 90 mm) = £1.15, *Shannon* (faceplate = £7.53), *Simcare* (plastic pressure plates, Surrey model: 25 or 32 mm or Standard model with attached flange for use with lightweight bags: 25, 32, or 38 mm = £6.70; stainless wire pressure frame, hook, lug, to fit 25, 32, 38, 44, or 51 mm flange) = £8.16; cotton facepiece = £20.31; pressure plates (25, 32, or 38 mm) = £4.63, *Ward* (celluloid colostomy cup with sponge or solid rim, small, medium, or large = £31.24, with sponge rubber or solid rim, belt fitting = £35.65; St Mark's shield, celluloid with 4 studs = £6.79)

SKIN PROTECTIVES, FILLERS, AND CLEANSERS

Balspray® (Bullen)
Aerosol. Net price 1 unit = £6.74
Bullen Karaya Gum Powder® (Bullen)
Powder. Net price 70 g = £4.34
Chiron® (Simcare)
Barrier cream (with antiseptic). Net price 52 g = £4.50
CliniShield Wipes® (CliniMed)
Barrier wipes. Net price 50 = £11.19
Comfeel® (Coloplast)
Barrier cream. Net price 60 g = £3.43
Protective film. Net price 30 sachets = £8.10; applicator = £3.79
Dansac® (Dansac)
Karaya paste. Net price 50 g = £2.36
Soft paste. Net price 50 g = £2.81
Day-Drop® (TVM)
Barrier Cream. Net price 50 g = £1.98
Derma-gard® (Simcare)
Protective skin wipes. Net price 50 = £13.18
Hollister® (Hollister)
Karaya paste. Net price 128 g = £6.24
Do not apply to severely excoriated skin

Karaya powder. Net price 71 g = £7.40

Skin gel. Net price 28 g = £5.42. Label: 15
Do not apply to severely excoriated skin

Orabase® (ConvaTec)

Paste, see section 12.3.1

Orahesive® (ConvaTec)

Powder (with adherent properties), see section 12.3.1

Payne® (Payne)

Barrier cream. Net price 50 g = £3.15

Pelican® (Pelican)

Paste (formerly Simpla® gel). Net price 1 pack = £5.89

Saltair® (Salts)

Karaya gum powder. Net price per puffer pack = £4.06

Ostomy cleansing soap (soap spirit). Net price 110-mL =
£2.44

Peri-Prep wipes. Net price 50 = £13.25

Seel-a-peel® (Simcare)

Paste. Net price 50 mL = £2.55

Simcare® (Simcare)

Karaya gum powder. Net price 100 g = £6.34

Karaya gum sheet. Net price 1 = £6.35

Stomahesive® (ConvaTec)

Paste. Net price 60 g = £6.32. For filling and sealing skin
creases

Stomosol® (DePuy)

Skin shield. Net price 50 = £7.45

Translet® (Rüsch)

Wipes. Net price 30 = £5.45

SKIN PROTECTORS

Bullen

Karaya gum washers, regular or extra hard. Net price 10
washers (2 inch diameter: 2 × 0.875 inch or 2 × 1.125
inch hole) = £11.80; 2.5 inch diameter: regular 2.5 × 1.25
inch or extra hard 2.5 × 1.5 inch hole = £13.68; 3 inch
diameter: 3 × 0.875 inch, 3 × 1.125 inch, 3 × 1.5 inch, or
3 × 2 inch hole = £15.68

CliniMed

Biotrol® skin protectors. Net price 20 × 20 cm, 5 =
£36.76; 10 × 10 cm or 10 cm diameter, 10 = £15.35

Coloplast

Protective sheets. Net price 10 non-sterile sheets (10 ¥
10 cm) = £18.31; 5 (15 ¥ 15 cm) = £31.02; 5 (20 ¥ 20
cm) = £38.60; 30 rings (10, 15, 20, 25, 30, 40, or 50 mm)
= £30.60

ConvaTec

Wafers. Net price 5 Stomahesive® wafers (100 ¥ 100 mm) =
£9.42; 3 (200 ¥ 200 mm) = £22.99; 10 Varihesive® wafers
(100 ¥ 100 mm) = £8.08

Dansac

Karaya rings. Net price 25 rings (22, 25, 32, 38, 50 or
63 mm) = £37.48

DePuy

Schacht rings. Net price 10 foam, colostomy or ileostomy
rings = £7.10

Drew

Washers. Net price 20 K-Seal® karaya gum washers
(small) = £8.53; large = £10.09

Hollister

Skin barrier. Net price 5 Hollister® skin barriers (4 × 4
inch) = £9.38; 5 (8 × 8 inch) = £28.53

Pelican

Protectors (formerly Simplaseel® wafers). Net price 10
(100 × 100 mm) = £16.85

Salts

Protectors. Net price 60 karaya gum washers (small) =
£6.80; 10 (large) = £11.08; 5 foam cushions (25, 32, 38,
or 51 mm) = £2.25; 5 dri pads (40 mm) = £2.28; 20
Cohesive® washers (small: 50 mm) = £28.80; 10 (large:
95 mm) = £19.05; 10 Realistic® washers (13, 19, 22, 25,
29, 32, or 38 mm) = £13.85; 1 Saltair® twinpack (small)
= £8.32; large = £11.65; 10 foam seals (as in twin packs)
= £1.70; 5 United® skin barrier wafers (10 × 10 cm) =
£9.03; 3 = £21.25; for Salger® pouches, 5 karaya washers
with foam (40 or 57 mm) = £11.79

Shannon

Protectors. Net price 1 foam sponge ring = 73p; 10
Kaygee® washers (2.5 inch base: 0.875 or 1.125 inch hole
or 2.75 inch base: 0.875 or 1.375 inch hole) = £6.60

Shaw

Protectors. Net price 5 Body Mould® squares (1.0, 1.25,
or 1.5 inch hole) = £9.65; 10 washers (1.0 or 1.25 inch
hole) = £8.90; 5 rings (1.0, 1.25, or 1.5 inch hole) =
£8.90; 12 Healwell® squares (1.0, 1.25 or 1.5 inch hole) =
£9.15; 12 rings (1.0, 1.25 or 1.5 inch hole) = £7.90

Simcare

Protectors. Net price 5 foam pads, white (76 mm
diameter: 25 mm hole) = £4.31; 76 mm diameter: 29, 32,
or 38 mm hole or 90 mm diameter: 32 or 38 mm hole =
£5.89; black (25 mm hole) = £5.51; 1 karaya gum sheet
(300 × 100 mm) = £6.35; 20 rings (19, 25, 32, 38, or 44
mm) = £21.17; karaya rings (19, 25, 32, 38, or 51 mm) =
£23.15; 10 Down's® adhesive karaya washers (51
mm base: 22 or 29 mm hole) = £10.31; 70 mm base: 22
or 29 mm hole = £12.71; 10 Redifit® karaya gum
washers (25, 32, 38, 44, or 51 mm) = £12.71; 20 Seel-a-
peel® squares (100 mm sq) = £36.22; 5 squares (150 mm
sq) = £22.31

STOMA CAPS AND DRESSINGS

Available from *Bullen* (1 stoma cap = £4.22), *Coloplast*
(100 Colocap® stomacaps = £95.70), *ConvaTec*
(Colodress Plus®, 30 stoma caps (19 mm hole cut-to-
size) = £30.66, *Dansac* (50 Dansac® Mini caps (30 or 44
mm) = £50.32), *Hollister* (50 stoma caps (51 or 76 mm)
= £50.82), *Salts* (30 stoma caps for Simplicity 1®
pouches = £30.43), *Simcare* (20 leisure pouches =
£21.46), *Steeper* (1 celluloid colostomy shield, 10cm
with 4 studs = £4.35; 12 waterproof material squares for
use with colostomy dressings (16.5 × 16.5 cm) = £2.93;
1 celluloid colostomy cup with solid rim and 4 studs =
£18.54; 1 celluloid cup with 4 studs and chute = £22.31;
2 zip fasteners fitted to colostomy belt = £7.29; 1
waterproof front fitted to colostomy belt = £6.01; 1 pair
woven understraps with buttonholed ends = £2.79; 1 sq
yd waterproof material = £2.84; 1 Donald Rose®
ileostomy/colostomy bath belt with internal chamber for
dressings and stud fastenings for adjustment = £18.07)

TUBING

Available from *Hollister* (10 urostomy drain tubes =
£21.42; 8 tubes for fitting to Lo-Profile® urostomy bags
= £19.93; for Premium®urostomy pouches, 10 drain tube
adaptors = £17.07), *Salts* (2 night tube adaptors = 85p),
Simcare (for Carshalton® urostomy pouches, 10
connectors = £3.71), *Steeper* (1 metal spring tubing clip
= £2.03)

Appendix 9: Cautionary and Advisory Labels for Dispensed Medicines

Numbers following the preparation entries in the BNF correspond to the code numbers of the cautionary labels that pharmacists are recommended to add when dispensing. It is also expected that pharmacists will counsel patients when necessary.

Counselling needs to be related to the age, experience, background, and understanding of the individual patient. The pharmacist should ensure that the patient understands how to take or use the medicine and how to follow the correct dosage schedule. Any effects of the medicine on driving or work, any foods or medicines to be avoided, and what to do if a dose is missed should also be explained. Other matters, such as the possibility of staining of the clothes or skin by a medicine should also be mentioned.

For some preparations there is a special need for counselling, such as an unusual method or time of administration or a potential interaction with a common food or domestic remedy, and this is indicated where necessary.

ORIGINAL PACKS. Many preparations are now dispensed in unbroken original packs that bear complete instructions for the patient or provide a leaflet addressed to the patient. These labels or leaflets should not normally be obscured or removed. Where it is known that such instructions are provided with an original pack intended for the patient no label has been listed under the preparation. Label 10 may be used where appropriate. Leaflets are available from various sources advising on the administration of preparations such as eye-drops, eye ointments, inhalers, and suppositories.

SCOPE OF LABELS. In general no label recommendations have been made for injections on the assumption that they will be administered by a health professional or a well-instructed patient. The labelling is not exhaustive and pharmacists are recommended to use their professional discretion in labelling new preparations and those for which no labels are shown.

Individual labelling advice is not given on the administration of the large variety of antacids. In the absence of instructions from the prescriber, and if on enquiry the patient has had no verbal instructions, the directions given under 'Dose' should be used on the label.

It is recognised that there may be occasions when pharmacists will use their knowledge and professional discretion and decide to omit one or more of the recommended labels for a particular patient. In this case counselling is of the utmost importance. There may also be an occasion when a prescriber does not wish additional cautionary labels to be used, in which case the prescription should be endorsed 'NCL' (no cautionary labels). The exact wording that is required instead should then be specified on the prescription.

Pharmacists have traditionally labelled medicines with various wordings in addition to those directions specified on the prescription. Such labels include 'Shake the bottle', 'For external use only', and 'Store in a cool place', as well as 'Discard . . . . days after opening' and 'Do not use after . . . .', which apply particularly to antibiotic mixtures, diluted liquid and topical preparations, and to eye-drops. Although not listed in the BNF these labels should continue to be used when appropriate; indeed, 'For external use only' is a legal requirement on external liquid preparations, while 'Keep out of the reach of children' is a legal requirement on all dispensed medicines.

It is the usual practice for patients to take standard tablets with water or other liquid and for this reason no separate label has been recommended.

The label or labels for each preparation are recommended after careful consideration of the information available. However, it is recognised that in some cases this information may be either incomplete or open to a different interpretation. The Executive Editor will therefore be grateful to receive any constructive comments on the labelling suggested for any preparation.

Recommended label wordings

Wordings which can be given as separate warnings are labels 1–19 and labels 29–33. Wordings which can be incorporated in an appropriate position in the directions for dosage or administration are labels 21–28. A label has been omitted for number 20.

If separate labels are used it is recommended that the wordings be used without modification. If changes are made to suit computer requirements, care should be taken to retain the sense of the original.

(1) Warning. May cause drowsiness
To be used on *preparations for children* containing antihistamines, or other preparations given to children where the warnings of label 2 on driving or alcohol would not be appropriate.

(2) Warning. May cause drowsiness. If affected do not drive or operate machinery. Avoid alcoholic drink
To be used on *preparations for adults that can cause drowsiness*, thereby affecting the ability to drive and operate hazardous machinery; label 1 is more appropriate for children. *It is an offence to drive while under the influence of drink or drugs.*

Some of these preparations only cause drowsiness in the first few days of treatment and some only cause drowsiness in higher doses.

In such cases the patient should be told that the advice applies until the effects have worn off. However many of these preparations can produce a slowing of reaction time and a loss of mental concentration that can have the same effects as drowsiness.

Avoidance of alcoholic drink is recommended because the effects of CNS depressants are enhanced by alcohol. Strict prohibition however could lead to some patients not taking the medicine. Pharmacists should therefore explain the risk and encourage compliance, particularly in patients who may think they already tolerate the effects of alcohol (see also label 3). Queries from patients with epilepsy regarding fitness to drive should be referred back to the patient's doctor.

Side-effects unrelated to drowsiness that may affect a patient's ability to drive or operate machinery safely include *blurred vision, dizziness, or nausea*. In general, no label has been recommended to cover these cases, but the patient should be suitably counselled.

(3) Warning. May cause drowsiness. If affected do not drive or operate machinery
To be used on *preparations containing monoamine-oxidase inhibitors*; the warning to avoid alcohol and dealcoholised (low alcohol) drink is covered by the MAOI treatment card.

(4) Warning. Avoid alcoholic drink
To be used on *preparations where a reaction such as flushing may occur if alcohol is taken* (e.g. metronidazole and chlorpropamide). Alcohol may also enhance the hypoglycaemia produced by some oral antidiabetic drugs but routine application of a warning label is not considered necessary.

(5) Do not take indigestion remedies at the same time of day as this medicine
To be used with label 25 on *preparations coated to resist gastric acid* (e.g. enteric-coated tablets). This is to avoid the possibility of premature dissolution of the coating in the presence of an alkaline pH.

Label 5 also applies to drugs such as ketoconazole where the absorption is significantly affected by antacids; the usual period of avoidance recommended is 2 to 4 hours.

(6) Do not take iron preparations or indigestion remedies at the same time of day as this medicine
To be used on *preparations containing ciprofloxacin, doxycycline, minocycline, and penicillamine*. These drugs chelate iron and calcium ions and are less well absorbed when given with iron or calcium-containing antacids. If necessary these incompatible preparations may be given about two hours apart.

(7) Do not take milk, iron preparations or indigestion remedies at the same time of day as this medicine
To be used on *preparations containing tetracyclines that chelate iron, calcium, and magnesium* and are thus less available for absorption; if it is necessary to give milk, iron or antacids, the usual period of avoidance is about 2 hours. Doxycycline and minocycline are less liable to form chelates and therefore only require label 6 (see above).

(8) Do not stop taking this medicine except on your doctor's advice
To be used on *preparations that contain a drug which is required to be taken over long periods without the patient necessarily perceiving any benefit* (e.g. antituberculous drugs).

Also to be used on *preparations that contain a drug whose withdrawal is likely to be a particular hazard* (e.g. clonidine for hypertension). Label 10 (see below) is more appropriate for corticosteroids.

(9) Take at regular intervals. Complete the prescribed course unless otherwise directed
To be used on *preparations where a course of treatment should be completed* to reduce the incidence of relapse, the development of resistance, or failure of treatment.

The preparations are antimicrobial drugs given by mouth. Very occasionally, some may have severe side-effects (e.g. diarrhoea in patients receiving clindamycin) and in such cases the patient may need to be advised of reasons for stopping treatment quickly and returning to the doctor.

(10) Warning. Follow the printed instructions you have been given with this medicine
To be used particularly on *preparations containing anticoagulants, lithium, monoamine-oxidase inhibitors, and oral corticosteroids*. The appropriate treatment card should be given to the patient and any necessary explanations given.

This label may also be used on other preparations to remind the patient of the instructions that have been given.

(11) Avoid exposure of skin to direct sunlight or sun lamps
To be used on *preparations that may cause phototoxic or photoallergic reactions* if the patient is exposed to ultraviolet radiation. Many drugs other than those listed (e.g. phenothiazines and sulphonamides) may on rare occasions cause reactions in susceptible patients. Exposure to high intensity ultraviolet radiation from sunray lamps and sunbeds is particularly likely to cause reactions.

(12) Do not take anything containing aspirin while taking this medicine
To be used on *preparations containing probenecid and sulphinpyrazone* whose activity is reduced by aspirin.

Label 12 should not be used for anticoagulants since label 10 is more appropriate.

(13) Dissolve or mix with water before taking
To be used on *preparations that are intended to be dissolved in water* (e.g. soluble tablets) or *mixed with water* (e.g. powders, granules) before use. In a few cases other liquids such as fruit juice or milk may be used.

(14) This medicine may colour the urine
To be used on *preparations that may cause the patient's urine to turn an unusual colour*. These include phenolphthalein (alkaline urine pink), tri-

amterene (blue under some lights), levodopa (dark reddish), and rifampicin (red).

(15)   Caution flammable: keep away from fire or flames
To be used on *preparations containing sufficient flammable solvent to render them flammable if exposed to a naked flame.*

(16)   Allow to dissolve under the tongue. Do not transfer from this container. Keep tightly closed. Discard eight weeks after opening
To be used on *glyceryl trinitrate tablets* to remind the patient not to transfer the tablets to plastic or less suitable containers.

(17)   Do not take more than . . . . in 24 hours
To be used on *preparations for the treatment of acute migraine* except those containing ergotamine, for which label 18 is used. The dose form should be specified, e.g. tablets or capsules.

It may also be used on preparations for which no dose has been specified by the prescriber.

(18)   Do not take more than . . . in 24 hours or . . . in any one week
To be used on preparations containing ergotamine. The dose form should be specified, e.g. tablets or suppositories.

(19)   Warning. Causes drowsiness which may continue the next day. If affected do not drive or operate machinery. Avoid alcoholic drink
To be used on *preparations containing hypnotics (or some other drugs with sedative effects) prescribed to be taken at night.* On the rare occasions (e.g. nitrazepam in epilepsy) when hypnotics are prescribed for daytime administration this label would clearly not be appropriate. Also to be used as *an alternative to the label 2 wording* (the choice being at the discretion of the pharmacist) *for anxiolytics prescribed to be taken at night.*

It is hoped that this wording will convey adequately the problem of residual morning sedation after taking 'sleeping tablets'.

(21)   . . . with or after food
To be used on *preparations that are liable to cause gastric irritation,* or *those that are better absorbed with food.*

Patients should be advised that a *small amount of food is sufficient.*

(22)   . . . half to one hour before food
To be used on some preparations (e.g. propantheline) *whose absorption is thereby improved.* Most oral antibiotics require label 23 instead (see below).

(23)   . . . an hour before food or on an empty stomach
To be used on *oral antibiotics whose absorption may be reduced by the presence of food and acid in the stomach.*

(24)   . . . sucked or chewed
To be used on *preparations that should be sucked or chewed.*
The pharmacist should use discretion as to which of these words is appropriate.

(25)   . . . swallowed whole, not chewed
To be used on *preparations that are enteric-coated or designed for modified-release.*

Also to be used on *preparations that taste very unpleasant or may damage the mouth* if not swallowed whole.

(26)   . . . dissolved under the tongue
To be used on *preparations designed for sublingual use.* Patients should be advised to hold under the tongue and avoid swallowing until dissolved. The buccal mucosa between the gum and cheek is occasionally specified by the prescriber.

(27)   . . . with plenty of water
To be used on *preparations that should be well diluted* (e.g. chloral hydrate), *where a high fluid intake is required* (e.g. sulphonamides), or *where water is required to aid the action* (e.g. methylcellulose). The patient should be advised that 'plenty' means at least 150 mL (about a tumblerful). In most cases fruit juice, tea, or coffee may be used.

(28)   To be spread thinly . . .
To be used on *external corticosteroid preparations.*

(29)   Do not take more than 2 at any one time. Do not take more than 8 in 24 hours
To be used on containers of dispensed *solid dose preparations containing paracetamol for adults when the instruction on the label indicates that the dose can be taken on an 'as required' basis.* The dose form should be specified, e.g. tablets or capsules.

This label has been introduced because of the serious consequences of overdosage with paracetamol.

(30)   Contains paracetamol
To be used on containers of dispensed *preparations containing paracetamol when the name on the label does not include the word 'paracetamol'.*

(31)   Contains aspirin and paracetamol
To be used on containers of dispensed *preparations containing aspirin and paracetamol (e.g. benorylate), when the name on the label does not include the words 'aspirin' and 'paracetamol'.*

(32)   Contains aspirin
To be used on containers of dispensed *preparations containing aspirin when the name on the label does not include the word 'aspirin'.*

(33)   Contains an aspirin-like medicine
To be used on containers of dispensed *preparations containing a salicylate derivative.*

Products and their labels

Products introduced or amended since publication of BNF No. 27 (March 1994) are <u>underlined</u>.
Proprietary names are in *italic*.
C = counselling advised; see BNF = consult product entry in BNF

Acarbose,
    C, administration, see BNF
Acebutolol, 8
Acemetacin, 21, C, driving
Acetazolamide, 3
Acetazolamide m/r, 3, 25
Acetylcysteine gran, 13
Achromycin, 7, 9, 23, C, posture
Acipimox, 21
Acitretin, 10 patient information
    leaflet, 21
Acrivastine, C, driving, alcohol, see
    BNF
Acrosoxacin, 2, 23
Actinac, 28
Acupan, 2, 14 (urine pink)
Acyclovir susp and tabs, 9
Adalat caps, 21, C, see BNF
Adalat LA, 25
Adalat Retard, 21, 25
Adcortyl external preps, 28
Adcortyl with Graneodin, 28
Adifax, 2
Adizem preps, 25
AeroBec, 8, C, dose
AeroBec Forte, 8, 10 steroid card,
    C, dose
Aerocrom, 8
Akineton, 2
Albendazole, 9
Alclometasone external preps, 28
Aldomet, 3, 8
Alfuzosin, 3, C, dose
Algitec, C, chew thoroughly
Alimix, C, administration
Allegron, 2
Allopurinol, 8, 21, 27
Alphodith, 10 patient information
    leaflet, 28
Alphosyl HC, 28
Aloxiprin, 12, 21
Alphaderm, 28
Alprazolam, 2
Alrheumat, 21
Alvedon, 30
Alvercol, 25, 27, C, administration,
    see BNF
Amantadine, C, driving
Ambaxin, 9
Aminophylline m/r, see preps
Amiodarone, 11
Amitriptyline, 2
Amitriptyline m/r, 2, 25
Amorolfine, 10 patient information
    leaflet
Amoxapine, 2
Amoxil, 9
*Amoxil dispersible tabs and
    sachets*, 9, 13
Amoxil Fiztab, 9, 10 patient
    information leaflet
Amoxil paed susp, 9, C, use of
    pipette
Amoxycillin, 9
Amoxycillin chewable tabs, 9, 10
    patient information leaflet
Amoxycillin dispersible tabs and
    sachets, 9, 13
Amphotericin loz, 9, 24, C, after food
Amphotericin mixt (g.i.), 9, C, use
    of pipette
Amphotericin mixt (mouth), 9, C,
    use of pipette, hold in mouth, after
    food
Amphotericin tabs, 9
Ampicillin, 9, 23
Ampiclox, 9, 23
Ampiclox Neonatal, 9, C, use of
    pipette
Amylobarbitone, 19
Amytal, 19

Anafranil, 2
Anafranil m/r, 2, 25
Androcur, 2, 21
Angettes-75, 32
Anhydrol Forte, 15
Anquil, 2
Antabuse, 2, C, alcohol reaction,
    see BNF
Antacids, see BNF dosage
    statements
Antepsin, 5, C, administration, see
    BNF
Anthranol preps, 28
Anticoagulants, oral, 10
    anticoagulant card
Antihistamines (see individual
    preparations)
Antipressan, 8
Anturan, 12, 21
Apisate, 25, C, driving
Apsin VK, 9, 23
Arelix, 21
Arpimycin, 9
Arpicolin, C, driving
Artane, C, before or after food,
    driving, see BNF
Arythmol, 21, 25
Arthrotec, 21, 25
Asacol, 5, 25
Ascorbic acid, effervescent, 13
Ascorbic acid tabs (500mg), 24
Asendis, 2
Aspav, 2, 13, 21, 32
Aspirin and papaveretum
    dispersible tabs, 2, 13, 21, also 32
    (if 'aspirin' not on label)
Aspirin dispersible tabs, 13, 21, also
    32 (if 'aspirin' not on label)
Aspirin effervescent, 13, also 32 (if
    'aspirin' not on label)
Aspirin e/c, 5, 25, also 32 (if 'aspirin'
    not on label)
Aspirin m/r, 25, also 32 (if 'aspirin'
    not on label)
Aspirin supps, 32 (if 'aspirin' not on
    label)
Aspirin tabs, 21, also 32 (if 'aspirin'
    not on label)
Aspirin, paracetamol and codeine
    tabs, 21, 29, also 31 (if 'aspirin'
    and 'paracetamol' not on label)
Astemizole, C, driving, alcohol, see
    BNF
Atarax, 2
Atenolol, 8
Ativan, 2 or 19
Atromid-S, 21
Augmentin, 9
Augmentin dispersible tabs, 9, 13
Auranofin, 21
Aureocort, 28
Aventyl, 2
Avloclor, 5, C, malaria prophylaxis,
    see BNF
Avomine, 2
Azapropazone, 11, 21, C, photo-
    sensitivity, see BNF
Azatadine, 2
Azathioprine, 21
Azithromycin, 5, 9, 23

Bacampicillin, 9
Baclofen, 2, 8
Bactrim, 9
Bactrim dispersible tabs, 9, 13
Baratol, 21
Baxan, 9
Becloforte preps, 8, 10 steroid card,
    C, dose
Beclomethasone external preps, 28

Beclomethasone inhalations, 8, 10
    steroid card (high-dose
    preparations only), C, dose
Becodisks, 8, C, dose
Becotide preps, 8, C, dose
Bedranol S.R., 8, 25
Bendogen, 21
Benemid, 12, 21, 27
Benoral susp and tabs, 21, 31
Benoral gran, 13, 21, 31
Benorylate, 21, 31
Benorylate gran, 13, 21, 31
Benperidol, 2
Benzhexol, C, before or after food,
    driving, see BNF
Benztropine, 2
Benzoin tincture, cpd, 15
Berkolol, 8
Beta-Adalat, 8, 25
Beta-Cardone, 8
Betahistine, 21
Betaloc, 8
Betaloc-SA, 8, 25
Betamethasone inj, 10 steroid card
Betamethasone tab, 10 steroid card,
    21
Betamethasone external preps, 28
Betamethasone scalp application,
    15, 28
Betaxolol tabs, 8
Bethanechol, 22
Bethanidine, 21
Betim, 8
Betnelan, 10 steroid card, 21
Betnesol injection, 10 steroid card
Betnesol tabs, 10 steroid card, 13,
    21
Betnovate external preps, 28
Betnovate scalp application, 15, 28
Betnovate-RD, 28
Bezafibrate, 21
Bezalip, 21
Bezalip-Mono, 21, 25
Biorphen, C, driving
Biperiden, 2
Bisacodyl tabs, 5, 25
Bisoprolol, 8
Blocadren, 8
Bolvidon, 2, 25
Bonefos, C, food and calcium, see
    BNF
Bradilan, 5, 25
Bricanyl SA, 25
Britiazim, 25
Britlofex, 2
Brocadopa, 14 (urine reddish), 21
Broflex, C, before or after food,
    driving, see BNF
Bromazepam, 2
Bromocriptine, 21, C, hypotensive
    reactions
Brompheniramine, 2
Brufen, 21
Brufen gran, 13, 21
Brufen Retard, 25, 27
Buccastem, 2, C, administration,
    see BNF
Budesonide external preps, 28
Budesonide inhalations, 8, 10
    steroid card (high-dose
    preparations only), C, dose
Buprenorphine, 2, 26
Burinex K, 25, 27, C, posture, see
    BNF
Buserelin nasal spray, C, nasal
    decongestants, see BNF
Buspar, C, driving
Buspirone, C, driving
Butacote, 5, 21, 25
Butobarbitone, 19

Dental Practitioners' Formulary

List of Dental Preparations

The following list has been approved by the appropriate Secretaries of State, and the preparations therein may be prescribed by dental practitioners on form FP14 (GP14 in Scotland).

Sugar-free versions, where available, are preferred.

Acyclovir Cream, BP
Acyclovir Oral Suspension, BP
Acyclovir Tablets 200 mg, BP
Amoxycillin Capsules, BP
Amoxycillin Oral Powder, DPF
Amoxycillin Oral Suspension, BP
Amoxycillin Tablets, Dispersible, DPF
Amphotericin Lozenges, BP
Amphotericin Oral Suspension, DPF
Ampicillin Capsules, BP
Ampicillin Oral Suspension, BP
Artificial Saliva, DPF
Ascorbic Acid Tablets, BP
Aspirin Tablets, Dispersible, BP[1]
Benzydamine Mouthwash, DPF
Benzydamine Oral Spray, DPF
Carbamazepine Tablets, BP
Carmellose Gelatin Paste, DPF
Cephalexin Capsules, BP
Cephalexin Oral Suspension, DPF
Cephalexin Tablets, BP
Cephradine Capsules, BP
Cephradine Oral Solution, DPF
Chlorhexidine Gluconate gels containing at least 1%
Chlorhexidine Mouthwash, DPF
Chlorhexidine Oral Spray, DPF
Chlorpheniramine Tablets, BP
Choline Salicylate Dental Gel, BP
Clindamycin Capsules, BP
Clindamycin Oral Suspension, Paediatric, DPF
Diazepam Oral Solution, BP
Diazepam Tablets, BP
Diflunisal Tablets, BP
Dihydrocodeine Tablets 30 mg, BP
Doxycycline Capsules 100 mg, BP
Ephedrine Nasal Drops, BP
Erythromycin Ethyl Succinate Oral Suspension, DPF
Erythromycin Ethyl Succinate Oral Suspension, Paediatric, DPF
Erythromycin Ethyl Succinate Tablets, DPF
Erythromycin Stearate Tablets, BP

Preparations in this list which are not included in the BP or BPC are described on next page

Erythromycin Tablets, BP
Fluconazole Capsules 50 mg, DPF
Fluconazole Oral Suspension 50 mg/5 mL, DPF
Hydrocortisone Cream 1%, BP
Hydrocortisone Lozenges, BPC
Hydrocortisone and Miconazole Cream, DPF
Hydrocortisone and Miconazole Ointment, DPF
Hydrogen Peroxide Mouthwash, DPF
Ibuprofen Oral Suspension, DPF[2]
Ibuprofen Tablets, BP
Lignocaine 5% Ointment, DPF
Menthol and Eucalyptus Inhalation, BP 1980[3]
Metronidazole Oral Suspension, DPF
Metronidazole Tablets, BP
Miconazole Oral Gel, DPF
Mouthwash Solution-tablets, DPF
Nitrazepam Tablets, BP
Nystatin Ointment, BP
Nystatin Oral Suspension, BP
Nystatin Pastilles, DPF
Oxytetracycline Capsules, BP
Oxytetracycline Tablets, BP
Paracetamol Oral Suspension 120 mg/5 mL, BP[4]
Paracetamol Tablets, BP
Paracetamol Tablets, Dispersible, DPF
Pethidine Tablets, BP
Phenoxymethylpenicillin Oral Solution, BP
Phenoxymethylpenicillin Tablets, BP
Povidone-iodine Mouthwash, DPF
Probenecid Tablets, BP
Promethazine Hydrochloride Tablets, BP
Promethazine Oral Solution, BP
Sodium Chloride Mouthwash, Compound, BP
Sodium Fluoride Oral Drops, DPF
Sodium Fluoride Tablets, DPF
Sodium Fusidate Ointment, BP
Sodium Perborate Mouthwash, DPF
Temazepam Capsules, DPF
Temazepam Oral Solution, BP
Temazepam Tablets, DPF
Tetracycline Capsules, BP
Tetracycline Tablets, BP
Thymol Glycerin, Compound, BP 1988[5]
Triamcinolone Dental Paste, BP
Vitamin B Tablets, Compound, Strong, BPC
Zinc Sulphate Mouthwash, DPF

---

1. BP 1993 has directed that when soluble aspirin tablets are prescribed, dispersible aspirin tablets should be dispensed
2. Ibuprofen Oral Suspension DPF is sugar free
3. This preparation does not appear in BP 1988
4. BP 1993 directs that when Paediatric Paracetamol Oral Suspension or Paediatric Paracetamol Mixture is prescribed and no strength stated Paracetamol Oral Suspension 120 mg/5 mL should be dispensed
5. This preparation does not appear in BP 1993

Details of DPF preparations

Preparations on the List of Dental Preparations which are not included in the BP or BPC are described as follows in the DPF.

Although brand names have sometimes been included for identification purposes preparations on the list should be prescribed by non-proprietary name.

PoM **Amoxycillin Oral Powder** (proprietary products: *Amoxil Sachets SF*), amoxycillin 750 mg and 3 g (as trihydrate)

PoM **Amoxycillin Tablets Dispersible** (proprietary products: *Amoxil Dispersible Tablets*, amoxycillin 500 mg (as trihydrate); *Flemoxin Solutab*, amoxycillin 375 mg and 750 mg (as trihydrate))

PoM **Amphotericin Oral Suspension** (proprietary product: *Fungilin Suspension*), amphotericin 100 mg/mL

Artificial Saliva, consists of sorbitol 1.8 g, carmellose sodium (sodium carboxymethylcellulose) 390 mg, dibasic potassium phosphate 48.23 mg, potassium chloride 37.5 mg, monobasic potassium phosphate 21.97 mg, calcium chloride 9.972 mg, magnesium chloride 3.528 mg, sodium fluoride 258 micrograms/60 mL, with preservatives and colouring agents (proprietary product: *Luborant*)

Benzydamine Mouthwash (proprietary product: *Difflam Oral Rinse*), benzydamine hydrochloride 0.15%

Benzydamine Oral Spray (proprietary product: *Difflam Spray*), benzydamine hydrochloride 0.15%

Carmellose Gelatin Paste (proprietary product: *Orabase Paste*), gelatin, pectin, carmellose sodium, 16.58% of each in a suitable basis

PoM **Cephalexin Oral Suspension**, cephalexin 125 mg and 250 mg/5 mL (may be powder for reconstitution or ready prepared)

PoM **Cephradine Oral Solution** (proprietary product: *Velosef Syrup*), cephradine 250 mg/5mL when reconstituted with water

Chlorhexidine Gel (proprietary product: *Corsodyl Dental Gel*), chlorhexidine gluconate 1%

Chlorhexidine Mouthwash (proprietary product: *Corsodyl Mouthwash*), chlorhexidine gluconate 0.2%

Chlorhexidine Oral Spray (proprietary product: *Corsodyl Spray*), chlorhexidine gluconate 0.2%

PoM **Clindamycin Oral Suspension, Paediatric** (proprietary product: *Dalacin C Paediatric Suspension*), clindamycin 75 mg (as hydrochloride palmitate)/5mL when reconstituted with purified water (freshly boiled and cooled)

PoM **Erythromycin Ethyl Succinate Oral Suspension** (proprietary product: *Erythroped, Erythroped SF, Erythroped Suspension Forte*), erythromycin 250 mg and 500 mg (as ethyl succinate)/5mL when reconstituted with water

PoM **Erythromycin Ethyl Succinate Oral Suspension, Paediatric** (proprietary products: *Erythroped PI, Erythroped PI SF*), erythromycin 125 mg (as ethyl succinate)/5mL when reconstituted with water

PoM **Erythromycin Ethyl Succinate Tablets** (proprietary product: *Erythroped A*), erythromycin ethyl succinate 500 mg

PoM **Fluconazole Capsules 50 mg** (proprietary product: *Diflucan*), fluconazole 50 mg

PoM **Fluconazole Oral suspension 50 mg/50 mL** (proprietary product: *Diflucan*), fluconazole 50 mg/50 mL when reconstituted with water

PoM **Hydrocortisone and Miconazole Cream** (proprietary product: *Daktacort Cream*), hydrocortisone 1%, miconazole nitrate 2%

PoM **Hydrocortisone and Miconazole Ointment** (proprietary product: *Daktacort Ointment*), hydrocortisone 1%, miconazole nitrate 2%

Hydrogen Peroxide Mouthwash consists of hydrogen peroxide solution 6% (≡ approx. 20 volumes), BP

PoM[1] **Ibuprofen Oral Suspension** (proprietary product: *Junifen Sugar Free*), ibuprofen 100 mg/5mL

1. For exemption, see p. 183.

Lignocaine 5% Ointment, lignocaine 5% in a suitable basis

PoM **Metronidazole Oral Suspension** (proprietary product: *Flagyl S*), metronidazole 200 mg (as benzoate)/5mL

Miconazole Oral Gel (proprietary product: *Daktarin Oral Gel*), miconazole 25 mg/mL

Mouthwash Solution-tablets, consist of tablets which may contain antimicrobial, colouring and flavouring agents in a suitable soluble effervescent basis to make a mouthwash suitable for dental purposes

PoM **Nystatin Pastilles** (proprietary product: *Nystan Pastilles*), nystatin 100 000 units

Paracetamol Tablets, Dispersible (proprietary product: *Panadol Soluble*), paracetamol 500 mg in an effervescent basis

Povidone-iodine Mouthwash (proprietary product: *Betadine Mouthwash*), povidone-iodine 1%

Sodium Fluoride Oral Drops, see section 9.5.3

Sodium Fluoride Tablets, see section 9.5.3

Sodium Perborate Mouthwash (proprietary product: *Bocasan Mouthwash*), sodium perborate 68.6%

PoM **Temazepam Capsules**, temazepam 10, 15, 20 and 30 mg

Note. Temazepam Capsules DPF are soft gelatin capsules

PoM **Temazepam Tablets**, temazepam 10 and 20 mg

Zinc Sulphate Mouthwash, consists of zinc sulphate lotion, BP. Directions for use: dilute 1 part with 4 parts of warm water

Note. May be difficult to obtain

Nurse Prescribers' List

Appendix NPF. List of preparations approved by the Secretary of State which may be prescribed on forms FP10(CN) and FP10(PN) by Nurses for National Health Service patients

Preparations on this list which are not included in the BP or BPC are described on p. 614

Medicinal preparations

Aqueous Cream, BP
Arachis Oil Enema, NPF
Aspirin Tablets, Dispersible, 300 mg, BP
Bisacodyl Suppositories, BP (includes 5-mg and 10-mg strengths)
Bisacodyl Tablets, BP
Calamine Cream, Aqueous, BP
Calamine Lotion, BP
Calamine Lotion, Oily, BP 1980
Carbaryl alcoholic lotions containing at least 0.5%
Carbaryl aqueous lotions containing at least 0.5%
Carbaryl shampoos containing at least 0.5%
Catheter Maintenance Solution, Chlorhexidine, NPF
Catheter Maintenance Solution, Mandelic Acid, NPF
Catheter Maintenance Solution, Sodium Chloride, NPF
Catheter Maintenance Solution, 'Solution G', NPF
Catheter Maintenance Solution, 'Solution R', NPF
Clotrimazole Cream 1%, BP
[1]Dextranomer Beads, NPF
[1]Dextranomer Paste, NPF
Dimethicone barrier creams containing at least 10%
Docusate Capsules, NPF
Docusate Enema, NPF
Docusate Enema, Compound, NPF
Docusate Oral Solution, NPF
Docusate Oral Solution, Paediatric, NPF
Emulsifying Ointment, BP
Glycerol Suppositories, BP
Hydrous Ointment, BP
Ispaghula Husk Granules, Effervescent, NPF
Ispaghula Husk Powder, Effervescent, NPF
Lactulose Solution, BP
Lignocaine Gel, BP
Lignocaine Ointment, NPF

Lignocaine and Chlorhexidine Gel, BP
Lindane Lotion, NPF
Lindane Shampoo, NPF
Magnesium Hydroxide Mixture, BP
Magnesium Sulphate Paste, BP
Malathion alcoholic lotions containing at least 0.5%
Malathion aqueous lotions containing at least 0.5%
Malathion shampoos containing at least 1%
Mebendazole Tablets, NPF sufficient to order on one prescription enough for a 100-mg dose for the oral treatment of enterobiasis in an adult or child over 2 years of age followed if necessary by a second 100-mg dose two weeks later
Miconazole Oral Gel, 15-g tube, DPF
Paracetamol Oral Suspension, BP (includes 120 mg/5 mL and 250 mg/5 mL strengths—both of which are available as sugar-free formulations)
Paracetamol Tablets, BP
Paracetamol Tablets, Soluble, NPF
Permethrin Cream, NPF
Permethrin Cream Rinse, NPF
Phenothrin Alcoholic Lotion, NPF
Phosphates Enema (Formula B), BP
Piperazine Citrate Elixir, BP
Piperazine and Senna Powder, NPF
Povidone–Iodine Aqueous Solution, NPF
Senna Granules, Standardised, BP
Senna Oral Solution, NPF
Senna Tablets, BP
Senna and Ispaghula Granules, NPF
Sodium Chloride Solution, Sterile, BP
Sodium Citrate Compound Enema, NPF
Sterculia Granules, NPF
Sterculia and Frangula Granules, NPF
Thymol Glycerin, Compound, BP 1988
Titanium Ointment, NPF
Zinc and Castor Oil Ointment, BP

1. Dextranomer Paste Pad Dressings, included as appliance in Part IXA of the Drug Tariff, are also prescribable

This list is currently only for the purposes of the **Nurse Prescribing demonstration scheme** which will operate in eight General Practitioner (GP) Fundholding practices and will involve nurses with a District Nurse (DN) or Health Visitor (HV) qualification. It constitutes an appendix to the BNF and as such is termed **'appendix NPF'**

Appliances and Reagents (including Wound Management Products)

Chemical Reagents

The following as listed in Part IXR of the Drug Tariff:

  Detection Tablets for Glycosuria
  Detection Tablets for Ketonuria
  Detection Strips for Glycosuria
  Detection Strips for Ketonuria
  Detection Strips for Proteinuria
  Detection Strips for Blood Glucose

Fertility (Ovulation) Thermometer as listed in Part IXA of the Drug Tariff

Film Gloves, Disposable, EMA as listed in Part IXA of the Drug Tariff

Elastic Hosiery including accessories as listed in Part IXA of the Drug Tariff

Hypodermic Equipment

The following as listed in Part IXA of the Drug Tariff:

  Hypodermic Syringes—U100 Insulin
  Hypodermic Syringe Carrying Case
  Screw cap to convert Hypodermic Syringe Carrying Case for use with Pre-set U100 Insulin Syringe
  Hypodermic Syringe—Single Use or Single-patient Use, U100 Insulin with Needle
  Hypodermic Needles—Sterile, Single-use
  Lancets—Sterile, Single-use
  Needle Clipping Device

Incontinence Appliances as listed in Part IXB of the Drug Tariff

Pessaries, Ring as listed in Part IXA of the Drug Tariff

Stoma Appliances and Associated Products as listed in Part IXC of the Drug Tariff

Urethral Catheters as listed in Part IXA of the Drug Tariff

Urine Sugar Analysis Equipment as listed in Part IXA of the Drug Tariff

Wound Management and Related Products

(including bandages, dressings, gauzes, lint, stockinette, etc)

The following as listed in Part IXA of the Drug Tariff:

  Absorbent Cottons
  Absorbent Cotton Gauzes
  Absorbent Cotton and Viscose Ribbon Gauze, BP 1988
  Absorbent Lint, BPC
  Arm Slings
  Cellulose Wadding, BP 1988
  Cotton Conforming Bandage, BP 1988
  Cotton Crêpe Bandage, BP 1988
  Crêpe Bandage, BP 1988
  Elastic Adhesive Bandage, BP
  Elastic Web Bandages
  Gauze and Cellulose Wadding Tissue, BP 1988
  Gauze and Cotton Tissues
  Heavy Cotton and Rubber Elastic Bandage, BP
  High Compression Bandages (Extensible)
  Knitted Polyamide and Cellulose Contour Bandage, BP 1988
  Knitted Viscose Primary Dressing, BP, Type 1
  Multiple Pack Dressing No. 1
  Multiple Pack Dressing No. 2
  Open-wove Bandage, BP 1988, Type 1
  Paraffin Gauze Dressing, BP
  Perforated Film Absorbent Dressing
  Polyamide and Cellulose Contour Bandage, BP 1988
  Povidone–Iodine Fabric Dressing, Sterile
  Skin Closure Strips, Sterile
  Sterile Dressing Packs
  Stockinettes
  Surgical Adhesive Tapes
  Suspensory Bandages, Cotton
  Swabs
  Titanium Dioxide Elastic Adhesive Bandage, BP
  Triangular Calico Bandage, BP 1980
  Vapour-permeable Adhesive Film Dressing, BP
  Vapour-permeable Waterproof Plastic Wound Dressing, BP, Sterile
  Wound Management Dressings (including gel, colloid and foam)
  Zinc Paste Bandages (including both plain and with additional ingredients)

In the Drug Tariff Appliances and Reagents which may **not** be prescribed by Nurses are annotated Ⓝ

This list is currently **only** for the purposes of the **Nurse Prescribing demonstration scheme** which will operate in eight General Practitioner (GP) Fundholding practices and will involve nurses with a District Nurse (DN) or Health Visitor (HV) qualification.

Details of NPF preparations

Preparations on the Nurse Prescribers' List which are not included in the BP or BPC are described as follows in the pilot edition of the Nurse Prescribers' Formulary which has been produced for the Nurse Prescribing demonstration scheme.

Although brand names have sometimes been included for identification purposes preparations on the list should be prescribed by non-proprietary name.

Arachis Oil Enema, (proprietary product: *Fletchers' Arachis Oil Retention Enema*), arachis oil

Carbaryl alcoholic lotions, (proprietary products: *Carylderm Lotion*; *Suleo-C Lotion*), carbaryl 0.5% in an alcoholic basis

Carbaryl aqueous lotions, (proprietary products: *Clinicide Lotion*, carbaryl 0.5%; *Derbac C Liquid*, carbaryl 1%), carbaryl 0.5-1% in an aqueous basis

Carbaryl shampoos, (proprietary products: *Carylderm Shampoo*, carbaryl 1%; *Derbac C Shampoo*, carbaryl 0.5%; *Suleo-C Shampoo*, carbaryl 0.5%), carbaryl 0.5-1% in a shampoo basis

Catheter Maintenance Solution, Chlorhexidine, (proprietary products: *Uro-Tainer Chlorhexidine*; *Uriflex C*), chlorhexidine 0.02%

Catheter Maintenance Solution, Mandelic Acid, (proprietary product: *Uro-Tainer Mandelic Acid*), mandelic acid 1%

Catheter Maintenance Solution, Sodium Chloride, (proprietary products: *Uro-Tainer Sodium Chloride*; *Uriflex-S*), sodium chloride 0.9%

Catheter Maintenance Solution, 'Solution G', (proprietary products: *Uro-Tainer Suby G*, *Uriflex G*), citric acid 3.23%, magnesium oxide 0.38%, sodium bicarbonate 0.7%, disodium edetate 0.01%

Catheter Maintenance Solution, 'Solution R', (proprietary products: *Uro-Tainer Solution R*, *Uriflex R*), citric acid 6%, gluconolactone 0.6%, magnesium carbonate 2.8%, disodium edetate 0.01%

Dextranomer Beads, (proprietary product: *Debrisan Beads*), dextranomer

Dextranomer Paste, (proprietary product: *Debrisan Paste*), dextranomer in a soft paste basis

Dimethicone barrier creams, (proprietary products: *Conotrane Cream*, dimethicone '350' 22%; *Savlon Nappy Rash Cream*, dimethicone '1000' 10%; *Siopel Barrier Cream*, dimethicone '1000' 10%; *Vasogen Barrier Cream*, dimethicone 20%), dimethicone 10-22%

Docusate Capsules, (proprietary product: *Dioctyl Capsules*), docusate sodium 100 mg

Docusate Enema, (proprietary product: *Norgalax Micro-enema*) docusate sodium 120 mg in 10 g

Docusate Enema, Compound, (proprietary product: *Fletchers' Enemette*), docusate sodium 90 mg, glycerol 3.78g/5 mL with macragol and sorbic acid

Docusate Oral Solution, (proprietary product: *Dioctyl Oral Solution*), docusate sodium 50 mg/5 mL

Docusate Oral Solution, Paediatric, (proprietary product: *Dioctyl Paediatric Oral Solution*), docusate sodium 12.5 mg/5 mL

Ispaghula Husk Granules, Effervescent, (proprietary product: *Fybogel Granules*), ispaghula husk 3.5g/sachet

Ispaghula Husk Powder, Effervescent, (proprietary product: *Regulan Powder*), ispaghula husk 3.6 g/6.4-g sachet

Lignocaine Ointment, (proprietary product: *Xylocaine Ointment*), lignocaine 5%

Lindane Lotion, (proprietary product: *Quellada Lotion*), lindane 1%

Lindane Shampoo, (proprietary product: *Quellada Application PC*), lindane 1%

Malathion alcoholic lotions, (proprietary products: *Prioderm Lotion*; *Suleo-M Lotion*), malathion 0.5% in an alcoholic basis

Malathion aqueous lotions, (proprietary product: *Derbac-M Lotion*), malathion 0.5% in an aqueous basis

Malathion shampoos, (proprietary product: *Prioderm Cream Shampoo*), malathion 1% in a shampoo basis

Mebendazole Tablets, (proprietary product: *Ovex Tablets*), mebendazole 100 mg

Paracetamol Tablets, Soluble, (proprietary product: *Panadol Soluble*), paracetamol 500 mg in an effervescent basis

Permethrin Cream, (proprietary product: *Lyclear Dermal Cream*), permethrin 5%

Permethrin Cream Rinse, (proprietary product: *Lyclear Cream Rinse*), permethrin 1%

Phenothrin Alcoholic Lotion, (proprietary product: *Full Marks Lotion*), phenothrin 0.2% in a basis containing isopropyl alcohol

Piperazine and Senna Powder, (proprietary product: *Pripsen Oral Powder*), piperazine phosphate 4 g, sennosides 15.3 mg/sachet

Povidone–Iodine Aqueous Solution, (proprietary product: *Betadine Antiseptic Solution*), povidone–iodine 10%

Senna Oral Solution, (proprietary product: *Senokot Syrup*), sennosides 7.5 mg/5 mL

Senna and Ispaghula Granules, (proprietary product: *Manevac Granules*), senna fruit 12.4%, ispaghula 54.2%

Sodium Citrate Compound Enema, (proprietary products: *Micolette Micro-enema*; *Micralax Micro-enema*; *Relaxit Micro-enema*), sodium citrate 450 mg with glycerol, sorbitol and an anionic surfactant

Sterculia Granules, (proprietary product: *Normacol Granules*), sterculia 62%

Sterculia and Frangula Granules, (proprietary product: *Normacol Plus Granules*), sterculia 62%, frangula (standardised) 8%

Titanium Ointment, (proprietary product: *Metanium Ointment*), titanium dioxide 20%, titanium peroxide 5%, titanium salicylate 3%, titanium tannate 0.1%

Index of Manufacturers

Hospital manufacturing units—see p 624

Abbott
Abbott Laboratories Ltd,
Abbott House, Norden Rd,
Maidenhead, Berks SL6 4XE.
(0628) 773355

A&H
Allen & Hanburys Ltd,
Stockley Park West, Uxbridge,
Middx UB11 1BT.
081-990 3001

Alcon
Alcon Laboratories (UK) Ltd,
Imperial Way, Watford, Herts
WD2 4YR.
(0923) 246133

Alembic Products
Alembic Products Ltd,
Unit 4, Brymau 2 Estate,
River Lane, Saltney,
Chester, Cheshire CH4 8RQ.
(0244) 680147

Allerayde
Allerayde,
Queens Head Court,
42 Kirk Gate, Newark,
Notts NG24 1AB.
(0636) 613444

Allergan
Allergan Ltd,
Coronation Rd, High
Wycombe, Bucks HP12 3SH.
(0494) 444722

Alpha
Alpha Therapeutic UK Ltd,
Howlett Way, Fison Way
Industrial Estate, Thetford,
Norfolk IP24 1HZ.
(0842) 764260

Amgen
Amgen Ltd,
240 Cambridge Science Park,
Milton Rd, Cambridge
CB4 4WD.
(0223) 420305

Antigen
Antigen Pharmaceuticals Ltd,
Trafalgar House,
Union St, Southport,
Merseyside PR9 0QS.
(0704) 545608

APS
Approved Prescription Services
Ltd,
see Berk.

Armour
Armour Pharmaceutical Co. Ltd,
RPR House,
52 St. Leonards Rd,
Eastbourne, East Sussex
BN21 3YG.
(0323) 410200

Ashbourne
Ashbourne Pharmaceuticals Ltd,
Victors Barns, Hill Farm,
Brixworth, Northampton
NN6 9DQ.
(0604) 882190

ASTA Medica
ASTA Medica Ltd,
168 Cowley Rd, Cambridge
CB4 4DL.
(0223) 423434

Astra
Astra Pharmaceuticals Ltd,
Home Park Estate,
Kings Langley,
Herts WD4 8DH.
(0923) 266191

Astra Tech
Astra Tech Ltd,
PO Box 13, Stroud, Glos
GL5 3DL.
(0453) 791763

Aurum
Aurum Pharmaceuticals Ltd
48 High Street, Billingshurst,
West Sussex RH14 9NY.
(0403) 786781

Bailey, Robert
Robert Bailey & Son plc,
Dysart St, Great Moor,
Stockport, Cheshire
SK2 7PF.
061-483 1133

Baker Norton
Division of Norton Healthcare
see Norton.

Bard
C. R. Bard International Ltd,
Forest House, Brighton Rd,
Crawley, West Sussex
RH11 9BP.
(0293) 27888

Baxter
Baxter Healthcare Ltd,
Caxton Way, Thetford, Norfolk
IP24 3SE.
(0842) 767000

Bayer
Bayer plc,
Pharmaceutical Business
Group, Bayer House,
Strawberry Hill, Newbury,
Berks RG13 1JA.
(0635) 39000

Bayer Diagnostics
Bayer Diagnostics,
Ames Technicon, Evans House,
Hamilton Close, Houndmills,
Basingstoke,
Hants RG21 2YE.
(0256) 29181

Baypharm
see Bayer.

Becton Dickinson
Becton Dickinson UK Ltd,
Between Towns Rd,
Cowley, Oxford,
Oxon OX4 3LY.
(0865) 748844

Beecham
Beecham Research,
see SmithKline Beecham.

Beecham Products
see SmithKline Beecham
Healthcare.

Beiersdorf
Beiersdorf UK Ltd,
Yeomans Drive, Blakelands,
Milton Keynes,
Bucks MK14 5LS.
(0908) 211444

Bell and Croyden
John Bell and Croyden,
54 Wigmore St, London
W1H 0AU.
071-935 5555

Bencard
see SmithKline Beecham.

Bengué
Bengué & Co. Ltd.
see Syntex.

Berk
Berk Pharmaceuticals,
Brampton Rd, Hampden Park,
Eastbourne, East Sussex
BN22 9AG.
(0323) 501111

Beta
Beta Medical Products Ltd,
Valley Lodge, Bakewell Rd,
Matlock, Derbyshire
DE4 3BN.
(0629) 582198

BHR
BHR Pharmaceuticals Ltd,
41 Centenary Business Centre,
Hammond Close,
Attleborough Fields, Nuneaton,
Warwickshire CV11 6RY.
(0203) 353742

Bio Diagnostics
Bio Diagnostics Ltd,
Upton Industrial Estate,
Rectory Rd, Upton-upon-
Severn, Worcs WR8 0XL.
(0684) 592262

Biocare
Biocare International Inc.
Belvoir House, Chapel St,
Haconby, Lincs
PE10 0UP.
(0778) 570441

Bioglan

Bioglan Laboratories Ltd,
1 The Cam Centre,
Wilbury Way, Hitchin,
Herts SG4 0TW.
(0462) 438444

Bio-Medical

Bio-Medical Services,
BMS Laboratories Ltd,
River View Rd, Beverley,
North Humberside HU17 0LD.
(0482) 860228

Biorex

Biorex Laboratories Ltd,
2 Crossfield Chambers,
Gladbeck Way, Enfield, Middx
EN2 7HT. 081-366 9301

Biotest

Biotest (UK) Ltd,
Unit 21A Monkspath Business
Park, Highlands Rd, Shirley,
Solihull, West Midlands
B90 4NZ.
021-733 3393

Blake

Thomas Blake & Co,
The Byre House, Fearby,
Nr. Masham, North Yorkshire
HG4 4NF.
(0765) 689042

BM Diagnostics

Boehringer Mannheim
(Diagnostics & Biochemicals)
Ltd,
Bell Lane, Lewes, East Sussex
BN7 1LG.
(0273) 480444

Body's Care

Body's Care Centre Ltd,
631 London Rd,
Westcliffe-on-Sea, Essex
SS0 9PE.
(0702) 337339

Boehringer Ingelheim

Boehringer Ingelheim Ltd,
Ellesfield Ave, Bracknell, Berks
RG12 4YS.
(0344) 424600

Boehringer Mannheim

Boehringer Mannheim UK
(Pharmaceuticals) Ltd,
Simpson Parkway, Kirkton
Campus, Livingston, West
Lothian EH54 7BH.
(0506) 412512

Boots

The Boots Co. plc,
1 Thane Rd West, Nottingham
NG2 3AA.
(0602) 492900

BPL

Bio Products Laboratory,
Dagger Lane, Elstree, Herts
WD6 3BX.
081-905 1818

Braun

B. Braun (Medical) Ltd,
Braun House, 13–14
Farmbrough Close, Aylesbury
Vale Industrial Park, Aylesbury,
Bucks
HP20 1DQ.
(0296) 393900

Brevet

Brevet Hospital Products,
Unit 17, Barncoose Industrial
Estate, Wilson Way,
Redruth, Cornwall TR15 3RQ.
(0209) 219097

Bristol-Myers

Bristol-Myers Squibb
Pharmaceuticals Ltd,
141–149 Staines Rd, Hounslow,
Middx TW3 3JA.
081-572 7422

Britannia

Britannia Pharmaceuticals Ltd,
Forum House, 41–75 Brighton
Rd, Redhill, Surrey RH1 6YS.
(0737) 773741

BritCair

BritCair Ltd,
Division of CV Laboratories
Ltd,
Gordon House, Gordon Rd,
Aldershot, Hants GU11 1LD.
(0252) 333314

David Bull

David Bull Laboratories,
Spartan Close, Tachbrook Park,
Warwick CV34 6RS.
(0926) 451515

Bullen

C. S. Bullen Ltd,
3–7 Moss St, Liverpool L6 1EY.
051-207 6995

Bullen & Smears

Bullen & Smears Ltd,
99 Kempston St, Liverpool
L3 8HE.
051-207 1239

Burgess

Edwin Burgess Ltd,
see Leo.

Cabot

see Solco Basle.

Cambmac

Cambmac Instruments Ltd,
Pembroke Ave, Waterbeach,
Cambridge CB5 9PY.
(0223) 441144

Cambridge

Cambridge Laboratories,
Richmond House,
Old Brewery Court,
Sandyford Rd,
Newcastle upon Tyne NE2 1XG.
091-261 5950

Camp

Camp Ltd,
Northgate House,
Staple Gardens, Winchester,
Hants SO23 8ST.
(0962) 855248

Cantassium

The Cantassium Company,
Larkhall Laboratories,
225 Putney Bridge Rd,
London SW15 2PY.
081-874 1130

Chancellor

Chancellor Group Ltd,
see Consolidated.

Charwell

Charwell Pharmaceuticals Ltd,
Charwell House, Wilsom Rd,
Alton, Hants GU34 2TJ.
(0420) 84801

Chefaro

Chefaro Proprietaries Ltd,
see Organon.
(0223) 420956

Chugai

Chugai Pharma UK Ltd,
Mulliner House, Flanders Rd,
Turnham Green, London
W4 1NN
081-742 0777

Ciba

CIBA Laboratories,
Wimblehurst Rd, Horsham,
West Sussex RH12 4AB.
(0403) 272827

CIBA Vision

CIBA Vision Ophthalmics,
Flanders Rd, Hedge End,
Southampton SO3 3LG.
(0489) 785399

Cilag

Cilag Ltd,
PO Box 79, Saunderton, High
Wycombe, Bucks HP14 4HJ.
(0494) 563541

Cirrus

Cirrus Associates,
Little Hintock,
Kington Magna,
Gillingham, Dorset SP8 5EW.
(0747) 838165

Clement Clarke

Clement Clarke International
Ltd,
Airmed House, Edinburgh Way,
Harlow, Essex CM20 2ED.
(0279) 414969

CliniFlex

CliniFlex Ltd,
see CliniMed.

CliniMed

CliniMed Ltd,
Cavell House, Knaves Beech
Way, Loudwater, High
Wycombe, Bucks HP10 9QY.
(0628) 850100

Clintec

Clintec Nutrition Ltd,
Shaftesbury Court,
18 Chalvey Park, Slough,
Berks SL1 2HT.
(0753) 550800

Colgate-Palmolive
Colgate-Palmolive Ltd,
Guildford Business Park,
Middleton Rd, Guildford,
Surrey GU2 5LZ.
(0483) 302222

Coloplast
Coloplast Ltd,
Peterborough Business Park,
Peterborough PE2 0FX.
(0733) 239898

Consolidated
Consolidated Chemicals Ltd,
Abbey Rd,
The Industrial Estate,
Wrexham, Clwyd LL13 9PW.
(0978) 661351

ConvaTec
ConvaTec Ltd,
Harrington House, Milton Rd,
Ickenham, Uxbridge, Middx
UB10 8PU.
(0895) 678888

Co-Pharma
Co-Pharma Ltd,
Talbot House, Church St,
Rickmansworth, Herts
WD3 1DE.
(0923) 710934

Cow & Gate
Cow & Gate Nutricia Ltd,
Newmarket Ave,
White Horse Business Park,
Trowbridge, Wilts BA14 0XQ.
(0225) 768381

Cox
A. H. Cox & Co Ltd,
Whiddon Valley, Barnstaple,
Devon EX32 8NS.
(0271) 311257

CP
CP Pharmaceuticals Ltd,
Ash Rd North, Wrexham
Industrial Estate, Wrexham,
Clwyd LL13 9UF.
(0978) 661261

Credenhill
Credenhill Ltd,
10 Cossall Industrial Estate,
Ilkeston, Derbys DE7 5UG.
(0602) 320144

Crookes
Crookes Healthcare Ltd,
PO Box 94, 1 Thane Rd West,
Nottingham NG2 3AA.
(0602) 507431

Cupal
Cupal Ltd,
Pharmaceutical Laboratories,
King St, Blackburn, Lancs
BB2 2DX.
(0254) 580321

Cupharma
Cupharma Ltd,
145B Hughenden Rd, High
Wycombe, Bucks HP13 5PN.
(0494) 522114

Cusi
Cusi (UK) Ltd,
Cusi House, Lion Lane,
Haslemere, Surrey GU27 1JL.
(0428) 661078

Cussons
Cussons (UK) Ltd,
Kersal Vale, Manchester
M7 0GL.
061-792 6111

Cutter
see Bayer.

Cuxson
Cuxson, Gerrard & Co. (IMS)
Ltd,
Oldbury, Warley, West Midlands
B69 3BB.
021-552 1355

Cyanamid
see Lederle.

Daniels
Richard Daniel & Son Ltd,
Mansfield Rd, Derby DE1 3RE.
(0332) 40671

Dansac
Dansac Ltd,
Pembroke Ave, Waterbeach,
Cambridge, CB5 9PY.
(0223) 441144

Davis & Geck
see Lederle.

DDC
DDC (London) Ltd,
158 Notting Hill Gate, London
W11 3GQ.
071-229 4224

DDD
DDD Ltd,
94 Rickmansworth Rd,
Watford, Herts WD1 7JJ.
(0923) 229251

DDSA
DDSA Pharmaceuticals Ltd,
310 Old Brompton Rd, London
SW5 9JQ.
071-373 7884

De Vilbiss
De Vilbiss Health Care UK Ltd,
Airlinks, Spitfire Way, Heston,
Middx TW5 9NR.
081-756 1133

De Witt
E. C. De Witt & Co Ltd,
Tudor Rd, Manor Park,
Runcorn, Cheshire WA7 1SZ.
(0928) 579029

Delandale
Delandale Laboratories Ltd,
see Lorex.

Dental Health
Dental Health Products Ltd,
Broughton House, 33 Earl St,
Maidstone, Kent ME14 1PF.
(0622) 762269

DePuy
DePuy Healthcare,
Millshaw House, Manor Mill
Lane, Leeds LS11 8LQ.
(0532) 706000

Dermal
Dermal Laboratories Ltd,
Tatmore Place, Gosmore,
Hitchin, Herts SG4 7QR.
(0462) 458866

Dermalex
see Sanofi Winthrop.

DF
Duncan, Flockhart & Co Ltd,
Division of Glaxo Laboratories
Ltd
see Glaxo.

Dista
Dista Products Ltd,
see Lilly.

Dow Corning
Dow Corning Ltd,
Kings Court, 185 Kings Rd,
Reading, Berks RG1 4EX.
(0734) 596888

Downs
see Simcare.

Drew
John Drew (London) Ltd,
433 Uxbridge Rd, Ealing,
London W5 3NT.
081-992 0381

Du Pont
Du Pont Pharmaceuticals Ltd,
Avenue One, Letchworth
Garden City, Herts SG6 2HU.
(0462) 482648

Dumex
Dumex Ltd,
Tring Business Centre,
Upper Icknield Way,
Tring, Herts HP23 4JX.
(0442) 890090

Duphar
Duphar Laboratories Ltd,
Gaters Hill, West End,
Southampton SO3 3JD.
(0703) 472281

Durbin
B & S Durbin Ltd,
240 Northolt Rd, South Harrow,
Middx HA2 8DU.
081-422 1303

Dylade
see Fresenius .

Eastern
Eastern Pharmaceuticals Ltd,
Coomb House, 7 St Johns Rd,
Isleworth, Middx TW7 6NA.
081 569 8174

Elan
Elan Pharma Ltd,
see P-D.

Elida Gibbs
Elida Gibbs Ltd,
Coal Rd, Seacroft, Leeds
LS14 2AR.
(0532) 737473

Ellis
Ellis, Son & Paramore Ltd,
Spring Street Works,
Sheffield S3 8PB.
(0742) 738921

EMS
EMS Medical Ltd,
Unit 3, Stroud Industrial Estate,
Oldends Lane, Stonehouse, Glos
GL10 2DG.
(0453) 791791

EuroCetus
EuroCetus UK Ltd,
Salamander Quay West,
Park Lane, Harefield, Middx
UB9 6NY.
(0895) 824087

Euroderma
Euroderma Ltd,
The Old Coach House,
34 Elm Rd, Chessington,
Surrey KT9 1AW.
081-974 2266

Evans
Evans Medical Ltd,
Evans House, Regent Park,
Kingston Rd, Leatherhead,
Surrey KT22 7PQ.
(0372) 364000

Everfresh
Everfresh Natural Foods,
Gatehouse Close, Aylesbury,
Bucks HP19 3DE.
(0296) 25333

Farillon
Farillon Ltd,
Ashton Rd, Harold Hill,
Romford, Essex RM3 8UE.
(0708) 379000

Farley
Farley Health Products Ltd,
Torr Lane, Plymouth PL3 5UA.
(0752) 24151

Farmitalia Carlo Erba
Farmitalia Carlo Erba Ltd,
see Pharmacia

Ferraris
Ferraris Development &
Engineering Co Ltd,
26 Lea Valley Trading Estate,
Angel Rd, Edmonton, London
N18 3JD.
081-807 3636

Ferring
Ferring Pharmaceuticals Ltd,
Greville House, Hatton Rd,
Feltham, Middx TW14 9PX.
081-893 1543

Fisons
Fisons plc,
Pharmaceutical Division,
Coleorton Hall, Ashby Rd,
Coleorton, Coalville, Leics
LE67 8GP.
(0509) 634000

FoodWatch
FoodWatch Health Products Ltd,
Pollards Yard, Wood St,
Taunton, Somerset
TA1 1UP.
(0823) 325023

Forley
Forley Ltd,
54 Hillbury Ave, Harrow,
Middx HA3 8EW.
081-665 9169

Fournier
Fournier Pharmaceuticals Ltd,
19–20 Progress Business
Centre, Whittle Parkway,
Slough SL1 6DQ.
(0628) 660552

Fox
C. H. Fox Ltd,
22 Tavistock St, London
WC2E 7PY
071-240 3111

FP
Family Planning Sales Ltd,
28 Kelburne Rd, Cowley,
Oxford OX4 3SZ.
(0865) 772486

Fresenius
Fresenius Ltd,
6–8 Christleton Court, Stuart
Rd, Manor Park, Runcorn,
Cheshire WA7 1ST.
(0928) 579444

Fry
Fry Surgical International Ltd,
Unit 17, Goldsworth Park
Trading Estate, Woking, Surrey
GU21 3BA.
(0483) 721404

Galderma
Galderma (UK) Ltd,
Leywood House, Woodside Rd,
Amersham, Bucks HP6 6AA.
(0494) 432606

Galen
Galen Ltd,
Seagoe Industrial Estate,
Craigavon, Northern Ireland
BT63 5UA.
(0762) 334974

Garnier
Laboratoires Garnier, Golden
Ltd,
PO Box 5, Pontyclun, Glam
CF7 8XW.
(0443) 237456

Geigy
Geigy Pharmaceuticals,
see Ciba.

Geistlich
Geistlich Sons Ltd,
Newton Bank, Long Lane,
Chester CH2 3QZ.
(0244) 347534

General Designs
General Designs Ltd,
PO Box 38, Kingston, Surrey
KT2 7YP.
081-336 2323

Generics
Generics (UK) Ltd,
12 Station Close, Potters Bar,
Herts EN6 1TL.
(0707) 644556

GF Supplies
see Nutricia.

Glaxo
Glaxo Laboratories Ltd,
Stockley Park West, Uxbridge,
Middx UB11 1BT.
081-990 9444

Glenwood
Glenwood Laboratories Ltd,
Jenkins Dale, Chatham, Kent
ME4 5RD.
(0634) 830535

Gluten Free Foods Ltd
Gluten Free Foods Ltd,
8 Queen Anne St, London
W1M 9LD.
071-255 2446

Goldshield
Goldshield Pharmaceuticals Ltd,
Bensham House, Bensham
Lane, Thornton Heath, Surrey
CR7 7EQ.
081-684 3664

Graseby Medical
Graseby Medical Ltd,
Colonial Way, Watford, Herts
WD2 4LG.
(0923) 246434

Henleys
Henleys Medical Supplies Ltd,
Brownfields, Welwyn Garden
City, Herts AL7 1AN.
(0707) 333164

Hillcross
Hillcross Pharmaceuticals,
Primrose Mill, Harrison St,
Briercliffe, Burnley BB10 2HP.
(0282) 830042

Hoechst
Hoechst UK Ltd,
Pharmaceutical Division,
Hoechst House, Salisbury Rd,
Hounslow, Middx TW4 6JH.
081-570 7712

Hollister
Hollister Ltd,
Rectory Court, 42 Broad St,
Wokingham, Berks RG11 1AB.
(0734) 775545

**Hospital Management &
Supplies**
Hospital Management and
Supplies Ltd,
Salthouse Rd, Brackmills,
Northampton, NN4 7UF.
(0604) 704600

Hough
Hough, Hoseason & Co. Ltd,
22 Chapel St, Levenshulme,
Manchester M19 3PT.
061-224 3271

Hypoguard
Hypoguard Ltd,
Dock Lane, Melton,
Woodbridge, Suffolk IP12 1PE.
(03943) 7333

IATRO
IATRO Medical Systems,
Unit F-15, Lanterns Court,
22 Millharbour, London
E14 9TU.
071-987 7889

Immuno
Immuno Ltd,
Arctic House, Rye Lane, Dunton
Green, Nr Sevenoaks, Kent
TN14 5HB.
(0732) 458101

IMS
International Medication
Systems (UK) Ltd,
Foster Ave,
Woodside Park Estate,
Dunstable,
Beds LU5 5TA.
(0582) 475005

Incare
Incare Medical Products,
see Hollister.

Innovex
Innovex Medical,
see Novex.

Intercare
Intercare Products Ltd,
7 The Business Centre,
Molly Millars Lane,
Wokingham, Berks RG11 2QZ.
(0734) 790345

Invicta
see Pfizer.

Iolab
Iolab,
The Braccans,
London Rd, Bracknell,
Berks RG12 2AT.
(0344) 864070

ISIS
ISIS Products Ltd,
Gough Lane, Bamber Bridge,
Preston, Lancs PR5 6AQ.
(0772) 628311

J&J
Johnson & Johnson Patient Care
Ltd,
Coronation Rd, Ascot, Berks
SL5 9EY.
(0344) 872626

Jackson
Ernest Jackson & Co. Ltd,
Crediton, Devon EX17 3AP.
(03632) 2251

Jacobs
The Jacobs Bakery Ltd,
Suttons Business Park, Earley,
Reading, Berks RG6 1AZ.
(0734) 492000

Janssen
Janssen Pharmaceutical Ltd,
Grove, Wantage, Oxon
OX12 0DQ.
(0235) 777333

JLB
JLB Textiles Ltd,
Unit 2B, St Columb Industrial
Estate, St Columb Major,
Cornwall TR9 6SF.
(0637) 880065

JRJ
JRJ Trading Co,
Unit 4, West Burrowfield,
Welwyn Garden City, Herts
AL7 4TW.
(0707) 390251

K & K-Greeff
K & K-Greeff Ltd,
Suffolk House, George St,
Croydon CR9 3QL.
081-686 0544

K/L
K/L Pharmaceuticals Ltd,
25 Macadam Place, South
Newmoor Industrial Estate,
Irvine KA11 4HP.
(0294) 215951

K Pharm
K Pharmaceuticals,
see Norton.

Kendall
The Kendall Company (UK)
Ltd,
2 Elmwood, Chineham Business
Park, Crockford Lane,
Basingstoke, Hants RG24 0WG.
(0256) 708880

Kendall-Lastonet
see Kendall.

Knoll
Knoll Ltd,
Fleming House, 71 King St,
Maidenhead, Berks SL6 1DU.
(0628) 776360

Kyowa Hakko
Kyowa Hakko UK Ltd,
CP House, 97–107 Uxbridge
Rd, Ealing, London W5 5TL.
081-840 4600

LAB
Laboratories for Applied
Biology Ltd,
91 Amhurst Park, London
N16 5DR.
081-800 2252

Laerdal
Laerdal Medical Ltd,
Laerdal House, Goodmead Rd,
Orpington, Kent BR6 0HX.
(0689) 76634

Lagap
Lagap Pharmaceuticals Ltd,
37 Woolmer Way, Bordon,
Hants GU35 9QE.
(0420) 478301

Lamberts
Lamberts (Dalston) Ltd,
Dalston House, Hastings St,
Luton, Beds LU1 5BW.
(0582) 400711

Lederle
Lederle Laboratories,
Cyanamid House, Fareham Rd,
Gosport, Hants PO13 0AS.
(0329) 224000

Leo
Leo Laboratories Ltd,
Longwick Rd, Princes
Risborough, Aylesbury, Bucks
HP27 9RR.
(0844) 347333

LifeScan
LifeScan,
Enterprise House, Station Rd,
Loudwater, High Wycombe,
Bucks HP10 9UF.
(0494) 442211

Lilly
Eli Lilly & Co Ltd,
Dextra Court, Chapel Hill,
Basingstoke, Hants RG21 2SY.
(0256) 473241

Link
Link Pharmaceuticals Ltd,
Node Court,
Drivers End, Codicote,
Herts SG4 8TR.
(0438) 821086

Lipha
Lipha Pharmaceuticals Ltd,
Harrier House, High St,
West Drayton, Middx UB7
7QG. (0895) 449331

Lorex
Lorex Pharmaceuticals Ltd,
Lunar House, Globe Park,
Marlow, Bucks SL7 1LW.
(0628) 488011

Loveridge
J. M. Loveridge plc,
Southbrook Rd, Southampton
SO9 3LT.
(0703) 228411

Loxley
Loxley Medical,
Unit 5D, Carnaby Industrial
Estate, Bridlington, North
Humberside YO15 3QY.
(0262) 603979

LRC
LRC Products Ltd,
North Circular Rd, Chingford,
London E4 8QA.
081-527 2377

Lundbeck
Lundbeck Ltd,
Sunningdale House, Caldecott
Lake Business Park, Caldecott,
Milton Keynes MK7 8LF.
(0908) 649966

3M
3M Health Care Ltd,
3M House, Morley St,
Loughborough, Leics LE11 1EP.
(0509) 611611

Macfarlan Smith
Macfarlan Smith Ltd,
Wheatfield Rd, Edinburgh
EH11 2QA.
031-337 2434

Marlen
Marlen (UK) Ltd,
Unit F4C,
Keighley Business Centre,
South St, Keighley,
West Yorkshire BD21 1AG.
(0535) 610300

Martindale
Martindale Pharmaceuticals Ltd,
Bampton Rd, Harold Hill,
Romford, Essex RM3 8UG.
(0708) 386660

Medac
Medac GmbH,
Fehlandtstraße 3,
D-2000 Hamburg 36, Germany.
(010 49 40) 3509020

Medasil
Medasil (Surgical) Ltd,
Medasil House, Hunslet Rd,
Leeds LS10 1AU.
(0532) 433491

Medic-Aid

Medic-Aid Ltd,
Hook Lane, Pagham, Sussex
PO21 3PP.
(0243) 267321

Medipharma

Medipharma Laboratories Ltd,
Medipharma House, 468 Street
Lane, Leeds LS17 6HA.
(0532) 663048

Mediplus

Mediplus Ltd,
Guildmaster Works,
Desborough Rd, High
Wycombe, Bucks HP11 2QA.
(0494) 536222

MediSense

MediSense Britain Ltd,
PO Box 2159, Coleshill,
Birmingham B46 1HZ.
(0675) 467044

Medix

Medix Ltd,
Medix House, Catthorpe,
Lutterworth, Leics LE17 6DB.
(0788) 860366

Medo

Medo Pharmaceuticals Ltd,
see Schwarz.

Mepra-pharm

Mepra-pharm,
Brent House, Kenton Rd,
Harrow, Middx HA3 8DA.
081-907 4332

Merck

E. Merck Pharmaceuticals,
Winchester Rd, Four Marks,
Alton, Hants GU34 5HB.
(0420) 564011

Merieux

Merieux UK,
Clivemont House, Clivemont
Rd, Maidenhead, Berks SL6
7BU.
(0628) 785291

Merrell

Marion Merrell Dow Ltd,
Lakeside House, Stockley Park,
Uxbridge, Middx UB11 1BE.
081-848 3456

Milupa

Milupa Ltd,
Milupa House, Uxbridge Rd,
Hillingdon, Middx UB10 0NE.
081-573 9966

MMG

MMG (Europe) Ltd,
157 Redland Rd, Bristol
BS6 6YE.
(0272) 736883

Molnlycke

Molnlycke Ltd,
Southfields Rd, Dunstable, Beds
LU6 3EJ.
(0582) 600211

Monmouth

Monmouth Pharmaceuticals,
3/4 Huxley Rd, The Surrey
Research Park, Guildford,
Surrey GU2 5RE.
(0483) 65299

Morson

Thomas Morson
Pharmaceuticals,
see MSD.

MSD

Merck Sharp & Dohme Ltd,
Hertford Rd, Hoddesdon, Herts
EN11 9BU.
(0992) 467272

Napp

Napp Laboratories Ltd,
Cambridge Science Park, Milton
Rd, Cambridge CB4 4GW.
(0223) 424444

Nationwide Ostomy

Nationwide Ostomy Supplies
Ltd,
North West House, 62 Oakhill
Trading Estate, Walkden,
Manchester M28 5PT.
(0204) 709255

Nestlé

Nestlé Co. Ltd,
St. George's House, Croydon
CR9 1NR.
081-686 3333

Network Management

Network Management Ltd,
Christy Estate, North Lane,
Aldershot, Hants GU12 4QP.
(0252) 29911

Neutrogena

Neutrogena (UK) Ltd,
Neutrogena House, Century
Point, Halifax Rd, Cressex,
High Wycombe, Bucks HP12
3SL.
(0494) 474787

Nordic

Nordic Pharmaceuticals Ltd,
see Ferring.
081-898 8665

Norgine

Norgine Ltd,
116 London Rd, Headington,
Oxford OX3 9BA.
(0865) 750717

Norma

Norma Chemicals Ltd,
see Wallace Mfg.

North West

North West Medical Supplies
Ltd,
Green Arms Rd, Bolton
BL7 0ND.
(0204) 852383

Norton

H. N. Norton & Co. Ltd,
Gemini House, Flex Meadow,
Harlow, Essex CM19 5TJ.
(0279) 426666

Novex

Novex Pharma Ltd,
Innovex House, Marlow Park,
Marlow, Bucks SL7 1TB.
(0628) 491500

Novo Nordisk

Novo Nordisk Pharmaceutical
Ltd,
Novo Nordisk House,
Broadfield Park, Brighton Rd,
Pease Pottage, Crawley, West
Sussex RH11 9RT.
(0293) 613555

Nutricia

Nutricia Dietary Products Ltd,
see Cow & Gate

Nycomed

Nycomed (UK) Ltd,
Nycomed House, 2111 Coventry
Rd, Sheldon, Birmingham
B26 3EA.
021-742 2444

Omnicare

The Omnicare Group Ltd,
Unit 7E, Blacknest Works,
Blacknest, Nr. Alton, Hants
GU34 4PX.
Dial 100 and ask for 'Freephone
Omnicare Oxygen'

Oral B Labs

Oral B Laboratories Ltd,
Gatehouse Rd, Aylesbury, Bucks
HP19 3ED.
(0296) 432601

Organon

Organon Laboratories Ltd,
Cambridge Science Park, Milton
Rd, Cambridge, CB4 4FL.
(0223) 423445

Organon-Teknika

Organon-Teknika Ltd,
see Organon
(0223) 423650

Ortho

Ortho Pharmaceutical Ltd,
see Cilag.

Owen Mumford

Owen Mumford Ltd,
Brook Hill, Woodstock, Oxford
OX7 1TU.
(0993) 812021

Oxford Nutrition

Oxford Nutrition Ltd,
PO Box 31, Oxford OX4 3UH.
(0865) 716323

Oxygen Therapy Co Ltd

The Oxygen Therapy Co Ltd,
Dumballs Rd, Cardiff
CF1 6JE.
0800 373580

Paines & Byrne

Paines & Byrne Ltd,
Brocades House, Pyrford Rd,
West Byfleet, Surrey KT14
6RA.
(0932) 355405

Panpharma
Panpharma Ltd,
Panpharma House, Repton
Place, White Lion Rd, Little
Chalfont, Amersham, Bucks
HP7 9LP. (0494) 766866

Parema
Parema Ltd,
Sullington Rd, Shepshed,
Loughborough, Leics
LE12 9JJ.
(0509) 502051

Payne
S G & P Payne,
Percy House, Brook St, Hyde,
Cheshire SK14 2NS.
061-367 8561

P-D
Parke-Davis Medical,
Lambert Court, Chestnut Ave,
Eastleigh, Hants SO5 3ZQ.
(0703) 620500

Pelican
Pelican Healthcare Ltd,
see Simpla
(0222) 747787

Penn
Penn Pharmaceuticals Ltd,
Tafarnaubach Industrial Estate,
Tredegar, Gwent, NP2 3AA.
(0495) 711711

Pennine
Pennine Healthcare,
Pontefract St, Ascot Drive
Industrial Estate, Derby
DE2 8JD.
(0332) 384489

Perstorp
Perstorp Pharma Ltd,
Wound-Care Division, Studio 1,
Intec 2, Wade Rd, Basingstoke,
Hants RG24 0NE.
(0256) 477868

Pfizer
Pfizer Ltd,
Sandwich, Kent CT13 9NJ.
(0304) 616161

Pharmacia
Pharmacia Ltd,
Davy Ave, Knowlhill,
Milton Keynes, MK5 8PH.
(0908) 661101

Pharmark
Pharmark,
4–5 Colman House, High St,
London SE20 9EX.
081-689 3969

Pharma-Plast
Pharma-Plast Ltd,
Thornhill Rd, North Moons
Moat, Redditch, Worcs
B98 9NL.
(0527) 64222

Pharmax
Pharmax Ltd,
Bourne Rd, Bexley, Kent
DA5 1NX.
(0322) 550550

Philip Harris
Philip Harris Medical Ltd,
Hazelwell Lane, Birmingham
B30 2PS.
021-433 3030

Pickles
J. Pickles & Sons,
Beech House, 62 High St,
Knaresborough, N. Yorks
HG5 0EA.
(0423) 867314

Portex
Portex Ltd,
Hythe, Kent CT21 5AB.
(0303) 260551

Porton
Porton Products Ltd,
1 Bath Rd, Maidenhead, Berks
SL6 4UH.
(0628) 771417

Procea
Procea,
Alexandra Road, Dublin 1.
Dublin 741741

Procter & Gamble
Procter & Gamble (Health &
Beauty Care) Ltd,
Rusham Park, Whitehall Lane,
Egham, Surrey TW20 9NW.
(0784) 434422

Procter & Gamble Pharm.
Procter & Gamble
Pharmaceuticals UK Ltd,
Lovett House, Lovett Rd,
Staines, Middx TW18 3AZ.
(0784) 495000

Quinoderm Ltd
Quinoderm Ltd,
Manchester Rd, Oldham, Lancs
OL8 4PB.
061-624 9307

Rand Rocket
Rand Rocket Ltd,
ABCare House, Hownsgill
Industrial Park, Consett,
County Durham DH8 7NU.
(0207) 591099

R & C
Reckitt & Colman Products Ltd,
Dansom Lane, Hull HU8 7DS.
(0482) 26151

Regent
Regent Laboratories Ltd,
Cunard Rd, London NW10 6PN.
081-965 3637

Renacare
Renacare Ltd,
Nunn Brook Rd, Huthwaite,
Sutton-in-Ashfield, Notts
NG17 2HU.
(0623) 555809

Rendell
W. J. Rendell Ltd,
Ickleford Manor, Hitchin,
Herts SG5 3XE.
(0462) 32596

Rhône-Poulenc Rorer
Rhône-Poulenc Rorer Ltd,
52 St Leonards Rd,
Eastbourne, East Sussex
BN21 3YG.
(0323) 721422

Richborough
see Pfizer.

Rima
Rima Pharmaceuticals Ltd,
214–216 St James's Rd,
Croydon, Surrey CR0 2BW.
081-683 1266

Robinsons
Robinson Healthcare,
Hipper House, Chesterfield,
Derbyshire S40 1YF.
(0246) 220022

RoC
Laboratoires RoC UK Ltd,
The Kirkgate, 19–31 Church St,
Epsom, Surrey KT17 4PF.
(0372) 749223

Roche
Roche Products Ltd,
PO Box 8, Welwyn Garden City,
Herts AL7 3AY.
(0707) 366000

Roche Consumer Health
see Roche.

Rona
see Lipha.

Roussel
Roussel Laboratories Ltd,
Broadwater Park, North Orbital
Rd, Uxbridge, Middx UB9 5HP.
(0895) 834343

RP Drugs
RP Drugs Ltd,
RPD House, Yorkdale
Industrial Park, Braithwaite St,
Leeds LS11 9XE.
(0532) 441400

Rüsch
Rüsch UK Ltd,
PO Box 138, Cressex Industrial
Estate, High Wycombe, Bucks
HP12 3NB.
(0494) 532761

Rybar
Rybar Laboratories Ltd,
see Shire.

Sallis
E. Sallis Ltd,
Vernon Works, Waterford St,
Old Basford, Nottingham
NG6 0DH.
(0602) 787841

Salts
Salt & Son Ltd,
Saltair House, Lord St,
Heartlands,
Birmingham B7 4DS.
021-359 5123

Sandoz
Sandoz Pharmaceuticals,
Frimley Business Park, Frimley,
Camberley, Surrey GU16 5SG.
(0276) 692255

Sanofi Winthrop
Sanofi Winthrop Ltd,
One Onslow St, Guildford,
Surrey GU1 4YS.
(0483) 505515

Sara Lee
Sara Lee Household & Personal
Care (UK) Ltd,
225 Bath Rd, Slough SL1 4AU.
(0753) 523971

Schering Health
Schering Health Care Ltd,
The Brow, Burgess Hill,
West Sussex RH15 9NE.
(0444) 232323

Schering-Plough
Schering-Plough Ltd,
Shire Park, Welwyn Garden
City, Herts AL7 1TW.
(0707) 363636

Scholl
Scholl Consumer Products Ltd,
475 Capability Green, Luton,
Beds LU1 3LU.
(0582) 482929

Schwarz
Schwarz Pharma Ltd,
Schwarz House, East St,
Chesham, Bucks HP5 1DG.
(0494) 772071

Scientific Hospital Supplies
Scientific Hospital Supplies
(UK) Ltd,
100 Wavertree Boulevard,
Wavertree Technology Park,
Liverpool L7 9PT.
051-228 1992

Scotia
Scotia Pharmaceuticals Ltd,
Units 26–29, Surrey Technical
Centre, The Research Park,
40 Occam Rd, Guildford, Surrey
GU2 5YH.
(0483) 304408

Searle
Searle Pharmaceuticals,
PO Box 53, Lane End Rd, High
Wycombe, Bucks HP12 4HL.
(0494) 521124

Serono
Serono Laboratories (UK) Ltd,
99 Bridge Rd East, Welwyn
Garden City, Herts AL7 1BG.
(0707) 331972

Servier
Servier Laboratories Ltd,
Fulmer Hall, Windmill Rd,
Fulmer, Slough SL3 6HH.
(0753) 662744

Seton
Seton Healthcare,
Seton Healthcare Group plc,
Tubiton House, Medlock St,
Oldham, Lancs OL1 3HS.
061-652 2222

Seton-Prebbles
see Seton.

Seven Seas
Seven Seas Ltd,
Hedon Rd, Marfleet, Hull
HU9 5NJ.
(0482) 75234

Seward
Seward Medical,
131 Great Suffolk St, London
SE1 1PP.
071-357 6527

Shannon
T. J. Shannon Ltd,
59 Bradford St, Bolton
BL2 1HT.
(0204) 21789

Shaw
A. H. Shaw and Partners Ltd,
Manor Rd, Ossett, West
Yorkshire WF5 0LF.
(0924) 273474

Sherwood
Sherwood Medical Industries
Ltd,
County Oak Way, Crawley, West
Sussex RH11 7YQ.
(0293) 534501

Shire
Shire Pharmaceuticals Ltd,
Fosse House, East Anton Court,
Icknield Way, Andover, Hants
SP10 5RG.
(0264) 333455

Sigma
Sigma Pharmaceuticals plc,
PO Box 233, Watford, Herts
WD2 4EW.
(0923) 250201

Simcare
Simcare,
Peter Rd, Lancing, West Sussex
BN15 8TJ.
(0903) 761122

Simpla
Simpla Plastics Ltd,
Cardiff Business Park, Cardiff
CF4 5WF.
(0222) 747000

Sinclair
Sinclair Pharmaceuticals Ltd,
Borough Rd, Godalming, Surrey
GU7 2AB.
(0483) 426644

S&N
Smith & Nephew Medical Ltd,
PO Box 81, 101 Hessle Rd, Hull
HU3 2BN.
(0482) 25181

S&N Pharm.
Smith & Nephew
Pharmaceuticals Ltd,
Bampton Rd, Harold Hill,
Romford, Essex RM3 8SL.
(0708) 349333

SK&F
Smith Kline & French
Laboratories,
see SmithKline Beecham.

SmithKline Beecham
SmithKline Beecham
Pharmaceuticals,
SmithKline Beecham plc,
Mundells, Welwyn Garden
City, Herts AL7 1EY.
0800 616482

SmithKline Beecham Health-care
SmithKline Beecham
Consumer Healthcare,
St Georges Ave, Weybridge,
Surrey KT13 0DE.
(0932) 822000

SNBTS
Scottish National Blood
Transfusion Service,
Protein Fractionation Centre,
21 Ellen's Glen Rd,
Edinburgh EH17 7QT.
031-664 2317

Spodefell
Spodefell Ltd,
5 Inverness Mews, London
W2 3QJ.
071-229 9125

Squibb
E. R. Squibb & Sons Ltd,
see Bristol-Myers.

Stafford-Miller
Stafford-Miller Ltd,
Broadwater Rd, Welwyn Garden
City, Herts AL7 3SP.
(0707) 331001

STD Pharmaceutical
STD Pharmaceutical Products,
Fields Yard, Plough Lane,
Hereford HR4 0EL.
(0432) 353684

Steeper
Steeper (Orthopaedic) Ltd,
Unit 4D, Mead Rise,
Temple Gate, Bristol BS3 4RP.
(0272) 717436

Steriseal
Steriseal Ltd,
Thornhill Rd, Redditch, Worcs
B98 9NL.
(0527) 64222

Sterling Health
Sterling-Winthrop Group Ltd,
see Sanofi Winthrop.

Sterwin
see Sanofi Winthrop.

Stiefel
Stiefel Laboratories (UK) Ltd,
Holtspur Lane, Wooburn Green,
High Wycombe, Bucks
HP10 0AU.
(0628) 524966

Storz
Storz Ophthalmics,
see Lederle.

Stuart
see Zeneca.

Syntex
Syntex Pharmaceuticals Ltd,
Syntex House, St. Ives Rd,
Maidenhead, Berks SL6 1RD.
(0628) 33191

Terumo
Terumo Europe N.V.
1st Floor Offices,
62 Mount Pleasant Rd,
Tunbridge Wells,
Kent TN1 1RB.
(0892) 526331

Thackraycare
see DePuy.

Thames
see Consolidated.

Thornton & Ross
Thornton & Ross Ltd,
Linthwaite Laboratories,
Huddersfield HD7 5QH.
(0484) 842217

Tillomed
Tillomed Laboratories Ltd,
Unit 2, Campus 5, Letchworth
Business Park, Letchworth
Garden City, Herts SG6 2JF.
(0462) 480344

Timesco
Timesco of London,
176 Pentonville Rd, London
N1 9JP.
071-278 0712

Torbet
Torbet Laboratories Ltd,
Broughton House, 33 Earl St,
Maidstone, Kent ME14 1PF.
(0622) 762269

Tosara
Tosara Products Ltd,
Baldoyle Industrial Estate,
Grange Rd, Dublin 13.
Dublin 321199

Typharm
Typharm Ltd,
14 Parkstone Rd, Poole, Dorset
BH15 2PG.
(04254) 79711

UCB Pharma
UCB Pharma Ltd,
Star House, 69 Clarendon Rd,
Watford, Herts WD1 1DJ.
(0923) 211811

Ultra
Ultra Laboratories Ltd,
Trinity Trading Estate, Tribune
Drive, Sittingbourne, Kent
ME10 2PG.
(0795) 70953

Ultrapharm
Ultrapharm Ltd,
PO Box 18, Henley-on-Thames,
Oxon RG9 2AW.
(0491) 578016

Unigreg
Unigreg Ltd,
Enterprise House, 181 Garth Rd,
Morden, Surrey SM4 4LL.
081-330 1421

Unipath
Unipath Ltd,
Norse Rd, Bedford
MK41 0QG.
(0234) 347161

Universal
Universal Hospital Supplies,
313 Chase Rd, London N14
6JA.
081-882 6444

Uno Plast
Uno Plast Ltd,
The Wykeham Industrial Estate,
Moorside Rd, Winchester, Hants
SO23 7RX.
(0962) 841777

Upjohn
Upjohn Ltd,
Fleming Way, Crawley,
West Sussex RH10 2LZ.
(0293) 531133

Vernon-Carus
Vernon-Carus Ltd,
Penwortham Mills, Preston,
Lancs PR1 9SN.
(0772) 744493

Vestar
Vestar Ltd,
51 Cambridge Place, Hills Rd,
Cambridge CB2 1NS.
(0223) 461380

Vestric
Vestric Ltd,
West Lane, Runcorn, Cheshire
WA7 2PE.
(0928) 717070

Vitabiotics
Vitabiotics Ltd,
Vitabiotics House, 3 Bashley
Rd, London NW10 6SU.
081-963 0999

Vitaflo
Vitaflo Ltd,
6 Moss St, Paisley PA1 1BJ.
0800 515174

Vitalograph
Vitalograph Ltd,
Maids Moreton House,
Buckingham MK18 1SW.
(0280) 822811

Vygon
Vygon (UK) Ltd,
Bridge Rd, Cirencester, Glos
GL7 1PT.
(0285) 67051

H G Wallace
H G Wallace Ltd,
Colchester, Essex CO2 8JH.
(0206) 795133

Wallace Mfg
Wallace Manufacturing
Chemists Ltd,
Randles Rd, Knowsley
Industrial Park, Merseyside
L34 9HX.
051-549 1255

Wanskerne
Wanskerne Ltd,
31 High Cross St, St. Austell,
Cornwall PL25 4AN.
(0726) 69500

Ward
Ward Surgical Appliance Co
Ltd,
57A Brightwell Ave, Westcliffe-
on-Sea, Essex SS0 9EB.
(0702) 354064

WBP
WB Pharmaceuticals Ltd,
see Boehringer Ingelheim.

Welfare Foods
see Nutricia.

Welland
Welland Medical Ltd,
7 Brunel Centre, Newton Rd,
Crawley, West Sussex
RH10 2TU.
(0293) 615455

Wellcome
The Wellcome Foundation Ltd,
Wellcome Medical Division,
Crewe Hall, Crewe, Cheshire
CW1 1UB.
(0270) 583151

Whitehall
Huntercombe Lane South,
Taplow, Maidenhead, Berks
SL6 0PH.
(0628) 669011

Willis
S. R. Willis & Sons Ltd,
176 Albion Rd, London N16
9JR. 071-254 7373

Windsor
see Boehringer Ingelheim.

W-L
Warner Lambert UK Ltd,
see P-D.

Wyeth
Wyeth Laboratories,
Huntercombe Lane South,
Taplow, Maidenhead, Berks
SL6 0PH
(0628) 604377

Yamanouchi
Yamanouchi Pharma Ltd,
Yamanouchi House, Pyrford Rd,
West Byfleet, Surrey
KT14 6RA.
(0932) 345535

Zeal
G. H. Zeal Ltd,
8 Lombard Rd, Merton, London
SW19 3UU.
081-542 2283

Zeneca
Zeneca Pharma,
King's Court, Water Lane,
Wilmslow, Cheshire SK9 5AZ.
(0625) 535999

Zyma
Zyma Healthcare,
Mill Rd, Holmwood, Dorking,
Surrey RH5 4NU.
(0306) 742800

Hospital Manufacturing Units

The following may be contacted for information on hospital units with facilities for the manufacture of 'special-order' products.

Addresses are listed by NHS regions

ENGLAND

East Anglian
Mr G. Hanson,
Regional Production Manager,
Pharmacy Department,
The Ipswich Hospital,
Heath Rd, Ipswich, Suffolk
IP4 5PD.
(0473) 712233 Extn 5603

Mersey
Dr M. G. Lee,
Regional Quality Control
Pharmacist,
Mersey RHA,
Hamilton House, 24 Pall Mall,
Liverpool L3 6AL.
051-236 4620 Extn 2133

North East Thames
Mr M. Lillywhite,
Regional Production
Pharmacist,
St. Bartholomew's Hospital,
West Smithfield, London
EC1A 7BE.
071-601 7477

North West Thames
Mr H. Stokoe,
Regional Technical Pharmacist,
North West Thames Regional
Pharmaceutical Service,
40 Eastbourne Terr, London
W2 3QR.
071-262 8011 Extn 3291

North Western
Mr M.D. Booth,
Production & Aseptic Services
Manager,
Stockport Pharmaceuticals,
Stepping Hill Hospital,
Stockport, Cheshire SK2 7JE.
061-419 5657

Northern
Mr P. W. McKenzie,
Regional Technical Services
Pharmacist,
Pharmacy Department,
Newcastle General Hospital,
Westgate Rd,
Newcastle upon Tyne NE4 6BE.
091-273 8811 Extn 22479

Oxford
Ms Ruth Dolton,
Director,
Mandeville Medicines,
Stoke Mandeville Hospital,
Aylesbury, Bucks HP21 8AL.
(0296) 315501

South East Thames
Mr J. Cheetham,
Principal Pharmacist,
Guy's Hospital,
St. Thomas' St, London
SE1 9RT.
071-955 5000 Extn 5378/3712

South West Thames
Mr S. J. Riley,
Regional Production
Pharmacist,
Pharmacy Department,
Lanesborough Wing,
St. George's Hospital,
Blackshaw Rd, Tooting, London
SW17 0QT.
081-725 1770

South Western
Mr C. W. Lewis,
Director,
Manorpark Pharmaceuticals,
Blackberry Hill Hospital,
Manor Rd, Bristol BS16 2EW.
(0272) 754852

Trent
Mr P. W. Golightly,
Regional Drug Information
Pharmacist,
Royal Infirmary,
Leicester, Leics LE1 5WW.
(0533) 523218

Wessex
Dr E. Brierley,
Regional Manufacturing Unit,
Queen Alexandra Hospital,
Cosham, Portsmouth, Hants
PO6 3LY.
(0705) 324625

West Midlands
Mr M. Phillips,
Regional Quality Control
Pharmacist, Pharmacy
Department, City Hospital,
Dudley Rd, Birmingham
B18 7QH.
021-507 5236

Yorkshire
Mr E. Holt,
Principal Pharmacist,
Production Unit,
The Royal Infirmary,
Acre St, Lindley, Huddersfield,
West Yorks HD3 3EA.
(0484) 422191 Extn 2421

NORTHERN IRELAND

Mrs S. Millership,
Central Pharmaceutical
Production Unit,
EHSSB Distribution Centre,
Boucher Cres, Belfast
BT12 7HU.
(0232) 667799 Extn 4742

SCOTLAND

Mr J. Cook,
Principal Pharmacist—
Regional Production,
Tayside Pharmaceuticals,
Ninewells Hospital,
Dundee DD1 9SY.
(0382) 60111 Extn 2273

WALES

Specialist Principal Pharmacist,
Sterile Products Unit,
Pharmacy Department,
University Hospital of Wales,
The Heath, Cardiff CF4 4XW.
(0222) 747747 Extn 3114

Index

Where an entry is followed by more than one page reference, the principal reference is printed in **bold** type. Proprietary (trade) names are printed in *italic* type.